Nurse Practitioner Certification Exam Prep

SIXTH EDITION

Nurse Practitioner Certification Exam Prep

SIXTH EDITION

Margaret A. Fitzgerald,

DNP, FNP-BC, NP-C, FAANP, CSP, DCC, FAAN, FNAP
Founder, Fitzgerald Health Education Associates
North Andover, Massachusetts
Family Nurse Practitioner
Greater Lawrence Family Health Center
Lawrence, Massachusetts

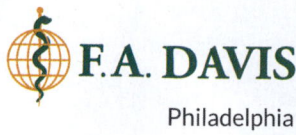

F.A. DAVIS

Philadelphia

F. A. Davis Company
1915 Arch Street
Philadelphia, PA 19103
www.fadavis.com

Printed in the United States of America

Last digit indicates print number: 10 9 8 7 6 5 4 3 2

Publisher: Susan Rhyner
Manager of Project and eProject Management: Catherine Carroll
Content Project Manager: Amanda Minutola
Design & Illustration Manager: Carolyn O'Brien

As new scientific information becomes available through basic and clinical research, recommended treatments and drug therapies undergo changes. The author(s) and publisher have done everything possible to make this book accurate, up to date, and in accord with accepted standards at the time of publication. The author(s), editors, and publisher are not responsible for errors or omissions or for consequences from application of the book, and make no warranty, expressed or implied, in regard to the contents of the book. Any practice described in this book should be applied by the reader in accordance with professional standards of care used in regard to the unique circumstances that apply in each situation. The reader is advised always to check product and prescribing information for changes and new information regarding dose and contraindications before administering any drug. Caution is especially urged when using new or infrequently ordered drugs.

Library of Congress Cataloging-in-Publication Data

Names: Fitzgerald, Margaret A., author.
Title: Nurse practitioner certification exam prep /
Margaret A. Fitzgerald.
Description: Sixth edition. | Philadelphia, PA : F.A. Davis Company, [2021] |
Includes bibliographical references and index.
Identifiers: LCCN 2016053464 | ISBN 9780803677128
| MESH: Nursing Care—methods | Family Nursing | Nurse
Practitioners | Certification | Examination Questions
Classification: LCC RT120.F34 | NLM WY 18.2 | DDC 610.73076—dc23
LC record available at https://lccn.loc.gov/2016053464

Dedication

With much admiration and great affection, and on behalf of the NP community, I dedicate this book to Dr. Loretta Ford, co-founder of the NP profession. We thank you for your vision and commitment to improving the health of our nation. We honor your work and give thanks as well to your beloved husband, the late Mr. Bill Ford, whom you described as "the wind beneath your wings." One of the greatest joys of my many years of work with the NP community, and that of my husband and business partner, Marc Comstock, has been counting you and Bill as dear friends. Happy 100th Birthday (December 28, 2020)

Contributor

Kara L. Ashley, M.Ed.
Northeast Association of Learning Specialists
West Hartford, CT

Acknowledgments

This book represents a sum of the efforts of many people.

I thank my family, especially my husband, and business partner, Marc Comstock, for their support and patience as they lived through this experience.

I thank the staff of Fitzgerald Health Education Associates for sharing me with this project for many months.

I thank the patients and staff of the Greater Lawrence (MA) Family Health Center, where I have practiced for more than 30 years, as they continue to serve as a source of inspiration as I developed this book. Gracias.

I thank Susan Rhyner, Amanda Minutola, and the F.A. Davis staff for their ongoing encouragement.

Last, but not least, I thank the tens of thousands of nurse practitioners who, over the years, have participated in the Fitzgerald Health Education Associates Nurse Practitioner Certification and continuing education programs. Your eagerness to learn, thirst for knowledge, dedication to success, and commitment to excellence in health-care provision continue to inspire me. I am privileged to be part of your professional development.

Preface

The scope of practice of the nurse practitioner (NP) is wide, encompassing the care of the young, the old, the sick, and the well. This book has been developed to help the NP develop the knowledge and skills to successfully enter NP practice and earn certification, an important landmark in professional achievement.

This book represents a perspective on learning and practice developed during my years of practice at the Greater Lawrence (MA) Family Health Center and as an NP and professional speaker. In addition, my experiences throughout the years of helping thousands of NPs achieve professional success through conducting Fitzgerald Health Education Associates NP Certification and Advance Practice Update Courses influenced the development and presentation of the information held within.

This book is not intended to be a comprehensive clinical text; rather, it is meant to be a source to reinforce learning and a guide for the development of the knowledge base and critical thinking skills needed for safe, entry-level NP practice. The reader is encouraged to answer the questions given in each section and then check on the accuracy of the responses. The discussion section is intended to enhance learning through highlighting the essentials of primary care NP practice. The numerous tables can serve as a quick-look resource, not only as the NP prepares for entry to practice and certification but also in the delivery of ongoing care.

—MARGARET A. FITZGERALD, DNP, FNP-BC, NP-C, FAANP, CSP, FAAN, DCC, FNAP
Founder
Fitzgerald Health Education Associates, LLC
North Andover, Massachusetts
Family Nurse Practitioner
Greater Lawrence (MA) Family Health Center
Lawrence, Massachusetts

question. Bear in mind how the pathophysiology of the condition affects the presentation and treatment.

In clinical practice, you would likely gather more information than is given in a scenario in one of the test questions. During the certification examination, you have to decide on the best response given the information in front of you by applying sound clinical judgment.

Decide whether extra information found in a particularly long answer is pertinent to the question and not simply a distractor.

When keeping in mind major information about presenting issues, pharmacology, and best practices, it can be easy to lose sight of important little words—words such as *but, however, despite, except,* and *if.* These are common cuing words that tell you that things may not always be as simple as they appear. These words can indicate a shift, a possible contradiction or contraindication, and a conditional situation or scenario. Pay attention to these words. A careful test taker can use these words to construct a strategy for answering the question. For example, in a question that reads, "All of the following are symptoms of 'X' except," you can treat this as a mini true/false question. You will be given three or four "true" choices and one "false" choice. That false choice is your answer. On a related note, be wary of options that include extreme words, such as "always," "never," "all," "best," "worst," and "none." Seldom is anything absolute in health care.

In addition, look at the information presented and then ask yourself, "Is this question a test of the ability to gather subjective or objective information? Is this question a test of the ability to develop a working diagnosis or to plan a course of intervention, or evaluation of response to care?" This thinking helps focus your thought process as you choose the answer. Read each question and all responses thoroughly and carefully so that you mark your choice only after you are sure you understand the concept being tested in the question. Answering a question quickly might lead to choosing a response that contains correct information about a given condition but might not be the correct response for that particular question. As you use this book to help develop your knowledge base, deciding on the best answer will become increasingly easy.

Remaining mindful of a conceptual framework that works for you can aid question comprehension and accuracy in your answering. If you are mathematically or visually minded, a good strategy might be to think of the question as a math problem or scientific equation with (patient) + (presentation) + (context) = (best action). Consolidating and storytelling work for people who need to "talk through" answers and their thinking to find the best result. Turn the question into a story and predict the ending before you look at the possible answers. When in doubt, process of elimination can be a useful exercise. By eliminating wrong answers, you can narrow down your choices by rereading the question with the remaining possibilities in mind.

With the strategies we have covered here, let's look at the following test item:

> You see 18-year-old Sam, who was seen approximately 36 hours ago at a local walk-in center for treatment of ear pain. Sam was diagnosed with (L) acute otitis media, and an appropriate dose of amoxicillin, to be taken bid, was prescribed. Today, Sam states that he has taken three amoxicillin doses since the medication was prescribed but continues to have discomfort in the affected ear. The left tympanic membrane is red and immobile.

This is an action-oriented question, directing you to consider Sam's care and chief complaint. Based on the scenario presented, you can assume the following:

■ Because no chronic health problems are mentioned, implied is that Sam is a young adult who is typically in good health.

■ Acute otitis media (AOM) is a common episodic illness usually caused by *Streptococcus pneumoniae, Haemophilus influenzae, Moraxella catarrhalis,* or respiratory virus.

■ A first-line antimicrobial for AOM treatment is amoxicillin. When given in a sufficient dose, this antibiotic is effective against *S pneumoniae* and both *H influenzae* and *M catarrhalis* that do not produce β-lactamase. Nearly all *M catarrhalis* and about 30% of *H influenzae* isolates produce β-lactamase, rendering amoxicillin ineffective. Clavulanate is a β-lactamase inhibitor, and when given in conjunction with amoxicillin is an effective treatment option when AOM fails to respond to amoxicillin alone.

TEST TAKING TIP
On high-level tests, the difference between the best answer and the distractor answers will not always be clear.

TEST TAKING TIP
Remember: Test questions are designed to have one best answer but often contain more than one possibly correct answer.

TEST TAKING TIP
Remember: Multiple-choice tests do not lend themselves to plentiful extraneous detail.

TEST TAKING TIP
Identifying the verb in the question can help you determine the purpose of the question.

■ As inflammation and purulent exudate forms in the middle ear, a small space rich with pain receptors, otalgia is an expected finding in AOM. This usually resolves after 2 to 3 days of antimicrobial therapy.

■ Tympanic membrane immobility is a cardinal sign of AOM that despite antimicrobial therapy does not resolve for many weeks. A patient report of otalgia is also needed to make the AOM diagnosis.

The following answer choices are given:

A. Advise Sam to discontinue the current antimicrobial and start a course of amoxicillin with clavulanate.

B. Perform tympanocentesis and send a sample of the exudate for culture and sensitivity.

C. Have Sam return in 24 hours for reevaluation.

D. Recommend that Sam take an appropriate dose of ibuprofen as needed for discomfort for the next 2 to 3 days.

Which answer included the best course of action for Sam? Let's review the answers to see which one is correct and why.

A. Advise Sam to discontinue the current antimicrobial and start a course of amoxicillin with clavulanate.

• Choosing this response infers amoxicillin treatment failure. AOM antimicrobial treatment failure is usually defined, however, as persistent otalgia with fever after 72 hours of therapy. Sam has taken fewer than 3 days of therapy, an interval too short to assign continued symptoms to ineffective antimicrobial therapy. In addition, there is no report of Sam's condition worsening in the short time since he was initially seen. Therefore, prescribing an antimicrobial with a broader spectrum activity, such as amoxicillin/clavulanate, is not warranted at this time. This is an excellent example of how critical it is to have a knowledge base that includes the standards of evidence-based practice.

B. Perform tympanocentesis and send a sample of the exudate for culture and sensitivity.

• AOM treatment is based on empirical antimicrobial therapy in which the clinician chooses an agent with activity against the most likely organisms in a given condition, bearing in mind the most common resistant pathogens. Tympanocentesis is indicated only with treatment failure after 10 to 21 days of antimicrobial therapy with a second-line agent, with the goal of detecting a significantly resistant organism; at that point, culture and sensitivity of middle ear exudate would be appropriate, usually with referral to otolaryngology to have this procedure done. With fewer than 2 days of treatment, tympanocentesis is not indicated.

C. Have Sam return in 24 hours for reevaluation.

• If Sam's condition worsens in the next day, reevaluation is prudent. However, choosing this option ignores Sam's complaint of pain.

D. Recommend that Sam take an appropriate dose of ibuprofen as needed for discomfort for the next 2 to 3 days.

• Choosing option D infers that treating Sam's pain is the most appropriate intervention. This is the best response and the correct answer.

Now consider this question: **Which of the following best describes asthma?** No clinical scenario is presented; the question simply asks for a definition of a pathological state. When considering the options, the test taker must recall that asthma is a chronic inflammatory disease of the airways involving an increase in bronchial hyperresponsiveness. This condition leads to a potentially reversible decrease in the FEV_1-to-FVC ratio and is an example of how the NP boards often include questions on the clinical presentation of pathophysiology. This type of answer lends itself well to becoming a "true/false" question. As you read each answer, ask yourself whether a choice is true or false. You are looking for the "true" answer. If answers seem partially true, or true sometimes, select the one that is mostly true, most of the time.

Here are your answer choices:

A. Intermittent airway inflammation with occasional bronchospasm

B. A disease of bronchospasm leading to airway inflammation

C. Chronic airway inflammation with superimposed bronchospasm

D. Relatively fixed airway obstruction

Let's again look at the choices and reveal the correct answer.

A. Intermittent airway inflammation with occasional bronchospasm

• Because asthma is a chronic, not intermittent, inflammatory airway disease, this option is incorrect.

B. A disease of bronchospasm leading to airway inflammation

• Because asthma is a chronic inflammatory airway disease that leads to airway hyperresponsiveness, this option is incorrect.

C. Chronic airway inflammation with superimposed bronchospasm
- This option most closely matches the definition of asthma and is the best option.

D. Relatively fixed airway obstruction
- Because the airway obstruction in asthma is largely reversible, this option is incorrect. This answer is more descriptive of chronic obstructive pulmonary disease.

Develop a Plan of Review Study That Works for You

With test design in mind, it is time to think about planning an effective study strategy. As you learned in your graduate studies, there are many "right" ways to study. The most important factors to your success, regardless of learning style, depend on an organized and purposeful study plan. This issue of time needed for certification preparation is unique to each examination candidate. That said, one of the major pitfalls in study is the failure to put aside the time to prepare. Map out the demands on your time in the first months after completing your NP program, including work hours, family, personal and professional commitments, as well as time you have perhaps set aside for some well-deserved downtime. After doing this, set up a schedule of study time, allotting a greater amount of time to areas of knowledge deficit and less to areas in which you only need to refresh your knowledge base. Make sure you cover all areas listed as possible examination content.

> **TEST TAKING TIP**
> Plan your date for certification only after a period of well-planned, systematic, certification-focused study.

Start with reviewing the information on the examination content. Make a list of the areas in which you feel your knowledge base is secure and in which just reviewing material to refresh your memory will likely suffice. Then make a second list in which you identify areas of weaknesses and areas in which you need to concentrate your review. If you have taken an NP review course, you are likely aware that the content of certain parts of the program were truly review, whereas other sections helped to point out areas in which you needed to expand on your knowledge base. Knowing on which areas to best concentrate your study helps you decide how to allocate your study time.

As you study, please keep in mind that the NP certification examination tests your ability to answer the following questions:

- ***Why*** is a patient at risk for a problem?
- ***How*** has a clinical problem developed?
- ***What*** is the most likely clinical presentation of the condition?
- ***Why*** is a given intervention effective?
- ***How*** does that intervention work?
- ***What*** is the most likely clinical outcome?
- ***Why*** is this clinical problem of significance to the overall health-care system?

A poor approach to preparing for the examination and practice is to memorize information so you know what to do but not why you are doing it. A better approach to preparing for the examination and practice is to understand concepts and apply knowledge so you know what to do and why you are doing it. Using this book will help greatly in building your knowledge base so that you are able to apply information to answer questions to help you in your pursuit of certification. In addition, the Fitzgerald Health Education Associates *NP Certification Examination Review and Advanced Practice Update* prepares you in the why, how, and what of NP practice, as well as helps to prepare you for success on the NP boards.

As you work through practice questions, and do this only after working on building your knowledge base, make a note next to each with words or symbols that indicate how certain you are of your answer. For some, you will be "sure" or "confident" that an answer is correct; for others you may be "mostly" or "somewhat sure"; and for others, you are likely offering a best guess. After you score your pretest, examine how your answers match up with your predicted performance. If you marked yourself "confident" on an item you got wrong, start by studying the question and answer choices carefully to glean the possible reasons you might have selected the wrong answer for that particular question. Ask yourself the following:

- Did I understand the context properly?
- If I read the context properly, did I misinterpret or misread the question?
- Was there unfamiliar content or vocabulary that led me to an incorrect conclusion?
- What was it about the distractors that distracted me?
- What is lacking in my knowledge base that caused me to answer the question incorrectly?

If you correctly answered a question for which you were not completely certain of the best answer, ask yourself what information in the context, action, or answer choices helped to lead you in the right direction. Frequent pretesting will not only help you to become more comfortable on test day, it can also help you to be more effective at unlocking a question.

When studying for the NP boards, some people will work best alone, whereas others benefit from collaborating with a study group. Participating in study groups can be helpful and a terrific way to share information and resources. Alternatively, study groups can yield a poor return on time invested if all members are not similarly committed. Study groups can meet in person or virtually, such as via Skype, Zoom, Google, or other similar groups. The following are some guidelines for forming a successful study group:

- All group members must treat attendance and participation as they would any other professional commitment, such as work or school.
- Well in advance, set a schedule, place, and time to meet, as well as a topic for the meeting.
- Plan a start and end time, with a clear objective for the session.
- Study groups usually work best when a group member volunteers to research and present information on a subject on a predetermined schedule. The presentation is typically followed by a discussion of the issue and a review of sample examination questions and rationales for the correct response.
- The leader of a given session should also assume responsibility for keeping the discussion on track, facilitating the efficient use of time and resources.

To help avoid the group deteriorating into a chat session, plan for a short period of socialization following high-yield study sessions. Here is an example of a session planned by a successful study group with three members, Sarah, Ben, and Helena.

The session will start promptly at 7 p.m. and end at 9 p.m., with the objective of identifying the risk factors, clinical presentation, assessment, and intervention in community-acquired pneumonia in the adult. Sarah is the presenter and also group leader for the evening and is responsible for keeping us on track. A social period from 9 to 9:30 p.m. will follow. We will meet at Helena's apartment. Ben is responsible for refreshments.

> **TEST TAKING TIP**
> Once you have secured your knowledge base, you are ready to move on to high-quality practice examinations.

Whenever possible, try to create a study situation that will mimic the actual test. Set a timer and be mindful of pacing yourself. *During the test, expect to answer about 60 to 70 or more multiple-choice questions per hour.* This means you will likely be spending less than a minute, on average, on each question. Some questions take only a few seconds, whereas others require more time for thought. Check yourself at 15- or 20-minute intervals to determine whether you are progressing at an acceptable rate, setting a number of questions that you should have answered by a certain time.

How to Manage Nerves During Review and On Test Day

Everyone who sits for one of the certification examinations is anxious to some degree. This anxiety can be a helpful emotion, focusing the NP certification candidate on the task at hand: studying and successfully sitting for this important examination, a tangible end-product of the candidate's graduate or postgraduate education. When excessive, however, anxiety can get in the way of success. Stress yields anxiety, anxiety yields stress; one can be viewed as the product of the other. The stress of preparing for an important examination triggers the sympathetic nervous system to undergo Seyle's three phases of the general adaptation syndrome: alarm, resistance, and exhaustion. In the alarm stage, perhaps triggered by contemplating the preparation needed to achieve certification success, the hypothalamus activates the autonomic nervous system, triggering the pituitary and the body defenses, resulting in a heightened sense of awareness of surroundings, alertness, and focus. At this level of arousal, studying for and taking a test often yield great results.

> **TEST TAKING TIP**
> A well-prepared examination candidate is highly focused on what needs to be done to be successful on the examination.

Distractions can be filtered out; extraneous information can be discarded in favor of the essentials. During the examination, anxiety and knowledge intersect; information retrieval is facilitated, and examination questions are fluidly processed. Difficult examination items are usually put in perspective, with the test taker recognizing that most items were answered with relative ease. The NP certification candidate emerges from the test feeling challenged but confident.

Although a moderate amount of anxiety is natural, and even useful, many candidates can find themselves struggling with anxiety that is causing physical or emotional distress. The process of completing a rigorous course of graduate education and study can result in a protracted period of stress. Now, the formerly helpful stress leads to the second stage of the general adaptation syndrome, resistance, in which epinephrine is released to help counteract or escape from the stressor. At that time, the feeling of milder anxiety present in the first stage gives way to a sense of greater nervousness, often accompanied by uncomfortable physical sensations such as dry mouth, tachycardia, and tremor. Studying or test taking becomes difficult; information retrieval is inhibited. This stage is mentally and physically taxing and, if left unchecked, can lead to exhaustion, complicating the challenging task of successfully completing the certification examination. Although the reaction is most severe at the time of the test, most people who have severe test-taking anxiety have a similar, although milder, reaction with the deep study needed to prepare for a critical examination such as NP certification.

The following scenario describes a person with a problematic case of studying-testing anxiety:

The NP certification examination candidate is having a tough day, with a work shift that stretched for 3 unexpected hours and an unusually long commute, all following a poor night's sleep as a result of a noisy neighborhood party. To counteract this, the candidate drank a few extra cups of strong coffee and drank an "energy drink," really nothing more than a can of sugar and caffeine. She also skipped lunch and made a quick trip to a fast-food restaurant for some fries as a snack. Studying was part of today's plan, however, so she sits down to prepare for the examination with great intentions of reviewing critical information. Surrounded by great stacks of study material, the NP candidate thinks about what might be on the examination and ponders the wide scope and knowledge base needed to be successful. Now the candidate becomes aware of a dry mouth and tight feeling in the throat. Determined, she sits down and decides to study about antimicrobial therapy. The words on the page seem to blur when the candidate tries to read about the spectrum of activity of an antibiotic; then, having difficulty keeping this information straight, she decides to skip that and focuses on memorizing a few antibiotic dose ranges, information that is unlikely to be on the boards. Even with repeated tries, the NP candidate cannot keep this information at hand and now becomes even more anxious, feeling tension in the back of her neck and a rapidly beating heart. The candidate now tries a few practice examination questions but answers three questions about the appropriate use of antimicrobial therapy in acute otitis media incorrectly. Now, even the thought of sitting for the examination causes the NP candidate to freeze.

In an ideal world, we could all control schedules and set aside vast periods of calm, focused review. Life, however, is complicated. Although developing a study schedule is important, rescheduling study time is likely a good idea when a day has been particularly difficult. Trying to learn when exhausted and stressed by other influences is often counterproductive. Certain scents can be helpful for putting the NP candidate in the right frame of mind to study, particularly under less-than-ideal conditions. These include basil, cinnamon, lemon, and peppermint for mental alertness and chamomile, lavender, and orange for relaxation.

Learning a relaxation technique to use before studying or test taking can help you start your review session with a clear mind and shift your focus from whatever events or stress your day may have contained. You can also employ these same techniques on test day to help center yourself if you feel overwhelming anxiety begin to creep in. Start the session by reading or repeating a positive message about being successful on the examination.

Eat a light but nourishing meal containing complex carbohydrates, fruits or vegetables, and high-quality protein to feed the body and mind. Avoid refined sugars and excessive fat intake, which can sap energy and derail quality study.

The NP candidate's anxiety started when pondering the wide range of possible topics on the certification examination. Starting the session by studying a narrowly focused topic with a specific outcome goal rather than simply studying might have averted this. Setting up a system of study can enhance the success of a study session further. One method is the SQ4R system, in which one surveys the study information to establish goals; formulates questions about the information; and then reads to answer these questions, followed by reciting the responses to the original questions and reviewing to see whether the original goals were met. Study and test-taking

> **TEST TAKING TIP**
> Avoid excessive amounts of caffeinated beverages prior to studying for the boards, which can add to anxious feelings.

anxiety can also be tamed with the help of a learning specialist who can work with the NP candidate to develop the needed skills. Learning specialists can usually be contacted through the academic support centers at universities.

How to Manage Test Day

You have devoted years of study and months of preparation to this day, and this very thought can be daunting. Approaching test day with an empowered mindset can help alleviate fears and prepare you for what lies ahead. Let's assume you have devoted a large amount of time to a purposeful and organized study regimen, and you are starting to think about the test day itself. Coaches often advise their athletes to avoid anything new on game day. You will be wise to heed this advice as well. This is not the time to change your diet, caffeine intake, medications, or sleep schedule.

> **TEST TAKING TIP**
>
> The test environment will be different from what you are used to, so try to keep your routines as close to "normal" for you as possible.

Visit the Web site of the certifying body to learn all that you can about test center rules, what you are and are not allowed to bring to the test site, and information about pacing and breaks. Usually the testing agency has a "test drive" video of what to expect with the examination software and the like. On test day, leave yourself plenty of time to arrive at your test center, get settled, and enter the test without feeling rushed. Be sure to have a government-issued photo ID as well as copies of all confirmation numbers and e-mails from the test center or organization. Expect that video surveillance will be used in test centers to limit fraud and ensure security. At many test centers, you will be asked to empty your pockets and place all personal items in a locker provided for your use.

> **TEST TAKING TIP**
>
> Expect that the topics you studied will be presented in random order on the test.

As part of your review, you should have some practice pacing yourself as you answer the test questions. Remember, you will have about 1 minute per test item. Do not get bogged down on a question or questions part of the way through the examination. If you are stumped by a question, use the testing software's highlighting option to mark the question, answer the question to the best of your ability, and move on, with a plan to return to this item at the end of the test. Do not be surprised if you highlight more questions earlier in the examination and less as you progress and are more comfortable with the test format and your brain is "warmed up." Remind yourself that you have answered many questions with relative ease. Finish all of the questions that you can answer and then come back later to process the problematic questions.

A question on diabetes mellitus follows one on hypertension and can be preceded by a question on women's health. A question on a teen will be followed by a question on an older adult.

Preparing for and taking the NP certification examination takes focus, determination, and courage. You have devoted years of study and months of preparation to this endeavor. Approaching test day with an empowered mindset can help alleviate fears and prepare you for what lies ahead. Emphasize context and adaptive expertise over memorization, become a master at "unlocking" test questions, and be honest with yourself about your learning style and study habits as you prepare to set yourself up for the best outcome.

Consider these clinical practice and certification tips as you prepare:

■ **Remember that common disease occurs commonly and that the uncommon presentation of a common disease is more common than the common presentation of an uncommon disease.**

- The fundamental tools of NP practice include the ability to procure comprehensively yet succinctly the information needed to develop accurate diagnoses.
- Gathering the needed subjective and objective information in the care of a person with common acute, episodic, and chronic health problems is the most important skill the NP can develop.
- Develop the skill of taking a thorough yet concise health history that is pertinent to the patient's presenting complaint or health problem.
- As you proceed through the history, recall the rationale behind each question you ask and how a given response impacts the possible etiology of the patient's health problem.
- Know how to perform a thorough yet succinct symptom analysis. It is during this process that the detective work of diagnosis starts.
- Use the physical examination to confirm the findings of the health history.

■ **Remember that the physical examination is guided by the health history, not the other way around.**

- The NP has the responsibility of arriving at a diagnosis, developing a treatment plan, and providing ongoing evaluation of response to treatment.
- To maximize your experience in your clinical rotations, learn to recognize the typical presentation for the 20 most common health problems that present to your practice site, including chief complaint and physical examination findings, differential diagnosis, needed diagnostics, intervention, and ongoing evaluation.
- Armed with this information, you can focus your study on a thorough knowledge of the assessment and treatment of these conditions.
- As an adult learner, carrying this applied learning to the boards helps make your NP education come alive.

Using these principles as you study for your NP boards will increase your likelihood of success with certification as well as your transition to NP practice. Best wishes—the world is waiting for the contributions that you will bring!

References

Mastering tests. https://firstyear.mit.edu/tutoring-support/study-tips/mastering-tests
Nugent P, Vitale B. *Test Success: Test-Taking Techniques for Beginning Nursing Students*. 6th ed. Philadelphia, PA: F.A. Davis; 2012.
Sefcik D. *How to Study for Standardized Tests*. Sudbury, MA: Jones & Bartlett; 2012.
Taking multiple choice exams. http://people.uwec.edu/ivogeler/multiple.htm
Test-taking strategies. https://xcasc.byu.edu/testtaking-strategies

Health Promotion and Disease Prevention

2

Select Topics in Health Promotion and Disease Prevention

Primary Prevention

Primary prevention measures include activities provided to individuals to prevent the onset or acquisition of a given disease. The goal of primary prevention measures is to spare individuals the suffering, burden, and cost associated with the clinical condition: primary prevention is the first level of health care. An example is health-protecting education and counseling, such as encouraging the use of car restraints and bicycle helmets, counseling about safer sexual practices, and providing information on accident and fall prevention. Given its focus on preventing illness or injury, primary prevention is usually viewed as the most effective form of health care.

Immunizations and chemoprophylaxis are also examples of primary prevention measures. Active immunization through the use of vaccines provides long-term protection from disease. In herd or community immunity, a significant portion of a given population has immunity against an infectious agent; the likelihood that the susceptible portion of the group would become infected is minimized (Fig. 2-1). Passive immunity is provided when a person receives select antibodies, usually via the administration of immune globulin (IG), after exposure to an infective agent. This immunity is temporary and requires the patient to present after exposure; the protection provided by IG usually starts within hours of receiving the doses and lasts a number of months. The use of vaccines to produce lasting disease protection is preferred to passive immunization through the use of IG. Another example of passive immunity is the acquisition of disease protection provided from the mother to the unborn child via the placenta.

Secondary Prevention

Secondary prevention measures include activities provided to identify and treat asymptomatic persons who have risk factors for a given disease or in preclinical disease.

Other examples of secondary prevention activities include screening for clinical conditions with a protracted asymptomatic period, such as a blood pressure measurement to detect hypertension and a lipid profile to detect hyperlipidemia (Table 2-1).

> **CLINICAL CONCEPT**
>
> Examples of secondary prevention include screening examinations for preclinical evidence of cancer, such as mammography, colonoscopy, and cervical examination with a Pap test.

Tertiary Prevention

Tertiary prevention measures are part of the management of an established disease. The goal of tertiary prevention is to minimize disease-associated complications and the negative health effects of the established clinical conditions. Examples include medications and lifestyle modification to normalize blood glucose levels in individuals with diabetes mellitus and in conjunction with the treatment of heart failure, aimed at improving or minimizing disease-related symptoms.

Discussion Sources

Centers for Disease Control and Prevention. Prevention. https://www.cdc.gov/pictureofamerica/pdfs/picture_of_america_prevention.pdf

National Institute of Allergy and Infectious Diseases (NIAID). Community immunity. https://www.nih.gov/about-nih/what-we-do/nih-almanac/national-institute-allergy-infectious-diseases-niaid

Section 1: Preventive Services Recommended by the USPSTF

The U.S. Preventive Services Task Force (USPSTF) recommends that clinicians discuss these preventive services with eligible patients and offer them as a priority. All these services have received an "A" or a "B" (recommended) grade from the Task Force. Refer to the endnotes for each recommendation for population-specific clinical considerations.

Recommendation	Adults		Special Populations	
	Men	Women	Pregnant Women	Children/ Adolescents
Abdominal Aortic Aneurysm, Screening[1]	✓			
Alcohol Misuse Screening and Behavioral Counseling	✓	✓	✓	
Aspirin for the Prevention of Cardiovascular Disease[2]	✓	✓		
Bacteriuria, Screening[3]			✓	
BRCA-Related Cancer in Women, Screening[4]		✓		
Breast Cancer, Preventive Medications[5]		✓		
Breast Cancer, Screening[6]		✓		
Breastfeeding, Counseling[7]		✓	✓	
Cervical Cancer, Screening[8]		✓		
Chlamydial Infection, Screening[9]		✓	✓	
Colorectal Cancer, Screening[10]	✓	✓		
Congenital Hypothyroidism, Screening[11]				✓
Depression in Adults, Screening[12]	✓	✓		
Diabetes Mellitus, Screening[13]	✓	✓		
Falls in Older Adults, Counseling, Preventive Medication, and Other Interventions[14]	✓	✓		
Folic Acid Supplementation to Prevent Neural Tube Defects, Preventive Medication[15]		✓		
Gestational Diabetes Mellitus, Screening[16]			✓	
Gonococcal Ophthalmia Neonatorum, Preventive Medication[17]				✓
Gonorrhea, Screening[18]		✓		
Hearing Loss in Newborns, Screening[19]				✓
Hepatitis B Virus Infection in Pregnant Women, Screening[20]			✓	
Hepatitis C Virus Infection in Adults, Screening[21]	✓	✓	✓	✓
High Blood Pressure in Adults, Screening	✓	✓		
HIV Infection, Screening[22]	✓	✓	✓	✓
Intimate Partner Violence and Elderly Abuse, Screening[23]		✓		
Iron Deficiency Anemia, Prevention[24]				✓
Iron Deficiency Anemia, Screening[25]			✓	
Lipid Disorders in Adults, Screening[26]	✓	✓		
Lung Cancer, Screening[27]	✓	✓		
Major Depressive Disorder in Children and Adolescents, Screening[28]				✓
Obesity in Adults, Screening[29]	✓	✓		
Obesity in Children and Adolescents, Screening[30]				✓
Osteoporosis, Screening[31]		✓		
Phenylketonuria (PKU), Screening[32]				✓
Sexually Transmitted Infections, Counseling[33]	✓	✓		✓
Sickle Cell Disease in Newborns, Screening[34]				✓
Skin Cancer, Counseling[35]	✓	✓	✓	✓
Syphilis Infection (Pregnant Women), Screening			✓	
Tobacco Use in Adults, Counseling and Interventions[36]	✓	✓	✓	
Tobacco Use in Children and Adolescents, Primary Care Interventions[37]				✓
Visual Impairment in Children Ages 1 to 5, Screening[38]				✓

FIGURE 2-1 Preventive services recommended by the U.S. Preventive Services Task Force (USPSTF).

http://www.ahrq.gov/professionals/clinicians-providers/guidelines-recommendations/guide/section1.html

Continued

Section 1: Preventive Services Recommended by the USPSTF (continued)

[1] One-time screening by ultrasonography in men aged 65 to 75 who have ever smoked.

[2] When the potential harm of an increase in gastrointestinal hemorrhage is outweighed by a potential benefit of a reduction in myocardial infarctions (men aged 45 to 79 years) or in ischemic strokes (women aged 55 to 79 years).

[3] Pregnant women at 12 to 16 weeks gestation or at first prenatal visit, if later.

[4] Refer women whose family history is associated with an increased risk for deleterious mutations in BRCA1 or BRCA2 genes for genetic counseling and evaluation for BRCA testing.

[5] Engage in shared, informed decision making and offer to prescribe risk-reducing medications, if appropriate, to women aged 35 years and older without prior breast cancer diagnosis who are at increased risk.

[6] Biennial screening mammography for women aged 50 to 74 years. Note: The Department of Health and Human Services, in implementing the Affordable Care Act, follows the 2002 USPSTF recommendation for screening mammography, with or without clinical breast examination, every 1 to 2 years for women aged 40 and older.

[7] Interventions during pregnancy and after birth to promote and support breastfeeding.

[8] Screen with cytology every 3 years (women aged 21 to 65) or co-test (cytology/HPV testing) every 5 years (women aged 30 to 65).

[9] Sexually active women 24 and younger and other asymptomatic women at increased risk for infection. Asymptomatic pregnant women 24 and younger and others at increased risk.

[10] Adults aged 50 to 75 using fecal occult blood testing, sigmoidoscopy, or colonoscopy.

[11] Newborns.

[12] When staff-assisted depression care supports are in place to assure accurate diagnosis, effective treatment, and follow-up.

[13] Asymptomatic adults with sustained blood pressure greater than 135/80 mm Hg.

[14] Provide intervention (exercise or physical therapy and/or vitamin D supplementation) to community-dwelling adults 65 years and older at increased risk for falls.

[15] All women planning or capable of pregnancy take a daily supplement containing 0.4 to 0.8 mg (400 to 800 µg) of folic acid.

[16] Asymptomatic pregnant women after 24 weeks of gestation.

[17] Newborns.

[18] Sexually active women, including pregnant women 25 and younger, or at increased risk for infection.

[19] Newborns.

[20] Screen at first prenatal visit.

[21] Persons at high risk for infection and adults born between 1945 and 1965.

[22] All adolescents and adults aged 15 to 65 years and others who are at increased risk for HIV infection and all pregnant women.

[23] Asymptomatic women of childbearing age; provide or refer women who screen positive to intervention services.

[24] Routine iron supplementation for asymptomatic children aged 6 to 12 months who are at increased risk for iron deficiency anemia.

[25] Routine screening in asymptomatic pregnant women.

[26] Men aged 20 to 35 and women over age 20 who are at increased risk for coronary heart disease; all men aged 35 and older.

[27] Asymptomatic adults aged 55 to 80 years who have a 30 pack-year smoking history and currently smoke or have quit smoking within the past 15 years.

[28] Adolescents (aged 12 to 18 years) when systems are in place to ensure accurate diagnosis, psychotherapy, and follow-up.

[29] Patients with a body mass index of 30 kg/m^2 or higher should be offered or referred to intensive, multicomponent behavioral interventions.

[30] Screen children aged 6 years and older; offer or refer for intensive counseling and behavioral interventions.

[31] Women aged 65 years and older and women under age 65 whose 10-year fracture risk is equal to or greater than that of a 65-year-old white woman without additional risk factors.

[32] Newborns.

[33] All sexually active adolescents and adults at increased risk for STIs.

[34] Newborns.

[35] Children, adolescents, and young adults aged 10 to 24 years.

[36] Ask all adults about tobacco use and provide tobacco cessation interventions for those who use tobacco; provide augmented, pregnancy-tailored counseling for those pregnant women who smoke.

[37] Provide interventions to prevent initiation of tobacco use in school-aged children and adolescents.

[38] Screen children aged 3 to 5 years.

FIGURE 2-1–cont'd

TABLE 2-1 Secondary Prevention Principles

PRINCIPLE	COMMENT
Prevalence is sufficient to justify screening.	Routine mammography is appropriate in women but not men.
Health problem has significant effect on quality or quantity of life.	Target diseases for secondary prevention include hypertension, type 2 diabetes mellitus, dyslipidemia, and certain cancers.
The target disease has a long asymptomatic period. The natural history of the disease, or how the disease unfolds without intervention, is known.	Treatment is available for the target disease. Providing treatment alters the disease's natural history.
A population-acceptable screening test is available.	The test should be safe, be available at a reasonable cost, and have reasonable sensitivity and specificity.

Source: Principles of screening. https://wiki.cancer.org.au/policy/Principles_of_screening

QUESTIONS

1. An example of a primary prevention measure for a 78-year-old man with chronic obstructive pulmonary disease (COPD) is:

   A. reviewing the use of prescribed medications.

   B. conducting a home survey to minimize fall risk.

   C. checking FEV_1 (force expired volume at 1 second) to FVC (forced vital capacity) ratio.

   D. ordering a fecal occult blood test (FOBT).

2. Which of the following is an example of a primary prevention activity in a 76-year-old woman with osteoporosis?

   A. bisphosphonate therapy

   B. calcium supplementation

   C. ensuring adequate illumination in the home

   D. use of a back brace

3. Secondary prevention measures for a 78-year-old man with COPD whose medications include an inhaled corticosteroid, long-acting beta-2 agonist, and theophylline, include:

   A. screening for mood disorders.

   B. administering influenza vaccine.

   C. obtaining a serum theophylline level.

   D. advising about appropriate use of car passenger restraints.

4. Tertiary prevention measures for a 69-year-old woman with heart failure include:

   A. administering pneumococcal vaccine.

   B. adjusting therapy to minimize dyspnea.

   C. surveying skin for precancerous lesions.

   D. reviewing safe handling of food.

5. Which of the following products provides passive immunity?

   A. hepatitis B immune globulin (HBIG)

   B. measles, mumps, and rubella (MMR) vaccine

   C. pneumococcal conjugate vaccine

   D. influenza vaccine

6. Active immunity is defined as:

   A. resistance developed in response to an antigen.

   B. immunity conferred by an antibody produced in another host.

   C. the resistance of a group to an infectious agent.

   D. defense against disease acquired naturally by the infant from the mother.

7. Which of the following is usually viewed as the most cost-effective form of health care?

   A. primary prevention

   B. secondary prevention

   C. tertiary prevention

   D. cancer-reduction measures

8. An 18-year-old woman with allergic rhinitis presents for primary care. She is sexually active with a male partner and is 1 year post-coitarche; during that time she had two sex partners. An example of a primary prevention activity for this patient is:

   A. screening for sexually transmitted infection (STI).
   B. counseling about safer sexual practices.
   C. prescribing therapies for minimizing allergy.
   D. obtaining a liquid-based Papanicolaou (Pap) test.

9. When a critical portion of a population is immunized against a contagious disease, most members of the group, even the unimmunized, are protected against that disease because there is little opportunity for an outbreak. This is known as _____ immunity.

   A. passive
   B. humoral
   C. epidemiological
   D. community

For answers and rationales, see end of chapter.

Influenza and Its Burden

Overview

An individual who presents with an abrupt onset of signs and symptoms including fever, myalgia, headache, malaise, nonproductive cough, sore throat, and rhinitis typically has uncomplicated influenza illness, more commonly known as "the flu." Children with influenza commonly have acute otitis media, nausea, and vomiting in addition to the aforementioned signs and symptoms. Although the worst symptoms in most uncomplicated cases resolve in about 1 week, the cough and malaise often persist for 2 or more weeks.

Rarely, influenza virus infection has been associated with encephalopathy, transverse myelitis, myositis, myocarditis, pericarditis, and Reye syndrome.

Mode of Transmission

Influenza viruses spread from person to person largely via respiratory droplets from an infected person, primarily through a cough or sneeze. In an immunocompetent adult, the influenza virus has a short incubation period, with a range of 1 to 4 days (average of 2 days). Adults pass the illness on 1 day before the onset of symptoms and continue to remain infectious for approximately 5 days after the onset of the illness. Children remain infectious for 10 or more days after the onset of symptoms and can shed the virus before the onset of symptoms. People who are immunocompromised can remain infectious for up to 3 weeks.

Complications and At-Risk Groups

Historically, the risks for complications, hospitalizations, and deaths from influenza have been higher among adults older than age 65 years, young children, and individuals of any age with certain underlying health conditions than among healthy older children and younger adults. In children younger than 5 years, hospitalization rates for influenza-related illness have ranged from approximately 500/100,000 for children with high-risk medical conditions to 100/100,000 for children without high-risk medical conditions. Hospitalization rates for influenza-related illness among children younger than 24 months are comparable to rates reported among adults older than 65 years. Influenza strains such as H1N1, an influenza A virus also known as swine flu,

CLINICAL CONCEPT

Individuals with ongoing health problems such as pulmonary or cardiac disease, young children, and pregnant women also have increased risk of influenza-related complications including pneumonia.

and H5N1, an influenza A virus also known as avian flu, appear to cause a greater disease burden in younger adults.

Immunization

Considering these factors, influenza, regardless of the viral strain, is not just a bad cold, but rather a potentially serious illness with significant morbidity and mortality risk across the life span. Even in the absence of complications, this viral illness typically causes many days of incapacitation and suffering and the risk of death. Over the past several flu seasons, vaccine effectiveness has typically ranged between 40% and 50%, with ongoing effort for a target of approximately 70% efficacy. The injectable vaccine does not contain live virus and is not shed; there is no risk of transmitting an infectious agent to household contacts. Influenza vaccine should only be delayed in the presence of moderate-to-severe illness with or without fever, which is the general rule for all immunizations.

While universal influenza immunization has been recommended for all aged 6 months and older for a number of years, members of certain at-risk groups should, in particular, be targeted for this vaccine. These include persons who live with or care for persons at high risk for influenza-related mortality and morbidity. Persons who provide essential community services should be considered for vaccination to minimize disruption of essential activities during influenza outbreaks. Students and other people in institutional or other group-living situations should be encouraged to receive the vaccine to minimize the risk of an outbreak in a relatively closed community. If supply of influenza vaccines is limited, certain groups at highest risk of influenza complication or transmission should be prioritized for immunization (Box 2-1).

> **CLINICAL CONCEPT**
>
> Because of the change in the respiratory and immune system normally present during pregnancy, influenza is five times more likely to cause serious disease in a pregnant woman when compared with a nonpregnant woman.

Most influenza vaccines are the quadrivalent form, providing protection against two influenza type A and two influenza type B strains. (See Box 2-1 for details on candidates for each vaccine.) The influenza vaccine should not be delayed to procure a specific vaccine preparation if an appropriate one is already available.

Two special influenza immunization situations bear mention. Children younger than 9 years who are receiving initial influenza immunization need two doses of vaccine separated by 4 or more weeks. Pregnant women should be immunized against influenza; the vaccine can be given regardless of pregnancy trimester.

Women who are immunized against influenza during pregnancy are able to pass a portion of this protection on to the unborn child, providing important protection during the first 6 months of life. Flu vaccine is also safe to give during lactation. Current recommendations advise that most individuals who are allergic to eggs can safely receive influenza vaccine (see Box 2-1).

In the northern hemisphere, the optimal time to receive any influenza vaccine is usually in the fall months, at least 1 month prior to the anticipated onset of the flu season; this timing is 6 months later in the southern hemisphere. The influenza

---

BOX 2-1 Advisory Committee on Immunization Practices (ACIP) Recommendations on Influenza Immunization

Routine influenza vaccination is recommended for all persons aged 6 months and older.

Although everyone should get a flu vaccine each flu season, certain patient populations are at high risk of having serious flu-related complications or live with or care for people at high risk for developing flu-related complications. Populations include:

- All children aged 6 through 59 months and adults 50 years and older.
- Adults and children who have chronic pulmonary (including asthma) or cardiovascular (except isolated hypertension), renal, hepatic, neurological, hematological, or metabolic disorders (including diabetes mellitus).
- Persons who are immunocompromised due to any cause.
- Women who are or will be pregnant during the influenza season.
- Children and adolescents (aged 6 months to 18 years) who receive aspirin- or salicylate-containing medications and who might be at risk for experiencing Reye syndrome after influenza virus infection.

Continued

BOX 2-1 Advisory Committee on Immunization Practices (ACIP) Recommendations on Influenza Immunization–cont'd

- Residents of nursing homes and other long-term care facilities.
- American Indians/Alaska Natives.
- Persons who are extremely obese (body mass index ≥40 kg/m^2).
- Health-care personnel, employees of nursing homes and long-term care facilities who have contact with patients, and students in these professions who will have contact with patients.
- Household contacts (including children) and caregivers of children aged ≤59 months and adults aged ≥50 years, particularly contacts of children aged less than 6 months.
- Household contacts and caregivers of persons with medical conditions that put them at high risk for severe complications from influenza.

All children aged 6 months to 8 years who receive a seasonal influenza vaccine for the first time should receive two doses spaced ≥4 weeks apart.

There are a variety of vaccines currently available to protect against influenza.

- Trivalent inactivated vaccine (IIV3) in standard dose administered intramuscularly approved for all aged ≥6 months who have no other contraindications. This is the typical "flu shot." A quadrivalent inactivated vaccine (IIV4) is also available intramuscularly or intradermally. A needle-free option via jet injector is also available for adults 18 to 64 years.
- Intradermal IIV4 in a lower dose when compared to standard flu vaccine administered intramuscularly (9 mcg rather than 15 mcg of each strain per dose) in a smaller volume (0.1 mL rather than 0.5 mL) approved for use in adults aged 18 to 64 years, with a preferred injection site over the deltoid.
- Inactivated IIV3 containing a greater dose of antigen when compared to standard flu vaccine (60 mcg rather than 15 mcg per dose) approved for use in adults aged ≥65 years
- Live, attenuated influenza vaccine, quadrivalent (LAIV4) via nasal spray: a flu vaccine made with live, weakened flu viruses that is given as a nasal spray. The viruses in the nasal spray vaccine do not cause the flu. LAIV4 is approved for use in healthy individuals, excluding pregnant women, aged 2 through 49 years.
- A trivalent cell culture-based inactivated influenza vaccine (ccIIV3), which is indicated for persons ≥4 years.
- A recombinant hemagglutinin vaccine (RIV3 or RIV4), which is indicated for persons aged ≥18 years.
- An adjuvanted trivalent inactivated influenza vaccine (aIIV3) administered intramuscularly for persons ≥65 years.

The following recommendations apply when considering influenza vaccination of persons who have or report a history of egg allergy:

1. Persons who have experienced only hives following exposure to egg should receive influenza vaccine. Any licensed and recommended influenza vaccine that is otherwise appropriate for the patient's age and health status may be used.
2. People who report having had reactions to egg involving angioedema, respiratory distress, lightheadedness, or recurrent emesis, or people who required epinephrine or other emergency medical intervention, may similarly receive any licensed and recommended influenza vaccine (e.g., appropriate IIV, RIV4, or LAIV4) that is otherwise appropriate for the patient's age and health status. The selected vaccine should be administered in an inpatient or outpatient medical center (including but not necessarily limited to hospitals, clinics, health departments, and physician offices). Vaccine administration should be supervised by a health-care provider who is able to recognize and manage severe allergic conditions.
3. People who are able to eat lightly cooked egg (e.g., scrambled egg) without a reaction are unlikely to be allergic. Egg-allergic people might tolerate egg in baked products (e.g., bread or cake). Tolerance to egg-containing foods does not exclude the possibility of egg allergy. Egg allergy can be confirmed by a consistent medical history of adverse reactions to eggs and egg-containing foods, plus skin and/or blood testing for immunoglobulin E directed against egg proteins.
4. Providers should consider observing all patients for 15 minutes after vaccination to decrease the risk of injury should they experience syncope.
5. A previous severe allergic reaction to influenza vaccine, regardless of the component suspected to be responsible, is a contraindication to future receipt of influenza vaccine.

Source: Grohskopf LA, Sokolow LZ, Broder KR, et al. Prevention and control of seasonal influenza with vaccines: Recommendations of the Advisory Committee on Immunization Practices–United States, 2018-19 influenza season. MMWR. 2018;67(3):1–20. https://www.cdc.gov/mmwr/volumes/67/rr/rr6703a1.htm?s_cid=rr6703a1_w

vaccine is given annually, and its contents are reflective of the viruses anticipated to cause influenza for the upcoming flu season.

Although select antiviral medications, including oseltamivir (Tamiflu), carry indications for the post-exposure prevention of influenza, all have a less favorable adverse reaction profile than influenza vaccine; these products are also significantly more expensive with greater risk for treatment failure. Active immunization against influenza A and B is the preferred method of disease prevention. Baloxavir marboxil (Xofluza) is a first-in-class polymerase acidic endonuclease inhibitor approved for the treatment of flu in patients 12 years and older; however, it is not currently approved for postexposure prophylaxis.

Discussion Sources

Centers for Disease Control and Prevention. Influenza (flu). https://www.cdc.gov/flu/index.htm

Centers for Disease Control and Prevention. Influenza vaccination information for health care workers. https://www.cdc.gov/flu/healthcareworkers.htm

Centers for Disease Control and Prevention. Influenza antiviral medications. https://www.cdc.gov/flu/professionals/antivirals/index.htm

QUESTIONS

10. When advising a patient about injectable influenza immunization, the nurse practitioner (NP) considers the following about the use of this vaccine:

    A. Its use is not recommended in sickle cell anemia.

    B. Its use is limited to children older than 2 years.

    C. Its use is limited because it contains live virus.

    D. Its use is recommended for virtually all members of the population.

11. A middle-aged man with COPD who is about to receive injectable influenza vaccine should be advised of the following:

    A. It is more than 90% effective in preventing influenza.

    B. Its use is contraindicated in the presence of select common health conditions including COPD.

    C. Localized reactions such as soreness and redness at the site of the immunization are fairly common.

    D. A short, intense, flu-like syndrome typically occurs after immunization.

12. A 44-year-old woman with asthma presents asking for a "flu shot." She is seen today for an urgent care visit, is diagnosed with a lower urinary tract infection, and is prescribed trimethoprim-sulfamethoxazole. She is without fever or gastrointestinal upset with stable respiratory status. You inform her that she:

    A. should return for the immunization after completing her antibiotic therapy.

    B. would likely develop a significant reaction if immunized today.

    C. can receive the immunization today.

    D. is not a candidate for any form of influenza vaccine.

13. Which of the following statements is most accurate regarding the use of antiviral agents for postexposure prophylaxis against influenza?

    A. Antivirals are not indicated for postexposure prophylaxis.

    B. The use of antivirals is less expensive than vaccines for prevention of flu.

    C. Antivirals have a higher risk of adverse effects compared to vaccination.

    D. When properly timed, using an antiviral is nearly 100% effective in preventing influenza.

14. Which of the following statements best describes antiviral use such as oseltamivir (Tamiflu) in the care of patients with or at risk for influenza?

    A. Initiation of therapy early in acute influenza illness can help minimize the severity of disease when the illness is caused by a nonresistant viral strain.

    B. The primary indication is in preventing influenza A during outbreaks.

    C. The drugs are active only against influenza B.

    D. The use of these medications is an acceptable alternative to the influenza vaccine.

15. All of the following are considered high-risk populations for serious flu-related complications except:

    A. children between 6 and 59 months.

    (B.) those of Asian ethnicity.

    C. adults with renal dysfunction.

    D. those who are extremely obese.

16. The most common mode of influenza virus transmission is via:

    A. contact with a contaminated surface.

    (B.) respiratory droplet.

    C. saliva contact.

    D. skin-to-skin contact.

17. In an immunocompetent adult, the length of incubation for the influenza virus is on average: *— healthy/normal*

    A. less than 24 hours.

    (B.) 1 to 4 days.

    C. 4 to 7 days.

    (D.) more than 1 week.

18. Influenza protection options for a 68-year-old man with hypertension, dyslipidemia, and type 2 diabetes mellitus include receiving:

    A. live attenuated influenza vaccine via nasal spray.

    (B.) high-dose trivalent inactivated vaccine (IIV3) via intramuscular injection.

    C. IIV4 via jet injector.

    D. appropriate antiviral medication at the initial onset of influenza-like illness.

19. Which of the following should not receive vaccination against influenza?

    A. a 19-year-old with a history of hive-form reaction to eating eggs

    B. a 24-year-old woman who is 8 weeks pregnant

    (C.) a 4-month-old infant who was born at 32 weeks of gestation

    D. a 28-year-old woman who is breastfeeding a 2-week-old infant

20. A healthy 6-year-old girl presents for care. Her parents request that she receive vaccination for influenza and report that she has not received this vaccine. How many doses of influenza vaccine should she receive this flu season?

    A. 1

    (B.) 2

    C. 3

    D. 4

21 to 24.   Match the appropriate influenza vaccination preparation to each of the following individuals. *(Some choices may be used more than once; some questions may have multiple answers.)*

    ___B___   21. A healthy 67-year-old man

    ___b___   22. A 12-year-old boy with asthma

    ___D___   23. A 42-year-old woman with severe egg allergy

    ___B___   24. A healthy 12-month-old infant

        A. LAIV4 (intranasal)

        B. IIV4 (intramuscular)

        C. IIV3, high dose (intramuscular)

        D. Recombinant influenza vaccine (RIV3, intramuscular)

For answers and rationales, see end of chapter.

Measles, Mumps, and Rubella and Their Burden

Overview

Rubella typically causes a relatively mild, 3- to 5-day illness with little risk of complication to the person infected. However, when rubella is contracted during pregnancy, the effects on the fetus can be devastating. Measles can cause severe illness with serious sequelae, including encephalitis and pneumonia; sequelae of mumps include orchitis and possible decreased male fertility.

Mode of Transmission

MMR are typically transmitted from person-to-person contact via respiratory droplets. Outbreaks of measles, mumps, or rubella typically occur when an infected individual reaches a community where groups of people are unvaccinated. Measles are still common in many parts of the world, including Europe, Asia, the Pacific, and Africa. Travelers to these areas can bring the disease to the United States and start an outbreak, primarily affecting unvaccinated individuals. Currently, approximately 1 in 10 children do not receive the MMR vaccine in the United States, largely due to parents declining the vaccine.

Complications and At-Risk Groups

Given that an initial MMR dose is given at age 12 months, infants (aged less than 12 months) are among the highest risk groups. In addition, all individuals, regardless of age, who have not received MMR vaccine or without a history of these illnesses are at risk.

Rubella typically causes a relatively mild, 3- to 5-day illness with little risk of complication to the person infected. When rubella is contracted during pregnancy, however, the effects on the fetus can be devastating. Immunizing the entire population against rubella exploits herd or community immunity and protects pregnant women from contracting rubella, therefore eliminating the risk of congenital rubella syndrome.

Measles can cause severe illness in any age group, though those younger than 5 years are more likely to suffer from severe complications.

Encephalitis can lead to convulsions, resulting in intellectual disabilities, while ear infections can cause permanent hearing loss. In pregnancy, measles can lead to premature birth and a low-birth-weight baby.

The sequelae of mumps include orchitis and possible decreased fertility; the fertility issue is more severe in males. Other possible complications can include encephalitis and meningitis as well as permanent loss of hearing.

> **CLINICAL CONCEPT**
> About 1 in 20 children develop pneumonia as a complication of measles, the most common cause of death from measles in young children.

Measles, Mumps, and Rubella Vaccine

The MMR vaccine contains live but weakened (attenuated) virus. A quadrivalent vaccine, protecting against measles, mumps, rubella, and varicella (chickenpox), is also available and usually used to immunize younger children (approved for use in children 12 months to 12 years).

- Two immunizations are recommended for children, starting with the first dose between 12 and 15 months of age and the second dose at 4 through 6 years of age. The second dose can be given earlier as long as it is a month apart from the first dose.
- For infants 6 to 11 months who will be traveling internationally, one dose of MMR should be given. If the dose was given before 1 year of age, the child should receive two additional doses of MMR (separated by at least 28 days).
- Adults who do not have evidence of immunity should also get at least one dose of MMR. Adults born in 1957 or earlier are considered immune as a result of having had these diseases (native or wild infection); vaccine against these three formerly common illnesses was unavailable until the 1960s.

As with all vaccines, giving additional doses to patients with an unclear immunization history is safe. (Download the latest Centers for Disease Control and Prevention [CDC] recommended adult, child, adolescent, and "catch-up" immunization schedules from the CDC Web site—see Discussion Sources.) Health-care professionals should have documented evidence of immunity (e.g., written documentation of adequate vaccination, laboratory evidence of immunity, or laboratory confirmation of measles). In practice, titers are rarely needed to confirm immunity. In the absence of documented evidence, two doses of MMR vaccine should be given at least 28 days apart.

During outbreaks, anyone without evidence of immunity should be brought up to date on MMR vaccination. An additional dose of MMR can be considered, even in the presence of previously documented completed MMR vaccine series, during outbreaks of measles and mumps.

Patients with a history of anaphylactic reaction to neomycin or gelatin should not receive MMR. The MMR vaccine is safe to use during lactation, but its use during pregnancy is discouraged because of the theoretical but unproven risk of congenital rubella syndrome from the live virus contained in the vaccine. The MMR vaccine is well tolerated; there have been rare reports of mild, transient adverse reactions such as rash and sore throat.

There has been speculation on the link between MMR vaccine and autism, primarily based on a small case series published in 1998 by Wakefield and colleagues. Despite the small sample size ($N = 12$) and poor study design, the study received wide publicity, and MMR vaccination rates dropped. The National Academy of Sciences conducted a review of all the evidence related to the MMR vaccine and autism. This independent panel examined completed studies, ongoing studies, published medical and scientific articles, and expert testimony to assess whether or not there was a link between autism and the MMR vaccine. The groups concluded that the evidence reviewed did not support an association between autism and the MMR vaccine. Although the preservative thimerosal, a mercury derivative, has been mentioned as a possible autism contributor, the MMR vaccine licensed for use in the United States does not contain this preservative.

Discussion Sources

Centers for Disease Control and Prevention. Vaccines and immunizations. https://www.cdc.gov/vaccines/index.html

Centers for Disease Control and Prevention. Recommended child and adolescent immunization schedule for ages 18 years or younger, United States. https://www.cdc.gov/vaccines/schedules/hcp/imz/child-adolescent.html

Centers for Disease Control and Prevention. Catch-up immunization schedule for persons aged 4 months–18 years who start late or who are more than 1 month behind, United States. https://www.cdc.gov/vaccines/schedules/hcp/imz/catchup.html

Centers for Disease Control and Prevention. Measles vaccination. https://www.cdc.gov/vaccines/vpd/measles/index.html

Centers for Disease Control and Prevention. Rubella (German measles) vaccination. https://www.cdc.gov/vaccines/vpd/rubella/index.html

Centers for Disease Control and Prevention. Mumps vaccination. https://www.cdc.gov/vaccines/vpd/mumps/index.html

QUESTIONS

25. When considering the diseases of MMR and the MMR vaccine, the NP considers the following:

    A. Patients born before 1957 have a high likelihood of immunity against these diseases because of a history of natural infection.

    B. Considerable mortality and morbidity occur with all three diseases.

    C. The virus is shed after vaccine administration.

    D. The use of the MMR vaccine is often associated with protracted arthralgia.

26. Which of the following is true about the MMR vaccine?

    A. It contains inactivated virus.

    B. Its use is contraindicated in patients with a history of egg allergy.

    C. Revaccination of an immune person is associated with risk of significant systemic allergic reaction.

    D. Two doses given at least 1 month apart are recommended for adults who have not been previously immunized.

27. A 22-year-old man is starting a job in a college health center and needs proof of German measles, measles, and mumps immunity. He received childhood immunizations and supplies documentation of MMR vaccination at age 1.5 years. Your best response is to:

    A. obtain rubella, measles (rubeola), and mumps titers.

    B. give MMR immunization now.

    C. advise him to obtain IG if he has been exposed to measles or rubella.

    D. advise him to avoid individuals with skin rashes.

28. Concerning the MMR vaccine, which of the following is true?

   A. The link between use of the MMR vaccine and childhood autism has been firmly established.

   B. There is no credible scientific evidence that the MMR vaccine increases the risk of autism.

   C. The use of the combined vaccine is associated with increased autism risk, but giving the vaccine's three components as separate vaccines minimizes this risk.

   D. The vaccine contains thimerosal, a mercury derivative.

29. Assuming all of the following individuals are not immune to MMR, which of the following is not recommended to receive the MMR vaccination?

   A. a 1-year-old boy with a history of hive-form reaction to egg ingestion

   B. a 24-year-old woman who is 20 weeks pregnant

   C. a 4-year-old girl who was born at 32 weeks of gestation

   D. a 32-year-old woman who is breastfeeding a 2-week-old

30 to 32. Indicate (Yes or No) whether it is helpful to administer an extra dose of MMR vaccine during the following outbreaks:

   N   **30.** Rubella

   Y   **31.** Measles

   Y   **32.** Mumps

For answers and rationales, see end of chapter.

Pneumococcal Disease and Its Burden

Overview

Pneumococcal disease, caused by the gram-positive diplococcus *Streptococcus pneumoniae,* results in significant mortality and morbidity.

> **CLINICAL CONCEPT**
>
> Pneumococcal disease can include sinusitis, acute otitis media, pneumonia, septicemia, and meningitis.

Approximately 900,000 people in the United States will get pneumococcal pneumonia each year, with 400,000 requiring hospitalization. An estimated 3,700 individuals die each year from invasive pneumococcal disease (meningitis and septicemia). Over 95% of pneumococcal deaths occur in adults.

At-Risk Groups

The latest recommendations from the Advisory Committee on Immunization Practices (ACIP) on pneumococcal vaccination established three levels of risk: average, increased, and highest.

- Average risk: those younger than 65 years of age without any chronic medical conditions; no pneumococcal vaccination needed.
- Increased risk: those 19 to 65 years old, cigarette smokers, or those with chronic medical conditions (e.g., diabetes, lung disease, cardiovascular disease, liver disease, or kidney disease [except end-stage kidney disease or nephrotic syndrome]) but without immune compromise. Vaccination is recommended.
- Highest risk: those 65 years and older or with immune compromised conditions, including those due to disease (e.g., malignancy, HIV, end-stage kidney disease), iatrogenic causes (e.g., chronic use of systemic corticosteroids, immunomodulators, transplant recipients), or functional or anatomic asplenia. Vaccination is recommended.

Pneumococcal Vaccine

The pneumococcal polysaccharide vaccine (Pneumovax, PPSV23) contains purified polysaccharide from 23 of the most common *S pneumoniae* serotypes. Pneumococcal conjugate vaccine (Prevnar, PCV13) contains purified capsular polysaccharide from 13 serotypes of pneumococcus. Both vaccines are used in older adults (65 years and older) as well as younger adults at high risk of infection. Use of PCV13 is associated with greater immunogenicity when compared with PPSV23, but it does not provide protection against as many pneumococcal serotypes.

PCV13 has been routinely used in childhood for a number of years. PPSV23 is not licensed for use in children younger than age 2 years. For those 65 years and older who have not yet received pneumococcal vaccine, individuals should receive PCV13 followed by PPSV23 at least 1 year later. If an initial PPSV23 vaccine was received at age 65 years or older, a repeat dose of PPSV23 is not required.

For younger adults in the increased risk category, individuals should receive PPSV23 followed by PCV13 at least 1 year later, and finally a second dose of PPSV23 at age 65 years (and at least 1 year following PCV13 and at least 5 years following the first PPSV23 dose).

In the highest risk category, those 65 years and older should receive PCV13 followed by PPSV23 at least 1 year later. Younger adults with highest-risk conditions (e.g., immunocompromised) should receive PCV13 followed by PPSV23 8 or more weeks later. Revaccination with PPSV23 5 years after the first PPSV23 dose is recommended for individuals in this risk group who are younger than age 65 years, as they are at greatest risk of having a rapid decline in antibody levels, including those with sickle cell disease, splenectomy, chronic renal failure, nephrotic syndrome, immunocompromise, generalized malignancy, or on immunosuppressing medications. At age 65 years, a final dose of PPSV23 should be administered (at least 5 years from the previous dose) for those who received PPSV23 at an earlier age.

This immunization, with initial and repeat vaccination, is generally well tolerated (Table 2-2).

Whatever the form used, the pneumococcal vaccine primarily protects against invasive disease such as meningitis and septicemia associated with pneumonia and disease caused by *S pneumoniae*; this organism is the leading cause of death from community-acquired pneumonia (CAP) in the United States. The PPSV23 vaccine protects from approximately 90% of the bacteremic disease associated with the pathogen, whereas the conjugate form (PCV13) is protective against approximately 70% of the bacteremic disease associated with the pathogen. These immunizations are ineffective, however, against pneumonia and invasive disease caused by other infectious agents, including *Mycoplasma pneumoniae*, *Chlamydophila* (formerly *Chlamydia*) *pneumoniae*, *Legionella* species, and select gram-negative respiratory pathogens such as *Haemophilus influenzae*, *Moraxella catarrhalis*, and *Klebsiella pneumoniae*.

Protection from invasive pneumococcal disease in a person living with HIV warrants special mention; the risk of pneumococcal infection is up to 100 times greater in people living with HIV than in other adults of similar age. Similar to the highest-risk category, once the diagnosis of HIV infection is made, the patient should receive both PCV13 and PPSV23 vaccines as soon as possible; PCV13 is given first, followed by PPSV23 8 weeks later. A second dose of PPSV23 should be administered at least 5 years after the initial dose, and a third dose should be administered at age 65 years (and at least 5 years from the previous dose) if the person was younger than age 65 years at the time of the second PPSV23 dose.

Discussion Sources

Centers for Disease Control and Prevention. PCV13 (pneumococcal conjugate) vaccine. https://www.cdc.gov/vaccines/vpd /pneumo/downloads/pneumo-vaccine-timing.pdf

Centers for Disease Control and Prevention. Ask the experts: Pneumococcal vaccines (PCV13 and PPSV23). http://www.immunize .org/askexperts/experts_pneumococcal_vaccines.asp

TABLE 2-2 Pneumococcal Vaccine Adverse Reactions

Local Reactions Including Pain, Redness	30%–50%
Fever, myalgia	Polysaccharide PPSV23 (Pneumovax)–valent polysaccharide vaccine) = Uncommon, <1%
	Conjugate PCV13 (Prevnar)-valent conjugate vaccine = 11%–40% in children, significantly less in adults with adverse reaction profile similar to 23-valent polysaccharide vaccine
Severe, potentially life threatening	Rare

Source: Updated recommendations for prevention of invasive pneumococcal disease among adults using the 23-valent pneumococcal polysaccharide vaccine (PPSV23). MMWR. 2010;59(34):1102–1106. https://www.cdc.gov/mmwr/preview/mmwrhtml/mm5934a3.htm

QUESTIONS

33. When advising an adult patient about pneumococcal immunization, the NP considers the following about the vaccine:

    A. The vaccine contains inactivated bacteria.

    B. Its use is contraindicated in individuals with lower airway disease.

    C. It protects against community-acquired pneumonia caused by atypical pathogens.

    D. Its use is seldom associated with significant adverse reactions.

34. Which of the following is an example of invasive pneumococcal disease?

    A. pneumonia

    B. acute otitis media

    C. meningitis

    D. sinusitis

35. Which of the following would not be a candidate for an initial dose of the pneumococcal vaccine?

    A. a healthy 66-year-old man

    B. a 34-year-old woman who smokes half a pack of cigarettes per day

    C. a 32-year-old woman in her first trimester of pregnancy

    D. a 56-year-old man with type 2 diabetes mellitus

36. All of the following patients received PPSV23 more than 5 years ago. Who is a candidate for receiving a second dose of PPSV23 immunization at this time?

    A. a 45-year-old man who is a cigarette smoker

    B. a 66-year-old woman with a 10-year history of COPD who received PCV13 1 year ago

    C. a 35-year-old man with moderate persistent asthma

    D. a 57-year-old woman with atrial fibrillation

37 to 40. Identify whether the item has the characteristics of 23-valent PPSV23, 13-valent PCV13, or both.

    _13_ 37. Routinely used in early childhood

    _13_ 38. Use is associated with greater immunogenicity

    both 39. Routinely used in all well adults aged 65 years or older

    _23_ 40. Not licensed for use in children younger than 2 years of age

41. A 28-year-old adult presents who recently found out he is living with HIV. The NP recommends:

    A. vaccination with PPSV23 now and revaccination with PPSV23 at age 65 years.

    B. vaccination with PCV13 now and revaccination with PPSV23 in 8 weeks.

    C. vaccination with PCV13 now and revaccination with PPSV23 in 5 years.

    D. no vaccination needed until age 65 years.

42. Which of the following is recommended for a 65-year-old woman in generally good health who has not received any form of pneumococcal vaccine?

    A. PCV13 only

    B. PPSV23 only

    C. PCV13 now and PPSV23 in 1 year

    D. PPSV23 now and PCV13 in 8 weeks

For answers and rationales, see end of chapter.

Hepatitis A and Its Burden

Overview

Hepatitis A infection is caused by hepatitis A virus (HAV), a small RNA virus. Transmission through the fecal-oral route is the primary means of HAV transmission in the United States. Often, a member of a household or someone who lives in close contact with others introduces the infection into the group. HAV replicates in the liver, is excreted in bile, and is shed in stool.

Jaundice, when present, occurs about 1 week after the onset of symptoms; jaundice is not found in most cases, but once it occurs, the amount of HAV in the stool diminishes.

Fecal-contaminated water supplies are the most common source of infection. Adequate chlorination and purification of municipal water, as recommended in the United States, kills HAV before it enters the water supply. Effective methods to inactivate HAV include heating or cooking foods to temperatures greater than 185°F (greater than 85°C) for 1 minute or disinfecting surfaces with a 1:100 dilution of sodium hypochlorite, the active component of household bleach, in tap water. For travel to developing nations, the traveler should be advised to avoid foods that are usually eaten raw, including fruits, many vegetables, and shellfish from contaminated waterways. Thorough food cooking largely eliminates this risk. In the majority, hepatitis A typically causes a self-limiting infection with a very low mortality rate. HAV infection does not become chronic. However, co-infection with hepatitis A and C, with hepatitis A and B, or acute hepatitis A in addition to a chronic liver disease can lead to a rapid deterioration in hepatic function. See Chapter 8 for more information on the clinical presentation, diagnostics, and treatment of hepatitis.

> **CLINICAL CONCEPT**
> Peak infectivity in acute hepatitis A occurs during the 2-week period before the onset of jaundice or elevation of liver enzymes, when concentration of virus in the stool is highest.

At-Risk Groups

In developing countries with limited pure water, most children contract this disease by age 5 years; more than 70% of children younger than age 6 years will have few or no symptoms during HAV infection.

In North America, adults 20 to 39 years old account for nearly 50% of the reported cases; in the United States, nearly half of all reported hepatitis A cases have no specific risk factor identified. Among adults with identified risk factors, the majority of cases are among men who have sex with other men, persons who use illegal drugs, and international travelers.

Prevention and Immunization

ACIP recommends all children to be vaccinated against HAV starting at 1 year of age. Priority candidates for immunization against HAV include individuals who have a significant risk for acquisition or transmission of hepatitis A, including people who reside in or travel to areas in which the disease is endemic, food handlers, sewage workers, animal handlers, day-care attendees and workers, long-term care residents and workers, military personnel, and health-care workers.

Injection drug users also benefit from the vaccine. HAV is rarely transmitted sexually or from needle sharing; rather, injection drug users often live in conditions that facilitate the oral-fecal transmission of HAV.

Co-infection with hepatitis A and C, co-infection with hepatitis A and B, or acute hepatitis A in addition to chronic liver disease, including all forms of fatty liver disease, can lead to a rapid deterioration in hepatic function; these individuals should be immunized against hepatitis A. If a person who has a clotting factor disorder and is receiving clotting factor concentrates does not have documentation of HAV immunity, that person should also be immunized.

Any person anticipating close personal contact, such as a household member or caregiver, with an international adoptee during the first 60 days after arrival in the United States from a country with high or intermediate endemicity is also encouraged to be immunized; the HAV vaccine should be given at least 2 weeks prior to the arrival of the adoptee if possible.

The following additional populations should be immunized against HAV: men who have sex with men, persons working with HAV-infected primates or with HAV in a research laboratory setting, and anyone who requests HAV protection.

HAV vaccine, which does not contain live virus, is usually well tolerated without systemic reaction. A variety of formulas are available with different numbers of doses recommended, dependent on the clinical situation. Consult the CDC vaccine schedules to ensure proper vaccination.

Treatment for HAV is largely supportive. There is no chronic form of the infection. (See Chapter 8.) With HAV exposure, IG or HAV vaccine can be given within 2 weeks to minimize the risk of hepatitis A infection. Postexposure prophylaxis can be considered for children less than 12 months, immunocompromised individuals, those with chronic liver disease, and for those whom the vaccine is contraindicated. Anti-HAV IG is preferred over the vaccine in these populations as well as for those older than 40 years of age. If IG is unavailable, then the vaccine can be used (unless contraindicated). IG is a product derived from pooled blood that contains preformed antibodies against the virus and has an outstanding safety profile.

CLINICAL CONCEPT

Past HAV infection confers lifelong immunity.

Discussion Source

Centers for Disease Control and Prevention. Viral hepatitis: hepatitis A information. https://www.cdc.gov/hepatitis/hav/index.htm

QUESTIONS

43. Of the following, the most common route of HAV transmission is:

A. needle sharing.

B. raw shellfish ingestion.

C. ingestion of contaminated food or water.

D. exposure to blood and body fluids.

44. When answering questions about the HAV vaccine, the NP considers that it:

A. contains live virus.

B. should be offered to adults who frequently travel to countries where the disease is endemic.

C. is contraindicated for use in children younger than age 6 years.

D. usually confers lifelong protection after a single injection.

45. Usual treatment for an adult with acute hepatitis A includes:

A. interferon-alfa therapy.

B. high-dose ribavirin.

C. parenteral acyclovir.

D. supportive care.

46. Peak infectivity of persons with hepatitis A usually occurs:

A. before the onset of jaundice.

B. at the time of maximum elevation of liver enzymes.

C. during the recovery period.

D. at the time of maximum disease-associated symptoms.

47. In the United States, what proportion of all reported hepatitis A cases have no specific risk factor identified?

A. approximately 25%

B. approximately 50%

C. approximately 75%

D. nearly 100%

48. Which of the following represents the food or beverage that is least likely to be contaminated with HAV?

A. a lettuce salad

B. a bowl of hot soup

C. a plate of peeled mango

D. a glass of iced tea

49. A 62-year-old man is recently diagnosed with nonalcoholic fatty liver disease. He does not recall ever having HAV infection, and his immunization history does not show vaccination for HAV. The NP correctly recommends:

A. that titers should be ordered to check for past HAV infection.

B. a single dose of HAV vaccine.

C. a two-dose series of HAV vaccine.

D. that no HAV vaccine is needed as it is contraindicated due to his age.

50. You see a 27-year-old man who has had no immunizations "since I was a little kid" and has no vaccination record. He states that he ate at a restaurant last week that was later reported to have a worker identified as being infected with the HAV. He is healthy and shows no sign of infection but is concerned about contracting the HAV. You recommend that he receive:

A. HAV vaccine today.

B. HAV IG within the next week.

C. HAV vaccine plus IG today.

D. no intervention at this time; monitor for HAV infection symptoms and receive an antiviral if symptoms manifest.

51. When answering questions about the HAV vaccine, you consider that all of the following are true except:

A. It generally is well tolerated.

B. It should be offered to individuals who frequently travel to developing countries.

C. It is a recommended immunization for health-care workers.

D. It contains live HAV virus.

52. When discussing the use of IG with a 60-year-old woman who was recently exposed to HAV, you consider that:

A. IG is derived from pooled donated blood.

B. the product must be used within 1 week of exposure to provide protection.

C. its use in this situation constitutes an example of active immunization.

D. a short, intense, flu-like illness often occurs after its use.

For answers and rationales, see end of chapter.

Hepatitis B and Its Burden

Overview

The hepatitis B virus (HBV) is caused by the small double-stranded DNA HBV that contains an inner core protein of hepatitis B core antigen (HBcAg) and an outer surface of hepatitis B surface antibody (HBsAg). The virus is usually transmitted through an exchange of blood and body fluids, including semen, vaginal secretions, and saliva, via percutaneous and mucosal exposure.

Acute hepatitis B is a serious illness that can lead to acute hepatic failure, particularly in patients with underlying liver disease including chronic hepatitis and fatty liver disease. Approximately 5% to 10% of adults with hepatitis B infection develop chronic hepatitis B. Although usually appearing clinically well, a person with chronic hepatitis B continues to be able to transmit the virus. Chronic hepatitis B is a potent risk factor for the development of hematoma or primary hepatocellular carcinoma and hepatic cirrhosis. See Chapter 8 for clinical presentation, diagnostics, and treatment options for hepatitis B.

> **CLINICAL CONCEPT**
> HBV has a long incubation period with symptoms occurring an average of 90 days after exposure but could range from 60 to 150 days.

At-Risk Groups

Groups at particular risk for HBV acquisition include sex partners of people with acute or chronic HBV infection, sexually active persons who have one or more sex partners and/or a new partner, men who have sex with men, injection drug users, household contacts of persons with chronic HBV infection, patients receiving hemodialysis, residents and staff of facilities for people with developmental disabilities, and travelers to or adoptees from countries with intermediate or high prevalence of HBV infection.

Additional at-risk groups include health-care and public safety workers at risk for occupational exposure to blood or body fluids. Individuals with type 1 and 2 diabetes mellitus are considered at higher risk for HBV acquisition when in settings such as a hospital, an assisted-living facility, or a long-term care facility where blood sugars are checked using common equipment and without proper technique. Infants born to mothers with HBV infection are at particular risk for HBV acquisition via the placenta, during birth, and/or via breast milk. Without intervention, approximately 40% of infants born to mothers with HBV will develop chronic hepatitis B, and approximately one-fourth of the infected infants will go on to die of chronic liver disease.

Prevention and Immunization

Hepatitis B infection can be prevented by limiting percutaneous and mucosal exposure to blood and body fluids and through immunization. Recombinant HBV vaccine, which does not contain live virus, is well tolerated but is contraindicated in those who have a history of anaphylactic reaction to baker's yeast (Table 2-3). As with all vaccines, immunization against HBV should be delayed in the face of serious or life-threatening illness. See the Centers for Disease Control and Prevention Web site for additional information on the HBV vaccine dosing schedule across the life span.

The HBV vaccine became available in 1982; however, universal childhood vaccination started in 1991, and as a result one major at-risk group is adults born before that date who have not been offered the vaccine. Health-care and public safety workers are recommended to be HBV immunized; receiving this vaccine is often a requirement of employment. Additional groups who should be encouraged to receive HBV vaccine include persons with chronic liver disease and those living with HIV. Because of an increased risk of developing chronic HBV, unvaccinated adults with diabetes mellitus type 1 or 2 should also be encouraged to receive HBV vaccine. All other persons seeking protection from HBV infection, whether acknowledging specific HBV risk, are candidates for immunization.

Infants who become infected perinatally with HBV have an estimated 25% lifetime chance of developing hepatocellular carcinoma or cirrhosis. As a result, all pregnant women should be screened for HBsAg at the first prenatal visit, regardless of HBV vaccine history. Because the HBV vaccine is not 100% effective and perinatal transmission is possible, a woman could have carried HBV before becoming pregnant.

Women at particularly high risk for new HBV acquisition during pregnancy should be retested for HBsAg in later pregnancy. In cases in which maternal HBsAg status is unknown, a situation common in

TABLE 2-3 Personal Immunization Contraindications

ANAPHYLACTIC REACTION HISTORY	IZ TO AVOID
Neomycin	IPV, MMR, varicella
Streptomycin, polymyxin B, neomycin	IPV, vaccinia (smallpox)
Baker's yeast	Hepatitis B
Gelatin, neomycin	Varicella zoster
Gelatin	MMR

Abbreviations: *MMR, measles, mumps, and rubella; IPV, inactivated polio vaccine; IZ, immunization*

children who have been adopted internationally, consideration should be given to testing the child for evidence of perinatal acquisition of HBV infection.

About 90% to 95% of adolescents and adults who receive the HBV vaccine develop HBsAb (anti-HBs) after completing the series, implying protection from the virus. About 98% of healthy term infants achieve seroprotection with vaccination. HBsAb testing should be considered, however, to confirm the development of HBV protection in individuals with a high risk for infection (e.g., select health-care workers with anticipated high levels of blood and body fluid exposure, infants born to HBsAg-positive mothers, and sex partners of HBsAg-positive persons) and individuals at risk for poor immune response (e.g., dialysis patients, immunosuppressed patients, and persons living with HIV).

Booster doses of HBV vaccine are recommended only in certain circumstances, including for infants born to HBsAg-positive mothers, health-care providers, hemodialysis patients, and other immunocompromised persons. For these high-risk individuals, a booster dose should be administered when the anti-HBs level is less than 10 mIU/mL. For patients receiving hemodialysis, the need for booster doses should be assessed by annual testing for antibody to HBsAg (anti-HBs or HBsAb). For other immunocompromised persons (e.g., people living with HIV, hematopoietic stem cell transplant recipients, and persons receiving chemotherapy), annual testing and booster doses should be considered with an ongoing risk of exposure. Ongoing serological surveillance in the immunocompetent population is not recommended.

Postexposure prophylaxis is effective in preventing HBV infection. In a person with documentation of a complete HBV vaccine series and who did not receive postvaccination testing, a single HBV vaccine booster dose should be given with exposure to a nonoccupational known HBsAg-positive source. A person who is in the process of being vaccinated but who has not completed the vaccine series should receive the appropriate dose of HBIG and should complete the vaccine series.

Unvaccinated persons should receive HBIG and hepatitis B vaccine as soon as possible after HBV exposure, preferably within 24 hours after exposure. Testing for HIV, hepatitis A, and hepatitis C should also be offered; where applicable, postexposure prophylaxis should be offered. Owing to the complexity of care, intervention for the person with possible HBV occupational exposure should be done in consultation with experts in the area.

> **CLINICAL CONCEPT**
> Routine testing for the presence of HBsAb after immunization is not generally recommended in infants, children, or adults.

Discussion Sources

Centers for Disease Control and Prevention. Hepatitis B questions and answers for health professionals. http://www.cdc.gov/hepatitis/hbv/hbvfaq.htm

Schillie S, Vellozzi C, Reingold A, et al. Prevention of hepatitis B virus infection in the United States: Recommendations of the Advisory Committee on Immunization Practices. *MMWR Recomm Rep*. 2018;67(R1):1–31. http://www.cdc.gov/mmwr/preview/mmwrhtml/rr5516a1.htm?s_cid=rr5516a1_e

QUESTIONS

53. Concerning HBV vaccine, which of the following is true?

    A. The vaccine contains live, whole HBV.

    B. Adults should routinely have testing for protective HBV titers measured after three doses of vaccine.

    C. The vaccine should be offered during treatment for sexually transmitted diseases in unimmunized adults.

    D. Serological testing for HBsAg should be done before hepatitis B vaccination is initiated in adults.

54. In which of the following groups is routine HBsAg screening recommended?

    A. hospital laboratory workers

    B. adults who have received the hepatitis B vaccine series

    C. pregnant women

    D. college students

55. You see a 45-year-old man who has been sexually active with a man diagnosed with acute hepatitis B within the past week. He has not received the HBV vaccine and has no history of acute or chronic hepatitis B. You advise that he should: (*Choose all that apply.*)

A. be advised that there is no particular interventional post-HBV exposure therapy.

B. consider additional STI testing.

C. be tested for HBsAb.

D. consider receiving HBIG and start the hepatitis B immunization series.

56. HBV vaccine should not be given to a person with a history of anaphylactic reaction to:

A. eggs.

B. baker's yeast.

C. neomycin.

D. streptomycin.

57. Risks associated with chronic hepatitis B include all of the following except:

A. hepatocellular carcinoma.

B. cirrhosis.

C. continued ability to transmit the organism.

D. cholelithiasis.

58. Jason is a healthy 19-year-old who presents for primary care. According to his immunization record, he received two doses of HBV vaccine 1 month apart at age 16 years. Which of the following best describes his HBV vaccination needs?

A. He should receive a single dose of HBV vaccine now.

B. A three-dose HBV vaccine series should be started during today's visit.

C. He has completed the recommended HBV vaccine series.

D. He should be tested for HBsAb, and further immunization recommendations should be made according to the test results.

59. All of the following individuals have not received vaccination against HBV. The vaccine should not be given in which of the following patients?

A. a 35-year-old man with multiple sclerosis

B. a 25-year-old woman with a past history of Guillain-Barré syndrome

C. a 48-year-old woman with systemic lupus erythematosus

D. a 28-year-old man who is acutely ill with bacterial meningitis

60. A major HBV at-risk group is adults born before the year that widespread use of the vaccine in childhood began. What year was this?

A. 1972

B. 1986

C. 1991

D. 1998

61. You see Harold, a 25-year-old man who recently had multiple sexual encounters including receptive anal intercourse without condom use with a male partner who has chronic hepatitis B. Harold provides documentation of receiving a properly timed hepatitis B immunization series. In addition to counseling about safer sexual practices and additional STI testing, you also advise that Harold:

A. needs to repeat his hepatitis B immunization series.

B. receive a single dose of HBV vaccine.

C. be tested for HBsAb.

D. should receive HBIG and a single dose of the hepatitis B immunization series.

For answers and rationales, see end of chapter.

Varicella-Zoster Virus and Its Burden

Overview

Varicella-zoster virus (VZV) causes the highly contagious, systemic disease commonly known as chickenpox; VZV infection typically presents with 300 to 500 vesicular lesions, body aches, fever, itch, and fatigue. The varicella virus is transmitted via respiratory droplets and contact with open lesions. Chickenpox can be serious, especially in infants, adults, and individuals of all ages who are immunocompromised. The greatest rate of mortality from varicella is in adults 30 to 49 years old, pregnant women, and infants. Varicella complications commonly include infected skin lesions and, less commonly but more seriously, pneumonia, sepsis, and encephalitis.

Prior to the availability of the VZV vaccine, chickenpox was a prevalent childhood illness. As a result, nearly all adults born before 1980 will have evidence of varicella immunity due to having had chickenpox. A history of naturally occurring chickenpox, also known as wild varicella infection, usually confers lifetime immunity. Reinfection is, on rare occasion, seen in immunocompromised patients, however. More often, reexposure causes an increase in antibody titers without causing disease. A late chickenpox complication is zoster, also known as shingles. (See section on zoster and its prevention.)

Varicella Vaccine

The varicella vaccine is routinely administered to children on or after their first birthday with a repeat dose usually given between ages 4 and 6 years.

In particular, health-care workers, family contacts of immunocompromised patients, and day-care workers should be targeted for varicella vaccine, as should adults who are in environments with a high risk of varicella transmission, such as college dormitories, military barracks, and long-term care facilities. Pregnant women should be assessed for evidence of varicella immunity. Women who do not have evidence of immunity should receive the first dose of varicella vaccine on completion or termination of pregnancy and before discharge from the health-care facility. The second dose should be administered 4 to 8 weeks after the first dose.

The varicella vaccine is highly protective against severe, invasive varicella. Mild cases of chickenpox are occasionally reported even after immunization, however. Because this is a live, attenuated virus vaccine, it should be used with caution in certain clinical situations (Table 2-4).

> **CLINICAL CONCEPT**
>
> Older children and adults with no history of varicella infection or previous immunization should receive two varicella immunizations 4 to 8 weeks apart.

Evidence of immunity to varicella includes documentation of age-appropriate vaccination with VZV vaccine, laboratory evidence of immunity or laboratory confirmation of disease, birth in the United States before 1980, or the diagnosis or verification of a history of varicella disease or herpes zoster by a health-care provider. Among adults born before 1980 with an unclear or negative varicella history, most are also seropositive. Confirming varicella immunity through varicella titers, even in the presence of a history of varicella infection, should be done in health-care workers because of their risk of exposure and potential transmission of the disease.

For healthy children and adults without evidence of varicella immunity, vaccination within 3 to 5 days of exposure to varicella is beneficial in preventing or modifying the disease. Studies have shown that vaccination administered within 3 days of exposure to rash is at least 90% effective in preventing varicella, whereas vaccination within 5 days of exposure to rash is approximately 70% effective in preventing varicella and 100% effective in modifying severe disease. For individuals without evidence of immunity who have contraindications for vaccination but are at risk for severe disease and complications, use of varicella-zoster immune globulin (VZIG) is recommended for postexposure prophylaxis.

Complications of Varicella Zoster: Zoster (Shingles)

After having chickenpox, VZV can lie dormant in sensory nerve ganglia. Later reactivation causes shingles, a painful, vesicular-form rash in a dermatomal pattern. About 15% of individuals who have

TABLE 2-4 Live, Attenuated Virus Vaccines

Vaccine prepared from live microorganisms or viruses cultured under adverse conditions leading to loss of virulence but retention of their ability to induce protective immunity.

LIVE ATTENUATED VIRUS VACCINE EXAMPLES	PRECAUTIONS FOR USE IN SPECIAL POPULATIONS
MMR (measles, mumps, rubella)	Pregnancy because of theoretical risk of passing virus to unborn child
Varicella (chickenpox)	
Intranasal influenza virus vaccine (FluMist)*	Immune suppression, with the exception of HIV, because of potential risk of becoming ill with virus
Zoster (Zostavax)**	For direction on giving live virus vaccines in children and adults living with HIV, clarification from the CDC immunization guidelines should be followed.
Rotavirus vaccine (oral vaccine only given to young infants)	Use contraindicated in infants diagnosed with severe combined immunodeficiency (SCID)

*Please check on the latest recommendations on the use of FluMist, as these have varied year-to-year, at https://www.cdc.gov/vaccines/hcp/.
**Seldom use with limited availability.*

had chickenpox develop shingles during their lifetime. Shingles rates are markedly reduced in individuals who have received varicella vaccine compared with individuals who have had wild or native VZV disease. The virus is present in the vesicles seen in shingles. If an individual without varicella immunity comes in contact with shingles skin lesions, that individual could contract chickenpox. An individual with shingles cannot transmit shingles to another person.

About one in three people in the United States will develop shingles. The risk of shingles increases with age (particularly in persons older than 50 years), though those with compromised immune systems are also at higher risk. High-risk individuals include those with malignancies such as leukemia or lymphoma, those living with HIV, as well as those taking immunosuppressive medications (e.g., systemic corticosteroids). Though shingles is not a life-threatening condition, certain complications can severely impact quality of life.

The severity and duration of postherpetic neuralgia are greater for older adults, further emphasizing the need to ensure the older adult population is vaccinated. Lesions occurring around the eye (ophthalmic shingles) can cause painful eye infections and permanent vision loss. Other, less common complications can include encephalitis, facial paralysis, or hearing and balance problems.

CLINICAL CONCEPT

The most common serious shingles complication is postherpetic neuralgia, which is characterized by severe and debilitating pain that persists for weeks or months after the lesions have resolved.

Zoster Vaccine

There are two vaccines currently available for shingles. Zostavax (ZVL) is a live vaccine that was approved in 2006 and has been shown to provide protection for about 5 years. It is given as a single dose to adults 60 years and over. Since Zostavax is a live virus vaccine, it is contraindicated for those with immunosuppression or immunodeficiency (including those living with HIV, taking immunosuppressive medications, undergoing radiation or chemotherapy, or who have leukemia or lymphoma) as well as during pregnancy. Shingrix (RZV) is a recombinant zoster vaccine that became available in 2017 and is the preferred vaccine by ACIP due to its greater immunogenicity, less contraindications, and potentially longer duration of protection. The vaccine is recommended for immunocompetent adults 50 years and older and is given in two doses separated by 2 to 6 months. Individuals who already received Zostavax should also receive Shingrix for full protection against shingles. The zoster vaccine should still be given to individuals who have had shingles, though vaccination should be delayed until an acute episode of shingles resolves, usually within 8 weeks after the onset of lesions.

Discussion Sources

Centers for Disease Control and Prevention. Varicella vaccination information for healthcare professionals. https://www.cdc.gov
/vaccines/vpd/varicella/hcp/index.html
Centers for Disease Control and Prevention. Shingles (herpes zoster) vaccination. https://www.cdc.gov/vaccines/vpd/shingles/index.html

QUESTIONS

62. Which of the following statements is correct about the varicella vaccine?

    A. It contains killed VZV.

    B. The use of the vaccine is associated with an increase in reported cases of shingles.

    C. Varicella vaccine should be offered to adults who were born in the United States prior to 1980 and report a childhood history of chickenpox.

    D. Although highly protective against invasive varicella disease, mild cases of chickenpox have been reported in immunized individuals.

63. For which of the following patients should an NP order varicella antibody titers?

    A. a 14-year-old with an uncertain immunization history

    B. a health-care worker who reports having had varicella as a child

    C. a 22-year-old woman who received two varicella immunizations 6 weeks apart

    D. a 72-year-old with shingles

64. A woman who has been advised to receive VZIG asks about its risks. You respond that IG is a:

    A. synthetic product that is well tolerated.

    B. pooled blood product that often transmits infectious disease.

    C. blood product obtained from a single donor.

    D. pooled blood product with an excellent safety profile.

65. Maria is a 28-year-old healthy woman who is 6 weeks pregnant. Her routine prenatal laboratory testing reveals she is not immune to varicella. She voices her intent to breastfeed her infant for at least 6 months. Which of the following represents the best advice for Maria?

    A. She should receive VZV vaccine once she is in her second trimester of pregnancy.

    B. Maria should be advised to receive two doses of properly timed VZV vaccine after giving birth.

    C. Once Maria is no longer breastfeeding, she should receive one dose of VZV vaccine.

    D. A dose of VZIG should be administered now.

66. How is the varicella virus most commonly transmitted?

    A. droplet transmission

    B. contact with inanimate reservoirs

    C. contact transmission

    D. water-borne transmission

67. All of the following are potentially serious complications associated with shingles except:

    A. condyloma acuminatum.

    B. postherpetic neuralgia.

    C. permanent vision loss.

    D. encephalitis.

68 to 71. Indicate (Yes or No) whether each of the following individuals is eligible to receive the Shingrix vaccine.

    _____ **68.** A 57-year-old man who reports he never had chickenpox as a child

    _____ **69.** A 33-year-old woman who is trying to conceive her first child

———— **70.** A 62-year-old man living with HIV

———— **71.** A 66-year-old who received the Zostavax vaccine 1 year ago

72. Which of the following statements regarding Shingrix and Zostavax is false?

A. Zostavax contains live virus, while Shingrix does not.

B. Both Shingrix and Zostavax are given as a single dose.

C. Shingrix induces greater immunogenicity compared to Zostavax.

D. There are more contraindications with Zostavax compared with Shingrix.

For answers and rationales, see end of chapter.

Tetanus, Diphtheria, and Pertussis and Their Burden

Overview

Tetanus (lockjaw) infection is caused by *Clostridium tetani,* an anaerobic, gram-positive, spore-forming rod. This organism is usually found in soil, particularly if it contains manure, and enters the body through a deep, soil-contaminated wound. The end point can be a life-threatening systemic disease characterized by painful muscle weakness and spasm (lockjaw) with at least a 10% mortality rate.

Diphtheria, caused by *Corynebacterium diphtheriae,* a gram-negative bacillus, is typically transmitted from person-to-person contact via respiratory droplets or cutaneous lesion. This organism causes a severe illness involving the respiratory tract, including the appearance of pseudomembranous pharyngitis and possible airway obstruction. Owing to high immunization rates, a confirmed case of diphtheria has not been reported in the United States for more than a decade.

Pertussis (also known as whooping cough) is caused by the gram-negative organism *Bordetella pertussis.* The disease is highly contagious and spreads via respiratory droplets from coughing and sneezing.

The infection is characterized by a paroxysmal cough (a series of severe, vigorous coughs during a single expiration) that often makes it difficult to breathe. Following a coughing fit, the individual often needs to take deep breaths resulting in the high-pitched "whooping" sound. While pertussis can affect individuals at any age, the disease most often affects infants and young children and can be fatal, particularly in infants less than 1 year old. Following infection, it can take 1 to 3 weeks for signs and symptoms to appear. Early signs resemble the common cold and include runny nose, nasal congestion, sneezing, mild fever, and mild cough. Symptoms worsen over the next week or two to include thick mucus accumulating in the airways causing uncontrollable coughing. Prolonged coughing episodes can provoke vomiting and result in a red or blue face and cause extreme fatigue. If left untreated, adverse outcomes from pertussis can lead to pneumonia, seizures, brain damage, or death.

> **CLINICAL CONCEPT**
>
> Many infants are infected with pertussis by older siblings, parents, or caregivers who might be unaware that they have the disease.

Immunization

There are currently three types of vaccines used in the prevention of these three diseases:

- DTaP (diphtheria and tetanus toxoids and acellular pertussis vaccine)—indicated for those 2 months to 6 years of age
- Tdap (tetanus toxoid, reduced diphtheria toxoid, and acellular pertussis vaccine)—indicated for those 7 years and older
- Td (tetanus and diphtheria toxoids vaccine)—used as a booster dose every 10 years

In the developed world, tetanus and diphtheria are uncommon infections because of widespread immunization. Because protective titers wane over time, and adults are frequently lacking up-to-date immunization, most cases of tetanus occur in adults older than 50 years.

A primary series of three tetanus vaccine injections sets the stage for long-term immunity. A booster tetanus dose every 10 years is recommended, but protection is probably present for 20 to 30 years after a primary series. Using Td vaccine rather than tetanus toxoid (TT vaccine, discontinued in 2013) for primary series and booster doses in adulthood also assists in keeping diphtheria immunity.

Early childhood tetanus and diphtheria immunizations also include acellular pertussis vaccine, providing protection for this highly contagious, cough-transmitted illness. Children receive a five-dose series of DTaP given at ages 2, 4, 6, and 15 to 18 months and at 4 to 6 years. This confers approximately 98% effectiveness against pertussis within the first year after the fifth dose, though effectiveness declines over time. A single dose of Tdap during adulthood provides additional protection from pertussis. For adults receiving initial immunization, a series of three vaccine doses is needed. Two of the three can be Td, and one should be Tdap. Rarely have cases of tetanus occurred in persons with a documented primary tetanus series.

To protect newborns from pertussis, one booster dose of Tdap is recommended for pregnant women for each pregnancy, regardless of prior Tdap vaccine history. All household members and caregivers should also be up to date on their immunization against pertussis. Given the contagious nature of pertussis, herd immunity against this disease requires greater than 90% of individuals in the community to be immunized.

The use of tetanus and diphtheria with or without acellular pertussis immunizations is well tolerated and produces few adverse reactions. A short-term, localized area of redness and warmth is quite common and is not predictive of future problems with tetanus immunization.

When a patient presents with a clean minor wound and an unclear tetanus immunization history or inadequate tetanus immunization (0 to 2 doses), a dose of tetanus vaccine should be provided. In the presence of all other wounds and an unclear or inadequate tetanus immunization history (0 to 2 doses), a dose of tetanus vaccine with tetanus immunoglobulin (TIG), an example of passive immunization, is advised. With TIG use, temporary immunity is provided.

Postexposure prophylaxis should be considered for those with close contacts to individuals infected with diphtheria or pertussis. For close contacts, especially household contacts, to diphtheria, a diphtheria booster dose appropriate for age should be given as well as antimicrobial therapy (one dose of benzathine penicillin G injection or a 7- to 10-day course of oral erythromycin). For pertussis, postexposure antimicrobial use is recommended for all household contacts of a pertussis case, as well as individuals following exposure to an infectious pertussis case who are at high risk of developing severe pertussis or who have close contact with others at high risk of developing severe pertussis. High-risk individuals include infants, women in their third trimester of pregnancy, and all persons with preexisting health conditions that can exacerbate a pertussis infection (e.g., immunocompromised or asthma). Antimicrobial therapy can include the macrolides or trimethoprim-sulfamethoxazole (TMP-SMX) (see Chapter 18 for more details).

> **CLINICAL CONCEPT**
> After exposure to pertussis, all unimmunized or underimmunized contacts should receive an age-appropriate dose of DTaP or Tdap vaccine.

Discussion Sources

Centers for Disease Control and Prevention. About diphtheria. http://www.cdc.gov/diphtheria/about/index.html

Centers for Disease Control and Prevention. Tetanus. https://www.cdc.gov/vaccines/pubs/pinkbook/tetanus.html

Centers for Disease Control and Prevention. Ask the experts: Diphtheria, tetanus, pertussis. http://www.immunize.org/askexperts /experts_per.asp

Liang JL, Tiwari T, Moro P, et al. Prevention of pertussis, tetanus, and diphtheria with vaccines in the United States: recommendations of the Advisory Committee on Immunization Practices (ACIP). *MMWR Recomm Rep.* 2018;67(2):1–44. https://www.cdc .gov/mmwr/volumes/67/rr/rr6702a1.htm

QUESTIONS

73. An 18-year-old man without acute or chronic health problems presents for health care. He has no primary tetanus immunization series documented. Which of the following represents the immunization needed?

   A. three doses of diphtheria, tetanus, and acellular pertussis (DTaP) vaccine 2 months apart

   B. tetanus IG now and two doses of tetanus-diphtheria (Td) vaccine 1 month apart

   C. tetanus, diphtheria, and acellular pertussis (Tdap) vaccine now with a dose of Td vaccine in 1 and 6 months

   D. Td vaccine as a single dose

74. Which wound presents the greatest risk for tetanus infection?

   A. a puncture wound obtained while gardening

   B. a laceration obtained while trimming raw beef

    C. a human bite

    D. an abrasion obtained by falling on a sidewalk

75. A 50-year-old man with hypertension and dyslipidemia presents for a primary care visit. He states, "It has been at least 10 years since my last tetanus shot." He should be immunized with:

    A. Td.

    B. tetanus IG.

    C. Tdap.

    D. none of the above, owing to his concomitant health problems.

76. Problems after tetanus, diphtheria, and pertussis immunization typically include:

    A. localized reaction at the site of injection.

    B. myalgia and malaise.

    C. low-grade fever.

    D. diffuse rash.

77. Infection with *Corynebacterium diphtheriae* usually causes:

    A. a diffuse rash.

    B. meningitis.

    C. pseudomembranous pharyngitis.

    D. a gastroenteritis-like illness.

78. The organism that causes pertussis is primarily spread via:

    A. contact with a contaminated surface.

    B. respiratory droplets.

    C. blood contact.

    D. skin-to-skin contact.

79. At which age is a child at greatest risk of death from pertussis?

    A. younger than 1 year

    B. 2 to 4 years

    C. 5 to 10 years

    D. older than 10 years

80. Susan is in her second trimester of pregnancy. Her records show that she last received the Tdap vaccine 2 years ago during her last pregnancy. The NP recommends:

    A. a Tdap vaccination during the third trimester.

    B. a Tdap vaccination soon after delivery.

    C. a Td booster immediately.

    D. a Td booster in 8 years.

81. To ensure a newborn is protected from pertussis, is it important that the Tdap immunization status is up to date for:

    A. all children in the household younger than 10 years of age.

    B. the mother and all children in the household younger than 5 years of age.

    C. any immunocompromised household members.

    D. all members of the household and anyone who will be in close contact with the newborn.

82. For a 3-year-old who is up to date with recommended immunizations and was exposed to pertussis, postexposure prophylaxis can include treatment with:

A. a beta-lactam.

B. a macrolide.

C. a systemic antifungal.

D. an additional dose of DTaP.

83. One year after completing the five-dose series of DTaP, approximately _____ of children are protected against pertussis.

A. 45%

B. 67%

C. 80%

D. 98%

84. Effective herd immunity against pertussis requires _____ of the population to be up to date on pertussis immunization.

A. 30%

B. 50%

C. 75%

D. greater than 90%

85 to 87. Indicate (Yes or No) which of the following should receive the Tdap vaccine.

_____ **85.** The partner of a woman in the first trimester of pregnancy who provides documentation of receiving Tdap 4 years ago

_____ **86.** A 67-year-old who received the Td vaccine 5 years ago and is anticipated to be the caregiver of a newborn granddaughter

_____ **87.** A 34-year-old man who remembers getting a "tetanus shot" shortly after college about 12 years ago but cannot recall the exact vaccine used

For answers and rationales, see end of chapter.

Stages of Change Model

Possessing information about methods for disease prevention and health maintenance is an important part of patient education. Knowledge of harmful conduct alone does not ensure a change in behavior; NPs need to consider many factors in patient counseling and education (Box 2-2).

In providing ongoing health care, the NP should maintain an attitude that the patient is capable of changing and achieving improved health. Change occurs dynamically and often unpredictably. A commonly used change framework is based on the work of Prochaska and DiClemente and is known as the Stages of Change Model/Transtheoretical Model (TTM). In this model, five stages of preparation for change are reported:

■ Precontemplation: The patient is not interested in change and might be unaware that the problem exists or minimizes the problem's impact.

■ Contemplation: The patient is considering change and looking at its positive and negative aspects. The person often reports feeling "stuck" with the problem, unable to figure out how to change to solve or minimize the health issue.

■ Preparation: The patient exhibits some change behaviors or thoughts and often reports feeling that he or she does not have the tools to proceed.

■ Action: The patient is ready to go forth with change, often takes concrete steps to change, but is often inconsistent with following through.

■ Maintenance/relapse: The patient learns to continue the change and has adopted and embraced the healthy habit. Relapse can occur, however, and the person learns to deal with backsliding.

BOX 2-2 Orderly Approach to Patient Education and Counseling

■ Assess the patient's knowledge base about factors contributing to the problem.

■ Evaluate the contribution of the patient's belief system to the problem.

■ Ask the patient about perceived barriers to action and supporting factors.

■ Match teaching to the patient's perception of the problem.

■ Inform the patient about the purpose and benefit of an intervention.

■ Give the patient an anticipated time of onset of effect of a therapy.

■ Suggest small rather than large changes in behavior.

■ Give accurate, specific information.

■ Consider adding new positive behaviors, rather than attempting to discontinue established behaviors.

■ Link desired behavior with established behavior.

■ Give a strong, personalized message about the seriousness of the health risk.

■ Ask for a commitment from the patient.

■ Use a combination of teaching strategies, such as visual, oral, and written methods.

■ Strive for an interdisciplinary approach to patient education and counseling, with all members of the team giving the same message.

■ Maintain frequent contact with the patient to monitor progress.

■ Expect gains and periodic setbacks.

Source: Freda MC. Issues in patient education. J Midwifery Womens Health. *2004;49(3). http://www.medscape.com/viewarticle/478283_3*

CLINICAL CONCEPT

With relapse, an important message to convey to the patient is that he or she was successfully able to make the change once and can do it again and that the patient is continuing to learn how to change behavior.

As a health counselor, the NP provides a valuable role in continually "tapping" the patient with a message of concern about health and safety, helping to move the person in the precontemplation stage to the contemplation stage. After the patient is at this stage, presenting treatment options and support for change is a critical part of the NP's role. During action and maintenance stages, the NP needs to be positive and encouraging, even with the occasional relapse.

Using statements that begin with "we" convey the message that the NP is there to help facilitate success.

Discussion Source

Substance Abuse and Mental Health Services Administration. *Enhancing Motivation for Change in Substance Abuse Treatment.* Rockville, MD: U.S. Department of Health and Human Services; 1999. Treatment Improvement Protocol (TIP) Series 35. HHS Publication (SMA) 13-4212. https://www.ncbi.nlm.nih.gov/books/NBK64967/

QUESTIONS

88. When working with a middle-aged man with a body mass index of 33 kg/m² who is considering weight reduction, an NP considers that one of the first actions should be to:

    A. add an exercise program while minimizing the need for dietary changes.

    B. ask the patient about what he believes contributes to his weight issues.

    C. refer the patient to a nutritionist for diet counseling.

    D. ask the patient for a commitment to lose weight.

89. A sedentary, obese 52-year-old woman is diagnosed with hypertension and states, "It is going to be too hard to diet, exercise, and take these pills." What is the least helpful response to her statement?

    A. "Try taking your medication when you brush your teeth."

    B. "You really need to try to improve your health."

    C. "Tell me what you feel will get in your way of improving your health."

    D. "Could you start with reducing the amount of salty foods in your diet?"

90. During an office visit, a 38-year-old woman states, "I drink way too much but do not know what to do to stop." According to the Stages of Change Transtheoretical Model, her statement is most consistent with a person at the stage of:

   A. precontemplation.

   B. contemplation.

   C. preparation.

   D. action.

91. During an office visit, a 48-year-old man who smokes two packs of cigarettes per day states, "My kids are begging me to quit. My dad smoked and died when he was 80. I am not sure what all the fuss is about." According to the Stages of Change Transtheoretical Model, his statement is most consistent with a person at the stage of:

   A. precontemplation.

   B. contemplation.

   C. preparation.

   D. action.

92. Linda is a 52-year-old woman who presents for a follow-up visit for hypertension, type 2 diabetes mellitus, and dyslipidemia. She has a 50 pack-year cigarette smoking history, quit smoking 6 months ago, and now reports smoking about 10 cigarettes per day for the past 2 weeks while being particularly stressed during her 78-year-old mother's recent serious illness. Linda states, "I give up. I guess I cannot quit." Which of the following is the most appropriate response to Linda's statement?

   A. "Do you think your mother's illness was a trigger for your smoking?"

   B. "Can we work on a plan to help you to get back to being smoking free?"

   C. "Once your mom is well again, you should try quitting again."

   D. "You sound really discouraged about this."

For answers and rationales, see end of chapter.

Tobacco Use

Tobacco use poses a tremendous health hazard; tobacco-related diseases result in a significant burden to public health and health-care costs.

Effective treatments exist, however, that can significantly increase rates of long-term abstinence.

Treatment of tobacco use and dependence guidelines from the Agency for Healthcare Research and Quality (AHRQ) offer the following recommendations for smoking cessation:

- Clinicians and health-care delivery systems must consistently identify and document tobacco use status and treat every tobacco user seen in a health-care setting. Brief tobacco dependence treatment is effective.
- Clinicians should offer every patient who uses tobacco at least the brief treatments shown to be effective. An example of a brief intervention includes the "5 As": Ask, Advise, Assess, Assist, Arrange (Table 2-5). This strategy should be used with all tobacco users, including individuals with no current desire to quit, because this can serve as a motivating factor in future attempts to discontinue tobacco use.
- Individual, group, and telephone counseling can be helpful, and their effectiveness increases with treatment intensity. Two components of counseling—practical counseling (problem-solving/skills training) and social support—are especially effective, and clinicians should use these when counseling those patients making an attempt to quit. Telephone quit-line counseling has been shown to be effective with diverse populations and has broad reach. Clinicians and health-care delivery systems should ensure patient access to quit lines and promote quit-line use.

Tobacco-dependence treatments are effective across a broad range of populations. Clinicians should encourage every patient willing to make a quit attempt to use the counseling treatments and appropriate

> **CLINICAL CONCEPT**
> Tobacco dependence is a chronic disease that often requires repeated intervention and multiple attempts to quit.

TABLE 2-5 Five As

Ask about tobacco use	Identify and document tobacco use status for every patient at every visit.
Advise to quit	In a clear, strong, and personalized manner, urge every tobacco user to quit.
Assess willingness to make a quit attempt	Is the tobacco user willing to make a quit attempt at this time?
Assist in quit attempt	For the patient willing to make a quit attempt, offer FDA-approved medication and provide or refer for counseling or additional treatment to help the patient quit.
	For patients unwilling to quit at the time, provide interventions designed to increase future quit attempts.
Arrange follow-up	For the patient willing to make a quit attempt, arrange for follow-up contacts, beginning within the first week after the quit date.
	For patients unwilling to or uninterested in making a quit attempt at the time, address tobacco dependence and willingness to quit at next clinic visit.

Source: Treating Tobacco Use and Dependence. *Rockville, MD: Agency for Healthcare Research and Quality; April 2013. http://www.ahrq.gov /professionals/clinicians-providers/guidelines-recommendations/tobacco/clinicians/update/index.html*

medications. Numerous effective medications are available for tobacco dependence, and clinicians should encourage their use by all patients attempting to quit smoking—except when medically contraindicated or with specific populations for which there is less evidence of effectiveness (i.e., pregnant women, smokeless tobacco users, light smokers, and adolescents). These medications to enhance success in smoking cessation include nicotine replacement therapy (NRT) (e.g., patch, gum, inhaler, nasal spray, and lozenge) and medications to reduce the desire to smoke (bupropion [Zyban, Wellbutrin] and varenicline [Chantix]).

> **CLINICAL CONCEPT**
>
> The use of electronic cigarettes is not considered a safe or effective aid in smoking cessation.

The use of these medications reliably increases long-term smoking abstinence rates. Generally, the risk associated with the use of these medications is less than that associated with continued tobacco use. Adverse effects occasionally attributed to the use of smoking cessation medications are sometimes actually a result of nicotine withdrawal. The U.S. Food and Drug Administration (FDA) added a warning, however, regarding the use of varenicline: specifically, depressed mood, agitation, changes in behavior, suicidal ideation, and suicide have been reported in patients attempting to quit smoking while using varenicline. Patients should tell their health-care provider about any history of psychiatric illness before starting this medication; clinicians should also ask about mental health history before starting this medication. Close monitoring for changes in mood and behavior should continue through this therapy.

Counseling and medication are effective when used by clinicians as solo interventions for treating tobacco dependence. The combination of counseling and medication is more effective, however, than either alone. Clinicians should encourage all individuals making a quit attempt to use both counseling and medication. For an individual who is not interested in quitting smoking, motivational intervention is often helpful and should be provided at every clinical visit.

Treatments for tobacco dependence are clinically effective and highly cost effective relative to interventions for other clinical disorders. Providing insurance coverage for these treatments increases quit rates. Insurers and purchasers should ensure that all insurance plans include the counseling and medication identified as effective in the AHRQ guidelines as covered benefits.

Discussion Source

Tobacco Use and Dependence Guideline Panel. *Treating Tobacco Use and Dependence: 2008 Update.* Rockville, MD: U.S. Department of Health and Human Services; 2008. http://www.ncbi.nlm.nih.gov/books/NBK63952

QUESTIONS

93. The components of brief intervention for treating tobacco use include:

    A. Ask, Advise, Assess, Assist, Arrange.

    B. Advise, Intervene, Counsel, Follow Up, Prescribe.

    C. Document, Counsel, Caution, Describe, Demonstrate.

    D. Advise, Describe, Confer, Prescribe, Document.

94. A brief intervention that provides motivation to quit tobacco use should be:

    A. used at every clinical visit that the tobacco user has, regardless of reason for the visit.

    B. offered when the tobacco user voices concern about the health effects of smoking.

    C. applied primarily during visits for conditions that are clearly related to or exacerbated by tobacco use, such as respiratory tract disease.

    D. when the clinician is conducting a comprehensive health assessment, such as with the annual physical examination.

95. The use of FDA-approved pharmacological intervention in tobacco use:

    A. makes little difference in smoking cessation rates.

    B. reliably increases long-term smoking abstinence rates.

    C. is helpful but generally poorly tolerated.

    D. poses a greater risk to health than continued tobacco use.

96. You see a 48-year-old patient who started taking Chantix 4 weeks ago to aid in smoking cessation. Which of the following is the most important question to ask during today's visit?

    A. "How many cigarettes a day are you currently smoking?"

    B. "On a scale of 0 to 10, how strong is your desire to smoke?"

    C. "Have you noticed any changes in your mood?"

    D. "Are you having any trouble sleeping?"

For answers and rationales, see end of chapter.

QUESTION ANSWERS AND RATIONALES

Select Topics in Health Promotion and Disease Prevention

1. Correct: B. conducting a home survey to minimize fall risk.
Primary prevention is the first level of health care and includes activities provided to individuals to prevent the onset or acquisition of a given disease or injury. Though this often involves immunization against infectious diseases, primary prevention can also include education and counseling on disease prevention and conducting home surveys to minimize the risk of accidents (B).
Incorrect:
Secondary prevention measures include activities provided to identify and treat asymptomatic persons who have risk factors for a given disease or are in preclinical disease. This can involve screening for cancer, such as ordering FOBT to screen for colorectal cancer (D). Tertiary prevention measures are part of the management of

an established disease. For a patient with COPD, this can include assessing respiratory function (C) and reviewing current medications (A).

2. Correct: C. ensuring adequate illumination in the home
Primary prevention is the first level of health care and includes activities provided to individuals to prevent the onset or acquisition of a given disease or injury. Adequate illumination is important in reducing the risk of falls and injury, improper administration of medicines, and so on, and is considered a primary prevention measure (C). This is particularly important in the elderly population as they are at higher risk of fractures and more likely to be taking multiple medications.
Incorrect:
Tertiary prevention measures are part of the management of an established disease. Bisphosphonate therapy (A), calcium supplementation (B), and the use of a back

brace (D) are all part of the management of this patient's osteoporosis and are thus considered tertiary prevention measures.

3. **Correct: A. screening for mood disorders.**
Secondary prevention measures include activities provided to identify and treat asymptomatic persons who have risk factors for a given disease or are in preclinical disease. These measures typically involve screening tests, such as screening for mood disorders (A) and cancer.
Incorrect:
Immunizations (B) and advising about the appropriate use of car passenger restraints (D) are aimed to prevent disease or injury and are considered primary prevention measure. Obtaining a serum theophylline level (C) is part of the management plan for the patient's COPD diagnosis and thus is a tertiary prevention measure.

4. **Correct: B. adjusting therapy to minimize dyspnea.**
Tertiary prevention measures are part of the management of an established disease. A tertiary prevention measure for this patient with heart failure can include evaluating and adjusting therapy to minimize dyspnea (B).
Incorrect:
Immunization (A) and reviewing the safe handling of food (D) are both aimed to prevent disease and illness and are considered primary prevention measures. Screening for cancer, such as surveying skin for precancerous lesions (C), is a secondary prevention measure.

5. **Correct: A. hepatitis B immune globulin (HBIG)**
Passive immunity is provided when a person receives select antibodies produced in another host, usually via the administration of IG, after exposure to an infective agent (A). This type of immunity is not preferred as passive immunity is only temporary and requires the patient to present following exposure to an infecting agent.
Incorrect:
Active immunity can be acquired through vaccination (B, C, D) or following an active infection. Active immunity via vaccination is preferred over passive immunity as active immunity provides long-term protection from the disease.

6. **Correct: A. resistance developed in response to an antigen.**
Active immunity is defined as resistance developed through exposure to an antigen (A). Active immunity can be acquired through vaccination or following an active infection.
Incorrect:
Passive immunity is acquired when a person receives select antibodies produced in another host. This can be through administration of antibodies (i.e., IG) (B) or naturally by a fetus or infant from the mother (D). The resistance of a group to an infectious agent describes an aspect of herd immunity (C), which can be accomplished when a certain percentage of the population has active immunity (either through vaccination or following infection) against an infecting agent.

7. **Correct: A. primary prevention**
The goal of primary prevention is to prevent a disease or injury before it happens. In this manner, it is the most cost-effective approach to health care as it eliminates all the costs associated with treating the disease (A).
Incorrect:
Though not as cost-effective as primary prevention measures, secondary prevention measures are also cost-effective in health care, particularly if screening is performed to identify disease at early stages where treatment and recovery are possible (B). Tertiary prevention is often considered a failure of primary prevention measures and is the costliest approach to care (C). "Cancer-reduction measures" is a nondefined term, though any management approaches for an established disease can be considered part of tertiary prevention measures (D).

8. **Correct: B. counseling about safer sexual practices.**
The goal of primary prevention is to prevent a disease or injury before it happens. Educating the patient about safer sexual practices is important in reducing the risk for sexually transmitted diseases (B).
Incorrect:
Screening for STIs (A) and performing a Pap test (D) are both part of secondary prevention measures to potentially detect/identify already established diseases. Prescribing medication to minimize allergy (C) can be part of the patient's management plan for allergic rhinitis and is considered a tertiary prevention measure.

9. **Correct: D. community**
In herd or community immunity (D), a significant portion of a given population has immunity against an infectious agent; the likelihood that the susceptible portion of the group would become infected is minimized.
Incorrect:
Passive immunity is provided when a person receives select antibodies produced in another host (A), usually via the administration of IG. Humoral immunity is an aspect of immunity mediated by antibodies in body fluids (or humors) (B). Epidemiological immunity is not a defined term (C).

Influenza and Its Burden

10. **Correct: D. Its use is recommended for virtually all members of the population.**
The injectable inactivated influenza vaccine (IIV3 or IIV4) is the traditional "flu shot" that is approved for use in virtually all members of the population 6 months of age and older (D). It does not contain live virus and so can be used in pregnant women and patients with compromised immunity.
Incorrect:
IIV3 or IIV4 can be used for generally all individuals 6 months and older (B). There are no special precautions for its use in patients with sickle cell anemia (A), and the vaccine does not contain live virus (C), and so virus is not shed following vaccination.

11. Correct: C. Localized reactions such as soreness and redness at the site of the immunization are fairly common.

The most common adverse effect of the flu shot is soreness and redness at the site of immunization, though this typically resolves after a short period of time. Local redness is generally expected with all vaccines when an immunogenic substance is injected into tissue.

Incorrect:

Current estimates of influenza vaccine effectiveness generally range between 40% and 50% (A). The vaccine is not contraindicated for any common health conditions, such as COPD (B), and can even be administered to individuals with mild-to-moderate illness and those currently taking antimicrobial therapy. A short, intense illness following immunization can occur, though this is a very rare reaction to the vaccine (D).

12. Correct: C. can receive the immunization today.

For this patient with mild-to-moderate illness and who is generally stable, she is eligible to receive the influenza vaccine even while taking antimicrobial therapy (C).

Incorrect:

Influenza vaccination can be given to individuals with mild-to-moderate illness (D) as well as those on antimicrobial therapy (A). Current illness does not increase the risk of severe adverse reactions of the vaccine (B). The vaccine should be used with precautions for those with moderate-to-severe illness with or without fever and those with egg allergies other than hives (e.g., angioedema, respiratory distress, lightheadedness, or recurrent emesis).

13. Correct: C. Antivirals have a higher risk of adverse effects compared to vaccination.

Though antivirals can be used for postexposure prophylaxis in individuals exposed to the influenza virus, this method is not preferred over vaccination due to higher costs and greater risk of adverse effects when compared to vaccination (C).

Incorrect:

Certain antivirals are approved for use in postexposure prophylaxis (A), though this is not the preferred method to prevent influenza. Antiviral treatment is more expensive compared to vaccination (B) and still has a high rate of treatment failure (D).

14. Correct: A. Initiation of therapy early in acute influenza illness can help minimize the severity of disease when the illness is caused by a nonresistant strain.

Antivirals can be effective in reducing the duration and severity of influenza, particularly when taken soon after the onset of symptoms (less than 48 hours) (A).

Incorrect:

Oseltamivir is indicated for the treatment or prevention of influenza caused by either influenza A or B strains (B, C). Though antivirals can be effective in preventing flu, the preferred method is vaccination due to lower cost, lower risk of adverse effects, and higher effectiveness (D).

15. Correct: B. those of Asian ethnicity.

Though everyone 6 months and older should receive the influenza vaccine, certain patient populations are considered to be at a higher risk of serious influenza-related complications. However, those of Asian ethnicity are not considered to be among this high-risk group (B).

Incorrect:

Those considered at high risk of influenza-related complications include young children (6 to 59 months) (A) and older adults (50 years and older), any person who is immune compromised, those with chronic health disorders (including respiratory, renal, and hepatic) (C), American Indians/Alaskan Natives, and the extremely obese (D), among others.

16. Correct: B. respiratory droplet.

Though the influenza virus can live on surfaces for a short while, the most common method of transmission is person-to-person via respiratory droplet (B), primarily following a cough or sneeze.

Incorrect:

The most common mode of transmission of influenza virus is via respiratory droplet. Transmission can occur more rarely through contaminated surface (A) or saliva contact (C). The virus cannot be spread through skin-to-skin contact (D).

17. Correct: B. 1 to 4 days.

For the immunocompetent adult, the incubation period for influenza is relatively short and between 1 and 4 days. Adults can be contagious from 1 day before the start of symptoms to approximately 5 days after the onset of symptoms.

18. Correct: B. high-dose trivalent inactivated vaccine (IIV3) via intramuscular injection.

Appropriate vaccines for adults 65 years and older include inactivated influenza vaccine (standard or high-dose formulation, IIV3 or IIV4) given via intramuscular injection (B). An adjuvanted vaccine (aIIV3) is also approved for older adults.

Incorrect:

For adults 65 years and older, the live attenuated influenza virus (LAIV4) is not appropriate (approved for those 2 through 49 years) (A), nor are vaccines delivered via a jet injector (approved for those 18 to 64 years) (C). Use of an antiviral for prophylaxis is not preferred over vaccination, particularly in an older adult with chronic medical conditions (D).

19. Correct: C. a 4-month-old infant who was born at 32 weeks of gestation

Influenza vaccination is generally recommended for all individuals aged 6 months and older. Therefore, the 4-month-old infant would not be administered the vaccine (C). All persons in close contact with the infant should be strongly recommended to get vaccinated to protect the infant from the flu.

Incorrect:

For those with only a hive-form reaction to eggs, immunization with any age-appropriate vaccine is acceptable (A). Vaccination is also recommended at any time during pregnancy (B), as well as for nursing mothers (D), as this can provide some protection to the child through passive immunity.

20. Correct: B. 2

ACIP recommends that all children aged 6 months to 8 years who are receiving the influenza vaccine for the first time should receive two doses spaced at least 4 weeks apart (B).

21 to 24. Matching Questions

21. Correct: B. IIV4 (intramuscular) or C. IIV3, high dose (intramuscular)

For patients aged 65 years and older, the high-dose IIV3 can be used and might induce a greater immunogenic response compared to the standard dose vaccine. When high-dose vaccine is not available, the IIV3 or IIV4 are appropriate choices, as well as the adjuvanted vaccine (aIIV3).

22. Correct: B. IIV4 (intramuscular)

For children 6 months and older, the IIV3 or IIV4 are preferred for immunization. Though LAIV4 is approved for use in children 2 years and older, the American Academy of Pediatrics gives preference to injectable inactivated vaccines as these might offer better protection compared to LAIV4.

23. Correct: D. Recombinant influenza vaccine (RIV3, intramuscular)

Individuals with mild allergic reaction (e.g., hives) can receive any age-appropriate influenza vaccine. Those with more severe reactions (e.g., angioedema, respiratory distress, lightheadedness, or recurrent emesis) might benefit from the RIV3 vaccine.

24. Correct: B. IIV4 (intramuscular)

For a 12-month-old, IIV3 or IIV4 (standard dose) are appropriate choices for vaccination.

Measles, Mumps, and Rubella and Its Burden

25. Correct: A. Patients born before 1957 have a high likelihood of immunity against these diseases because of a history of natural infection.

The MMR vaccine was not available until the 1960s. Those born before 1957 are considered to be immune to these diseases as a result of having these diseases through native or wild infection (A).

Incorrect:

Though measles and mumps can be associated with severe complications, rubella often leads to a mild illness of 3 to 5 days with little risk of complications in otherwise healthy individuals (B). The vaccine contains live but weakened virus that is not shed following vaccination (C). The MMR vaccine is generally safe and well tolerated with only mild, transient adverse reaction, such as rash or sore throat (D).

26. Correct: D. Two doses given at least 1 month apart are recommended for adults who have not been previously immunized.

Adults who do not have evidence of immunity to MMR should get immunized. The full effect of the MMR vaccine occurs after administration of two doses given at least 28 days apart (D).

Incorrect:

The MMR vaccine contains live but weakened virus (A). It is safe to use in individuals with egg allergy (B) but is contraindicated for those with a history of anaphylactic reaction to neomycin or gelatin. The vaccine is safe to give to individuals with an unclear immunization history (C).

27. Correct: B. give MMR immunization now.

Two doses at least 28 days apart are needed for the full effect of the MMR vaccine. Since this individual supplied evidence of obtaining one dose, the second dose should be given immediately (B).

Incorrect:

With available documentation of his immunization record, titers are not needed (and rarely performed in the clinical setting) to confirm immunity (A). Active immunity through vaccination is preferred over short-term passive immunity through the use of IG for disease prevention (C). Avoiding individuals with skin rashes is impractical for an individual working in the college health center (D).

28. Correct: B. There is no credible scientific evidence that the MMR vaccine increases the risk of autism.

Following the publication by Wakefield and colleagues on a possible link between MMR vaccine and autism, the National Academy of Sciences conducted an extensive review and found no such link (B). The authors of the Wakefield et al. paper were later found guilty of ethical violations, and several inconsistencies were identified in the study. Unfortunately, the stigma of autism with MMR vaccine (and vaccination in general) remains.

Incorrect:

There is no credible evidence linking autism with MMR vaccine use (A). Based on Wakefield's flawed data, one theoretical approach to limit the risk of autism was to separate the vaccine into its individual components (C). Thimerosal, a mercury derivative, might have an association with autism; however, this preservative is not contained in the MMR vaccine (D).

29. Correct: B. a 24-year-old woman who is 20 weeks pregnant

The MMR live virus vaccine should be used with caution during pregnancy (B). This is based on a theoretical but unproven risk of congenital rubella syndrome from the live virus vaccine.

Incorrect:

The MMR vaccine is safe to use among individuals with egg allergy (A) or during lactation (D) and can be administered to children beginning at 1 year of age (or from 6 to 11 months of age if traveling internationally) (C). The vaccine is contraindicated in individuals with a history of anaphylactic reaction to neomycin or gelatin.

30 to 32. Yes or No

30. Correct: **No**

31. Correct: **Yes**

32. Correct: **Yes**

During outbreaks of measles and mumps, administration of an extra dose of MMR vaccine can be considered to ensure protection against these diseases that can have severe complications. The same consideration is not needed during rubella outbreaks, as for most individuals, this is typically a mild disease of short duration with little risk of complications.

Pneumococcal Disease and Its Burden

33. Correct: **D. Its use is seldom associated with significant adverse reactions.**

The pneumococcal vaccines are generally safe and well tolerated, even with revaccination (D). The most common adverse reactions are local injection site reactions, including pain and redness, which are often mild and transient.

Incorrect:

Neither pneumococcal vaccines contain inactivated bacteria (A). PPSV23 contains purified pneumococcal polysaccharide from 23 serotypes, while PCV13 contains purified capsular polysaccharide from 13 serotypes. The vaccines are recommended for patients with lower airway disease, such as asthma and COPD (B). The vaccine only protects against infections caused by certain serotypes of S pneumoniae and will not prevent infection caused by atypical pathogens (C).

34. Correct: **C. meningitis**

Invasive pneumococcal disease is defined as a pneumococcal infection confirmed by the isolation of S pneumoniae from a normally sterile site. This can include the cerebral spinal fluid (meningitis) (C) or the blood (septicemia).

Incorrect:

Noninvasive pneumococcal disease occurs in areas that are not normally sterile. These can include the sinuses (sinusitis, D), middle ear (otitis media, B), and inner lining of the airways (pneumonia, A).

35. Correct: **C. a 32-year-old woman in her first trimester of pregnancy**

An important aim of primary prevention for health-care providers is to recognize high-risk patient populations who are eligible for immunization. In addition to the elderly, patients with a variety of risk factors are eligible for pneumococcal vaccination. However, pregnancy is not among those factors; thus, pregnancy is not an indication for either pneumococcal vaccine (C).

Incorrect:

Pneumococcal vaccination is indicated for all adults 65 years and older (A) as well as those with certain risk factors for infection and complications, including tobacco users (B), and those with diabetes mellitus (D); chronic heart, lung, or liver disease; or alcoholism. Immunocompromised patients would also be eligible for vaccination.

36. Correct: **B. a 66-year-old woman with a 10-year history of COPD who received PCV13 1 year ago**

For those at increased risk and younger than 65 years, a single dose of PPSV23 should be given followed by a dose of PCV13 once they reach 65 years of age, and then a second dose of PPSV23 at least 1 year later. Among the patients listed, the 66-year-old woman is the only one eligible for the second dose of PPSV23 as she has received the first dose over 5 years ago and received PCV13 1 year prior.

Incorrect:

Those at increased risk of pneumococcal disease include adults 19 to 64 years of age and tobacco users; those with diabetes mellitus; chronic heart, lung, or liver disease; or alcoholism. These individuals should receive one dose of PPSV23 prior to age 65 years, and then a dose of PCV13 at age 65 years (and at least 1 year from the first PPSV23 vaccination) and a second dose of PPSV23 1 year later (and at least 5 years from the first PPSV23 dose). For those at increased risk and younger than 65 years (A, C, D), a second dose of PPSV23 is not needed until after age 65 years (and 1 year following PCV13 vaccination).

37 to 40. Identify

37. Correct: **PCV13**

38. Correct: **PCV13**

39. Correct: **Both**

40. Correct: **PPSV23**

PCV13 (which replaced the seven-valent vaccine, PCV7) is routinely used in early childhood for protection against pneumococcal disease. The purified capsular polysaccharide vaccine provides greater immunogenicity when compared to PPSV23. Though PPSV23 provides protection against a greater number of serotypes compared to PCV13, it is not approved for use in children younger than 2 years of age. Both vaccines are currently approved for use in adults 65 years and older, with PCV13 recommended to be given first followed by PPSV23 at least 1 year later for those who had not previously been vaccinated against pneumococcal disease.

41. Correct: **B. vaccination with PCV13 now and revaccination with PPSV23 in 8 weeks.**

For those at highest risk of pneumococcal disease, such as those living with HIV, the initial vaccination regimen should include PCV13 first followed by PPSV23 at least 8 weeks later (B). A second dose of PPSV23 should be

given 5 years following the first dose, and revaccination with PPSV23 can be performed after age 65 years.
Incorrect:
For younger adults living with HIV, pneumococcal vaccination is recommended with PCV13 initially and then PPSV23 at least 8 weeks later (A, C, D). Other patient populations in the highest risk group include those with congenital or acquired immunodeficiencies, cerebrospinal fluid (CSF) leaks, cochlear implants, sickle cell disease, congenital or acquired asplenia, chronic renal failure, generalized malignancies, solid organ transplant, and iatrogenic immunosuppression.

42. **Correct: C. PCV13 now and PPSV23 in 1 year**
For those 65 years and older who have not received any pneumococcal vaccination, the recommended schedule is to first receive one dose of PCV13 followed by PPSV23 at least 1 year later.
Incorrect:
Both pneumococcal vaccines should be administered in adults over 65 years who had not previously received the pneumococcal vaccine (A, B). PCV13 should be given first, followed by PPSV23 at least 1 year later (D).

Hepatitis A and Its Burden

43. **Correct: C. ingestion of contaminated food or water.**
The most common mode of transmission of hepatitis A is via the fecal-oral route. This can happen when an infected person prepares food without properly washing hands after using the toilet (thus contaminating the food) or drinking water or using ice contaminated with the virus (more common in endemic countries). Hepatitis B, C, and D are transmitted by contacting the blood or body fluids of an infected individual.
Incorrect:
HAV replicates in the liver, is excreted in the bile, and is shed in stool. Thus, contact or exchange of blood or body fluids is not a typical mode of transmission for this virus (A, D). HAV is rarely transmitted sexually or from needle sharing. Rather, illegal drug users (injection and noninjection users) often live in conditions that facilitate HAV transmission. Eating raw shellfish that was harvested from contaminated waters can transmit HAV; however, this is a less common occurrence than other modes of transmission (B).

44. **Correct: B. should be offered to adults who frequently travel to countries where the disease is endemic.**
In addition to all children getting vaccinated against HAV starting at 12 months of age, the vaccine should be offered to adults at increased risk of infection. This includes individuals who are traveling to or working in countries where HAV is endemic (B). Optimally, the vaccine should be given 4 to 6 weeks prior to traveling to endemic areas.
Incorrect:
The vaccine does not contain live virus and is safe to administer to pregnant women and immunocompromised individuals (A). Children should get vaccinated

at 12 months of age (C), and a two-dose series of the single antigen vaccine can be used to optimize protection (D).

45. **Correct: D. supportive care.**
HAV infection typically results in a mild, self-limiting infection, and treatment is largely supportive (D).
Incorrect:
Antivirals (e.g., acyclovir or ribavirin) are not indicated for the treatment of HAV infection (B, C). Interferon-alfa is also not recommended for management of this infection (A). Postexposure prophylaxis can include the use of anti-HAV IG, though this is reserved for certain patient populations.

46. **Correct: A. before the onset of jaundice.**
The concentration of virus in stool is highest in the 2-week period prior to the onset of jaundice.
Incorrect:
Peak infectivity occurs in the 2-week period before the onset of jaundice, which is before liver enzymes are most elevated (B) and symptoms are most apparent (D). Once jaundice occurs, the level of HAV in the stool diminishes (C).

47. **Correct: B. approximately 50%**
Key risk factors for HAV infection in the United States include men who have sex with men, illegal drug users, and travelers to areas where HAV is endemic. However, about 50% of HAV cases have no specific risk factor identified (B).

48. **Correct: B. a bowl of hot soup.**
Cooking foods to temperatures greater than 185°F (greater than 85°C) is an effective method to inactivate HAV. Among the answer choices, the bowl of hot soup will not likely include active HAV (B).
Incorrect:
HAV is more likely to be transmitted through raw food (A, C) or contaminated water or other cold beverages (D) than with properly cooked foods. The virus is inactivated by cooking foods to temperatures greater than 185°F (greater than 85°C).

49. **Correct: C. a two-dose series of HAV vaccine.**
For individuals with chronic hepatic disease (such as nonalcoholic fatty liver disease), vaccination with the two-dose series (single antigen vaccine) is recommended (C). This is due to a higher risk of a rapid decline in liver function, especially in the presence of concomitant infection with hepatitis B or hepatitis C.
Incorrect:
Titers are rarely needed to confirm prior infection, and the vaccine should simply be given when prior HAV infection is uncertain (A). A two-dose series of the HAV vaccine is needed for optimum protection (B), and there is no contraindication for vaccine use in older adults.

50. **Correct: A. HAV vaccine today.**
For individuals who might have been exposed to HAV, postexposure prophylaxis with the HAV vaccine (A) is recommended for healthy individuals over 12 months of

age. IG can be considered for those 40 years and older given increased risk of more severe manifestations of infection. Both of these treatments are most effective if given within 2 weeks of exposure.

Incorrect:

IG (B, C) can be considered for postexposure prophylaxis in individuals 40 years and older when administered within 2 weeks of the suspected exposure to virus. The HAV vaccine given today would be recommended (D) to protect against HAV infection, and the patient should be strongly encouraged to receive the second dose for long-term immunity.

51. Correct: D. it contains live HAV virus.

The HAV vaccine does not contain live virus (D) and is administered as a two-dose series, given about 6 to 12 months apart.

Incorrect:

The HAV vaccine is generally well tolerated (A). It should be offered to anyone who is at higher risk of HAV infection or transmitting the infection, including individuals who are traveling to endemic areas (B), health-care workers (C), food handlers, sewage workers, and long-term care residents and workers.

52. Correct: A. IG is derived from pooled donated blood.

IG is a product derived from pooled blood (A) that contains preformed antibodies against the virus.

Incorrect:

Postexposure prophylaxis for individuals exposed to HAV includes the HAV vaccine for anyone over 12 months of age. For those over age 40 years, IG should also be offered given the higher risk of complications in older adults. Postexposure prophylaxis is most effective when given within 2 weeks of exposure to the virus (B). IG provides short-term passive immunization (C) and is generally well tolerated (D). Immunization with HAV vaccine should be encouraged for long-term immunity to HAV.

Hepatitis B and Its Burden

53. Correct: C. The vaccine should be offered during treatment for sexually transmitted diseases in unimmunized adults.

The HBV vaccine can be offered to any unimmunized adult and given to any adult seeking protection against HBV. Those who present for treatment of sexually transmitted diseases can be at higher risk of HBV and should be strongly encouraged to get vaccinated (C).

Incorrect:

The HBV vaccine is a recombinant vaccine that does not contain live virus and is generally well tolerated (A). Over 90% of those who complete the HBV vaccine series achieve seroprotection; thus, it is not necessary to routinely perform titers to ensure the presence of HBsAb (B). Titers can be checked in certain individuals, including health-care workers, infants born to HBsAg-positive mothers, hemodialysis patients, and sex partners of HBsAg-positive individuals. Testing for

HBsAg is not required prior to initiating the HBV vaccine series (D).

54. Correct: C. pregnant women

As the HBV vaccine is not 100% effective, it is important to screen pregnant women for the presence of an active HBV infection (C) to protect the fetus/newborn from infection. Without intervention, approximately 40% of infants born to HBsAg-positive mothers will develop chronic HBV infection.

Incorrect:

Health-care providers, including hospital laboratory workers, should be tested for the presence of HBsAb following vaccination to ensure seroprotection against HBV (A). Routine screening for active infection (acute or chronic) in those who have completed the vaccination series (B) as well as college students (D) is not needed.

55. Correct: B. consider additional STI testing; and D. consider receiving HBIG and start the hepatitis B immunization series.

For an individual who has not been immunized against HBV and has been exposed to an HBsAg-positive source, postexposure prophylaxis should include HBIG and the HBV vaccine as soon as possible (preferably within 24 hours of exposure) (D). Postexposure prophylaxis is particularly effective given the long incubation period of the virus (about 90 days on average). Testing for other STIs, including HIV, hepatitis A, and hepatitis C, should also be offered for this patient (B).

Incorrect:

Postexposure prophylaxis with HBIG and HBV vaccine is effective in reducing the risk of infection (A). Testing for HBsAb is not needed as this patient was not vaccinated and does not have a history of prior HBV infection (C), and testing would not impact the postexposure prophylaxis strategy.

56. Correct: B. baker's yeast.

The HBV vaccine is generally well tolerated, but it is contraindicated in individuals who have a history of anaphylactic reaction to baker's yeast (B). If a person is able to eat bread, then he or she likely does not have an allergy to baker's yeast.

Incorrect:

There are no warnings or precautions on the use of the HBV vaccine among individuals with allergic reactions to eggs (A), neomycin (C), or streptomycin (D).

57. Correct: D. cholelithiasis.

Acute hepatitis B is a serious illness that predominantly impacts the liver. There is no association of HBV infection and cholelithiasis (or the development of gallstones) (D). Risk factors for gallstones can include older age, genetic factors, pregnancy, diabetes mellitus, dyslipidemia, certain medications, and diet and lifestyle factors.

Incorrect:

Chronic HBV infection is a potent risk factor for the development of certain liver diseases, including hematoma or primary hepatocellular carcinoma (A) and hepatic cirrhosis (B). Although usually appearing clinically well, a person with chronic hepatitis B continues to be able to transmit the virus (C), primarily through an exchange of blood or body fluids.

58. **Correct: A. He should receive a single dose of HBV vaccine now.**

When the three-dose series of HBV vaccine is interrupted after the second dose, the third dose should be given immediately to complete the series. The entire series will not need to be repeated.

Incorrect:

The HBV vaccination usually requires a three- or four-dose series (a two-dose option is available for 11- to 15-year-olds only). Thus, his series is not complete (C), and he should receive the final dose immediately. When a series is interrupted, it is not necessary to repeat the full series (B). Testing for HBsAb is rarely needed in immunocompetent individuals and those without risk for HBV infection (D).

59. **Correct: D. a 28-year-old man who is acutely ill with bacterial meningitis**

When considering immunization for nearly all vaccines, vaccination should be withheld for individuals with moderate-to-severe acute illness, such as bacterial meningitis (D).

Incorrect:

Vaccines in general can be administered to individuals with mild illness, including those taking antimicrobial therapy. The HBV vaccine can be administered to those with multiple sclerosis (A), systemic lupus erythematosus (C), and a history of Guillain-Barré syndrome (B).

60. **Correct: C. 1991**

Universal childhood vaccination against HBV began in 1991 (C). Therefore, those born before this date comprise a major risk group for HBV and are generally candidates for HBV vaccination.

61. **Correct: B. receive a single dose of HBV vaccine.**

For those who have documentation of completing the HBV vaccine series, postexposure prophylaxis following exposure to an HBsAg-positive source includes a single booster dose of HBV vaccine (B).

Incorrect:

A single booster dose is recommended for postexposure prophylaxis for an individual who has already completed the HBV series. It is not necessary to repeat the entire series (A) or test for the presence of HBsAb (C). HBIG and the HBV vaccine are used for postexposure prophylaxis among individuals with no history of HBV vaccination or those who have not completed the entire HBV vaccine series (D).

Varicella-Zoster Virus and Its Burden

62. **Correct: D. Although highly protective against invasive varicella disease, mild cases of chickenpox have been reported in immunized individuals.**

The varicella vaccine provides effective protection against severe and invasive varicella infection. However, mild cases of chickenpox have been reported in individuals who had been immunized (D).

Incorrect:

The varicella vaccine is a live attenuated virus vaccine (A) and should be used with caution in certain situations, particularly in individuals with compromised immune systems or during pregnancy. Those who received the varicella vaccine have a lower rate of shingles compared to those who had wild or native varicella infection (B). Those with documented immunity to varicella do not need varicella immunization, while those born prior to 1980 are assumed to have immunity to varicella (C).

63. **Correct: B. a health-care worker who reports having had varicella as a child**

Antibody titers are not routinely needed in immunocompetent individuals to check for immunity against varicella. For health-care professionals, titers should be considered to ensure immunity as they are at higher risk of exposure to varicella and have a higher potential to transmit the infection to others (B).

Incorrect:

Varicella antibody titers are not routinely needed. For an adolescent with an uncertain immunization history, the vaccine should be simply given without the need for titers (A). Titers are not needed to confirm seroprotection following immunization in immunocompetent adults (C). For a person with shingles, the person must have already been infected with varicella in the past (and thus immune to varicella), which has now reemerged to cause shingles (D).

64. **Correct: D. pooled blood product with an excellent safety profile.**

IG is a pooled blood product that provides safe, effective, short-term passive immunity to an individual (D). VZIG should be considered for postexposure prophylaxis in individuals without evidence of immunity but with contraindication to vaccination and who are at high risk of severe disease and complications.

Incorrect:

IG is a pooled blood product, and thus is not from a single donor (C) or a synthetic product (A). It is very safe to use with low risk of disease transmission (B).

65. **Correct: B. Maria should be advised to receive two doses of properly timed VZV vaccine after giving birth.**

Since the varicella vaccine is a live attenuated virus vaccine, there is a theoretical risk of passing the virus to the unborn child. Therefore, vaccination should wait until the completion of pregnancy, with the first dose given immediately after birth and the second dose 4 to 8 weeks later (B).

Incorrect:

It is not recommended to give the varicella vaccine during pregnancy due to a theoretical risk of passing the virus to the unborn child (A, D). The first dose can be given immediately after the completion of pregnancy because there is little risk of passing the active virus in breast milk as the virus is not shed during lactation (C). There is no contraindication of the vaccine during lactation.

66. **Correct: A. droplet transmission**
Transmission of varicella virus can be achieved through droplet transmission or contact with open lesions. Droplet transmission occurs more frequently (A).
Incorrect:
The most common mode of transmission of varicella virus is through droplet transmission. Skin contact of open lesions can also transmit the virus, though this occurs less frequently (C). Contact with contaminated surfaces (B) and water-borne transmission (D) are not typical modes of transmission for this virus.

67. **Correct: A. condyloma acuminatum.**
Condyloma acuminatum, or genital warts, is caused by human papillomavirus and is not a complication of shingles (A).
Incorrect:
Shingles is associated with several serious and debilitating complications. The most common is postherpetic neuralgia, which is characterized by severe pain that can last weeks to months after resolution of lesions (B). Ophthalmic shingles can increase the risk of eye infection and permanent vision loss (C). Encephalitis (D) and meningitis are also complications of shingles, though these occur more rarely.

68 to 71. Yes or No

68. **Correct: Yes**

69. **Correct: No**

70. **Correct: Yes**

71. **Correct: Yes**
Shingrix is generally recommended for all individuals over age 50 years regardless of prior history of chickenpox (68). The vaccine does not contain live virus and is safe to use in individuals with compromised immunity, such as those living with HIV (70). Shingrix is encouraged in those who have already been vaccinated with Zostavax to maximize protection against shingles (71). The vaccine is not indicated for women under the age of 50 years who are pregnant or trying to conceive (69).

72. **Correct: B. Both Shingrix and Zostavax are given as a single dose.**
Shingrix is administered as a two-dose regimen separated by 2 to 6 months, while Zostavax is given as a single dose.
Incorrect:
Though Zostavax and Shingrix are indicated for the prevention of shingles, ACIP gives preference to Shingrix as it induces greater immunogenicity following the two-dose regimen and potentially provides protection for a longer duration (C). Zostavax contains live virus and is contraindicated among those with immunosuppression,

immunodeficiency, or during pregnancy (A, D). Shingrix is a recombinant vaccine that does not contain live vaccine and is not contraindicated in those with compromised immune systems.

Tetanus, Diphtheria, and Pertussis and Their Burden

73. **Correct: C. tetanus, diphtheria, and acellular pertussis (Tdap) vaccine now with a dose of Td vaccine in 1 and 6 months**
Persons older than 18 years of age who have never been vaccinated against pertussis, tetanus, or diphtheria should receive a series of three vaccinations containing tetanus and diphtheria toxoids, which includes one dose of Tdap (C). The preferred schedule is a single dose of Tdap, followed by a dose of Td at least 4 weeks after Tdap and another dose of Td 6 to 12 months later.
Incorrect:
For this patient, only one dose of acellular pertussis is needed for protection against pertussis, and so three doses of DTaP are not necessary (A). Additionally, DTaP is indicated for those under 7 years of age, with older individuals using the Tdap vaccine. Tetanus IG is not needed as the patient does not present with an injury consistent with a high risk for tetanus (B). This individual requires protection against pertussis, which will not be provided with the Td vaccine (D). A three-dose series of tetanus and diphtheria toxoids ensures adequate protection against these diseases.

74. **Correct: A. a puncture wound obtained while gardening**
Infection with *Clostridium tetani*, the cause of tetanus, most likely occurs following a deep wound that is contaminated with soil, particularly if it contains manure (A). A deep puncture wound would also provide an anaerobic environment for the bacteria to grow.
Incorrect:
Shallow injuries, such as a bite, abrasion, or laceration, would not provide the anaerobic environment for the bacteria to grow (C, D). Bite wounds are associated with a high risk of bacterial infection but are not associated with tetanus. Tetanus is also more likely with a wound contaminated with soil that contains the tetanus-causing bacteria, rather than a wound from a kitchen accident (B).

75. **Correct: C. Tdap**
Adults should receive a tetanus booster vaccination every 10 years. To prevent the spread of pertussis, all adults should receive one dose of Tdap in place of Td (C).
Incorrect:
Without prior documentation of receiving the Tdap vaccine once in adulthood, all adults should have one booster dose of Td replaced with Tdap to protect against pertussis (A). The tetanus IG is reserved for those with an unclear immunization history and with an injury that places the individual at high risk of tetanus. This patient presents with no injury and so tetanus IG is not needed (B). The

Tdap vaccine is not contraindicated for persons with hypertension or dyslipidemia (D).

76. **Correct: A. localized reaction at the site of injection.**
The DTaP and Tdap vaccines are generally well tolerated and produce few adverse reactions, even in children. As with all vaccines, when an immunologically active substance is administered into the tissue via injection, a localized reaction including redness and pain can occur at the site of injection (A).
Incorrect:
The vaccines are generally well tolerated with few adverse reactions. Fever is not common following vaccination, even in children (C). Diffuse rash (D) and myalgia and malaise (B) have not been associated with this vaccine.

77. **Correct: C. pseudomembranous pharyngitis**
Diphtheria, caused by the gram-negative *Corynebacterium diphtheriae*, is characterized by a severe respiratory tract infection that can include pseudomembranous pharyngitis and airway obstruction (C). The bacteria are spread through respiratory droplets or cutaneous lesions. Due to high vaccination rates, diphtheria is seldom encountered in the United States but is more prevalent in other parts of the world.
Incorrect:
Diphtheria most typically causes a severe respiratory tract infection. The disease is not commonly associated with a diffuse rash (A), meningitis (B), or gastroenteritis-like illness (D).

78. **Correct: B. respiratory droplets.**
Pertussis is a highly contagious disease that is primarily spread person-to-person via respiratory droplets from coughing or sneezing (B). Frequently, younger children and infants get the infection from contact with older siblings and adults who do not realize they have the disease.
Incorrect:
Pertussis is primarily spread via respiratory droplets from coughing and sneezing. Contact with contaminated surfaces (A), blood contact (C), and skin-to-skin contact (D) are not typical or viable modes of transmission for this disease.

79. **Correct: A. younger than 1 year**
Though pertussis can occur in people at any age, it most often affects infants and young children, with the highest risk for mortality among children younger than 1 year of age (A).
Incorrect:
The greatest risk of death from pertussis occurs in those younger than 1 year of age. Older children and adults (B, C, D) can still get a serious infection from the bacteria leading to prolonged violent coughing fits accompanied by vomiting and fatigue.

80. **Correct: A. a Tdap vaccination during the third trimester.**
Women during pregnancy are recommended to have a Tdap dose with each pregnancy regardless of previous Td or Tdap vaccination history (A). This helps to ensure the newborn is protected from pertussis. Additionally, prior to the baby's birth, all household members and caregivers should be up to date on pertussis immunization.
Incorrect:
The Tdap vaccine should be given to women at each pregnancy, regardless of prior Td or Tdap vaccination history. The vaccine should be given preferably in the third trimester rather than waiting after delivery (B). The vaccine is given primarily for protection against pertussis, so a Td booster is not needed since her last Tdap dose was 2 years ago (C). With the Tdap dose given during this pregnancy, her next Td dose would not be needed until 10 years later in the absence of another pregnancy (D).

81. **Correct: D. all members of the household and anyone who will be in close contact with the newborn.**
Newborns are particularly vulnerable to serious pertussis infection, and children younger than 1 year of age are at highest risk of death from pertussis. Thus, to protect the newborn from infection, all members of the household as well as any caregivers and others in close contact with the child should be up to date on immunization (D).
Incorrect:
To protect a newborn from pertussis, all individuals in close contact with the child, including household members and caregivers, should be up to date on immunization. This recommendation is not limited to younger children (A), mothers (B), and immunocompromised members of the household (C).

82. **Correct: B. a macrolide.**
Postexposure prophylaxis for someone exposed to pertussis can include antimicrobial treatment with a macrolide (erythromycin, clarithromycin, or azithromycin) or TMP-SMX (for children older than 2 months and a history of hypersensitivity to macrolides).
Incorrect:
A beta-lactam is not recommended (A) and an antifungal agent will not be effective (C) for treatment or postexposure prophylaxis of pertussis. As the child is up to date on immunization, an additional DTaP dose is not needed (D).

83. **Correct: D. 98%**
Vaccine effectiveness against pertussis reaches 98% within the first year following the fifth dose of DTaP. This effectiveness declines over time; thus, one dose of Tdap is recommended for adults to boost immunity against pertussis.
Incorrect:
The five-dose series of DTaP confers a vaccine effectiveness of 98% against pertussis (A, B, C).

84. **Correct: D. greater than 90%**
Herd immunity is the measure of protection against a contagious disease due to a certain percentage of the population (herd) having immunity (either through

vaccination or following wild or native infection). Given the highly contagious nature of pertussis, herd immunity against this infection requires a threshold of about 92% to 94% of the population to be immunized. Thus, this emphasizes the importance of ensuring that all individuals remain up to date on pertussis immunization to protect the most vulnerable in the population, particularly young children.

Incorrect:
Over 90% of the population needs to be immunized against pertussis to confer herd immunity (A, B, C).

85 to 87. Yes or No

85. Correct: **No**

86. Correct: **Yes**

87. Correct: **Yes**
Adults are recommended to substitute one booster dose of Td with Tdap to confer protection against pertussis. The woman who received Tdap 4 years ago does not need another dose of Tdap (75). The 34-year-old should receive the Tdap vaccine to ensure protection against pertussis (77). Pregnant women should also receive a Tdap dose with each pregnancy to protect the newborn child. All household members and caregivers of newborns should be up to date on pertussis vaccination (76).

Stages of Change Model

88. Correct: **B. ask the patient about what he believes contributes to his weight issues.**
For a patient in the contemplation stage of behavioral change, it is important for the NP to help identify barriers to change and develop a plan to overcome those barriers. Asking the patient to identify what contributes to his weight issues will help to move the patient from contemplation to preparation by developing an individualized plan to reduce weight (B).

Incorrect:
For a patient at the early contemplation stage, it is important to first identify barriers to change in order to address the health issue. By first having the patient identify what he believes is contributing to his weight issues, the NP can now develop a plan (e.g., diet, exercise) to address these issues (A, C) in the preparation stage. A commitment to lose weight would be more appropriate at a later stage once the plan is set (D).

89. Correct: **B. "You really need to try to improve your health."**
Generalized statements about improving her health are not useful, and they do not offer helpful advice on how to improve health (B). Statements should help to encourage the patient that she does have the ability to change and improve her health. She is likely well aware that she needs to improve her health, and a statement like this will only add to her frustration.

Incorrect:
For a patient who may feel overwhelmed with changing behavior, it can be helpful to first offer small suggestions

to change. This can include tips on remembering when to take a medication (A) or making a small change in diet (D). It is also important to understand what the patient feels are barriers to change that can improve health (C) and to provide encouraging feedback that change is possible, even in small steps over time.

90. Correct: **B. contemplation.**
Contemplation is the stage at which an individual recognizes a need to change but is unable to determine how to make a change. This is consistent with the woman in this example who recognizes that she has a drinking problem but does not know what to do to change (B).

Incorrect:
Precontemplation is the stage where an individual does not wish to change or does not even recognize there is a problem that needs to change. This would be demonstrated by this individual if she did not see a need to limit her drinking (A). The stage of preparation follows contemplation and involves some change in behavior or thoughts (e.g., trying to cut the number of drinks each day in half but is not always successful) (C). During the action stage, the individual takes concrete steps toward change but can be inconsistent with follow-through (e.g., enrolling in group counseling) (D).

91. Correct: **A. precontemplation.**
Precontemplation is the stage at which an individual does not wish to change or does not even recognize there is a problem that needs to change. This is consistent with this individual who does not see a need to quit smoking (A).

Incorrect:
Contemplation is the stage at which an individual recognizes a need to change but is unable to determine how to make a change (B). This could be illustrated by a patient asking about smoking cessation tools. The stage of preparation follows contemplation and involves some change behavior or thoughts (e.g., deciding to wait until after lunch before having the first cigarette) (C). During the action stage, the individual takes concrete steps toward change (e.g., using a nicotine replacement transdermal patch) (D).

92. Correct: **A. "Do you think your mother's illness was a trigger for your smoking?"**
This patient is in the maintenance/relapse stage where the individual learns to continue the change but can also experience relapses. During a relapse, it is important to convey the message that she was successful once in making the change and can do it again. However, it will be important to help her realize the cause of the relapse so that she can continue to learn the process of change. This can be accomplished by asking her to identify the trigger when she expresses thoughts of giving up ("I guess I cannot quit.") (A).

Incorrect:
During a relapse, it is important to have the individual identify the cause of the relapse in order to learn

from the experience and continue with the change. This should be done prior to starting on a new plan to change (B). For individuals during a relapse, restarting the change behavior should occur as soon as possible and not be based on a possible future event ("Once your mom is well again"), as this delays or can even eliminate the opportunity for change (C). The NP needs to be positive and encouraging even during a relapse (D).

Tobacco Use

93. **Correct: A. Ask, Advise, Assess, Assist, Arrange.**
An example of a brief intervention when evaluating a patient who is a tobacco user includes the "5 As." This intervention involves: (1) Ask about tobacco use (document tobacco use status at every patient visit); (2) Advise to quit (done in a clear, strong, and personalized manner); (3) Assess willingness to make a quit attempt; (4) Assist in quit attempt (offer medication and provide or refer counseling as appropriate); and (5) Arrange follow-up (for those who are willing and unwilling to make a quit attempt).

94. **Correct: A. used at every clinical visit that the tobacco user has, regardless of reason for the visit.**
The brief intervention is most effective when it is done consistently at every visit, regardless of the reason for the visit (A).
Incorrect:
Brief interventions should be done at every office visit for greatest effectiveness. If the brief intervention is reserved for only certain visits, such as annual exams (D), sick visits related to respiratory disease (C), or only when the patient expresses concern (B), the brief intervention would be performed too infrequently to be effective in eliciting a quit attempt.

95. **Correct: B. reliably increases long-term smoking abstinence rates.**
Several FDA-approved medications are approved to assist in smoking cessation and include nicotine replacement therapy as well as medications that decrease the desire to smoke (bupropion and varenicline). The appropriate use of these medications has been demonstrated to reliably increase the rate of long-term smoking abstinence (B).
Incorrect:
Current FDA-approved medications can improve the probability of long-term smoking abstinence (A). The risks associated with these medications are less than the risk of continued smoking (D). Though adverse effects are associated with the use of these agents, these are sometimes related to nicotine withdrawal and not the medication itself (C). Varenicline should be used with caution as it is associated with depressed mood, agitation, changes in behavior, suicidal ideation, and suicide.

96. **Correct: C. "Have you noticed any changes in your mood?"**
Varenicline use has been associated with depressed mood, agitation, changes in behavior, suicidal ideation, and suicide in some patients attempting to quit smoking. Though all of the questions are reasonable for this patient, mood screening is most important, since this is an issue of patient safety and minimizing the risk of self-harm (C).
Incorrect:
All of the questions are reasonable during the assessment of this patient following 4 weeks of varenicline therapy (A, B, D). These questions can help to assess adjustment to therapy or address adverse effects of treatment. However, due to the association of mood change and suicidal ideation with varenicline use, an assessment of changes in mood is most important after 4 weeks of medication use.

Neurological Disorders 3

Cranial Nerves

Knowledge of the cranial nerves (CNs) is critical for performing an accurate neurological assessment. Because these are paired nerves arising largely from the brainstem, a unilateral CN dysfunction is common, often reflecting a problem in the ipsilateral cerebral hemisphere. See Figure 3-1 and Table 3-1.

Cranial Nerve Mnemonic

A commonly used mnemonic for identifying and remembering the cranial nerves is **O**n **O**ld **O**lympus **T**owering **T**ops, **A** **F**inn **A**nd **G**erman **V**iewed **S**ome **H**ops. The details of the cranial nerves are as follows:

CN I—**O**lfactory: You have one nose, where CN I resides. Its function contributes to the sense of smell.

CN II—**O**ptic: You have two eyes, where you will find CN II. The function of this CN is vital to vision and visual fields and, in conjunction with CN III, pupillary reaction.

CN III—**O**culomotor: CN III, the eye (oculo) movement (motor) nerve, works with CNs IV and VI (abducens, which helps the eyeball abduct or move). The actions of these CNs are largely responsible for the movement of the eyeball and eyelid.

CN IV—**T**rochlear: This nerve innervates the superior oblique muscle of the eye.

CN V—**T**rigeminal: Three (tri) types of sensation (temperature, pain, and tactile) come from this three-branched nerve that covers three territories of the face. For normal corneal reflexes to be present, the afferent limb of the first division of CN V and the effect limb of CN VII need to be intact.

CN VI—**A**bducens: As mentioned, this nerve helps the eyeball to move inward or abduct.

CN VII—**F**acial: Dysfunction of this nerve gives the characteristic findings of Bell's palsy (facial asymmetry, drooping mouth, absent nasolabial fold, impaired eyelid movement).

CN VIII—**A**uditory or vestibulocochlear: When this nerve does not function properly, hearing (auditory) or balance is impaired (vestibulocochlear). Rinne's test is part of the evaluation of this CN.

CN IX—**G**lossopharyngeal: The name of this CN provides a clue that its function affects the tongue (glosso) and throat (pharynx). Along with CN X, the function of this nerve is critical to swallowing, palate elevation, and gustation.

CN X—**V**agus: This CN is involved in parasympathetic regulation of multiple organs, including sensing aortic pressure and regulating blood pressure, slowing heart rate, and regulating taste and the digestive rate.

CN XI—**A**ccessory or **S**pinal root of the accessory: The function of this CN can be tested by evaluating shoulder shrug and lateral neck rotation.

CN XII—**H**ypoglossal: The function of this CN is tested by noting the movement and protrusion of the tongue.

Discussion Source

Loyola University Medical Education Network. The cranial nerves. http://www.meddean.luc.edu/lumen/MedEd/GrossAnatomy/h_n/cn/cn1/mainframe.htm

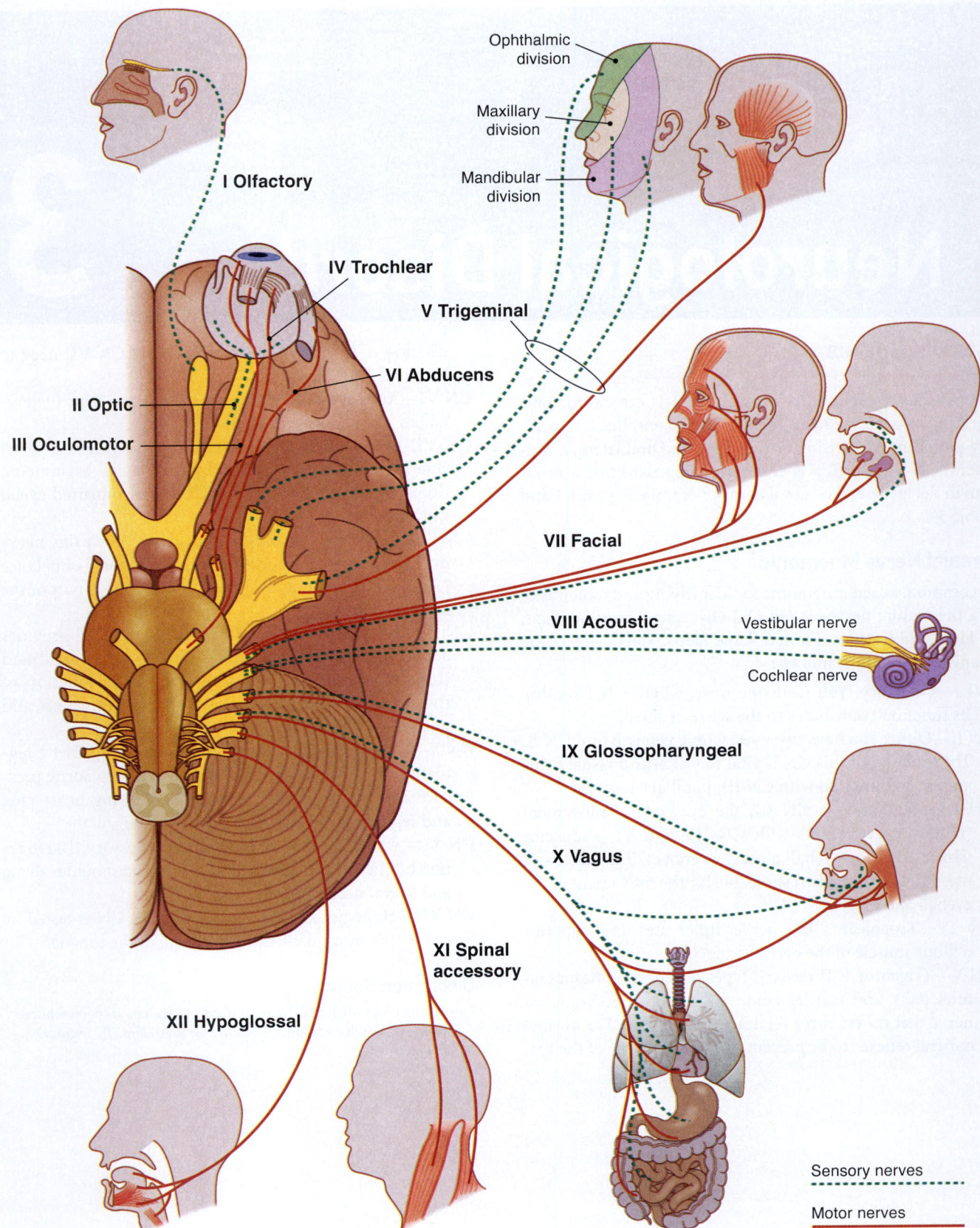

FIGURE 3-1 Origin of cranial nerves.

Dillon, PM. Nursing Health Assessment: A Critical Thinking, Case Studies Approach. 2nd ed. Philadelphia, PA: F.A. Davis; 2007.

TABLE 3-1 Cranial Nerves

I	II	III	IV	V	VI	VII	VIII	IX	X	XI	XII
Olfactory	Optic	Oculomotor	Trochlear	Trigeminal	Abducens	Facial	Acoustic	Glossopharyngeal	Vagus	Spinal accessory	Hypoglossal
Smell	Vision	Eyelid and eyeball movement	Innervates superior oblique, turns eye downward and laterally	Chewing, face and mouth, touch and pain	Turns eye laterally	Controls most facial expressions, secretion of tears and saliva, taste	Hearing, equilibrium, sensation	Taste, senses carotid blood pressure	Senses aortic blood pressure, slows heart rate, stimulates digestive organs, taste	Controls trapezius and sternocleidomastoid, controls swallowing movements	Controls tongue movements
Oh	Oh	Oh	To	Touch	And	Feel	A	Great	Vein	Ah	Heaven!
On	Old	Olympus	Towering	Tops	A	Finn	And	German	Viewed	Some	Hops!
Oh	Once	One	Takes	The	Anatomy	Final	All	Good	Vacations	Are	Heavenly

QUESTIONS

1. Assessing vision and visual fields involves testing CN:
   A. I.
   B. II.
   C. III.
   D. IV.

2. You perform extraocular movement (EOM) testing on a middle-aged patient. He is unable to move his eyes upward and inward. This indicates a possibility of paralysis of CN:
   A. II.
   B. III.
   C. V.
   D. VII.

3. Loss of corneal reflex is in part seen in dysfunction of CN:
   A. III.
   B. IV.
   C. V.
   D. VI.

4 to 6. Match the CN with the appropriate function or test.
   _____ **4.** CN I
   _____ **5.** CN VII
   _____ **6.** CN IX
   A. tongue and throat, swallowing
   B. sense of smell
   C. facial asymmetry, drooping mouth (Bell's palsy)

For answers and rationales, see end of chapter.

Bell's Palsy

Overview

Bell's palsy, also known as idiopathic facial paralysis (IFP), is an acute paralysis of CN VII (in the absence of brain dysfunction) that is seen without other signs and symptoms. Bell's palsy is the most common neurological disorder affecting the cranial nerves and is more common in adults, individuals with diabetes, and pregnant women.

Though the exact cause is unknown, the condition is believed to result from inflammation of the cranial nerve within the temporal bone, presumably related to mechanical compression. Bell's palsy is often linked to viral infections, including herpes simplex virus, herpes zoster, Epstein-Barr virus, cytomegalovirus, HIV, and select bacterial infections such as Lyme disease.

> **CLINICAL CONCEPT**
> With Bell's palsy, some individuals will experience additional symptoms, including taste disturbances, otalgia, ocular pain, and/or tingling or numbness of the cheek and mouth.

Clinical Presentation

The patient who presents with Bell's palsy usually reports a history of sudden onset of unilateral facial paralysis including the inability to raise the eyebrow or smile on the affected side as well as decreased lacrimation in the affected eye with difficulty closing the affected eyelid. Given to facial flaccidity, the patient will often report inadvertently biting the inside of the affected cheek as the tissue catches between the molars when chewing. However, swallowing is unaffected as is the ability to move the jaws to chew food. The remaining neurological examination is normal, including visual fields, extraocular movements, and sense of smell.

For most people, Bell's palsy is temporary, and symptoms usually start to improve within a few weeks, with complete recovery by 6 months. A small percentage of people will have permanent symptoms.

Bell's Palsy: Differential Diagnosis

The differential diagnosis in Bell's palsy includes other conditions in which unilateral facial paralysis is noted, including stroke, facial tumor (i.e., facial nerve or parotid gland), and/or brain tumor. With the aforementioned conditions, while facial nerve involvement is often noted, there are significant abnormalities in the neurological examination, including altered EOM, hemiparesis (weakness on one side of the body), visual field defects, and other motor or sensory symptoms if other cranial nerves are involved; onset of these abnormalities can range from sudden onset in stroke to more gradual onset, such as in malignancies. Lyme disease should be considered (particularly for those in the Northeast United States), as well as Guillain-Barré syndrome, basilar meningitis, herpes zoster, HIV, leukemia/lymphoma, malignant otitis externa, and osteomyelitis of the skull, among others. Herpes zoster ophthalmicus that involves CN VII can cause facial paralysis similar to Bell's palsy, though other signs will likely be associated with zoster infection, including influenza-like illness, low-grade fever, and dermatomal pain during the prodromal phase followed by the development of a unilateral rash.

Diagnostic Testing

The diagnosis of Bell's palsy is arrived at clinically through history of present illness (HPI) and physical examination, and additional tests are often performed to help rule in or rule out other reasons for unilateral facial paralysis. If the diagnosis is doubtful or signs and symptoms last longer than 6 to 8 weeks, additional diagnostic testing is needed. The term *Bell's palsy* is used to describe only acute (sudden onset), unilateral, peripheral, lower motor-neuron facial nerve paralysis in the absence of central nervous system disease.

Diagnostic approaches that can be used to determine the cause of the symptoms include electromyography (to measure electrical activity of the facial muscle in response to stimulation); imaging scans to rule out tumor or head injury are typically ordered only when there is uncertainty of the diagnosis or there are other abnormalities in HPI or physical examination; imaging scans are, therefore, not ordered routinely. Appropriate testing for Lyme disease should be obtained in a patient presenting with signs and symptoms of unilateral facial nerve paralysis; this is a rare finding noted in secondary stage Lyme disease.

Treatment

Guidelines from the American Academy of Neurology (AAN) strongly recommend the use of systemic oral corticosteroids such as oral prednisone to treat new-onset Bell's palsy to increase the probability of recovery of facial function. There is little evidence to support late use; optimal effect is seen when the corticosteroid is started within 72 hours of symptom onset.

With ocular involvement, such as impaired eye closure and abnormal tear flow, an eye-care professional should be consulted. The use of tear substitutes, lubricants, and eye protection is often needed to reduce the risk of corneal drying and foreign-body exposure to the eye until those protective functions return with recovery. Facial physical therapy is an option, particularly with incomplete recovery. See Figure 3-2.

> **CLINICAL CONCEPT**
> Current evidence demonstrates questionable benefit with the use of antivirals such as acyclovir or valacyclovir as part of Bell's palsy therapy.

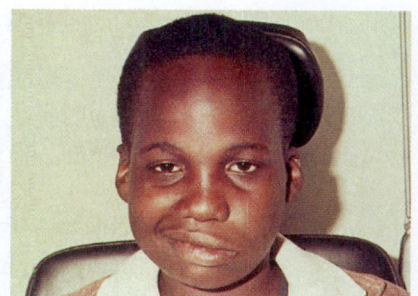

FIGURE 3-2 Bell's palsy.
Dillon, PM. Nursing Health Assessment: The Foundation of Clinical Practice. 3rd ed. Philadelphia, PA: F.A. Davis; 2016.

Discussion Sources

Anderson P. New AAN guideline on Bell's palsy. Medscape. http://www.medscape.com/viewarticle/774056

Gronseth GS, Paduga R; American Academy of Neurology. Evidence-based guideline update: steroids and antivirals for Bell palsy: report of the Guideline Development Subcommittee of the American Academy of Neurology. *Neurology*. 2012;79:2209–2213.

Lo BM. Bell palsy empiric therapy. Medscape. https://emedicine.medscape.com/article/2018337-overview

QUESTIONS

7. You examine a 29-year-old woman, Cecilia, who reports a sudden onset of right-sided facial asymmetry. She is unable to close her right eyelid tightly, frown, or smile on the affected side. She states, "I was fine last night when I went to bed and woke up like this." Her health history and physical examination are otherwise unremarkable. Her medications include a multivitamin daily and a progestin implant for contraception. She is not a smoker. This presentation likely represents paralysis of CN:

   A. III.

   B. IV.

   C. VII.

   D. VIII.

8. Which represents the most appropriate diagnostic test for Cecilia, the patient in question 7?

   A. complete blood cell count with white blood cell (WBC) differential

   B. Lyme disease testing

   C. computed tomography (CT) scan of the head with contrast medium

   D. blood urea nitrogen and creatinine levels

9. In prescribing a systemic corticosteroid for a patient with Bell's palsy, the nurse practitioner (NP) considers that its use:

   A. has not been shown to be helpful in improving outcomes in this condition.

   B. should be initiated as soon as possible after the onset of facial paralysis.

   C. is likely to help minimize ocular symptoms.

   D. may prolong the course of the disease.

10. Bell's palsy is also known as:

   A. Lyme disease.

   B. facial nerve palsy.

   C. idiopathic facial paralysis.

   D. facial asymmetry syndrome.

11. A 46-year-old man diagnosed with Bell's palsy and being treated with a systemic corticosteroid asks the NP about the use of an antiviral medication as he read online that an antiviral can help to "cure the disease." The NP correctly responds:

   A. an antiviral can be considered though the benefit has not been established in clinical studies.

   B. the toxicity associated with antivirals will outweigh any benefit of treatment.

   C. antivirals can be considered if symptoms do not improve after 4 weeks.

   D. antiviral treatment is contraindicated when taking a systemic corticosteroid.

12. A 35-year-old normotensive woman with a history of bilateral tubal ligation presents with a 6-month history of gradual bilateral facial nerve paralysis, difficulty swallowing, altered EOMs, and diminished deep tendon reflexes (DTRs) in all four extremities. The NP considers:

   A. immediate initiation of systemic corticosteroids.

   B. antiviral treatment with acyclovir.

   C. making a prompt referral to neurology.

   D. obtaining a C-reactive protein (CRP) level.

For answers and rationales, see end of chapter.

Primary and Secondary Headache

Overview

The primary headaches, including migraine, tension-type, and cluster, are the most common chronic pain syndromes seen in health care (Table 3-2). These conditions result in significant suffering. The pathophysiology of primary headaches has not been well explained but is likely multifactorial with the intersection of genetic factors and environmental or lifestyle triggers. There is also a strong correlation between migraine and motion sickness, though the exact mechanism for this relationship is unknown.

MIGRAINE AND TENSION-TYPE HEADACHE

These headaches are discussed in tandem as they likely share a common pathophysiology and respond to similar treatments. In addition, patients will often report moving across a "headache continuum," reporting migraine symptoms at times and tension-type headache at other times. Significant headache family history is usually reported with either headache type.

Clinical Presentation

The clinical presentation of the two most common primary headache types, migraine with or without aura and tension-type headache, differs (Table 3-3). In tension-type headache, cephalgia (head pain) is usually described as a pressing, nonpulsatile pain, mild to moderate in intensity, and usually bilateral in location. Classically, tension-type headache presents in a band-like pattern, often with mild nausea but not vomiting, and photophobia or phonophobia is reported, but not both. In migraine, headache is described as usually at a unilateral location, although occasionally bilateral, with a pulsating quality, moderate to severe in intensity, and aggravated by normal activity such as walking or other lighter physical activity. Photo- and phonophobia are reported, as well as nausea and often vomiting. Patients with migraine or tension-type headache typically report a strong family history of either headache type and are more likely to be female.

> **CLINICAL CONCEPT**
> Development of the appropriate diagnosis is critical to caring for patients with headache.

Migraine without aura affects about 80% of persons with migraine. On careful questioning, many patients report a migraine warning, such as agitation, jitteriness, disturbed sleep, or unusual dreams, prior to the onset of the typical unilateral throbbing headache. (See Table 3-3 for diagnostic criteria.) Migraine with aura is found in about 20% of patients with migraine disorders. The aura is a recurrent neurological symptom that arises from the cerebral cortex or brainstem. Typically, the aura develops over 5 to 20 minutes, lasts less than 1 hour, and is accompanied or followed by unilateral cephalgia. Patients who have migraines with aura do not have more severe headaches than patients without aura, but the former patients are more likely to be offered a fuller range of therapies.

Despite the existence of specific criteria, clinicians frequently misdiagnose headache. One reason for error is the nature of these diagnostic criteria. The International Headache Society (IHS) criteria do not include all symptoms frequently observed in episodes of migraine. Consequently, migraine associated with muscle or neck pain, which is not an IHS migraine diagnostic criterion, is often diagnosed as tension-type

TABLE 3-2 Headache: Primary Versus Secondary

PRIMARY HEADACHE	SECONDARY HEADACHE
Not associated with other diseases, likely complex interplay of genetic, developmental, and environmental risk factors	Associated with or caused by other conditions, generally does not resolve until specific cause is diagnosed and addressed
Migraine, tension-type, cluster	Intracranial issue such as brain tumor, intracranial bleeding, inflammation, viremia, or any condition that causes increased intracranial pressure

TABLE 3-3 Primary Headache: Clinical Presentation and Diagnosis

HEADACHE TYPE	HEADACHE CHARACTERISTICS
Tension-type headache	■ Lasts 30 minutes to 7 days (usually 1 to 24 hours) with two or more of the following characteristics: • Pressing, nonpulsatile pain • Mild to moderate in intensity • Usually bilateral location • Notation of 0 to 1 of the following (greater than 1 suggests migraine): nausea, photophobia, or phonophobia • Female-to-male ratio 5:4 • Significant family history of similar headache usually reported
Migraine without aura	■ Lasts 4 to 72 hours with two or more of the following characteristics: • Usually unilateral location, although occasionally bilateral • Pulsating quality, moderate to severe in intensity • Aggravation by normal activity such as walking, or causes avoidance of these activities ■ During headache, one or more of the following: • Nausea/vomiting, photophobia, phonophobia • Female-to-male ratio 2:1 • Positive family history in 70% to 90%
Migraine with aura	■ Migraine-type headache occurs with or after aura ■ Focal dysfunction of cerebral cortex or brainstem causes one or more aura symptoms to develop over 4 minutes, or two or more symptoms occur in succession ■ Symptoms include feeling of dread or anxiety, unusual fatigue, nervousness or excitement, GI upset, visual or olfactory alteration ■ No aura symptom should last greater than 1 hour. If this occurs, an alternative diagnosis should be considered ■ Positive family history in 70% to 90%
Cluster headache	■ Tendency of headache to occur daily in groups or clusters, hence the name "cluster headache" ■ Clusters usually last several weeks to months, then disappear for months to years ■ Usually occurs at characteristic times of year, such as vernal and autumnal equinox with one to eight episodes per day, at the same time of day. Common time is approximately 1 hour into sleep; the pain awakens the person (hence the term "alarm clock" headache) ■ Headache is often located behind one eye with a steady, intense ("hot poker in the eye" sensation), severe pain in a crescendo pattern lasting 15 minutes to 3 hours, with most in the range of 30 to 45 minutes. Pain intensity has helped earn the condition the name "suicide headache." Most often occurs with ipsilateral autonomic signs such as lacrimation, conjunctival injection, ptosis, and nasal stuffiness ■ Female-to-male ratio approximately 1:3 to 1:8 (depending on source) ■ Family history of cluster headache present in approximately 20%

Source: National Headache Foundation. The complete headache chart. http://www.headaches.org/2008/12/11/the-complete-headache-chart/

headache, and migraine associated with nasal symptoms such as rhinorrhea and nasal congestion, also not included as IHS diagnostic criteria, is diagnosed as a "sinus" headache. In both cases, these headaches are usually migraine in nature.

Diagnostic Testing

Headache is rarely the presenting symptom of a serious illness. The key points to consider in assessing a patient with headache are presented in Box 3-1 and Table 3-4. Migraine and tension-type headache diagnosis is made clinically, based on patient history, particularly history of similar or identical headache in

BOX 3-1 Helpful Observations in Patients With Acute Headache

- History of previous identical headaches
- Intact cognition
- Supple neck
- Normal neurological examination results
- Improvement in symptoms while under observation and treatment

TABLE 3-4 Headache "Red Flags" (SNOOP Mnemonic)

Consider diagnosis other than primary headache if headache "red flags" present.

	REPRESENTS	PRESENTATION	POSSIBLE CLINICAL CORRELATION
S	Presence of **s**ystemic symptoms	Systemic symptoms, including fever, unintended weight loss, others	Infection (meningitis, encephalitis), inflammation, metastatic disease, others
	Secondary headache risk factors	Secondary headache risk factors, including HIV, malignancy, pregnancy, anticoagulation, marked blood pressure elevation (greater than 180/120 mm Hg), others	Metastatic disease, intracerebral hemorrhages, others
N	**N**eurological signs, symptoms	Newly acquired neurological finding, including confusion, impaired alertness or consciousness, nuchal rigidity, papilledema, cranial nerve dysfunction, abnormal motor function, others	CNS infection/encephalitis, mass lesion, stroke, arteriovenous malformation, collagen vascular disease, others
O	**O**nset	Sudden, abrupt, or split-second (the "thunderclap" headache)	Subarachnoid hemorrhage (especially with thunderclap headache)
		Onset of headache with exertion, sexual activity, coughing, and sneezing is suggestive of increased intracranial pressure	Mass lesion
O	**O**nset (age at onset of headache)	Older (greater than 50 years), younger (less than 5 years)	Temporal arteritis (older), mass lesion (older or younger)
P	**P**rior headache history	Change in quality, frequency	Medication overuse, mass lesion, subdural hematoma
	Positional	Change in upright versus laying down; neck position	Intracranial hypotension, posterior fossa pathology, cervicogenic headache
	Papilledema	Visual problems	Encephalitis, meningitis, mass lesion

Sources: Dodick DW. Clinical clues and clinical rules: primary vs secondary headache. *Adv Stud Med. 2003;3:S550–S555; Merck Manual: Approach to the Patient with Headache.*
https://www.merckmanuals.com/professional/neurologic_disorders/headache/approach_to_the_patient_with_headache.html.

the past, and physical examination. Between primary headaches, the neurological examination is normal. During migraine or tension-type headache, the only acceptable changes in neurological examination are photophobia and/or phonophobia.

The question of whether to obtain neuroimaging with head CT or magnetic resonance imaging (MRI) to evaluate for underlying disease often arises in the care of a patient with nonacute primary headache. In the absence of a normal neurological examination, particularly in a patient who reports numerous episodes of similar headache, the results of neuroimaging yield little additional information but add significantly to health-care costs (Table 3-5). However, neuroimaging is considered in the presence of headache "red flags" to rule out other conditions that can contribute to the headache (see SNOOP mnemonic

TABLE 3-5 Head Computed Tomography Scan Versus Magnetic Resonance Imaging

CT SCAN	MRI
Rapid imaging (approximately 5 to 10 minutes; important if intracranial hemorrhage is suspected)	Longer procedure (approximately 45 minutes)
Exposes patient to ionizing radiation (cancer risk)	No exposure to ionizing radiation
Greater risk of allergic reaction to contrast agent (iodine)	Contrast agent less likely to cause allergic reaction (gadolinium)
Can be used in patients with implantable devices	Cannot be used in patients with implantable devices
Better at detecting acute hemorrhage and bone abnormalities	Better at detecting small and subtle lesions
Less cost	More expensive

CLINICAL CONCEPT

Patients who have migraine without aura are often misdiagnosed as having tension-type headaches and are often not offered appropriate headache therapy.

in Table 3-4). In older adults with new-onset headache, especially if different from previous headache, a CRP test can be ordered to rule out giant cell arteritis. A visual examination can be considered, especially in those with visual complaints leading up to or during headache.

Treatment

Abortive/Acute Therapy

Headache treatment should start with identifying and reducing headache triggers. Lifestyle modification is a highly effective and often underused headache therapy (Box 3-2). In addition, abortive or acute headache therapy should be offered. Consideration should be given for coexisting migraine and tension-type headache; acute or abortive headache therapies are often helpful in treating both headache types.

Choosing an abortive agent for a migraine or tension-type headache involves consideration of many factors. These medications are available in many forms (i.e., oral, parenteral, nasal spray, or rectal suppository). Following are examples of the medications and the available routes of administration:

■ The selective serotonin receptor agonists, better known as the triptans, are a medication class specifically used for the relief of migraine headache. These agents are often effective in reducing migraine-related symptoms, such as photophobia and phonophobia, but are more limited in complete relief of migraine pain. Adjunctive therapy is often used for pain relief, typically with an NSAID. Because of a potential vasoconstrictor effect, triptan use is contraindicated in patients with Prinzmetal angina, with established or high risk for coronary artery disease, with uncontrolled hypertension, in pregnant women, or with recent ergot use. Because of the risk of serotonin syndrome, triptans should be used with caution with monoamine oxidase inhibitors (MAOIs), high-dose selective serotonin reuptake inhibitors (SSRIs), or selective serotonin and norepinephrine reuptake inhibitors (SNRIs). (Frovatriptan [Frova®] is one triptan that is not contraindicated with concomitant use of MAOIs.)
  • Triptans are available in various types, including rapid-onset triptans (effect within minutes to a few hours depending on route; e.g., sumatriptan [Imitrex®], rizatriptan [Maxalt®]) and slow-onset triptans (effect up to 24 hours; e.g., naratriptan [Amerge®], zolmitriptan [Zomig®]). Triptans are available in oral, IV, melt tablets, transdermal, and intranasal formulations. Melt tablets (orally dissolving tablets) offer convenience for those with nausea or without water to swallow a pill. However, these formulations are absorbed through the gastrointestinal (GI) tract and not the buccal surface and thus do not necessarily have a faster onset of action compared to pills. Although triptans are specifically labeled for use in migraine, their effectiveness in severe tension-type headache lends further support to the hypothesis of a shared mechanism in migraine and tension-type headache.
■ The oral 5-HT-1F agonist class (-ditan suffix, lasmiditan) is helpful in the treatment of migraine with or without aura and noted to improved pain as well as nausea and sensitivity to light and sound. Nausea,

BOX 3-2 Lifestyle, Health Status, Medication, and Dietary Triggers in Migraine and Tension-Type Headache

A comprehensive headache treatment plan includes minimizing or eliminating triggers whenever possible.

Lifestyle, Health Status, and Medication Triggers

- Menses, ovulation, or pregnancy
- Birth control/hormone replacement (estrogen and/or progestin/progesterone) therapy
- Illness of virtually any kind, whether acute or chronic
- Intense or strenuous activity/exercise
- Sleeping too much/too little/jet lag
- Fasting/missing meals
- Bright or flickering lights
- Excessive or repetitive noises
- Odors/fragrances/tobacco smoke
- Weather/seasonal changes
- High altitudes
- Medications
- Stress/stress letdown

Dietary Triggers

- Sour cream
- Ripened cheeses (cheddar, Stilton, Brie, Camembert)
- Sausage (bologna, salami, pepperoni, summer sausage, hot dogs)
- Pizza
- Chicken liver pâté
- Herring (pickled or dried)
- Any pickled, fermented, or marinated food
- Monosodium glutamate (MSG) (soy sauce, meat tenderizers, seasoned salt)
- Freshly baked yeast products, sourdough bread
- Chocolate
- Nuts or nut butters
- Broad beans, lima beans, fava beans, snow peas
- Onions
- Figs, raisins, papayas, avocados, red plums
- Citrus fruits
- Bananas
- Caffeinated beverages (tea, coffee, cola, sports and energy drinks)
- Alcoholic beverages (wine, beer, whiskey, others)
- Aspartame/phenylalanine-containing foods or beverages

Sources: The Migraine Trust. Common triggers. https://www.migrainetrust.org/about-migraine/trigger-factors/common-triggers/; Cleveland Clinic. Headaches and food. https://my.clevelandclinic.org/health/articles/9648-headaches-and-food

photophobia, and phonophobia are often referred to as most bothersome symptoms (MBS) in migraine trials. This drug class is known to have a sedative effect and should not be taken within 8 hours of driving or operating machinery. In addition, this medication should not be taken with other medications or substances that are potential depress the central nervous system, including alcohol, due to risk of cumulative sedative effect. This medication class is classified as a controlled substance, schedule V. Aside from sedation, this medication class is generally well tolerated, though cost is considerable. As a result, the oral 5-HT-1 agonists are typically used when other less expensive medications are ineffective and/or not tolerated.

- The oral calcitonin gene-related peptide receptor agonists (-gepant suffix, rimegepant, ubrogepant) is indicated in the treatment of migraine with or without aura and noted to improved pain as well as MBS. The medication class should be avoided with concomitant use of strong CYP3A4 inhibitors; dose adjustment is advised with less potent 3A4 inhibitors. A higher cost option, this is a generally well-tolerated drug class. This drug class is added to migraine therapy when less expensive medications are ineffective and/or not tolerated.

- Ergotamines are ergot derivatives that act as 5-HT$_{1A}$ and 5-HT$_{1D}$ receptor agonists and do not alter cerebral blood flow. Because of the potential vasoconstrictor effect, ergot use should be avoided in the presence of coronary artery disease and pregnancy. Ergotamines are available in various forms, including oral and sublingual tablets, suppositories, injectables, and nasal sprays; examples include dihydroergotamine mesylate (Migranal®, D.H.E. 45®) and ergotamine tartrate with caffeine (Migergot®). These products are helpful in the treatment of migraine but not tension-type headache.
- NSAIDs can be highly effective in tension-type and migraine headache. These products inhibit prostaglandin and leukotriene synthesis and are most helpful when used at the first sign of headache, when GI upset is not a significant issue. A rapid-onset NSAID such as ibuprofen in high doses with booster doses is advised. Plain naproxen (Naprosyn®) has a relatively slow onset of analgesic activity, whereas naproxen sodium (Aleve®, Anaprox®) is associated with a significantly more rapid onset of pain relief. Acetaminophen and aspirin can also provide relief in migraine and tension-type headache but provide less analgesic effect. Adding an analgesic such as an NSAID to the use of a triptan yields improved pain control in many migraineurs. An example of a combined triptan/NSAID product is Treximet® (sumatriptan with naproxen sodium). Regular, long-term use of analgesics can increase the risk of rebound or medication overuse headaches. Ibuprofen and naproxen have a lower risk of analgesic rebound headache compared with aspirin and acetaminophen, while combination over-the-counter (OTC) products (caffeine, aspirin, and acetaminophen [Excedrin Migraine®]) are common causes of rebound headaches.
- Fioricet® is a combination medication consisting of caffeine, butalbital, and acetaminophen. Caffeine enhances the analgesic properties of acetaminophen, and butalbital's barbiturate action enhances select neurotransmitter action, helping to relieve migraine and tension-type headache pain. With infrequent use, this product offers an inexpensive and generally well-tolerated headache treatment and can be particularly useful for those for which a triptan is contraindicated. Frequent or excessive use of Fioricet® should be discouraged because of the potential for barbiturate dependency from butalbital and analgesic rebound headache from the acetaminophen component of the product.
- Excedrin Migraine® is an OTC aspirin, acetaminophen, and caffeine combination product that is approved by the U.S. Food and Drug Administration (FDA) for migraine therapy and is effective in tension-type headache. Its advantages include ease of patient access to the product, excellent adverse effect profile, and low cost; the product is available as a branded form as well as a less costly generic. With regular, long-term use of acetaminophen or the combination product, there is a higher risk of rebound headache compared to other analgesics (e.g., NSAIDs).
- Neuroleptics are a class of medications historically used to treat major mental health disorders; this class of drugs is also known as the first-generation antipsychotics. Examples of neuroleptics are prochlorperazine (Compazine®) and promethazine (Phenergan®). Because of their antiemetic effect, these products are occasionally used as adjuncts in migraine therapy. Because these drugs generally are highly sedating, using them in the clinician's office can make it difficult for patients to return home. Use should be limited to 3 days a week because of the risk of extrapyramidal movements (EPMs). Other antiemetics used in migraine include the 5-HT$_3$ antagonists such as ondansetron (Zofran®), a nonsedating antiemetic option that is helpful if the patient needs to return quickly to work or other responsibilities. Metoclopramide (Reglan®), a prokinetic agent that is generally well tolerated with infrequent use, is helpful in relieving milder GI symptoms; this drug should not be used on a frequent or daily basis because of EPM risk.

> **CLINICAL CONCEPT**
>
> Other methods of pain control should be attempted prior to prescribing opioids in any chronic, recurring pain condition.

- Use of systemic corticosteroids such as prednisone is helpful with intractable or severe migraine, status migrainosus, and cluster headache. Owing to the well-known adverse effects of this drug class, corticosteroid use for this purpose is not recommended more often than once a month. Examples of corticosteroid types and doses include prednisone 20 mg QID for 2 days.
- Opioids such as hydrocodone and oxycodone provide analgesia and are on occasion prescribed for migraine rescue. These products are sedating and potentially habituating in addition to being substances of potential abuse.

Route of Therapy

The route of medication for the treatment of headache should also be considered. Oral products generally take one-half to 1 hour before there is significant relief of pain. These products are best suited for patients with headache and with no to minimal GI distress. As with all migraine therapies, oral medications should be used as soon as possible after the onset of symptoms. The use of oral products to manage headache is the least expensive option and facilitates patient self-care. Whenever possible, oral medications should be used.

Injectable products (e.g., sumatriptan [Imitrex®] and dihydroergotamine [D.H.E. 45®, Migranal®], ketorolac [Torodol®]) have a rapid onset of action, usually within 15 to 30 minutes. These products are best suited for patients with rapidly progressing headache accompanied by significant GI upset. Sumatriptan is available as a self-injector for patient administration. Injectables are usually the most expensive treatment option.

Dihydroergotamine is usually given intravenously for severe migraine along with parenteral hydration, requiring a visit to either urgent or emergency care. While a helpful option, treatment that encourages self-care should be the goal.

Select triptans (sumatriptan [Imitrex®], zolmitriptan [Zomig®], others) and the ergot derivative dihydroergotamine (Migranal®) are available as nasal sprays, have a similarly rapid onset of action, and are tolerable in the presence of GI upset. Analgesics (aspirin, acetaminophen) or antiemetics (prochlorperazine [Compazine®], promethazine [Phenergan®], and ondansetron hydrochloride [Zofran®]) can be used for pain control or treatment of GI upset, respectively.

Prophylactic/Prevention Medications

Use of prophylactic or prevention therapy for migraine and tension-type headache should be considered if abortive or acute headache therapy is used frequently or if inadequate symptom relief is obtained from appropriate use of these therapies. The goal of headache prophylactic/prevention therapy is a minimum of a 50% reduction in the number of headaches, along with easier-to-control headaches that respond more rapidly to standard therapies and likely require less medication. About two-thirds of all patients with primary headache who are candidates for prevention therapy reach these goals.

Before headache prophylaxis is initiated, headache-provoking medications, such as estrogen, progestin/progesterone therapy, and vasodilators, should be eliminated or limited, if possible. Lifestyle modifications should be implemented to minimize headache risk. These include common headache triggers such as inadequate sleep, not attending to hydration needs, and ingestion of fermented foods. (See Box 3-2.)

Most standard headache prevention medication agents work through a variety of mechanisms, and 1 to 2 months of use are needed before an effect is seen. With all of these medications, the prescriber should be well informed of the adverse effect profile and contraindications for each medication class. These medications have been studied primarily in migraine prophylaxis, but their use in prevention of tension-type headache has also been noted. This stems from the common pathophysiology of both headaches.

> **CLINICAL CONCEPT**
> Patients, while working with the health-care provider, can consider tapering prophylaxis once headaches are better controlled and lifestyle modifications are in place to minimize headache risk.

Beta blockers are commonly used in migraine and tension-type headache prevention, though the exact mechanism of how this drug class works is not clear. Metoprolol and propranolol have the strongest evidence demonstrating preventive effects; however, atenolol and nadolol also demonstrate some effectiveness. Current evidence-based guidelines do not support the use of any calcium channel blockers including verapamil for this purpose.

Select antiepileptic drugs (AEDs), such as divalproex sodium, sodium valproate, and topiramate, have also demonstrated effectiveness in preventing migraines. These drugs have multiple modes of action on the central nervous system that likely impact the pathophysiology of migraines. However, the AED lamotrigine is not recommended for migraine prevention because evidence indicates that this agent is ineffective. Most headache prophylaxis is prescribed to women during the reproductive years; the majority of AEDs have well-documented teratogenic effects. Careful patient counseling about this risk coupled with ensuring the use of a highly effective contraceptive method are in order.

Select antidepressants, including the tricyclic antidepressants (TCAs) such as nortriptyline and amitriptyline, as well as the selective SNRIs, including venlafaxine, can also be considered for migraine prophylaxis. TCAs have also been well studied for the prevention of tension-type headache and can be considered a first-line option for this purpose. Calcitonin gene-related peptide (CGRP) inhibitors are a more recently available class of agents that are effective in migraine prevention.

CGRP is a small neuropeptide found at the ends of nerves and embedded in blood vessels and can play a role in vasodilation and pain signaling. Several monoclonal antibodies that block CGRP or its receptor have been developed to prevent migraine episodes. CGRP inhibitors include fremanezumab (Ajovy®), erenumab (Aimovig™), and galcanezumab (Emgality®). These are administered via subcutaneous injection (given monthly or every 3 months), though oral formulations of CGRP inhibitors are also in development. CGRP monoclonal antibodies have demonstrated efficacy in reducing the frequency of chronic and episodic migraines, with a substantial proportion of patients experiencing a greater than 50% reduction in migraine days. These agents also remain effective in patients who failed prior preventive treatments for migraine. These agents generally work rapidly (within 1 or 2 weeks) with few adverse effects, though the drug class is quite expensive.

Evidence supports the use of certain herbal preparations, vitamins, and minerals for the prevention of migraine headaches. The strongest evidence supports the use of *Petasites* (butterbur) for migraine prevention, although riboflavin, magnesium, and feverfew can also be helpful. Coenzyme Q10 (CoQ10) and estrogen supplementation, in particular during the premenstrual week, can also be considered for migraine prevention, although the evidence is weaker to support their use. Nutritional supplement use for headache prevention during pregnancy and lactation has not been well studied and is not advised.

CLUSTER HEADACHE

Overview

Cluster headaches, also known as migrainous neuralgia, are most common in middle-aged men, particularly men with heavy alcohol and tobacco use. Although cluster headache is the only primary headache type more common in men than in women, more recent study reveals that the condition is likely underdiagnosed in women.

Clinical Presentation

Cluster headaches involve severe or very severe, strictly unilateral pain (orbital, supraorbital, or temporal pain) that can last 15 to 180 minutes with a frequency ranging from once a day to eight times daily. Headaches are often accompanied by one or more of the following symptoms: conjunctival injection, lacrimation, nasal congestion, rhinorrhea, forehead and facial sweating, miosis, ptosis, or eyelid edema.

> **CLINICAL CONCEPT**
>
> Sometimes called the "suicide headache" because of the severity of the associated pain, cluster headache occurs periodically in clusters (hence its name) of several weeks.

Diagnostic Testing

Similar to migraine and tension-type headache, the diagnosis is largely clinical with a history of attacks consistent with the periodicity and rhythmicity of cluster headaches being essential for the diagnosis. Laboratory tests and imaging studies are not useful in confirming a cluster headache diagnosis but can be used to exclude other causes of headache, particularly in the presence of red flag signs and symptoms (see Table 3-4).

Treatment

Treatment includes a reduction of triggers, such as tobacco and alcohol use, and initiation of prophylactic therapy and appropriate abortive therapy. In cluster headache, abortive treatments can include high-flow oxygen therapy, triptans, ergot alkaloids, and local anesthetics, including lidocaine nasal spray. Preventive/prophylactic agents can include the use of calcium channel blockers, mood stabilizers (e.g., lithium), and anticonvulsants.

SECONDARY HEADACHES

Overview

Secondary headaches are caused by an underlying disease process. Implied in secondary headaches is that the condition will usually not resolve until the underlying process is treated or resolves. Causes of secondary headache can include severe hypertension, infection of the head and neck, head trauma and hematoma, malignancy, or intracerebral hemorrhage. One common and self-limiting cause of secondary headache is select viral illness (viremia) such as influenza; in this situation, the headache ends when the underlying viral illness resolves.

Clinical Presentation

Aside from viremia, the person with secondary headache presents with an abnormal neurological examination. Often, secondary headache is associated with increased intracranial pressure (ICP). The headache in ICP is usually reported as worst upon awakening, which is when brain swelling is the most severe. The pain is less intense as the day progresses and as the pressure lessens, in contrast to a tension-type headache, which usually worsens as the day goes on.

Diagnostic Testing

A thorough medical history and physical examination can often aid in the diagnostic process and differentiate between primary and secondary headache. Identification of headache red flags is critical in the diagnostic process (see SNOOP mnemonic in Table 3-4).

Treatment

Because intervention is guided by the underlying cause, establishing the appropriate diagnosis in all forms of secondary headache is critical.

Discussion Sources

Chawla J. Migraine headache. Medscape. https://emedicine.medscape.com/article/1142556-overview

Institute for Clinical Systems Improvement (ICSI). *Diagnosis and Treatment of Headache*. Bloomington, MN: ICSI; 2011.

Robbins L, Ludwig F, Bassett B. Clinical pearls for treating headache patients. Chicago Headache Clinic. http://chicagoheadacheclinic.com/pdf/Clinical_Pearls_for_Treating_Headache_Patients.pdf

Silberstein SD, Holland S, Freitag F, et al. Evidence-based guideline update: pharmacologic treatment for episodic migraine prevention in adults. Report of the Quality Standards Subcommittee of the American Academy of Neurology and the American Headache Society. *Neurology*. 2012;78:1337–1345.

> **CLINICAL CONCEPT**
>
> With suspected secondary headache, expert consultation is typically required, with the possible exception of secondary headache associated with viremia, which is usually self-limiting.

QUESTIONS

13. A 27-year-old man presents with a 5-week history of recurrent headaches that awaken him during the night. The pain is severe, lasts about 1 hour, and is located behind his left eye. Additional symptoms include lacrimation and nasal discharge. His physical examination is within normal limits, and he is currently headache-free. This clinical presentation is most consistent with:

    A. migraine without aura.

    B. migraine with aura.

    C. cluster headache.

    D. increased ICP.

14. A 22-year-old woman presents with a 3-year history of recurrent, unilateral, pulsating headaches with vomiting and photophobia. The headaches, which generally last 3 hours, can be minimized by resting in a dark room. She can usually tell that she is going to get a headache. She explains, "I see little 'squiggles' before my eyes for about 15 minutes before the headache starts." Her physical examination is unremarkable. This presentation is most consistent with:

    A. tension-type headache.

    B. migraine without aura.

    C. migraine with aura.

    D. cluster headache.

15. Indicators that a headache can be the presenting symptom of a serious underlying illness and consideration for neuroimaging include all of the following except:

    A. similar headaches that occur periodically in clusters.

    B. increasing frequency and severity of headaches.

    C. headache causing confusion, dizziness, and/or lack of coordination.

    D. sudden, abrupt onset.

16. Prophylactic treatment for migraine headaches in a 28-year-old woman with no chronic health problems who uses a levonorgestrel-releasing intrauterine device (LNG-IUD) for contraception includes the use of:

    A. nortriptyline.

    B. ergot derivative.

    C. naproxen sodium.

    D. clonidine.

17. Among the following beta blockers, which is the preferred agent to use in preventing migraine head-ache in a 40-year-old woman with a history of bilateral tubal ligation and no history of airway disease?

A. acebutolol

B. carvedilol

C. atenolol

D. propranolol

18. Antiepileptic drugs useful for preventing migraine headaches include all of the following except:

A. divalproex.

B. valproate.

C. lamotrigine.

D. topiramate.

19. Evidence supports the use of all of the following vitamins and supplements for migraine prevention except:

A. butterbur.

B. riboflavin.

C. feverfew.

D. ginkgo biloba.

20. You are examining a 65-year-old man who has a history of acute coronary syndrome (ACS) and migraine. Which of the following agents represents the best choice of acute headache (abortive) ther-apy for this patient?

A. verapamil

B. ergotamine

C. acetaminophen

D. sumatriptan

21. A 45-year-old man experiences rapidly progressing migraine headaches that are accompanied by sig-nificant GI upset. Appropriate acute headache (abortive) treatment includes all of the following except:

A. injectable sumatriptan.

B. dihydroergotamine nasal spray.

C. oral naproxen sodium.

D. zolmitriptan nasal spray.

22. With migraine, which of the following statements is true?

A. Migraine with aura is the most common form.

B. Most migraineurs are in ongoing health care for the condition.

C. The condition is equally common in both men and women.

D. The pain is typically described as pulsating.

23. In tension-type headache, which of the following is true?

A. Photophobia is seldom reported.

B. The pain is typically described as "pressing" in quality.

C. The headache is usually unilateral.

D. Physical activity usually makes the discomfort worse.

24 to 28.   Indicate if each of the following is a risk factor for cluster headaches (yes or no).

_____ 24. onset at age 65 years or older

_____ 25. heavy alcohol use

_____ 26. tobacco user

_____ **27.** male gender

_____ **28.** recent increase in life stressors

29. Which of the following is most specific for abortive therapy of cluster headaches?

A. NSAIDs

B. supplemental oxygen

C. opioids

D. neuroleptics

30. Which of the following oral agents has the most rapid analgesic onset?

A. plain naproxen (Naprosyn®)

B. liquid ibuprofen (Motrin®, Advil®)

C. immediate-release diclofenac (Voltaren®)

D. enteric-coated naproxen (Naproxen EC®)

31. Triptans should be used with caution with the concomitant use of:

A. high-dose SSRI.

B. calcium channel blockers.

C. fluoroquinolones.

D. high-dose statin.

32. Limitations associated with the use of butalbital with acetaminophen and caffeine (Fioricet®) include its:

A. energizing effect.

B. GI upset profile.

C. high rate of rebound headache if used frequently.

D. low clinical efficacy.

33. The use of neuroleptics such as prochlorperazine (Compazine®) and promethazine (Phenergan®) in headache therapy should be limited to less than three times per week because of their:

A. habituation potential.

B. EPM risk.

C. ability to cause rebound headache.

D. activating effect.

34. Which of the following statements about ergotamines is false?

A. This drug class is effective in the treatment of tension-type headaches.

B. They act as 5-HT_{1A} and 5-HT_{1D} receptor agonists.

C. With its use, this drug class carries a potential vasoconstrictor effect.

D. Use should be avoided in the presence of coronary artery disease.

35. With appropriately prescribed headache prophylactic therapy, the patient should be informed to expect:

A. virtual resolution of headaches.

B. no fewer but less severe headaches.

C. an approximately 50% reduction in the number of headaches.

D. that lifelong therapy is advised.

36. A 48-year-old woman presents with a monthly 4-day premenstrual migraine headache, poorly responsive to triptans and analgesics, and accompanied by vasomotor symptoms (hot flashes). The clinician considers prescribing all of the following except:

A. continuous monophasic combined oral contraceptive.

B. phasic combined oral contraceptive with a 7-day-per-month withdrawal period.

C. low-dose estrogen patch use during the premenstrual week.

D. triptan prophylaxis.

37. A first-line prophylactic treatment option for the prevention of tension-type headache is:

A. nortriptyline.

B. verapamil.

C. carbamazepine.

D. valproate.

38. A 47-year-old woman experiences occasional migraine with aura and reports improvement in photophobia and phonophobia with zolmitriptan use and a small reduction in headache pain. You consider prescribing the addition of which of the following to help improve her overall migraine symptoms?

A. gabapentin

B. topiramate

C. naproxen sodium

D. magnesium

39. A 68-year-old man presents with new-onset headaches. He describes the pain as bilateral frontal to occipital and most severe when he arises in the morning and when coughing. He feels much better by mid-afternoon. The history is most consistent with headache caused by:

A. vascular compromise.

B. increased ICP.

C. brain tumor.

D. tension with atypical geriatric presentation.

40. Short-term systemic corticosteroid therapy would be most appropriate in treating:

A. monthly tension-type headache.

B. migraines occurring on a weekly basis.

C. acute intractable or severe migraines and cluster headaches.

D. periodic migraines occurring during pregnancy.

41. When evaluating a patient with acute headache, all of the following observations would indicate the absence of a more serious underlying condition except:

A. onset of headache with exertion, coughing, or sneezing.

B. history of previous identical headache.

C. supple neck.

D. normal neurological examination results.

42. The more common secondary headache etiology includes all of the following except:

A. brain tumor.

B. intracranial bleeding.

C. cluster cephalalgia

D. viremia.

43 to 45. Match the female-to-male ratio for each type of primary headache listed:

_____ **43.** Tension-type headache

_____ **44.** Migraine without aura

_____ **45.** Cluster headache

      A. 1:3 to 1:8

      B. 2:1

      C. 5:4

46 to 48. Match each patient with the most appropriate triptan formulation.

_____ **46.** A 34-year-old man with rapid-onset migraine headache that typically lasts 3 to 4 hours with nausea but no vomiting

_____ **47.** A 44-year-old woman with a slowly developing migraine that typically lasts 6 to 8 hours with little GI upset

_____ **48.** A 38-year-old woman with rapid-onset migraine that is often accompanied with significant nausea and vomiting

    A. oral naratriptan

    B. oral sumatriptan

    C. intranasal zolmitriptan

49 to 54. Indicate the appropriate course of action (head CT scan, head MRI, or neither) for each of the following patients:

_____ **49.** A 45-year-old man who presents with a sudden, abrupt headache. Upon questioning, he appears somewhat confused with decreased alertness to his surroundings.

_____ **50.** A 48-year-old woman with a history of breast cancer who presents with a 3-month history of progressively severe headache and bulging optic disk.

_____ **51.** A 24-year-old man who presents in the emergency department (ED) following a motor vehicle accident. He exhibits confusion and falls in and out of consciousness.

_____ **52.** A 57-year-old woman with a prior history of a brain tumor that was removed 8 years ago. She complains of headaches that have been increasing in frequency and intensity over the past month.

_____ **53.** A 37-year-old man diagnosed with cluster-type headache 10 years ago that is consistently alleviated with high-dose oral NSAID and injectable triptan

_____ **54.** A 27-year-old woman with migraines occurring consistently for the past 10 years around 2 to 3 days prior to onset of menses, accompanied by photo-/phonophobia, nausea, and vomiting, with partial relief with ibuprofen; normal neurological examination

55. In counseling a patient who experiences migraines, you recommend all of the following lifestyle changes to minimize the risk of triggering a headache except:

    A. avoiding eating within 1 to 2 hours of morning awakening.

    B. limiting exposure to cigarette smoke.

    C. avoiding trigger physical activities.

    D. implementing strategies to reduce stress.

56. A 37-year-old woman complains of migraine headaches that typically occur within hours after eating in a restaurant. Potential triggers that can influence the onset and severity of migraine symptoms include all of the following except:

    A. cheese pizza.

    B. pickled or fermented foods.

    C. freshly baked yeast products.

    D. baked whitefish.

57. Which of the following is incorrect regarding the CGRP inhibitor class?

    A. dosed once monthly or quarterly

    B. used for prevention of migraines

    C. dosed by subcutaneous injection

    D. nearly eliminates migraines for over 50% of individuals

58. Which of the following is a likely candidate for the use of a CGRP inhibitor?

    A. A 57-year-old man who experiences a migraine about once every 2 to 3 months

    B. A 45-year-old woman who experiences about 15 migraine days per month despite propranolol therapy

C. A 32-year-old woman currently experiencing an acute migraine with severe GI upset and vomiting

D. A 46-year-old man with a history of cluster headaches for the past 7 years

59. Which of the following is most closely linked to migraines?

A. dyslipidemia

B. completing at least one full-term pregnancy

C. allergic reaction to shellfish

D. motion sickness

For answers and rationales, see end of chapter.

Bacterial Meningitis

Overview

Meningitis is an infection of the meninges, cerebrospinal fluid (CSF), and ventricles. The disease is typically defined further by its cause, such as bacterial (pyogenic), viral (aseptic), fungal, or other. In bacterial meningitis, the causative pathogens differ according to patient age and certain risk characteristics. Bacterial seeding usually occurs via hematogenous spread, when organisms can enter the meninges through the bloodstream from other parts of the body; the pathogen likely was asymptomatically carried in the nose and throat. Another mechanism of meningitis acquisition is local extension of an existing illness such as bacterial sinusitis or acute otitis media.

In cases that do not typically involve the pathogen *N meningitidis*, meningitis is not typically contagious from person to person. Congenital problems and trauma can provide a pathway via facial fractures or malformation (e.g., cleft lip or palate). Common pathogens in bacterial meningitis in adults include *Streptococcus pneumoniae* (gram-positive diplococci), *Neisseria meningitidis* (gram-negative diplococci), *Staphylococcus* species (gram-positive cocci), and *Haemophilus influenzae* type b (Hib; gram-negative coccobacilli). Infection with *H influenzae* type B rarely occurs in adults and is occurring less frequently even in children with universal vaccination of infants against this pathogen.

The issue of meningitis contagion needs to be addressed. *N meningitidis,* an organism normally carried in the oropharynx in about 5% to 10% of healthy adults and 60% to 80% of individuals in closed populations, such as military recruits, is transmitted through direct contact or respiratory droplets from infected people. Meningococcal disease most likely occurs within a few days of acquisition of a new strain, before the development of specific serum antibodies. Individuals acquire the infection if they are exposed to virulent bacteria and have no protective bactericidal antibodies. Smoking and concurrent upper respiratory tract viral infection diminish the integrity of the respiratory mucosa and increase the likelihood of invasive disease. Other risk factors include being younger than 20 years of age, living in a community setting, pregnancy (for meningitis caused by listeriosis), and having a compromised immune system. The incubation period of the organism averages 3 to 4 days (range 1 to 10 days), which is the period of communicability. Bacteria can be found for 2 to 4 days in the nose and pharynx and for up to 24 hours after starting antibiotics. Public health authorities should be contacted when a person presents with suspected or documented bacterial meningitis to provide expert consultation efforts to minimize disease spread, if possible.

Clinical Presentation

The clinical presentation of bacterial meningitis in an adult is usually reported to include the classic triad of fever, headache, and nuchal rigidity (stiff neck). In reality, less than 50% of the time does the disease present in this manner. Additional signs and symptoms include nausea, vomiting, photophobia, and/or change in mental status including drowsiness, confusion, delirium, or coma. New-onset seizures are occasionally reported. About one-fourth of adults with bacterial meningitis, with rapidly progressing illness, usually present for care within less than 24 hours of symptom onset. In addition, signs and symptoms of an underlying meningitis-associated condition, such as acute otitis media, sinusitis, or pneumonia are noted; under these circumstances, presentation for care is usually within a week of illness onset. In meningitis caused by *N meningitidis,* a purpura or a petechial rash is noted in about 50% of patients.

Brudzinski and Kernig signs, suggestive of nuchal rigidity and meningeal irritation, are often positive in children 2 years or older and adults with bacterial meningitis (see Figs. 3-3 and 3-4). The Brudzinski sign is elicited when passive neck flexion in a supine patient results in flexion of the knees and hips. The Kernig sign is elicited with the patient lying supine and the hip flexed at 90°. A positive sign is present when extension of the knee from this position elicits resistance or pain in the lower back or posterior thigh. Papilledema, or optic disk bulging, or absence of venous pulsations on funduscopic examination indicates increased ICP (Fig. 3-5).

In addition to bacterial meningitis, other diagnoses to consider as part of the differential include viral meningitis, medication-induced meningeal inflammation, meningeal carcinomatosis, central nervous system (CNS) vasculitis, stroke, and encephalitis.

Encephalitis, or inflammation of the brain, can cause flu-like symptoms, such as fever or severe headache, and can also result in confusion, seizures, and sensory or motor impairment. Encephalitis is more likely viral in origin and usually manifests with fewer meningeal signs.

Diagnostic Testing

To eliminate or support the diagnosis of bacterial meningitis, lumbar puncture with CSF evaluation should be considered as part of the evaluation of a febrile person who has altered findings on neurological examination. Pleocytosis, defined as a WBC count of more than 5 cells/mm³ of CSF, is an expected finding in meningitis caused by bacterial, viral, tubercular, fungal, or protozoan infection; an elevated CSF opening pressure is also a nearly universal finding with bacterial meningitis. The typical CSF response in bacterial meningitis includes a WBC median count of 1,200 cells/mm³ of CSF with 90% to 95% neutrophils; additional findings are a reduced CSF glucose amount below the normal level of about 40% of the plasma level, and an elevated CSF protein level. In viral or aseptic meningitis, CSF results include normal glucose level, normal to slightly elevated protein levels, and lymphocytosis. Further testing to ascertain the causative organism is warranted. Head CT or MRI should be considered before lumbar puncture is performed.

Neuroimaging with head CT or MRI offers little aid in making a meningitis diagnosis but can be used to exclude other conditions, such as brain abscess or mass, sinus or mastoid infection, or skull fracture. Imaging can also detect complications of meningitis such as hydrocephalus, cerebral infarct, or brain abscess. A lumbar puncture and initiation of antimicrobial therapy should not be delayed until neuroimaging is done for a patient with suspected meningitis.

Treatment

The first therapy in bacterial meningitis is its prevention through appropriate use of select vaccines. The pneumococcal conjugate vaccine (PCV13) results in over 90% effectiveness in preventing invasive disease, including meningitis, in healthy children, whereas the pneumococcal polysaccharide vaccine (PPSV23) has been shown to be 50% to 85% effective in preventing invasive disease in healthy adults by the serotypes covered in the vaccine. The Advisory Committee on Immunization Practices (ACIP) recommends that adults 65 years and older receive PCV13 and/or PPSV23 as part of routine vaccination (though younger adults with certain risk factors are eligible for pneumococcal vaccination; see Pneumococcal Disease and Its Burden section in Chapter 2).

Infection with Hib most commonly occurs in children younger than 2 years of age; thus, vaccination is recommended for all infants. Routine vaccination against Hib is not recommended in children older than 5 years and adults, as infection occurs rarely by this pathogen and immunity is already present. Some individuals at higher risk of infection can be considered for immunization, including those with anatomical or functional asplenia, sickle cell anemia, HIV, or immunosuppression.

In the United States, there are two kinds of meningococcal vaccines: meningococcal conjugate vaccine (MCV4 or Menactra®, Menveo®) and serogroup B meningococcal vaccine (MenB [Bexsero®, Trumenba®]). MCV4 can prevent four types of meningococcal disease, including two of the three types most common in the United States (serogroup C, Y, and W-135) and a type that causes epidemics in Africa (serogroup A); MenB offers protection against serogroup B. When given at recommended schedules, MCV4 is highly effective in preventing meningococcal infection caused by strains covered in the vaccines. MCV4 is recommended

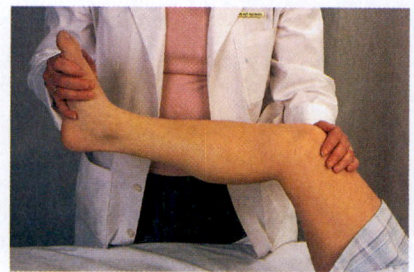

FIGURE 3-3 Kernig sign.
Dillon, PM. Nursing Health Assessment: The Foundation of Clinical Practice. 3rd ed. Philadelphia, PA: F.A. Davis; 2016.

CLINICAL CONCEPT

Patients with viral meningitis usually have less severe symptoms that have a gradual onset; skin rash is uncommon.

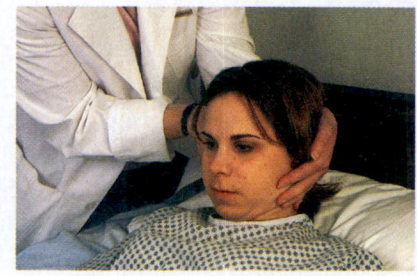

FIGURE 3-4 Brudzinski sign.
Dillon, PM. Nursing Health Assessment: The Foundation of Clinical Practice. 3rd ed. Philadelphia, PA: F.A. Davis; 2016.

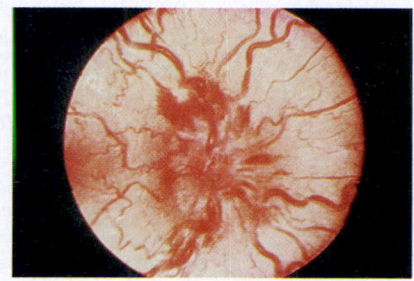

FIGURE 3-5 Bulging optic disk in papilledema.
Dillon, PM. Nursing Health Assessment: The Foundation of Clinical Practice. 3rd ed. Philadelphia, PA: F.A. Davis; 2016.

for all children as part of the routine preadolescent provider visit (11 to 12 years old) with a booster dose given at 16 years of age as immunity wanes after 5 years. For adolescents who do not receive the MCV4 vaccine prior to 16 years of age, a single dose can be administered (no booster needed). Students should receive the MCV4 vaccine within 5 years of starting college, and many colleges now require proof of immunization.

Other individuals at increased risk for whom routine vaccination is recommended are microbiologists who are routinely exposed to meningococcal bacteria, individuals who are functionally or surgically asplenic, individuals with immune system disorder, those living with HIV (if another indication for vaccination exists), people who are likely to travel to countries that have an outbreak of or have high endemicity of meningococcal disease, and people who might have been exposed to meningitis during an outbreak. High-risk groups should receive an initial dose followed by a booster after 8 weeks, then additional booster doses every 5 years.

Higher risk can be due to a serogroup B outbreak or certain medical conditions (including complement component deficiencies and functional or anatomical asplenia). The MenB vaccine should be given preferably between 16 and 18 years of age and can be given at the same time as the MCV4 booster dose.

The priority age group for receiving MenB vaccination is ages 16 to 23 years. Bexsero® is given as two doses (at 0 and ≥1 month after the first dose), while Trumenba® can be given either as a two-dose regimen (0 and 6 months) or three-dose regimen (0, 1 to 2 months, and 6 months; preferred regimen during an outbreak of serogroup B meningococcal disease).

Widespread or universal chemoprophylaxis is not recommended during a meningococcal meningitis outbreak. Chemoprophylaxis against meningococcal meningitis in the presence of an outbreak should

> ### CLINICAL CONCEPT
>
> Prudent clinical practice requires keeping abreast of current trends in causative pathogens and microbial resistance and seeking expert neurological, infectious disease, and public health consultation in this potentially life-threatening condition.

be considered for individuals in close contact, including household-type or closer contact when there is a potential for sharing glassware and dishes, and with patients in an endemic situation. Chemoprophylaxis has limited efficacy in interrupting transmission during an epidemic. Options include rifampin 600 mg PO every 12 hours for 2 days, and prophylaxis persisting for up to 10 weeks after treatment. Given rifampin's ability to induce cytochrome P450 isoenzymes, this medication should only be used after a complete inventory of all medications the patient could be taking has been conducted and no potential drug interactions identified. Other alternatives can include a single intramuscular dose of ceftriaxone 250 mg or a single dose of ciprofloxacin 500 to 750 mg. Immunization against *N meningitidis* can also be used in an outbreak; this option is helpful against current and future outbreaks. The choice of vaccine should be decided based on the serogroup causing the outbreak. However, these vaccines do not provide coverage against all strains within the serogroups, and effectiveness will largely depend on the particular outbreak strain(s).

Treatment of a patient with meningitis includes supportive care and use of the appropriate anti-infective agents. Empiric bacterial antimicrobial therapy will depend on findings from the Gram stain, culture, or other CSF testing to help identify the potential pathogen, and the feedback from expert consultation. Susceptibility results can also be used to guide appropriate treatment selection. Acyclovir is an option in aseptic meningitis, pending identification of the offending virus.

Discussion Sources

Centers for Disease Control and Prevention. Meningococcal disease. https://www.cdc.gov/meningococcal/about/index.html

Centers for Disease Control and Prevention. Prevention and control of meningococcal disease: recommendations of the Advisory Committee on Immunization Practices (ACIP). *MMWR.* 2013;62(RR02):1–22.

Centers for Disease Control and Prevention. Use of serogroup B meningococcal vaccines in adolescents and young adults: recommendations of the Advisory Committee on Immunization Practices, 2015. *MMWR.* 2015;64(41):1171–1176.

Centers for Disease Control and Prevention. Viral meningitis. https://www.cdc.gov/meningitis/viral.html

de Assis Acquino Gondim F. Meningococcal meningitis. Medscape. https://emedicine.medscape.com/article/1165557-overview

QUESTIONS

60. An 18-year-old college freshman is brought to the student health center with a chief complaint of a 3-day history of progressive headache and intermittent fever. On physical examination, he has positive Kernig and Brudzinski signs. The most likely diagnosis is:

A. viral encephalitis.

B. bacterial meningitis.

C. acute subarachnoid hemorrhage.

D. epidural hematoma.

61. Of the following, which is the least likely bacterial source to cause meningitis?

A. colonization of the skin

B. colonization of the nose and throat

C. extension of acute otitis media

D. extension of bacterial rhinosinusitis

62. Risk factors for bacterial meningitis include all of the following except:

A. being over 25 years of age.

B. living in a community setting.

C. having a current history of cigarette smoking.

D. using immunosuppressant drugs.

63. The average incubation period for the organism *N meningitidis* is:

A. 24 hours.

B. 3 to 4 days.

C. 12 to 14 days.

D. 21 days.

64. A 19-year-old college sophomore was diagnosed with meningococcal meningitis today. You speak to the school health officers about the risk to the other students on campus. You inform them that:

A. the patient does not have a contagious disease.

B. all students are at significant risk regardless of their degree of contact with the infected person.

C. only intimate partners are at risk.

D. individuals with household-type or more intimate contact are considered to be at risk.

65. When evaluating the person who has bacterial meningitis, the NP expects to find CSF results of:

A. low protein.

B. a predominance of lymphocytes.

C. glucose at about 30% of serum levels.

D. low opening pressure.

66. When evaluating a patient who has aseptic or viral meningitis, the NP expects to find CSF results of:

A. low protein.

B. a predominance of lymphocytes.

C. glucose at about 30% of serum levels.

D. low opening pressure.

67. Which of the following describes the Kernig sign?

A. Neck pain occurs with passive flexion of one hip and knee, which causes flexion of the contralateral leg.

B. Passive neck flexion in a supine patient results in flexion of the knees and hips.

C. Elicited with the patient lying supine and the hip flexed 90°, it is present when extension of the knee from this position elicits resistance or pain in the lower back or posterior thigh.

D. Headache worsens when the patient is supine.

68. Physical examination findings in papilledema include:

A. arteriovenous nicking.

B. macular hyperpigmentation.

    C. optic disk bulging.

    D. pupillary constriction.

69. Which of the following vaccines is not typically recommended for individuals over 5 years of age?

    A. PCV13

    B. Hib

    C. MCV4

    D. MenB

70. Which of the following signs and symptoms most likely suggests meningitis caused by *N meningitidis*?

    A. a purpura or petechial rash

    B. absence of fever

    C. development of encephalitis

    D. absence of nuchal rigidity

71. All of the following persons should receive a dose of the MCV4 meningococcal vaccine except:

    A. a 19-year-old who received a first dose at 12 years of age.

    B. a 22-year-old who has not received the vaccine and will be moving to a college dormitory.

    C. a 35-year-old who will be traveling to a country where meningococcal disease is hyperendemic.

    D. a 14-year-old who received a first dose of the same vaccine at 11 years of age.

72. Chemoprophylaxis for household contacts of an individual diagnosed with meningitis can include all of the following except:

    A. a single dose of ceftriaxone.

    B. multiple doses of rifampin.

    C. multiple doses of amoxicillin.

    D. a single dose of meningococcal conjugate vaccine (MCV4 or Menactra®).

73 to 75. Indicate (Yes or No) whether postexposure prophylaxis is needed for adult household contacts of an individual with the following conditions.

_____ **73.** Viral meningitis

_____ **74.** Bacterial meningitis associated with acute bacterial rhinosinusitis

_____ **75.** Bacterial meningitis with bacterial pneumonia

For answers and rationales, see end of chapter.

Multiple Sclerosis

Overview

Multiple sclerosis (MS), a recurrent, chronic demyelinating disorder of the CNS, is a disease characterized by episodes of focal neurological dysfunction, with symptoms occurring acutely, worsening over a few days, and lasting weeks, followed by a period of partial to full resolution.

    MS can occur at any age but most commonly affects people between the ages of 20 and 40 years. Women are about twice as likely to develop MS compared with men. Other risk factors include family history of MS, ethnicity (highest incidence in those of northern European ancestry), certain viral infections (e.g., Epstein-Barr), and the presence of another autoimmune disease (e.g., thyroid disease, type 1 diabetes, or inflammatory bowel disease). Observational studies have also identified vitamin D deficiency as a modifiable risk factor for MS, which might be related to a higher prevalence of MS among populations in higher latitudes.

    MS is usually classified into two forms: (1) relapsing, remitting MS (RRMS), in which episodes resolve with improvement of neurological function between exacerbations and minimal to no cumulative defects, and which accounts for approximately 85% of patients with the condition; and (2) primary progressive MS, in which episodes do not fully resolve, and there are cumulative defects. Most patients with RRMS enter a stage referred to as secondary progressive MS.

Clinical Presentation

Symptoms of MS can vary and depend on the location of affected nerve fibers.

Heat sensitivity is also common in persons with MS, with small increases in body temperature triggering or exacerbating MS symptoms. Early treatment of MS can delay progression of disease and prevent disability. Unfortunately, due to a nonspecific presentation, an MS diagnosis is often delayed from the initial onset of symptoms and not definitively reached until only after multiple evaluation, often by a variety of health-care providers.

The initial diagnosis of MS is often difficult to make because the signs of recurrent fatigue, muscle weakness, and other nonspecific signs and symptoms are often attributed to other diseases or simply to stress and fatigue. Head MRI can reveal demyelinating plaques, a typical finding in MS. However, these lesions can also be present with other conditions, such as lupus, migraines, or diabetes. Following diagnosis, MRI can be used to monitor disease progression in the brain and spinal cord. A lumbar puncture is conducted to evaluate for abnormal findings in the CSF and can help rule out viral infections or other conditions that can cause neurological symptoms similar to MS. Characteristic CSF findings include pleocytosis (increase in WBCs found in CSF fluid) with predominance of monocytes and abnormal protein levels, including a modest increase in total protein, a markedly increased gamma-globulin fraction, a high immunoglobulin G index, the presence of oligoclonal bands, and an increase in myelin basic protein. Evoked potential testing can contribute to the development of the diagnosis by detecting lesions or nerve damage in the optic nerves, brainstem, or spinal cord.

The McDonald criteria can be used to assist in the diagnosis of MS even after one attack and uses a combination of clinical, imaging (e.g., MRI), and paraclinical tests (i.e., CSF analysis, evoked potentials). Blood tests are usually normal in MS patients but can be used to exclude other conditions. As with other conditions that have a complex origin and complicated course, expert consultation should be sought when diagnosing suspected MS and caring for the patient with the condition.

Treatment

MS treatment generally falls into three categories: therapy for relapses, long-term disease-modifying medications, and symptomatic management. Triggers for MS exacerbations are varied but often include onset of a common infectious disease such as urinary tract infection; however, most exacerbations have no identifiable trigger. Management of exacerbations includes treatment of the underlying precipitating illness, if present, and systemic high-dose corticosteroids, such as methylprednisolone. Because most exacerbations improve without specific therapy, disagreement exists as to the utility of this treatment. This therapy seems to shorten the course of most exacerbations but does not seem to have an impact on long-term disease progression. Some clinicians opt for lower-dose corticosteroid therapy with variable results. When corticosteroids are contraindicated or MS exacerbation does not respond to this treatment, plasmapheresis can be used as a second-line option.

Immunomodulatory therapy with interferon beta-1b (Betaseron®, Extavia®), interferon beta-1a (Avonex®, Rebif®), or peginterferon beta-1a (Plegridy®) has been shown to significantly reduce the frequency of exacerbations and long-term disability in RRMS. Immunosuppressive therapy with mitoxantrone (Novantrone®) also has some utility in reducing the rate of progression. Natalizumab (Tysabri®) is a monoclonal antibody with considerable clinical efficacy in treating MS, but this medication carries a warning about progressive multifocal leukoencephalopathy (PML), a rare, destructive brain infection, associated with its use. Oral dimethyl fumarate (Tecfidera®) significantly decreases relapses and disease progression but is associated with a risk for PML, lymphopenia, and hepatotoxicity. Subcutaneous glatiramer acetate (Copaxone®) has been demonstrated to reduce the number of MS attacks by blocking the immune system's attack on myelin. Alemtuzumab (Lemtrada®) is a monoclonal antibody against cell surface glycoprotein CD52 with considerable efficacy. However, it comes with several boxed warnings, including immune thrombocytopenia, serious and life-threatening infusion reactions, and stroke. Ocrelizumab (Ocrevus®) is a monoclonal antibody directed against CD20-expressing B cells and can potentially cause life-threatening infusion reactions as well as increased risk for malignancies. Fingolimod (Gilenya®) is an

---

CLINICAL CONCEPT

Common MS signs and symptoms include weakness or numbness of a limb, monocular visual loss, diplopia, vertigo, facial weakness or numbness, sphincter disturbances, ataxia, and nystagmus.

CLINICAL CONCEPT

Expert consultation should be sought while providing care for the complex health-care needs of patients with MS.

oral medication that traps immune cells in lymph nodes. Because of associated bradycardia with this drug, patients should have their heart rate monitored for 6 hours following the first dose. Teriflunomide (Aubagio®), which inhibits the production of T and B cells, has been shown to reduce MS attacks and associated lesions. However, liver function must be closely monitored for patients taking this medication because it can cause serious liver damage.

Symptom management therapies are aimed at the specific needs of the individual patient and often include nondrug interventions, such as physical and occupational therapy, and management of urological problems such as altered bladder function.

Discussion Sources

Luzzio C. Multiple sclerosis. Medscape. http://emedicine.medscape.com/article/1146199

Rae-Grant A, Day GS, Marrie RA, et al. Practice guideline recommendation summary: disease-modifying therapies for adults with multiple sclerosis: Report of the Guideline Development, Dissemination, and Implementation Subcommittee of the American Academy of Neurology. *Neurology.* 2018;90:777–788.

QUESTIONS

76. The cause of MS is best described as:

A. a destructive process of the nerve fiber protecting myelin.

B. an intracranial viral infection.

C. inflammation of the brain and/or spinal cord.

D. an autoimmune disorder that destroys muscle fibers.

77. Common symptoms of MS, especially in earlier disease, include all of the following except:

A. numbness or weakness in one or more limbs.

B. double vision or blurring vision.

C. facial weakness or numbness.

D. symptoms improving in a warmer environment.

78. Risk factors for MS include all of the following except:

A. being older than 50 years of age.

B. female gender.

C. northern European ancestry.

D. autoimmune disease.

79 to 81. Match each diagnostic test with the expected finding for a patient with multiple sclerosis.

_____ **79.** MRI

_____ **80.** Analysis of CSF

_____ **81.** Evoked potential test

A. presence of oligoclonal bands

B. presence of demyelinating plaques

C. delays in timing of CNS response

82. Treatment options in MS to attenuate disease progression include:

A. interferon beta-1b.

B. methylprednisolone.

C. ribavirin.

D. phenytoin.

For answers and rationales, see end of chapter.

Parkinson's Disease

Overview

Parkinson's disease (PD) is a slowly progressive movement disorder that is largely caused by the loss of the pigmented dopaminergic neurons of the substantia nigra pars compacta. Additional pathological changes include the presence of Lewy bodies and Lewy neurites. The majority of changes occur in the basal ganglia in the base. Given that about 60% to 80% of dopaminergic neurons are lost prior to the onset of the motor dysfunction seen in PD, clinical presentation is a late, not early, manifestation of PD. Age at onset is usually in the sixth decade and older, but the onset can occur in much younger adults. PD is noted in approximately 1% of the adult population age 60 years and older.

Clinical Presentation

The diagnosis of PD is made by clinical evaluation and consists of a combination of four cardinal features: tremor at rest, rigidity, bradykinesia (slowness in the execution of movement), and postural instability. At least two of the first three listed must be present for the diagnosis (postural instability emerges in later disease).

Over time, an individual with PD will hold the arms rigidly at the sides with little movement during ambulation; forward falls are common. The parkinsonian gait usually consists of a series of rapid small steps; to turn, patients must take several small steps, moving forward and backward.

> **CLINICAL CONCEPT**
> Resting tremor of an upper limb is the most common initial sign of PD.

Whereas movement disorder is the PD hallmark, nonmotor signs can also be present in early PD. These can include excessive salivation, forgetfulness, constipation, and urinary retention. A reduced, altered sense of smell (hyposmia) is often one of the first symptoms, though this is often not noted by the patient until the disease is quite advanced.

Later stages of disease are characterized by more pronounced bradykinesia, including facial bradykinesia associated with a decreased blink rate and facial expression (i.e., mask-like facies) as well as balance issues. Mood disorders are common among those with PD, and routine screening for depression and anxiety should be performed. Though signs of cognitive dysfunction can appear early in disease, dementia typically occurs later in the disease process (8 or more years after the onset of motor function findings). Hallucinations can occur in later disease, particularly when associated with Lewy body disease.

Patients with an onset of PD before age 40 years should be tested for Wilson's disease. Other diagnoses to consider include Alzheimer's disease, cardioembolic stroke, dementia with Lewy bodies, Huntington's disease, lacunar syndrome, and normal pressure hydrocephalus.

Diagnostic Testing

The diagnosis of PD is made clinically, based on patient history and physical examination. With classic presentation, no additional testing is required. Additional testing, including brain imaging such as MRI, electromyography, or lumbar puncture, is usually ordered in conjunction with expert neurological consultation and is aimed at ruling in or out other diagnoses.

Treatment

Treatment of PD is aimed at reducing symptoms and providing neuroprotection. Because PD is characterized by an alteration in the dopaminergic pathway, dopamine agonists such as ropinirole (Requip®) and pramipexole (Mirapex®) are usually the early disease treatment of choice, in part because of a proposed neuroprotective effect and a better adverse effect profile than levodopa. Levodopa, a metabolic precursor of dopamine, continues to be used to minimize symptoms but tends to be less effective with more adverse effects as the disease progresses; most patients who take levodopa for more than 5 to 10 years develop dyskinesia. Levodopa is often given with carbidopa in the fixed-dose combination known as Sinemet® or Parcopa®. Monoamine oxidase-B (MAO-B) inhibitors, such as selegiline (Eldepryl®, Zelapar®) or rasagiline (Azilect®), can also be considered in early disease, as these agents help increase levodopa's half-life by reducing its metabolism.

Exercise and physical therapy should be encouraged to improve gait, balance, initiation of movement, and functional independence. Some evidence suggests a neuroprotective effect of exercise, and vigorous exercise in midlife possibly reduces the risk of development of PD.

Amantadine (Symmetrel®) is an antiviral drug with time-limited (usually less than 1 year) antiparkinsonian benefits, but it can be used in later stages of the disease to help reduce dyskinesias. Catechol-O-methyltransferase (COMT) inhibitors including tolcapone (Tasmar®) and entacapone (Comtan®) are clinically helpful because these medications increase the half-life of levodopa by reducing its metabolism. Apomorphine (Apokyn®) is an injectable-only dopamine agonist that can be used in advanced Parkinson disease as a rescue therapy for the treatment of hypomobility or "off" periods. Other medications used in the treatment of PD include anticholinergics, such as benztropine (Cogentin®) and trihexyphenidyl (Artane®), to help with tremor; however, this class of drugs is well known to cause dry mouth, urinary retention, and altered mentation, particularly in older adults. In view of the complexity of prescribing for PD and medication choices, the NP should be well versed in these products and seek expert neurological consultation.

> **CLINICAL CONCEPT**
>
> As PD progresses after several months to years, patients often develop variability in response to treatment about 4 to 5 hours after taking a dose of medication.

With early treatment of PD (e.g., levodopa), the individual typically experiences a stable and sustained response throughout the day. This is known as motor fluctuations, often referred to as "on" and "off" periods. During an "on" period, a person can move with relative ease. An "off" period describes times when a person has more difficulty with movement; this can be manifested either by significant difficulty in initiating movement or with uncontrolled body movements including dyskinesia. A common time for a person with Parkinson disease to experience an "off" period is toward the end of a levodopa-dosing period, when the drug seems to be "wearing off." This problem can usually be managed with medication adjustment. Adding a COMT or MAO-B inhibitor can prolong the effect of levodopa as can using a higher dose of levodopa or dosing more frequently. Newer approaches include adding intermittent inhaled doses of levodopa (Inbrija™) or switching to a sustained-release formulation of levodopa/carbidopa. An enteral suspension of carbidopa/levodopa (Duopa™) that is infused into the jejunum by portable pump can also help reduce "off" times.

For most people with PD, "off" periods and dyskinesias can be managed with changes in medications. However, when medication adjustments do not improve mobility or when medications cause significant adverse effects, surgical treatment can be considered, especially with uncontrolled writhing movement (choreiform movement or dyskinesia) of the body or a limb. Pallidotomy (destruction of part of the globus pallidus interna) can be helpful in tremor, rigidity, bradykinesia, and levodopa-induced dyskinesias. Subthalamotomy, or ablation of part of the subthalamic nucleus, has shown promise in improving the cardinal features of PD as well as reducing dyskinesia. Deep brain stimulation surgery for PD is the preferred surgical option as it does not involve destruction of brain tissue and is reversible. This high-frequency electrostimulation process is helpful in making the "off" state more like movement in the "on" state, and this can improve levodopa-induced dyskinesias. As with other therapies, expert consultation should be sought, and all options should be thoroughly discussed with the patient before pursuing surgical intervention. Regular follow-up care is necessary to ensure motor and nonmotor symptoms are properly managed.

Clinicians should also consider management of psychiatric conditions associated with PD. Cholinesterase inhibitors such as rivastigmine (Exelon®) and donepezil (Aricept®) can be used to manage dementia. Anticholinergic agents should be avoided when possible, as these can impair cognitive function. Individuals with PD should be routinely screened for depression and treated accordingly. SSRIs are most commonly used, though research indicates that this class might have limited effect in patients with PD. Other options can include tricyclic antidepressants or SNRIs (e.g., venlafaxine). Antipsychotics can be considered for those experiencing hallucinations or delusions, a common adverse effect from antiparkinsonian medications. Pimavanserin (Nuplazid®) is approved for use in PD patients and does not affect the dopamine pathway. Other options include quetiapine and clozapine, though blood level monitoring is needed with use of clozapine. Typical antipsychotics should be avoided as they can exacerbate motor symptoms of PD.

Discussion Sources

Hauser RA. Parkinson disease. Medscape. https://emedicine.medscape.com/article/1831191-overview

Jankovic J, Poewe W. Therapies in Parkinson's disease. *Curr Opin Neurol.* 2012;25:433–447.

National Parkinson Foundation. Understanding Parkinson's. http://www.parkinson.org/understanding-parkinsons

QUESTIONS

83. PD is primarily caused by:

   A. degradation of myelin surrounding nerve fibers.

   B. loss of the pigmented dopaminergic neurons.

C. deterioration of neurons in the brainstem.

D. excessive production of acetylcholinesterase in the CSF.

84. Which of the following is most consistent with findings in patients with PD?

A. rigid posture with poor muscle tone

B. mask-like facies and continued cognitive function

C. tremor at rest and bradykinesia

D. excessive arm swinging with ambulation and flexed posture

85. The diagnosis of PD relies on findings of:

A. clinical evaluation of its cardinal clinical features.

B. head MRI or CT scan.

C. pleocytosis in the CSF.

D. a visual evoked potential test.

86. When considering treatment for PD, levodopa is typically used:

A. as prophylaxis for individuals at high risk of developing PD.

B. as a first-line treatment in early disease.

C. when there is inadequate response with a COMT inhibitor.

D. only after neuroablative surgery in advanced disease.

87. Other conditions to consider in the differential diagnosis of PD can include all of the following except:

A. Alzheimer's dementia.

B. normal pressure hydrocephalus.

C. Huntington's disease.

D. multiple sclerosis.

88 to 90. Match each type of procedure with its description in the treatment of PD.

_____ **88.** Subthalamotomy

_____ **89.** Pallidotomy

_____ **90.** Deep brain stimulation

    A. ablation of part of the globus pallidus interna

    B. destruction of part of the subthalamic nucleus

    C. high-frequency electrostimulation of the brain

91. Which of the following statements regarding "on" and "off" periods of PD is false?

A. A person can move with relative ease during an "on" period.

B. An "off" period typically occurs at the maximum serum concentration (C_{max}) following levodopa dosing.

C. Medication adjustment can usually minimize "off" periods.

D. Surgical treatment may be needed to manage dyskinesia during "off" periods.

92 to 94. Match each type of medication with the condition it can treat for patients with PD.

_____ **92.** SNRI (e.g., venlafaxine)

_____ **93.** Pimavanserin (Nuplazid®)

_____ **94.** Cholinesterase inhibitors (e.g., rivastigmine [Exelon®])

    A. dementia

    B. depression

    C. hallucinations

95. A 64-year-old man recently diagnosed with PD asks about exercising. He states, "I usually like to walk briskly around my neighborhood for 30 minutes at least four to five times a week." The NP responds:

A. Prolonged exercise should be avoided as this can hasten progression of disease.

B. Exercise should be limited to about 15 minutes every other day.

C. Exercise is encouraged and likely has a neuroprotective effect.

D. There is no evidence that exercise has any impact on PD.

For answers and rationales, see end of chapter.

Seizure Disorders

Overview

A seizure occurs when there is an imbalance between the inhibitory and excitatory forces within the brain, favoring excitation. Seizures can be either provoked, where there is a transient recognizable cause for the seizure (e.g., head trauma, brain tumor, electrolyte disturbance), or unprovoked, where there is no identifiable cause. Epilepsy is the most common cause of unprovoked seizures. A careful medical history and physical examination will help to assist in the diagnosis and determine what additional testing is needed.

Clinical Presentation

Knowledge of the presentation of common forms of seizures is critical (Table 3-6). The classification of what type of seizure disorder, and therefore the appropriate treatment, is derived largely from the patient's health history and description of the event, if witnessed.

Important aspects of history taking with the seizure event include:

■ Was a warning event present?
■ What actually happened during the seizure?
■ Did the patient relate to the environment?

TABLE 3-6 Description of Common Seizure Disorders

SEIZURE TYPE	DESCRIPTION OF SEIZURE	COMMENTS
Absence (petit mal)	Blank staring lasting 3 to 50 seconds accompanied by impaired level of consciousness	Usual age of onset 3 to 15 years
Myoclonic	Awake state or momentary loss of consciousness with abnormal motor behavior lasting seconds to minutes; one or more muscle groups causing brief jerking contractions of the limbs and trunk, occasionally flinging patient	Difficult to control; at least half also have tonic-clonic seizures. Usual age of onset 2 to 7 years
Tonic-clonic (grand mal)	Rigid extension of arms and legs followed by sudden jerking movements with loss of consciousness; bowel and bladder incontinence common with postictal confusion	Onset at any age; in adults, new onset may be found in brain tumor, after head injury, alcohol withdrawal
Simple partial or focal seizure (jacksonian)	Awake state with abnormal motor, sensory, autonomic, or psychic behavior; movement can affect any part of body, localized or generalized	Typical age of onset 3 to 15 years
Complex partial	Aura characterized by unusual sense of smell or taste, visual or auditory hallucinations, stomach upset; followed by vague stare and facial movements, muscle contraction and relaxation, and autonomic signs; can progress to loss of consciousness	Onset at any age

Source: Schacter SC. Types of seizures. Epilepsy Foundation. https://www.epilepsy.com/learn/types-seizures

- Does the patient have any recollection of the seizure?
- How did the patient feel after the seizure?
- How long was the recovery following the seizure?
- What is the frequency and duration of seizures?
- Is there a known trigger for a seizure?

When evaluating a patient with a reported seizure, other conditions to consider in the differential diagnosis can include cardioembolic stroke, frontal lobe epilepsy, idiopathic orthostatic hypotension, migraine, or transient global amnesia. Other conditions that can cause a seizure-like episode include syncope, certain metabolic conditions (e.g., hypoglycaemia, hyponatremia), transient ischemic attack (TIA), sleep disorder, paroxysmal dyskinesia, and psychiatric conditions (e.g., panic attack).

Diagnostic Testing

Diagnostic testing in seizure is aimed at revealing a potential, modifiable underlying cause. Prolactin level can be helpful when performed shortly after a seizure (within 20 minutes). Levels are typically elevated following a generalized tonic-clonic or complex partial seizure and can help to differentiate a seizure from a psychogenic nonepileptic seizure event.

Video-EEG monitoring can help further classify seizure type and establish a definitive diagnosis, especially when there is loss of consciousness. However, this procedure is costly and should therefore be limited to those with suspected pseudoseizures (i.e., nonepileptic event resulting from a psychological condition) or who do not respond to treatment. Expert consultation should be sought for the person with a suspected or documented seizure disorder.

CLINICAL CONCEPT

For those experiencing unprovoked seizures, an electroencephalograph (EEG) can be used to help confirm a diagnosis of epilepsy.

Treatment

The goal of treatment is to prevent seizures with minimal adverse effects. The type of seizure directs the treatment of a seizure disorder. Often, with a single seizure with a known provocation, such as alcohol withdrawal or severe sleep deprivation, the treatment is focused on avoiding the seizure trigger. For unprovoked seizures, expert knowledge of the indications and adverse effects of antiepileptic medications is needed before therapy is initiated or continued.

Numerous seizure therapies include standard or older products such as phenytoin, carbamazepine, clonazepam, ethosuximide, and valproic acid, and more recently developed AEDs, such as gabapentin, lamotrigine, and topiramate. Certain AEDs, including phenytoin and carbamazepine, are narrow therapeutic index (NTI) drugs. A certain amount of such drugs is therapeutic, and just slightly more than this amount is potentially toxic. Conversely, a slightly lower dose might not be therapeutic. Other NTI drugs include warfarin, theophylline, and digoxin. Many of these drugs have high levels of protein binding and undergo drug metabolism via hepatic enzyme pathways, such as cytochrome P-450 (CYP 450). Phenytoin is highly protein bound (greater than 90%); when taken with other highly protein-bound drugs, it can potentially be displaced from its protein-binding site, leading to increased free phenytoin and a risk of toxicity. Carbamazepine and phenytoin can increase the metabolic capacity of hepatic enzymes, which leads to more rapid metabolism of the drug and reduced levels of this and other drugs. Phenytoin use increases theophylline clearance by increasing CYP 450 enzyme activity. Concomitant use of theophylline and phenytoin can lead to altered phenytoin pharmacokinetics. The net result is that when phenytoin and theophylline are given together, levels of both drugs can decrease by 40%. When taken with birth control pills, carbamazepine induces estrogen metabolism, potentially leading to contraceptive failure. The prescriber should be familiar with the drug interactions of all AEDs and monitor therapeutic levels and for adverse reactions.

The majority of patients can achieve seizure-free status with pharmacotherapy. For patients with refractory epilepsy, surgery can be considered and can actually be curative in a large majority of patients. Lobectomy and lesionectomy are two of the more common procedures and are typically performed following epileptic zone mapping via video-EEG.

Individuals with seizures are restricted from driving, though these driving restrictions vary from state to state. Typically, a seizure-free period must be met before driving restriction is lifted, and this can vary from 3 months to a year or more.

Commercial drivers are often required to have a 5-year seizure-free period prior to operating a motor vehicle. Health-care providers should be aware of local laws regarding seizures and driving restrictions and comply with reporting to their state Department of Motor Vehicles when required (either by the patient or provider).

Discussion Sources

Indiana University School of Medicine, Division of Clinical Pharmacology. P450 drug interaction table: abbreviated clinically relevant table. http://medicine.iupui.edu/clinpharm/ddis/clinical-table/

Jankovic SM, Dostic M. Choice of antiepileptic drugs for the elderly: possible drug interactions and adverse effects. *Expert Opin Drug Metab Toxicol.* 2012;8:81–91.

Ko DY. Epilepsy and seizures. Medscape. https://emedicine.medscape.com/article/1184846-overview

QUESTIONS

96 to 99. Match each type of seizure with its most appropriate description.

_____ **96.** Myoclonic

_____ **97.** Absence (petit mal)

_____ **98.** Tonic-clonic (grand mal)

_____ **99.** Simple partial or focal

    A. blank staring lasting 3 to 50 seconds, accompanied by impaired level of consciousness

    B. awake state with abnormal motor and psychic behavior lasting seconds

    C. rigid extension of arms and legs, followed by sudden jerking movements with loss of consciousness

    D. brief, jerking contractions of arms, legs, trunk, or all of these

100. Which of the following antiepileptic medications is least likely to cause a significant drug-drug interaction?

    A. carbamazepine

    B. phenytoin

    C. gabapentin

    D. clonazepam

101. Which of the following medications requires ongoing therapeutic monitoring of drug levels?

    A. topiramate

    B. phenytoin

    C. gabapentin

    D. lamotrigine

102. Which of the following statements about potential drug interactions with phenytoin is false?

    A. Phenytoin increases theophylline clearance by increasing CYP 450 enzyme activity.

    B. When taken with other highly protein-bound drugs, the free phenytoin concentration can increase to toxic levels.

    C. Phenytoin can increase the metabolic capacity of hepatic enzymes, thus leading to reduced drug levels.

    D. When phenytoin and theophylline are given together, the result is a higher concentration of both drugs than when given separately.

103. The most common cause of new-onset unprovoked seizure is:

    A. cardioembolic stroke.

    B. epilepsy.

    C. psychogenic condition.

    D. hypoglycemia.

104. A 34-year-old mother of two daughters is being evaluated following a new-onset seizure that caused a momentary loss of consciousness. Before being discharged, she asks if she can still drive her car. The NP responds that:

    A. driving restrictions will likely be placed if there is a repeat episode.

    B. she can drive as long as it is locally and for short distances.

C. driving is restricted until a seizure-free period is achieved that is determined by state law.

D. driving is restricted until a seizure-free period of 1 year.

105. When evaluating a patient with a new-onset unprovoked seizure, the most important aspect of the diagnostic evaluation is:

A. patient history.

B. serum CRP.

C. head MRI.

D. a complete blood count (CBC).

For answers and rationales, see end of chapter.

Transient Ischemic Attack and Stroke

Transient Ischemic Attack Overview

A TIA is an acute neurological event in which all signs and symptoms, including numbness, weakness, and flaccidity, and visual changes, ataxia, or dysarthria, resolve usually within minutes, but certainly by 24 hours after onset. In suspected TIA, if neurological changes persist beyond 24 hours, the diagnosis of stroke should be considered.

Risk factors include carotid artery disease and other forms of atherosclerosis; structural cardiac problems, such as valvular problems that lead to increased risk of embolization; and hypercoagulable conditions, such as antiphospholipid antibody and combined oral contraceptive use. Nonmodifiable risk factors include older age, male gender, prior history of TIA, sickle cell disease, and African American ethnicity.

> **CLINICAL CONCEPT**
> TIA should be considered a "stroke warning."

Clinical Presentation

A TIA can last from a few minutes to several hours, and presentation can be highly variable depending on the area of the brain affected. However, the signs and symptoms often resemble those of an early stroke. These can include unilateral weakness, numbness, or paralysis of the face or limb, slurred or garbled speech, blindness or diplopia in one or both eyes, dizziness and loss of balance, and a sudden-onset severe headache. When evaluating a patient with suspected TIA, other conditions to consider in the differential diagnosis include carotid artery dissection, meningitis, MS, stroke, hypoglycemia, seizure, and subarachnoid hemorrhage.

Diagnostic Testing

Given that TIA episodes can typically last only minutes in duration, a careful patient history is critically important from the patient as well as any witnesses to the episode to help in establishing the diagnosis. The patient and/or witness history in TIA should report any changes in speech, behavior, gait, memory, or movement. Laboratory testing is largely done to rule in or out other possible conditions and can include blood glucose, CBC, and serum electrolytes as well as coagulation studies and 12-lead ECG. Imaging of the brain with MRI or CT should be performed within 24 hours of symptom onset. Vascular imaging should also be performed by Doppler ultrasonography, CT angiography (CTA), or magnetic resonance angiography (MRA). CTA and MRA are useful in evaluating the vessels of both the brain and neck.

Treatment

Management of TIA is aimed at reducing the short- and long-term risks for stroke. Intervention includes minimizing risk factors through lifestyle modification (e.g., smoking cessation; diet; exercise; and cardiovascular and cerebrovascular disease risk reduction such as aggressive treatment of dyslipidemia, hypertension, and diabetes mellitus) and long-term antiplatelet therapy (e.g., aspirin or clopidogrel). For those at high risk of stroke or whose TIA is associated with cardioembolism (e.g., related to atrial fibrillation or valvular disease), anticoagulation therapy, such as direct oral anticoagulant (DOAC) or warfarin use, can be considered in addition to antiplatelet therapy.

Stroke Overview

Stroke is the fifth leading cause of death and the leading cause of disability in the United States. Acute stroke is caused by a sudden loss of blood circulation to an area of the brain that results in neurological dysfunction. Ischemic stroke occurs when there is a blockage of a cerebral artery preventing blood flow, while a hemorrhagic stroke occurs when a blood vessel bursts or leaks blood into the surrounding brain tissue. Both types of stroke can present similarly, though hemorrhagic stroke is more commonly associated with nausea, vomiting, headache, and sudden change in consciousness. Risk factors are similar to those listed for TIA with the highest frequency of stroke occurring in older adults, men, and those with African ancestry. Other potential risks for stroke include trauma to the head and neck, high torsion of the neck (e.g., high-impact sports, roller coasters), high-velocity chiropractic manipulation, and certain positions during surgery (e.g., beach-chair position).

Coagulopathies can predispose individuals to excessive bleeding and hemorrhagic stroke, including antiphospholipid antibody, inherited disorders leading to factor VII, VIII, IX, X, and XIII deficiency, as well as factor V Leiden mutation. Women with inherited coagulopathies should avoid estrogen-containing contraceptives (e.g., combined oral contraceptives) as this can increase the risk of thrombosis and stroke. Expert consultation is needed for these patients with pregnancy. Often low molecular weight heparin is prescribed to minimize clot risk and maximize pregnancy success.

About 80% of strokes are due to cerebral ischemia, about 15% are due to cerebral hemorrhage, and 5% are due to subarachnoid hemorrhage; in younger adults, carotid artery dissection can cause stroke, accounting for about 5% of all strokes.

If blood flow is not restored, the ischemic tissue will be compromised, and the ischemia evolves into a cerebral infarction, often with devastating long-term consequences. If acute stroke is suspected, the patient must undergo emergency neuroimaging and be evaluated for thrombolytic or revascularization therapy in the appropriate health-care setting.

> **CLINICAL CONCEPT**
>
> Acute stroke should be thought of as a "brain attack," in which a portion of the brain is acutely ischemic, a potentially reversible condition if blood flow is reestablished.

Clinical Presentation

Stroke should be considered for any patient presenting with acute neurological deficit and altered level of consciousness. Acute stroke is often thought of as manifesting with sudden-onset unilateral limb weakness and motor dysfunction. Although these findings are often part of the clinical presentation, other findings, such as changes in hearing and vision, seizure, and head and neck pain, are often noted (Table 3-7). Signs and symptoms can vary considerably depending on the area of the brain affected, and typically a combination of symptoms is present.

Diagnostic Testing

Immediate brain imaging is essential to confirm a hemorrhagic or ischemic stroke. When utilizing neuroimaging for stroke, a head CT scan is helpful in identifying acute cerebral hemorrhage, whereas MRI is a more sensitive test in the acute phase of ischemic stroke.

CT or MRA is helpful in showing stenosis or occlusion in the brain-supplying vessels. There is evidence supporting the use of MRA to also screen patients with a strong family history (i.e., two or more first-degree relatives) of intracranial aneurysm given the high mortality rate of aneurysmal rupture. Carotid ultrasound, echocardiogram, and cerebral angiogram can help to identify or rule out concomitant and contributing conditions as well as identify the possible source of the blood clot. An echocardiogram can be used to find the source of clots in the heart that may have traveled to the brain to cause a stroke. A transesophageal echocardiogram can be used to obtain clear, detailed ultrasound images of the heart and any blood clots that are present.

Treatment

Because atherosclerosis is a major contributor to stroke risk, prevention of the condition should be aimed at reducing atherosclerotic risk through control of hypertension, dyslipidemia, and diabetes mellitus. Patients with a history of ischemic stroke are also at high risk for another cerebrovascular event, myocardial infarction, and sudden cardiac death, and benefit from aggressive measures to reduce atherosclerotic risk.

The goal of treatment in acute stroke is to restore blood circulation to the brain (for ischemic stroke) and control bleeding and provide supportive therapy (for hemorrhagic stroke). For ischemic stroke, fibrinolytic therapy with alteplase (Activase®) can restore blood flow in some patients when administered within 3 to 4.5 hours of stroke onset.

TABLE 3-7 Acute Stroke Presentation

SIGN/SYMPTOM	CLINICAL PRESENTATION
Alteration in consciousness	Stupor
	Confusion
	Agitation
	Memory loss
	Delirium
	Seizures
	Coma
Headache	Intense or unusually severe, often with sudden onset, usually described as having different characteristics compared with patient's typical primary headache
	Altered level of consciousness or neurological deficit
	Unusual or severe neck or facial pain
Aphasia, facial weakness or asymmetry	Paralysis of facial muscles (e.g., noted when patient speaks or smiles)
	May be on same side (ipsilateral) or opposite side (contralateral) to limb paralysis
Altered coordination	Incoordination, weakness, paralysis, or sensory loss of one or more limbs (usually one-half of the body and in particular the hand)
	Ataxia (poor balance, clumsiness, or difficulty walking)
Visual loss	Monocular or binocular
	Report of partial loss of the field
Miscellaneous	Vertigo
	Diplopia
	Unilateral hearing loss
	Nausea, vomiting
	Photophobia
	Phonophobia

Sources: Yew KS, Cheng EM. Diagnosis of acute stroke. Am Fam Phys. 2015;91;528–536. https://www.aafp.org/cfp/2015/0415/p528.html; Jauch EC. Ischemic stroke clinical presentation. Medscape. https://emedicine.medscape.com/article/1916852-clinical#b3

Secondary prevention against ischemic stroke should include antiplatelet therapy with aspirin or aspirin with extended-release dipyridamole (Aggrenox®); if these options are not tolerated or in the presence of peripheral arterial or multivessel atherosclerotic disease, clopidogrel (Plavix®) should be prescribed. These agents inhibit platelet activation through different mechanisms of action. When stroke originates from cardiac embolus, usually due to atrial fibrillation, oral anticoagulation with a DOAC therapy or warfarin should be started. Though DOACs tend to be more costly compared to warfarin, this drug class has the advantages of predictable pharmacokinetics, fewer drug interactions, and no requirement for routine therapeutic monitoring. Examples of DOACs used for the prevention of stroke include dabigatran (Pradaxa®), rivaroxaban (Xarelto®), apixaban (Eliquis®), and edoxaban (Savaysa®). Warfarin therapy is an alternative to DOAC therapy, albeit with the need for ongoing laboratory monitoring to reach a goal international normalized ratio (INR) of 2 to 3.

For those with hypertension who have had a stroke, appropriate antihypertensive medications should be initiated to try to get the patient to goal. For secondary stroke prevention, guidelines from the American College of Cardiology/American Heart Association (ACC/AHA) recommend a blood pressure goal of less than 130/80 mm Hg. Agents recommended to decrease blood pressure after stroke include thiazide diuretics (e.g., hydrochlorothiazide [HCTZ]), calcium antagonists, angiotensin-converting enzyme (ACE) inhibitors, and angiotensin receptor blockers (ARBs). Combination therapy that uses lower doses of medications can provide enhanced efficacy with decreased frequency of adverse effects.

Discussion Sources

Cruz-Flores S. Stroke anticoagulation and prophylaxis. Medscape. http://emedicine.medscape.com/article/1160021-overview#aw2aab6b3

Internet Stroke Center. Emergency stroke evaluation and diagnosis. http://www.strokecenter.org/wp-content/uploads/2011/08/Emergency-Stroke-Evaluation-Diagnosis.pdf

Nanda A. Transient ischemic attack. Medscape. http://emedicine.medscape.com/article/1910519-overview

QUESTIONS

106. Risk factors for TIA include all of the following except:

    A. atrial fibrillation.

    B. carotid artery disease.

    C. combined oral contraceptive use.

    D. pernicious anemia.

107. A TIA is characterized as an episode of reversible neurological symptoms that can last

    A. 1 hour.

    B. 12 hours.

    C. 24 hours.

    D. 48 hours or more.

108. When providing ongoing care for a patient with a recent TIA, you consider that:

    A. long-term antiplatelet therapy is likely indicated.

    B. this person has a relatively low risk of future stroke.

    C. women present with this disorder more often than men.

    D. rehabilitation will be needed to minimize the effects of the resulting neurological insult.

109 to 111. Rank the following causes of stroke from most common (1) to least common (3):

_____ 109. Cerebral hemorrhage

_____ 110. Cerebral ischemia

_____ 111. Subarachnoid hemorrhage

112 to 114. Match each type of stroke with its most common underlying cause.

_____ 112. Cerebral hemorrhage

_____ 113. Cerebral ischemia

_____ 114. Subarachnoid hemorrhage (SAH)

        A. atherosclerosis

        B. ruptured cerebral aneurysm

        C. hypertension

115. Antiplatelet agents commonly used in secondary prevention of stroke include all of the following except:

    A. aspirin.

    B. clopidogrel.

    C. aspirin plus extended-release dipyridamole.

    D. rivaroxaban.

116. Which of the following conditions is least likely to contribute to an increased risk of ischemic or hemorrhagic stroke?

A. hyperlipidemia

B. diabetes mellitus

C. Crohn's disease

D. hypertension

117 to 123. When considering the diagnosis of acute stroke, which of the following can be part of the presentation? (Answer yes or no.)

_____ **117.** partial loss of visual field

_____ **118.** unilateral hearing loss

_____ **119.** facial muscle paralysis

_____ **120.** vertigo

_____ **121.** diplopia

_____ **122.** headache

_____ **123.** ataxia

124. Acute cerebral hemorrhage is best identified with which of the following imaging techniques?

A. transesophageal echocardiogram

B. CT scan

C. cerebral angiogram

D. MRA

125. The use of a DOAC for secondary prevention of stroke is most useful for:

A. all individuals who experience a first episode of TIA.

B. any individual with a stroke history.

C. those with hemorrhagic stroke only.

D. those with ischemic stroke and cardioembolic conditions.

126. You see a 25-year-old woman with a known factor V Leiden mutation who asks about contraceptives. You suggest all of the following except:

A. combined oral contraceptive.

B. LNG-IUD.

C. copper-containing IUD.

D. levonorgestrel implant.

127. Which of the following patients would you consider neuroimaging with MRA to screen for the presence of a cerebral aneurysm?

A. a 67-year-old man with a 35 pack-year smoking history and hypertension

B. a 48-year-old woman with type 2 diabetes mellitus, dyslipidemia, and history of acute coronary syndrome

C. a 33-year-old woman with factor V Leiden mutation taking combined oral contraceptive

D. a 46-year-old with four first-degree relatives with subarachnoid hemorrhage

128 to 132. You see a 54-year-old man who is a current smoker and has a history of hypertension, type 2 diabetes mellitus, and dyslipidemia. In considering stroke prevention, indicate if each of the following statements is true or false.

_____ **128.** An acceptable blood pressure goal is less than 130/80 mm Hg.

_____ **129.** An appropriate A1c target for this individual is less than 8.5%.

_____ **130.** A statin is contraindicated for this patient.

_____ **131.** Appropriate first-line antihypertensive medications can include thiazide diuretic, ACE inhibitor or ARB, or calcium channel blocker

_____ **132.** He should be initiated on a DOAC.

For answers and rationales, see end of chapter.

Giant Cell Arteritis

Overview

Giant cell arteritis (GCA) is an autoimmune vasculitis involving medium and large vessels with resulting arterial inflammation that affects just part of an artery with sections of normal artery in between. GCA has historically been known as temporal arteritis; this term is considered inaccurate as more than only the temporal artery can be involved. In GCA, inflammation and swelling of the arteries cause decreased blood flow resulting in the condition's associated symptoms.

This condition is most common in patients 50 to 85 years old; average age at onset is 70 years, and it is more common in women of European ancestry than any other group. GCA and polymyalgia rheumatica are thought to represent two parts of a spectrum of disease and are often found together.

Clinical Presentation

Physical examination of suspected GCA should include head and neck, ophthalmic, and neurological examination as well as vital signs and blood pressure in both arms. GCA typically presents with a severe unilateral headache that usually develops over a few days. For the person with a primary headache type such as migraine or tension-type headache, the cephalalgia reported in GCA is described as different in character, often with a stabbing quality not noted in most primary headaches.

> **CLINICAL CONCEPT**
>
> GCA-associated headache is usually reported as being located in the frontal, vertex, or occipital area, rather than in the temporal area.

Often there is also a history of recent-onset respiratory tract symptoms (cough, sore throat, hoarseness). Jaw claudication, that is, pain in the jaw, is usually reported as well as acute reduction or change in vision. Approximately 50% of patients with GCA experience visual symptoms, including transient visual blurring, diplopia, eye pain, or sudden loss of vision; transient repeated episodes of blurred vision are usually reversible, but sudden loss of vision is an ominous sign and is almost always permanent. Occasionally, and most often noted in the frail older adult, there is a change in mental status and less report of headache.

In GCA, extracranial branches of the carotid artery are often involved; this results in a tender or nodular, pulseless vessel, usually the temporal artery. Those with mild GCA frequently complain of fatigue and generalized muscle aches and pain, which can be mistaken for polymyalgia rheumatica (PMR). Among patients with GCA, about 50% to 70% also have associated PMR, which is characterized by aching in the proximal portions of the extremities and trunk. This typically involves morning stiffness of the neck, shoulder girdle, and hip girdle that gets worse with exertion and can be severe and debilitating.

Diagnostic Testing

Diagnosis of GCA should include a confirmatory arterial biopsy as this is the standard for diagnosis. Because the disease frequently skips portions of the vessel, biopsy specimens of multiple vessel sites should be obtained. Color duplex ultrasonography of the temporal arteries has been used as an alternative or complement to superficial temporal artery biopsy. This technique has a high specificity when a classic halo sign is observed about the vessel, but results are user dependent.

CRP and erythrocyte sedimentation rate (ESR), although nonspecific tests of inflammation, are usually markedly elevated in GCA. One of these tests is usually done prior to arterial biopsy to confirm the presence of an inflammatory process. Head CT and MRI are not first-line diagnostic approaches as the brain is typically unaffected by GCA.

Treatment

Treatment of GCA helps minimize the risk of blindness, which is one of the most serious complications of the disease, and also serves to minimize pain. As soon as the diagnosis is made, indeed, even as the GCA diagnostic process is ongoing, high-dose systemic corticosteroid therapy should be initiated. This therapy typically involves prednisone, 40 to 60 mg per day (or up to 80 to 100 mg/day when neurological or visual symptoms are present) until the disease appears to be under control, followed by a careful dose reduction until the lowest dose that can maintain clinical response can be determined. This dose is continued for 6 months to 2 years. When symptoms have been stable, and the corticosteroid therapy is to be discontinued, a slow taper with close monitoring is warranted because of the risk of adrenal suppression and/or disease resurgence. GI cytoprotection with misoprostol or a proton pump inhibitor and bone protection with a bisphosphonate plus calcium/vitamin D supplement should also be provided to minimize these corticosteroid-related adverse effects. Low-dose aspirin (81 mg per day) can also be considered to reduce the risk of stroke.

Corticosteroid-sparing agents, such as methotrexate, azathioprine, cyclophosphamide, and cyclosporine, can be helpful in reducing adverse effects associated with long-term systemic corticosteroid therapy. However, data are lacking on the effectiveness of these agents in treating GCA. Tocilizumab (Actemra®), a monoclonal antibody targeting interleukin-6 (IL-6), has been approved for the treatment of GCA. When given in combination with a tapering course of systemic corticosteroids, patients achieved more rapid remission and a greater rate of sustained remission compared to a tapered corticosteroid regimen only after 26 weeks. Tocilizumab is administered as a subcutaneous injection once weekly, though dosing every other week can also be considered. Expert consultation with neurology, ophthalmology, and/or rheumatology should be considered in GCA diagnosis and treatment.

Discussion Sources

Barraclough K, Mallen CD, Helliwell T, et al. Diagnosis and management of giant cell arteritis. *Br J Gen Pract.* 2012;62:329–330.

Charlton R. Optimal management of giant cell arteritis and polymyalgia rheumatic. *Ther Clin Risk Manag.* 2012;8:173–179.

Seetharaman M. Giant cell arteritis (temporal arteritis). Medscape. http://emedicine.medscape.com/article/332483-overview

QUESTIONS

133. Risk factors for GCA include all of the following except:

A. older age.

B. female gender.

C. osteoarthritis.

D. European ancestry.

134. In examining a 65-year-old woman who is undergoing evaluation for GCA, the NP considers the condition's clinical presentation is influenced by the disease's pathophysiology. Which of the following statements is false regarding GCA?

A. It results in inflammation of temporal and other arteries.

B. Normal arterial sections can be found in between affected sections.

C. It primarily impacts smaller-sized vessels.

D. GCA can result in a finding of a tender and/or nodular, pulseless vessel.

135. Mrs. Lewis is a 74-year-old woman with well-controlled hypertension. She is taking HCTZ and presents with a 3-day history of unilateral throbbing headache with difficulty chewing because of jaw pain. On physical examination, you find a tender, pulseless, noncompressible temporal artery. Blood pressure (BP) is 160/88 mm Hg, apical pulse is 98 bpm, and respiratory rate is 22/min; the patient is visibly uncomfortable. The optimal technique to confirm a diagnosis of GCA is:

A. to check serum creatine kinase (CK).

B. biopsies of likely affected arteries.

C. CT scan of the head without contrast.

D. MRI of the head.

136. Therapeutic intervention for Mrs. Lewis should include:

A. systemic corticosteroid therapy.

B. addition of an ACE inhibitor to her antihypertensive regimen.

  C. warfarin therapy.

  D. initiation of topiramate (Topamax®) therapy.

137. Headache associated with GCA is least likely to occur in the:

  A. frontal area.

  B. temporal area.

  C. vertex.

  D. occipital area.

138. For a patient receiving standard therapy for GCA, the use of all of the following concomitant therapies should be considered except:

  A. aspirin.

  B. nitrate.

  C. bisphosphonate and calcium/vitamin D.

  D. a proton pump inhibitor.

139. Concomitant disease often seen with GCA includes:

  A. polymyalgia rheumatica.

  B. acute pancreatitis.

  C. psoriatic arthritis.

  D. reactive arthritis.

140. One of the most serious complications of GCA is:

  A. hemiparesis.

  B. arthritis.

  C. blindness.

  D. uveitis.

For answers and rationales, see end of chapter.

QUESTION ANSWERS AND RATIONALES

Cranial Nerves

1. Correct: B. II.
CN II is the optic nerve that conveys visual information from the retina (B).
Incorrect:
CN I is the olfactory nerve that is responsible for the sense of smell (A). CN III is the oculomotor nerve involved in movement of the eye but not in transmitting visual information (C). CN IV is the trochlear nerve that is also involved in eye movement but not vision (D).

2. Correct: B. III.
The oculomotor nerve works with CNs III, IV, and VI and is largely responsible for movement of the eye and eyelid. CN III is involved in precise movement of the eyes for visual tracking or fixation on an object (B).
Incorrect:
CN II is involved in transmitting visual information from the eye but not eye movement (A). CN V is responsible for temperature, pain, and tactile sensations over areas of

the face (C). CN VII is responsible for facial movement involved in expressions (D).

3. Correct: C. V.
For normal corneal reflexes, the afferent limb of the first division of CN V and the effect limb of CN VII need to be intact (C).
Incorrect:
CN III is involved in precise movement of the eyes for visual tracking or fixation on an object (A). CN IV and CN VI are both involved in eye movement but not vision (B, D).

4 to 6. Matching Questions

4. Correct: B. sense of smell

5. Correct: C. facial symmetry, drooping mouth (Bell's palsy)

6. Correct: A. tongue and throat, swallowing
CN I is the olfactory nerve; it impacts the sense of smell or olfaction (4). CN VII is the facial nerve

involved in facial expression. Paralysis of CN VII is associated with Bell's palsy that is characterized by drooping mouth and facial asymmetry (5). CN IX is the glossopharyngeal nerve that is involved in multiple functions including movement of the tongue and throat as well as swallowing (6).

Bell's Palsy

7. Correct: C. VII.
This is a typical presentation for Bell's palsy, which is associated with dysfunction of CN VII (C). Patients with Bell's palsy will frequently have an unremarkable medical history with sudden development of symptoms.
Incorrect:
CN VII is involved in facial movement and expression. CN III and CN IV are involved in movement of the eye but not facial muscles (A, B). CN VIII is involved in hearing and balance (D).

8. Correct: B. Lyme disease testing
The diagnosis of Bell's palsy is largely a clinical one derived from patient history and physical examination. Since facial nerve paralysis is possible, though rarely, with Lyme disease, testing for this disease can be considered, especially for patients in the Northeast United States (B).
Incorrect:
No specific diagnostic tests are available to identify Bell's palsy, and blood tests would not be helpful in the diagnostic process (A, D). Imaging of the head is not typically required, though it should be considered when there is uncertainty with the diagnosis and to rule out other conditions, such as malignancy (C).

9. Correct: B. should be initiated as soon as possible after the onset of facial paralysis.
The use of systemic corticosteroids is recommended for the treatment of Bell's palsy. Treatment should begin as soon as possible (preferably within 1 week of the onset of symptoms) to increase the chance of recovery of facial function (B).
Incorrect:
Systemic corticosteroids have been shown to improve recovery of Bell's palsy when started soon after symptom onset (A). Treatment can decrease the duration of symptoms (D). Systemic corticosteroids will not specifically address ocular symptoms (eyelid closure, decreased lacrimation) (C) and so localized measures should be used during the recovery process (i.e., eye lubrication drops and eye protection).

10. Correct: C. idiopathic facial paralysis.
Bell's palsy is also called idiopathic facial paralysis (IFP) and is the most common cause of unilateral facial paralysis (C).
Incorrect:
Facial nerve palsy is a general term that can be used to describe a spectrum of conditions resulting in facial paralysis (B). Lyme disease can be associated with unilateral facial nerve palsy, but this is a separate condition from Bell's palsy (A). Facial asymmetry syndrome is not a defined syndrome (D).

11. Correct: A. an antiviral can be considered though the benefit has not been established in clinical studies.
According to the AAN, antivirals can be considered for new-onset Bell's palsy, though the benefit of such treatment has not been established in clinical studies (A).
Incorrect:
Antivirals that can be considered for the treatment of Bell's palsy, such as valacyclovir, are generally well tolerated with low toxicity risk and might provide some benefit when administered soon after symptom onset (B). If there is a decision to start an antiviral, treatment should be initiated as soon as possible and not delayed (C). Antivirals can be used concomitantly with systemic corticosteroids and are not contraindicated in those situations (D).

12. Correct: C. making a prompt referral to neurology.
This patient presents with a prolonged history of very concerning symptoms that are likely not related to Bell's palsy or Lyme disease. Thus, without a clear etiology, a prompt referral to neurology will be the most appropriate course of action (C).
Incorrect:
Though systemic corticosteroids are indicated for treatment of Bell's palsy, this patient presentation suggests a condition beyond Bell's palsy (A). Similarly, the symptoms are not consistent with a viral infection (e.g., herpes zoster); thus, antiviral therapy would not be appropriate (B). The C-reactive protein test is a generalized test to measure inflammation and is not specific to any particular disease. It would not be helpful in the diagnostic process (D).

Primary and Secondary Headache

13. Correct: C. cluster headache.
Cluster headaches are characterized by severe unilateral pain, often over the eye, and accompanied by lacrimation and rhinorrhea (C). The pain frequently occurs about 1 hour into sleep and is sometimes called the "alarm clock" headache.
Incorrect:
The patient description is most consistent with a cluster headache. Migraine with and without aura are best described as a pulsating headache often associated with photophobia and phonophobia as well as nausea and vomiting (A, B). Headache associated with increased intracranial pressure is usually worse upon awakening from a night's sleep when brain swelling is most severe and becomes less intense as the day progresses (D).

14. Correct: C. migraine with aura.
The pulsating quality of the headache with vomiting and photophobia most likely indicate migraine headache. The presence of a warning sign of an impending headache suggests migraine with aura (C).

Incorrect:

The pulsating quality of the headache suggests a migraine headache, while the warning sign of an impending headache suggests the presence of aura (B). Tension-type headaches are nonpulsatile in nature, typically bilateral, and mild to moderate in intensity (A). Cluster headache would be consistent with a report of headaches occurring in groups during the day and often accompanied with lacrimation and rhinorrhea (D).

15. **Correct: A. similar headaches that occur periodically in clusters.**

A secondary headache caused by a serious underlying illness can often be detected by evaluating for headache "red flags" and using the SNOOP mnemonic. When a patient reports experiencing similar headaches in the past, this is a reassuring finding that a new underlying illness is not involved (A). Headaches that occur in clusters would suggest a primary headache condition of cluster headache.

Incorrect:

The SNOOP mnemonic can be used to help identify warning signs of a serious underlying illness causing the headache disorder. These red flags can include a change in headache frequency and severity (B) as well as onset of headache (D). Headaches that cause neurological changes such as confusion, dizziness, or lack of coordination should also be evaluated for an underlying cause (C).

16. **Correct: A. nortriptyline.**

Prophylactic agents can be used to reduce the frequency of migraines and allow migraine treatments to be more effective. The most common prophylactic agents include beta blockers, antiepileptic drugs, and tricyclic antidepressants, such as nortriptyline (A). Nortriptyline is better tolerated than amitriptyline.

Incorrect:

Ergot derivatives and NSAIDs (such as naproxen sodium) can be used as abortive treatments of migraines but not for prophylaxis (B, C). Clonidine, an alpha blocker, is not recommended for migraine prophylaxis (D).

17. **Correct: D. propranolol**

Metoprolol and propranolol have the greatest evidence supporting their use for migraine prophylaxis. In the absence of airway disease, a noncardioselective agent is recommended, such as propranolol (D). In patients with a history of asthma or COPD, a cardioselective agent such as metoprolol is preferred.

Incorrect:

Acebutolol has shown limited benefit in migraine prevention (A). Atenolol and carvedilol might provide some benefit in this patient, but these agents have not been studied as extensively in migraine prevention as propranolol (B, C).

18. **Correct: C. lamotrigine.**

Though antiepileptic drugs can be effective in migraine prevention, studies demonstrate that lamotrigine is ineffective in this purpose and should be avoided for migraine prevention (C).

Incorrect:

Though lamotrigine provides no benefit in migraine prophylaxis, other antiepileptic agents, such as divalproex, valproate, and topiramate, have demonstrated effectiveness for this purpose (A, B, D).

19. **Correct: D. ginkgo biloba.**

Though certain herbal supplements, vitamins, and minerals have demonstrated some effectiveness in preventing migraines, ginkgo biloba is not among them (D).

Incorrect:

Supplements that can be used to prevent migraines include butterbur (A), feverfew (C), riboflavin (B), and magnesium.

20. **Correct: C. acetaminophen**

For patients with a history of coronary artery disease, the use of agents with vasoconstrictor properties should be avoided. Analgesics, such as NSAIDs or acetaminophen, can be effective in relieving pain caused by migraines (C). Patients should be aware of the risk of rebound headache with frequent, long-term use of acetaminophen.

Incorrect:

For a patient with a history of ACS, vasoconstrictor agents should be avoided for the treatment of acute headache. These would include the triptans (D) and ergot derivatives (B). Calcium channel blockers, such as verapamil, are not recommended for the treatment or prevention of migraines (A).

21. **Correct: C. oral naproxen sodium.**

For a patient experiencing nausea and vomiting due to migraine, oral medications should be avoided as these will not likely be tolerated. Among the answer choices, the oral naproxen should be avoided for this patient (C).

Incorrect:

Oral medications should be avoided in migraine patients who are experiencing severe GI upset. Several other options are available for abortive treatment of acute migraine, including injection (A), nasal spray (B, D), and transdermal patches. Melt tablets can also be considered, though these medications are absorbed through the GI tract.

22. **Correct: D. The pain is typically described as pulsating.**

For migraines, the classical description of the pain is a pulsating quality.

Incorrect:

Migraine without aura is the more common form of migraine, affecting about 80% of those with migraine (A). Most individuals who suffer from migraines are not receiving ongoing care for their condition (B). Migraines are more common in women, with a female-to-male ratio of 2:1 for those with migraine without aura (C).

23. **Correct: B. The pain is typically described as "pressing" in quality.**

For those with tension-type headache, the pain is often described as a pressing, nonpulsatile pain (B).

Incorrect:

Photophobia is a common trait with all headache types (A). For tension-type headache, the pain is usually bilateral (C), and physical activity can sometimes improve pain (D). In migraines, physical activity will typically worsen pain.

24 to 28. Yes or No

24. Correct: No

25. Correct: Yes

26. Correct: Yes

27. Correct: Yes

28. Correct: No

Cluster headaches occur most commonly among middle-aged men (27), particularly those who report heavy alcohol use (25) or tobacco users (26). Onset of a new headache after age 65 years would indicate a red flag for a secondary headache and require further evaluation (24). An increase in stress would more likely result in the development of tension-type headaches rather than cluster headache (28).

29. Correct: B. supplemental oxygen

Abortive treatment of cluster headache can include the use of triptans, ergot derivatives, and analgesics. However, a therapy specific for cluster headaches is the use of high-flow oxygen therapy (B).

Incorrect:

Though analgesics such as NSAIDs and opioids can be used to treat pain associated with primary headaches, these approaches are not specific for cluster headaches (A, C). The use of opioids should also be reserved for when other analgesic approaches are unsuccessful. Neuroleptics are not indicated for the treatment of cluster headache (D).

30. Correct: B. liquid ibuprofen (Motrin®, Advil®)

Selection of an appropriate NSAID should take into account onset of action in addition to analgesic effect. Among the answer choices, liquid ibuprofen offers the most rapid onset of action and is gentle on the upper GI tract (B).

Incorrect:

Plain naproxen and enteric-coated naproxen have a relatively slow onset of action (A, D), while naproxen sodium provides a more rapid onset of pain relief. Diclofenac also has a delayed onset of action, reaching peak plasma concentration over 2 hours after oral dosing (C).

31. Correct: A. high-dose SSRI.

Triptans work as a selective serotonin receptor agonist, thus allowing for an increased uptake of serotonin. Triptans should be used with caution with high-dose SSRI therapy due to a risk of serotonin syndrome (A).

Incorrect:

Triptans should be avoided or used with caution among patients taking high-dose SSRI therapy or MAOIs. There

is no warning on triptan use concomitantly with calcium channel blockers (B), fluoroquinolones (C), or high-dose statin therapy (D).

32. Correct: C. high rate of rebound headache if used frequently.

With occasional use, Fioricet® can provide an effective and well-tolerated treatment for migraine and tension-type headaches. However, due to the acetaminophen component, rebound headache is possible with frequent, long-term use of this product (C). Also, barbiturate dependency can develop with excessive use due to the butalbital component.

Incorrect:

Fioricet® can provide effective relief of headaches with occasional use (D). It is not associated with an energizing effect (A) and is generally well tolerated (B).

33. Correct: B. EPM risk.

Due to their antiemetic effects, the neuroleptics are sometimes used as adjunctive therapy in migraine therapy. However, use should be limited to 3 days per week because of the risk of EPMs (B). Other antiemetics that can be considered are ondansetron and metoclopramide, though the latter is also associated with EPM risk.

Incorrect:

The neuroleptics are not associated with habituation potential (A) or an activating effect (D). Rebound headache is a concerning risk with excessive use of acetaminophen or aspirin but not the neuroleptics (C).

34. Correct: A. This drug class is effective in the treatment of tension-type headaches.

Ergotamines can be an effective option for the treatment of migraines and cluster headaches. However, they are not recommended in the treatment of tension-type headaches (A).

Incorrect:

Ergotamines act as 5-HT_{1A} and 5-HT_{1D} receptor agonists and do not alter cerebral blood flow (B). These agents do have a potential for vasoconstrictor effect and so their use is contraindicated in the presence of coronary artery disease and pregnancy (C, D).

35. Correct: C. an approximately 50% reduction in the number of headaches.

The goals of headache prophylaxis therapy are to achieve at least a 50% reduction in headache frequency and to have headaches that are more easily managed with standard therapies (C). With traditional agents, 1 to 2 months of treatment is needed before an effect is seen. Once migraines are better controlled, the patient can consider tapering prophylaxis treatment, especially if lifestyle modifications are also put in place to minimize headache risk.

Incorrect:

A realistic goal of headache prophylaxis therapy is to reduce headache frequency by 50%; complete resolution of headaches is not a likely or realistic result (A). In addition to fewer headaches, the severity can be diminished, and headaches are more easily managed with standard therapies (B). Once migraines are better controlled, patients can consider tapering therapy rather than lifelong treatment (D).

36. Correct: D. triptan prophylaxis.

Menses and ovulation can be potential triggers for migraine headaches. Estrogen supplementation, particularly during the premenstrual week, can be considered for migraine prevention. Triptans, however, are used as abortive therapy and not prophylaxis (D).

Incorrect:

Several approaches can be used for estrogen supplementation as migraine prevention, including the use of combined oral contraceptives (A, B) or a low-dose estrogen transdermal patch (C) during the premenstrual week.

37. Correct: A. nortriptyline.

In observational studies for the prevention of tension-type headaches, tricyclic antidepressants, such as nortriptyline, have been most studied and can be considered as a first-line therapy for this purpose.

Incorrect:

Antiepileptics, such as valproate and carbamazepine, have been well studied for the prevention of migraine headaches and can be used for this purpose (C, D). However, they are not well studied for tension-type headache prevention. Calcium channel blockers, such as verapamil, are not recommended for headache prevention (B).

38. Correct: C. naproxen sodium

Triptans can be an effective option for relief of migraine-associated symptoms, such as phonophobia and photophobia. However, this class has a more limited effect on migraine pain relief and will often require adjunctive therapy with an analgesic. NSAIDs, such as naproxen sodium, can be used for this purpose (C).

Incorrect:

A first-line option for relief of migraine pain includes the NSAIDs, such as naproxen sodium. Antiepileptics, such as gabapentin and topiramate, can be considered for prophylaxis but not for treatment of acute migraine (A, B). Supplementation with magnesium can also be considered for prophylaxis but not abortive therapy (D).

39. Correct: B. increased ICP.

The presentation is most consistent with ICP, which is characterized by worst pain upon awakening when brain swelling is most severe (B). The pain gradually subsides as the day progresses.

Incorrect:

A new-onset headache in an elderly individual is a possible warning sign of a secondary headache that requires further evaluation. A headache that is worst upon awakening and gradually subsides during the day is most consistent with ICP. Tension-type headaches typically worsen as the day goes on (D). Though vascular compromise and brain tumor are less likely causes of the headache, evaluations are needed to rule these out (A, C).

40. Correct: C. acute intractable or severe migraines and cluster headaches.

Systemic corticosteroids can be considered for patients with intractable or severe migraine pain or with cluster headache (C). Because of adverse effects, these agents should not be used more than once per month.

Incorrect:

Systemic corticosteroids can be considered for severe migraines or cluster headaches but are not an appropriate option for tension-type headache (A). These agents should not be used more frequently than once per month (B). Systemic corticosteroids should be used with caution during pregnancy due to safety profile and potential effects on the newborn (e.g., possible increased risk of asthma) (D). Other safer options should be considered prior to the use of corticosteroid therapy.

41. Correct: A. onset of headache with exertion, coughing, or sneezing.

When evaluating a patient with headache, the healthcare provider should assess for the presence of any "red flags" that can indicate a more serious underlying illness. The SNOOP mnemonic can be used in the evaluation, and a key finding includes headache onset that is sudden or abrupt or headache that occurs with exertion, coughing, or sneezing (A).

Incorrect:

Individuals with a primary headache will typically have normal neurological examination findings and a supple (able to bend) neck (C, D). A history of previous, identical headaches is a reassuring finding that there is not a more serious underlying illness present (B).

42. Correct: C. cluster cephalalgia

Cluster cephalalgia, also known as cluster headache, is a primary headache disorder and is not associated with an underlying disease process.

Incorrect:

Increased ICP is the most common cause of secondary headache symptoms. Increased ICP is characterized by headache pain that is worst upon awakening (when brain swelling is most severe) and slowly resolves as the day progresses. Common causes of increased ICP include the presence of a brain tumor (A), intracranial bleeding (e.g., stroke or trauma) (B), inflammation, and viremia (D). The presence of headache "red flags" suggests further evaluation of the patient is needed, including imaging studies.

43 to 45. Matching Questions

43. Correct: C. 5:4

44. Correct: B. 2:1

45. Correct: A. 1:3 to 1:8

Females are more likely to have migraine without aura and tension-type headaches, while males are more likely to experience cluster headaches. For migraines without aura, females are approximately twice as likely as men to experience these headaches (44), while for tension-type headaches, the female-to-male ratio is closer to 5:4 (43).

The gender ratio for cluster headaches varies considerably depending on the epidemiological study, but the general female-to-male ratio ranges from 1:3 to 1:8 (45).

46 to 48. Matching Questions

46. Correct: **B. oral sumatriptan**

47. Correct: **A. oral naratriptan**

48. Correct: **C. intranasal zolmitriptan**

When considering a triptan medication for abortive migraine treatment, it is important to match the type of triptan with the patient and migraine characteristics. For patients with rapid-onset migraines of shorter duration, a rapid-onset triptan such as sumatriptan is most appropriate as it will be effective when the migraine is most debilitating (46). Similarly, for patients with migraines that are slower onset and longer duration, a triptan with a slow onset, such as naratriptan, will be more effective (47). Oral formulations are appropriate for patients without GI upset and vomiting. Otherwise, injection or intranasal formulations can be considered (48).

49 to 54. Matching Questions

49. Correct: **head CT scan**

Head imaging is indicated for this patient. Due to the rapid onset of neurological signs, a head CT scan would be preferred as it is a faster process than MRI and is better at detecting subarachnoid hemorrhage.

50. Correct: **head MRI**

For progressively severe headache over a period of months, head imaging is indicated. Due to a prior history of cancer, MRI would be preferred as it does not expose the patient to ionizing radiation.

51. Correct: **head CT scan**

A head CT scan would be indicated to detect acute hemorrhage due to head trauma.

52. Correct: **head MRI**

Head imaging is indicated for this patient due to the progressive nature of the headaches and prior history of cancer. MRI is preferred as it does not expose the patient to ionizing radiation and is better at detecting small and subtle lesions.

53. Correct: **neither**

Cluster headache is a primary headache and does not require head imaging studies.

54. Correct: **neither**

The presentation is consistent with premenstrual migraine, a primary headache, and does not require head imaging. The patient should consider initiating migraine prophylaxis.

55. Correct: **A. avoiding eating within 1 to 2 hours of morning awakening.**

In preventing and managing headaches, lifestyle modifications can be an important part of decreasing the burden of migraines. Avoiding triggers is an essential part of these changes. Though fasting or missing meals can be a trigger of migraines, eating within 1 to 2 hours after awakening is not a likely trigger for migraines (A).
Incorrect:
Common triggers of migraines include menses/ovulation, odors/fragrances/tobacco smoke (B), acute or chronic illness, intense or strenuous physical activity (C), bright or flickering lights, excessive or repetitive noises, medications, and stressful situation or stress letdown (D).

56. Correct: **D. baked whitefish.**

Certain foods can act as triggers for migraines. Though pickled or dried fish (e.g., herring) can be a trigger for migraines, a baked whitefish is not a typical migraine trigger (D).
Incorrect:
Common triggers for migraine can include pickled or fermented foods (B), ripened cheeses, pizza (A), freshly baked yeast products (C), foods containing MSG, dried fruits (e.g., raisins), and caffeinated beverages, among others.

57. Correct: **D. nearly eliminates migraines for over 50% of individuals**

CGRP inhibitors represent the latest class used in the prevention of migraines. Though these agents are not expected to eliminate migraines, the majority of recipients experience a reduction in migraine frequency by at least 50% (D).
Incorrect:
CGRP inhibitors are dosed via subcutaneous injection (C) and are administered once monthly or every 3 months (A). They are indicated for the prevention of migraines (B) and not for abortive treatment of acute migraine.

58. Correct: **B. A 45-year-old woman who experiences about 15 migraine days per month despite propranolol therapy**

The CGRP inhibitors are indicated for individuals with episodic (4 to 14 migraine days per month) and chronic migraine (15 or more migraine days per month) for the prevention of migraine. The ideal candidates for CGRP inhibitors are those who experience multiple migraine days per month, particularly if standard headache prophylactic medications have been ineffective, as these agents are effective in decreasing migraine episodes by more than 50%. Among those listed, the patient with 15 migraine days per month would be the best candidate for CGRP inhibitor therapy for migraine prevention (B).
Incorrect:
CGRP inhibitors are used for migraine prevention and not treatment of acute migraine (C). This class is best used for those who experience multiple migraine days per month rather than the rare or occasional migraine (A). These agents are not approved for the prevention of cluster headaches (D).

59. Correct: **D. motion sickness**

There is a strong genetic component for the development of migraine as 70% to 90% of those who experience migraines report a family history of migraines. Individuals who experience migraines frequently report being susceptible to motion sickness, though the exact mechanism of this association in not known (D).

Incorrect:

There is a strong association between motion sickness and migraines. There is no such known relationship between migraines and dyslipidemia (A), pregnancy history (B), and allergy to shellfish (C).

Bacterial Meningitis

60. **Correct: B. bacterial meningitis.**

The classic presentation of bacterial meningitis includes fever, headache, and nuchal rigidity. The presence of Kernig and Brudzinski signs helps to support this diagnosis (B).

Incorrect:

Viral encephalitis typically presents with fewer meningeal signs, while viral meningitis presents with less severe and slower onset of symptoms compared to bacterial meningitis (A). Acute subarachnoid hemorrhage is frequently associated with severe, sudden-onset headache, such as the "thunderclap" headache that can be accompanied by nausea, vomiting, and photophobia (C). Epidural hematoma would be considered with a patient report of head trauma that could cause bleeding within the skull (D). This condition would normally be accompanied by severe headache, nausea, and possible seizures.

61. **Correct: A. colonization of the skin**

The most likely causes of bacterial meningitis include an extension of acute infection and colonization of the nose and throat. Among the answer choices, skin colonization is the least likely source of bacterial meningitis (A).

Incorrect:

The extension of acute infections, particularly acute otitis media (C) and rhinosinusitis (D), is a common cause of bacterial meningitis. Colonization of the nose and throat with virulent bacteria can also contribute to the development of this disease (B). Meningitis occurs when the bacteria enter the bloodstream and cross into the meninges.

62. **Correct: A. being over 25 years of age.**

A major risk factor for bacterial meningitis is being under age 20 years (A). Hence, vaccination against meningitis is focused on older children and adolescents.

Incorrect:

Other key risk factors for bacterial meningitis include living in a community setting (e.g., college campuses) (B), cigarette smoking (C), having a current viral upper respiratory tract infection, and immunosuppression (D).

63. **Correct: B. 3 to 4 days.**

Knowing the incubation period of *N meningitidis* is important to counsel and treat patients as well as to work with public health officials in identifying the possible source of infection as well as other individuals who

might have been exposed to the pathogen and at risk for infection. The typical incubation period for this organism is 3 to 4 days (B).

64. **Correct: D. individuals with household-type or more intimate contact are considered to be at risk.**

Transmission of *N meningitidis* is typically person to person through either direct contact or respiratory droplets from an infected individual. Those at risk of infection include household-like contacts (e.g., those who eat and drink in the same dwelling) or more intimate contacts (D). Chemoprophylaxis is recommended for these high-risk individuals.

Incorrect:

Meningitis caused by *N meningitidis is* a contagious disease that is spread through direct contact or respiratory droplets (A). Those at high risk of infection are limited to household-type contacts and those with more intimate contact with the infected individual (C) and would not include the entire college campus (B).

65. **Correct: C. glucose at about 30% of serum levels.**

For a patient with bacterial meningitis, CSF findings would typically include elevated WBCs with a predominance of neutrophils, a glucose level below the normal amount of approximately 40% plasma level (C), and elevated protein level.

Incorrect:

A higher protein level in CSF is a typical finding during bacterial meningitis, as well as a predominance of neutrophils (A). Lymphocytes are predominant during viral meningitis along with a normal level of glucose (B). An elevated opening pressure is a nearly universal finding in meningitis (D).

66. **Correct: B. a predominance of lymphocytes.**

For a patient with viral or aseptic meningitis, CSF findings would typically include elevated WBCs with a predominance of lymphocytes (B).

Incorrect:

In viral or aseptic meningitis, CSF findings typically include a normal glucose level (approximately 40% of serum levels) (C), normal to slightly elevated protein levels (A), and elevated opening pressure (a near universal finding for meningitis) (D).

67. **Correct: C. Elicited with the patient lying supine and the hip flexed 90°, it is present when extension of the knee from this position elicits resistance or pain in the lower back or posterior thigh.**

The Kernig sign, Brudzinski sign, and nuchal rigidity are important indicators for meningitis, though they are not absolutely predictive of this condition. The Kernig sign is elicited by placing the patient in a supine position and flexing the hip at 90°. A positive Kernig sign is indicated if there is resistance or pain in the lower back or posterior thigh (C). This is caused by severe stiffness of the hamstrings that makes it difficult to straighten the leg. The positive sign can indicate the presence of spinocerebellar lesions and would require further evaluation for a definitive diagnosis.

Incorrect:

The Brudzinski sign is positive when passive neck flexion in a supine patient results in flexion of the knees and hips and is also an indication of spinocerebellar lesions possibly caused by meningitis (B). The other two answer choices are not associated with any clinical examination for meningitis (A, D).

68. **Correct: C. optic disk bulging.**

Papilledema, or optic disc bulging, is a possible finding in meningitis that would indicate elevated intracranial pressure (C).

Incorrect:

Arteriovenous nicking observed during a retinal examination is most frequently found in individuals with chronic hypertension (A). Pupillary constriction, or narrowing of the pupil, can be caused by various factors, including excessive lights or certain medications, and is not an indicator for meningitis (D). Macular hyperpigmentation is not related to meningitis and is possibly genetic in origin (B).

69. **Correct: B. Hib**

The Hib vaccine series is typically completed prior to age 5 years. As infection with *H influenzae* type B is rare among older children and adults (who likely have gained immunity against this pathogen), the vaccine is not routinely recommended for anyone over 5 years of age (B). Individuals with certain risk factors for infection can be considered for immunization.

Incorrect:

The two meningococcal vaccines, MCV4 and MenB, are recommended during adolescence (C, D). The pneumococcal vaccine, PCV13, is recommended universally in young children as well as the elderly (65 years and older) and those between 2 and 64 years with certain risk factors for infection (A).

70. **Correct: A. a purpura or petechial rash**

An indication of meningitis caused by *N meningitidis* is the presence of a purpura or petechial rash, which develops in about 50% of these patients (A). The rash is not vascular in origin and will not blanch with pressure.

Incorrect:

Nuchal rigidity and fever are common findings in bacterial meningitis and would not be used to differentiate infection caused by *N meningitidis* versus other pathogens (B, D). Encephalitis is more likely to occur with viral infection (C).

71. **Correct: D. a 14-year-old who received a first dose of the same vaccine at 11 years of age.**

The preferred timing for the MCV4 vaccine is a first dose between 11 and 12 years of age and a booster dose at least 5 years later. The 14-year-old should wait until at least age 16 years to receive the booster dose (D).

Incorrect:

The 19-year-old is eligible to receive a booster dose as it has been at least 5 years since the primary dose was given (A). For those who did not receive the MCV4 vaccine during adolescence, the vaccine can be given for those at high risk of infection, including those living in a community setting (B) or traveling to areas with high endemic levels of disease (C).

72. **Correct: C. multiple doses of amoxicillin.**

Prevention of meningitis following possible exposure can include administration of the meningococcal vaccine (preferably matched with the infecting strain) or antimicrobial treatment. However, amoxicillin is not a recommended antimicrobial agent for this purpose (C).

Incorrect:

Chemoprophylaxis can include a dose of vaccine (D) or antimicrobial therapy with ceftriaxone (A), rifampin (B), or ciprofloxacin.

73 to 75. Yes or No

73. **Correct: No**

74. **Correct: No**

75. **Correct: No**

Postexposure prophylaxis in adults can be considered for household or more intimate contacts of an individual with bacterial meningitis caused by *N meningitidis*. Postexposure prophylaxis is not used in cases of viral meningitis or streptococcal meningitis (73). Pneumonia and acute bacterial rhinosinusitis are not likely to be caused by *N meningitidis* (more likely caused by *S pneumoniae*); therefore, postexposure prophylaxis would not be needed (74, 75).

Multiple Sclerosis

76. **Correct: A. a destructive process of the nerve fiber protecting myelin.**

MS is a recurrent, chronic disorder that involves demyelination of nerve fibers of the CNS (A). Symptoms of MS can vary depending on the location of the affected nerve fibers.

Incorrect:

Intracranial viral infection is the most common cause of encephalopathy, or inflammation of the brain, which is characterized by flu-like illness along with fever, headache, and potentially neurological signs and symptoms (B, C). MS involves degradation of nerve fibers and is not an autoimmune disorder that destroys muscle cells as seen in myositis (D).

77. **Correct: D. symptoms improving in a warmer environment.**

Symptoms of MS can vary considerably depending on the location of the affected nerve fibers. A common symptom is heat sensitivity, as small increases in body temperature can trigger or exacerbate symptoms (D).

Incorrect:

Common symptoms of MS include weakness or numbness of a limb (A), monocular vision loss, diplopia (B), vertigo, facial weakness or numbness (C), sphincter disturbances, ataxia, and nystagmus.

78. **Correct: A. being older than 50 years of age.**
Although MS can affect individuals at any age, the disease most commonly affects people between 20 and 40 years old (A).
Incorrect:
Risk factors for MS include female gender (B), family history of MS, northern European ancestry (C), certain viral infections, and presence of another autoimmune disease (D). There is also evidence linking MS with vitamin D deficiency and those living in higher latitudes.

79 to 81. Matching Questions

79. **Correct: B. presence of demyelinating plaques**

80. **Correct: A. presence of oligoclonal bands**

81. **Correct: C. delays in timing of CNS response**
Several diagnostic approaches are used to make a definitive diagnosis of MS. Analysis of CSF will typically find pleocytosis, elevated protein level, elevated gamma-globulin fraction, high immunoglobulin G index, and the presence of oligoclonal bands (80). MRI can help reveal the presence of demyelinating plaques on nerve fibers, which is the typical finding in MS (79). Evoked potential test is used to measure CNS response to stimuli, and a delay in response would indicate the presence of lesions or nerve damage (81).

82. **Correct: A. interferon beta-1b.**
Immunomodulatory therapy is often used to reduce the frequency of MS exacerbations and slow down disease progression. These disease-modifying therapies can include interferon beta-1b (A), interferon beta-1a, as well as several monoclonal antibodies and other agents aimed at reducing the autoimmune response. However, these agents are commonly associated with serious and life-threatening adverse events and should be selected based on expert consultation.
Incorrect:
Systemic corticosteroids, such as methylprednisolone, can be used to treat an acute exacerbation of MS. These agents tend to shorten the exacerbation but have little impact on overall disease progression (B). Antiviral agents (e.g., ribavirin) and phenytoin are not indicated for the management of MS (C, D).

Parkinson's Disease

83. **Correct: B. loss of the pigmented dopaminergic neurons.**
PD is largely caused by the loss of the pigmented dopaminergic neurons in the midbrain (B). Additional pathological changes include the presence of Lewy bodies and Lewy neurites that can contribute to dementia and psychosis.

Incorrect:
PD is not associated with degradation of myelin surrounding nerve fibers as in seen in patients with MS (A). The loss of neurons in PD is found in the midbrain rather than the brainstem (C). PD is not associated with an overproduction of acetylcholinesterase (D).

84. **Correct: C. tremor at rest and bradykinesia**
The diagnosis of PD is made by clinical evaluation and consists of a combination of four cardinal features: tremor at rest, rigidity, bradykinesia, and postural instability (C). Postural instability is typically found later in the disease process, while tremor at rest is the most common early sign of PD.
Incorrect:
PD is associated with a flexed posture rather than a rigid posture (A). Diminished facial expression and mask-like facies are also found in PD, though diminished cognitive function, even in early disease, is a typical trait (B). The parkinsonian gait involves having the arms remain rigid at the sides with little movement with ambulation (D).

85. **Correct: A. clinical evaluation of its cardinal clinical features.**
The diagnosis of PD is made by clinical evaluation and consists of a combination of four cardinal features: tremor at rest, rigidity, bradykinesia, and postural instability (A). Additional diagnostic testing can be done primarily to rule in or out other possible diagnoses.
Incorrect:
Additional diagnostic testing is not required to make a diagnosis of PD. Head MRI or CT scan can be used to detect for lesions (e.g., MS) or malignancies (B). Pleocytosis in the CSF as well as a delayed response in a visual evoked potential test are consistent with a diagnosis of MS (C, D).

86. **Correct: B. as a first-line treatment in early disease.**
Levodopa has traditionally been the first treatment of choice in early disease management of PD (B). However, long-term use of this agent is associated with serious adverse events, such as dyskinesia. Other treatment options in early disease management include the use of dopamine agonists that have a better safety profile than levodopa.
Incorrect:
There is no prophylaxis treatment available to prevent PD (A). COMT inhibitors are typically used concomitantly with levodopa as these agents can extend the half-life of levodopa (C). Levodopa is not reserved for advanced disease but can be used as first-line therapy following the PD diagnosis (D).

87. **Correct: D. multiple sclerosis.**
MS is not usually associated with the key findings of PD, namely, tremor at rest, rigidity, bradykinesia, or postural instability (D). MS episodes can include limb numbness or weakness, monocular vision loss, diplopia, facial

weakness or numbness, ataxia, and nystagmus. MS episodes typically occur in a more rapid manner than the gradual progressive nature of PD.

Incorrect:

Cognitive decline associated with Alzheimer's dementia can mimic that of PD (A). A high prevalence of depression is also observed in both Alzheimer's dementia and PD. Normal pressure hydrocephalus, caused by elevated levels of CSF, presents with a gradual progressive disorder that can include abnormal gait, urinary incontinence, and dementia (B). Huntington's disease, a genetic disorder that affects neurons in the basal ganglia and cortex, can initially present with mild chorea (i.e., fidgetiness) but is replaced in later disease with parkinsonian symptoms of bradykinesia, rigidity, and postural instability (C).

88 to 90. Matching Questions

88. Correct: B. destruction of part of the subthalamic nucleus

89. Correct: A. ablation of part of the globus pallidus interna

90. Correct: C. high-frequency electrostimulation of the brain

Surgical procedures for PD can be considered when medical treatments are inadequate or associated with significant adverse effects or for those with uncontrolled choreiform movement or dyskinesia. Neuroablative treatment can include pallidotomy (destruction of part of the globus pallidus interna) (89) as well as subthalamotomy (destruction of part of the thalamus) (88). These procedures can be effective in reducing Parkinson's motor symptoms as well as correcting dyskinesia. Deep brain stimulation that uses high-frequency electrostimulation offers an alternative with promising results and without destruction of brain tissue (90).

91. Correct: B. An "off" period typically occurs at the maximum serum concentration (C_{max}) following levodopa dosing.

As Parkinson disease progresses, patients often develop variability in response to treatment with "off" periods occurring toward the end of the levodopa dosing period. This is typically well beyond the C_{max} of levodopa (B).

Incorrect:

As PD progresses, patients will experience motor fluctuations that vary from "on" periods where there is ease of movement (A) and "off" periods where movement is more difficult. Medication adjustment can help to minimize the "off" periods, including higher or more frequent dosing of levodopa or using a sustained-release formulation (C). For patients who experience dyskinesia during "off" periods, neuroablative surgery or deep brain stimulation therapy can be considered (D).

92 to 94. Matching Questions

92. Correct: B. depression

93. Correct: C. hallucinations

94. Correct: A. dementia

Depression is a common comorbidity among patients with PD, and routine evaluation for depression is important. Treatment can include SNRIs or tricyclic antidepressants (92). Hallucinations and delusions can emerge as a consequence of antiparkinson medications. Pimavanserin is indicated to treat hallucinations in patients with PD (93). Cholinesterase inhibitors can be considered to slow the progression of dementia in patients with PD (94).

95. Correct: C. Exercise is encouraged and likely has a neuroprotective effect.

Exercise and physical therapy should be encouraged to improve gait, balance, initiation of movement, and functional independence. There is also a growing body of evidence that suggests exercise has a neuroprotective effect that might slow the progression of disease (C). Additional studies suggest that vigorous exercise in mid-life might even reduce the risk of development of PD.

Incorrect:

Exercise and physical therapy should be encouraged in patients with PD, as they can offer many benefits in reducing the signs of PD and slow progression (A). The amount and type of exercise should be based on the patient's health status and exercise tolerance (B). Some research has indicated that exercise can have a neuroprotective effect during PD (D).

Seizure Disorders

96 to 99. Matching Questions

96. Correct: D. brief, jerking contractions of arms, legs, trunk, or all of these

97. Correct: A. blank staring lasting 3 to 50 seconds, accompanied by impaired level of consciousness

98. Correct: C. rigid extension of arms and legs, followed by sudden jerking movements with loss of consciousness

99. Correct: B. awake state with abnormal motor and psychic behavior lasting seconds

When examining a patient with new-onset seizure disorder, it is critical to recognize the different types of seizures as this will help guide further patient assessment and management. A myoclonic seizure can be in the awake state or with temporary loss of consciousness and include brief jerking of the limbs, trunk, or all of these (96). A petit mal seizure is characterized by a short period of blank staring followed by a period of impaired consciousness (97). Seizures that involve an awake state with abnormal motor and psychic behavior are most likely due to a simple partial or focal seizure (99). Tonic-clonic seizures are characterized by rigid extension of arms followed by sudden jerking motions and loss of consciousness (98).

100. Correct: C. gabapentin

Newer antiepileptic medications are generally preferred over older drugs because of less likelihood of drug-drug interaction as well as a broader therapeutic index. Newer medications include gabapentin (C), lamotrigine, and topiramate.

Incorrect:

Older antiepileptic drugs can cause significant drug-drug interactions through their impact on the CYP 450 pathway. These older medications include phenytoin (B), carbamazepine (A), and valproate (D). Phenytoin can lead to a diminished level of theophylline when given together, while carbamazepine can induce estrogen metabolism, leading to contraceptive failure. Phenytoin and carbamazepine also have a narrow therapeutic index, and monitoring of serum drug levels is often necessary to ensure a safe and effective level is achieved.

101. Correct: B. phenytoin

Certain AEDs, including phenytoin and carbamazepine, have narrow therapeutic indexes where certain serum concentrations of such drugs is therapeutic (B); however, a drug level just slightly more than this amount is potentially toxic, while a drug level slightly lower might not have any therapeutic effect. Because of the careful balance between concentrations that are effective versus toxic or ineffective, therapeutic drug level monitoring is required to ensure safe and effective dosing of these medications.

Incorrect:

Newer antiepileptic medications have broader therapeutic indexes that do not require monitoring of drug levels. Newer agents also have less potential for drug-drug interactions and are often the preferred choice over older medications. These include topiramate (A), gabapentin (C), and lamotrigine (D).

102. Correct: D. When phenytoin and theophylline are given together, the result is a higher concentration of both drugs than when given separately.

Phenytoin and carbamazepine are strong CYP 450 enzyme inducers and will increase clearance of drugs that are metabolized by CYP 450. Concomitant dosing of phenytoin with theophylline will result in a decrease in levels of both drugs by as much as 40% (D).

Incorrect:

Phenytoin is a strong CYP 450 enzyme inducer and can lead to increased clearance of drugs that are substrates of this hepatic enzymatic pathway, such as theophylline (A, C). Phenytoin is also highly protein bound and, when taken with other highly protein-bound drugs, can be displaced from its binding site and result in higher and potentially toxic concentrations (B).

103. Correct: B. epilepsy.

Seizures can be either provoked, where there is a transient recognizable cause for the seizure, or unprovoked, where there is no identifiable cause. Epilepsy is the most common cause of unprovoked seizures (B).

Incorrect:

When evaluating a patient who experienced a seizure-like episode, it is important to consider other conditions as part of the differential diagnosis. These can include cardioembolic stroke (A), hypoglycemia (D), or psychiatric conditions (e.g., panic attack) (C). Seizure-like episodes due to these conditions would not be considered unprovoked as they are caused by a transient recognizable event.

104. Correct: C. driving is restricted until a seizure-free period is achieved that is determined by state law.

For individuals who experience seizures, driving is restricted until a seizure-free period is achieved (C). This can vary from 3 months to 1 year or more based on state law and other factors.

Incorrect:

Following a seizure, driving is restricted until a seizure-free period is achieved (A, B). This can vary from 3 months to a year or more, based on state law (D). The state Department of Motor Vehicles must be notified by either the patient or the health-care provider. Thus, health-care providers must be aware of local laws regarding driving restrictions in patients with seizures.

105. Correct: A. patient history.

A careful and thorough patient health history that provides an accurate description of the seizure event is critical in understanding the type of seizure experienced, which will be important in guiding additional diagnostic testing and management approaches (A). Important aspects of the seizure episode can include warning signs of the seizure, what happened during the seizure, duration and frequency of seizure, and recovery following the seizure.

Incorrect:

Following a seizure episode, a careful patient history is critical in guiding evaluation and management of the patient. Blood tests such as CRP (B), a measure of inflammation, or CBC (D) are not helpful in the evaluation of seizure. However, serum prolactin levels taken soon after the seizure (within 20 minutes) can help to differentiate an epileptic seizure from a nonepileptic seizure event. A head MRI is also not recommended or helpful in the diagnosis of seizure but can be used to rule in or out other conditions (C). An EEG is often used to help confirm a diagnosis of epilepsy.

Transient Ischemic Attack and Stroke

106. Correct: D. pernicious anemia.

Risk factors for TIA can include atherosclerotic conditions, structural cardiac problems, and conditions that lead to a hypercoagulable state. Pernicious anemia is not a known risk factor for TIA (D).

Incorrect:

Carotid artery disease often associated with atherosclerosis can increase the risk of TIA and stroke (B). Atrial fibrillation and the use of estrogen-containing contraceptives can lead to a hypercoagulable state increasing the risk of TIA (A, C). Prevention of TIA involves making lifestyle modifications that can minimize these risk factors.

107. Correct: C. 24 hours.
A TIA episode typically lasts only a few minutes but can persist for up to 24 hours, and the effects are fully reversible once the episode ends (C). For episodes lasting longer than 24 hours, a stroke diagnosis should be considered.
Incorrect:
In most cases, the symptoms of a TIA will resolve within an hour or two; however symptoms can last up to 24 hours in rare cases (A, B). When symptoms persist beyond 24 hours, this is usually indicative of a stroke and not TIA (D).

108. Correct: A. long-term antiplatelet therapy is likely indicated.
Long-term management of TIA aims to reduce the risk of future TIA episodes and stroke. Antiplatelet therapy with aspirin, aspirin plus extended-release dipyridamole, or clopidogrel, is recommended for secondary prevention of stroke (A). If the TIA is associated with a cardioembolic condition (e.g., atrial fibrillation or valvular disorder), then the addition of an anticoagulant such as warfarin should be considered as well.
Incorrect:
Individuals who experience a TIA are usually at increased risk of stroke and, thus, preventive measures are needed as part of ongoing care (B). TIA and stroke are more common among men than women (C). The effects of TIA are fully reversible, so rehabilitation is not needed following an episode (D).

109 to 111. Matching Questions

109. Correct: 2

110. Correct: 1

111. Correct: 3
The majority of strokes are due to cerebral ischemia, accounting for about 80% of all strokes (110). Cerebral hemorrhage is the cause of about 15% of strokes (109), with the remaining 5% caused by subarachnoid hemorrhage (111).

112 to 114. Matching Questions

112. Correct: C. hypertension

113. Correct: A. atherosclerosis

114. Correct: B. ruptured cerebral aneurysm
Cerebral ischemia is the most common type of stroke and is frequently caused by atherosclerotic disease that forms an occlusion in a cerebral blood vessel (113). The most common cause of cerebral hemorrhage is hypertension, though other causes can include head trauma, drug abuse, and arteriovenous malformation (112). SAH occurs when there is bleeding between the arachnoid and pia mater. The most common cause of

spontaneous SAH is a rupture of an aneurysm, though head trauma can also cause SAH (114).

115. Correct: D. rivaroxaban.
Rivaroxaban is a direct oral anticoagulant (DOAC) that can be used for secondary prevention following stroke associated with a thromboembolism (D). The medication is not considered an antiplatelet.
Incorrect:
The most common antiplatelets used in secondary prevention of stroke include aspirin or the combination of aspirin plus extended-release dipyridamole (A, C). For those who cannot tolerate aspirin, clopidogrel can be used as an alternative antiplatelet agent (B).

116. Correct: C. Crohn's disease
Crohn's disease is an autoimmune condition that primarily affects the GI tract. It has not been implicated in increasing the risk of any type of stroke (C).
Incorrect:
Ischemic stroke is most frequently the result of atherosclerotic disease, which is associated with hyperlipidemia and diabetes mellitus (A, B). The most common reason for hemorrhagic stroke is hypertension (D).

117 to 123. Yes or No

117. Correct: Yes

118. Correct: Yes

119. Correct: Yes

120. Correct: Yes

121. Correct: Yes

122. Correct: Yes

123. Correct: Yes
In addition to the unilateral limb weakness and motor dysfunction commonly associated with stroke, the presentation of stroke can be highly variable depending on the extent of damage and the area of brain affected. Vision problems can include partial loss of visual field as well as double vision (diplopia) (117, 121). Unilateral hearing loss and facial muscle paralysis (often on one side) are also common findings (118, 119). Signs that affect balance and coordination can occur frequently (120, 123). A severe, sudden-onset headache can be a sign of hemorrhagic stroke (122).

124. Correct: B. CT scan
A head CT scan is the imaging technique of choice to detect an acute cerebral hemorrhage (B).
Incorrect:
A transesophageal echocardiogram is useful in imaging the heart and detecting the presence of blood clots, such as due to valvular disease or atrial fibrillation (A). A cerebral angiogram can also be useful in identifying the source of a blood clot (C). MRA is most useful in detecting the presence of stenosis or occlusion of cerebral blood vessels (D). This technique is also valuable in detecting the presence of aneurysms that might be at risk of rupture.

125. Correct: D. those with ischemic stroke and cardio-embolic conditions.

Direct oral anticoagulants can be a practical alternative to warfarin for secondary prevention of stroke. Anticoagulant therapy is most useful among patients with ischemic stroke and cardioembolic conditions, such as valvular disease or atrial fibrillation, that can increase the risk of blood clot development (D).

Incorrect:

Anticoagulant therapy is not recommended for all patients with a TIA, though antiplatelets are recommended to minimize future stroke risk (A). Anticoagulation therapy can be considered for patients with a history of TIA that is associated with a cardioembolic condition (e.g., atrial fibrillation). Anticoagulants such as warfarin or DOACs are not recommended for all stroke patients (B), particularly those with a history of hemorrhagic stroke (C), as this can increase bleeding risk and intracranial hemorrhage.

126. Correct: A. combined oral contraceptive.

Factor V Leiden mutation is a coagulopathy that increases the risk of thrombosis. The use of estrogen-containing products should be avoided as this can accelerate the formation of abnormal blood clots. Combined oral contraceptive contains estrogen and should not be recommended for this patient (A).

Incorrect:

Progesterone-only contraceptives, such as LNG-IUD, implant, or pills, are safe to use in patients with known coagulopathies (B, D). The copper-containing IUD is also an appropriate choice as it does not involve the release of hormone (C).

127. Correct: D. a 46-year-old with four first-degree relatives with subarachnoid hemorrhage

Though a ruptured aneurysm is associated with high mortality, it occurs infrequently, and routine screening by MRA is not indicated for all patients who are at increased risk for stroke. However, those with a strong family history of subarachnoid hemorrhage (i.e., two or more first-degree relatives) are at high risk for a ruptured aneurysm and should be considered for screening via MRA (D).

Incorrect:

The smoker with hypertension is at higher risk of hemorrhagic stroke (A), while the individual with diabetes mellitus and dyslipidemia is at higher risk of ischemic stroke (B). However, there is no indication to screen these patients for aneurysm. The woman with factor V Leiden mutation who is taking a combined oral contraceptive is at high risk of developing a thrombosis but, again, is not indicated for screening via MRA (C). She should be switched to a progesterone-only contraceptive to decrease thrombosis risk.

128 to 132. True or False

128. Correct: True

129. Correct: False

130. Correct: False

131. Correct: True

132. Correct: False

For this patient, reducing the risk of stroke will involve addressing each of his comorbidities to minimize the risk of atherosclerosis. In addition to counseling on smoking cessation, medications should be optimized to attain established goals for diabetes mellitus, dyslipidemia, and hypertension. According to the latest hypertension guidelines from AHA/ACC, the blood pressure goal for a patient with diabetes mellitus is less than 130/80 mm Hg (128). First-line agents can include one or a combination of thiazide diuretic, calcium channel blocker, or ACE inhibitor or ARB (131). A statin is recommended as first-line therapy to treat dyslipidemia, and it is not contraindicated in this patient according to the information provided (130). Generally, an A1c of less than 7% is acceptable for most patients with type 2 diabetes mellitus, though this value can be higher in the elderly or frail patient (129). There is no indication for the use of anticoagulant therapy in this patient (132).

Giant Cell Arteritis

133. Correct: C. osteoarthritis.

GCA is most commonly found in older adults and is more common in women than men. The presence of osteoarthritis is not a risk factor for GCA (C).

Incorrect:

In addition to older adults and female gender (A, B), there is a greater incidence of GCA among individuals of European descent, particularly those of Scandinavian origin (D).

134. Correct: C. It primarily impacts smaller-sized vessels.

GCA is characterized by vasculitis that primarily impacts medium- to larger-sized blood vessels (C).

Incorrect:

GCA is caused by inflammation of medium- to larger-sized vessels, including the temporal artery as well as extracranial branches of the carotid artery (A). The inflammation often impacts segments of the artery with normal sections appearing between affected sections (B). This is the rationale of why multiple biopsies are needed to make the diagnosis of GCA. The inflammation can often result in a tender or nodular, pulseless vessel (D).

135. Correct: B. biopsies of likely affected arteries.

Initial diagnostic tests for GCA can include ESR and CRP, which are nonspecific tests to check for the presence of inflammation. However, a definitive diagnosis of GCA will require biopsies of the affected artery (B).

Incorrect:

Imaging of the head with CT or MRI is not necessary for the diagnosis of GCA (C, D). These techniques can be used to help rule in or out other possible diagnoses that might be causing the symptoms. Color duplex ultrasonography can be used to complement findings from biopsy. Creatine kinase is not helpful in the diagnosis of GCA as it is used to detect skeletal muscle damage (A).

136. Correct: A. systemic corticosteroid therapy.

First-line treatment of GCA is long-term, high-dose systemic corticosteroid therapy, such as prednisone 40 to 60 mg/day (or higher when neurological or visual symptoms are present). Once the disease has stabilized, a careful dose reduction is performed until the lowest dose that can maintain clinical response can be determined. This dose is continued for 6 months to 2 years.

Incorrect:

The patient's elevated blood pressure is likely caused by the pain associated with GCA; thus, the addition of another antihypertensive medication is not needed at this time (B). Once the GCA symptoms are relieved, an adjustment to her antihypertensive medications can be considered if blood pressure remains elevated. Antiplatelet therapy, such as low-dose aspirin, can be used to prevent risk of stroke, though warfarin is not indicted for GCA (C). Topiramate is used in the prevention of primary headache, but it plays no role for this secondary headache (D).

137. Correct: B. temporal area.

Headaches associated with GCA do not typically encompass the temporal area (B).

Incorrect:

The characteristic headache associated with GCA most frequently involves the frontal (A), vertex (C), and occipital areas (D).

138. Correct: B. nitrate.

Concomitant medications are often used to prevent health risks associated with the condition or counter associated adverse effects of long-term corticosteroid therapy. However, nitrates, often used to treat angina, are not included among these medications.

Incorrect:

Low-dose aspirin is recommended for its antiplatelet effect and the prevention of stroke in these patients (A). Bisphosphonates, calcium, and vitamin D are used to prevent bone loss and development of osteoporosis associated with long-term corticosteroid therapy (C). A proton pump inhibitor is used for GI cytoprotection (D).

139. Correct: A. polymyalgia rheumatica.

Among patients with GCA, about 50% to 70% also have associated polymyalgia rheumatica, which is characterized by aching in the proximal portions of the extremities and trunk.

Incorrect:

Arteritis, inflammation of the artery, should not be confused with arthritis, which is inflammation of the joints and can involve an autoimmune process. Reactive arthritis occurs often in response to an infection (D), while psoriatic arthritis sometimes occurs in those with psoriasis (C). These conditions are not related to GCA, nor is acute pancreatitis or inflammation of the pancreas (B).

140. Correct: C. blindness.

Permanent blindness is a serious complication of GCA (C). Early signs of the disease can include transient visual blurring, diplopia, and eye pain. Sudden loss of vision is a worrisome sign as it can often be permanent. For patients suspected to have GCA (and even prior to biopsy results), corticosteroid therapy should be started as soon as possible to minimize the risk of permanent vision loss.

Incorrect:

Permanent vision loss is one of the most serious complications of GCA. The condition is not normally associated with hemiparesis (weakness on one side) (A), arthritis (B), or uveitis (inflammation of the eye) (D).

Skin Disorders

4

Skin Lesions

Identification of common dermatological lesions is important to safe clinical practice. In order to succeed in practice, the clinician must speak "the language of dermatology." This includes learning key clinical concepts in dermatology, including being able to define key terms (Table 4-1).

- Primary skin lesions: These are skin lesions that have resulted from a disease process and have not been altered by outside manipulation, treatment, or the natural course of disease.
  - Example of a primary skin lesion: Vesicle, a fluid-filled lesion, diameter less than 1 cm, noted in varicella (chickenpox), herpes zoster (shingles), herpes simplex type 1 and type 2.
- Secondary skin lesions: These are skin lesions altered by outside manipulation, treatment, and/or the natural course of disease.
  - Example of a secondary skin lesion: Crust, a raised lesion caused by dried serum and blood remnants, develops when a vesicle ruptures.

In addition, see the following key assessment tips in caring for the person presenting with a dermatology problem. In addition to the typical history of present illness and symptom analysis, ask the following questions:

- Where is the oldest lesion, and when did it occur? Where is the newest lesion, and when did it occur?
  - This allows the examiner to assess the evolution of the skin lesions.
- Is the person otherwise well?
  - If otherwise well, the person likely has a condition limited to the skin such as rosacea, or keratosis pilaris.
- Is the person highly symptomatic but not systemically ill?
  - Often, the person with a skin condition is generally well but is highly symptomatic with itch, pain, or other complaint, such as eczema (itch), zoster (pain and itch).
- Is the person systemically ill?
  - The person who is systemically ill with fever, involuntary weight loss, fatigue, and a dermatological condition often has a serious condition with a dermatological manifestation such as systemic lupus erythematosus (SLE) or Lyme disease.
- What type of lesion or lesions are noted?
- What is the pattern of the lesions?
  - Identifying the type of lesion(s) and lesion pattern is critical to arriving at the correct diagnosis.

Discussion Sources

Czerkasij V. A strategy for learning dermatology. *J Nurse Pract.* 2010;6:555–556.

James WD, Elston DM, Treat JR, Rosenbach M, Neuhaus IM. *Andrews' Diseases of the Skin: Clinical Dermatology.* 13th ed. Philadelphia, PA: Elsevier; 2019.

TABLE 4-1 Skin Lesions

LESION	DESCRIPTION	EXAMPLE
Common Primary Skin Lesions		
Macule	Flat discoloration, usually less than 1 cm in diameter	Freckle
Patch	Flat area of skin discoloration, larger than a macule	Vitiligo
Papule	Raised lesion, less than 1 cm, may be the same or different color than the surrounding skin	Raised nevus
Vesicle	Fluid filled, less than 1 cm	Varicella
Plaque	Raised lesion, ≥1 cm, may be the same or different color than surrounding skin	Psoriasis
Purpura	Lesions caused by red blood cells leaving circulation and becoming trapped in skin	Petechiae, ecchymosis
Pustule	Vesicle-like lesion with purulent content	Impetigo, acne
Wheal	Circumscribed area of skin edema	Hive
Nodule	Raised lesion, ≥1 cm, usually mobile	Epidermal cyst
Bulla	Fluid filled, ≥1 cm	Blister with second-degree burn
Common Secondary Skin Lesions		
Excoriation	Marks produced by scratching	Seen in areas of pruritic skin diseases
Lichenification	Skin thickening resembling callus formation	Seen in areas of recurrent scratching
Fissure	Narrow linear crack into epidermis, exposing dermis	Split lip, athlete's foot
Erosion	Partial focal loss of epidermis; heals without scarring	Area exposed after bullous lesion opens
Ulcer	Loss of epidermis and dermis; heals with scarring	Pressure sore
Scale	Raised, flaking lesion	Dandruff, psoriasis
Atrophy	Loss of skin markings and full skin thickness	Area treated excessively with higher-potency corticosteroids
Terms Describing Patterns of Skin Lesions		
Annular	In a ring	Erythema migrans in Lyme disease
Confluent or coalescent	Multiple lesions blending together	Multiple skin conditions
Reticular	Net-like cluster	Multiple skin conditions
Dermatomal	Along a neurocutaneous dermatome	Herpes zoster
Linear	In streaks	Poison ivy

Source: James WD, Berger TG, Elston DM. Andrews' Diseases of the Skin: Clinical Dermatology. 12th ed. Philadelphia, PA: Elsevier; 2016.

QUESTIONS

1 to 10. Match the following descriptions to the correct lesion names.

_____ 1. Fluid-filled lesion of less than 1 cm in diameter

_____ 2. Flat discoloration less than 1 cm in diameter

_____ 3. Circumscribed area of skin edema

_____ 4. Narrow linear crack into epidermis, exposing dermis

_____ 5. Vesicle-like lesion with purulent content

_____ 6. Flat discoloration greater than 1 cm in diameter

_____ 7. Raised lesion, larger than 1 cm, may be the same or a different color from the surrounding skin

_____ 8. Loss of epidermis and dermis

_____ 9. Loss of skin markings and full skin thickness

_____ 10. Skin thickening usually found over pruritic or friction areas

    A. ulcer

    B. atrophy

    C. fissure

    D. wheal

    E. pustule

    F. patch

    G. plaque

    H. macule

    I. vesicle

    J. lichenification

11 to 15. Match the following descriptions with the correct distribution name.

_____ 11. Multiple lesions blending together

_____ 12. Net-like cluster

_____ 13. In a ring formation

_____ 14. In streaks

_____ 15. Along a neurocutaneous dermatome

    A. reticular

    B. linear

    C. annular

    D. confluent or coalescent

    E. dermatomal

16 to 17. Match the type of skin lesion with the correct definition.

_____ 16. Primary

_____ 17. Secondary

    A. resulting from a disease process and unaltered by outside manipulation, treatment, or the natural course of disease

    B. altered by outside manipulation, treatment, and/or the natural course of disease

For answers and rationales, see end of chapter.

Dermatology Pharmacology

TOPICAL MEDICATION DISPENSING

Knowledge of the amount of a cream or ointment needed to treat a dermatological condition with a topical medication is an important part of the prescriptive practice (Table 4-2).

TABLE 4-2 Topical Medication-Dispensing Formulas

	AMOUNT NEEDED FOR ONE APPLICATION	AMOUNT NEEDED IN TWICE-A-DAY APPLICATION FOR 1 WEEK	AMOUNT NEEDED IN TWICE-A-DAY APPLICATION FOR 1 MONTH
Hands, head, face, anogenital region	2 g	28 g	120 g (4 oz)
One arm, anterior or posterior trunk	3 g	42 g	180 g (6 oz)
One leg	6 g	84 g	320 g (12 oz)
Entire body	30–60 g	420–840 g (14–28 oz)	1.8–3.6 kg (60–120 oz or 3.75–7.5 lb)

Source: Habif TP, Dinulos JGH, Chapman MS, Zug KA. Skin Disease: Diagnosis and Treatment. 4th ed. Philadelphia, PA: Elsevier; 2017.

CLINICAL CONCEPT

Clinicians often write prescriptions for an inadequate amount of a topical medication with an insufficient number of refills, possibly creating a situation in which treatment fails because of an inadequate length of therapy.

Aside from providers not prescribing a sufficient amount of medication, patients often are confused as to how much of the cream or ointment to apply. A helpful way of teaching a patient the appropriate amount of a cream or ointment to apply on a problematic area of skin is to use the "fingertip unit" (FTU) method of measurement. One FTU is the amount of topical cream or ointment that is squeezed out from a standard tube along an adult's fingertip. A fingertip is from the very end of the finger to the first crease in the finger. Two FTUs is approximately 1 gram of a topical cream or ointment.

One FTU of a cream or ointment is enough to treat an area of skin twice the size of the palm of an adult's hand with the fingers together, or approximately 2% body surface area (BSA) for the average adult.

Discussion Sources

Habif TP, Campbell JL, Chapman SM, et al. *Skin Disease: Diagnosis and Treatment.* 3rd ed. Philadelphia, PA: Elsevier Saunders; 2011.
Henderson R. Fingertip units for topical steroids. https://patient.info/treatment-medication/steroids/fingertip-units-for-topical-steroids

QUESTIONS

18. How many grams of a topical cream or ointment are needed for a single application to the hands?

A. 1

B. 2

C. 3

D. 4

19. How many grams of a topical cream or ointment are needed for a single application to an arm?

A. 1

B. 2

C. 3

D. 4

20. How many grams of a topical cream or ointment are needed for a single application to the entire body?

A. 10 to 30

B. 30 to 60

C. 60 to 90

D. 90 to 120

21. One FTU can be expected to cover what percentage of BSA?

A. 2

B. 5

C. 10

D. 20

22. How many grams of a topical cream or ointment can be expected in two FTUs?

A. 1

B. 3

C. 5

D. 10

For answers and rationales, see end of chapter.

TOPICAL MEDICATION ABSORPTION

The safe prescription of a topical agent for patients with dermatological disorders requires knowledge of the best vehicle for the medication. Certain parts of the body, notably the face, axillae, and genital area, are quite permeable, allowing greater absorption of topical medication than less permeable areas, such as the extremities and trunk. In particular, the thickness of the palms of the hands and soles of the feet creates a barrier so that relatively little topical medication is absorbed when applied to these sites. Cutaneous drug absorption is typically inversely proportional to the thickness of the stratum corneum. Hydrocortisone absorption from the forearm is less than one-third of the amount that is absorbed from the forehead.

In general, the less viscous the vehicle containing a topical medication is, the less medication is absorbed. As a result, medication contained in a gel or lotion is absorbed in smaller amounts than medication contained in a cream or ointment. Topical medications in ointment form usually allow for maximal drug absorption. Besides enhancing absorption of the therapeutic agent, creams and ointments provide lubrication to the region, often a desirable effect in the presence of xerosis or lichenification.

Discussion Source

Robertson D, Maibach H. Dermatologic pharmacology. In: Katzung B, ed. *Katzung's Basic and Clinical Pharmacology.* 14th ed. New York, NY: McGraw-Hill Medical; 2018:1068–1086.

QUESTIONS

23. You write a prescription for a topical agent and anticipate the greatest rate of absorption when it is applied to the:

A. palms of the hands.

B. soles of the feet.

C. face.

D. abdomen.

24. You prescribe a topical medication and want it to have maximum absorption, so you choose the following vehicle:

A. gel.

B. lotion.

   C. cream.

   D. ointment.

25. Which of the following vehicles is preferred for maximum drug absorption when treating the antecubital fossa of the arm?

   A. gel

   B. lotion

   C. cream

   D. ointment

For answers and rationales, see end of chapter.

CLINICAL CONCEPT

Because of the risk of subcutaneous tissue atrophy, the super-high potency corticosteroids should not be used continuously for more than 3 weeks.

TOPICAL CORTICOSTEROIDS

Corticosteroids, whether topical or systemic (oral or parenteral), are a class of drugs often used to treat a variety of dermatological disorders, particularly conditions characterized by hyperproliferation, inflammation, and immunological involvement. Although corticosteroids exhibit their therapeutic effect through numerous mechanisms (including immunosuppressive and anti-inflammatory properties), their relative potency is based on vasoconstrictive activity; that is, the most potent topical steroids, such as betamethasone (class I), have significantly greater vasoconstricting action than the least potent agents, such as hydrocortisone (class VII) (Table 4-3).

TABLE 4-3 Examples of Topical Corticosteroid Potency

POTENCY/CLASS	TOPICAL CORTICOSTEROID
Low potency (Classes V to VII)	Hydrocortisone (0.5%, 1%, 2.5%)
	Fluocinolone acetonide 0.01% (Synalar®)
	Desonide (0.05%)
	Triamcinolone acetonide 0.025% (Aristocort®)
	Fluocinolone acetonide 0.025% (Synalar®)
	Hydrocortisone butyrate 0.1%
	Hydrocortisone valerate 0.2% (Westcort®)
	Triamcinolone acetonide 0.1%
Midrange potency (Classes III to IV)	Betamethasone dipropionate, augmented, 0.05% (Diprolene AF® cream)
	Mometasone furoate 0.1% (Elocon® ointment)
	Amcinonide (0.1%)
High potency (Class II)	Fluocinolone acetonide 0.2% (Synalar-HP®)
	Desoximetasone 0.25% (Topicort®)
	Fluocinonide 0.05% (Lidex®)
	Betamethasone dipropionate, augmented, 0.05% (Diprolene® gel, ointment)
Super-high potency (Class I)	Clobetasol propionate 0.05% (Temovate®)
	Halobetasol propionate 0.05% (Ultravate® 0.05%)

Source: Benson HA, Watkinson AC. Topical and Transdermal Drug Delivery: Principles and Practice. Hoboken, NJ: John Wiley & Sons; 2012:357–366.

The potency of the topical corticosteroid should be matched to the condition, with use of the higher potency agents (classes I to III) usually limited to more difficult-to-treat conditions including alopecia areata, hyperkeratotic/nummular eczema, lichen planus, and psoriasis.

Medium-potency topical corticosteroids (classes IV and V) are most often used for the treatment of atopic dermatitis, seborrheic dermatitis, and stasis dermatitis. Low-potency topical corticosteroid use (classes VI and VII) is usually limited to areas where the medication will be well absorbed as the affected dermal layer is thin, including diaper dermatitis, dermatitis on the face including the eyelids, perianal inflammation, or with intertrigo (skinfolds). To enhance the potency of a topical corticosteroid, an occlusive dressing can be used to cover the area after applying the topical agent. Low-, medium-, and high-potency topical corticosteroids should not be used continuously for longer than 3 months to avoid adverse effects including subcutaneous tissue atrophy.

Discussion Sources

James WD, Elston DM, Treat JR, Rosenbach M, Neuhaus IM. *Andrews' Diseases of the Skin: Clinical Dermatology.* 13th ed. Philadelphia, PA: Elsevier; 2019.

Robertson D, Maibach H. Dermatologic pharmacology. In: Katzung B, ed. *Katzung's Basic and Clinical Pharmacology.* 14th ed. New York, NY: McGraw-Hill Medical; 2018:1068–1086.

Stringer J. Adrenocortical hormones. In: Stringer J, ed. *Basic Concepts in Pharmacology.* 5th ed. New York, NY: McGraw-Hill Medical; 2017:185–188.

QUESTIONS

26. One of the mechanisms of action of a topical corticosteroid preparation is as:

    A. an antimitotic.

    B. an exfoliant.

    C. a vasoconstrictor.

    D. a humectant.

27. To enhance the potency of a topical corticosteroid, the prescriber recommends that the patient apply the preparation:

    A. to dry skin by gentle rubbing.

    B. and cover with an occlusive dressing.

    C. before bathing.

    D. with an emollient.

28. Which of the following is the least potent topical corticosteroid?

    A. betamethasone dipropionate 0.1% (Diprosone®)

    B. clobetasol propionate 0.05% (Cormax®)

    C. hydrocortisone 2.5%

    D. fluocinonide 0.05% (Lidex®)

29. What is the maximum recommended amount of time a low- to medium-potency topical corticosteroid can be used continuously in a non-intertriginous area to avoid adverse effects?

    A. 1 week

    B. 1 month

    C. 3 months

    D. 6 months

30. What is the maximum recommended amount of time a super-high potency topical corticosteroid can be used continuously to avoid adverse effects?

    A. 1 week

    B. 3 weeks

    C. 2 months

    D. 4 months

31 to 33.   Match each topical corticosteroid potency with its most appropriate use.

_____   **31.** Low potency

_____   **32.** Medium potency

_____   **33.** High potency

        A. seborrheic dermatitis

        B. psoriasis

        C. dermatitis involving the eyelids

For answers and rationales, see end of chapter.

ANTIHISTAMINES

Antihistamines prevent the action of formed histamine and can be used to control acute symptoms of itchiness and allergy. All antihistamines, whether administered orally, parenterally, or topically, work by blocking histamine-1 (H_1) receptor sites, preventing histamine from inducing or perpetuating inflammation.

Systemic antihistamines are usually divided into two groups: standard or first-generation products, such as a variety of commonly used oral products including diphenhydramine (Benadryl®) or chlorpheniramine (Chlor-Trimeton®), and newer or second-generation products, such as loratadine (Claritin®), desloratadine (Clarinex®), cetirizine (Zyrtec®), fexofenadine (Allegra®), and levocetirizine (Xyzal®). The first-generation antihistamines readily cross the blood-brain barrier, causing sedation; as a result, these medications should be used with appropriate caution and should not be taken during activities when risk of accident or injury is significant. Their anticholinergic activity can result in drying of secretions, visual changes, and urinary retention; the latter is most often a problem for older men with benign prostatic hyperplasia. The use of first-generation antihistamines by older adults, particularly in higher doses as a sleep aid, can result in negative cognitive effects. The second-generation antihistamines do not easily cross the blood-brain barrier, which results in lower rates of sedation. With little anticholinergic effect, the use of a product such as loratadine is likely to provide less drying of nasal secretions compared with diphenhydramine use but also will have less negative effect on cognition, particularly in older adults.

Discussion Source

Robertson DB, Maibach HI. Dermatologic pharmacology. In: Katzung B, ed., _Katzung's Basic and Clinical Pharmacology_. 14th ed. New York, NY: McGraw-Hill Medical; 2018:1068–1086.

QUESTIONS

34. Antihistamines exhibit their therapeutic effect by:

    A. inactivating circulating histamine.

    B. preventing the production of histamine.

    C. blocking activity at histamine receptor sites.

    D. acting as a procholinergic agent.

35. A possible adverse effect with the use of a first-generation antihistamine such as diphenhydramine in an 80-year-old man is:

    A. urinary retention.

    B. hypertension.

    C. tachycardia.

    D. urticaria.

36. Which of the following medications is likely to cause the most sedation?

    A. chlorpheniramine

    B. cetirizine

    C. fexofenadine

    D. loratadine

For answers and rationales, see end of chapter.

Impetigo

Overview

Impetigo is a contagious skin infection with a typical presentation of purulent skin lesions. Although most common among children in tropical or subtropical regions, the prevalence increases in northern climates during the summer months. Impetigo's peak incidence is among children 2 to 5 years old, although older children and adults can also be affected.

There is no gender or racial predilection for the condition. Impetigo skin lesions are nearly always caused by the gram-positive group A streptococci, *Staphylococcus aureus,* or a mix of both. Personal hygiene has an influence on impetigo disease incidence in that colonization with a given causative pathogen strain precedes the development of impetigo lesions by a mean duration of 10 days; inoculation of surface organisms into the skin by abrasions, minor trauma, or insect bites then ensues. In adults, minor skin injuries noted with shaving, particularly with a dull blade that was previously used by another person, are often the antecedent event to the development of impetigo.

Clinical Presentation

Impetigo usually occurs on exposed areas of the body; the infection most frequently affects the face and extremities. The lesions remain well localized but are frequently multiple and can be either bullous or nonbullous.

The lesions of nonbullous impetigo usually begin as papules that rapidly evolve into vesicles surrounded by an area of erythema. The pustules increase in size, breaking down in the next 4 to 6 days, forming characteristic thick crusts. About 70% of patients with impetigo have nonbullous lesions.

Bullous impetigo is usually caused by strains of *S aureus* that produce a toxin causing cleavage in the superficial skin layer. The causative pathogen is usually present in the nose before the outbreak of the cutaneous disease. The bullous lesions usually appear initially as superficial vesicles that rapidly enlarge to form a bulla or blister that is often filled with a dark or purulent liquid and can take on a pustular appearance. The bullae are typically well demarcated without any surrounding erythema. The lesion ruptures, and a thin, lacquer-like crust typically forms quickly. The pattern of the lesion often reflects autoinoculation with the offending organism. See Figure 4-1. In either form, the lesions heal slowly and leave depigmented areas. Systemic symptoms are not common but can include weakness, fever, and diarrhea.

Streptococcal strains can be transferred from the skin or impetigo lesions to the upper respiratory tract. Although regional lymphadenitis occurs, systemic symptoms are usually absent. Rarely, an impetigo lesion can become deeply ulcerated, with the resulting condition known as ecthyma. When evaluating suspected bullous impetigo, other conditions to consider in the differential diagnosis can include bullous erythema multiforme, bullous lupus erythematosus, herpes simplex virus, insect bites, Stevens-Johnson syndrome, thermal burn, toxic epidermal necrolysis, or varicella infection.

> **CLINICAL CONCEPT**
>
> Most cases of nonbullous impetigo are caused by staphylococci alone or in combination with streptococci.

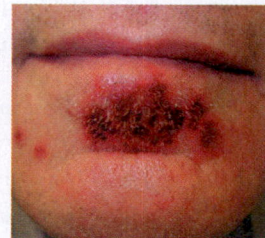

FIGURE 4-1 Impetigo.
Barankin B, Anatoli F. Derm Notes: Clinical Dermatology Pocket Guide. Philadelphia, PA: F.A. Davis; 2006.

Diagnostic Testing

Impetigo is usually diagnosed clinically, based on patient history, risk factors, and clinical presentation. Culture and susceptibility testing of the lesions is generally limited to select situations, such as during an impetigo outbreak in a closed community (e.g., in a day-care setting), suspected resistant lesion, or complicated disease.

Treatment

While impetigo will usually resolve without treatment within 1 to 2 weeks without scarring or sequelae, prescribing appropriate antimicrobial therapy helps accelerate resolution and improves comfort. In addition, treatment minimizes contagion.

Topical antimicrobial therapy is adequate for nonbullous impetigo with a single lesion or small area of involvement. First-line therapy can include mupirocin (Bactroban® or Centany®) or retapamulin (Altabax®) ointment. In mild disease, topical antimicrobial therapy is as effective as oral therapy and has a smaller risk for systemic adverse effects. Bacitracin and neomycin are less-effective topical treatments; use of these products is not recommended for the treatment of impetigo. Nearly three-quarters of individuals with impetigo have the nonbullous form.

Patients with bullous impetigo, who have numerous lesions, are not responding to or cannot tolerate topical agents, or during outbreaks affecting several people should receive oral antimicrobials effective against *S aureus* and *Streptococcus pyogenes*. *S aureus* currently accounts for most cases of bullous impetigo and for a substantial portion of nonbullous infections. Therefore, antimicrobials with a gram-positive spectrum of activity and stability in the presence of beta-lactamase, such as dicloxacillin or amoxicillin-clavulanate or a first-generation or second-generation cephalosporin such as cephalexin, are used as a first-line choice, particularly if methicillin-susceptible *S aureus* (MSSA) is considered to be the likely causative pathogen. Patients with extensive impetigo lesion distribution and/or who present with systemic symptoms should also receive oral antimicrobial therapy.

> **CLINICAL CONCEPT**
>
> Children with impetigo should be kept out of school or day care for 24 hours after initiation of antibiotic therapy, and family members should be checked for lesions.

Impetigo caused by methicillin-resistant *S aureus* (MRSA) is increasing in frequency. In addition, up to 10% of MRSA strains are now resistant to mupirocin. Oral doxycycline, a tetracycline form, can be helpful but should not be used in children younger than 11 years owing to the risk of staining of the permanent teeth. Additional therapeutic options include trimethoprim-sulfamethoxazole and clindamycin; the use of clindamycin is associated with an increased risk for *Clostridium difficile* infection (CDI). Most episodes of impetigo resolve without complication or need for a second-line agent.

Treatment of impetigo is important to minimize the risk of infectious transmission.

Discussion Sources

Bolaji RS, Dabade TS, Gustafson CJ, Davis SA, Krowchuk DP, Feldman SR. Treatment of impetigo: oral antibiotics most commonly prescribed. *J Drugs Dermatol.* 2012;11(4):489–494.

Gilbert DN, Chambers HF, Eliopoulos GM, Saag MS, Pavia AT. *The Sanford Guide to Antimicrobial Therapy.* 50th ed. Sperryville, VA: Antimicrobial Therapy, Inc.; 2020:57.

Lewis LS. Impetigo treatment and management. Medscape. https://emedicine.medscape.com/article/965254-treatment

Stevens DL, Bisno AL, Chambers HF, et al. Practice guidelines for the diagnosis and management of skin and soft tissue infections: 2014 update by the Infectious Diseases Society of America. *Clin Infect Dis.* 2014;59(2):e10–e52.

QUESTIONS

37. A mother brings in her 4-year-old otherwise well child with a 2- to 3-day history of increasing skin lesions. When considering a diagnosis of bullous impetigo, the nurse practitioner (NP) expects to find:

    A. complaint of intense itch.

    B. vesicular lesions in a scattered pattern.

    C. plaques in a dermatomal pattern.

    D. systemic symptoms such as fever and chills.

38. An examination of the 4-year-old child in the previous question reveals approximately 30 lesions on the lower extremities and abdomen. Appropriate treatment can include:

    A. topical mupirocin.

    B. oral erythromycin.

    C. oral doxycycline.

    D. oral cephalexin.

39. A 20-year-old man presents with a complaint of new-onset lesions on his chest that appeared within a few days after shaving his chest with a razor he found in the college dormitory. A finding most consistent with nonbullous impetigo is:

    A. scattered blisters 1 to 3 cm in diameter filled with a dark fluid.

    B. scaly patches with accompanying pruritus.

    C. scattered vesicles surrounded by an area of erythema.

    D. a linear pattern of purpura that do not blanch with pressure to the skin.

40. The likely causative organisms of nonbullous impetigo in a 6-year-old child include:

    A. *Haemophilus influenzae* and *Streptococcus pneumoniae*.

    B. group A streptococcus and *S aureus*.

   C. *Moraxella catarrhalis* and select viruses.

   D. *Pseudomonas aeruginosa* and select fungi.

41. The spectrum of antimicrobial activity of mupirocin (Bactroban®) includes:

   A. primarily gram-negative organisms.

   B. select gram-positive organisms.

   C. *Pseudomonas* species and anaerobic organisms.

   D. only organisms that do not produce beta-lactamase.

42. An impetigo lesion that becomes deeply ulcerated is known as:

   A. cellulitis.

   B. erythema.

   C. ecthyma.

   D. empyema.

43. First-line treatment of nonbullous impetigo with fewer than five lesions of 1 to 2 cm in diameter on the legs of a 9-year-old girl is:

   A. topical mupirocin.

   B. topical neomycin.

   C. oral cefixime.

   D. oral doxycycline.

44. An oral antimicrobial option for the treatment of methicillin-susceptible *S aureus* skin infection includes all of the following except:

   A. amoxicillin.

   B. dicloxacillin.

   C. cephalexin.

   D. trimethoprim-sulfamethoxazole (TMP-SMX).

45. A 5-year-old with bullous impetigo has been treated with topical mupirocin for 3 days without any improvement. Aside from discontinuing topical mupirocin therapy, what would you recommend as the next step in therapy?

   A. Prescribe topical retapamulin.

   B. Prescribe oral dicloxacillin.

   C. Prescribe oral TMP-SMX.

   D. Prescribe oral minocycline.

46. You see a kindergarten student with impetigo and advise that she can return to school _____ hours after initiating effective antimicrobial therapy.

   A. 24

   B. 48

   C. 72

   D. 96

For answers and rationales, see end of chapter.

Acne Vulgaris

Overview

Acne vulgaris is a common dermatological condition. Approximately 80% of teens and younger adults are affected with acne, with more than 20% having severe disease with subsequent scarring. In teens, due to the contributions of androgens, males are overrepresented in more severe acne. Only 15% of adolescents and young adults seek treatment for acne vulgaris, which affects this age group at a time in their lives when body image and social acceptance are usually of greater influence than they are at any other time of life. At least 15% of adults age 24 years or more, usually women, will continue to report problems with acne. By age 45 years, the prevalence of acne wanes.

Acne is caused by a combination of factors, including an increase in sebaceous activity that causes plugging of follicles and retention of sebum, allowing an overgrowth of the organism *Propionibacterium acnes*. This overgrowth allows an inflammatory reaction with the resulting wide variety of lesions, including open and closed comedones, pustules, and cysts.

Clinical Presentation

Acne vulgaris lesions are found in the areas of the skin where sebaceous follicles are most plentiful, including the face, upper chest, and back. See Figure 4-2. Occasionally the upper arms are also involved. While usually a condition where pain, itch, and other common complaints associated with skin conditions are usually not reported, larger lesions can cause localized tenderness, heat, and erythema. Systemic signs and symptoms such as fever and body aches are not reported. At the same time, the psychological burden of acne cannot be minimized.

Acne presentation is usually classified by severity and lesions noted:

- Mild acne: Presence of closed comedones ("whiteheads"), a few papulopustules ("pimples"), with or without open comedones ("blackheads")
- Moderate acne: Presence of closed comedones with inflammatory papules and pustules; greater number of lesions with evidence of more inflammation present than seen in mild acne, with or without open comedones ("blackheads")
- Severe or nodulocystic acne: Presence of comedones, inflammatory lesions, and large nodules or cysts, usually greater than 5 mm in diameter. Often scarring from previous lesions is evident.

Diagnostic Testing

Acne vulgaris is diagnosed clinically, based on patient history, risk factors, and clinical presentation. Given that a single bacterial organism is associated with the condition, culture and susceptibility testing of the lesions are not warranted. In women with particularly severe acne, consideration should be given to proceed with an evaluation for polycystic ovary syndrome (PCOS).

Treatment

When selecting acne treatment, therapeutic options should be based on the severity of acne (mild, moderate, or severe) (Table 4-4). In addition, the patient should be advised that about 4 to 6 weeks of therapy for nearly all acne therapies is needed prior to seeing significant clinical effect.

The need for follow-up visits with acne therapy is critical as patients often self-discontinue therapy without an adequate clinical trial. In addition, even with clinical response, acne is usually a recurrent condition, necessitating multiple rounds of treatment or chronic therapy.

Due to follicular plugging, the use of a keratolytic/comedolytic agent is advised in acne, regardless of its severity. Examples include tretinoin (Retin-A®), adapalene, and tazarotene. Less potent keratolytic products include salicylic 2.5% acne wash (Table 4-5). Individuals using a topical tretinoin should be advised to use sunscreen, as tretinoin has a photosensitizing effect that can increase the risk of sunburn

> **CLINICAL CONCEPT**
>
> With topical acne therapy, the product should be applied to the entire area where acne could occur, not simply as spot treatment for existing lesions.

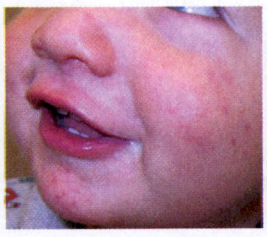 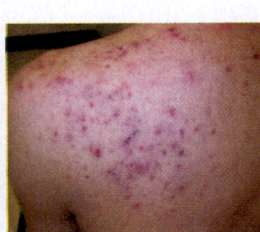 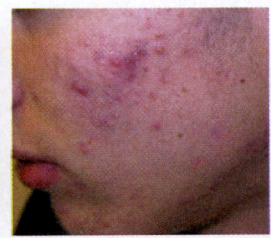 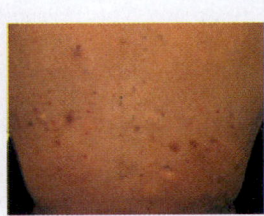

FIGURE 4-2 Acne vulgaris.
Barankin B, Anatoli F. Derm Notes: Clinical Dermatology Pocket Guide. Philadelphia, PA: F.A. Davis; 2006.

TABLE 4-4 Combined Acne Severity Classification

SEVERITY	DEFINITION
Mild acne	Fewer than 20 comedones, or
	Fewer than 15 inflammatory lesions, or
	Total lesion count fewer than 30
Moderate acne	20 to 100 comedones, or
	15 to 50 inflammatory lesions, or
	Total lesion count 30 to 125
Severe acne	More than five nodules, or
	Total inflammatory lesion count greater than 50, or
	Total lesion count greater than 125

Note: There is no universally agreed-upon system for grading acne.

Source: Liao DC. Management of acne. J Fam Pract. 2003;52:43–51.

TABLE 4-5 Acne Medications

ACNE MEDICATION	MECHANISM OF ACTION AND CONSIDERATIONS FOR USE
Benzoyl peroxide gel, cream, lotion, various concentrations	■ Antimicrobial against *P acnes* and comedolytic effects ■ Safe and effective, OTC availability ■ Lower-strength formulation often as effective as higher strength and likely to cause less skin irritation ■ Often given in combination with topical antibiotics, usually used with a keratolytic
Azelaic acid (Finacea®, Azelex®) 15% and 20% cream	■ Likely antimicrobial against *P acnes*, keratolytic, possibly alters androgen metabolism ■ Mild skin irritation with redness and dryness common with initial use, improves over time ■ Less potent, but less irritating than tretinoin preparations
Salicylic acid (2.5% solution, cream, lotion)	■ Keratolytic effect, unplugs pores and loosens dry, scaly, or thickened skin
Tretinoin (retinoic acid) gel, cream, various concentrations	■ Decreases cohesion between epidermal cells, keratolytic, increases epidermal cell turnover, transforms closed to open comedones
Adapalene (Differin®), tazarotene (Tazorac®), synthetic tretinoin	■ Mild skin irritation with redness and dryness common with initial use, improves over time; expect approximately 6 weeks of therapy before noting improvement ■ Photosensitizing; advise patient to use sunscreen
Oral antibiotics (doxycycline, most common; others include minocycline, clindamycin, erythromycin, azithromycin)	■ Antimicrobial against *P acnes*, anti-inflammatory ■ Indicated for treatment of moderate papular inflammatory acne, usually when topical therapy has been inadequate ■ Once skin clears (usually about 3 to 6 months), taper off slowly over a few months while adding topical antibiotic agents; rapid discontinuation results in return of acne ■ Long-term therapy is often needed ■ Protracted minocycline use associated with risk of skin pigmentation; use is discouraged

Continued

TABLE 4-5 Acne Medications—cont'd

ACNE MEDICATION	MECHANISM OF ACTION AND CONSIDERATIONS FOR USE
Topical antibiotics (clindamycin, erythromycin, tetracycline, others)	■ Antimicrobial against *P acnes*, anti-inflammatory ■ Indicated in treatment of mild to moderate inflammatory acne vulgaris; less effective than oral antibiotics; often given in combination with benzoyl peroxide
Combined estrogen-progestin hormonal contraceptives such as birth control pills, ring, or patch; spironolactone	■ Reduction in ovarian androgen production, decreased sebum production
Isotretinoin (Accutane®, Roaccutane®, Claravis®, Sotret®, Amnesteem®, Absorica®) capsules, various strengths	■ Likely inhibits sebaceous gland function ■ Indicated for treatment of cystic acne that does not respond to other therapies ■ Usual course of treatment is 4 to 6 months; discontinue when nodule count is reduced by 70%; repeat course only if needed after 6 months off drug ■ Adverse effects include cheilitis, conjunctivitis, hypertriglyceridemia, xerosis, photosensitivity, and potent teratogenicity; careful monitoring for mood destabilization and suicidal thoughts is an important part of patient care during isotretinoin use

Sources: Gilbert DN, Chambers HF, Eliopoulos GM, Saag MS, Pavia AT. *The Sanford Guide to Antimicrobial Therapy. 50th ed.* Sperryville, VA: Antimicrobial Therapy, Inc.; 2020:52; James WD, Berger TG, Elston DM. *Andrews' Diseases of the Skin: Clinical Dermatology. 12th ed.* Philadelphia, PA: Elsevier; 2016.

regardless of skin tone. Antibacterial agents are usually used and range from topical benzoyl peroxide, available over the counter (OTC) and most effective in milder acne, to prescription topical antimicrobials; these agents are most helpful in the treatment of pustular lesions. The mechanism of action of antibacterials in acne therapy is probably not based solely on their antimicrobial action but is likely in part a result of anti-inflammatory activity.

Hormonal therapy can be considered for females with acne, especially when other treatment options have had inadequate results. Combined oral contraceptive pills, which contain both estrogen and progestin, will help to suppress ovarian androgen production and can block the effect of androgens at the sebaceous glands. Alternatively, aldosterone antagonists, such as spironolactone, will reduce free testosterone levels and limit the effect of androgens at the sebaceous glands.

Isotretinoin (Accutane®) is effective in severe and/or cystic acne that does not respond to conventional therapy such as an adequate clinical trial of an oral antibiotic with a topical keratolytic. Although most patients who take isotretinoin have adverse effects related only to dry skin, the prescriber and patient need to be well aware of potentially serious problems associated with its use, including pseudotumor cerebri (idiopathic intracranial hypertension), hypertriglyceridemia, elevated hepatic enzymes, and cheilitis. The U.S. Food and Drug Administration (FDA) ruled that labeling for the use of isotretinoin be changed to reflect a possible connection between its use and altered mood. During isotretinoin treatment, the patient should be observed closely for symptoms of depression, such as sad mood, irritability, impulsivity, altered sleep, loss of interest or pleasure in previously enjoyable activities, change in weight or appetite, and new problems with school or work performance. In addition, the patient should be asked about suicidal ideation and altered mood at every office visit while taking the medication. Patients should stop isotretinoin use and they and/or their caregivers should contact the health-care professional right away if the patient has any of the previously mentioned symptoms. Simply discontinuing the offending medication might be insufficient, and further evaluation is likely needed.

Isotretinoin is also a potent teratogen; women taking the medication should have two negative pregnancy tests, including one on the second day of their normal menstrual period, before beginning the medication. In addition, women using isotretinoin should use two forms of highly effective contraception and have a pregnancy test done monthly during therapy. In addition, the woman taking isotretinoin should be advised to avoid pregnancy for 1 month after discontinuing the medication.

Acne-inducing drugs should be avoided, if possible. Certain medications, such as lithium and phenytoin (Dilantin®), often cannot be discontinued because of underlying health problems. Drug-induced acne can be treated with conventional therapy (see Table 4-5). See Table 4-6 for treatment recommendations for acne.

CLINICAL CONCEPT

Due to the adverse effect profile and the teratogenic potential, isotretinoin (Accutane) prescribing is limited to clinicians who have taken a course on the safer use of the medication.

TABLE 4-6 Treatment Recommendations for Acne

	MILD ACNE (COMEDONAL OR INFLAMMATORY/MIXED LESIONS)	MODERATE ACNE (COMEDONAL OR INFLAMMATORY/MIXED LESIONS)	SEVERE ACNE (INFLAMMATORY/MIXED AND/OR NODULAR LESIONS)
Initial treatment	Benzoyl peroxide (BP) or Topical retinoid	Topical combination therapy: BP + antibiotic or BP + retinoid or Retinoid + BP + antibiotic	Oral antibiotic + Topical combination therapy: BP + antibiotic or BP + retinoid or BP + retinoid + antibiotic or Oral isotretinoin
Initial treatment (alternative)	Topical combination therapy BP + antibiotic or BP + retinoid or BP + retinoid + antibiotic	Oral antibiotic + topical retinoid + BP or Topical retinoid + oral antibiotic + BP + topical antibiotic	
Inadequate response	Add BP or retinoid if not already prescribed or Change alternate topical retinoid concentration, type, and/or formulation or Consider topical dapsone	Consider alternate combination therapy or Consider change in oral antibiotic or Add combined oral contraceptive or oral spironolactone (females) or Consider oral isotretinoin	Consider changing oral antibiotic or Add combined oral contraceptive or oral spironolactone (females) or Consider oral isotretinoin

Source: Zaenglein AL, Pathy AL, Schlosser BJ, et al. Guidelines of care for the management of acne vulgaris. J Am Acad Dermatol. 2016;74:945–973.

Discussion Sources

Eichenfield LF, Krakowski AC, Piggott C, et al. Evidence-based recommendations for the diagnosis and treatment of pediatric acne. *Pediatrics.* 2013;131:S163. http://pediatrics.aappublications.org/content/pediatrics/131/Supplement_3/S163.full.pdf

Gilbert DN, Chambers HF, Eliopoulos GM, Saag MS, Pavia AT. *The Sanford Guide to Antimicrobial Therapy.* 50th ed. Sperryville, VA: Antimicrobial Therapy, Inc.; 2020:52.

James WD, Berger TG, Elston DM. *Andrews' Diseases of the Skin: Clinical Dermatology.* 12th ed. Philadelphia, PA: Elsevier; 2016:225–244.

Robertson DB, Maibach HI. Dermatologic pharmacology. In: Katzung B, ed. *Katzung's Basic and Clinical Pharmacology.* 14th ed. New York, NY: McGraw-Hill Medical; 2018:1068–1086.

U.S. Food and Drug Administration. Isotretinoin (marketed as Accutane) capsule information. https://www.fda.gov/Drugs/DrugSafety/ucm094305.htm

QUESTIONS

47. The use of which of the following medications contributes to the development of acne vulgaris?

A. lithium

B. propranolol

C. sertraline

D. clonidine

48. First-line therapy for mild acne vulgaris with closed comedones includes:

A. oral antibiotics.

B. isotretinoin.

    C. benzoyl peroxide.

    D. hydrocortisone cream.

49. When prescribing a topical retinoid such as tretinoin (Retin-A®), the NP advises the patient to:

    A. use it with an exfoliant to minimize irritating effects.

    B. use a sunscreen because the drug is photosensitizing.

    C. add a sulfa-based cream to enhance anti-acne effects.

    D. expect a significant improvement in acne lesions after approximately 1 week of use.

50. First-line treatment of moderate acne can include which of the following (more than one answer may be chosen)?

    A. benzoyl peroxide plus topical antimicrobial

    B. spironolactone (females)

    C. topical retinoid plus benzoyl peroxide

    D. oral isotretinoin

51. You see a 16-year-old boy with moderate acne who has been treated with a topical antimicrobial and topical retinoid for the past 6 months with an outstanding clinical response. You advise the teen that:

    A. the acne is fully resolved, and treatment can be discontinued.

    B. a slow taper of the topical antimicrobial can be attempted.

    C. the current treatment can be replaced with an oral antimicrobial.

    D. the topical retinoid can likely be discontinued.

52. You have initiated therapy for an 18-year-old man with acne vulgaris and have prescribed oral doxycy-cline. He returns in 3 weeks, complaining that his skin is "no better." Your next action is to:

    A. counsel him that at least 4 to 6 weeks of treatment are often needed before significant improvement is achieved.

    B. discontinue the doxycycline and initiate minocycline therapy.

    C. advise him that antibiotics are likely not an effective treatment for him and should not be continued.

    D. add a second antimicrobial agent such as TMP-SMX.

53. Who is the best candidate for isotretinoin (Accutane®) therapy?

    A. a 17-year-old patient with pustular lesions and poor response to benzoyl peroxide

    B. a 20-year-old patient with cystic lesions who has tried various therapies with minimal effect

    C. a 14-year-old patient with open and closed comedones and a family history of "ice pick" scars

    D. an 18-year-old patient with inflammatory lesions and improvement with tretinoin (Retin-A®)

54. In a 22-year-old woman using isotretinoin (Accutane®) therapy, the NP ensures follow-up tests to monitor for all of the following except:

    A. hepatic enzymes.

    B. triglyceride measurements.

    C. pregnancy.

    D. platelet count.

55. Leonard is an 18-year-old man who has been taking isotretinoin (Accutane®) for the treatment of acne for the past 2 months. Which of the following is the most important question for the clinician to ask at his follow-up office visit?

    A. "Are you having any problems remembering to take your medication?"

    B. "Have you noticed any dry skin around your mouth since you started using Accutane®?"

    C. "Do you notice any improvement in your skin?"

    D. "Have you noticed any recent changes in your mood?"

56 to 58. Match each of the following teenagers with the most appropriate category of acne severity.

_____ **56.** A 17-year-old with seven nodules and greater than 50 inflammatory lesions

_____ **57.** A 16-year-old with 15 comedones

_____ **58.** A 19-year-old with 30 comedones and total lesion count of approximately 75

     A. mild acne

     B. moderate acne

     C. severe acne

59. In a 13-year-old female patient with mild acne and who experiences an inadequate response to benzoyl peroxide treatment, an appropriate treatment option would be to:

     A. add a topical retinoid.

     B. add an oral antibiotic.

     C. consider referral for isotretinoin therapy.

     D. consider oral hormonal therapy.

60. The mechanism of action of combined oral contraceptives or spironolactone in acne treatment of an 18-year-old female with moderate acne is:

     A. an anti-inflammatory effect at lesions.

     B. a comedolytic effect.

     C. a reduction in circulating androgen level.

     D. a keratolytic effect.

61. A 22-year-old woman presents with moderate acne; she is currently taking phenytoin with excellent seizure control. The NP recommends which of the following to treat her acne?

     A. temporary discontinuation of phenytoin

     B. standard acne therapy

     C. referral for treatment with isotretinoin

     D. switch phenytoin to another antiepileptic medication

For answers and rationales, see end of chapter.

Bite Wounds

Overview

An estimated 50% of the population in an industrialized nation will sustain a bite wound at some time. At the same time, bite wounds should not be considered benign or inevitable. Approximately 80% of bite wounds are from dogs and cats, with the majority being household pets or otherwise known by the person who was bitten.

The most common victims of dog bites are children, with the bite most frequently occurring on the face or upper body. All bite wounds, regardless of origin, should be considered to carry bacterial infection risk. The risk of infection from bite wounds can vary from the relatively low rate with dog bites (approximately 5%) to the very high rate from cat bites (approximately 80%).

Intervention includes education to avoid further bites; a patient's history must include a complete documentation of events leading up to the bite.

Clinical Presentation

Initial assessment of the person, regardless of age, with a bite wound should include a multisystem survey to evaluate for additional injuries and ensure that problems with respiration and/or circulation are addressed first. In the majority of bite injuries from domesticated animals, the bite wound is the only injury. Dog bites can result in a laceration, puncture, crushing, or avulsion injury. Cat bites tend to cause puncture wounds as their sharp teeth penetrate through the skin, often trapping bacteria. Human bites tend to be more serious than domestic animal bites due to the nature and location of the bite, often occurring during an altercation, and risk of infection. A common human bite is the closed-fist injury where a flexed knuckle strikes a human tooth.

Diagnostic Testing

Bite wounds are usually assessed clinically without the need for additional testing. Routine culture and susceptibility testing of the wound is usually not indicated, unless during wound treatment there is concern for secondary infection.

Treatment

Initial therapy for all bite wounds should include vigorous wound cleansing with antimicrobial agents as appropriate and débridement if necessary. Starting short-term antimicrobial prophylactic therapy within 12 hours of the injury should be considered as directed by the location and origin of the bite wound, and tetanus immunization should be updated as needed (Table 4-7).

TABLE 4-7 Infectious Agents and Treatment in Bites

TYPE OF BITE	INFECTIVE AGENT	PROPHYLAXIS OR TREATMENT OF INFECTION
Bat, raccoon, skunk	Uncertain; streptococci and staphylococci from skin; significant rabies risk	For bacterial infection prevention/intervention Primary: Amoxicillin with clavulanate, 875 mg/125 mg BID or 500 mg/125 mg TID Alternative: Doxycycline, 100 mg BID Animal should be considered rabid, and patients should be given rabies immune globulin and vaccine and consider tetanus prophylaxis.
Cat	*Pasteurella multocida, S aureus*	Primary: Amoxicillin with clavulanate, 875 mg/125 mg BID 1000 mg/62.5 mg 2 tablets BID Alternative: cefuroxime, 0.5 g BID; doxycycline, 100 mg orally BID Switch to penicillin if *P multocida* is cultured from wound. Because 80% become infected, all wounds should be cultured and treated empirically.
Dog	*Pasteurella canis, S aureus,* streptococci, others	Primary: Amoxicillin with clavulanate, 875 mg/125 mg BID or 1000 mg/62.5 mg 2 tablets BID Alternative: Clindamycin, 300 mg QID, plus a fluoroquinolone; or clindamycin with TMP-SMX (children) Only 5% become infected. Treat only if bite is severe, or if significant comorbidity such as diabetes mellitus or immunosuppression.
Human	*Streptococcus viridans, Staphylococcus epidermidis, Corynebacterium, Eikenella corrodens, S aureus, Bacteroides* spp., *Peptostreptococcus*	Early, not yet infected: amoxicillin with clavulanate, 875 mg/125 mg BID for 5 days Later (3 to 24 hours, signs of infection): parenteral therapy with ampicillin with sulbactam, cefoxitin, others Penicillin allergy: Clindamycin with ciprofloxacin or TMP-SMX
Rat	*Streptobacillus moniliformis, Spirillum minus*	Primary: Amoxicillin with clavulanate, 875 mg/125 mg BID Alternative: doxycycline Rabies prophylaxis not indicated.
Pig or swine	Polymicrobial gram-positive cocci, gram-negative bacilli, anaerobes, *Pasteurella* spp.	Primary: Amoxicillin with clavulanate, 875 mg/125 mg BID Alternative: parenteral third-generation cephalosporin, others
Nonhuman primate	Herpesvirus simiae	Acyclovir or ganciclovir Valacyclovir (for postexposure prophylaxis)

TMP-SMX, trimethoprim-sulfamethoxazole.

Source: Gilbert DN, Chambers HF, Eliopoulos GM, Saag MS, Pavia AT. The Sanford Guide to Antimicrobial Therapy. 50th ed. Sperryville, VA: Antimicrobial Therapy, Inc.; 2020:53–54.

Surgical repair with percutaneous sutures can be performed for bites located on the face or scalp, simple wounds without underlying injury, and no immunocompromising conditions. As there is a higher risk of infection with surgical repair, wound closure should be avoided in immunocompromised individuals or wounds at high risk of infection.

The clinician should check with local authorities for information on rabies when a bite involves domestic pets; because the rabies risk in this situation is usually negligible, rabies prophylaxis is not indicated. In recent years, there has been an increase in cases of rabies domestically, primarily from bites by usually docile, often nocturnal wild animals that attack without provocation. These include bats, foxes, woodchucks, squirrels, and skunks. Human bites carry no rabies risk. If rabies prophylaxis is needed, this is often administered by or in conjunction with the local or regional public health authorities.

In all bite wounds, the patient's safety should be assessed. This is particularly important with human bites. If a child or other dependent person has been bitten by an adult, suspected abuse or neglect should be reported to the proper agency.

> **CLINICAL CONCEPT**
> Antimicrobial prophylaxis should be strongly considered for all cat bites, deep dog bite puncture wounds, bites involving an immunocompromised individual, hand wounds, and bites requiring surgical repair.

Discussion Sources

Ballentine JR. Human bites overview. emedicinehealth. http://www.emedicinehealth.com/human_bites/article_em.htm#human_bites_overview

Gilbert DN, Chambers HF, Eliopoulos GM, Saag MS, Pavia AT. *The Sanford Guide to Antimicrobial Therapy*. 50th ed. Sperryville, VA: Antimicrobial Therapy, Inc.; 2020:53–54.

QUESTIONS

62. A common infective agent in domestic pet cat bites is:

    A. viridans streptococcus species.

    B. *Pasteurella multocida*.

    C. *Bacteroides* species.

    D. *H influenzae*.

63. A 28-year-old woman presents to your practice with chief complaint of a cat bite sustained on her right ankle. Her pet cat had bitten her after she inadvertently stepped on its paw while she was in her home. Her cat is 3 years old, is up to date on immunizations, and does not go outside. Physical examination reveals pinpoint superficial puncture wounds on the right ankle consistent with the presenting history. She washed the wound with soap and water immediately and asks whether she needs additional therapy. Treatment for this patient's cat bite wound should include standard wound care with the addition of:

    A. oral erythromycin.

    B. topical bacitracin.

    C. oral amoxicillin-clavulanate.

    D. parenteral rifampin.

64. A 24-year-old man arrives at the walk-in center. He reports that while walking in the woods he was bitten on the ankle by a raccoon. The examination reveals a wound that is 1 cm deep on his right thigh. The wound is oozing bright red blood. Your next best action is to:

    A. administer high-dose parenteral penicillin.

    B. initiate antibacterial prophylaxis with oral amoxicillin.

    C. give rabies immune globulin and rabies vaccine.

    D. suture the wound after proper cleansing.

65. A significant rabies risk is associated with a bite from all of the following except:

    A. humans.

    B. foxes.

    C. bats.

    D. skunks.

66. You see a 33-year-old male with a minor dog bite on his hand. The examination reveals a superficial wound on the left palm. The dog is up to date on immunizations. In deciding whether to initiate antimicrobial therapy, you consider that _____ of dog bites become bacterially infected.

    A. 5%

    B. 20%

    C. 50%

    D. 75%

67. You see a 52-year-old woman who was bitten by a rat on her right hand while opening a dumpster. The examination reveals a wound approximately 1 cm deep that is oozing bright red blood. Treatment of this patient should include standard wound care with the addition of:

    A. rabies immune globulin.

    B. rabies vaccine.

    C. oral ciprofloxacin.

    D. oral amoxicillin-clavulanate.

68. You see a 28-year-old man who was involved in a fight approximately 1 hour ago with another adult. The patient states, "He bit me on the arm." Examination of the left forearm reveals an open wound consistent with this history. Your next best action is to:

    A. obtain a culture and susceptibility of the wound site.

    B. refer for rabies prophylaxis.

    C. irrigate the wound and débride as needed.

    D. close the wound with adhesive strips.

69. A 54-year-old man is brought in by the police to be evaluated for three human bites on his leg stemming from an altercation. He is alert, combative, and smells heavily of alcohol. Initial assessment should include:

    A. testing for blood alcohol content.

    B. waiting until the patient calms down for proper evaluation of the wounds.

    C. performing a multisystem survey to identify any other injuries.

    D. administration of antimicrobial prophylaxis.

For answers and rationales, see end of chapter.

Burn Wounds

Overview

Burn injuries are unfortunately common with nearly 500,000 Americans of all ages affected annually. Out of all who are burned, nearly 90% will be treated entirely as outpatients, with many presenting to urgent and primary care. Nearly one-half sustain burns from flame, approximately one-third from scalding by hot water, with the remaining burns caused by contact, electrical, chemical, and other reasons.

Among those requiring treatment at burn centers, the majority are male (68% versus 32% female), and the survival rate is very high at nearly 97%.

As with bites, burn intervention includes asking for a complete history of the events leading up to the injury to develop a plan for avoiding future events. In addition, education for burn avoidance for high-risk individuals for burn injury, such as children, elderly adults, and smokers, should be a routine part of primary care.

Clinical Presentation

Initial assessment of the person, regardless of age, with a burn injury should include a multisystem survey to evaluate for additional injuries and ensure that problems with respiration and/or circulation are addressed first. In the majority, the burn wound is the only injury.

> **CLINICAL CONCEPT**
> Approximately three-quarters of burn injuries occur in the home, with less than 10% in the workplace.

The burn should be assessed for the degree of skin and tissue injury:

■ First degree (*superficial*): Superficially red, somewhat painful, easily blanched, warm to touch
■ Second degree (*partial thickness*): Deeply red, blistered, swollen, hot to touch, raw, moist surface, very painful
■ Deep second degree (*deep partial thickness*): Involves deeper layers of dermis, appears white, does not blanch
■ Third degree (*full thickness*): Whitish, charred or translucent, not painful, affected area lacks pinprick sensation. However, third-degree burns are often surrounded by painful first- and second-degree burns.

It is important to estimate the BSA affected by the burn (Fig. 4-3). The palmar surface of the hand including the fingers represents a BSA of 1% throughout the life span and can provide a helpful guide in estimating the extent of a burn.

Diagnostic Testing

The burn diagnosis is made clinically by correlating health history with physical examination. Routine culture and susceptibility of the burn surface is not warranted. Indeed, the burn surface is likely sterile for the first 48 hours after injury. If infection ensues in a burn, consideration should be given for obtaining a culture and susceptibility.

Treatment

According to the American Burn Association, referral to a burn center for inpatient or outpatient care is recommended in the following situations:

■ Partial-thickness burns greater than 10% of total body surface area (TBSA), greater than 5% for children
■ Burns that involve the face, hands, feet, genitalia, perineum, major joints, and/or are circumferential
■ Third-degree burns in any age group
■ Electrical burns, including lightning injury
■ Chemical burns
■ Inhalation injury

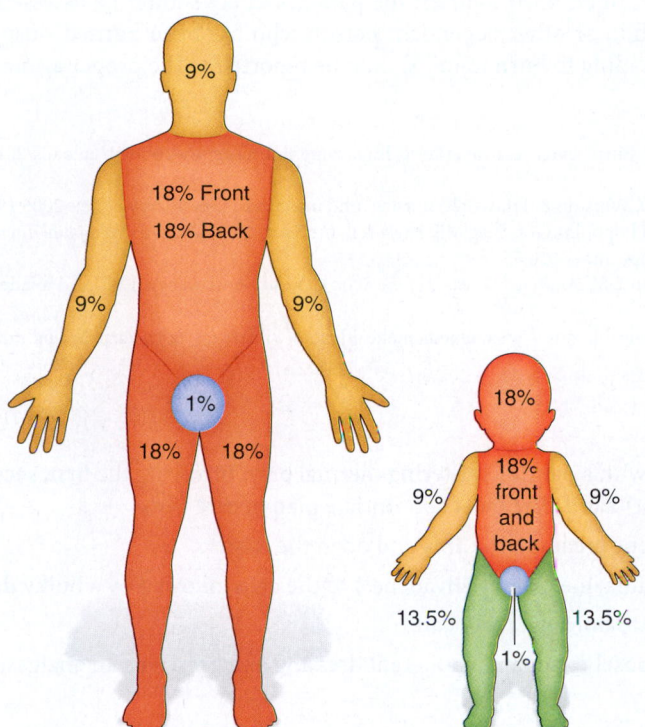

FIGURE 4-3 Rule of nines for calculating total burn surface area.
Capriotti T, Parker Frizzell J. Pathophysiology: Introductory Concepts and Clinical Perspectives. Philadelphia, PA: F.A. Davis; 2016.

■ Burn injury in patients with preexisting medical disorders that could complicate management, prolong recovery, or affect mortality, and/or significant concomitant injury
■ Burned children in hospitals without qualified personnel or equipment for the care of children
■ Burn injury in patients who will require special social, emotional, or rehabilitative intervention

Smaller (less than 10% of BSA), minor (second-degree or lower) burns not involving a high-function area such as the hand or foot and of minimal cosmetic consequence can be treated in the outpatient setting.

Gram-positive bacteria, such as *S aureus* or coagulase-negative streptococci, can colonize the burn area within 48 hours of injury unless a topical antimicrobial is used. Eventually, colonization with other gram-positive (e.g., enterococci) or gram-negative bacteria (i.e., *Pseudomonas aeruginosa*, *Escherichia coli*, *Klebsiella pneumoniae*) can occur. As a result, treatment options include prevention of infection by use of a topical antibiotic such as mafenide acetate (Sulfamylon®) or silver sulfadiazine (Silvadene®) or via specific dressings. One example of a lower-cost burn treatment is to use petroleum gauze dressing that provides protection to the affected area. Several commercially available dressings are available to help alleviate pain, provide antimicrobial coverage, and/or decrease healing time in burn therapy. These include absorptive dressings (e.g., Acquacel® Ag, DuoDERM®), nonabsorptive dressings (e.g., Xeroform®, Mepitel®, Acticoat™), or biocomposite dressings (e.g., Biobrane®). Systemic antibiotics for prophylaxis are generally not as effective as topical agents.

Outpatient management will require a capable family member or visiting nurse to evaluate, cleanse, and apply dressings to the wound. Patients should be educated on the proper method of changing dressings at home.

A follow-up visit should be scheduled the following day (within 24 hours) after the injury to assess pain management and the patient's competence with changing the dressing. Subsequent visits can be scheduled on a weekly basis until healing occurs, though daily assessments, particularly during the first week, might be needed if there is any concern the patient is not getting adequate care at home. Referral to a burn center or surgeon should be considered with wounds that worsen during the first 72 hours after injury or are causing significant scarring. Therapies to minimize scarring can include scar massage, compression garments, topical silicone, and corticosteroid injections. Occupational or physical therapy should be considered for patients with burns that extend over a joint that could lead to loss of function or range of motion.

In all burn injuries, the patient's safety should be assessed. In particular, for the child or other dependent person who has been burned, suspected abuse or neglect leading to burn injury should be reported to the proper agency.

> **CLINICAL CONCEPT**
>
> Ongoing monitoring with regular follow-up visits is needed to ensure adequate burn healing, while long-term follow-up care can include cosmetic or reconstructive surgery to diminish scarring or changes in pigmentation.

Discussion Sources

American Burn Association. Burn center referral criteria. http://ameriburn.org/wp-content/uploads/2017/05/burncenterreferral criteria.pdf

Church D, Elsayed S, Reid O, Winston B, Lindsay R. Burn wound infections. *Clin Microbiol Rev.* 2006:19:403–434.

Gilbert DN, Chambers HF, Eliopoulos GM, Saag MS, Pavia AT. *The Sanford Guide to Antimicrobial Therapy.* 50th ed. Sperryville, VA: Antimicrobial Therapy, Inc.; 2020:55.

James WD, Berger TG, Elston DM. *Andrews' Diseases of the Skin: Clinical Dermatology.* 12th ed. Philadelphia, PA: Elsevier; 2016:18–19.

Plantz SH. Burns. emedicinehealth. http://www.emedicinehealth.com/wilderness_burns/article_em.htm

QUESTIONS

70. A patient presents with a painful, blistering thermal burn involving the first, second, and third digits of his right (dominant) hand. The most appropriate plan of care is to:

  A. apply an anesthetic cream to the area and open the blisters.

  B. apply silver sulfadiazine cream (Silvadene®) to the area followed by a bulky dressing.

  C. refer the patient to burn specialty care.

  D. wrap the burn loosely with a nonadherent dressing and prescribe an analgesic agent.

71. Gram-negative bacteria that commonly cause burn wound infections include all of the following except:

  A. *P aeruginosa.*

  B. *E coli.*

C. *K pneumoniae.*

D. *H influenzae.*

72. Which of the following is the best option to prevent a burn wound infection in a 45-year-old otherwise well man with an approximately 8% BSA partial-thickness (second degree) burn on his trunk?

A. topical corticosteroid

B. topical silver sulfadiazine

C. oral erythromycin

D. oral moxifloxacin

73. You examine a patient with a red, tender thermal burn that involves the entire surface of the anterior right leg and that has excellent capillary refill. The estimated involved BSA is approximately:

A. 5%.

B. 9%.

C. 13%.

D. 18%.

74. A burn that is about twice as large as an adult's palmar surface of the hand including the fingers encompasses a BSA of approximately _____ %.

A. 1

B. 2

C. 3

D. 4

75 to 77. Match the following type of burn with the correct description.

_____ 75. First-degree burn

_____ 76. Second-degree burn

_____ 77. Third-degree burn

A. affected skin blanches with ease.

B. surface is raw and moist.

C. affected area is white and leathery.

78. A 45-year-old man with a second-degree burn on his upper thigh (2% BSA) is released for outpatient management of his burn wound. A follow-up visit should be scheduled within:

A. 24 hours.

B. 72 hours.

C. 1 week.

D. 3 weeks.

For answers and rationales, see end of chapter.

Atopic Dermatitis

Overview

Atopic dermatitis, or eczema, is one manifestation of a type I hypersensitivity reaction. This type of reaction results from immunoglobulin E (IgE) antibodies occupying receptor sites on mast cells. This causes a degradation of the mast cell and subsequent release of histamine, resulting in vasodilation, mucous gland stimulation, and tissue swelling. See Figure 4-4.

The atopy subgroup includes many common clinical conditions, such as allergic rhinitis, atopic dermatitis, allergic gastroenteropathy, and allergy-based asthma. Atopic diseases have a strong familial component

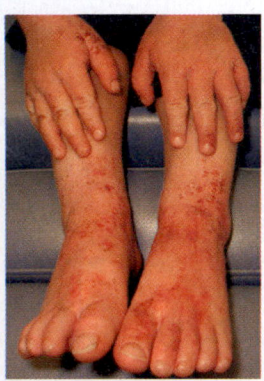

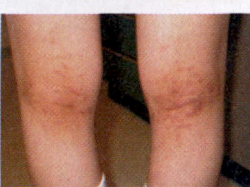

FIGURE 4-4 Atopic dermatitis.
Barankin B, Anatoli F. Derm Notes: Clinical Dermatology Pocket Guide. Philadelphia, PA: F.A. Davis; 2006.

CLINICAL CONCEPT

Type I hypersensitivity reactions are usually divided into two subgroups: atopy and anaphylaxis.

and tend to cause localized rather than systemic reactions. Individuals with atopic disease are often able to identify allergy-inducing agents. Allergic contact dermatitis is a form of eczematous dermatitis. Common causes of contact dermatitis include exposure to metals including nickel, rubber additives to shoes and gloves, some toiletries, and topical medications.

Clinical Presentation

A key symptom of atopic dermatitis is pruritus (itching). The disease typically has an intermittent course with flares and remissions occurring. The primary physical findings in atopic dermatitis include xerosis (dry skin), lichenification (from repeated rubbing or scratching the itchy skin lesions noted with eczema), and eczematous lesions. The eczematous changes and morphology can occur at various body sites and will depend on the age of the patient (i.e., infant, child, or adult). For example, in the infant and child, atopic dermatitis usually involves the face and neck; this distribution is rarely seen in the older child or adult. In any age, the flexor surfaces such as the antecubital fossa and popliteal space are involved, but the groin and axillary regions are spared.

Criteria for the diagnosis of atopic dermatitis include the presence of itching and subsequent scratching plus three or more of the following: red or inflamed rash, presence of excessive dryness/scaling, and location in skinfolds of arms or legs. With severe outbreaks, vesicles are often present. Additional findings include early age at initial onset (0 to 5 years). In infants and toddlers with atopic dermatitis, the diaper area, owing to the occlusive, damp environment, is usually spared.

When making a diagnosis of atopic dermatitis, other conditions to consider in the differential include lichen simplex chronicus, nummular dermatitis, plaque psoriasis, scabies, seborrheic dermatitis, and tinea corporis.

Diagnostic Testing

The diagnosis of atopic dermatitis is made clinically based on patient history and clinical presentation. The results of skin culture do not add to diagnosis or treatment, as this will typically lead to a finding of normal skin flora. With difficult-to-treat atopic dermatitis, particularly in the presence of concomitant allergic rhinitis and/or asthma, testing for specific allergens will occasionally prove helpful.

Treatment

Treatment for atopic dermatitis includes avoiding offending agents, minimizing skin dryness by limiting soap and water exposure, and using lubricants consistently. In general, the patient should be encouraged to treat the skin with care because it tends to be sensitive; the person with atopic dermatitis has an abnormal skin barrier that allows for loss of water and resulting dryness. When flares occur, the skin eruption is caused largely by histamine release. Oral antihistamines, topical and systemic corticosteroids, or both are typically used to control flares. Cool, wet dressings made from a clean cloth with cool water or Burow's solution (Domeboro®), a liquid preparation containing aluminum sulfate, acetic acid, precipitated calcium carbonate, and water, can be applied to the affected area for 30 minutes to provide significant symptom relief; application of an intermediate-potency topical corticosteroid is usually needed to control acute symptoms. After control of acute symptoms is achieved, the topical corticosteroid of lowest potency that yields the desired effect should be used (see Table 4-3).

Pimecrolimus (Elidel®) and tacrolimus (Protopic®) are immunomodulators that are helpful in the treatment of atopic dermatitis and offer an additional, noncorticosteroid option for atopic dermatitis. These products block T-cell stimulation by antigen-presenting cells and inhibit mast cell activation. Tacrolimus and pimecrolimus should be used only as labeled and only if other prescription and supportive treatments have failed to work or cannot be tolerated. These products should not be used in children younger than age 2 years. Crisaborole (Eucrisa®) is a topical phosphodiesterase-4 (PDE-4) inhibitor approved for mild-to-moderate atopic dermatitis in adults and children as young as 2 years of age. The ointment should be applied twice daily and is generally safe and well tolerated.

Several biological therapies are being used for the treatment of atopic dermatitis, including dupilumab (Dupixent®), a monoclonal antibody approved for the treatment of moderate-to-severe atopic dermatitis and delivered via subcutaneous injection. Given the cost of biologics, this class of therapy is usually limited to use when standard therapy has failed or is contraindicated in the treatment of atopic dermatitis.

Itch (pruritus) is a distressing symptom; many patients say it is more bothersome than pain. Pruritus is a cardinal symptom of many forms of dermatitis. Histamine contributes to the development of itching; the use of an antihistamine can provide relief. Pruritus tends to be worse at night, often causing sleep disturbance. In particular, providing the patient with a bedtime dose of antihistamine can yield tremendous relief from itching and improve sleep. Cetirizine (Zyrtec®) and levocetirizine are less-sedating antihistamines that are metabolites of hydroxyzine. Topical antihistamines have demonstrated little effect and are not recommended for atopic dermatitis.

> **CLINICAL CONCEPT**
> Oral hydroxyzine (Atarax®) and doxepin usually provide better relief of itching than other antihistamines.

Discussion Sources

James WD, Berger TG, Elston DM. *Andrews' Diseases of the Skin: Clinical Dermatology.* 12th ed. Philadelphia, PA: Elsevier; 2016:62–69.

Ong PY. Atopic dermatitis. In: Kellerman RD, Rakel DP, eds. *Conn's Current Therapy 2019.* Philadelphia, PA: Saunders; 2019:940–943.

Robertson D, Maibach H. Dermatologic pharmacology. In: Katzung, B, ed. *Katzung's Basic and Clinical Pharmacology.* 14th ed. New York, NY: McGraw-Hill Medical; 2018:1068–1086.

QUESTIONS

79. A mother brings to the clinic her 3-year-old daughter, who presents with dry red patches on her face around the eyes. The mother has observed her daughter constantly rubbing the area, which has caused swelling around the eyes. Physical examination is consistent with atopic dermatitis. The NP considers that this is a diagnosis that:

    A. requires a skin culture to confirm contributing bacterial organisms.

    B. should be supported by a biopsy of the affected area.

    C. necessitates obtaining peripheral blood eosinophil level.

    D. is usually made by clinical assessment alone.

80. Type I hypersensitivity reactions, such as atopic dermatitis, involve the action of which antibodies binding to receptor sites on mast cells?

    A. IgG

    B. IgM

    C. IgE

    D. IgA

81. During type I hypersensitivity reactions, histamine released from degraded mast cells causes all of the following except:

    A. vasodilation.

    B. mucous gland stimulation.

    C. enhanced sebum production.

    D. tissue swelling.

82. The most important aspect of skin care for individuals with atopic dermatitis is:

    A. frequent bathing with antibacterial soap.

    B. consistent use of medium-potency to high-potency topical steroids.

    C. application of lubricants.

    D. treatment of dermatophytes.

83. One of the most common trigger agents for contact dermatitis is:

    A. exposure to nickel.

    B. use of fabric softener.

    C. bathing with liquid body wash.

    D. eating spicy foods.

84. A common site for atopic dermatitis in teens or adults is on the:
   A. dorsum of the hand.
   B. face.
   C. neck.
   D. flexor surfaces.

85. A common site for atopic dermatitis in an infant is:
   A. the diaper area.
   B. the face.
   C. the neck.
   D. the posterior trunk.

86. In counseling a patient with atopic dermatitis, you suggest all of the following can be used to alleviate symptoms of a flare except:
   A. the use of oral antihistamines.
   B. applying a heating pad on the affected region for 30 minutes.
   C. the use of topical corticosteroids.
   D. applying cool, wet dressings made from a clean cloth and water to the affected area.

87 to 89. Match each description with the correct condition.
_____ 87. Atopic dermatitis
_____ 88. Scabies
_____ 89. Seborrheic dermatitis
   A. chronic, recurrent condition of greasy, scaly lesions on the scalp and nasolabial folds
   B. red, itchy, scaly skin appearing on the elbows
   C. new-onset vesicular lesions appearing along the waistline

90. The mechanism of action of pimecrolimus (Elidel®) in the treatment of atopic dermatitis is as:
   A. an immunomodulator.
   B. an antimitotic.
   C. a mast cell activator.
   D. an exfoliant.

91. When counseling a patient about the use of tacrolimus (Protopic®) or pimecrolimus (Elidel®), you mention that:
   A. this is the preferred atopic dermatitis treatment in infants.
   B. there is a possibility of increased cancer risk with its use.
   C. the product is used interchangeably with topical corticosteroids.
   D. the product is a potent antihistamine.

92. You see a 34-year-old man with atopic dermatitis localized primarily on the arms who complains of severe itching. The condition becomes worse at night and interferes with his sleep. You recommend:
   A. taking a bedtime dose of antihistamine.
   B. taking a bedtime dose of acetaminophen.
   C. taking a hot shower prior to bedtime.
   D. applying a warm compress to the affected areas 30 minutes prior to bedtime.

93. For which of the following patients with atopic dermatitis would the use of dupilumab (Dupixent®) be most appropriate?

   A. an 11-month-old with moderate disease on the face

   B. a 45-year-old with mild disease that responds well to cool compresses

   C. a 9-year-old with severe atopic dermatitis on legs and arms with only partial response to topical low-potency corticosteroids

   D. a 37-year-old with moderate disease on the legs with little response to medium-potency topical corticosteroids

For answers and rationales, see end of chapter.

Herpes Zoster

Overview

Herpes zoster infection, commonly known as shingles, is an acutely painful condition caused by the varicella-zoster virus, the same agent that causes chickenpox. The virus lies dormant in the dorsal root ganglia of a dermatome. When activated, the characteristic blistering lesions form.

Anyone who has had chickenpox is at risk for shingles, whereas recipients of varicella-zoster immunization have virtually no risk. Given that the varicella (chickenpox) vaccine started to be used widely in the United States in 1995, nearly everyone born prior to that date has a history of chickenpox and, therefore, is vulnerable to shingles. (See Chapter 2 for more information about chickenpox and the varicella vaccine.)

Shingles is usually seen in adults age 50 years and over, patients who are immunocompromised, and individuals with some other underlying health problem. When shingles is seen in younger adults, the possibility of immunocompromise should be considered. During the acute attack, the chickenpox (varicella-zoster) virus is shed; patients can transmit this infection.

Shingles is not communicable from person to person. Most patients with this condition will have only one episode; a significant percentage will have repeat episodes. Scarring and postherpetic neuralgia (PHN) are problematic sequelae of shingles.

Clinical Presentation

The clinical presentation of zoster is fairly characteristic. Prior to the onset of the skin lesions, the patient will report a 1- to 2-day prodrome (range 1 to 10 days, average 48 hours) with mild, nonspecific symptoms such as generalized body aches prior to the skin eruption, often accompanied by itch, burning, or other painful sensation where the lesion will eventually erupt. Depending on where on the body the zoster outbreak occurs, this prodrome often provides a clinical challenge as the pain location can be on the head, thorax, or lumbar sacral area.

The resulting pain is burning, throbbing, or stabbing; intense itch is also occasionally described. The thoracic dermatomes are the most commonly involved sites, followed by the lumbar dermatomes. Occasionally, regional lymphadenopathy is noted. See Figure 4-5. The rash usually resolves within 14 to 21 days with slowly developing crusting of lesions. Often, there is resulting scarring and/or changes in pigmentation at the site of the lesion.

Shingles involving the ocular dermatome (cranial nerve V, herpes zoster ophthalmicus [HZO]), accounting for approximately 10% to 15% of all patients with the condition, bears special mention. The prodromal symptoms are noted in and around the eye, and the clinical presentation usually includes a profound unilateral conjunctivitis, iritis, lid retraction, and ptosis. Expert ophthalmological consultation should be promptly sought to confirm the diagnosis of HZO and to provide careful treatment and follow-up to minimize the risk of vision loss.

CLINICAL CONCEPT

Zoster's characteristic blistering lesions, occurring along a dermatome, usually not crossing the midline, erupt after the prodrome.

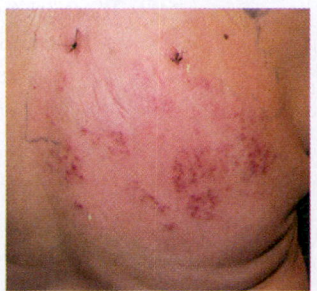
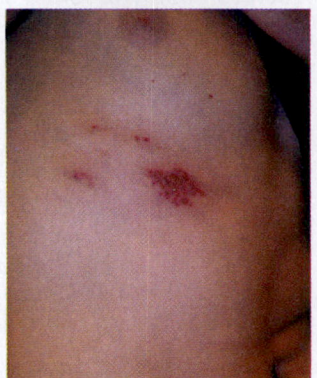

FIGURE 4-5 Herpes zoster (shingles). *Barankin B, Anatoli F. Derm Notes: Clinical Dermatology Pocket Guide. Philadelphia, PA: F.A. Davis; 2006.*

Diagnostic Testing

Diagnosis of shingles is usually straightforward because of its characteristic lesions. If confirmation is needed, a Tzanck smear reveals giant multinucleated cells, a finding in all herpetic infections.

Initiating antiviral therapy with high-dose acyclovir (Zovirax®), valacyclovir (Valtrex®), or famciclovir (Famvir®), preferably within the first 72 hours of herpes zoster outbreak, helps limit the severity of the lesions and minimizes the risk of PHN and scarring. During the acute stage of shingles, systemic corticosteroids are often prescribed along with antivirals. This combination therapy usually results in more rapid resolution of pain but not of zoster lesions.

Adequate analgesia should be offered to a person with shingles. Using topical agents such as topical lidocaine gel 5%, Burow's solution with a high-potency NSAID or opioid, or a combination of these helps provide considerable relief. In the case of shingles involving a body part where clothing could rub against the lesions, applying petroleum jelly (Vaseline) with a loose dressing, with the aim of protecting the rash from the friction of clothing, is often helpful in relieving the pain or itch associated with the condition.

The patient with shingles should also be monitored for superinfection of lesions. Because of the risk of complication and possible compromise of vision, expert consultation should be sought if herpes zoster involves a facial or ocular dermatome (see earlier discussion). When other areas of the body are involved, specialty consultation is usually not warranted.

PHN is defined as pain persisting at least 1 month after the rash has healed. Risk factors for the development of PHN include the site of initial involvement, with greatest risk if the outbreak involves the trigeminal or brachial plexus region; moderate risk with a thoracic outbreak; and lower risk with jaw, neck, sacral, and lumbar involvement. Additional risks include severe rash and intense prodromal pain.

The incidence of PHN increases dramatically with age, with only 4% of adults 30 to 50 years old reporting PHN and approximately 50% of adults older than 80 years reporting a shingles outbreak. Once the PHN pain is established, it can be difficult to alleviate, even with opioid medications. Tricyclic antidepressants (e.g., amitriptyline, nortriptyline), gabapentin (Neurontin®), pregabalin (Lyrica®), and topical lidocaine patches can offer some relief and are often used in the treatment of postherpetic neuralgia. Topical capsaicin can also be helpful although this needs to be applied at least five times daily.

Prevention

There are two vaccines currently available for shingles. Zostavax® (ZVL) is a live vaccine that was approved in 2006 and has been shown to provide protection for about 5 years and is about 50% effective in preventing shingles. It is given as a single dose to adults 60 years and older. Since Zostavax® is a live virus vaccine, it is contraindicated for those with immunosuppression or immunodeficiency (including those living with HIV, taking immunosuppressive medications, undergoing radiation or chemotherapy, or with leukemia or lymphoma) as well as during pregnancy. Shingrix (RZV) is a recombinant zoster vaccine that has become more recently available and is the preferred vaccine by the Advisory Committee on Immunization Practices (ACIP) due to its greater immunogenicity with nearly 100% efficacy in preventing shingles, less contraindications, and potentially longer duration of protection. The vaccine is recommended for immunocompetent adults 50 years and older and is given in two doses separated by 2 to 6 months. ZVL is no longer used.

The zoster vaccine should still be given to individuals who have had shingles, though vaccination should be delayed until an acute episode of shingles resolves, usually within 8 weeks after the onset of lesions.

> **CLINICAL CONCEPT**
> Individuals who already received Zostavax® should also receive Shingrix® for full protection against shingles.

Discussion Sources

James WD, Berger TG, Elston DM. *Andrews' Diseases of the Skin: Clinical Dermatology.* 12th ed. Philadelphia, PA: Elsevier; 2016:372–376.

Janniger CK. Herpes zoster. Medscape. http://emedicine.medscape.com/article/1132465-overview

McElveen WA. Postherpetic neuralgia. Medscape. http://emedicine.medscape.com/article/1143066-overview

QUESTIONS

94. A 48-year-old woman living with HIV presents with a chief complaint of a 2-day history of painful, itchy rash on her trunk consistent with the diagnosis of shingles. The NP expects to find:

   A. linear vesicular lesions that do not cross the midline and are distributed over the posterior thorax.

   B. generalized vesicular lesions with crusting.

C. scattered umbilicated lesions over the posterior thorax.

D. slightly raised honey-colored plaques on the anterior thorax.

95. A diagnosis of herpes zoster is typically made:

A. clinically.

B. following a Tzanck smear.

C. following culture and susceptibility testing.

D. with biopsy of the lesion.

96. Shingles most commonly involve the dermatomes of the:

A. legs and pubic area.

B. face.

C. upper arms and shoulders.

D. thorax.

97. When caring for an adult with an outbreak of shingles, you advise that:

A. there is no known treatment for this condition.

B. during outbreaks, the chickenpox (varicella) virus is shed.

C. although they are acutely painful, the lesions heal well without scarring or lingering discomfort.

D. this condition commonly strikes young and old alike.

98. Analgesia options for a patient with shingles can include all of the following except:

A. topical lidocaine gel 5% with oral acetaminophen.

B. Burow's solution with a high-potency oral NSAID.

C. applying a protective dressing with petroleum jelly and short-term use of an oral opioid.

D. fentanyl transdermal patch and a topical medium-potency corticosteroid on the affected area.

99. Risk factors for the development of PHN include:

A. age younger than 50 years at the time of the outbreak.

B. severe prodromal symptoms.

C. lumbar location of lesions.

D. low volume of lesions.

100. Treatment options in PHN include all of the following except:

A. injectable methylprednisolone.

B. oral pregabalin.

C. oral nortriptyline.

D. topical lidocaine.

101. All of the following are potentially serious complications associated with shingles except:

A. condyloma acuminatum.

B. PHN.

C. permanent vision loss.

D. encephalitis.

102 to 105. Indicate (Yes or No) whether each of the following individuals is eligible to receive the Shingrix vaccine.

_____ **102.** A 57-year-old man who reports he never had chickenpox as a child

_____ **103.** A 33-year-old woman who is trying to conceive her first child

_____ **104.** A 62-year-old man living with HIV

_____ **105.** A 66-year-old who received the Zostavax vaccine 1 year ago

106. Which of the following statements regarding Shingrix and Zostavax® is false?

    A. Zostavax® contains live virus while Shingrix does not.

    B. Both Shingrix and Zostavax® are given as a single dose.

    C. Shingrix induces greater immunogenicity compared to Zostavax®.

    D. There are more contraindications with Zostavax® compared with Shingrix.

For answers and rationales, see end of chapter.

Onychomycosis

Overview

Onychomycosis, or dermatophytosis of the nail, is found in the toenails or fingernails and can involve the nail matrix, nail bed, and/or nail plate. While onychomycosis is not a life-threatening condition, this is a chronic disfiguring disorder where nail discomfort is commonly reported. In addition, the psychological stress of having an altered nail appearance is considerable.

> **CLINICAL CONCEPT**
>
> Particularly with comorbid conditions such as diabetes mellitus, onychomycosis complications can include cellulitis, osteomyelitis, and tissue necrosis.

Clinical Presentation

The patient with onychomycosis usually presents after many months of altered nail appearance and often after trying a number of home or over-the-counter remedies without success. The nails are dull, thickened, and lusterless with a pithy consistency. Parts of the nail often break off.

In distal lateral subungual onychomycosis, the nail has a yellow-white appearance due to subungual hyperkeratosis and onycholysis. Endonyx onychomycosis has a milky white discoloration of the nail plate but without subungual hyperkeratosis. Total dystrophic onychomycosis is characterized by a thickened, opaque, and yellow-brown nail. Other conditions that can mimic onychomycosis include contact dermatitis, nail psoriasis, traumatic onycholysis, and lichens planus.

Diagnostic Testing

Because trauma and other conditions can cause a similar appearance, confirmation of the diagnosis with microscopic examination for hyphae of the nail scrapings mixed with potassium hydroxide (KOH) is important, although it has a high rate of false-negative results. Fungal cultures should be obtained from pulverized nail scrapings or clippings. Newer approaches involve polymerase chain reaction (PCR) analysis to detect fungal DNA from infected nails. Dermoscopy can be used to help differentiate distal subungual onychomycosis from traumatic injury. In fungal infection, there would be an irregular margin with yellow-white spikes that project into the proximal nail plate.

Treatment

Oral antifungals such as itraconazole (Sporanox®), terbinafine (Lamisil®), and fluconazole (Diflucan®) offer well-tolerated, effective treatment for fingernail and toenail fungal infections. These medications can be used in pulse cycles, with times of drug use alternating with abstinent periods. An example of pulse dosing in onychomycosis therapy is itraconazole, 400 mg daily, for the first week of the month for 2 months to treat the fingernails and for 3 months to treat the toenails. The products are held within the nail matrix for months after therapy; this produces effective treatment at a considerably reduced cost compared with constant therapy. In addition, all oral antifungals have hepatotoxic potential and can cause an increase in hepatic enzyme levels. Pulse therapy reduces this risk considerably, though a transient but clinically insignificant increase in hepatic enzyme levels can occur. For patients taking oral antifungal medications, complete blood count (CBC) and hepatic enzyme levels should be evaluated every 4 to 6 weeks. Oral agents such as griseofulvin require months of therapy with a high rate of relapse.

The use of itraconazole is limited due to a number of clinically significant drug-drug interactions. Itraconazole is a potent inhibitor of cytochrome P450 3A4, a pathway also used by up to 50% of all prescription drugs including diazepam, digoxin, anticoagulants, and certain HIV protease inhibitors. Its use is contraindicated with concomitant use of several medications, including ergotamines, cisapride, lovastatin, simvastatin, and ticagrelor, and should be used with caution with many other medications. In addition, fluconazole is a cytochrome P450 2CP inhibitor, a pathway also used by drugs such as carbamazepine, some benzodiazepines, and calcium channel blockers. The concomitant use of these antifungals with the aforementioned medications can lead to significant drug interactions. Terbinafine has significantly less drug interaction potential.

Laser therapy has been used to treat onychomycosis, though compelling evidence on its efficacy is still lacking. Photodynamic therapy has demonstrated some beneficial effects though well-controlled studies are still needed. Surgical approaches can include mechanical, chemical, or surgical nail aversion and can be considered as adjunctive therapy for those taking oral antifungal treatment.

Topical treatments often prove to be ineffective because the antifungal agent is held within the nail matrix. Nail lacquers consist of an antifungal agent (e.g., ciclopirox or amorolfine) in a clear, stable, film-forming lacquer vehicle. When applied to the nails, these products provide a hard, clear, water-resistant film containing the antifungal agent. However, the effectiveness of these products in treating nail fungal infections is limited, usually helpful when a small percentage of the nail is impacted, and typically poorer than oral antifungal agents. Topical over-the-counter creams and medications, such as Vicks VapoRub®, thymol oil, and tree tea oil, are usually not effective as the nails are too thick and hard for external applications to penetrate to the site of infection.

Discussion Sources

Gilbert DN, Chambers HF, Eliopoulos GM, Saag MS, Pavia AT. *The Sanford Guide to Antimicrobial Therapy*. 50th ed. Sperryville, VA: Antimicrobial Therapy, Inc.; 2020:132.

James WD, Berger TG, Elston DM. *Andrews' Diseases of the Skin: Clinical Dermatology*. 12th ed. Philadelphia, PA: Elsevier; 2016:285–318.

Robertson D, Mailbach H. Dermatologic pharmacology. In: Katzung B, ed. *Katzung's Basic and Clinical Pharmacology*. 14th ed. New York, NY: McGraw-Hill Medical; 2018:1068–1086.

Tosti A. Onychomycosis. Medscape. http://emedicine.medscape.com/article/1105828-overview

QUESTIONS

107. Characteristics of onychomycosis include all of the following except:

A. it is readily diagnosed by clinical examination.

B. nail hypertrophy.

C. brittle nails.

D. white to yellow nail discoloration.

108. Oral antifungal treatment options for onychomycosis include all of the following except:

A. itraconazole.

B. fluconazole.

C. metronidazole.

D. terbinafine.

109. When considering pulse dosing of fluconazole, all of the following are accurate except that it:

A. reduces the risk of adverse effects.

B. reduces the cost of treatment.

C. shortens the duration of treatment.

D. alternates periods of treatment with abstinent periods.

110. When prescribing pulse dosing with an oral antifungal for the treatment of fingernail fungus, the clinician realizes that:

A. a transient but clinically insignificant increase in hepatic enzymes is occasionally seen with its use.

B. drug-induced leukopenia is a common problem.

C. the patient needs to be warned about excessive bleeding because of the drug's antiplatelet effect.

D. its use is contraindicated in the presence of iron deficiency anemia.

111. When considering laser therapy for the treatment of onychomycosis, the NP realizes that:

A. its benefits have been clearly demonstrated in clinical trials.

B. there is a lack of compelling evidence supporting its use.

C. this technique is more effective than oral antifungal therapy.

D. laser therapy is contraindicated with concomitant topical antifungal therapy.

112. Diagnostic tests that can be used to support a diagnosis of onychomycosis include all of the following except:

A. potassium hydroxide test of nail scrapings.

B. fungal culture of pulverized nail scrapings.

C. blood culture.

D. dermoscopy.

113. In counseling a patient on the use of topical products to treat nail fungal infections, the NP considers that:

A. nail lacquers, such as ciclopirox olamine 8% solution (Penlac®), offer similar effectiveness to oral antifungals.

B. some herbal products, such as tea tree oil, can be an effective alternative to oral agents.

C. topical products have limited penetration through the nail matrix to reach the site of infection.

D. cream-based products are more effective than gel-based products in treating nail fungal infections.

For answers and rationales, see end of chapter.

Scabies

Overview

Scabies is a communicable skin disease caused by infestation with a host-specific mite. To achieve contagion, close personal, skin-to-skin contact is needed. Contact with used, unwashed bedding and clothing from an affected person also can result in infection.

Clinical Presentation

The scabies lesions often start with the characteristic burrows but in most cases progress to a vesicular or papular form, usually with excoriation caused by scratching.

The patient's age contributes to where scabies lesions are found, in that the older adult often has excoriated lesions on the back, while infants and younger children commonly have lesions on the palms and soles. Nodular lesions are often seen, especially in younger children. Scaling, crusting, and excoriation can also be seen, particularly in scabies infestation that has been present for a number of weeks.

> **CLINICAL CONCEPT**
> The mites that cause scabies tend to burrow in areas of warmth, such as the finger webs, axillary folds, belt line, areolae, scrotum, penis, and under the breasts, with lesions developing and clustering in these areas.

Diagnostic Testing

The diagnosis of scabies is made clinically by health history and physical examination, noting the characteristic lesions and their distribution. The diagnosis can be confirmed by microscopic examination of skin scrapings, where the mites, larvae, ova, and feces are identified.

Treatment

Permethrin (Elimite®) lotion is the preferred method of treatment for scabies. The lotion must be left on for 8 to 14 hours to be effective; at that time, the patient should shower or bathe.

Despite effective therapy, individuals with scabies often have a significant problem with pruritus after permethrin treatment because of the presence of dead mites and their waste trapped in the skin, which causes an inflammatory reaction. This debris is eliminated from the body over a few weeks; the distress of itchiness passes at that time. Oral antihistamines, particularly for nighttime use, and low-potency to medium-potency topical corticosteroids should be offered to help with this problem (see Table 4-3). In the past, lindane (Kwell®) was used, but the use of this product presents potential problems with neurotoxicity and a resulting seizure risk and lower efficacy. Lindane should not be used by pregnant women, children, and elderly patients.

Bedclothes and other items used by a person with scabies must be either washed in hot water or placed in the clothes dryer for a normal cycle. Alternatively, items can be placed in plastic storage bags for at least 1 week because mites do not survive for more than 3 to 4 days without contact with the host.

Discussion Sources

Barry M. Scabies. Medscape. http://emedicine.medscape.com/article/1109204-overview

Gunning K, Pippitt K, Kiraly B, et al. Pediculosis and scabies: treatment update. *Am Fam Physician*. 2012;86(86):535–541.

James WD, Berger TG, Elston DM. *Andrews' Diseases of the Skin: Clinical Dermatology*. 12th ed. Philadelphia, PA: Elsevier; 2016:445–447.

QUESTIONS

114. A 78-year-old resident of a long-term care facility complains of generalized itchiness at night that disturbs her sleep. Her examination is consistent with scabies. Which of the following do you expect to find on examination?

    A. excoriated papules on the interdigital area

    B. annular lesions over the buttocks

    C. vesicular lesions in a linear pattern

    D. honey-colored crusted lesions that began as vesicles

115. In counseling a patient with scabies, the NP recommends all of the following methods to eliminate the mite from bedclothes and other items except:

    A. washing items in hot water.

    B. running items through the clothes dryer for a normal cycle.

    C. soaking items in cold water with bleach for at least 1 hour.

    D. placing items in a plastic storage bag for at least 1 week.

116. Which of the following represents the most accurate patient information when using permethrin (Elimite®) for treating scabies?

    A. To avoid systemic absorption, the medication should be applied over the body and rinsed off within 1 hour.

    B. The patient should notice a marked reduction in pruritus within 48 hours of using the product.

    C. Itch often persists for a few weeks after successful treatment.

    D. It is a second-line product in the treatment of scabies.

117. When advising the patient about scabies contagion, you inform her that:

    A. mites can live for many weeks away from the host.

    B. close personal contact with an infected person is usually needed to contract this disease.

    C. casual contact with an infected person is likely to result in infestation.

    D. bedding used by an infected person must be destroyed.

118. The use of lindane (Kwell®) to treat scabies is discouraged because of its potential for:

    A. hepatotoxicity.

    B. neurotoxicity.

    C. nephrotoxicity.

    D. pancreatitis.

For answers and rationales, see end of chapter.

Psoriasis Vulgaris

Overview

Psoriasis vulgaris is a chronic skin disorder caused by accelerated mitosis and rapid cell turnover, which lead to decreased maturation and keratinization. This process prevents the dermal cells from "sticking" together, allowing for a shedding of cells in the form of characteristic silvery scales and leaving an underlying red plaque. Genetic and immunological factors contribute to the development of psoriasis; there is likely an environmental and emotional factor where psoriasis often flares or worsens during extremes in weather as well as with physical or psychological stress. Psoriasis is more common in women, a characteristic of other autoimmune diseases.

Psoriasis severity is classified by BSA involved.

- Mild: Less than 2% BSA involved
- Moderate: 3% to 10% of BSA involved
- Severe: Greater than 10% BSA involved

> **CLINICAL CONCEPT**
>
> Forcible removal of psoriatic plaques can result in pinpoint bleeding, known as the Auspitz sign.

Clinical Presentation

Psoriasis is typically found in extensor surfaces; the lesions are most often found in plaques over the elbows and knees (see Fig. 4-6). The scalp and other surfaces are occasionally involved.

This is a common but not specific sign of psoriasis, as it is found with other dermatological conditions such as seborrheic dermatitis. Psoriasis vulgaris is the most common type and can involve the scalp, extensor surfaces, genitals, umbilicus, and lumbosacral and retroauricular regions. Plaque psoriasis commonly encompasses the extensor surfaces of the knees, elbows, scalp, and trunk. Guttate psoriasis mainly affects the trunk and typically appears 2 to 3 weeks following an upper respiratory tract infection caused by group A beta-hemolytic streptococci. Psoriasis can involve the ocular region and result in conjunctivitis, conjunctival hyperemia, corneal dryness, and blepharitis. One in five individuals with psoriasis will develop psoriatic arthritis.

Other conditions to consider in the differential diagnosis can include blepharitis, allergic contact dermatitis, cutaneous squamous cell carcinoma, lichen planus, nummular dermatitis, onychomycosis, pityriasis rosea, and seborrheic dermatitis.

Diagnostic Testing

The diagnosis of psoriasis is made by patient history, risk factors including family history of psoriasis, and physical examination. In cases with suspected psoriatic arthritis, testing can be done to differentiate this condition with rheumatoid arthritis and gout. With psoriatic arthritis, rheumatoid factor is negative, erythrocyte sedimentation rate is normal, and uric acid level can be elevated (which can cause some confusion with gout). X-rays of the joints can also be helpful in making a diagnosis of psoriatic arthritis. Findings suggestive of psoriatic arthritis include pencil-in-cup deformity and joint-space narrowing in the interphalangeal joints.

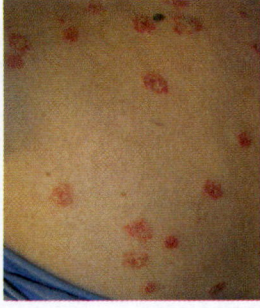 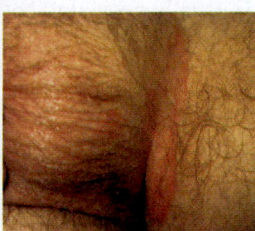 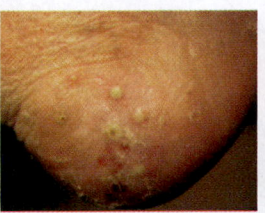 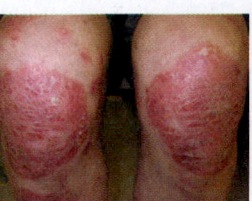

FIGURE 4-6 Psoriasis.
Barankin B, Anatoli F. Derm Notes: Clinical Dermatology Pocket Guide. Philadelphia, PA: F.A. Davis; 2006.

Treatment

Topical corticosteroids are the first-line treatment choice for mild psoriasis and when a limited area is affected. These agents have anti-inflammatory and mild antimitotic activity, which allows for regression of psoriatic plaques. A common psoriasis treatment plan is to use a medium-potency to high-potency drug for short periods until the plaques resolve and then to use a lower-potency product three to four times a week to maintain remission. Ocular corticosteroid solutions can be used with ophthalmic involvement. As with all dermatoses, consistent use of high-potency topical steroids is discouraged because of potential risk of skin atrophy, telangiectasia formation, corticosteroid-induced acne, and striae. In addition, the extensive use of topical corticosteroids leads to significant systemic absorption and potential subclinical adrenal function suppression. Tar preparations can be helpful, but these products have a low level of patient acceptance because of their messiness and odor. Coal tar is available OTC and can be found in shampoos, lotions, creams, or foams.

Additional treatment options include use of anthralin (Drithocreme®), a topical antimitotic, and calcipotriene, a topical vitamin D_3 derivative. Although offering effective psoriasis therapy, these products are significantly more expensive than topical corticosteroids and tars. Use should be reserved for corticosteroid-resistant conditions. Tazarotene is a topical retinoid prodrug that can control cell proliferation of the epithelial tissue and has some anti-inflammatory and immunomodulatory activity.

If psoriasis is generalized, covering more than 30% of BSA, treatment with topical products is difficult and expensive. Ultraviolet A light exposure three times per week is highly effective but is associated with an increase in skin cancer risk and photoaging. For severe, recalcitrant psoriasis, cyclosporine, methotrexate (particularly with arthritis), systemic retinoids, and newer biological agents such as tumor necrosis factor (TNF) modulators etanercept (Enbrel®), infliximab (Remicade), or adalimumab (Humira®) are also used. TNF-α is a proinflammatory cytokine that amplifies inflammation through various pathways and has been implicated in psoriasis pathogenesis. TNF-α antagonists bind to the cytokine and block its proinflammatory action. Although these biological agents can be effective in treating psoriasis, they are associated with significant adverse effects, including injection site and infusion reactions, infection, and reactivation of latent tuberculosis. The risk of infection is highest in patients with predisposing conditions, such as diabetes, heart failure, or concomitant use of immunosuppressive drugs. Other agents include the phosphodiesterase-4 enzyme inhibitor apremilast (Otezla®) for moderate-to-severe plaque psoriasis, as well as a growing list of interleukin inhibitors (secukinumab [Cosentyx®], ixekizumab [Taltz®], brodalumab (Siliq™], and ustekinumab [Stelara®]). Referral to a dermatology specialist is warranted when a patient has severe disease or has milder disease but fails to respond to standard therapy.

Discussion Sources

James WD, Berger TG, Elston DM. *Andrews' Diseases of the Skin: Clinical Dermatology.* 12th ed. Philadelphia, PA: Elsevier; 2016:185–198.

Meffert J, O'Connor RE. Psoriasis. Medscape. http://emedicine.medscape.com/article/1943419-overview

Robertson D, Maibach H. Dermatologic pharmacology. In: Katzung, B, ed. *Katzung's Basic and Clinical Pharmacology.* 14th ed. New York, NY: McGraw-Hill Medical; 2018:1068–1086.

Taheri A, Feldman SR. Biologics in practice: how effective are biologics? *Dermatologist.* 2012;20(11):34–37.

Weger W. Current status and new developments in the treatment of psoriasis and psoriatic arthritis with biological agents. *Br J Pharmacol.* 2010;160:810–820.

QUESTIONS

119. Psoriasis vulgaris is a chronic skin disease caused by:

    A. bacterial colonization.

    B. absence of melanin.

    C. accelerated mitosis.

    D. type I hypersensitivity reaction.

120. You examine a patient with a classic presentation of psoriasis vulgaris and expect to find the following lesions:

    A. lichenified areas in flexor areas.

    B. well-demarcated plaques on the knees.

C. greasy lesions throughout the scalp.

D. vesicular lesions over the upper thorax.

121. Psoriatic lesions arise from:

A. decreased skin exfoliation.

B. rapid skin cell turnover, leading to decreased maturation and keratinization.

C. inflammatory changes in the dermis.

D. lichenification.

122. When considering a diagnosis of psoriatic arthritis, all of the following tests can be helpful in differentiating from other conditions except:

A. rheumatoid factor.

B. erythrocyte sedimentation rate.

C. X-ray.

D. dual-energy X-ray absorptiometry.

123. Treatment options in generalized psoriasis vulgaris include all of the following except:

A. psoralen with ultraviolet A light (PUVA) therapy.

B. methotrexate.

C. cyclosporine.

D. systemic corticosteroids.

124. Which of the following is most accurate regarding the Auspitz sign?

A. This sign is specific for psoriasis vulgaris.

B. The sign is seen only in patients with psoriasis with concomitant psoriatic arthritis.

C. The sign is observed when pinpoint bleeding occurs when scales are forcibly removed.

D. The sign is needed to confirm a diagnosis of psoriasis.

125. The most appropriate use of biological agents in the management of psoriasis is:

A. as preventive therapy in those at high risk of disease.

B. for treatment of mild disease on a small affected area.

C. for treatment of moderate disease that responds well to methotrexate.

D. for treatment of moderate-to-severe disease with inadequate response to other medications.

126. For severe, recalcitrant psoriasis that affects more than 30% of the body, all of the following treatments are recommended except:

A. methotrexate.

B. topical anthralin (Drithocreme®).

C. TNF modulators.

D. cyclosporine.

127. The use of TNF modulators for the treatment of psoriasis is associated with an increased risk for:

A. gastrointestinal disorders.

B. nephrotoxicity.

C. QTc prolongation.

D. reactivation of latent tuberculosis.

For answers and rationales, see end of chapter.

Seborrheic Dermatitis

Overview

Seborrheic dermatitis is a chronic, recurrent skin condition found in areas with a high concentration of sebaceous glands, such as the scalp, eyelid margins, nasolabial folds, ears, and upper trunk. See Figure 4-7. Numerous theories are proposed for its cause. Seborrheic dermatitis is most likely caused by an inflammatory reaction to *Malassezia* species (formerly *Pityrosporum* species), a yeast form that is present on the scalp of all humans. Further supporting this hypothesis is the fact that seborrhea is often found in patients who are immunocompromised or chronically ill (e.g., elderly adults and people with Parkinson disease). *Malassezia* organisms are likely a cofactor linked to T-cell depression, increased sebum levels, and an activation of the alternative complement pathway.

Clinical Presentation

Lesions can be distributed over the oily and hair-bearing areas of the head, neck, and chest. Lesions can range from mild, patchy scaling to widespread distribution with thick, adherent crusts. Scaling can be present over red, inflamed skin with hypopigmentation, oozing, and crusting.

Diagnostic Testing

Diagnosis is usually made clinically based on a history of waxing and waning in severity and the distribution of lesions. Laboratory testing is not typically needed, though a fungal culture can be performed to rule out tinea capitis in children.

Treatment

Skin lesions associated with seborrhea usually respond to topical antifungals such as ketoconazole, further supporting the hypothesis that fungi contribute to the disease process. Class IV or lower corticosteroid creams, lotions, or solutions are also helpful during a seborrheic flare (see Table 4-3); topical immune modulators such as pimecrolimus and tacrolimus, sulfur or sulfonamide combinations, and propylene glycol offer additional treatment options. Coal tar shampoo can be used as a keratolytic. The use of lubricants such as petroleum jelly can help remove stubborn lesions so that the lesions can be exposed to antifungal therapy (e.g., selenium sulfide or ketoconazole shampoo). However, excessively oily or greasy products should not be used to treat the scalp as patient adherence to these products is low. Systemic ketoconazole or fluconazole is occasionally used if seborrheic dermatitis is severe or unresponsive. Biological agents are not indicated for the treatment of seborrheic dermatitis.

As with any skin condition, high-potency topical corticosteroid use is discouraged because of the risk of subcutaneous atrophy, telangiectatic vessels, and other problems. Although seborrhea usually worsens in the winter and improves in the summer, exposing lesions to sunlight is not recommended because of the potential increase in skin cancer risk and photoaging.

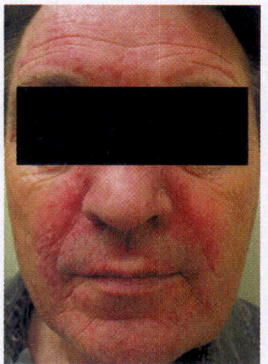
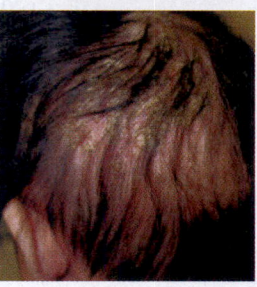

FIGURE 4-7 Seborrheic dermatitis. *Barankin B, Anatoli F. Derm Notes: Clinical Dermatology Pocket Guide. Philadelphia, PA: F.A. Davis; 2006.*

> **CLINICAL CONCEPT**
>
> In young children, cradle cap is a common form of seborrhea, while the diaper area is usually spared.

Discussion Sources

Schmidt JA. Seborrheic dermatitis: a clinical practice snapshot. *Nurse Pract.* 2011;36(8):32–37.
Selden ST. Seborrheic dermatitis. Medscape. http://emedicine.medscape.com/article/1108312-overview

QUESTIONS

128. Seborrheic dermatitis is most likely caused by:

A. accelerated mitosis of skin cells.

B. colonization of skin by *S aureus*.

C. an inflammatory reaction to *Malassezia* species on skin.

D. exposure to excessive ultraviolet (UV) radiation.

129. Which of the following best describes seborrheic dermatitis lesions?

  A. flaking lesions in the antecubital and popliteal spaces

  B. greasy, scaling lesions in the nasolabial folds

  C. intensely itchy lesions in the groin folds

  D. silvery lesions on the elbows and knees

130. Among the following, who is at greatest risk of developing seborrheic dermatitis?

  A. a 15-year-old boy residing in a rural setting

  B. a 34-year-old woman who smokes two packs per day (PPD)

  C. a 48-year-old male truck driver

  D. a 72-year-old man with Parkinson's disease

131. In counseling a patient with seborrheic dermatitis on the scalp about efforts to clear lesions, you advise her to:

  A. use ketoconazole shampoo.

  B. apply petroleum jelly nightly to the affected area.

  C. coat the area with high-potency corticosteroid cream three times a week.

  D. expose the lesions periodically to heat by carefully using a hair dryer.

132. A 64-year-old man with seborrhea mentions that his skin condition is "better in the summer when he gets outside more and much worse in the winter." You respond:

  A. sun exposure is a recommended therapy for the treatment of this condition.

  B. although sun exposure is noted to improve the skin lesions associated with seborrhea, its use as a therapy is potentially associated with an increased rate of skin cancer and photoaging.

  C. the lower humidity in the summer months noted in many areas of North America contributes to the improvement in seborrheic lesions.

  D. use high-potency topical corticosteroids during the winter months, tapering these off for the summer months.

133. You see a 67-year-old man with seborrheic dermatitis that has failed to respond to treatment with ketoconazole shampoo. An appropriate second-line treatment option can include all of the following except:

  A. oral fluconazole.

  B. a topical immune modulator.

  C. topical propylene glycol.

  D. TNF-α inhibitor.

134. All of the following regarding seborrheic dermatitis in a young child are accurate except:

  A. most frequently occurs on the scalp.

  B. requires referral to an infectious disease specialist for a child under 2 years of age.

  C. the condition is usually self-limiting.

  D. the diaper area is typically spared.

For answers and rationales, see end of chapter.

Skin Cancer

Overview

As with any area of dermatology, accurate diagnosis of a condition depends on knowledge of the description of the lesion and its most likely site of occurrence. The most potent risk factor for any skin cancer is sun exposure; patients should be instructed on sun avoidance.

Sunscreen use likely does little to minimize malignant melanoma risk. However, a history of five or more blistering sunburns before the age of 20 years can increase the risk of malignant melanoma by 80%.

Clinical Presentation

Skin examination has the benefit of enabling the examiner to detect premalignant lesions (e.g., actinic keratoses and other precursor lesions to squamous cell carcinoma including keratoacanthoma) and malignant lesions.

Malignant melanoma is a malignancy that arises from melanocytes, cells that make the pigment melanin, and is the most common fatal dermatological malignancy. "ABCDE" is a mnemonic for assessing malignant melanoma (see Fig. 4-8):

A = Asymmetric with nonmatching sides
B = Borders are irregular
C = Color is not uniform; brown, black, red, white, blue
D = Diameter usually larger than 6 mm, or the size of a pencil eraser
E = Evolving lesions, either new or changing (most melanomas manifest as new lesions)

The characteristics of basal cell carcinoma (BCC) include a long latency period and low metastatic risk. Depending on lesion location, untreated BCC can lead to significant deformity and possibly altered function. See Figure 4-9. As a result, early recognition and intervention are recommended. To help with BCC, remember the mnemonic "PUT ON" (sunscreen):

P = Pearly papule
U = Ulcerating
T = Telangiectasia
O = On the face, scalp, pinnae
N = Nodules = slow growing

Compared with BCC, squamous cell carcinoma (SCC) tends to grow more rapidly and has a low but significant metastatic risk. See Figure 4-10. SCC can arise spontaneously or from a preexisting, precancerous lesion including actinic keratosis or, less commonly, keratoacanthoma. Although difficult to distinguish from BCC by skin examination alone, the mnemonic "NO SUN" can help with the identification of early SCC lesions:

N = Nodular
O = Opaque

> **CLINICAL CONCEPT**
> The consistent use of high sun protection factor (SPF) sunscreen is critical and helps reduce, but not eliminate, the risk of squamous or basal cell carcinoma.

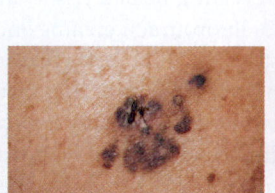 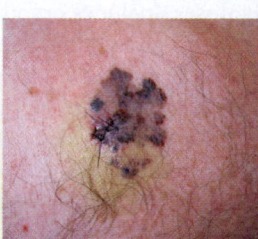 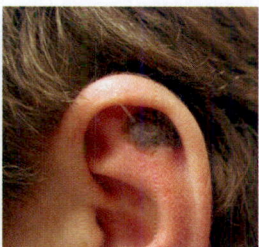 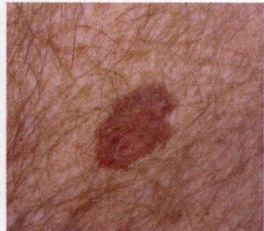

FIGURE 4-8 Melanoma.
Barankin B, Anatoli F. Derm Notes: Clinical Dermatology Pocket Guide. Philadelphia, PA: F.A. Davis; 2006.

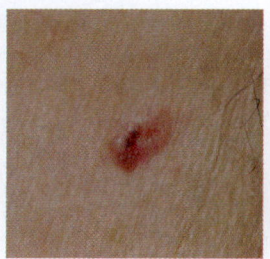 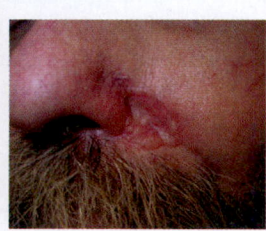 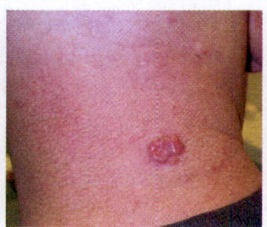 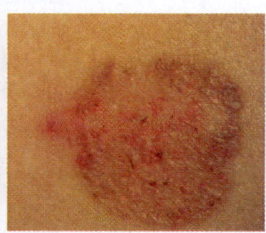

FIGURE 4-9 Basal cell carcinoma.
Barankin B, Anatoli F. Derm Notes: Clinical Dermatology Pocket Guide. Philadelphia, PA: F.A. Davis; 2006.

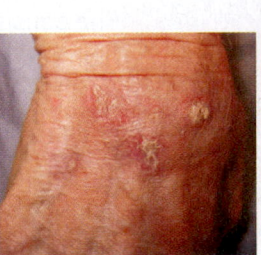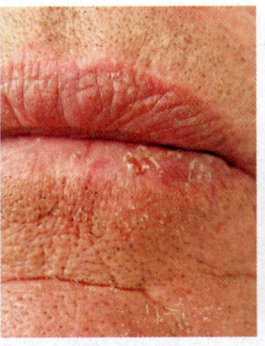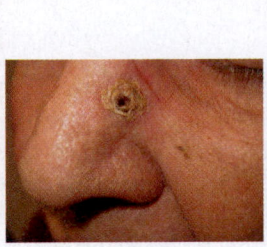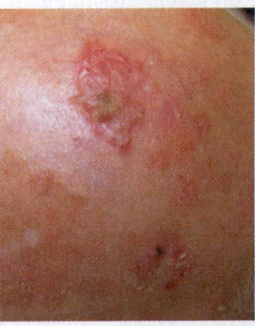

FIGURE 4-10 Squamous cell carcinoma.

Barankin B, Anatoli F. Derm Notes: Clinical Dermatology Pocket Guide. Philadelphia, PA: F.A. Davis; 2006.

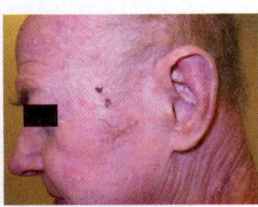

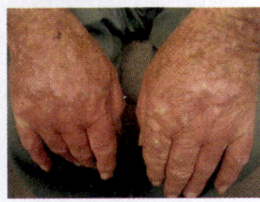

FIGURE 4-11 Actinic keratoses (AK; solar keratoses).

Barankin B, Anatoli F. Derm Notes: Clinical Dermatology Pocket Guide. Philadelphia, PA: F.A. Davis; 2006.

S = Sun-exposed areas
U = Ulcerating
N = Nondistinct borders

Later lesions often include scale and firm margins.

Actinic keratoses are UV-induced skin lesions that can evolve into SCC at a rate of approximately 1 in 100 (see Fig. 4-11). Actinic keratoses begin as small rough patches that appear to be superficially attached to the skin and are often more easily felt than seen; the lesions are often best identified by rubbing the examining finger over the affected area and appreciating the sandpaper-like quality. Over time, the lesions enlarge, typically 3 to 10 mm in diameter, and usually become scaly and red, although color can vary. Commonly, the patient with actinic keratoses will describe having scratched off the lesion in an attempt to remove, but noting the affected area quickly crusts over and the lesion recurs.

Diagnostic Testing

Although the aforementioned mnemonics are helpful in identifying these lesions, diagnosis of cutaneous malignancy requires a biopsy. Intervention depends on biopsy results and final diagnosis.

Treatment

Treatment of actinic keratoses, also known as solar keratoses, includes cryotherapy with liquid nitrogen. This causes destruction of the lesions with resulting crust for about 2 weeks, revealing healed tissue and usually an excellent cosmetic outcome. Alternatives include the use of 1% to 5% fluorouracil creams once a day for 2 to 3 weeks until the lesions become crusted over. As another alternative, 5% fluorouracil cream can be used once a day for 1 to 2 days weekly for 7 to 10 weeks. This regimen yields a similar therapeutic outcome without crusting or discomfort. Additional options include 5% imiquimod cream, topical diclofenac gel, and photodynamic therapy (PDT) with topical delta-aminolevulinic acid. Ingenol mebutate gel (Picato®) offers a faster treatment option of actinic keratoses, ranging from a 2-day dosing regimen (0.05% gel in trunk and extremities) to a 3-day dosing regimen (0.015% gel on face and scalp). Resurfacing with chemical peels and laser are additional destructive treatment options for actinic keratoses treatment.

Skin cancer therapy is usually surgical, involving removal of the lesion with a reasonable "clean" or disease-free margin. Mohs micrographic surgery is recommended in the presence of skin tumors with aggressive histological patterns or invasive features.

Intervention in malignant melanoma is based on additional factors including lesion removal, staging, and sentinel node biopsy results. With all skin cancers, expert consultation with dermatology is advised.

Discussion Sources

de Oliveira ECV, da Motta VRV, Pantoja PC, et al. Actinic keratosis—review for clinical practice. *Int J Dermatol.* 2019;58:400–407.

James WD, Berger TG, Elston DM. *Andrews' Diseases of the Skin: Clinical Dermatology.* 12th ed. Philadelphia, PA: Elsevier; 2016:676, 680–698.

CLINICAL CONCEPT

Nonsurgical options in BCC and SCC include destruction of the lesion with cryotherapy, electrodesiccation with curettage, focal radiation, and topical cancer chemotherapy.

Mancuso JB, Maruthi R, Wang SQ, Lim HW. Sunscreens: an update. *Am J Clin Dermatol*. 2017;18:643-650.
Ortel B, Bolotin D. Cancer of the skin. In: Bope ET, Kellerman RD, eds. *Conn's Current Therapy 2018*. Philadelphia, PA: Elsevier; 2018:932.
Spencer JM, Actinic keratosis. Medscape. http://emedicine.medscape.com/article/1099775-overview

QUESTIONS

135. A 49-year-old man presents with a skin lesion suspicious for malignant melanoma. You describe the lesion as having:

A. deep black-brown coloring throughout.

B. sharp borders.

C. a diameter of 3 mm or less.

D. variable pigmentation.

136. The use of sunscreen has minimal impact on reducing the risk of which type of problematic skin lesions?

A. squamous cell carcinoma

B. basal cell carcinoma

C. malignant melanoma

D. precancerous skin lesions such as actinic keratosis

137. A 72-year-old woman presents with a newly formed, painless, pearly, ulcerated nodule with relatively smooth borders and overlying telangiectasis on the upper lip. This most likely represents:

A. an actinic keratosis.

B. a BCC.

C. an SCC.

D. molluscum contagiosum.

138. Which of the following represents the most effective, highest yield method of cancer screening?

A. skin examination

B. stool examination for occult blood

C. pelvic examination

D. chest radiography

139. Which of the following is most worrisome for malignant melanoma?

A. a 45-year-old man with a mole on his upper abdomen who reports, "I cannot remember when I did not have this."

B. a 28-year-old woman who reports, "I have a new mole that just showed up on my neck a few weeks ago."

C. a 68-year-old man who reports, "I had a mole on my shoulder for years but now it is much smaller."

D. a 50-year-old woman with a 1-year history of a flaky patch of skin on her hand that "bleeds a little when I pick at it, then comes right back."

140. The most common sites for SCC and BCC include the:

A. palms of hands and soles of feet.

B. pelvic and lumbar regions.

C. abdomen.

D. face and rim of the external ear.

141. A 56-year-old truck driver presents with a new nodular, opaque lesion with nondistinct borders on his left forearm. This most likely represents:

A. an actinic keratosis.

B. an SCC.

    C. a BCC.

    D. a malignant melanoma.

142. Risk factors for malignant melanoma include:

    A. Asian ancestry.

    B. history of blistering sunburn.

    C. family history of psoriasis vulgaris.

    D. presence of atopic dermatitis.

143. Definitive diagnosis of skin cancer requires:

    A. skin examination.

    B. computed tomography (CT) scan.

    C. biopsy.

    D. serum antigen testing.

144. Nonsurgical options for the treatment of SCC and BCC include all of the following except:

    A. cryotherapy.

    B. electrodissection with curettage.

    C. topical cancer chemotherapy.

    D. oral hydroxyurea.

145. A skin biopsy result indicates the presence of malignant melanoma for a 53-year-old woman. Your next best step is to:

    A. perform excision of the entire lesion.

    B. apply electrodissection with curettage to the affected area.

    C. initiate treatment with an appropriate topical cancer chemotherapy.

    D. obtain consultation with a skin cancer expert to direct the next best action.

146. A skin lesion associated with actinic keratoses can be described as:

    A. a slightly rough, pink or flesh-colored lesion on the forehead.

    B. a well-defined, slightly raised, red, scaly plaque in a skinfold.

    C. a blistering then crusting lesion along a dermatome.

    D. a crusting lesion along flexor aspects of the fingers.

147. Treatment options for actinic keratoses include topical:

    A. vitamin D–derivative cream.

    B. fluorouracil.

    C. acyclovir.

    D. ketoconazole.

148. Recommended nonpharmacological options to treat actinic keratosis include all of the following except:

    A. a chemical peel.

    B. cryotherapy.

    C. laser resurfacing.

    D. Mohs micrographic surgery.

For answers and rationales, see end of chapter.

Warts

Overview

Verruca vulgaris lesions are also commonly known as warts. Transmitted by direct person-to-person contact, a variety of human papillomaviruses (HPVs) cause most nongenital warts. These include:

- Flat cutaneous warts: HPV-3, HPV-10
- Common warts: HPV-2, HPV-7
- Plantar warts: HPV-1, HPV-2, HPV-4

While many HPV types, especially HPV-16 and HPV-18, are known to be oncogenic, the HPV forms that cause warts do not have malignancy potential. (See Chapter 9 for information on genital warts.)

Clinical Presentation

Common warts are described as hyperkeratotic papules with rough, irregular surfaces. These occur most commonly on the hands and feet and can range in size from 1 mm to 1 cm. Plantar warts initially present as small papules that progress to deep, well-defined, round lesions with a rough keratotic surface. Lesions are often surrounded by a smooth area of calloused skin and can be painful due to deep growth. Flat warts, as the name suggests, are characterized by flat or slightly elevated lesions that can be smooth or slightly hyperkeratotic. These can appear in a group of a few lesions to hundreds of lesions that coalesce, and most commonly appear on the face, hands, and shins.

Several other conditions should be considered when making the differential diagnosis. Warts that are particularly large and refractory to conventional therapies might be due to verrucous carcinoma, a rare type of carcinoma that occurs on the plantar surface. Other conditions can include actinic keratosis, cutaneous SCC, lichen planus, molluscum contagiosum, and seborrheic keratosis.

Diagnostic Testing

Warts are usually diagnosed clinically. Lesion biopsy is warranted when the diagnosis is in question.

Treatment

There are a myriad of treatments available, both OTC and prescription only, and requiring clinician visit or with patient-directed care (Table 4-8). Surgical excision is rarely indicated. Intervention is warranted if warts interfere with function, such as with painful plantar warts on the soles of the feet, or if the lesions are cosmetically problematic and not resolving with standard therapy.

> **CLINICAL CONCEPT**
>
> "Watch and wait" therapy, where no treatment is prescribed, is also appropriate, as most warts will self-resolve within 12 to 24 months.

TABLE 4-8 Treatment Options for Warts

TREATMENT	INSTRUCTIONS FOR USE	COMMENTS
Liquid nitrogen	Apply to achieve a thaw time of 20 to 45 seconds Two freeze-thaw cycles may be administered every 2 to 4 weeks until lesion is gone	Usually good cosmetic results Can be painful, requires multiple treatments
Keratolytic agents (Cantharidin®, Occlusal-HP®, DuoFilm®, Duoplant®, Virasal®, others)	Apply as directed until lesions resolve	Often needs long-term (up to 6 months or more) therapy before resolution; multiple cycles often needed Well tolerated With plantar warts, pare down lesion, then apply 40% salicylic acid plaster, changing every 5 days

Continued

TABLE 4-8 Treatment Options for Warts—cont'd

TREATMENT	INSTRUCTIONS FOR USE	COMMENTS
Podophyllum resin (podofilox)	Patient applies three times a week for 4 to 6 weeks	Multiple cycles often needed Skin irritation common
Tretinoin	Apply BID to flat warts for 4 to 6 weeks	Needs consistent treatment for optimal results
Imiquimod (Aldara®)	Frequency and duration of use depend on wart location	Immunomodulator Low rate of wart recurrence
Laser therapy	Used to dissect lesions	Needs 4 to 6 weeks to granulate tissue Best reserved for treatment-resistant warts

Source: Long MC. Warts (verrucae). In: Bope ET, Kellerman RD, eds. Conn's Current Therapy 2019. *Philadelphia, PA: Elsevier; 2019:1041–1044.*

Discussion Sources

Dall'oglio F, D'Amico V, Nasca MR, Micali G. Treatment of cutaneous warts: an evidence-based review. *Am J Clin Dermatol.* 2012;13:73–96.

Long MC. Warts (verrucae). In: Bope ET, Kellerman RD, eds. *Conn's Current Therapy 2018.* Philadelphia, PA: Elsevier; 2018:1017–1020.

QUESTIONS

149. When counseling a person who has a 2-mm verruca-form lesion on the hand, you advise that:

    A. a variety of bacteria are the most common cause of these lesions.

    B. lesions usually resolve without therapy in 12 to 24 months.

    C. there is a significant risk for future dermatological malignancy.

    D. surgical excision is the treatment of choice.

150. The mechanism of action of imiquimod is as:

    A. an immunomodulator.

    B. an antimitotic.

    C. a keratolytic.

    D. an irritant.

151. Among the most common HPV types associated with cutaneous, nongenital warts are:

    A. 1, 2, and 4.

    B. 6 and 11.

    C. 16 and 18.

    D. 31 and 33.

152. The HPV responsible for nongenital warts is mainly passed through:

    A. contact with infected surfaces.

    B. exposure to saliva from infected person.

    C. person-to-person contact.

    D. exposure to infected blood.

153. A 53-year-old man presents with a large wart-like lesion on the sole of his foot that developed over the past 3 months. Treatment with an OTC salicylic acid medication has had no effect on the lesion. The lesion is round, about 2 cm in diameter, and has a rough keratotic surface. A possible diagnosis to consider is:

A. flat wart.

B. common wart.

C. verrucous carcinoma.

D. plaque psoriasis.

For answers and rationales, see end of chapter.

Cellulitis and Abscess

Cellulitis Overview

Cellulitis is an acute infection of the subcutaneous tissue and skin, typically starting with a skin wound, such as an insect bite, surgical incision, abrasion, or other cutaneous trauma. Cellulitis is most commonly found in the extremities. The causative pathogen of cellulitis is usually a gram-positive organism such as group A beta-hemolytic streptococci and *S aureus*. Rarely, particularly in immunocompromised individuals, certain gram-negative organisms are the causative agent.

Clinical Presentation

The clinical presentation of cellulitis includes a history of skin and tissue trauma, often relatively mild such as an abrasion or insect bite on the affected extremity. This can progress to a warm, red, painful, edematous area with sharply demarcated borders, local lymphangitis, and lymphadenitis. Rarely, tissue necrosis occurs. See Figure 4-12.

Other conditions to consider when making the differential diagnosis include erythema migrans, herpes zoster, septic arthritis or bursitis, and osteomyelitis. Noninfectious conditions can include contact dermatitis, acute gout, drug reaction, or insect bite. Signs of cellulitis on the lower extremity that include edema should raise concern for deep venous thrombosis, which can be detected with ultrasound evaluation.

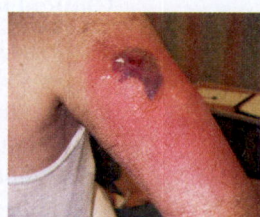

FIGURE 4-12 Cellulitis.
Barankin B, Anatoli F. Derm Notes: Clinical Dermatology Pocket Guide. Philadelphia, PA: F.A. Davis; 2006.

Diagnosis

For uncomplicated cellulitis, in the absence of systemic signs, there is usually no need for diagnostic testing if there is a limited area affected with minimal pain. In complicated disease and evidence of systemic toxicity, additional tests should include CBC with differential, blood culture, creatinine, bicarbonate, creatine phosphokinase, C-reactive protein, and other diagnostics as needed.

> **CLINICAL CONCEPT**
> Severe or complicated cellulitis can result in systemic symptoms such as fever, malaise, chills, lymphangitic spread, and pain disproportionate to examination findings.

Treatment

Treatment for cellulitis involves the choice of a systemic antimicrobial agent with significant gram-positive coverage (in streptococcal and staphylococcal infection); resistant pathogens, including MRSA, must be considered. Treatment options for cellulitis when MRSA risk is considered low include dicloxacillin, cephalexin, or azithromycin (if patient is penicillin allergic). With significant MRSA risk, or when cellulitis surrounds an area of furunculosis or abscess, treatment should be aimed at MRSA and streptococcal infection (see next section on abscess).

Inpatient treatment with parenteral therapy is recommended for certain patient populations, including those with systemic inflammatory response syndrome (SIRS), hemodynamic instability, or mental status changes, and/or those who are immunocompromised. With effective antimicrobial treatment, clinical improvement should be observed within 48 to 72 hours.

With lower-extremity cellulitis in patients with edema, obesity, diabetes mellitus, eczema, and venous insufficiency, there is a higher risk of recurrence. Clinicians should examine the interdigital toe spaces and treat fissuring, scaling, or maceration to eradicate colonization by potential pathogens. Antimicrobial prophylaxis to minimize the relapse risk with recurrent cellulitis is an option; therapy with an appropriate antibacterial is usually used for a protracted period of time, including weeks to months.

In addition to antimicrobial treatment, other actions can help facilitate resolution of cellulitis, including applying warm compresses to the affected area, keeping the affected limb rested, and elevating the affected area when possible. Cellulitis with draining wounds or abscess should undergo incision and drainage to aid resolution.

Abscess Overview

Caused by organisms that are normally found on the skin, a cutaneous abscess is a skin and soft tissue infection that results in a localized collection of purulent fluid. Prior to a cutaneous abscess forming, there is typically a history of trauma to the skin that allows the causative organism to enter the dermal soft tissue. Contributors to abscess formation include dermal bacterial overgrowth, immunosuppression, and impaired circulation.

Clinical Presentation

The most common cause of skin abscess is *S aureus* (either MSSA or MRSA), which accounts for about 75% of abscesses. The clinical presentation of a cutaneous abscess is usually as a cutaneous and soft tissue lesion with a collection of pus within the dermis or subcutaneous space. This results in a painful, erythematous nodule that can have a surrounding area of cellulitis. Spontaneous drainage of purulent material can occur, though systemic symptoms are not typical.

Because a community-acquired methicillin-resistant *S aureus* (CA-MRSA) lesion often has a dark or black center, the condition has often been attributed to a spider bite. In reality, spider bites are uncommon, usually occurring only when the arachnid is trapped in clothing or a shoe. In addition, few spider species have the capability of causing a significant bite.

Found primarily in the U.S. Midwest and Southeast, the brown recluse hibernates during the winter, so bites, which are generally painless, occur between March and October. The term *recluse* depicts a shy creature that typically hides in shoes, boxes, and other small, enclosed spaces. A single spider is occasionally spotted outside of its native region, having traveled in a suitcase or box. Only a small proportion of brown recluse spider bites become necrotic. When this occurs, a characteristic pattern known as the "red, white, and blue" sign follows, with a central purple-to-gray discoloration surrounded by a white ring of blanched skin and a large red halo. If necrosis occurs, a black eschar will form.

Other conditions to consider when making the differential diagnosis can include epidermoid cyst, folliculitis, nodular lymphangitis, and myiasis.

> **CLINICAL CONCEPT**
>
> In particular, the brown recluse spider, or *Loxosceles reclusa*, can cause a necrotizing bite and is often blamed for lesions that are actually caused by CA-MRSA.

Diagnostic Testing

An abscess diagnosis is usually made clinically, and laboratory testing is not typically required in otherwise healthy individuals with uncomplicated infection. Blood and abscess culture and susceptibility testing can be considered in certain situations, such as severe infection, presence of systemic signs, history of recurrent or multiple abscesses, treatment failure, extremes of age, and presence of underlying comorbidities (e.g., immunosuppression, diabetes, or malignancy).

Treatment

The choice of therapy for skin abscess must take into consideration issues of antimicrobial resistance and minimizing unnecessary antimicrobial use. In an afebrile patient with a cutaneous abscess less than 5 cm in diameter, the first-line treatment of community-acquired skin and soft tissue infection is incision, drainage, and localized care such as warm soaks. A wound culture and susceptibility testing should be obtained to help guide treatment. If the abscess is equal to or greater than 5 cm in diameter, antimicrobial therapy should be added to the aforementioned localized treatment.

Given that the antimicrobials effective against MSSA (certain cephalosporins, penicillins, penicillin with beta-lactamase inhibitor combinations, and select macrolides) are ineffective in CA-MRSA, documentation of the organism's resistance profile can help direct therapy. Most strains of CA-MRSA remain susceptible to TMP-SMX (Bactrim®), doxycycline, or clindamycin.

Linezolid (Zyvox®) is another effective, albeit expensive, oral treatment option, which is usually reserved for use with more severe infections, in patients with comorbidities, or when the aforementioned medications are not tolerated or are ineffective. When parenteral treatment is needed, commonly used management options include linezolid, vancomycin, and daptomycin.

Newer, albeit expensive, options include telavancin, dalbavancin, oritavancin, and ceftaroline. Oritavancin is given as a single dose, while dalbavancin is administered as two weekly doses to offer a more convenient option for outpatient care of more severe infection.

In the presence of intact GI function, parenteral antimicrobial therapy for the treatment of skin and soft tissue infection offers little advantage but does incur considerably more cost and inconvenience for the patient.

Although TMP-SMX is usually active against CA-MRSA, its coverage against streptococcus is uncertain. If the causative pathogen of the skin and soft tissue infection is unclear and streptococcal infection is considered a possibility, such as is seen in cellulitis or erysipelas that has accompanied a cutaneous abscess, then the antimicrobial choice should be aimed at medications that provide coverage against staphylococci and streptococci. In this situation, using TMP-SMX with a beta-lactam such as a cephalosporin is recommended.

Discussion Sources

Gilbert DN, Chambers HF, Eliopoulos GM, Saag M, Pavia AT. *The Sanford Guide to Antimicrobial Therapy*. 50th ed. Sperryville, VA: Antimicrobial Therapy, Inc.; 2020:55, 86.

Stevens DL. Bacterial diseases of the skin. In: Bope ET, Kellerman RD, eds. *Conn's Current Therapy 2018*. Philadelphia, PA: Elsevier; 2018:924–927.

QUESTIONS

154. A 62-year-old woman presents 2 days after noticing what she believed was a "bug bite" on her left lower leg. During this time, the area has become increasingly painful, with redness and heat. Examination reveals a tender warm, red, edematous area with sharply demarcated borders, approximately 7 cm in diameter. The patient is otherwise healthy with no fever. This most likely represents:

A. contact dermatitis.

B. an allergic reaction.

C. cellulitis.

D. erysipelas.

155. Which of the following statements is most accurate regarding cellulitis?

A. Insect bites, abrasion, or other skin trauma can be the origin of the skin injury that leads to cellulitis.

B. Cellulitis most often occurs on the chest and abdomen.

C. Tissue necrosis is a common complication of cellulitis.

D. Cellulitis often occurs spontaneously without any identifiable skin wound.

156. The most common causative organisms in cellulitis are:

A. *E coli* and *H influenzae*.

B. *Bacteroides* species and other anaerobes.

C. group A beta-hemolytic streptococci and *S aureus*.

D. pathogenic viruses.

157. Which of the following is the best treatment option for cellulitis when risk of infection with a methicillin-resistant pathogen is considered low?

A. dicloxacillin

B. amoxicillin

C. metronidazole

D. TMP-SMX

158. A 63-year-old male with a history of type 2 diabetes and BMI of 34 kg/m² presents with cellulitis on his left lower leg. He has a temperature of 101.7°F (38.7°C) and reports a 2-day history of headache and fatigue with nausea and one episode of vomiting. He is tolerating sips of fluids. Which of the following is the most appropriate treatment option?

    A. oral dicloxacillin

    B. oral TMP-SMX

    C. parenteral linezolid

    D. parenteral ciprofloxacin

159. You see a 36-year-old man with no chronic health problems who presents with two furuncles, each about 4 cm in diameter, on the right anterior thigh. These lesions have been present for 3 days, slightly increasing in size during this time. He has no fever or other systemic symptoms. You advise the following:

    A. incision and drainage of the lesion.

    B. a systemic antibiotic empirically.

    C. a topical antibiotic.

    D. aspiration of the lesion contents and prescription of a systemic antibiotic based on culture results.

160. A 45-year-old otherwise well woman was treated as an inpatient for a serious skin and soft tissue infection with parenteral linezolid and now is being seen on day 3 of her illness and is being discharged to home. She is feeling better and appears by examination to be clinically improved. Culture results reveal MRSA, susceptible to TMP-SMX, linezolid, daptomycin, vancomycin, and clindamycin and resistant to cephalothin and erythromycin. Her antimicrobial therapy should be completed with:

    A. oral cephalexin.

    B. oral TMP-SMX.

    C. parenteral vancomycin.

    D. oral linezolid.

161 to 167.   Answer the following questions true or false.

_____ 161. Skin lesions infected by CA-MRSA often occur spontaneously on intact skin.

_____ 162. CA-MRSA is most commonly spread from one person to another via airborne pathogen transmission.

_____ 163. All CA-MRSA strains are capable of causing necrotizing infection.

_____ 164. The mechanism of resistance of MRSA is via the production of beta-lactamase.

_____ 165. If a skin and soft tissue infection does not improve in 48 to 72 hours with antimicrobial therapy, infection with a resistant pathogen is likely the cause.

_____ 166. Most acute-onset necrotic skin lesions reported in North America are caused by spider bites.

_____ 167. In an adult with BMI greater than 40 kg/m² who is being treated with TMP-SMX for CA-MRSA skin and soft tissue infection, the recommended dose is two tablets BID.

For answers and rationales, see end of chapter.

Angular Cheilitis

Overview

Various oral and perioral infections are caused by *Candida* species, including angular cheilitis, also known as angular stomatitis, perlèche, or cheilosis.

In addition, physical characteristics can increase the risk for angular cheilitis, such as in an older adult who has a loss of vertical facial dimension because of loss of teeth, allowing for overclosure of the mouth; the resulting skinfolds create a suitable environment for *Candida* growth. See Figure 4-13.

Clinical Presentation

The characteristic findings in angular cheilitis include erythema with painful cracking, scaling, and ulceration at the corner of the mouth. Intermittent bleeding at the site of the lesions is common. Often, the patient will report that the condition came on suddenly. At the same time, most patients will delay presenting for treatment with a health-care provider and have attempted a number of home remedies and OTC products without success.

Diagnostic Testing

The diagnosis of angular cheilitis is usually made clinically by correlating health history, risk factors, and clinical presentation. In angular cellulitis, culture of the affected area is not required. Lesion biopsy is seldom indicated unless the diagnosis is in question.

Treatment

Topical antifungals such as nystatin or miconazole offer a reasonable first-line treatment for perioral and oral candidiasis. With particularly recalcitrant conditions and failure of topical therapy, oral antifungals (e.g., fluconazole) are occasionally needed. Treatment of the underlying condition is critical, as is maintenance of skin integrity through hygienic practices and skin lubrication. After angular cheilitis has responded to treatment and resolved, keeping the area moisturized with petroleum jelly or other moisturizer product is helpful in preventing its recurrence.

Discussion Sources

Devani A, Barankin B. Answer: can you identify this condition? 3. Angular cheilitis. *Can Fam Physician*. 2007;53(6):1022–1023. http://www.ncbi.nlm.nih.gov/pmc/articles/PMC1949217

Murchison DF. Lip sores, lip inflammation, and other changes (cheilitis). Merck Manual Consumer Version. https://www.merckmanuals.com/home/mouth-and-dental-disorders/lip-and-tongue -disorders/lip-sores,-lip-inflammation,-and-other-changes

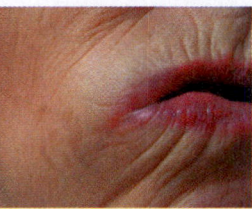
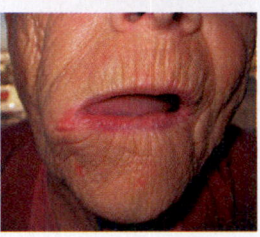

FIGURE 4-13 Angular cheilitis.
Barankin B, Anatoli F. Derm Notes: Clinical Dermatology Pocket Guide. Philadelphia, PA: F.A. Davis; 2006.

> **CLINICAL CONCEPT**
>
> A major candidiasis risk factor is an immunocompromised state, whether resulting from advanced age, malnutrition, or HIV infection.

QUESTIONS

168. An 88-year-old community-dwelling man who lives alone has limited mobility because of osteoarthritis. Since his last office visit 2 months ago, he has lost 5% of his body weight and has developed angular cheilitis. You expect to find the following on examination:

A. fissuring and cracking at the corners of the mouth.

B. marked erythema of the hard and soft palates.

C. white plaques on the lateral borders of the buccal mucosa.

D. raised, painless lesions on the gingival.

169. A common cause of angular cheilitis is infection by:

A. *E coli*.

B. *S pneumoniae*.

C. *Candida* species.

D. *Aspergillus* species.

170. Risk factors for angular cheilitis in adults include all of the following except:

A. advanced age.

B. HIV infection.

C. alteration of facial vertical dimension due to loss of teeth.

D. history of excessive dermal solar exposure.

171. First-line therapy for angular cheilitis therapy includes the use of:

   A. metronidazole gel.

   B. hydrocortisone cream.

   C. topical nystatin.

   D. oral ketoconazole.

For answers and rationales, see end of chapter.

Lyme Disease

Overview

Lyme disease is a multisystem infection caused by *Borrelia burgdorferi*, a tick-transmitted spirochete. Although original reports of this disease, also known as Lyme borreliosis, were clustered through select areas of the United States, primarily in the Northeast and Mid-Atlantic states, it has now been diagnosed in every state. The disease's name comes from the town of Old Lyme, Connecticut, where it was first diagnosed after a community epidemic of rash and arthritis. Lyme disease is the most common vector-borne disease in the United States.

Overdiagnosis of Lyme disease is a problem, as is the issue of significant but understandable anxiety about any tick exposure. In addition, not all ticks are infected, with rates varying from 15% to 65% in areas where Lyme disease is endemic. An infected tick must feed on the human host for more than 24 hours to transmit the spirochete that causes Lyme disease.

Clinical Presentation

Lyme disease is typically divided into three stages:

- *Stage 1* (early localized disease): This is a mild flu-like illness, often with a single annular lesion with central clearing (erythema migrans). The lesion is rarely pruritic or painful. Signs and symptoms can resolve in 3 to 4 weeks without treatment.
- *Stage 2* (early disseminated infection): Typically months later, the classic rash can reappear with multiple lesions, usually accompanied by arthralgias, myalgia, headache, and fatigue. Less commonly, cardiac manifestations such as heart block and neurological findings such as acute facial nerve paralysis (Bell's palsy) and aseptic meningitis can also be present. Individuals with Bell's palsy should undergo careful examination and serological testing for Lyme disease. Regression of Lyme disease symptoms can occur without treatment.
- *Stage 3* (late persistent infection): Starting approximately 1 year after the initial infection, musculoskeletal signs and symptoms usually persist, ranging from joint pain with no objective findings to frank arthritis with evidence of joint damage. Neuropsychiatric symptoms can appear, including memory problems, depression, and neuropathy.

Diagnostic Testing

Serum testing for *B burgdorferi* by enzyme-linked immunosorbent assay and a confirmatory Western blot assay for IgM antibodies help to support the clinical diagnosis of Lyme disease; IgM antibodies decline to low levels after 4 to 6 months of illness, whereas IgG is noted about 6 to 8 weeks after onset of symptoms and often persists at low levels despite successful treatment. This two-tier approach is recommended due to a high frequency of false-negative and false-positive results with enzyme immunoassays. Additional laboratory tests are usually not helpful as CBC is normal. Careful correlation of patient history and physical examination and astute interpretation of laboratory diagnostics are critical to prevent overdiagnosing and underdiagnosing Lyme disease.

> **CLINICAL CONCEPT**
>
> If a tick bite occurs, a single 200-mg dose of doxycycline taken orally appears to be effective in reducing Lyme disease risk if the tick is engorged and the patient lives in or has visited a Lyme-endemic area.

Treatment

Effective antimicrobials for treatment of Lyme disease include doxycycline, cefuroxime axetil (Ceftin®), amoxicillin, and select macrolides. The clinician needs to be aware of the latest recommendation for dosage and duration of treatment with these products; recommendations include treatment for 14 to 21 days for earlier disease and up to 28 days with more advanced disease. Ceftriaxone, given parenterally, can also be considered in later disease and in the presence of complications (e.g., carditis, facial paralysis, arthritis). Most adults with Lyme disease recover in weeks with appropriate treatment, although some have a late relapse. Expert consultation with infectious disease is advised.

Prevention of Lyme disease includes avoiding areas with known or potential tick infestation, wearing long-sleeved shirts and long pants, and using insect repellents. Inspecting the skin and clothing for ticks with appropriate tick removal is also helpful.

Observation is also a reasonable option given the low rate of infection after a tick bite, particularly with a nonengorged tick bite received in low-risk areas.

Discussion Sources

Barbour A. Symptoms, diagnosis and treatment of Lyme disease. American Lyme Disease Foundation. http://www.aldf.com/lyme-disease/

Centers for Disease Control and Prevention. Lyme disease. http://www.cdc.gov/lyme/

Gilbert DN, Chambers HF, Eliopoulos GM, Saag MS, Pavia AT. *The Sanford Guide to Antimicrobial Therapy*. 50th ed. Sperryville, VA: Antimicrobial Therapy, Inc.; 2020:60.

QUESTIONS

172. A 29-year-old woman has a sudden onset of right-sided facial asymmetry. She is unable to close her right eyelid tightly or frown or smile on the affected side. Her examination is otherwise unremarkable. This likely represents paralysis of cranial nerve:

    A. III.

    B. IV.

    C. VII.

    D. VIII.

173. Which of the following represents the most important diagnostic test for the patient in the previous question?

    A. CBC with white blood cell differential

    B. serum testing for *B burgdorferi* infection

    C. CT scan of the head with contrast enhancement

    D. serum protein electrophoresis

174. To transmit the bacterium that causes Lyme disease, an infected tick must feed on a human host for at least:

    A. 5 minutes.

    B. 30 minutes.

    C. 2 hours.

    D. 24 hours.

175. Lyme disease is caused by the bacterium:

    A. *Borrelia burgdorferi.*

    B. *Bacillus anthracis.*

    C. *Corynebacterium striatum.*

    D. *Treponema pallidum.*

176. Which of the following findings is often found in a person with stage 1 Lyme disease?

    A. peripheral neuropathic symptoms

    B. high-grade atrioventricular heart block

    C. Bell's palsy

    D. single painless annular lesion

177. Which of the following findings is often found in a person with stage 2 Lyme disease?

　A. peripheral neuropathic symptoms

　B. atrioventricular heart block

　C. conductive hearing loss

　D. macrocytic anemia

178. Stage 3 Lyme disease, characterized by joint pain and neuropsychiatric symptoms, typically occurs how long after initial infection?

　A. 1 month

　B. 4 months

　C. 1 year

　D. 5 years

179. Preferred antimicrobials for the treatment of adults with Lyme disease include all of the following except:

　A. a tetracycline.

　B. an aminoglycoside.

　C. a cephalosporin.

　D. a penicillin.

180. Which of the following would not be recommended to prevent Lyme disease when visiting a Lyme-endemic area?

　A. Wear long pants and long-sleeved shirts.

　B. Use insect repellent.

　C. If a tick bite occurs, wait until after consulting a health-care provider before removing the insect.

　D. If a tick bite occurs and the tick is engorged, seek health care so that a single dose of doxycycline can be prescribed.

For answers and rationales, see end of chapter.

Bed Bugs (*Cimex lectularius*)

Overview

Bed bugs (*Cimex lectularius*) are parasitic insects belonging to the family Cimicidae and are typically less than 1 cm in length and reddish-brown in color. Bed bug infestations have been increasing worldwide, likely because of increased resistance to insecticides, such as pyrethroid insecticides, and a ban on the use of dichlorodiphenyltrichloroethane (DDT).

　　These parasites can be found in furniture, floorboards, carpeting, peeling paint, areas of clutter, or other small spaces. Bed bugs do not have a preference for clean or unsanitary environments; these insects are found even in pristine homes and hotels: the pests only need a warm host and hiding places. The insects come out at night to feed on the blood of a host, with peak feeding times just before dawn. They are typically attracted to body heat, carbon dioxide, vibration, sweat, and odor. While certainly an uncomfortable condition, bed bugs are not known to transmit disease.

Clinical Presentation

Bed bug bites are usually red (often with a darker red spot in the middle), itchy, arranged in a rough line or in a cluster, and located on the face, neck, arms, and hands.

　　Seldom will a person be aware of the bite taking place as the insect injects an anaesthetic and anticoagulant to facilitate the blood meal.

CLINICAL CONCEPT

A bed bug bite closely resembles a flea or mosquito bite and often appears in a "breakfast, lunch, and dinner" pattern, in that the parasite will bite in one location, then move laterally to bite again, and repeat the action for the third bite.

Repeated exposure to bed bug bites can lead to skin reactions. Cutaneous reactions can include macules, papules, wheals, vesicles, bullae, and nodules. These reactions are typically self-limited and resolve within 1 to 2 weeks.

Diagnostic Testing

The diagnosis of bed bug bites is made clinically with no special diagnostic testing required. If bed bug bites are suspected, the home should be thoroughly inspected. The inspection is best performed at night when the insects are active. Signs for the presence of bed bugs include dark specks typically found along the mattress seams, light brown empty exoskeletons, or bloody smears on bed sheets (caused by crushing an engorged bed bug during sleep).

Treatment

Treatment of bites is not usually required. If a secondary infection occurs, treat with an antiseptic lotion or topical antibiotic. For allergic reactions or significant distress from bed bug bites from itch, topical corticosteroids or oral antihistamines can be helpful. A disseminated bullous eruption with systemic reaction caused by bed bug bites might occur, but this is rare and is usually self-limiting, requiring symptomatic treatment only, and resolves in 1 to 2 weeks.

Eliminating bed bugs can be difficult because they can live for weeks without feeding. If bed bugs are present in a home, professional extermination is recommended. A combination of pesticides and nonchemical treatments is usually used. Nonchemical treatments can include vacuuming crevices of floors, beds, and furniture where the insects are usually present, washing clothes and other items in hot water (at least 120°F), placing items in a clothes dryer at medium to high heat for at least 20 minutes, or freezing items, preferably in a freezer that is set for 0°F (−17°C), for at least 4 days.

Discussion Source

Studdiford JS, Conniff KM, Trayes KP, Tully AS. Bedbug infestation. *Am Fam Physician*. 2012;86:653–658.

QUESTIONS

181. All of the following characteristics about bed bugs are true except:

    A. they can be found in furniture, carpeting, and floorboards.

    B. their peak feeding time is at dawn.

    C. during feeding, they are attracted to body heat and carbon dioxide.

    D. they usually are found in unsanitary environments.

182. All of the following statements are true regarding skin reactions to bed bugs except:

    A. skin reactions are more common with repeated exposure to bed bug bites.

    B. skin reactions can typically involve papules, macules, or wheals.

    C. allergic reactions can be treated with topical corticosteroids.

    D. systemic skin reactions frequently occur following an initial exposure to bed bug bites.

183. You see a 42-year-old woman with a cluster of red, itchy spots on her left arm. She informs you that she recently stayed at a hotel that she later discovered was infested with bed bugs. You advise her that:

    A. she should immediately begin a regimen of oral antibiotics.

    B. the reaction is usually self-limiting and should resolve in 1 to 2 weeks.

    C. given that bed bug bites are usually not itchy; an alternative diagnosis should be considered.

    D. she should wash all of her clothes in cold water.

184. Signs that bed bugs are present in a home include all of the following except:

    A. small drops of fresh blood on floorboards.

    B. blood smears on bed sheets.

    C. presence of light brown exoskeletons.

    D. dark specks found along mattress seams.

185. Nonchemical means to eliminate bed bugs can include all of the following except:

    A. vacuuming crevices.

    B. washing bedding and other items in hot water.

    C. isolating the infested area from any hosts for 1 week.

    D. running bedding and other items in a dryer on high heat for at least 20 minutes.

For answers and rationales, see end of chapter.

Rosacea

Overview

The cause of rosacea is unknown, although inflammation plays a critical role in pathogenesis. Several organisms on the skin have been implicated in the development of rosacea. The *Demodex* species of mites that normally inhabit human hair follicles tend to prefer skin regions affected by rosacea. Bacterial species, such as *Helicobacter pylori* and *S aureus*, and yeast (*Malassezia* species) are also thought to contribute to the development of rosacea and would explain the effects of antimicrobials in the treatment of rosacea. Triggers for rosacea flares can be varied and specific for individual patients and can include UV/sunlight exposure, hot/cold exposure, exercise, stress, coffee, chocolate, caffeine, alcohol, spicy foods, and certain cosmetic products or medications.

Clinical Presentation

Rosacea is a common condition characterized by symptoms of facial flushing and a spectrum of clinical signs, including erythema, telangiectasia, and inflammatory papulopustular eruptions resembling acne. The symptoms of rosacea are usually intermittent but can progressively lead to permanently flushed skin and, in some cases, permanent telangiectasia.

    Rosacea can be classified into four subtypes with treatment selection guided by this classification:

- Erythematotelangiectatic type: Involves central facial flushing often accompanied by burning or stinging
- Papulopustular rosacea: Typically affects middle-aged women who present with a red central portion of their face that contains erythematous papules surmounted by pinpoint pustules
- Phymatous rosacea: Defined by marked skin thickenings and irregular surface nodularities of the nose, chin, forehead, one or both ears, and/or the eyelids
- Ocular rosacea: Includes a variety of manifestations, including blepharitis, conjunctivitis, inflammation of the lids, and conjunctival telangiectasias

Diagnostic Testing

The diagnosis of rosacea is made clinically by carefully correlating history and physical examination. No specific testing is required.

Treatment

The goal of treatment is to minimize the signs and symptoms of the disease. Prior to initiating therapy for rosacea, the triggers for rosacea should be identified and lifestyle modifications should be made to minimize exposure to these triggers. The daily use of sunscreen is recommended for all patients with rosacea.

    For erythematotelangiectatic and papulopustular rosacea, nonablative lasers can be effective in remodeling the dermal connective tissue and improving the epidermal barrier. Typically, one to three treatment sessions with a pulsed dye laser are needed to achieve the best results. Though this can reduce telangiectasia, it will not improve facial erythema associated with rosacea. For phymatous rosacea, mechanical dermabrasion, laser peel, and surgical shave techniques can be used to achieve cosmetic improvements.

    Effective treatment of rosacea can involve a combination of topical and oral medications. Topical treatments for rosacea include antimicrobials, immunosuppressants, and acne products. Metronidazole gel (0.75% or 1%) is commonly used as a first-line agent. Other topical antimicrobial options include erythromycin and clindamycin.

> **CLINICAL CONCEPT**
>
> Patients with rosacea should also avoid the use of astringents, toners, menthols, camphor, exfoliants, waterproof cosmetics that require solvents for removal, or products containing sodium laurel sulfate.

Acne products can be effective for patients with papules, pustules, and the phymatous and glandular types of rosacea. Topical products can include azelaic acid, sulfacetamide products, benzoyl peroxide, or retinoid-like agents (i.e., isotretinoin and tretinoin). Dapsone can be considered in patients with severe, refractory rosacea or those who cannot take isotretinoin. Tacrolimus ointment (Protopic®) can be helpful in reducing itching and inflammation. Tacrolimus should only be considered after other treatment options have failed. Use of topical medium-potency and high-potency corticosteroids on the face should be avoided because it can produce rosacea-like symptoms or worsen preexisting rosacea. Topical alpha agonists (i.e., brimonidine [Mirvaso®], oxymetazoline [Rhofade™]) have been approved for the treatment of erythema associated with rosacea. These agents have demonstrated significant improvement in facial redness after 1 month of use. Topical ivermectin (Soolantra®) cream can be used for treating inflammatory lesions associated with rosacea. Its exact mechanism of action is unknown but is believed to have an anti-inflammatory effect.

Oral medications can also be considered, often in combination with topical agents. Oral antibiotics are used more for their anti-inflammatory properties than for their antimicrobial activity.

Oral antibiotic options include minocycline, doxycycline, tetracycline, metronidazole, or erythromycin. Oral isotretinoin can also be useful in patients whose rosacea does not respond to other therapies. However, the patient and provider need to be aware of potentially serious adverse effects associated with its use (see Table 4-5).

> **CLINICAL CONCEPT**
>
> For those with ocular rosacea, an oral antimicrobial is preferred for treatment.

Discussion Sources

Baldwin HE. Diagnosis and treatment of rosacea: state of the art. *J Drugs Dermatol.* 2012;11:725–730.
Van Onselen J. Rosacea: symptoms and support. *Br J Nurs.* 2012;21:1252–1255.

QUESTIONS

186. All of the following organisms have been implicated in the development of rosacea except:

    A. viruses.

    B. bacteria.

    C. yeast.

    D. mites.

187. Patients with rosacea are recommended to use a daily:

    A. sunscreen.

    B. astringent.

    C. exfoliant.

    D. menthol gel.

188 to 190. Match each type of rosacea with the most appropriate first-line treatment option.

_____ 188. Ocular rosacea with blepharitis

_____ 189. Phymatous rosacea on the nose and chin

_____ 190. Erythematotelangiectatic rosacea on the cheeks

    A. surgical shave technique

    B. oral antimicrobial

    C. nonablative laser therapy

    D. medium-potency topical corticosteroid

191. Which of the following would not be an appropriate choice of oral antimicrobial treatment for rosacea?

    A. metronidazole

    B. levofloxacin

    C. erythromycin

    D. doxycycline

For answers and rationales, see end of chapter.

QUESTION ANSWERS AND RATIONALES

Skin Lesions

1 to 10. Matching Questions

1. Correct: I. vesicle

2. Correct: H. macule

3. Correct: D. wheal

4. Correct: C. fissure

5. Correct: E. pustule

6. Correct: F. patch

7. Correct: G. plaque

8. Correct: A. ulcer

9. Correct: B. atrophy

10. Correct: J. lichenification

A macule is a primary skin lesion less than 1 cm in diameter associated with a flat area of discoloration as seen with a freckle (2). When the area is larger than 1 cm, it is called a patch (6). A wheal, generally observed with hives, is a circumscribed area of skin edema (3). A fissure is associated with a narrow linear crack into the epidermis as observed with athlete's foot (4). A vesicle is a fluid-filled lesion of less than 1 cm (1). When the vesicle is filled with purulent content, such as observed with acne and impetigo, it is called a pustule (5). A plaque, as observed with psoriasis, consists of a raised lesion of at least 1 cm in diameter and can be the same or a different color than the surrounding skin (7). An ulcer is characterized by the loss of the top layers of skin as seen with pressure sores (8). Atrophy is the loss of full skin thickness as seen with excessive use of high-potency topical corticosteroids (9). Lichenification is the development of thickened skin that resembles callus formation (10).

11 to 15. Matching Questions

11. Correct: D. confluent or coalescent

12. Correct: A. reticular

13. Correct: C. annular

14. Correct: B. linear

15. Correct: E. dermatomal

A confluent or coalescent pattern includes multiple lesions blending together, as typically seen with eczema (11). Reticular consists of a net-like arrangement of lesions as seen in livedo reticularis (12). Annular describes lesions that occur in a ring, as seen with the "bulls-eye" pattern with erythema migrans in Lyme disease (13). A linear pattern consists of lesions that appear in streaks, such as a rash caused by exposure to poison ivy (14). A dermatomal pattern occurs when lesions appear along a neurocutaneous dermatome as observed with shingles (15).

16 to 17. Matching Questions

16. Correct: A. resulting from a disease process and unaltered by outside manipulation, treatment, or the natural course of disease

17. Correct: B. altered by outside manipulation, treatment, and/or the natural course of disease

Primary skin lesions are those that result from a disease process and have been unaltered in any way (16). Secondary skin lesions have been altered by outside manipulation, treatment, and/or the natural course of the disease, such as the development of a crust after a vesicle ruptures (17).

Topical Medication Dispensing

18. Correct: B. 2

When prescribing a topical medication, knowing the appropriate amount of medication needed will help to ensure patients have a sufficient amount of medication to complete a treatment regimen. A single application to the hands requires approximately 2 grams of cream or ointment (B). Therefore, 28 grams would be needed for a 1-week supply if medication needs to be applied twice per day.

Incorrect:

The recommended amount for a single application to the hands is 2 grams. An amount less than this will provide inadequate coverage (A) and more than this amount will be excessive (C, D).

19. Correct: C. 3

Approximately 3 grams of a medication cream or ointment will be needed for a single application to the arm (C). If treated twice daily, a sufficient 1-month supply of medication would require 180 grams (6 ounces).

Incorrect:

The recommended amount for a single application to an arm is 3 grams. An amount less than this will provide inadequate coverage (A, B) and more than this amount will be excessive (D).

20. Correct: B. 30 to 60

One application of topical cream or ointment would require 30 to 60 grams of medication (B). A 1-week supply, if treated twice daily, would require 420 to 840 grams (14 to 28 ounces) for a sufficient supply of medication.

The recommended amount for the entire body is 30 to 60 grams. An amount less than this will provide inadequate coverage (A) and more than this amount will be excessive (C, D).

21. Correct: A. 2

An FTU can be used to help educate patients on the proper amount of cream or ointment to use during treatment. One FTU is the amount of topical cream or ointment that is squeezed out from a standard tube along an adult's fingertip. One FTU is enough to treat an area of skin twice the size of the flat of an adult's palm with the fingers together, or approximately 2% BSA for the average adult (A).

Incorrect:

One FTU can be expected to adequately cover 2% BSA (around an area of skin twice the size of the flat of an adult's palm with the finger together). Approximately 2.5 FTUs are needed to cover 5% BSA (B), 5 FTUs are needed to cover 10% BSA (C), and 10 FTUs are needed to cover 20% BSA (D).

22. **Correct: A. 1**

One FTU is the amount of topical cream or ointment that is squeezed out from a standard tube along an adult's fingertip. A fingertip is from the very end of the finger to the first crease in the finger. Two FTUs are approximately 1 gram of a topical cream or ointment (A).

Incorrect:

Two FTUs are approximately 1 gram of cream or ointment. Six FTUs are needed for 3 grams (B), 10 FTUs are needed for 5 grams (C), and 20 FTUs are need for 10 grams of cream or ointment (D).

Topical Medication Absorption

23. **Correct: C. face.**

When considering medication absorption through the skin, it is important to recognize that the degree of drug absorption is inversely proportional to the thickness of the stratum corneum, or the outermost layer of the epidermis consisting primarily of dead cells. Of the answer choices, the face contains the thinnest layer of the stratum corneum and would, thus, result in the highest degree of medication absorption (C).

Incorrect:

The face represents a part of the body where skin absorption is most efficient. The thickness found in the soles of the feet (B), palms of the hand (A), and abdomen (D) acts as a barrier to medication absorption.

24. **Correct: D. ointment.**

In general, the more viscous the vehicle containing the medication, the greater the medication absorption. Ointment, which is generally a semisolid preparation of hydrocarbons and can leave a greasy protective film on the skin, offers the greatest absorption among the vehicle choices (D).

Incorrect:

Gels and lotions are less viscous vehicles compared with ointments and result in reduced medication absorption (A, B). Gels tend to liquify on contact with skin and have a drying property, which can be useful in hairy areas. Creams consist of an oil and water emulsion and have less viscosity compared to ointments (C). These tend to spread easily and will not leave the skin feeling greasy like ointments.

25. **Correct: D. ointment**

Greater absorption of medication occurs with greater viscosity of the vehicle. Therefore, when treating an area with thickened skin, such as the antecubital fossa, an ointment is preferred for maximum medication absorption and lubrication properties (D).

Incorrect:

Ointment is the preferred vehicle for maximal medication absorption on areas of thickened skin. Less viscous vehicles, such as gels (A), lotions (B), and creams (C), will result in less medication absorption.

Topical Corticosteroids

26. **Correct: C. a vasoconstrictor.**

Topical corticosteroids have a number of activities, including immunosuppressive and anti-inflammatory activity. However, the potency of these agents is based on their vasoconstrictive activity (i.e., the narrowing of the blood vessels as a result of contraction of the muscle walls lining the vessel) (C).

Incorrect:

Corticosteroids are characterized by their vasoconstrictor activity. These agents are not normally associated with antimitotic activity (i.e., blocking cell division) (A), as an exfoliant (i.e., removal of dead skin) (B), and a humectant (i.e., preserving moisture in the skin) (D).

27. **Correct: B. and cover with an occlusive dressing.**

One method to increase the exposure and potency of the topical corticosteroid is to cover the area with an occlusive dressing following application of the agent (B). Occlusive dressings typically contain a waxy coating that provide an air- and watertight seal over the skin that increases the penetration of medication into the skin.

Incorrect:

An occlusive dressing is the best approach to increase the potency of a topical corticosteroid. Applying the medication before bathing is not recommended as this will limit the time of exposure to the medication before it is washed away (C). An emollient will act as a barrier on the skin to limit drug penetration (D). Applying the medication to dry skin will not necessarily enhance the potency (A).

28. **Correct: C. hydrocortisone 2.5%**

Topical corticosteroids are divided into potency classes that range from high and super-high potency (classes I to III) to low potency (classes VI and VII). Hydrocortisone 2.5% belongs to the low-potency class (C).

Incorrect:

Betamethasone dipropionate 0.1% is considered a mid-range potency agent (A), while clobetasol propionate 0.05% (B) and fluocinonide 0.05% (D) are higher-potency agents.

29. **Correct: C. 3 months**

A low- to high-potency corticosteroid agent should not be used continuously for longer than 3 months due to the risk of adverse effects (C). One common adverse effect seen with high-potency corticosteroids is subcutaneous tissue atrophy.

30. **Correct: B. 3 weeks**

A super-high potency corticosteroid agent should not be used continuously for longer than 3 weeks due to a risk of subcutaneous tissue atrophy (B). If a longer duration is needed, the steroid can be gradually tapered to avoid rebound symptoms and then treatment can resume following a period of at least 1 week without steroid.

31 to 33. Matching Questions

31. Correct: **C. dermatitis involving the eyelids**

32. Correct: **A. seborrheic dermatitis**

33. Correct: **B. psoriasis**

Low-potency agents are usually limited to use in areas where the medication will be well absorbed as the affected dermal layer is thin. This can include conditions such as diaper dermatitis and dermatitis on the face including the eyelids (31). Medium-potency agents are most often used for the treatment of conditions such as atopic dermatitis, seborrheic dermatitis, and stasis dermatitis (32). High- and super-high-potency agents are usually limited to more difficult-to-treat conditions including alopecia areata, eczema, lichen planus, and psoriasis (33).

Antihistamines

34. Correct: **C. blocking activity at histamine receptor sites.**

Antihistamines primarily work by blocking histamine-1 receptor sites, thus preventing the action of histamine (C).

Incorrect:

Antihistamines do not inactivate circulating histamine (A), nor do they prevent the production of histamine (B). Antihistamines, particularly the first-generation agents, have an anticholinergic effect that contributes to many of the adverse effects associated with these agents (D).

35. Correct: **A. urinary retention.**

First-generation antihistamines are associated with anticholinergic effects, which can be more pronounced among older adults. These effects can include visual changes, urinary retention (A), constipation, and cognitive dysfunction.

Incorrect:

First-generation antihistamines are not recommended for use in older adults due to clinically significant anticholinergic effects. These effects do not typically include hypertension (B), tachycardia (C), or urticaria (D).

36. Correct: **A. chlorpheniramine**

The first-generation antihistamines, such as chlorpheniramine, are able to cross the blood-brain barrier and are associated with sedation as well as cognitive dysfunction in older adults (A).

Incorrect:

Second-generation antihistamines do not readily cross the blood-brain barrier and are not associated with sedation. Members of this class include cetirizine (B), fexofenadine (C), and loratadine (D).

Impetigo

37. Correct: **B. vesicular lesions in a scattered pattern.**

Bullous impetigo is characterized by a single lesion or multiple scattered lesions that can first appear as superficial vesicles that rapidly enlarge to form bullae or blisters filled with dark or purulent fluid (B).

Incorrect:

Bullous impetigo is not associated with intense itching (A). Lesions can develop in a scattered pattern and not as plaques along a neurocutaneous dermatome, such as observed with herpes zoster (C). Though systemic symptoms are possible in more severe disease, this is not a common occurrence with bullous impetigo (D).

38. Correct: **D. oral cephalexin.**

For bullous impetigo, an oral antimicrobial is preferred over a topical agent, especially when lesions are spread over a large area of the body. First-line agents can include cephalexin (D), doxycycline, or clindamycin. However, doxycycline should be avoided in children younger than 11 years because of a risk of staining permanent teeth.

Incorrect:

For this patient with extensive bullous impetigo, an oral antimicrobial is preferred over topical agents (A). Erythromycin is not recommended due to a high rate of resistance by the causative pathogens to the macrolides (B). Doxycycline should be avoided in young children because of the risk of staining permanent teeth (C).

39. Correct: **C. scattered vesicles surrounded by an area of erythema.**

Nonbullous impetigo typically begins as the presence of papules that rapidly evolve into vesicles surrounded by an area of erythema (C).

Incorrect:

The presence of blisters filled with a dark or purulent fluid is more likely to be consistent with bullous impetigo (A). A presentation of scaly patches with pruritus is more consistent with another dermatological condition, such as nummular eczema (B). The presence of purpura (small blood-filled lesions) is consistent with petechiae (D).

40. Correct: **B. group A streptococcus and *S aureus*.**

Knowing the most likely causative pathogens is critical in selecting the appropriate therapy. Impetigo is most likely caused by the gram-positive pathogens group A streptococcus and *S aureus* (B). Methicillin-resistant *S aureus* is increasingly the cause of impetigo, which can limit the selection of effective therapy.

Incorrect:

The most likely causative pathogens of bullous and nonbullous impetigo are gram-positive bacteria. Gram-negative bacteria, such as *H influenzae* and *P aeruginosa*, are less frequently implicated in these infections (A, D), as are fungal and viral pathogens (C, D)

41. Correct: **B. select gram-positive organisms.**

Skin infections are most commonly caused by gram-positive organisms. Mupirocin can be used to treat select skin infections as it exhibits activity against pathogenic gram-positive species, including *S pyogenes* and *S aureus* (B). However, resistance to mupirocin has emerged by *S aureus*, and up to 10% of clinical isolates exhibit resistance in the United States.

42. **Correct: C. ecthyma.**
On the rare occasion, an impetigo lesion can become deeply ulcerated. This condition is known as ecthyma (C).
Incorrect:
Cellulitis is an acute infection of the subcutaneous tissue and skin that presents with a warm, red, edematous area with sharply demarcated borders (A). Erythema refers to skin redness that can be caused by injury, infection, or inflammation (B). Empyema refers to the collection of purulent fluid in the pleural cavity, often as a result of pneumonia (D).

43. **Correct: A. topical mupirocin.**
Treatment of nonbullous impetigo that involves a few lesions on a small affected area can be treated with a topical antimicrobial. The treatment of choice includes mupirocin or retapamulin (A).
Incorrect:
A topical antimicrobial is appropriate for mild cases of nonbullous impetigo that involve a few lesions or a small area of skin. OTC antimicrobials (e.g., neomycin, polymyxin B) are not as effective as prescription medications and should not be used for treatment (B). For bullous impetigo or more serious cases of nonbullous impetigo, oral antimicrobial therapy would be appropriate. However, cephalexin, rather than cefixime, is the recommended cephalosporin for treatment (C). Doxycycline should be avoided in children younger than 11 years as it can stain the permanent teeth (D).

44. **Correct: A. amoxicillin.**
Treatment of skin infections should include an antimicrobial with gram-positive activity and that is stable in the presence of beta-lactamase. Amoxicillin exhibits activity against select gram-positive bacteria but will get degraded in the presence of beta-lactamase (A). The addition of clavulanate can protect the antimicrobial from degradation.
Incorrect:
First-line oral antimicrobials for impetigo include dicloxacillin (B), cephalexin (C), and TMP-SMX (D), as well as clindamycin, oxacillin, and amoxicillin-clavulanate.

45. **Correct: C. Prescribe oral TMP-SMX.**
Bullous impetigo should be initially treated with oral antimicrobial therapy and not a topical agent. Nonetheless, in the presence of treatment failure and a strong likelihood of infection caused by MRSA, an agent with activity against this pathogen should be chosen. TMP-SMX is an appropriate option for a young child (C).
Incorrect:
A topical agent is not preferred for the treatment of bullous impetigo (A). With suspicion of MRSA infection, dicloxacillin would not be an appropriate choice as the pathogen is resistant to this agent (B). Minocycline, a member of the tetracycline family, should also be avoided in children younger than 11 years as it can stain the permanent teeth (D).

46. **Correct: A. 24**
Impetigo is highly contagious and is spread through skin-to-skin contact as well as contaminated towels, clothing, and so on, that have contacted infected skin. Children with impetigo should not return to school or day care until after 24 hours of initiating antimicrobial therapy (A). Family members and other close contacts should also be evaluated for possible lesions.
Incorrect:
The recommended amount of time a child with impetigo should remain away from contact with other children is 24 hours after initiating antimicrobial therapy. In most cases, waiting longer than this is typically not necessary as the child will no longer be contagious (B, C, D).

Acne Vulgaris

47. **Correct: A. lithium**
Certain medications have been associated with the development of acne. Among these include lithium (A) and phenytoin, though the exact mechanism of inducing acne is not known. Acne-inducing medications should be discontinued when possible. Otherwise, standard acne medications can be used for therapy.
Incorrect:
Certain medications can contribute to the development of acne. However, propranolol (B), sertraline (C), and clonidine (D) have not been implicated in inducing acne.

48. **Correct: C. benzoyl peroxide.**
For mild acne, benzoyl peroxide offers an inexpensive and effective initial treatment option (C). Topical application provides both antimicrobial and comedolytic effects. The products are generally safe and well tolerated, particularly at lower concentrations, and are available OTC.
Incorrect:
Oral antibiotics can be considered for moderate-to-severe acne (A). Isotretinoin can also be considered for moderate-to-severe acne and usually after other treatment options have failed (B). Hydrocortisone cream is not a recommended treatment for acne (D).

49. **Correct: B. use a sunscreen because the drug is photosensitizing.**
Topical tretinoin has a photosensitizing effect. This can increase the risk of sunburn regardless of skin tone. Thus, the use of a sunscreen is recommended (B).
Incorrect:
The use of an exfoliant with tretinoin might actually increase skin irritation (A). Sulfa-based products are not generally recommended for acne as they have demonstrated minimal clinical effect (C). As with all acne products, 4 to 6 weeks of consistent use of treatment are generally needed to see improvement in symptoms (D).

50. **Correct: A. benzoyl peroxide plus topical antimicrobial; and C. topical retinoid plus benzoyl peroxide**
According to American Academy of Dermatology guidelines, first-line treatment of moderate acne can

include combination topical therapy, which can include benzoyl peroxide plus either a topical antimicrobial (A) or topical retinoid (C), or a combination of all three of these types of therapies.

Incorrect:
Hormonal therapy with a combined oral contraceptive or spironolactone can be considered in females with inadequate response to first-line medications (B). Hormonal therapy would be added to the current medication regimen. Similarly, oral isotretinoin can be considered for individuals who fail other therapies (D).

51. Correct: B. a slow taper of the topical antimicrobial can be attempted.
Though this patient has responded well to treatment, there is a high risk of recurrence if treatment is discontinued. However, the topical antimicrobial can be gradually tapered by using the product on a less frequent basis (B). The topical retinoid should be continued to prevent recurrence.

Incorrect:
Treatment with the retinoid should not be discontinued due to a risk of recurrence (A, D). For patients with a good response to topical antimicrobial, there is no need to switch to an oral antimicrobial agent (C).

52. Correct: A. counsel him that at least 4 to 6 weeks of treatment are often needed before significant improvement is achieved.
As with all acne medications, 4 to 6 weeks of consistent use are typically needed before any significant improvement in symptoms is observed (A). Treatment should continue as prescribed.

Incorrect:
Significant improvements in acne symptoms usually need at least 4 to 6 weeks of consistent treatment. A period of 3 weeks of treatment is too early to determine the effectiveness of antimicrobial treatment (C). Switching to another antimicrobial is not necessary at this point in his treatment (B, D). Minocycline is also not recommended for long-term treatment as it can lead to changes in skin pigmentation. Combination oral antimicrobial therapy is not a recommended treatment option for acne (D).

53. Correct: B. a 20-year-old patient with cystic lesions who has tried various therapies with minimal effect
Isotretinoin should be reserved for individuals with moderate-to-severe acne and who have had an inadequate response to multiple prior therapies. Of the individuals listed, the 20-year-old would most likely benefit as the patient has severe acne and failed various prior therapies (B).

Incorrect:
The 17-year-old should step up therapy to combination topical therapy before considering the use of isotretinoin (A). For the 14-year-old, there is no information on whether the patient has tried other therapies and the response to those therapies, and so isotretinoin would not be considered at this point (C). For the 18-year-old

with improvement with tretinoin, the patient should continue with the current therapy and would not be considered for isotretinoin therapy (D).

54. Correct: D. platelet count.
Individuals taking isotretinoin should be closely monitored for serious adverse effects as well as ensure females are utilizing two forms of highly effective birth control. However, the drug does not impact platelet counts and would not require monitoring of this aspect (D).

Incorrect:
Though effective in treating severe acne, isotretinoin is associated with serious adverse effects, including hypertriglyceridemia (B), elevated hepatic enzymes (A), and cheilitis. The treatment is also a potent teratogen; thus, females taking the medication should be advised to use two types of highly effective contraception methods and have pregnancy tests done monthly during therapy (C).

55. Correct: D. "Have you noticed any recent changes in your mood?"
There is an association with the use of isotretinoin with mood destabilization and suicidal thoughts. Though all of the answer choices are relevant questions to ask this patient during a follow-up visit, the most important question would relate to any changes to his mood as monitoring for suicidal thoughts is a critical part of patient care (D).

Incorrect:
The most important aspect of the follow-up visit is to evaluate for any mood changes or suicidal thoughts. Other aspects are also relevant, including medication adherence (A), less serious adverse effects (C), and clinical response (B). However, assessment of patient safety and potential for self-harm is the priority.

56 to 58. Matching Questions

56. Correct: C. severe acne

57. Correct: A. mild acne

58. Correct: B. moderate acne
Though there is no universal system to categorize the severity of acne, general principles can be used to evaluate patients and guide the most appropriate course of treatment. Mild acne typically involves less than 20 comedones or up to 30 total lesions (57). Moderate acne can involve 30 to 125 total lesions, 20 to 100 comedones, or 15 to 50 inflammatory lesions (58). The most severe form of acne will have 5 or more nodules, over 125 total lesions, or over 50 inflammatory lesions (56).

59. Correct: A. add a topical retinoid.
For mild acne, step-up therapy from benzoyl peroxide can include combination topical therapy with the addition of either a topical retinoid or a topical antimicrobial (A).

Incorrect:
An oral antibiotic or hormonal therapy would not normally be considered for a patient with mild acne but should be reserved for those with moderate to severe

acne, often after inadequate response to various topical treatment options (B, D). Similarly, isotretinoin would not be a recommended option for mild acne (C).

60. **Correct: C. a reduction in circulating androgen level.**
Combined oral contraceptive pills suppress ovarian androgen production and can block the effect of androgens at the sebaceous glands (C). Aldosterone antagonists, such as spironolactone, will reduce free testosterone levels and limit the effect of androgens at the sebaceous glands.
Incorrect:
Hormonal therapy does not have comedolytic (B) or keratolytic (D) effects, and it does not impact inflammation at the site of lesions (A).

61. **Correct: B. standard acne therapy**
Though phenytoin has been implicated in the development of acne, it is in the best interest of the patient to continue with phenytoin therapy as it provides excellent seizure control for this patient. Therefore, standard acne treatment should be initiated based on current recommendations, such as combination topical treatment (B).
Incorrect:
Since the patient has a good response to phenytoin, the drug should not be discontinued or switched to another agent (A, D). Isotretinoin should be reserved for individuals with moderate-to-severe acne who have failed prior therapies. Thus, this option would not be recommended for this patient as she has not yet been treated with acne medication (C).

Bite Wounds

62. **Correct: B. *Pasteurella multocida*.**
Cat bites are associated with high rates of infection due to the puncture-like wounds associated with these bites. The most common pathogens associated with cat bites are *P multocida* and *S aureus*.
Incorrect:
H influenzae is not normally associated with bite wounds (D). *Bacteroides* species and *Streptococcus viridans* are more typically associated with human bites (A, C).

63. **Correct: C. oral amoxicillin-clavulanate.**
Cat bites are associated with high rates of infection, and antimicrobial prophylaxis is recommended. Oral amoxicillin-clavulanate is the most common recommended antimicrobial for prophylaxis and treatment of local infections caused by dog, cat, or human bites (C).
Incorrect:
In considering prophylaxis for a cat bite, topical agents would not be effective in treating the puncture wound typically found with these types of bites (B). Oral agents are preferred to parenteral administration (D), and the macrolides are not recommended in these situations (A).

64. **Correct: C. give rabies immune globulin and rabies vaccine.**
A bite from a normally docile animal, especially during a daytime encounter with a nocturnal animal, raises a high suspicion of rabies. Patients should immediately receive rabies immune globulin and rabies vaccine as well as tetanus prophylaxis (C).
Incorrect:
The priority of the patient with a bite from an animal with suspected rabies is to provide rabies immune globulin and rabies vaccine. Prophylaxis for bacterial infection can also be considered, which can include oral amoxicillin-clavulanate (A, B). Depending on the type of wound, suturing can be delayed until an infection is ruled out (D).

65. **Correct: A. humans.**
Human bites carry no risk of rabies (A). Therefore, rabies immune globulin and rabies vaccine should not be considered for individuals with a human bite.
Incorrect:
Any mammalian carnivore and omnivore can transmit rabies. The most common animals in the United States to transmit rabies include foxes (B), bats (C), skunks (D), and raccoons.

66. **Correct: A. 5%**
Dog bites are associated with a relatively low rate of infection at approximately 5% (A). Infection is much more likely with cat bites (80%). The risk of infection will also depend on factors including the type of wound (i.e., puncture versus laceration) as well as patient status (e.g., immunocompromised). For patients at high risk of infection from a dog or cat bite, oral amoxicillin-clavulanate can be given for prophylaxis.

67. **Correct: D. oral amoxicillin-clavulanate.**
The preferred antimicrobial for prophylaxis following a rat bite is oral amoxicillin-clavulanate. Doxycycline can also be considered, particularly in the presence of penicillin allergy.
Incorrect:
There is a very low risk of rabies from a rat bite; thus, treatment with rabies immune globulin and rabies vaccine is not needed (A, B). The preferred antimicrobial for prophylaxis is amoxicillin-clavulanate and not a fluoroquinolone (C).

68. **Correct: C. irrigate the wound and débride as needed.**
As with all bite wounds, initial treatment should include vigorous wound cleansing and débridement if necessary (C). This will help to reduce the risk of infection. The use of antimicrobial prophylaxis can also be considered depending on the type of wound.
Incorrect:
Culture and susceptibility testing is not needed for the patient who presents soon after a human bite (A). This can be considered later in the disease process with signs of acute infection that do not respond to first-line antimicrobial therapy, or if there is suspicion of secondary infection. Human bites carry no risk of rabies (B). Closure of simple wounds should involve suturing rather than adhesion strips (D). However, delayed wound

closure can be considered to reduce the risk of infection in patients where there is a higher risk.

69. **Correct: C. performing a multisystem survey to identify any other injuries.**
For the patient with a human bite wound stemming from a possible altercation, initial assessment should include a multisystem survey to evaluate for additional injuries (C). This is to ensure that more serious conditions, such as respiration and/or circulation issues, are addressed first.
Incorrect:
Priority assessment of the patient with a human bite is to ensure more serious conditions are not present. A multisystem survey should not be delayed until the patient calms down, particularly if the patient is at risk for respiratory or cardiac distress (B). The use of antimicrobial prophylaxis can be considered but is not a priority (D). Testing for blood alcohol content is also not a priority (A).

Burn Wounds

70. **Correct: C. refer the patient to burn specialty care.**
Certain types of burns will require immediate referral to a burn specialty clinic to improve short- and long-term outcomes, including loss of function and range of motion. This includes burns that involve the face, hands, feet, genitalia, perineum, and major joints (C).
Incorrect:
Burns to the hand, especially the dominant hand, require immediate referral to a burn specialty clinic to prevent loss of function. Immediate application of creams and dressings and opening the blisters are not recommended procedures (A, B, D) without prior evaluation by a burn specialist.

71. **Correct: D. *H influenzae.***
Bacteria can colonize a burn area within 48 hours of injury. Knowing the most likely causative pathogens of infection is important in guiding appropriate prophylactic therapy. Several gram-positive and gram-negative pathogens can cause infection at burn sites. However, *H influenzae*, normally found in respiratory tract infections, is not a typical pathogen of these infections (D).
Incorrect:
Common gram-negative bacteria that cause infection at burn areas include *P aeruginosa* (A), *E coli* (B), and *K pneumoniae* (C). Gram-positive pathogens can include *S aureus* and coagulase-negative streptococci.

72. **Correct: B. topical silver sulfadiazine**
Topical agents are preferred over systemic antimicrobials for prevention of burn wound infections when limited areas are affected. The preferred first-line agent from the list provided is topical silver sulfadiazine (B), although other treatment options exist.
Incorrect:
Topical agents are preferred over systemic antimicrobials for the prevention of burn wound infections (C, D).

Topical corticosteroids are not recommended for treatment of burn wounds and do not exhibit an antimicrobial effect to prevent infection (A).

73. **Correct: B. 9%.**
When managing a patient with a burn wound, it is important to estimate the affected BSA of the injury. The rule of nines can be used to get an estimate of the BSA (see Fig. 4-3). The anterior or posterior surface of a lower limb is approximately 9% BSA, while the anterior or posterior surface of an upper limb is 4.5%. The posterior or anterior surface of the trunk is 18%, while the head and neck is 9% BSA. A patient with a burn over the entire anterior surface of a leg would have an estimated BSA of 9% affected by the burn (B).

74. **Correct: A. 1**
In addition to the rule of nines, another method to estimate the BSA of burns, particularly for smaller areas, is to have the palmar surface of the hand including the fingers represent 1% BSA (A). This is accurate throughout the life span and can be particularly useful in estimating BSA in young children.

75 to 77. Matching Questions

75. **Correct: A. affected skin blanches with ease.**

76. **Correct: B. surface is raw and moist.**

77. **Correct: C. affected area is white and leathery.**
First-degree burns typically involve the superficial layers of the skin and present with red, warm skin that is easily blanched (75). Second-degree burns can be partial thickness or deep partial thickness and present with deeply red, blistered, swollen skin that is raw, moist, and very painful (76). Third-degree or full-thickness burns can present with white, charred, or leathery-looking skin (77).

78. **Correct: A. 24 hours.**
Close monitoring of a patient with a burn wound is imperative in ensuring proper wound healing, early detection of infection, and adequate pain management. During outpatient management of a burn wound, a follow-up visit should be scheduled the following day (within 24 hours) to assess if the patient's pain is being properly managed and to evaluate the patient's or caretaker's competence with changing the wound dressing (A). Depending on the findings, daily assessments might be needed if there is any concern the patient is not getting adequate care at home, particularly during the first week after injury.

Atopic Dermatitis

79. **Correct: D. is usually made by clinical assessment alone.**
A diagnosis of atopic dermatitis is made clinically on the bases of patient history and clinical presentation (D). Criteria include the presence of itching and subsequent scratching and at least three of the following: red or inflamed rash, presence of excessive dryness/scaling, and location in skinfolds of arms or legs.

Incorrect:

Atopic dermatitis is related to a type I hypersensitivity reaction and not a bacterial infection. A skin culture for atopic dermatitis will not be useful and will usually find normal skin flora (A). The diagnosis is made clinically without the need for additional tests such as a skin biopsy (B) or peripheral blood eosinophil level (C).

80. **Correct: C. IgE**

Knowing the pathophysiology of a disease can be helpful in understanding proper management. Atopic dermatitis is associated with a type I hypersensitivity reaction resulting from immunoglobulin E (IgE) antibodies occupying the receptor sites on mast cells (C). The mast cells then degrade and release histamine, resulting in vasodilation, mucous gland stimulation, and tissue swelling.

81. **Correct: C. enhanced sebum production.**

Type I hypersensitivity reactions result from the release of histamine from degraded mast cells. This causes a number of physiological effects. However, increased sebum production, typically observed in the development of acne, is not related to these reactions (C).

Incorrect:

The release of histamine from mast cells can cause a number of physiological effects, including vasodilation (A), mucous gland stimulation (B), and tissue swelling (D). These are the hallmarks of a type I hypersensitivity reaction.

82. **Correct: C. application of lubricants.**

The most important aspect of management of atopic dermatitis is treating the skin as if it is sensitive. This can involve avoiding offending agents to the skin and minimizing skin dryness by limiting soap and water exposure. The use of skin lubricants can be effective in maintaining skin moisture (C).

Incorrect:

Exposure to soap and water should be limited in patients with atopic dermatitis as this will contribute to drying the skin (A). Topical corticosteroids are used to treat flares of the disease but are not part of routine maintenance of skin (B). Dermatophytes are associated with a fungal infection and are not involved in the disease process of atopic dermatitis (D).

83. **Correct: A. exposure to nickel.**

Common causes of contact dermatitis include exposure to metals including nickel (A), rubber additives to shoes and gloves, some toiletries, and topical medications.

Incorrect:

Allergic contact dermatitis is a type of eczematous dermatitis and can be triggered by exposure to a number of substances including certain metals, rubber additives, and topical medications. It is not normally triggered by exposure to fabric softener (B), bathing with liquid body wash (C), or eating spicy foods (D).

84. **Correct: D. flexor surfaces.**

Knowing the most common sites of skin lesions can be helpful in making the differential diagnosis. Atopic dermatitis in infants commonly appears on the face. However, this rarely occurs in older children and adults, where skin on flexor surfaces is most frequently affected (D).

Incorrect:

At any age, atopic dermatitis can affect flexor surfaces, such as the antecubital fossa and popliteal space, though the groin and axillary regions are spared. The face is rarely affected in older children and adults (B), though this is a common site in infants. The dorsum of the hand and the neck are not frequently involved (A, C).

85. **Correct: B. the face.**

Knowing the most common sites of skin lesions can be helpful in making the differential diagnosis. Atopic dermatitis in infants commonly appears on the face, though this rarely occurs in older children and adults.

Incorrect:

The diaper area is often spared in infants due to the moist occlusive environment (A). Though atopic dermatitis can occur on the neck (C) and trunk (D) of infants, it occurs less frequently at these locations than on the face.

86. **Correct: B. applying a heating pad on the affected region for 30 minutes.**

During a flare, a cool, moist environment (such as with a clean wet cloth or dressings) can help alleviate symptoms. A heating pad will contribute to drying of the skin and likely exacerbate symptoms; thus, its use should be avoided (B).

Incorrect:

Management of an atopic dermatitis flare can include the use of cool, wet dressings to keep the area moist (D). Topical corticosteroids as well as oral antihistamines can also be used to help alleviate symptoms (A, C).

87 to 89. Matching Questions

87. **Correct: B. red, itchy, scaly skin appearing on the elbows**

88. **Correct: C. new-onset vesicular lesions appearing along the waistline**

89. **Correct: A. chronic, recurrent condition of greasy, scaly lesions on the scalp and nasolabial folds**

Understanding the pathophysiology of skin lesions, including location and onset, is pertinent in making the differential diagnosis. The appearance of red, itchy skin on the flexor surfaces is characteristic of atopic dermatitis (87). Scabies, caused by a host-specific mite, typically appear in areas of warmth, such as axillary folds and the beltline (88). Seborrheic dermatitis most commonly occurs in areas with a high concentration of sebaceous glands, such as the forehead and nasolabial folds (89).

90. **Correct: A. an immunomodulator.**

Pimecrolimus and tacrolimus act as immunomodulators that block T-cell stimulation and inhibit mast cell activation (A). These can provide a useful noncorticosteroid option for the treatment of atopic dermatitis.

Incorrect:

Pimecrolimus will inhibit mast cell activation, not promote activation (C). It is not used as an exfoliant (D), and it does not block cell division (B).

91. **Correct: B. there is a possibility of increased cancer risk with its use.**

Pimecrolimus and tacrolimus have been associated with an increased, albeit low, risk of cancer and should only be used as labeled and only if there is an inadequate response with other therapies (B).

Incorrect:

Pimecrolimus and tacrolimus are immunomodulators, not antihistamines (D), and should not be used in children younger than 2 years (A). These agents offer a noncorticosteroid option for the treatment of atopic dermatitis but are not used interchangeably (C). Due to increased cancer risk, these agents should be used only when other therapies have provided inadequate response.

92. **Correct: A. taking a bedtime dose of antihistamine.**

Itch associated with atopic dermatitis is often described as the most bothersome symptom of the condition and can often be worst at nighttime. A bedtime dose of antihistamine can often provide relief from itching and improve sleep (A).

Incorrect:

A dose of acetaminophen might help with pain but will not relieve itching associated with atopic dermatitis (B). Heat and hot showers are not recommended for atopic dermatitis as these can further dry out the skin and exacerbate the condition (C, D).

93. **Correct: D. a 37-year-old with moderate disease on the legs with little response to medium-potency topical corticosteroids**

Dupilumab is approved for the treatment of moderate-to-severe atopic dermatitis in adults and children older than 12 years of age. Therefore, this biologic is appropriate to use in the 37-year-old with moderate disease and inadequate response with topical corticosteroid therapy (D).

Incorrect:

Dupilumab should not be used in children younger than 12 years of age (A, C). The agent would also not be needed in the 45-year-old with mild disease that is effectively managed with nonpharmacological therapy (B).

Herpes Zoster

94. **Correct: A. linear vesicular lesions that do not cross the midline and are distributed over the posterior thorax.**

A characteristic finding of herpes zoster is the development of blistering lesions that occur along a dermatome that usually does not cross the midline (A). Lesions are accompanied by an intense, painful, throbbing itch.

Incorrect:

Lesions associated with herpes zoster typically form along a dermatome in a linear fashion and are not generalized (B) or scattered (C). Generalized vesicular lesions with crusting are more likely to occur with dermatitis herpetiformis. Scattered umbilicated lesions are more consistent with molluscum contagiosum, of which individuals living with HIV are at greater risk depending on degree of immunosuppression. Early in the disease, the lesions are vesicular and clear, but eventually they cloud, rupture, and crust as the disease progresses, with plaques appearing later in the disease process. Slightly raised honey-colored plaques are more characteristic of nonbullous impetigo (D).

95. **Correct: A. clinically.**

The diagnosis of herpes zoster is usually a clinical diagnosis due to the characteristic type of lesions associated with the disease (A).

Incorrect:

If confirmation of herpes zoster is needed, a Tzanck smear can be performed, which will reveal giant multinucleated cells consistent with all herpetic infections (B). As a viral infection, culture and susceptibility testing is not useful (C) and a biopsy is not needed for diagnosis (D).

96. **Correct: D. thorax.**

Recognizing the characteristic distribution of lesions can be an important aspect in determining a correct diagnosis. Lesions associated with herpes zoster typically occur in a linear fashion along a dermatome. The most common site of lesions is on the thorax (D), though other body sites are possible.

Incorrect:

The most common site for lesions is on the thorax. Other common sites include the lumbar region as well as the face (B), where ophthalmic involvement can be particularly concerning. Lesions on the arms and legs are less common (A, C).

97. **Correct: B. during outbreaks, the chickenpox (varicella) virus is shed.**

Though shingles is not communicable from person to person, the chickenpox virus can be shed during an acute episode (B).

Incorrect:

Antivirals can be used to treat and minimize the severity of herpes zoster symptoms and are most effective when given early in the disease process, ideally within the first 72 hours of the outbreak (A). Long-term effects of shingles include scarring as well as PHN, characterized by intense pain that can linger for months after lesions resolve (C). The disease most commonly affects older adults as well as immunocompromised individuals (D).

98. Correct: D. fentanyl transdermal patch and a topical medium-potency corticosteroid on the affected area.
Topical corticosteroids are not indicated for the management of shingles' symptoms. Transdermal fentanyl, a highly potent opioid, is also not recommended (D) for this condition though short-term use of lower-potency oral opioids can be considered.
Incorrect:
Several treatment options can be considered to minimize the pain associated with shingles. Topical lidocaine (A) can offer relief as well as Burow's solution with an NSAID (B). A protective dressing with petroleum jelly over the affected area will prevent friction rub from clothing on sensitive areas, while short-term use of an oral opioid (C) will also provide relief.

99. Correct: B. severe prodromal symptoms.
PHN is a serious complication of herpes zoster that can last for several months following resolution of lesions. A risk factor for PHN is the presence of severe prodromal pain (B).
Incorrect:
Risk factors for PHN include location of lesions along the trigeminal or brachial plexus regions, with a lower risk in the jaw, neck, and lumbar regions (C). Risk also increases with age (A) as well as with greater severity of the rash (D).

100. Correct: A. injectable methylprednisolone.
Systemic corticosteroids are not indicated for the management of PHN (A).
Incorrect:
Several treatment options can be considered for relief of PHN symptoms. These include the use of tricyclic antidepressants (e.g., nortriptyline [C]), gabapentin, and pregabalin (B). Topical medications can include lidocaine (D) or capsaicin, though several applications of capsaicin will be needed for best effect.

101. Correct: A. condyloma acuminatum.
Condyloma acuminatum, or genital warts, is caused by human papillomavirus and is not a complication of shingles (A).
Incorrect:
Shingles is associated with several serious and debilitating complications. The most common is PHN, which is characterized by severe pain that can last weeks to months after resolution of lesions (B). Ophthalmic shingles can increase the risk of eye infection and permanent vision loss (C). Encephalitis (D) and meningitis are also complications of shingles, though these occur more rarely.

102 to 105. Yes or No
102. Correct: Yes
103. Correct: No

104. Correct: Yes
105. Correct: Yes
Shingrix is generally recommended for all individuals over age 50 years regardless of prior history of chickenpox (102). The vaccine does not contain live virus and is safe to use in individuals with compromised immunity, such as those living with HIV (104). Shingrix is encouraged in those who have already been vaccinated with Zostavax® to maximize protection against shingles (105). The vaccine is not indicated for men or women under the age of 50 years (103).

106. Correct: B. Both Shingrix and Zostavax® are given as a single dose.
Shingrix is administered as a two-dose regimen separated by 2 to 6 months, while Zostavax® is given as a single dose (B).
Incorrect:
Though Zostavax® and Shingrix are indicated for the prevention of shingles, ACIP gives preference to Shingrix as it induces greater immunogenicity following the two-dose regimen and potentially provides protection for a longer duration (C). Zostavax® contains live virus and is contraindicated among those with immunosuppression, immunodeficiency, or who are pregnant (A, D). Shingrix is a recombinant vaccine that does not contain live vaccine and is not contraindicated in those with compromised immune systems.

Onychomycosis

107. Correct: A. it is readily diagnosed by clinical examination.
It can often be challenging to differentiate onychomycosis from traumatic injury or another condition. Therefore, laboratory testing or other techniques are needed to confirm the diagnosis before initiating treatment (A).
Incorrect:
Characteristic findings of onychomycosis include the presence of a white-to-yellow nail on a finger or toe (D), nail hypertrophy (B), and brittle nails (C).

108. Correct: C. metronidazole.
Oral antifungal therapy is the first-line treatment for onychomycosis. Metronidazole is an antibacterial and antiprotozoan agent that would not be effective in the treatment of this fungal infection (C).
Incorrect:
Oral antifungal agents include itraconazole (A), fluconazole (B), terbinafine (D), and posaconazole.

109. Correct: Correct: C. shortens the duration of treatment.
Pulse dosing alternates periods of treatment with abstinent periods, such as treating only the first week of the month for 2 to 3 months. This is effective since the antifungal agent remains in the nail matrix for months after treatment. Pulse dosing, however, does not necessarily shorten the duration of therapy (C).

Incorrect:

Pulse dosing alternates periods of treatment with abstinent periods (D). There are several advantages to pulse dosing, including reducing the risk of drug-related adverse effects with the use of abstinent periods (A). These regimens can also decrease the overall cost of treatment compared to continuous treatment regimens as less total drug is used (B).

110. **Correct: A. a transient but clinically insignificant increase in hepatic enzymes is occasionally seen with its use.**

    Antifungal agents are associated with hepatotoxicity, and liver enzymes should be monitored every 4 to 6 weeks. Pulse dosing can be used to decrease the risk of drug-related adverse effects, though a transient increase in liver enzymes can still occur (A).

    Incorrect:

    Though the azole antifungal agents are associated with several clinically significant drug-drug interactions, they are not typically associated with leukopenia (B) or exhibit an antiplatelet effect (C). These agents are also not contraindicated in the presence of iron deficiency anemia (D).

111. **Correct: B. there is a lack of compelling evidence supporting its use.**

    Nonpharmacological treatment options can be considered for the treatment of onychomycosis, usually as adjunctive therapy to oral antifungal treatment. These techniques can include surgery, laser therapy, or photodynamic therapy. However, there is a lack of compelling evidence supporting the use of laser therapy for this indication, and well-controlled clinical trials are needed (B).

    Incorrect:

    There is a lack of compelling evidence supporting the use of laser therapy for onychomycosis (A). If this technique is used, it should be utilized as adjunctive therapy along with oral antifungal treatment (C). Laser therapy is not contraindicated with concomitant topical antifungal treatment (D).

112. **Correct: C. blood culture.**

    Laboratory tests are needed to confirm a diagnosis of onychomycosis prior to initiating antifungal treatment. However, as the fungus does not spread into the circulatory system, a blood culture would not be useful in the diagnostic process (C).

    Incorrect:

    Laboratory tests to differentiate fungal infection from trauma or other conditions can include detecting hyphae in nail scrapings mixed with potassium hydroxide (A) or performing a fungal culture of pulverized nail scrapings (B). Dermoscopy will also reveal white-to-yellow spikes protruding into the proximal nail plate that is characteristic of onychomycosis (D).

113. **Correct: C. topical products have limited penetration through the nail matrix to reach the site of infection.**

    The use of topical antifungal agents is not preferred over oral systemic medications as these products will not fully penetrate the nail matrix to the site of infection (C). These products can be considered for mild infections or as adjunctive therapy with oral antifungal treatment.

    Incorrect:

    Topical antifungal treatments are not as effective as oral treatment regardless of the vehicle used in the topical agent (A, D). Topical OTC medications and herbal treatments are generally not effective as they will not penetrate the nail matrix to the site of infection (B).

Scabies

114. **Correct: A. excoriated papules on the interdigital area**

    Lesions associated with scabies are best characterized as vesicular or popular with excoriation due to scratching the area (A). The mites tend to burrow in areas of warmth, including finger webs, axillary folds, and the belt line. In older adults, the back and shoulder are often affected.

    Incorrect:

    Annular lesion is a nonspecific characteristic but can be due to Lyme disease (B). Vesicular lesions in a linear pattern are more likely to be caused by herpes zoster or a possible phytodermatitis (C). Honey-colored crusted lesions are likely the result of nonbullous impetigo (D).

115. **Correct: C. soaking items in cold water with bleach for at least 1 hour.**

    The most effective methods to kill the mites are to use heat or to starve them. Soaking clothes in bleach can be effective in reducing bacterial count but is not as effective in eliminating mite burden (C).

    Incorrect:

    Heat and starvation are effective methods to kill mites in clothing and other items. Techniques can include washing in hot water (A), running items through a cycle in a clothes dryer (B), or placing items in a plastic storage bag for at least 1 week (D).

116. **Correct: C. Itch often persists for a few weeks after successful treatment.**

    Permethrin is an effective first-line agent for the treatment of scabies. However, since the dead mites and their waste are trapped in the burrows in the skin, patients will often report pruritus for weeks afterward as the wastes are slowly eliminated from the skin (C). Pruritus can be alleviated with the use of an oral antihistamine or low- to medium-potency topical corticosteroid.

    Incorrect:

    Permethrin lotion is an effective first-line treatment of scabies (D). The lotion should be left on the skin for 8 to 14 hours to be effective (A). Pruritus can last for weeks following effective treatment (B).

117. **Correct: B. close personal contact with an infected person is usually needed to contract this disease.**

    Person-to-person spread of scabies usually requires close personal, skin-to-skin contact (B). Scabies can also be spread through the use of infected, unwashed bedding or clothing.

Incorrect:

Close personal contact is needed to spread scabies from person to person (C). The mites typically survive only 3 to 4 days away from the host, and so placing clothing and bedding in a storage bag for a week will kill the mites (A). Washing bedding in hot water or running it through a normal cycle in the dryer will also eliminate the mites (D).

118. **Correct: B. neurotoxicity.**

Lindane was once used for the treatment of scabies. However, its use is now discouraged as it has been associated with neurotoxicity and a risk for seizures (B).

Incorrect:

Lindane is associated with neurotoxicity. The product is not typically associated with clinically significant hepatotoxicity (A), nephrotoxicity (C), or pancreatitis (D).

Psoriasis Vulgaris

119. **Correct: C. accelerated mitosis.**

The primary cause of psoriasis vulgaris is accelerated mitosis along with rapid cell turnover leading to decreased maturation and keratinization (C).

Incorrect:

Psoriasis is not caused by bacterial colonization, though this is seen in the development of impetigo (A). The absence of melanin is affiliated with vitiligo (B). Atopic dermatitis is caused by a type I hypersensitivity reaction (D).

120. **Correct: B. well-demarcated plaques on the knees.**

Psoriasis is most commonly identified by the presence of plaques over the extensor surfaces of the knees and elbows (B). The plaques form the characteristic silvery scales that shed and leave an underlying red plaque.

Incorrect:

Lichenification of the flexor regions is more consistent with eczema than psoriasis (A). Greasy lesions on the scalp and nasolabial folds can be found with seborrheic dermatitis (C). Vesicular lesions over the upper thorax are not consistent with psoriasis and are more likely to occur with herpes zoster infection, especially if the lesions occur along a dermatome (D).

121. **Correct: B. rapid skin cell turnover, leading to decreased maturation and keratinization.**

The primary cause of psoriasis vulgaris is accelerated mitosis along with rapid cell turnover leading to decreased maturation and keratinization (B).

Incorrect:

Psoriasis is not caused by decreased skin exfoliation, though keratolytic agents can be used to help soften and remove the scales for better penetration of topical medications (A). Inflammation does not play a major role in the development of psoriatic lesions (C), while lichenification is typically the result of repeated itching and rubbing of the skin to create a thickened, leathery patch (D).

122. **Correct: D. dual-energy X-ray absorptiometry.**

Psoriatic arthritis develops in approximately 20% of those with psoriasis. Diagnostic tests can be performed to differentiate psoriatic arthritis from other conditions, such as rheumatoid arthritis and gout. However, dual-energy x-ray absorptiometry is typically used to measure bone density and assess risk for osteoporosis and not arthritis (D).

Incorrect:

Typical findings in psoriatic arthritis that can help to differentiate it from other conditions include the absence of rheumatoid factor (A) and normal erythrocyte sedimentation rate (B). X-rays can be helpful in confirming the diagnosis (C), and characteristic findings can include the pencil-in-cup deformity.

123. **Correct: D. systemic corticosteroids.**

Topical steroids are the first-line treatment option for mild psoriasis and when the area affected is small. In more generalized disease, systemic medications are needed, though systemic corticosteroids are not a preferred therapy (D).

Incorrect:

Several options are available for the treatment of generalized psoriasis. Ultraviolet A light therapy can be effective though there is an increased risk of skin cancer and photoaging (A). Methotrexate provides an antimitotic effect that slows cell proliferation and development of plaques (B). Cyclosporine is an immunomodulator that demonstrates some beneficial effects in treating psoriasis (C).

124. **Correct: C. The sign is observed when pinpoint bleeding occurs when scales are forcibly removed.**

The Auspitz sign is described as pinpoint bleeding that occurs when scales are forcibly removed (C). This sign is commonly observed in patients with psoriasis but is not specific for the disease.

Incorrect:

The Auspitz sign is not specific for psoriasis as it is also seen in other dermatological conditions, such as seborrheic dermatitis (A). The sign is not required for diagnosis, as some individuals with psoriasis will not have the Auspitz sign (D). The sign can be present in patients with psoriasis with or without psoriatic arthritis (B).

125. **Correct: D. for treatment of moderate-to-severe disease with inadequate response to other medications.**

Treatment with biological agents should be reserved for patients with severe, recalcitrant psoriasis (D). Biological agents can include TNF-α inhibitors and interleukin inhibitors.

Incorrect:

Biological agents are not used as preventive therapy for individuals at high risk of psoriasis (A). Those with mild disease and/or psoriasis that affects a small area can be treated with topical medication, such as corticosteroids (B). Those patients who respond well to methotrexate should remain on that therapy without a need to switch to a biological agent (C).

126. Correct: B. topical anthralin (Drithocreme®).
Systemic medication is recommended for patients with severe, recalcitrant psoriasis or when the condition affects more than 30% of the body. The use of topical medications, such as topical anthralin, in cases where large areas are affected would be expensive and inconvenient (B).
Incorrect:
Systemic medications are preferred for severe psoriasis or when large areas are affected. Systemic medications can include methotrexate (A), cyclosporine (D), and biological agents such as TNF modulators (C) and interleukin inhibitors.

127. Correct: D. reactivation of latent tuberculosis.
Biological agents can be an effective option in the treatment of severe psoriasis and/or for patients who have an inadequate response to other therapies. However, these agents are associated with potentially serious adverse effects, such as injection site and infusion reactions, infection, and reactivation of latent tuberculosis (D).
Incorrect:
Biological agents are not typically associated with GI disorders (A), nephrotoxicity (B), or QTc prolongation (C).

Seborrheic Dermatitis

128. Correct: C. an inflammatory reaction to *Malassezia* species on skin.
Understanding the pathophysiology of disease is critical in guiding its management. Though the exact cause of seborrheic dermatitis is not known, evidence suggests that it is related to an inflammatory reaction to the presence of a particular species of yeast on the skin (C).
Incorrect:
Seborrheic dermatitis is not likely caused by accelerated mitosis of the skin cells, as is observed with psoriasis vulgaris (A). The presence of a particular species of yeast, rather than *S aureus*, on the skin is likely involved in the disease process (B). UV radiation can actually help the condition but is not recommended due to an increased risk of skin cancer and photoaging (D).

129. Correct: B. greasy, scaling lesions in the nasolabial folds
Recognizing the clinical presentation of disease is critical in making the differential diagnosis. The lesions associated with seborrheic dermatitis are best described as greasy and scaling, with a distribution concentrated on areas with a high concentration of sebaceous glands and hair follicles (B).
Incorrect:
Flaking lesions in the antecubital and popliteal spaces are more consistent with atopic dermatitis (A). Intensely itchy lesions in the groin folds are more likely associated with scabies or *Candida* infection (C), while silvery lesions on the elbows and knees best describe psoriasis vulgaris (D).

130. Correct: D. a 72-year-old man with Parkinson's disease
Knowing the epidemiology of disease as well as patient risk factors can be helpful in making the differential diagnosis. Seborrheic dermatitis occurs more frequently among the immunocompromised or chronically ill, such as elderly adults and those with Parkinson's disease (D).
Incorrect:
The elderly and those with Parkinson's disease are at higher risk of seborrheic dermatitis. Living in a rural setting (A), cigarette smoking (B), and truck drivers (C) are not risk factors for this condition.

131. Correct: A. use ketoconazole shampoo.
Appropriate treatment of seborrheic dermatitis on the scalp can include the use of ketoconazole shampoo for its antifungal effect (A). Coal tar shampoo can also be used as a keratolytic to soften and remove lesions from the scalp.
Incorrect:
Oily and greasy products are typically not recommended for treatment of the scalp due to low patient acceptance (B). High-potency corticosteroids are not recommended as this can cause subcutaneous atrophy of the area as well as excessive absorption of the corticosteroid (C). Use of a hair dryer has not been noted to be helpful for this condition (D).

132. Correct: B. although sun exposure is noted to improve the skin lesions associated with seborrhea, its use as a therapy is potentially associated with an increased rate of skin cancer and photoaging.
Seborrheic dermatitis generally improves in the summer as individuals are exposed to UV radiation from exposure to sunlight in greater amounts during the summer months. Though UV radiation can improve the condition, it is not recommended as therapy since it is associated with a higher risk of skin cancer and photoaging (B).
Incorrect:
Sun exposure is not recommended as therapy since it is associated with a higher risk of skin cancer and photoaging (A). Humidity does not play a role in the severity of symptoms (C), and high-potency topical corticosteroids are not recommended due to a risk of subcutaneous atrophy (D).

133. Correct: D. TNF-α inhibitor.
Biological agents, such as TNF-α inhibitors, are not indicated for the treatment of seborrheic dermatitis (D).
Incorrect:
When treatment with topical ketoconazole provides an inadequate response, other treatment options can include topical immune modulators such as

pimecrolimus or tacrolimus (B), propylene glycol (C), or sulfur or sulfonamide agents. For severe or unresponsive seborrhea, oral antifungal treatment with ketoconazole or fluconazole can be considered (A).

134. **Correct: B. requires referral to an infectious disease specialist for a child under 2 years of age.**
Seborrheic dermatitis in a young child, typically known as cradle cap, is usually a self-limiting condition that does not require referral to a specialist (B).
Incorrect:
In young children, seborrheic dermatitis is typically found on the scalp and is also known as cradle cap (A). This is often a self-limiting condition (C). Though the condition can occur on other parts of a young child's body, the diaper area is frequently spared (D).

Skin Cancer

135. **Correct: D. variable pigmentation.**
When evaluating a skin lesion for suspected malignant melanoma, the ABCDE mnemonic can be a useful tool. An indication of malignant melanoma is color that is not uniform throughout the lesion and can vary from brown, black, red, white, to blue (D).
Incorrect:
Using the ABCDE mnemonic, signs for malignant melanoma can include nonuniform coloring of the lesion (A), a diameter of at least 6 mm or about the size of a pencil eraser (C), as well as irregular borders (B). For suspected malignant melanoma, a biopsy should be performed to confirm the diagnosis.

136. **Correct: C. malignant melanoma**
Malignant melanoma is a malignancy that originates from melanocytes, and the risk of this type of cancer does not increase with exposure to sunlight. Thus, the use of sunscreen has little effect on reducing the risk of malignant melanoma (C).
Incorrect:
Sun exposure increases the risk of actinic keratosis (D), a premalignant lesion, as well as squamous cell carcinoma (A) and basal cell carcinoma (B). The consistent use of sunscreen can be beneficial in reducing the risk of these conditions.

137. **Correct: B. a BCC.**
A lesion description of a pearly, ulcerated nodule with small blood vessels (telangiectasis) is most consistent with a BCC (B). The location on the upper lip (or other sun-exposed areas) is also a common site for BCC lesions.
Incorrect:
Actinic keratosis typically has more of a flat, glued-on appearance on the skin rather than ulcerated, pearly nodule (A). SCC is possible, though this type of cancer is better characterized by irregular borders (C). A biopsy would be needed to confirm the diagnosis. Molluscum contagiosum is caused by a pox virus and would not typically appear as a single lesion (D).

138. **Correct: A. skin examination.**
Examination of the skin is the most effective method of cancer screening since it can detect cancer at the earliest stage of disease (A).
Incorrect:
Stool examination for occult blood can be used to detect colorectal cancer, but bleeding associated with these cancers typically occurs in later stages of disease (B). Pelvic examination for gynecological malignancies has low sensitivity and specificity and would detect cancer, such as ovarian cancer, in late stages (C). Similarly, utilizing a chest radiograph to identify lung cancer would detect cancer at later stages of disease (D).

139. **Correct: B. a 28-year-old woman who reports, "I have a new mole that just showed up on my neck a few weeks ago."**
The ABCDE mnemonic can be a helpful tool when assessing skin lesions for malignant melanoma. Evolving lesions, such as a new lesion or one increasing in size, would be a concerning sign, such as that reported by the 28-year-old woman (B).
Incorrect:
Lesions that have been present for years and/or that are decreasing in size would not be concerning when evaluating for malignant melanoma (A, C). The woman who presents with a flaky patch of skin more likely presents with actinic keratosis, which can be a precursor of SCC (D).

140. **Correct: D. the face and rim of the external ear.**
SCC and BCC occur most frequently on areas of skin that are most exposed to sunlight. These areas include the face and outer ear (D). Sunscreen with a high SPF is recommended to decrease the risk of these skin cancers.
Incorrect:
Sun-exposed areas are most at risk of developing SCC and BCC. Other areas are less likely to develop these types of skin cancer, including the palms of hands and soles of feet (A), pelvic and lumbar region (B), and abdomen (C).

141. **Correct: B. an SCC.**
When evaluating a lesion for SCC, the "NO SUN" mnemonic can be a helpful tool. This type of skin cancer is characterized by a nodular, opaque appearance on sun-exposed areas and nondistinct borders (B).
Incorrect:
Actinic keratosis is best described as scaly flat patches on the skin (A). BCC has a pearly, ulcerating appearance, often with small vessel involvement (C). Malignant melanoma is characterized as asymmetrical, irregular borders with a nonuniform color that can vary from brown, black, red, white, to blue (D).

142. **Correct: B. history of blistering sunburn.**
A key risk factor for malignant melanoma is a history of blistering sunburns (B). Having five or more blistering sunburns before the age of 20 years can increase the risk of malignant melanoma by 80%.

Incorrect:
An increased risk of malignant melanoma has not been established for those of Asian ancestry (A) or with the presence of other dermatological conditions such as psoriasis vulgaris (C) or atopic dermatitis (D).

143. Correct: C. biopsy.
As with virtually all cancers, histological examination via biopsy is required for a definitive diagnosis (C).
Incorrect:
Skin examination is critical in screening patients for skin cancer (A), though a biopsy is required for a definitive diagnosis. CT scan (B) or serum antigen testing (D) are not indicated for the diagnosis of skin cancer.

144. Correct: D. oral hydroxyurea.
There are several nonsurgical techniques that can be used for destruction of an SCC or BCC lesion. However, oral hydroxyurea, used for several other types of cancer such as leukemia, ovarian cancer, and head and neck cancer, is not typically used for SCC or BCC as nonsystemic techniques are preferred (D).
Incorrect:
Nonsurgical options for the treatment of SCC or BCC can include destruction of the lesion via cryotherapy (A), electrodissection with curettage (B), focal radiation, and topical cancer chemotherapy (C).

145. Correct: D. obtain consultation with a skin cancer expert to direct the next best action.
Malignant melanoma is a potentially fatal condition due to a risk of metastasis. As such, patients with malignant melanoma should be referred for expert consultation to determine the next best course of action (D).
Incorrect:
Malignant melanoma can be a life-threatening condition requiring expert consultation. Other types of skin cancer with a low risk of metastasis, such as SCC and BCC, can be treated without referral to a specialist. Nonsurgical approaches can include cryotherapy, electrodissection with curettage (B), or the use of a topical cancer chemotherapy (C). Alternatively, surgical excision of the lesion can be performed (A).

146. Correct: A. a slightly rough, pink or flesh-colored lesion on the forehead.
Actinic keratoses typically form on sun-exposed areas of skin and are best described as slightly rough, pink or flesh-colored lesions (A). They can sometimes be detected by running the finger over an area and feeling for small rough spots with a sandpaper-like quality.
Incorrect:
A plaque in the skinfold would likely not be actinic keratosis as the area is not exposed to sunlight (B). A blistering then crusting lesion along a dermatome more likely describes lesions associated with herpes zoster (C). The flexor aspect of the fingers is an uncommon site for these types of lesions (D).

147. Correct: B. fluorouracil.
Several topical agents can be used for the treatment of actinic keratoses. These include fluorouracil (B), imiquimod, ingenol mebutate, or diclofenac. Photodynamic therapy with delta-aminolevulinic acid is another option.
Incorrect:
Vitamin D–derivative cream is often used for the treatment of psoriasis vulgaris (A). Actinic keratoses are not caused by a viral or fungal infection and so would not benefit from treatment with acyclovir (C) or ketoconazole (D).

148. Correct: D. Mohs micrographic surgery.
Mohs surgery is typically reserved for skin tumors with aggressive histological patterns or invasive features. This would not be an approach used for the removal of actinic keratoses (D).
Incorrect:
Treatment options for actinic keratoses can include chemical peels (A), cryotherapy (B), or laser resurfacing (C).

Warts

149. Correct: B. lesions usually resolve without therapy in 12 to 24 months.
When considering treatment of a wart, a "watch and wait" approach is appropriate as most warts will resolve in 12 to 24 months as the host immune system eventually controls the virus (B).
Incorrect:
Warts are caused by HPV and not by bacteria (A). Viruses that cause warts do not cause malignancies, while viruses that cause cancer (e.g., HPV-16 and HPV-18) do not typically cause warts. Therefore, the development of warts is not an indication of future dermatological malignancy (C). Topical treatment is the preferred first-line therapy for warts (D). Surgical excision is reserved for cases where standard therapy has failed, the warts interfere with normal function, or the warts are cosmetically problematic.

150. Correct: A. an immunomodulator.
Imiquimod works as an immunomodulator (A). There is typically a low rate of recurrence with this product as it helps to boost the immune system to keep the virus in check.
Incorrect:
Imiquimod is not considered an irritant for the treatment of warts (D). Keratolytic agents are also used for the treatment of warts and can include cantharidin and salicylic acid (C). Antimitotic agents can disrupt skin growth and include retinoic acid derivatives, such as tretinoin (B).

151. Correct: A. 1, 2, and 4.
Common HPV types that cause nongenital warts are HVP types 1, 2, and 4 (A). These typically cause plantar warts.

Incorrect:

HPV types 6 and 11 are more commonly found with genital warts (B), while HPV types 16 and 18 are associated with oral and esophageal cancers (C). HPV types 31 and 33 are less commonly found and can contribute to the development of cervical and genitourinary cancers (D).

152. Correct: C. person-to-person contact.

The spread of HPV that causes nongenital warts is passed through direct person-to-person contact (C).

Incorrect:

For HPV types that cause nongenital warts, the virus stays localized and so would not be contained in the blood or saliva for spread (B, D). The virus is primarily passed through direct person-to-person contact rather than contact with infected surfaces (A).

153. Correct: C. verrucous carcinoma.

Verrucous carcinoma should be considered for abnormally large warts on the plantar surface that do not respond to conventional therapy (C).

Incorrect:

Common warts typically range in size from 1 mm to 1 cm and usually respond well to standard therapies (B). Flat warts can be smooth or slightly hyperkeratotic and usually appear in groups of lesions, sometimes in groups of hundreds of lesions (A). Plaque psoriasis typically appears on the elbows and knees (D).

Cellulitis and Abscess

154. Correct: C. cellulitis.

The characteristic signs of cellulitis include a tender, warm, red, edematous area with sharply demarcated borders. Though other conditions can mimic aspects of this presentation, the most likely diagnosis based on presentation and patient history is cellulitis (C).

Incorrect:

Contact dermatitis is usually associated with pruritic lesions and the formation of vesicles, bullae, and oozing (A). Patients with erysipelas, which involves the superficial lymphatics, typically present with systemic symptoms such as fever, chills, malaise, and headache (D). Allergic reaction, such as due to a medication, typically results in a maculopapular rash that is more generalized and can be accompanied by pruritus (B).

155. Correct: A. Insect bites, abrasion, or other skin trauma can be the origin of the skin injury that leads to cellulitis.

The development of cellulitis typically occurs following trauma to the skin (A). This allows the pathogen entry into the skin to cause the acute infection.

Incorrect:

Cellulitis occurs most often on the extremities and not the chest or abdomen (B). Often, trauma or a wound to the area precedes the development of cellulitis (D). Tissue necrosis is a severe but rare complication of the disease (C).

156. Correct: C. group A beta-hemolytic streptococci and _S aureus_.

Skin infections of all types are most commonly caused by select gram-positive organisms such as group A beta-hemolytic streptococci and _S aureus_, which commonly colonize the skin (C).

Incorrect:

Skin infections of all types are most commonly caused by select gram-positive organisms. _E coli_ and _H influenzae_ are gram-negative organisms not typically implicated in skin infections (A). Anaerobes would be an unlikely cause of skin infections as they do not usually colonize the skin due to the unfavorable environment (B). Viruses are not implicated in cellulitis (D).

157. Correct: A. dicloxacillin.

Appropriate treatment of cellulitis with low risk of MRSA can include dicloxacillin (A) as it exhibits activity against streptococci and _S aureus_ and remains active in the presence of beta-lactamase.

Incorrect:

Amoxicillin will get degraded by beta-lactamase (B). Metronidazole is used for the treatment of infections caused by anaerobes and some parasitic infections (C). TMP-SMX is effective against some MRSA strains but not as effective against streptococci. Its use is not recommended when MRSA risk is low (D).

158. Correct: C. parenteral linezolid

This patient presents with multiple comorbidities and systemic symptoms with report of altered GI function, indicating a complicated infection. Parenteral therapy in an inpatient setting should be considered to prevent the risk of serious complications of infection. Linezolid is an appropriate choice as it exhibits activity against gram-positive pathogens, including MRSA (C).

Incorrect:

For complicated cellulitis, an antimicrobial agent with potency against streptococci, MSSA, and MRSA is needed to ensure optimal outcome. Dicloxacillin is not effective against MRSA (A), while TMP-SMX is not as effective against streptococci (B). _S aureus_ exhibits elevated rates of resistance against fluoroquinolones, and so these agents are not recommended for complicated cellulitis (D).

159. Correct: A. incision and drainage of the lesion.

First-line treatment of uncomplicated abscess in a patient presenting without systemic symptoms is incision and drainage with localized care (A). The use of antimicrobials can be considered when certain factors are present.

Incorrect:

For uncomplicated abscess in an otherwise well patient, incision and drainage is the first-line therapy. The use of a systemic antimicrobial can be considered based on the size and number of abscesses or the presence of patient risk factors for serious complications (B, D). Topical antimicrobials are not recommended for the treatment of an abscess (C). Aspiration is not preferred over incision and drainage.

160. Correct: B. oral TMP-SMX.

For this patient, switching to a less costly but equally effective antimicrobial is the best option. TMP-SMX offers the best choice as it is convenient and susceptibility results support its use (B).

Incorrect:

Resistance to cephalothin, a first-generation cephalosporin, suggests that this strain will have cross-resistance to the other first-generation agents, such as cephalexin (A). Parenteral vancomycin would be inconvenient in the outpatient setting and is more costly than TMP-SMX (C). Oral linezolid is convenient for outpatient treatment but is more expensive than TMP-SMX (D).

161 to 167. True or False

161. Correct: False

Cellulitis or abscesses caused by CA-MRSA (or other bacterial pathogens) typically require trauma or injury (e.g., abrasion, insect bite) to allow the pathogen entry in the skin to cause infection.

162. Correct: False

CA-MRSA is most frequently spread through direct skin-to-skin contact.

163. Correct: False

Many strains of MRSA are not capable of causing a necrotizing infection.

164. Correct: False

MRSA is usually resistant to multiple classes of antimicrobials and utilizes different mechanisms of action. For methicillin resistance, this typically involves the acquisition of a nonnative gene encoding a penicillin-binding protein that has a significantly lower affinity for beta-lactams.

165. Correct: False

Failure to improve after 48 to 72 hours of antimicrobial therapy might be an indication that the infection has invaded deeper tissue and is more difficult to eradicate. However, susceptibility testing can be considered to ensure an effective antimicrobial is being used for the infection.

166. Correct: False

Necrotizing spider bites are not very common, and many MRSA infections are mistaken for a spider bite.

167. Correct: True

Dosing of TMP-SMX should be based on total body weight for obese patients.

Angular Cheilitis

168. Correct: A. fissuring and cracking at the corners of the mouth.

Characteristic signs of angular cheilitis include erythema with painful cracking, scaling, and ulceration of the mouth. This patient also presents with major risk factors for the condition, including older age and malnutrition (A).

Incorrect:

Marked erythema of the hard and soft palates are non-specific oral findings (B). White plaques on the buccal mucosa can be indicative of oral candidiasis but are not suggestive of angular cheilitis (C). A raised, painless lesion is more likely due to oral cancer or a syphilitic sore (D).

169. Correct: C. *Candida* species.

Knowledge of the most likely causative pathogen is critical in selecting a safe and effective treatment regimen. Angular cheilitis is caused by a *Candida* infection (C).

Incorrect:

Angular cheilitis is not caused by gram-positive (*S pneumoniae*) or gram-negative (*E coli*) bacteria (A, B). The condition is also not caused by *Aspergillus*, a mold that more commonly is involved in pulmonary infections in immunocompromised individuals (D).

170. Correct: D. history of excessive dermal solar exposure.

Angular cheilitis is more likely to occur in individuals with compromised immunity as well as facial structure that creates a suitable environment for *Candida* growth. Excessive dermal solar exposure has not been implicated as a risk factor for this condition (D).

Incorrect:

Angular cheilitis is more common in individuals with compromised immunity, including those with advanced age as well as those living with HIV (A, B). An alteration of facial vertical dimension will result in skinfolds at the corner of the mouth that create a suitable environment for *Candida* growth (C).

171. Correct: C. topical nystatin.

A reasonable first-line treatment for angular cheilitis is the use of a topical antifungal agent, such as nystatin (C).

Incorrect:

Oral antifungal therapy can be considered in cases of treatment failure with a topical antifungal (D). Metronidazole gel is not effective against *Candida* infections (A), and hydrocortisone cream is not indicated for this condition (B).

Lyme Disease

172. Correct: C. VII.

This patient presents with the classic symptoms of Bell's palsy, which is a potential complication of Lyme disease. The condition is caused by paralysis of CN VII (C).

Incorrect:

CN III is the oculomotor nerve responsible for eye movement (A). CN IV is the trochlear nerve also involved in eye movement (B). CN VIII is the auditory or vestibulocochlear nerve involved in hearing and balance (D).

173. Correct: B. serum testing for *B burgdorferi* infection

With a suspicion of Lyme disease, a dual-tier approach should be used to confirm the diagnosis. This involves serum testing for *B burgdorferi* with an enzyme immunoassay followed by a Western blot to detect the presence of IgM or IgG antibodies (B).

Incorrect:

In Lyme disease, a CBC with differential is typically normal (A). A CT scan of the head would not detect any abnormalities (C), and a serum protein electrophoresis is not useful in Lyme disease diagnosis, though it can detect abnormal hemoglobin as in the thalassemias (D).

174. Correct: D. 24 hours.

Though Lyme disease is the most common vector-borne disease in the United States, concern for the disease with tick bites tends to be overblown as not all tick bites will result in Lyme disease. A tick needs to feed on a human for at least 24 hours before the spirochete is transmitted. Also, the percentage of ticks harboring the spirochete can range from 15% to 65%, depending on the region.

175. Correct: A. *Borrelia burgdorferi*.

Knowing the etiology of infection is critical in ensuring safe practice. Lyme disease is caused by the spirochete *B burgdorferi* (A).

Incorrect:

B anthracis is the pathogen responsible for anthrax (B). *C striatum* is an uncommon pathogen that causes pneumonia and septicemia, typically acquired in the hospital setting (C). *T pallidum* is the pathogen responsible for syphilis (D).

176. Correct: D. single painless annular lesion

When treating Lyme disease, it is important to recognize the stage of disease to ensure effective therapy. Stage 1 disease is typically characterized by mild flu-like illness and a single, painless annular lesion (D).

Incorrect:

Bell's palsy and cardiac manifestations can present in stage 2 disease (B, C). Stage 3 disease can include neuropsychiatric symptoms as well as neuropathy (A).

177. Correct: B. atrioventricular heart block

Stage 2 is characterized by rash with multiple lesions, cardiac manifestations, and neurological findings (e.g., Bell's palsy) (B). Stage 2 usually occurs months following the initial infection.

Incorrect:

Peripheral neuropathic symptoms are consistent with stage 3 disease (A). Conductive hearing loss and macrocytic anemia are not typically associated with Lyme disease (C, D).

178. Correct: C. 1 year

The timing of symptom development is critical in making a differential diagnosis. Stage 3 disease typically occurs 1 year after the initial infection and is associated with musculoskeletal signs and symptoms as well as neuropathy and neuropsychiatric symptoms (C).

179. Correct: B. an aminoglycoside.

Knowing the agents that belong to each antimicrobial class is essential to safe practice. The aminoglycosides (e.g., tobramycin, gentamicin, amikacin) are not recommended for the treatment of Lyme disease (B).

Incorrect:

Recommended treatment of Lyme disease can include doxycycline (a tetracycline) (A), cefuroxime axetil (a cephalosporin) (C), or amoxicillin (a penicillin) (D).

180. Correct: C. If a tick bite occurs, wait until after consulting a health-care provider before removing the insect.

Several steps can be taken to reduce the risk of Lyme disease when visiting an endemic area. However, when a tick bite occurs, it should be removed as soon as possible to prevent transmission of the spirochete (C). The tick needs to feed on a human host for at least 24 hours before the pathogen is transmitted.

Incorrect:

Steps to prevent tick bites can include wearing long pants and long-sleeved shirts (A) as well as using insect repellent (B). If an engorged tick is found attached to the skin, thus suggesting it has been feeding for a prolonged period of time, a dose of doxycycline can be used to prevent Lyme disease (D).

Bed Bugs (*Cimex lectularius*)

181. Correct: D. they usually are found in unsanitary environments.

When considering bed bugs, it is important to note that they do not have a preference for unsanitary conditions but can also be found in clean environments as well (D).

Incorrect:

Bed bugs can be found in small spaces including furniture, floorboards, carpeting, peeling paint, and areas of clutter (A). They tend to come out at night to feed, with the peak feeding time around dawn (B). Bed bugs are attracted to body heat and carbon dioxide to find a feeding host (C).

182. Correct: D. systemic skin reactions frequently occur following an initial exposure to bed bug bites.

Skin reactions usually occur after repeated exposure to bed bug bites and not following the initial exposure (D).

Incorrect:

Skin reactions, including allergic reactions, typically occur after repeated exposure to bed bug bites and not following the initial exposure (A). Treatment of allergic reactions can include the use of topical corticosteroids or oral antihistamines (C). Lesions associated with bed bug bites can include papules, macules, or wheals (B).

183. Correct: B. the reaction is usually self-limiting and should resolve in 1 to 2 weeks.

Bed bug bites are typically red and itchy. Treatment is not usually required as the reaction is self-limiting and resolves in 1 to 2 weeks (B). Topical agents can be used for symptomatic relief of itch if needed.

Incorrect:

Treatment with an antimicrobial is not needed for bed bug bites unless there is a sign of secondary infection (A). The bites on her arm are consistent with the red, itchy lesions of bed bug bites (C). To kill bed bugs in clothing, they should be washed in hot water or run through the dryer on medium-to-high heat (D).

184. **Correct: A. small drops of fresh blood on floorboards.**

There are several signs to look for when inspecting a home for bed bugs. Though the presence of blood smears on bed sheets is an obvious sign (and due to crushing engorged bed bugs during sleep), you would not expect to find fresh blood on floorboards (A).

Incorrect:

Signs of bed bugs include blood smears on the bed sheets (B), the presence of light brown exoskeletons (C), and dark specks usually along mattress seams (D).

185. **Correct: C. isolating the infested area from any hosts for 1 week.**

Bed bugs can survive for weeks without feeding on a host, so an area would need to be isolated for a prolonged period of time (C). For areas infested with bed bugs, the use of a professional exterminator is recommended.

Incorrect:

Heat is an effective technique for killing bed bugs and can include washing clothing and bedding in hot water or running items in a dryer on medium-to-high heat (B, D). Vacuuming crevices and small areas where bed bugs can hide is also effective in decreasing their numbers (A).

Rosacea

186. **Correct: A. viruses.**

A number of organisms that colonize the skin have been implicated in causing rosacea. However, viruses are not among these organisms (A).

Incorrect:

Bacterial species implicated in rosacea include *H pylori* as well as *S aureus* (B). Rosacea can also be caused by the *Malassezia* species of yeast (C) as well as the *Demodex* species of mites (D).

187. **Correct: A. sunscreen.**

An important part of managing rosacea is identifying triggers for the condition and implementing lifestyle modifications to minimize these triggers. Sunlight is a common trigger, and the daily use of sunscreen is recommended for all types of rosacea (A).

Incorrect:

In addition to sunlight, other possible triggers for rosacea can include diet as well as the use of astringents (B), exfoliants (C), menthols (D), camphor, and waterproof cosmetics that require solvents to remove.

188 to 190. Matching Questions

188. **Correct: B. oral antimicrobial**

189. **Correct: A. surgical shave technique**

190. **Correct: C. nonablative laser therapy**

For treatment of ocular rosacea, an oral antimicrobial is the preferred first-line treatment (188). Phymatous rosacea, typically associated with skin thickenings and irregular surface nodularities, can be best treated with surgical shave techniques, mechanical dermabrasion, or laser peel (189). Erythematotelangiectatic rosacea can benefit from initial treatment with nonablative laser therapy (190). Oral antimicrobial therapy can also be considered for phymatous and erythematotelangiectatic rosacea for its anti-inflammatory effect, though these agents are not necessarily first-line options. Topical medium- or high-potency corticosteroids on the face should be avoided as they can worsen symptoms.

191. **Correct: B. levofloxacin**

The fluoroquinolones, such as levofloxacin, are not recommended for the treatment of rosacea (B). This class of agents should be used sparingly as there is concern for resistance development.

Incorrect:

Oral antimicrobial options for the treatment of rosacea can include metronidazole (A), erythromycin (C), or doxycycline (D). These medications can be used in combination with topical agents when treating rosacea. Oral antimicrobial therapy is the preferred treatment for ocular rosacea.

Eye, Ear, Nose, and Throat Problems

5

Conjunctivitis

Overview

Conjunctivitis describes an inflammation of the bulbar and/or palpebral conjunctiva. It is most commonly caused by viral infection, less commonly by bacterial infection or allergens. With allergic conjunctivitis, symptoms occur due to common seasonal triggers and depend on time of year and geographical location, for example, trees, grasses, weed pollens, or molds. With perennial allergic symptoms, dust mites are implicated. Viral conjunctivitis is most often caused by adenovirus. When caused by viruses, upper respiratory infection (URI), rhinorrhea, and other common cold symptoms are noted. Significantly less common than viral conjunctivitis, suppurative or bacterial conjunctivitis is most often caused by *Staphylococcus aureus*, *Streptococcus pneumoniae*, *Haemophilus influenzae*, or atypical streptococci.

Clinical Presentation

Unilateral or bilateral conjunctival inflammation is found regardless of the conjunctivitis cause. Additional findings are dictated as to whether the cause is allergic, viral, or bacterial. With all forms, there should not be photophobia or change in pupillary response.

- Allergic conjunctivitis is usually characterized by bilateral conjunctival inflammation, clear eye discharge, with accompanying ocular itch (Fig. 5-1).
- Viral conjunctivitis is usually characterized by unilateral or bilateral conjunctival inflammation and clear eye discharge, and it is often noted in the presence of URI-like symptoms such as rhinorrhea and cough. While the eyes might feel slightly irritated, there is usually no itchiness.
- Suppurative or bacterial conjunctivitis is usually characterized by unilateral or bilateral conjunctival inflammation with clear to purulent discharge. The clinical presentation of conjunctivitis differs based on whether it is infective or allergic, though conjunctival inflammation is found in all types.

Ascertaining the likely cause is critical to the choice of appropriate treatment (see Table 5-1 for specifics).

Diagnostic Testing

The diagnosis of conjunctivitis is usually made clinically, using the health history and physical examination to identify the disease's cause and then guide treatment. During the clinical examination for all types of conjunctivitis, vision screening with the Snellen or other similar chart should be conducted and should be at the patient's baseline, not revealing visual changes. Point-of-service testing for adenovirus infection is available. In suppurative or bacterial conjunctivitis, ocular culture and sensitivity is usually only performed with treatment failure or if *Chlamydia trachomatous* infection is suspected.

Treatment

For infectious conjunctivitis, reinforce contagion risk, avoiding touching the eye(s), and the importance of hand hygiene.

- Viral conjunctivitis is usually self-limiting, resolving without specific treatment. No antibacterial therapy is necessary, as risk is low for superimposed bacterial infection.
- An ocular antimicrobial minimizes risk of contagion and shortens illness course in suppurative or bacterial conjunctivitis.
- Allergic conjunctivitis usually improves with the use of ocular and systemic antiallergy medications. (See Table 5-1.)

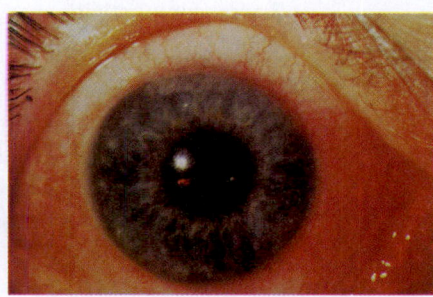

FIGURE 5-1 Acute allergic conjunctivitis.
Dillon P. Nursing Health Assessment: The Foundation of Clinical Practice. 3rd ed. Philadelphia, PA: F.A. Davis; 2016.

TABLE 5-1 Types of Conjunctivitis and Treatment

TYPE OF CONJUNCTIVITIS	TREATMENT
Suppurative or bacterial conjunctivitis (nongonococcal, nonchlamydial)	■ Primary: Fluoroquinolone (FQ) ocular solution (gatifloxacin, levofloxacin, moxifloxacin) ■ Alternative: Ocular polymyxin B plus trimethoprim solution ■ Avoid ocular tobramycin, gentamicin due to resistance risk
Allergic conjunctivitis	Nondrug therapies: ■ Avoid allergen ■ Cool eye compresses ■ Preservative-free artificial tears ■ Sunglasses to provide physical barrier from airborne allergens Drug therapies: ■ Control inflammatory mediators with ocular mast cell stabilizers (cromolyn), ocular antihistamine (olopatadine), oral antihistamines such as loratadine and other second-generation antihistamines

Discussion Sources

Gilbert DN, Chambers HF, Eliopoulos GM, Saag MS, Pavia AT. *The Sanford Guide to Antimicrobial Therapy.* 50th ed. Sperryville, VA: Antimicrobial Therapy, Inc.; 2020. https://webedition.sanfordguide.com/

Patel DS, Arunakirinathan M, Stuart A, Angunawela R. Allergic eye disease. *BMJ.* 2017;359;j4706. Doi: 10.1136/bmj.j4706.

QUESTIONS

1. A 29-year-old woman presents with a chief complaint of a red, irritated right eye for the past 48 hours with eyelids that were "stuck together" this morning when she awoke. Examination reveals injected palpebral and bulbar conjunctiva and reactive pupils; vision screen with the Snellen chart evaluation reveals 20/30 in the right eye (OD), left eye (OS), and both eyes (OU), and purulent eye discharge on the right only. This presentation is most consistent with:

   A. suppurative or bacterial conjunctivitis.

   B. viral conjunctivitis.

   C. allergic conjunctivitis.

   D. mechanical injury.

2. A 39-year-old man presents with a complaint of bilaterally itchy, red eyes with tearing that occurs intermittently throughout the year and is often accompanied by a rope-like eye discharge and clear nasal discharge. This is most consistent with conjunctival inflammation caused by:

   A. a bacterium.

   B. a virus.

   C. an allergen.

   D. an injury.

3. Common causative organisms of acute suppurative or bacterial conjunctivitis include all of the following except:

   A. *S aureus.*

   B. *H influenzae.*

   C. *S pneumoniae.*

   D. *Pseudomonas aeruginosa.*

4. Keeping in mind patterns of bacterial resistance, currently recommended treatment options in suppurative or bacterial conjunctivitis include an ophthalmological preparation containing:

   A. tobramycin.

   B. levofloxacin.

   C. gentamicin.

   D. azithromycin.

5. Treatment options in acute and recurrent allergic conjunctivitis include all of the following except:

   A. cromolyn ophthalmic drops.

   B. oral antihistamines.

   C. ophthalmological antihistamines.

   D. corticosteroid ophthalmic drops.

6. The most common virological cause of conjunctivitis is:

   A. coronavirus.

   B. adenovirus.

   C. rhinovirus.

   D. human papillomavirus.

7. Treatment of viral conjunctivitis can include:

   A. moxifloxacin ophthalmic drops.

   B. polymyxin B ophthalmic drops.

   C. oral acyclovir.

   D. cool artificial tear solution.

For answers and rationales, see end of chapter.

Ophthalmological Emergencies

Overview

Angle-closure glaucoma, anterior uveitis, retinal detachment, and ocular trauma are among the most common causes of ophthalmological emergencies seen in primary care. The role of the primary care nurse practitioner (NP) in ophthalmological emergencies is to identify and diagnosis these conditions in the at-risk patients in order to refer promptly to ophthalmological care (Table 5-2).

ANGLE-CLOSURE GLAUCOMA

Angle-closure glaucoma (ACG), sometimes called acute glaucoma, is caused by a sudden, marked increase in intraocular pressure (IOP). While ACG can occur without a known trigger, risk factors include female gender; use of select medications including topiramate, trimethoprim-sulfamethoxazole (TMP-SMX), hydrochlorothiazide; and medications with systemic anticholinergic effect (selective serotonin reuptake inhibitor, serotonin and norepinephrine reuptake inhibitor, tricyclic antidepressant, and others).

TABLE 5-2 Assessment of Select Ophthalmological Emergencies

	ANGLE-CLOSURE GLAUCOMA	ANTERIOR UVEITIS	RETINAL DETACHMENT	OCULAR TRAUMA
Is the vision affected?	Yes	Yes	Yes	Often affected
Is the eye painful?	Yes	Yes	Usually without pain	Yes
Is the eye red?	Yes	Yes	Usually not red	Yes
Is there eye discharge?	Yes, clear	Usually yes, clear	No	Usually yes, clear
Is there photophobia?	Yes	Yes	Usually no	Variable
Was there trauma?	No	No	Usually no	Yes

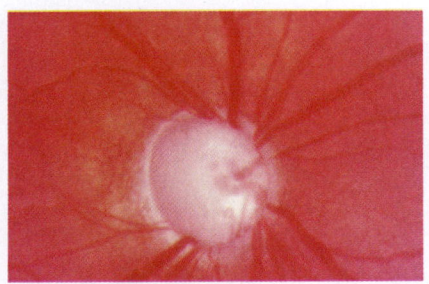

FIGURE 5-2 Glaucomatous cupping.
Dillon P. Nursing Health Assessment: The Foundation of Clinical Practice. 3rd ed. Philadelphia, PA: F.A. Davis; 2016.

Clinical Presentation

ACG clinical presentation usually includes acute-onset eye pain, eye redness with ciliary flush, hazy cornea, sluggish reactive pupil(s), photophobia, headache, nausea, and/or vomiting with changes in baseline vision. Drug-induced ACG usually presents bilaterally. On dilated eye examination, glaucomatous cupping is noted (Figs. 5-2 and 5-3).

Diagnostic Testing

Given ACG's pathophysiology, tonometry testing to document increased IOP (normal IOP: 8 to 22 mm Hg) is needed. While some emergency settings have a tonometer available, in many care settings, prompt referral to ophthalmology is needed for intraocular pressure evaluation.

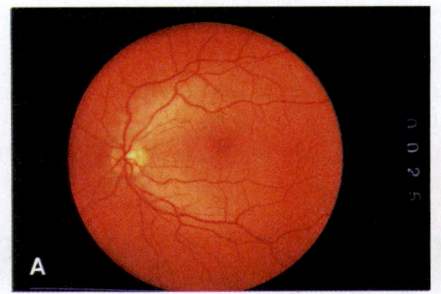 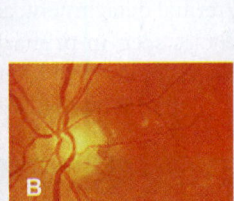 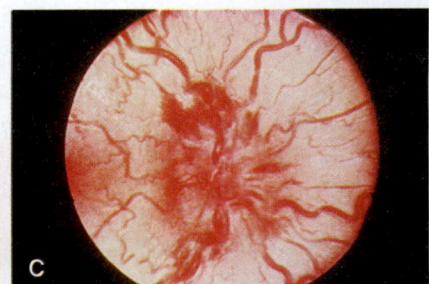

FIGURE 5-3 (A) Normal optic disk. (B) Low-grade hypertensive retinopathy. (C) Bulging optic disk in papilledema.
Dillon P. Nursing Health Assessment: The Foundation of Clinical Practice. 3rd ed. Philadelphia, PA: F.A. Davis; 2016.

Treatment

Treatment of ACG is aimed at promptly reducing intraocular pressure and the inflammation usually noted with the condition. This includes oral and ocular medications. (See Table 5-3.)

ANTERIOR UVEITIS

Anterior uveitis, also known as iritis, is the most common form of intraocular inflammation and involves the eye's anterior uveal tract, including the iris and ciliary body. Risk factors for this condition include a history of ocular trauma and, more commonly, an underlying autoimmune disease. Anterior uveitis is noted equally in males and females, most commonly in the fourth and fifth decades of life.

Clinical Presentation

Anterior uveitis usually presents with a rapid onset of unilateral, dully painful red eye, with discomfort often radiating to the temple and periorbital area, accompanied by visual change. The pupil is usually constricted, nonreactive, and irregularly shaped.

Diagnostic Testing

Diagnostic testing in anterior uveitis is usually focused on evaluation for underlying cause, including autoimmune inflammatory disease. As a result, HLA-B27 typing, erythrocyte sedimentation rate, antinuclear antibody, and/or rheumatoid factor testing are usually conducted. More than 50% of individuals with anterior uveitis are HLA-B27 serotype positive.

TABLE 5-3 Ophthalmological Emergencies and Treatment

CONDITION	RECOMMENDED TREATMENT
Angle-closure glaucoma	Prompt intraocular pressure lowering and inflammation relieving with select medications ■ Beta blockers via ocular drops ■ Alpha-2 agonists via ocular drops ■ Oral carbonic anhydrase inhibitors ■ Ocular, rarely systemic, corticosteroids ■ Miotic or cholinergic agents via ocular drops Further intervention as deemed necessary by ophthalmology
Anterior uveitis	■ Medications to assist in pupillary dilation, including corticosteroids, administered via ocular drops, by periocular injection, or systemically ■ Treatment of underlying autoimmune disease, if present
Retinal detachment	■ Laser photocoagulation or cryopexy (freezing procedure), vitrectomy, other surgical procedures
Ocular injury	■ Immediate referral to ophthalmology or emergency department for evaluation and intervention in ocular and additional injury, if present ■ Fluorescein staining to detect corneal injury; if protruding foreign body, stabilize rather than attempt to remove

Treatment

Aside from treating the anterior eye inflammation associated with the condition, anterior uveitis treatment includes intervention in the underlying autoimmune disease contributing to the condition. In addition to ophthalmological consultation, expert rheumatological input is usually warranted.

RETINAL DETACHMENT

Retinal detachment is usually caused by inflammatory and/or vascular abnormalities or injury that allows fluid to build up, encouraging the separation of the inner retinal layer from the retinal pigment epithelium. This condition requires prompt diagnosis and treatment in order to preserve vision.

Clinical Presentation

A sudden onset in unilateral decreased visual acuity and change in visual fields with the patient's description of "a curtain being pulled down" are common on retinal detachment. Additional findings include a report of new-onset light flashes, visual "floaters," and metamorphopsia (wavy visual field). In contrast to many ocular emergencies, the affected eye is typically not red or painful.

Diagnostic Testing

Retinal detachment is usually diagnosed by dilated eye examination, usually performed by an eye care specialist such as an ophthalmologist. Ocular ultrasound is increasingly used to support the diagnosis.

Treatment

Early diagnosis and treatment of retinal detachment are key to prevent permanent vision loss. While expert ophthalmological care is sought, no pressure should be put on the eyeball, and physical activity is kept to a minimum so as to not worsen the tear. Intervention is aimed at a procedure to seal the torn retina in place. A number of weeks of recovery prior to optimal vision return after the procedure is the norm; often, there is unfortunately a less than full vision recovery.

OCULAR INJURY

Ocular trauma usually involves injury to sclera or cornea and most commonly occurs following penetrating injury with a pellet gun or other foreign body, blunt trauma from a motor vehicle accident, or assault/fight. Accidental injury or injury from fighting are more common in males and will represent the majority of patients presenting with ocular trauma. Primary prevention of trauma to the eye includes the use of appropriate protective eyewear or face shield.

Clinical Presentation

Clinical presentation varies according to the provoking event and often includes additional trauma. Patient history reveals the cause of the injury. Ocular complaints include pain/discomfort, decreased visual acuity, and/or visual field alteration in the affected eye(s). The eye examination is usually consistent with injury and can include altered pupillary shape and response.

As with any injury, a thorough trauma survey examination should be conducted.

Diagnostic Testing

In ocular trauma, diagnostic testing varies by the underlying cause. Often, additional injury is present, which dictates diagnostic testing aimed at assessing cardiopulmonary status.

Treatment

Prompt referral to emergency and/or ophthalmological care is warranted in ocular injury. External pressure on the injured eye should be avoided. Vomiting and crying should be avoided, if possible, to avoid increasing intraocular pressure. A penetrating foreign body is best stabilized and left in place, leaving removal to ophthalmological experts.

Discussion Sources

Muchatuta MN. Iritis and uveitis. Medscape. http://emedicine.medscape.com/article/798323
Romaniuk VM. Ocular trauma and other catastrophes. *Emerg Med Clin North Am.* 2013;31:399–411.

QUESTIONS

8. All of the following are components of the classic ophthalmological emergency except:

A. eye pain.

B. nausea and vomiting.

C. red eye.

D. new-onset change in visual acuity.

9. Ms. Levine is a 48-year-old woman with hypertension and depression, taking an oral angiotensin-converting enzyme (ACE) inhibitor and sertraline, presenting with a sudden left-sided headache that is most painful in and behind her left eye. Her vision is blurred, and the left pupil is slightly dilated and poorly reactive. The left conjunctiva is markedly injected, with ciliary flush, and the eyeball is firm. Vision screen with the Snellen chart is 20/30 OD and 20/90 OS. The most likely diagnosis is:

A. unilateral herpetic conjunctivitis.

B. open-angle glaucoma (OAG).

C. angle-closure glaucoma.

D. anterior uveitis.

10. In caring for Ms. Levine, the most appropriate next action is:

A. prompt referral to an ophthalmologist.

B. to provide analgesia and repeat the evaluation when the patient is more comfortable.

C. to instill a corticosteroid ophthalmic solution.

D. to patch the eye and arrange for follow-up in 24 hours.

11. Johnathan is a 38-year-old man with spondyloarthropathy and presents with a new-onset right eye vision change accompanied by dull pain, tearing, and photophobia. The right pupil is small, irregular, and poorly reactive. Vision testing obtained by using the Snellen chart is 20/30 OS and 20/80 OD. He states he usually does not wear glasses and had a recent vision evaluation that was reported as normal. The most likely diagnosis is:

A. unilateral herpetic conjunctivitis.

B. OAG.

C. angle-closure glaucoma.

D. anterior uveitis.

12. Mrs. Sanchez is a 77-year-old woman with type 2 diabetes and history of bilateral cataract extraction who complains of new onset of "light flashes and floaters" with documented decreased visual acuity in her left eye. Examination reveals reduced visual field on the left and 20/30 vison on right, 20/90 vision on left with corrective lenses. The most likely diagnosis is:

A. OAG.

B. central retinal artery occlusion.

C. anterior uveitis.

D. retinal detachment.

13. For Mrs. Sanchez, the most appropriate next course of action is:

A. placement of an eye shield and follow-up in 48 hours.

B. to initiate treatment with an ophthalmic antimicrobial solution.

C. to initiate treatment with a corticosteroid ophthalmic solution.

D. immediate referral to an ophthalmologist.

14. A 45-year-old man presents with eye pain and redness. He reports that he was cutting a tree with a chain saw when some wood fragments hit his eye. You consider all of the following except:

   A. educating the patient on the use of appropriate eye protection for primary prevention of eye trauma.

   B. immediately removing any protruding foreign body from the eye.

   C. using fluorescein staining to detect small objects in the eye.

   D. prompt referral to an eye care specialist.

For answers and rationales, see end of chapter.

Primary Open-Angle Glaucoma

Overview

Primary open-angle glaucoma (POAG) results from elevated intraocular pressure caused by abnormal drainage of aqueous humor through the trabecular meshwork. POAG risk factors include African ancestry, diabetes mellitus, family history of POAG, history of certain eye trauma and uveitis, and advancing age.

POAG is often called "the silent thief of vision," as the slowly progressive peripheral vision loss is often not noticed by the patient until quite advanced. POAG is the second most common cause of irreversible blindness in North America.

Clinical Presentation

As mentioned, glaucoma, either open-angle or angle-closure, is primarily a problem with excessive intraocular pressure. As a result, the optic disk and cup are "pushed in," creating the classic finding often called *glaucomatous cupping*. This creates a cup-to-disk ratio of greater than 0.3 or asymmetry of cup-to-disk ratio of 0.2 or more (see Fig. 5-2). The cup-to-disc ratio compares the diameter of the physiological cup portion of the optic disc with the total diameter of the optic disc. One analogy to better understand the cup-to-disc ratio is the ratio of a donut hole to a donut, where the donut hole represents the cup with the surrounding area representing the disc.

CLINICAL CONCEPT

The three Ps of POAG are:

- Preventable (with periodic screening for preclinical disease)
- Painless (Unlike many vision-threatening conditions, POAG does not cause eye discomfort.)
- Permanent (Resulting peripheral vision loss is irreversible.)

TABLE 5-4 Treatment Options in Glaucoma

CHRONIC, PRIMARY OPEN-ANGLE GLAUCOMA (POAG) INTERVENTION	ACUTE, ANGLE-CLOSURE INTERVENTION
■ Reduce production of intraocular fluid	■ Prompt ophthalmological referral
• Topical beta-adrenergic antagonists	■ Therapeutic goal = Relief of acute intraocular pressure rise
• Topical alpha$_2$-agonist	• Reduce production of intraocular fluid
• Topical carbonic anhydrase inhibitors	• Topical beta-adrenergic antagonists
■ Increase fluid outflow	• Topical alpha$_2$-agonist
• Prostaglandin analogues	• Topical carbonic anhydrase inhibitors
• Miotic or cholinergic agents	– Increase fluid outflow
■ Surgical intervention if needed to attain normal pressures	• Prostaglandin analogues
• Trabeculoplasty	• Miotic or cholinergic agents
• Trabeculectomy	■ Surgical intervention when intraocular pressure normalized
• Photocoagulation	• Laser peripheral iridectomy
• Drainage implants	

Source: Mayo Clinic Staff. Glaucoma. https://www.mayoclinic.org/diseases-conditions/glaucoma/symptoms-causes/syc-20372839

If the cup fills 3/10 of the disc, the ratio will be 0.3 or normal; if it fills 7/10 of the disc, the ratio is 0.7, or abnormally large. A large cup-to-disc ratio is one of the hallmarks of untreated glaucoma.

Diagnostic Testing

The diagnosis of POAG is confirmed by tonometry and reveals increased intraocular pressure to greater than 25 mm Hg. A comprehensive eye examination including measurement of intraocular pressure should be conducted by an eye care provider for high-risk patients, including those with type 2 diabetes mellitus, African ancestry, advancing age, history of select ocular trauma or uveitis, and/or family history of POAG every 1 to 2 years. Early glaucoma detection and treatment help to avoid vision loss.

Treatment

Medication treatment options for primary open-angle or angle-closure glaucoma are therapeutically aimed at lowering IOP through a variety of methods, including ocular topical medications and, on occasion, surgery (Table 5-4).

Discussion Source

Mayo Clinic Staff. Glaucoma. https://www.mayoclinic.org/diseases-conditions/glaucoma/symptoms-causes/syc-20372839

QUESTIONS

15. Which of the following is a common vision problem in the person with untreated POAG?
    A. peripheral vision loss
    B. blurring of near vision
    C. difficulty with distant vision
    D. need for increased illumination

16. POAG is primarily caused by:
    A. hardening of the lens.
    B. elevated intraocular pressure.
    C. degeneration of the optic nerve.
    D. hypotension in the anterior maxillary artery.

17. Which of the following is most likely to be found on the funduscopic examination in a patient with untreated POAG?
    A. excessive cupping of the optic disk
    B. arteriovenous nicking
    C. papilledema
    D. flame-shaped hemorrhages

18. Risk factors for POAG include all of the following except:
    A. African ancestry.
    B. type 2 diabetes mellitus.
    C. advanced age.
    D. blue eye color.

19. Key diagnostic findings in POAG include which of the following?
    A. intraocular pressure greater than 25 mm Hg
    B. papilledema
    C. cup-to-disk ratio less than 0.3
    D. sluggish pupillary response

20. Who is at highest risk for the development of POAG?
    A. a 22-year-old woman of Asian ancestry with type 1 diabetes mellitus
    B. a 54-year-old man of European ancestry with bilateral cataracts
    C. a 68-year-old man of African ancestry with type 2 diabetes mellitus
    D. a 36-year-old woman of Native American ancestry with asthma

21. Treatment options for POAG include all of the following topical ocular agents except:
    A. beta-adrenergic antagonists.
    B. α_2-agonists.
    C. prostaglandin analogues.
    D. mast cell stabilizers.

For answers and rationales, see end of chapter.

Eyelid Disorders

Overview

The three most commonly encountered eyelid disorders are hordeolum (Fig. 5-4), chalazion (Fig. 5-5), and blepharitis. Risk factors and clinical presentation help differentiate these conditions and direct therapeutics (Table 5-5).

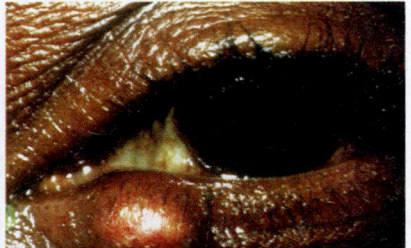

FIGURE 5-4 Hordeolum.
Dillon P. Nursing Health Assessment: The Foundation of Clinical Practice. 3rd ed. Philadelphia, PA: F.A. Davis; 2016.

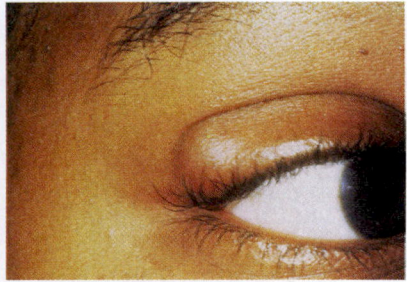

FIGURE 5-5 Chalazion.
Dillon P. Nursing Health Assessment: The Foundation of Clinical Practice. 3rd ed. Philadelphia, PA: F.A. Davis; 2016.

HORDEOLUM

Hordeolum (plural, hordeola) forms as a result of a staphylococcal infection of an eyelid hair follicle with resulting focal abscess. Recurrent lesions are common, especially in the presence of meibomian gland dysfunction.

Clinical Presentation

The patient typically presents with a chief complaint of a relatively sudden onset of a warm, painful, swollen, red lump on the eyelid. An internal hordeolum points toward conjunctival eye surface, whereas an external hordeolum is found on the lid margin. Cellulitis is a rare complication of the condition and is characterized by widespread eyelid redness, pain, and edema.

Diagnostic Testing

Hordeolum is diagnosed clinically, with no specific testing needed. Lesion culture and sensitivity is only obtained with failure to respond to standard therapy.

Treatment

While caused by a bacterial organism, fairly rapid resolution is seen with warm compress application, four times a day for 10 or more minutes. Antimicrobial therapy, ocular or systemic, is not warranted. In the rare occasion of treatment failure, expert ophthalmological consultation is advised.

CHALAZION

Chalazion (plural, chalazia) is a common eyelid condition that occasionally follows hordeolum. Its etiology is eyelid sebaceous gland obstruction and inflammation, but without infection.

Clinical Presentation

With a clinical presentation less acute when compared with hordeolum, chalazion presents with a slowly developing, nontender, hard, localized eyelid swelling without redness or heat. The upper or lower lid can be affected, and a single lesion is the rule.

TABLE 5-5 Common Eyelid Disorders and Their Treatment

CONDITION	RISK FACTORS	RECOMMENDED TREATMENT
Hordeolum ("stye")	Rosacea Male gender	■ Warm compresses to area for 10 minutes or more, four or more times a day until clear ■ Antimicrobials not needed or recommended
Chalazion	Rosacea Blepharitis Seborrhea History of prior chalazion	■ Warm compresses to area for 10 or more minutes, four or more times a day until clear ■ Antimicrobial use not needed or recommended
Blepharitis	Ocular rosacea Seborrheic dermatitis and/or psoriasis	■ Warm compresses to the eyelid(s) multiple times a day ■ Gentle cleansing of lid margin with diluted baby shampoo ■ Application of topical antibiotic (bacitracin) to lid margin

Diagnostic Testing

Chalazion is diagnosed clinically, with no specific testing needed. Given no infectious organism is involved, lesion culture and sensitivity is not advised.

Treatment

Chalazion resolution is usually seen with warm compress application, four times a day for 10 or more minutes. When chalazion does not resolve with standard therapy, lesion biopsy should be conducted to ensure the diagnosis is correct.

BLEPHARITIS

Blepharitis is caused by inflammation and/or staphylococcal colonization of the meibomian glands at the base of each eyelash. This condition is often seen with ocular rosacea, seborrheic dermatitis, and/or psoriasis, disorders that are usually associated with meibomian gland dysfunction.

Clinical Presentation

In blepharitis, the condition has usually been present for a number of weeks to months prior to presentation and includes lid redness, crusting, and flaking, often accompanied by a mild burning, itching, or grainy sensation. Untreated blepharitis can lead to permanent alterations of the eyelid margin and result in vision impairment.

Diagnostic Testing

Blepharitis is diagnosed clinically, with no specific testing needed. Lesion culture and sensitivity is not advised.

Treatment

Warm compresses to the eyelid(s) multiple times a day with the goal of reducing glandular congestion is the first-line treatment in blepharitis. Following the eye compresses, a gentle cleansing of the lid margin with diluted baby shampoo, usually applied with a cotton swab, to facilitate removal of crusts is helpful. Often this is sufficient. Application of a topical antibiotic such as bacitracin to the lid margin is helpful in minimizing bacterial colonization and its contributing inflammation. Given the contributing underlying causes are usually chronic diseases, long-term treatment is the rule.

Discussion Sources

Garrity J. Chalazion and hordeolum (stye). Merck Manual online. https://www.merckmanuals.com/professional/eye-disorders/eyelid-and-lacrimal-disorders/chalazion-and-hordeolum-stye

Gilbert DN, Chambers HF, Eliopoulos GM, Saag MS, Pavia AT. *The Sanford Guide to Antimicrobial Therapy*. 50th ed. Sperryville, VA: Antimicrobial Therapy, Inc.; 2020:13.

QUESTIONS

22. A 44-year-old man presents with a chief complaint of a "white bump that is a little sore" on the left eyelid. Examination reveals a 2-mm nondraining pustule on the lateral border of the left eyelid margin. The remainder of the ocular examination is within normal limits. This description is most consistent with:

    A. a chalazion.

    B. a hordeolum.

    C. blepharitis.

    D. cellulitis.

23. A 22-year-old woman presents with a "bump" on her right eyelid that has been present for a number of weeks. She states the lesion is not painful and is not draining. Examination reveals a 2-mm firm, nontender, nondraining swelling on the lateral border of the right eyelid margin. The remainder of the ocular examination is within normal limits. This presentation is most consistent with:

    A. a chalazion.

    B. a hordeolum.

    C. blepharitis.

    D. cellulitis.

24. First-line treatment for uncomplicated hordeolum is:

    A. topical corticosteroid applied to the lid margin.

    B. warm compresses multiple times a day to the affected area.

    C. referral to ophthalmology for incision and drainage.

    D. oral antimicrobial therapy with *S aureus* coverage.

25. A potential complication of hordeolum is:

    A. conjunctivitis.

    B. cellulitis of the eyelid.

    C. corneal ulceration.

    D. sinusitis.

26. Initial treatment for a chalazion is:

    A. topical fluoroquinolone.

    B. topical corticosteroid.

    C. warm compresses of the affected area.

    D. surgical excision.

27. A 37-year-old man presents complaining of a 3-day history of a burning, itchy eyelid. Examination reveals a red, crusty eyelid. This is most consistent with:

    A. a chalazion.

    B. a hordeolum.

C. blepharitis.

D. cellulitis.

28. Treatment for a blepharitis can include all of the following except:

A. topical antimicrobial.

B. intralesional corticosteroid injection.

C. warm compresses of the affected area.

D. gentle cleansing of the area with diluted baby shampoo.

For answers and rationales, see end of chapter.

Otitis Externa

Overview

Otitis externa (OE) is an inflammation or infection of the external auditory canal (EAC), the auricle, or both. OE risk factors include a history of recent ear canal trauma, usually after vigorous use of a cotton swab or other item to clean the canal, and conditions in which moisture is frequently held in the ear canal, such as with cerumen impaction and frequent swimming. Freshwater aural exposure presents more of a risk when compared to saltwater exposure. OE is most often caused by *P aeruginosa* and, less commonly with community-based infection, fungi such as *Candida* or *Aspergillus* species.

Clinical Presentation

When OE is fungal in origin, the clinical presentation typically includes a report of less pain but more itch; ear discharge is usually described as being thicker and white to gray in color. Additional OE findings include EAC inflammation, narrowing, and swelling, as well as a sensation of ear pressure fullness, and, less commonly, temporary decreased hearing.

Diagnostic Testing

The patient's history and physical examination, including otoscopy, usually provide sufficient information for the clinician to make the diagnosis of OE. Given that the organisms that cause OE are well known, ear canal culture is not recommended; antimicrobial therapy is based rather on anticipated pathogens that cause the condition. On rare occasion, Gram stain, and/or culture and sensitivity of ear canal discharge, are obtained with treatment failure.

> **CLINICAL CONCEPT**
>
> A hallmark OE finding is ear pain (otalgia), progressing over 1 to 2 days, on tragus palpation or with the application of traction to the pinna as well as purulent or serous, often foul-smelling, discharge from the ear canal.

Treatment

While seldom a life-threatening or serious illness, the person with OE is usually quite uncomfortable. As a result, pain management is key to OE treatment. See Table 5-6 for common treatments.

■ Effective topical therapies for otitis externa include otic suspension of an antimicrobial, such as a fluoroquinolone (ofloxacin or ciprofloxacin), or polymyxin B plus neomycin, with or without hydrocortisone solution; the addition of a topical corticosteroid will likely result in faster resolution of symptoms such as pain, canal edema, and canal erythema.

■ Additional treatment options containing acetic acid are effective but often not well tolerated due to discomfort with use.

■ When the ear canal is edematous to the point at which topical antimicrobial drops cannot be well distributed, an ear wick is usually inserted and left in place for 2 to 3 days.

■ Otic drops containing neomycin or aminoglycoside should not be used if tympanic membrane rupture is present or suspected.

■ Gentle ear irrigation should be considered to remove debris and facilitate aural canal contact with the antimicrobial, only if the tympanic membrane is intact.

■ Aural hygiene using gentle suction to remove debris can be helpful; irrigation in the presence of acute infection is usually not advocated.

■ Usually oral NSAIDs or acetaminophen are helpful and sufficient for pain management, particularly after the first 24 hours of antimicrobial therapy.

Otitis Externa Complications: Malignant or Necrotizing Otitis Externa

Malignant or necrotizing OE, with both terms commonly used interchangeably, is a complication that occurs in OE when the patient is immunocompromised. The infection invades the deeper soft tissue; osteomyelitis of the temporal bone is often seen in this rare condition. Presentation includes the usual features of OE and pain disproportionate to clinical findings. In suspected malignant OE, otolaryngology should be promptly consulted. Diagnostic imaging including computed tomography (CT) to depict bony erosion will usually be ordered. Additional imaging options include radionuclide bone scanning and gadolinium magnetic resonance imaging (MRI). Surgical débridement is typically needed. Parenteral antimicrobial therapy, usually with coverage against *Pseudomonas*, is usually warranted for this severe disease (see Table 5-6).

TABLE 5-6 Common Bacterial Ear, Nose, and Throat Infections: Etiology and Treatment

CONDITION	ETIOLOGY/CAUSATIVE ORGANISMS	TREATMENT	ADDITIONAL CLINICAL CONSIDERATIONS
Otitis externa (swimmer's ear)	*Pseudomonas* spp., anaerobes, *Staphylococcus epidermidis* Acute infection often *S aureus* Fungi rare etiology	Mild: Acetic acid plus propylene glycol with hydrocortisone otic drops Moderate-severe: Ciprofloxacin otic drops with hydrocortisone Alternative: Finafloxacin otic suspension (for *P aeruginosa* and *S aureus*)	Ear canal cleansing important Decrease risk of reinfection by use of eardrops of 1:2 mixture or white vinegar and rubbing alcohol after swimming
Malignant otitis externa in a person with diabetes mellitus, HIV/AIDS, on chemotherapy	*P aeruginosa* in more than 95%	First line Ciprofloxacin 400 mg IV q8h (or if very early infection, 750 mg po q8–12h). Prompt ENT consultation needed; no role for topical therapy	Surgical débridement usually needed; imaging to evaluate for osteomyelitis often indicated
Acute otitis media	*S pneumoniae*, *H influenzae*, *M catarrhalis*, viral or no pathogen (approximately 55% bacterial, *S pneumoniae* most common)	No systemic use antibiotics in prior month: Amoxicillin high dose 1,000 mg PO tid *or* Amoxicillin-clavulanate extended release 2,000/125 mg PO bid *or* Cefdinir 300 mg PO q12h or 600 mg PO q24h *or* Cefpodoxime proxetil 200 mg PO bid *or* Cefprozil 250 to 500 mg PO bid Systemic antibiotic use in the prior month: ■ Amoxicillin-clavulanate extended release 2,000/125 mg PO BID *or* ■ Ceftriaxone 1 to 2 g IV or IM q24h × 3 days	Consider drug-resistant *S pneumoniae* (DRSP) risk: Antimicrobial therapy in past 3 months, age less than 2 years, day-care attendance; HD amoxicillin usually effective in DRSP Length of therapy: age less than 2 years, 10 days; age 2 years or older, 5 to 7 days If allergy to beta-lactam drugs: TMP-SMX, clarithromycin, azithromycin; all less effective against DRSP compared with other options

Continued

TABLE 5-6 Common Bacterial Ear, Nose, and Throat Infections: Etiology and Treatment—cont'd

CONDITION	ETIOLOGY/CAUSATIVE ORGANISMS	TREATMENT	ADDITIONAL CLINICAL CONSIDERATIONS
		Duration of therapy if not mentioned, 5 to 7 days With beta-lactam allergy ■ β-lactam drug allergy: • If history is unclear or rash, effective oral cephalosporin acceptable (see previous list) • Avoid cephalosporins if IgE-mediated allergy, e.g., anaphylaxis	If penicillin allergy history is unclear or rash (no hive-form lesions), cephalosporins likely okay See Chapter 17 for additional information
Exudative pharyngitis	Most commonly: group A, C, G streptococcus; less commonly: *Fusobacterium,* Epstein-Barr virus, primary HIV, *Neisseria gonorrhoeae,* respiratory viruses	First-line for strep pharyngitis: penicillin V 500 mg PO × 10 days or benzathine penicillin 1.2 million units intramuscularly × 1 dose *or* cefdinir 300 mg PO bid × 5 to 10 days or 600 mg PO q24h × 10 days *or* cefpodoxime 100 mg PO bid × 5 days If penicillin allergy: clindamycin PO *or* azithromycin PO *or* clarithromycin PO Up to 35% *Streptococcus pyogenes* isolates resistant to macrolides such as azithromycin	Vesicular, ulcerative pharyngitis usually viral; only 10% of adult pharyngitis due to group A streptococcus No treatment recommended for asymptomatic group A streptococcus carrier For recurrent, culture-proven *S pyogenes,* primary treatment with cefdinir or cefpodoxime; alternative with amoxicillin-clavulanate or clindamycin

Source: Gilbert DN, Chambers HF, Eliopoulos GM, Saag MS, Pavia AT. The Sanford Guide to Antimicrobial Therapy. 50th ed. Sperryville, VA: Antimicrobial Therapy, Inc.; 2020:11, 49.

Discussion Sources

Gilbert DN, Chambers HF, Eliopoulos GM, Saag MS, Pavia AT. *The Sanford Guide to Antimicrobial Therapy*. 50th ed. Sperryville, VA: Antimicrobial Therapy, Inc.; 2020.

Nussenbaum B. Malignant otitis externa. Medscape. https://emedicine.medscape.com/article/845525-overview

Waitzman AA. Otitis externa. Medscape. http://emedicine.medscape.com/article/994550

QUESTIONS

29. A 27-year-old woman presents with otitis externa. Likely causative pathogens include all of the following except:

    A. *Pseudomonas* spp.

    B. *S epidermidis.*

    C. *S aureus.*

    D. *Moraxella catarrhalis.*

30. Which of the following individuals is least likely to develop OE?

    A. a 22-year-old who travels frequently by airplane

    B. a 32-year-old who frequently cleans the ear canals with a hair pin

    C. a 16-year-old who is on the high school varsity swim team

    D. a 36-year-old man with recurrent cerumen impaction

31. Appropriate antimicrobial therapy for uncomplicated OE in a 45-year-old with hypertension and dyslipidemia includes a course of:

    A. an oral macrolide.

    B. a parenteral cephalosporin.

    C. fluoroquinolone otic drops.

    D. aminoglycoside otic drops.

32. Physical examination findings in OE in a 38-year-old include:

    A. tympanic membrane immobility.

    B. increased ear pain with tragus pull.

    C. tympanic membrane erythema.

    D. tympanic membrane bullae.

33. An important risk factor for malignant/necrotizing OE includes:

    A. the presence of an immunocompromised condition.

    B. age younger than 21 years.

    C. a history of a recent URI.

    D. a complicated course of otitis media with effusion (OME).

34. Clinical presentation of malignant/necrotizing OE usually includes:

    A. foul-smelling discharge from the ear canal.

    B. pain disproportionate to the clinical presentation.

    C. increase in discomfort with manipulation of pinna.

    D. marked ear canal edema.

35. During a clinical visit with an NP where malignant OE is being considered, the next best steps in care include all of the following except:

    A. prompt otolaryngology consultation.

    B. oral or parenteral antimicrobial therapy.

    C. imaging to determine degree of bony erosion or other complications.

    D. use of analgesic otic drops.

For answers and rationales, see end of chapter.

Acute Otitis Media in Teens and Adults

Overview

Although often considered a disease limited to childhood, acute otitis media (AOM) still ranks among the most frequent diagnoses noted in acute or urgent care teen and adult office visits. (AOM in the child is covered in Chapter 18.)

Eustachian tube dysfunction usually precedes the development of AOM, allowing negative pressure to be generated in the middle ear; this negative pressure enables pharyngeal pathogens to be aspirated into the middle ear, and the infection takes hold. *S pneumoniae, H influenzae, M catarrhalis*, and various viruses contribute to the infectious and inflammatory process of the middle ear.

> **CLINICAL CONCEPT**
> Eustachian tube dysfunction is usually caused by a viral URI or untreated allergic rhinitis.

Clinical Presentation

AOM is a clinical diagnosis for which abnormalities in the otic examination such as tympanic membrane erythema, loss of tympanic membrane mobility, and visible bony landmarks are coupled with otalgia (ear pain) (Fig. 5-6).

Diagnostic Testing

Pneumatic otoscopy is occasionally performed to support the diagnosis, where limited to no tympanic membrane mobility is noted. Largely a clinical diagnosis, no additional specific diagnostic testing is usually needed in AOM. No middle ear or pharyngeal cultures are needed or recommended except for the rare occasion of AOM treatment failure.

Treatment

Common viruses that cause AOM include human rhinovirus, respiratory syncytial virus (RSV), adenovirus, and influenza virus. AOM caused by these viral agents usually resolves in 7 to 10 days with supportive care alone. While clinical guidelines that favor "watch and wait" therapy, where antimicrobial therapy is initiated only under certain circumstances and a significant percentage will resolve with supportive therapy only, have been well studied in pediatrics, adult AOM is usually treated with an antimicrobial.

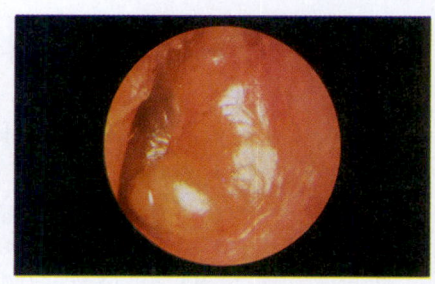

FIGURE 5-6 Acute otitis media (AOM). *Dillon P. Nursing Health Assessment: The Foundation of Clinical Practice. 3rd ed. Philadelphia, PA: F.A. Davis; 2016.*

Initial antimicrobial selection, given orally, in AOM will depend on whether the patients had recent prior antimicrobial use (within the past month), as one of the most potent risk factors for AOM caused by drug-resistant *S pneumoniae* (DRSP) is recent systemic antimicrobial use. Standard dose oral amoxicillin can be used if no prior antimicrobials have been used; otherwise, high-dose oral amoxicillin, high-dose oral amoxicillin-clavulanate, or certain oral cephalosporins are recommended for patients with recent systemic antimicrobial use. In beta-lactam allergy, select cephalosporins are usually acceptable if the reaction is limited to skin rash (see Table 5-6). Length of therapy is 5 to 7 days.

The use of oral over-the-counter (OTC) analgesics including ibuprofen or acetaminophen is usually sufficient to provide pain relief in AOM. (See Chapter 17 for further information on AOM in children.)

AOM Resolution and Prevention

With AOM recovery, tympanic membrane mobility, noted on pneumatic otoscopy, returns in about 1 to 2 weeks, and lymphadenopathy and tympanic membrane redness resolve, and the bony landmarks become visible. The cone of light typically is not noted. Serous fluid persists for 4 to 6 weeks in the middle ear, resulting in OME. Itching and crackling in the ear are common in patients with OME. Given that OME usually resolves in the previously mentioned time period after AOM, no particular therapy is indicated.

Avoiding conditions that can cause Eustachian tube dysfunction, such as URI, untreated or undertreated allergic rhinitis, tobacco use, and exposure to air pollution, can lead to a reduction in the occurrence of AOM.

Discussion Sources

Gilbert DN, Chambers HF, Eliopoulos GM, Saag MS, Pavia AT. *The Sanford Guide to Antimicrobial Therapy.* 50th ed. Sperryville, VA: Antimicrobial Therapy, Inc.; 2020:11.

Natal BL. Emergent management of acute otitis media. Medscape. http://emedicine.medscape.com/article/764006-overview

QUESTIONS

36 to 39. Indicate (Yes or No) which of the following viruses are implicated in causing AOM.

_____ **36.** RSV

_____ **37.** herpes simplex virus 2

_____ **38.** influenza virus

_____ **39.** rhinovirus

40 to 43. Indicate (Yes or No) which of the following bacteria are commonly implicated in causing AOM.

_____ **40.** *S pneumoniae*

_____ **41.** *H influenzae*

_____ **42.** *Escherichia coli*

_____ **43.** *M. catarrhalis*

44. Risk factors for AOM include all of the following except:

  A. URI.

  B. untreated allergic rhinitis.

  C. tobacco use.

  D. aggressive ear canal hygiene.

45. An 18-year-old high school senior presents with a 4-day history of left-sided otalgia and fullness, despite use of oral decongestants and ibuprofen. When considering a diagnosis of AOM, expected findings include:

  A. prominent tympanic membrane bony landmarks.

  B. tympanic membrane immobility.

  C. itchiness and crackling in the affected ear.

  D. submental lymphadenopathy on the affected side.

46. A 35-year-old man has a 3-day history of left ear pain that began after 1 week of URI symptoms. On physical examination, you find that he has AOM. He took an oral antimicrobial for the treatment of a skin and soft tissue infection 2 weeks ago. The most appropriate oral antimicrobial option for this patient is:

  A. standard-dose azithromycin.

  B. high-dose cephalexin.

  C. high-dose amoxicillin.

  D. standard-dose TMP-SMX.

47. A reasonable treatment option for AOM in an adult who reports a penicillin allergy, stating, "I just had a fine pink rash on my trunk," is:

  A. cefpodoxime.

  B. erythromycin.

  C. cephalexin.

  D. TMP-SMX.

48. Drug-resistant *S pneumoniae* is least likely to exhibit resistance to which of the following antimicrobial classes?

  A. advanced macrolides such as azithromycin

  B. tetracycline forms such as doxycycline

  C. first-generation cephalosporins such as cephalexin

  D. respiratory fluoroquinolones such as levofloxacin

49. Which of the following is absent in OME?

  A. fluid in the middle ear

  B. sensation of middle ear fullness

  C. fever

  D. itch

50. Treatment of OME usually includes:

  A. advising that this condition self-resolves.

  B. antimicrobial therapy.

  C. an antihistamine.

  D. a mucolytic.

For answers and rationales, see end of chapter.

Ménière's Disease, Ménière's Syndrome

Overview

Ménière's disease is an idiopathic condition, without a clearly identifiable underlying cause; Ménière's syndrome presents with identical signs and symptoms in which an underlying cause has been identified, such as lupus erythematosus or rheumatoid arthritis, resulting in an inflammatory response within the labyrinth. Both Ménière's disease and Ménière's syndrome are believed to result from idiopathic endolymphatic hydrops, a condition of increased hydraulic pressure within the inner ear endolymphatic system.

Clinical Presentation

The onset of Ménière's disease begins at early to middle adulthood with peak incidence in the 40- to 60-year-old age group, with this condition slightly more common in females.

Clinical presentation of Ménière's disease and Ménière's syndrome usually involves a history of episodes of vertigo with a sensation that the room is whirling about, often preceded by decreased hearing, low-tone roaring tinnitus, and a feeling of increased ear pressure. Particularly severe episodes are accompanied by nausea and vomiting. Attacks can last minutes to hours, with exhaustion often reported after the most severe symptoms have passed. Duration and frequency of attacks can vary, although common triggers include certain foods and drinks, mental and physical stress, and variations in the menstrual cycle.

> **CLINICAL CONCEPT**
>
> The following tetrad of symptoms must be present to make the Ménière's disease diagnosis, usually noted unilaterally:
>
> 1. Fluctuating hearing loss
> 2. Episodic vertigo
> 3. Tinnitus or ringing in the ears
> 4. Aural fullness

Diagnosis

Examination of a person with Ménière's disease typically reveals significant nystagmus or rhythmic oscillations of the eyes and slow movement toward one side, usually the side of the affected ear, with a rapid correction to the midline.

- The Weber tuning test result usually lateralizes to the unaffected ear, whereas the Rinne test shows that air exceeds bone conduction, a normal finding.
- Performing pneumatic otoscopy in the affected ear can elicit symptoms or cause nystagmus, whereas the same maneuver to the unaffected ear yields little response.
- High-frequency hearing loss is often noted by subjective and objective measures, often revealing diminished hearing.
- The Romberg test is positive, with the patient showing increased swaying and difficulty staying balanced when standing with the eyes closed.
- Additional findings include a positive Fukuda marching step test, in which a directional drift—usually toward the affected ear—is noted when the patient is asked to perform a march step with the eyes closed. This latter maneuver is often impossible for a patient with severe symptoms.
- The result of the Dix-Hallpike test (i.e., observation of horizontal or rotary nystagmus while moving a patient from sitting to supine with the head angled 45° to one side and then to the other) is occasionally also positive, indicating coexisting benign positional vertigo. Neuroimaging is usually not warranted, unless the examination reveals additional findings, or the diagnosis is unclear.

Treatment

Treatment of Ménière's disease is aimed at minimizing or preventing symptoms with a variety of medications, usually given orally:

- Antihistamines such as meclizine (Antivert, Bonine) or antiemetics can minimize overall symptoms.
- Benzodiazepines can be used to help reinforce rest and minimize anxiety associated with severe symptoms; these options do not treat the underlying condition.
- Thiazide diuretics decrease fluid pressure load in the inner ear and can be used to prevent, but not treat, attacks; these medications do not help after the attack has been triggered.
- Systemic corticosteroids also have been shown to be helpful, likely because of their anti-inflammatory properties, causing a reduction in endolymph pressure and potentially ameliorating vertigo, tinnitus, and hearing loss.

When standard therapy is ineffective and severe symptoms persist, expert consultation is warranted. A variety of treatment options are available and usually reserved for patients with frequent, severely debilitating episodes that are unresponsive to other, less radical therapies; options include endolymphatic sac decompression, vestibular neurectomy, and surgical or chemical labyrinthectomy. The possible risk of permanent hearing loss with these interventions must be reviewed with the patient. In Ménière's syndrome, symptomatic treatment and intervention for the underlying cause are warranted.

Discussion Sources

Li JC. Meniere disease (idiopathic endolymphatic hydrops). Medscape. https://emedicine.medscape.com/article/1159069-overview

Lustig LR. Meniere disease (Meniere's disease; endolymphatic hydrops). Merck Manual online. http://www.merckmanuals.com/professional/ear_nose_and_throat_disorders/inner_ear_disorders/menieres_disease.html?qt=&sc=&alt=

QUESTIONS

51 to 53. Indicate whether each case represents Ménière's disease (D) or Ménière's syndrome (S):

_____ **51.** A 44-year-old woman with a history of head trauma after a motor vehicle accident

_____ **52.** A 55-year-old woman who has osteoarthritis of the knees

_____ **53.** A 27-year-old woman with rheumatoid arthritis who remains significantly symptomatic despite optimized therapy

54. Which of the following is true concerning Ménière's disease?

A. Neuroimaging helps locate the offending cochlear lesion.

B. Associated high-frequency hearing loss is common.

C. This is largely a diagnosis of exclusion.

D. Tinnitus is rarely reported.

55 to 59. Indicate (Yes or No) whether each of the following clinical findings would be present in a patient with Ménière's disease.

_____ **55.** The Weber tuning test lateralizes to the affected ear.

_____ **56.** The Rinne test reveals that air exceeds bone conduction.

_____ **57.** Pneumatic otoscopy in the affected ear can elicit symptoms or cause nystagmus.

_____ **58.** The Romberg test is negative.

_____ **59.** The Fukuda marching step test is positive.

60. When evaluating a patient with Ménière's disease, the procedure of observing for nystagmus while moving the patient from sitting to supine with the head angled 45° to one side and then the other is called the:

A. Romberg test.

B. Dix-Hallpike test.

C. Rinne test.

D. Fukuda test.

61. Prevention and prophylaxis in Ménière's disease include all of the following except:

A. avoiding ototoxic drugs.

B. protecting the ears from loud noise.

C. limiting sodium intake.

D. restricting fluid intake.

62 to 65. Match the following to the lettered descriptions:

_____ **62.** Dizziness

_____ **63.** Vertigo

_____ **64.** Nystagmus

_____ **65.** Tinnitus

    A. perception that the person or the environment is moving

    B. subjective perception of altered equilibrium

    C. rhythmic oscillations of the eyes

    D. perception of abnormal hearing or head noises

For answers and rationales, see end of chapter.

Anterior Epistaxis

Overview

Anterior epistaxis (nosebleed) is most common in children under 10 years of age and in adults between the ages of 45 and 65 years; it is more common in males than females. Most commonly caused by localized nasal mucosa dryness during the winter months and by trauma, epistaxis is rarely caused by a coagulation disorder or uncontrolled hypertension.

Clinical Presentation

Approximately 90% of nosebleeds can be visualized in the anterior portion of the nasal cavity. There is no particular degree of blood pressure elevation known to trigger epistaxis.

Diagnostic Testing

Epistaxis is a clinical diagnosis with no particular testing needed. Less commonly, clotting studies are ordered to reveal the possibility of an underlying bleeding disorder, usually when epistaxis does not respond to standard therapy.

Treatment

Most episodes of epistaxis can be easily managed with firm pressure to the area superior to the nasal alar cartilage or an "entire nose pinched closed" position by the patient for a minimum of 10 minutes. Second-line measures for epistaxis management include nasal packing and/or the use of topical antifibrinolytic agents (thrombin) with or without topical vasoconstrictors. Nasal cautery is occasionally used in recurrent or refractory epistaxis. In the presence of anticoagulant use including warfarin, direct oral anticoagulants (DOACs) such as rivaroxaban (*Xarelto*), apixaban (*Eliquis*), and others, second-line management is often needed. For refractory cases that do not respond to second-line therapy, consider an otolaryngology consult for possible surgical intervention.

Discussion Sources

Fatakia A, Winters R, Amedee RG. Epistaxis: a common problem. *Ochsner J.* 2010;10:176–178. http://www.ncbi.nlm.nih.gov/pmc/articles/PMC3096213

Shukla PA, Chan N, Duffis EJ, et al. Current treatment strategies for epistaxis. *J Neurointerv Surg.* 2013;5:151–156. https://www.ncbi.nlm.nih.gov/pubmed/22231278

QUESTIONS

66. Who is most likely to present with anterior epistaxis?

    A. a 72-year-old woman, blood pressure of 178/102, who ran out of blood pressure medication 3 days ago

    B. a 32-year-old woman with Von Willebrand's disease

    C. a 42-year-old man who works outdoors during the months of December to March in the northeastern United States

    D. a 30-year-old with nasal polyps

67. First-line intervention for anterior epistaxis includes:

    A. nasal packing.

    B. application of topical thrombin or vasoconstrictor.

    C. firm pressure in an "entire nose pinched" position for a minimum of 10 minutes.

    D. chemical cauterization.

68. In an older adult with refractory epistaxis resistant to standard therapies, an underlying diagnosis occasionally found is:

    A. poorly controlled type 2 diabetes mellitus.

    B. accelerated hypertension.

    C. acute bacterial sinusitis.

    D. thrombocytopenia.

69. A 55-year-old man with atrial fibrillation who is taking multiple medications including DOAC presents with anterior epistaxis. He fails to respond to first-line therapy. Additional therapeutic approaches include all of the following except:

    A. initiating systemic prothrombotic therapy.

    B. nasal packing.

    C. nasal cautery.

    D. topical antifibrinolytic agents.

For answers and rationales, see end of chapter.

Allergic Rhinitis

Overview

Allergic rhinitis (AR) is due to genetic-environmental interactions in which a person with a genetic predisposition to allergens has environmental exposure that causes the immune system to shift to an allergenic state, with histamine and inflammatory mediator release. Upon reexposure to an allergen, that a person has been sensitized to (development of allergen-specific IgE antibodies), an allergic response will occur with release of histamine and inflammatory mediators from the mast cells.

Clinical Presentation

Allergic rhinitis causes a classic constellation of symptoms including sneezing; nasal, pharyngeal, and ocular itch; nasal congestion; rhinorrhea; and postnasal drip, in any combination.

Diagnostic Testing

Allergic rhinitis is a clinical diagnosis made from correlating the AR history with the physical examination findings. In the majority, testing to identify the specific allergic trigger is not warranted, especially if the patient responds well to standard therapy. More in-depth testing, such as skin or serological testing to pinpoint environmental allergens, is usually done when desensitization therapy, requiring specialty consultation, is being considered.

Treatment

As with any allergic disorder, first-line therapy is avoidance of the allergen or, at minimum, reduction in exposure. Total allergen avoidance is usually impossible. AR is triggered by indoor and outdoor aeroallergens. Dust mites are the most common trigger of perennial allergy symptoms. Pets, cockroaches, and mold spores are other indoor allergens found to cause nasal and ocular allergy symptoms. Pollens (e.g., trees, grasses, and ragweed) are major triggers in seasonal allergic rhinitis and allergic conjunctivitis (see Fig. 5-1).

    Pharmacotherapy in AR includes medications designed to relieve and/or to control symptoms (Figs. 5-7 and 5-8). Medications used to control allergy symptoms ("controllers") include intranasal corticosteroids, leukotriene modifiers, and mast cell stabilizers. Medications that are used to acutely relieve symptoms ("relievers") include antihistamines, decongestants, and, in severe cases, oral corticosteroids (Table 5-7). Acupuncture is also used when nonpharmacological therapy is desired.

ARIA Classification

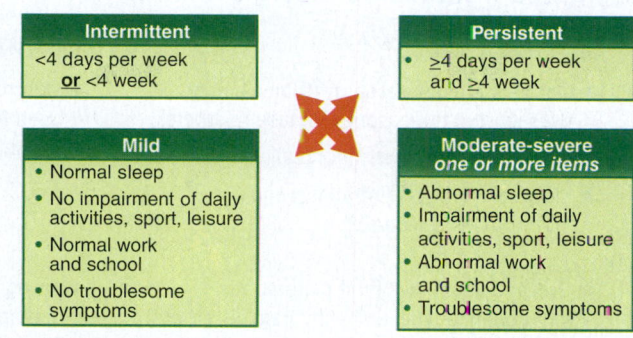

Intermittent	Persistent
<4 days per week **or** <4 week	• ≥4 days per week and ≥4 week

Mild	Moderate-severe *one or more items*
• Normal sleep • No impairment of daily activities, sport, leisure • Normal work and school • No troublesome symptoms	• Abnormal sleep • Impairment of daily activities, sport, leisure • Abnormal work and school • Troublesome symptoms

Symptoms reported prior to treatment

FIGURE 5-7 ARIA classification.
Adapted from Bousquet J, Van Cauwenberge P, Khaltaev N. Allergic rhinitis and its impact on asthma. J Allergy Clin Immunol. 2001;108 (suppl):S147–S334.

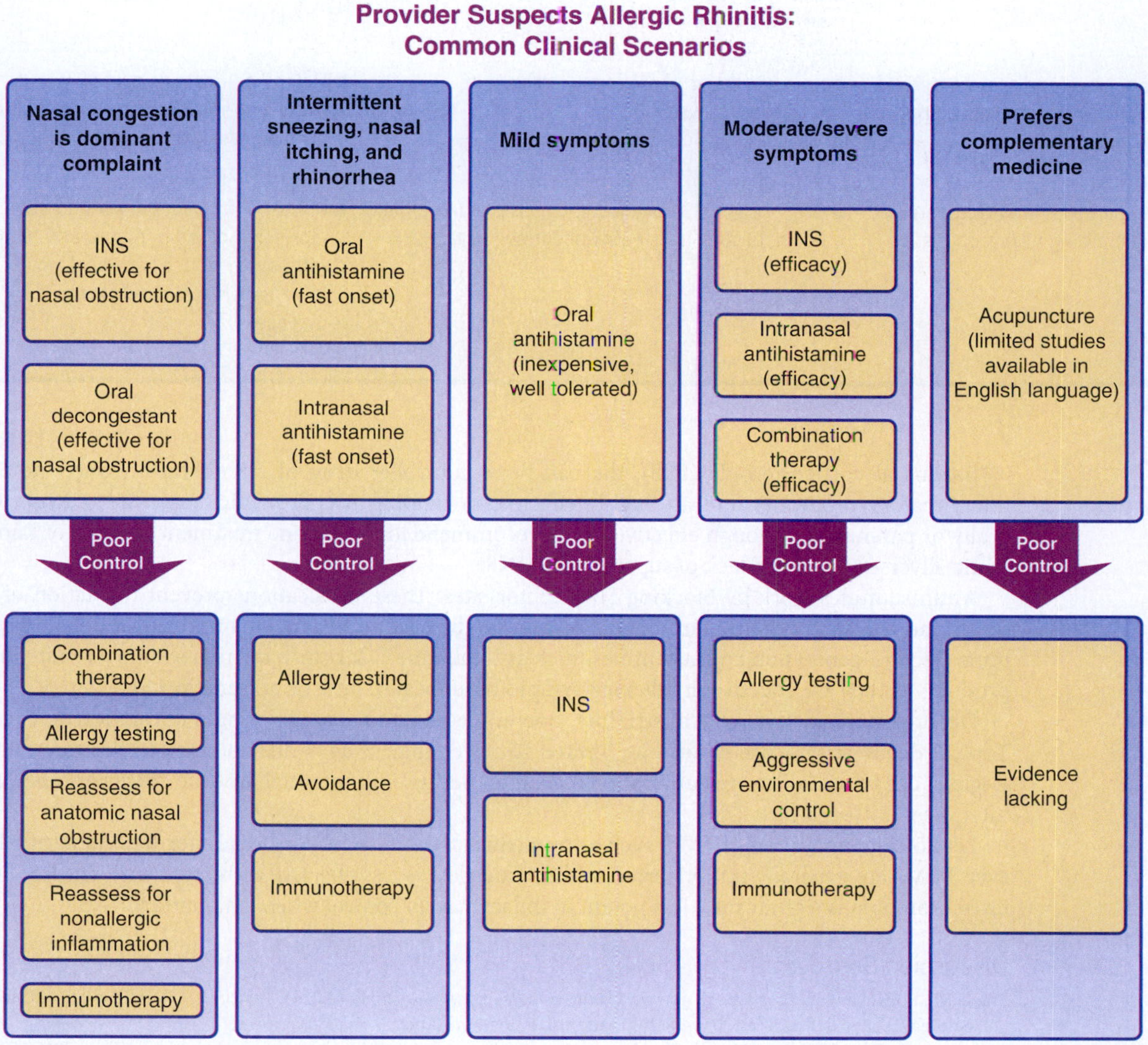

Provider Suspects Allergic Rhinitis: Common Clinical Scenarios

Nasal congestion is dominant complaint	Intermittent sneezing, nasal itching, and rhinorrhea	Mild symptoms	Moderate/severe symptoms	Prefers complementary medicine
INS (effective for nasal obstruction)	Oral antihistamine (fast onset)	Oral antihistamine (inexpensive, well tolerated)	INS (efficacy)	Acupuncture (limited studies available in English language)
Oral decongestant (effective for nasal obstruction)	Intranasal antihistamine (fast onset)		Intranasal antihistamine (efficacy)	
			Combination therapy (efficacy)	

Poor Control →

Combination therapy Allergy testing Reassess for anatomic nasal obstruction Reassess for nonallergic inflammation Immunotherapy	Allergy testing Avoidance Immunotherapy	INS Intranasal antihistamine	Allergy testing Aggressive environmental control Immunotherapy	Evidence lacking

FIGURE 5-8 INS, intranasal corticosteroids. Common allergic rhinitis clinical scenarios and treatment guidance from the American Academy of Otolaryngology–Head and Neck Surgery.
Seidman MD, Gurgel RK, Lin SY, et al. Clinical practice guideline: allergic rhinitis. Otolaryngol Head Neck Surg. 2015;152(suppl 1):S1–S43.
http://oto.sagepub.com/content/152/1_suppl/S1.long

TABLE 5-7 Medications Used in the Treatment of Allergic Rhinitis

THERAPEUTIC GOAL	INTERVENTION	COMMENT
Controller therapy to prevent formation of inflammatory mediators	■ Corticosteroid nasal spray (triamcinolone [Nasacort®], fluticasone [Flonase®], others) ■ Leukotriene modifiers (montelukast [Singulair®]) ■ Mast cell stabilizer (intranasal and optic cromolyn [NasalCrom®])	■ Controller therapy usually needs to be used for a few days to 2 weeks before maximum effect noted; little effect on acute symptoms
Rescue therapy by inactivating formed inflammatory mediators	■ Oral antihistamines (first generation [chlorpheniramine, diphenhydramine, others], second generation [loratadine, cetirizine, fexofenadine, levocetirizine, others]) ■ Antihistamine nasal spray (azelastine [Astelin®] nasal spray) ■ Antihistamine optic drops (ketotifen [Zaditor®] optic drops) ■ Short-term oral corticosteroids if needed for severe allergic symptoms	■ Using only antihistamine rescue therapy usually not as effective on overall disease control as consistent use of controller therapy with rescue therapy as an adjunct
Rescue therapy and symptom relief by minimizing nasal discharge	■ Anticholinergic nasal spray (ipratropium bromide [Atrovent®]) ■ Antihistamine nasal spray (Astelin®, others)	■ Helpful adjuncts as part of rescue therapy for patient with bothersome profuse nasal discharge
Rescue therapy and symptom relief by minimizing nasal congestion	■ Oral and nasal decongestants (alpha-adrenergic agonists such as pseudoephedrine [Sudafed®])	■ Potential for vasoconstriction and increased blood pressure and heart rate; avoid or use with caution in hypertension, cardiovascular disease

Intranasal corticosteroids (INS), the backbone controller drug of AR therapy, exhibit potent anti-inflammatory properties and are highly effective in treating AR. Systemic corticosteroid use, whether orally or parenterally, though effective, is not recommended for routine treatment because of known systemic adverse effects and lack of superiority to INS.

Antihistamines work by blocking H_1 receptor sites. These medications prevent the action of formed histamine, a potent inflammatory mediator, and can be used to treat acute or breakthrough allergy symptoms. Second-generation antihistamines, such as loratadine (Claritin®), are preferred over first-generation products as they are effective in relieving symptoms and cause little or no sedation.

Decongestants act as vasoconstrictors, opening edematous nasal passages and relieving congestion. Topical decongestant use should be limited to fewer than 5 days due to risk of rebound congestion. Regular use of oral decongestants is to be avoided because of potential adverse effects and potential for tolerance.

Leukotriene modifiers (LTMs) such as montelukast can also be considered for treatment of AR. However, LTMs are generally not preferred as this drug class is less effective compared with an INS. Similarly, nasal cromolyn is significantly less potent in inflammation control when compared to INS.

Discussion Sources

Brozek JL, Bousquet J, Agache I, et al. *Allergic Rhinitis and Its Impact on Asthma (ARIA) Guidelines—2016 Revision.* https://www.euforea.eu/sites/default/files/2018-08/2017_aria_2016_revision_2.pdf

Seidman MD, Gurgel RK, Lin SY, et al. Clinical practice guidelines: allergic rhinitis. *Otolaryngol Head Neck Surg.* 2015;152(suppl 1): S1–S43. http://oto.sagepub.com/content/152/1_suppl/S1.long

Wallace D, Dykewicz M. Diagnosis and management of rhinitis: an updated practice parameter. Joint Task Force on Practice Parameters (AAAAI, ACAAI and the Joint Council of Allergy, Asthma and Immunology). *J Allergy Clin Immunol.* 2008;122:S1–S84.

QUESTIONS

70. A 45-year-old man who works as a landscaper has seasonal AR. He asks you when the pollen count is likely to be the lowest. You respond:

A. "Early in the morning."

B. "During breezy times of the day."

C. "After a rain shower."

D. "When the sky is overcast."

71 to 74. Match each allergen with the appropriate characteristic. *(An answer can be used more than once.)*

_____ **71.** Pollens

_____ **72.** Pet dander

_____ **73.** Dust mites

_____ **74.** Mold spores

       A. most common perennial allergen

       B. most common seasonal allergen

       C. common indoor allergen

75. You prescribe a nasal corticosteroid for a 28-year-old woman with perennial AR. When advising her about the onset of symptom relief, the NP states that she will notice improvement:

A. immediately with the first spray.

B. in 1 to 2 days.

C. in a few days to a week.

D. in 2 or more weeks.

76. Which of the following medications is most appropriate for AR therapy in an acutely symptomatic 24-year-old machine operator?

A. nasal cromolyn

B. oral diphenhydramine

C. flunisolide nasal spray

D. oral loratadine

77. Antihistamines work primarily through:

A. vasoconstriction.

B. action on the histamine-1 (H_1) receptor sites.

C. inflammatory mediation.

D. peripheral vasodilation.

78. Decongestants work primarily through:

A. vasoconstriction.

B. action on the H_1 receptor sites.

C. inflammatory mediation.

D. peripheral vasodilation.

79. Which of the following medications affords the best relief of acute nasal itch?

A. anticholinergic nasal spray

B. oral decongestant

C. corticosteroid nasal spray

D. oral antihistamine

80. Which of the following medications affords the best relief of acute nasal congestion?
    A. anticholinergic nasal spray
    B. oral leukotriene modifier
    C. nasal decongestant
    D. oral antihistamine

81. Which of the following medications is preferred to treat acute rhinorrhea associated with AR?
    A. anticholinergic nasal spray
    B. oral antihistamine
    C. corticosteroid nasal spray
    D. oral leukotriene modifier

82. Ipratropium bromide (Atrovent®) helps control nasal secretions through:
    A. antihistaminic action.
    B. anticholinergic effect.
    C. vasodilation.
    D. vasoconstriction.

83. Oral decongestant use should be discouraged in patients with:
    A. AR.
    B. migraine headache.
    C. cardiovascular disease.
    D. chronic bronchitis.

84. Cromolyn's mechanism of action is as:
    A. an anti-immunoglobulin E antibody.
    B. a vasoconstrictor.
    C. a mast cell stabilizer.
    D. a leukotriene modifier.

85. In the treatment of AR, a leukotriene modifier should be used as:
    A. an agent to relieve nasal itch.
    B. an inflammatory inhibitor.
    C. a rescue drug.
    D. an intervention in acute inflammation.

86. Allergen subcutaneous or oral immunotherapy should be considered in all of the following except:
    A. when allergy symptoms are controlled with environmental management.
    B. when allergy symptoms persist despite optimal use of appropriate medications.
    C. when there is a desire to reduce the use of allergy medications.
    D. to prevent progression or development of asthma.

87. Which of the following is most appropriate for the treatment of moderate-to-severe AR when symptoms are not controlled with intranasal antihistamine?
    A. initiation of daily oral corticosteroids
    B. single dose of a long-acting parenteral or intramuscular corticosteroids
    C. initiation of daily intranasal corticosteroids
    D. immediate initiation of allergy immunotherapy

For answers and rationales, see end of chapter.

Antibiotic Allergy

Overview

The penicillins, including penicillin, amoxicillin, dicloxacillin, ampicillin, others, and the cephalosporins, with the *ceph* or *cef* prefix, are known as the beta-lactam antibiotics, since all share a beta-lactam ring in their molecular structure. The beta-lactams are the most commonly prescribed antimicrobial class as well as the class with the highest rate of allergic reaction.

Conventional practice is to assume that a patient with allergy to penicillin will also react to the cephalosporins. When select cephalosporins are eliminated, the cross-allergy rate is likely less than 1% with the use of the second-, third-, and fourth-generation cephalosporins, such as cefprozil (Ceftin®), cefuroxime, cefpodoxime (Vantin®), ceftazidime, and ceftriaxone (Rocephin®), and slightly higher with the use of the first-generation cephalosporins, including cephalexin (Keflex®) and cefadroxil (Duricef®). While about 10% of the population report penicillin allergy, the most common form of antibiotic allergy, this is likely a significant overestimation of this condition's prevalence.

Clinical Presentation

The most common clinical presentation of beta-lactam allergy is an immunoglobulin E (IgE)-mediated type I reaction including rapid-onset maculopapular skin eruptions, urticaria, and pruritus with more severe reactions involving respiratory symptoms with cough and bronchospasm and cardiovascular compromise including tachycardia and hypotension. The reaction's onset can occur rapidly after drug ingestion, particularly if the patient has been sensitized to the antibiotic by previous exposure. A less common form of beta-lactam allergy includes a hypersensitivity syndrome characterized by fever, eosinophilia, and other extracutaneous manifestations.

Diagnostic Testing

The initial diagnosis is developed on a history of select antibiotic exposure and the resulting clinical presentation of the previously mentioned signs and symptoms. If the history is consistent with a severe, rapid-onset IgE-mediated-type response, referral for allergy testing is the most prudent course; this approach should also be considered if the penicillin allergy history is unclear. When allergy testing is undertaken, confirmation of the presence or absence of penicillin or cephalosporin allergy, as well as allergy to other antibiotic classes, is important. With a history of less severe reactions, clinical judgment is warranted. Diagnostic testing can include skin testing as well as immunoassays.

Treatment

As with all allergic disorders, avoidance of the allergen is the first-line therapy. In the presence of an acute allergic reaction to a beta-lactam, particularly with anaphylaxis, the offending antibiotic should be promptly discontinued and treatment for anaphylaxis initiated. See Chapter 14 for details.

Allergic reactions to other antibiotic classes can also occur, though typically less frequently than reactions to beta-lactams. TMP-SMX can cause both immediate and delayed reactions. Delayed reactions can range from mild maculopapular exanthema and fixed drug eruptions to serious manifestations (i.e., anaphylaxis, Stevens-Johnson syndrome, or toxic epidermal necrolysis). Allergic reactions to fluoroquinolones (less than 2%) and macrolides (less than 3%) are uncommon. At the first sign of any drug-induced allergic reaction, the patient should stop taking the offending medication and seek appropriate health care.

In the person with history of penicillin allergy, whether to prescribe a cephalosporin or not requires careful data gathering on the exact reaction that occurs after penicillin use. In addition, input from evaluation by an allergist on safe antimicrobial use is valuable. When seeing a patient who reports being allergic to virtually all antibiotics, referral to allergy and immunology for antibiotic allergy testing is critical to confirm what medications are safe to use if the patient presents with an infectious disease when such therapy is warranted.

Discussion Sources

Har D, Solensky R. Penicillin and beta-lactam hypersensitivity. *Immunol Allergy Clin North Am.* 2017;37:643–662.

Norton AE, Konvinse K, Phillips EJ, Broyles AD. Antibiotic allergy in pediatrics. *Pediatrics.* 2018;141(5):e20172497. doi:https://doi.org/10.1542/peds.2017-2497

Thong BYH. Update on the management of antibiotic allergy. *Allergy Asthma Immunol Res.* 2010;2:77–86.

Zagursky RJ, Pichichero ME. Cross-reactivity in beta-lactam allergy. *J Allergy Clin Immunol Pract.* 2018;6(1):72–81.e1.

QUESTIONS

88. Which of the following medications is not a penicillin form?

   A. amoxicillin

   B. ampicillin

   C. dicloxacillin

   D. imipenem

89. A cutaneous reaction nearly always occurs with the use of oral amoxicillin in the presence of infection with:

   A. human herpes virus type 1.

   B. human papillomavirus type 11.

   C. adenovirus type 20.

   D. Epstein-Barr virus (EBV).

90. In a person with a well-documented history of systemic cutaneous reaction without airway impingement following penicillin use, the use of which of the following cephalosporins is most likely to result in an allergic response?

   A. cephalexin

   B. cefprozil

   C. cefuroxime

   D. cefpodoxime

91. Which of the following antimicrobial classes is associated with the highest rate of allergic reaction?

   A. the macrolides

   B. the beta-lactams

   C. the fluoroquinolones

   D. the sulfonamides

92. A 36-year-old man presents for his initial visit to become a patient in a primary care practice. He is generally in good health with a history of hyperlipidemia and is currently taking an HMG-CoA reductase inhibitor (statin). He reports that he is "allergic to just about every antibiotic" and reports a variety of reactions including diffuse urticaria, gastrointestinal upset, and fatigue but without respiratory involvement. He is unclear as to which antibiotics have caused these reactions and states that much of what he knows is from his mother who "told me I always got sicker instead of better when I took an antibiotic." His last use of an antimicrobial was more than 10 years ago when he was treated for a "sinus infection" and was without reaction and does not recall the name of this medication. The next most appropriate step in his care is to:

   A. advise the patient to obtain a more detailed history of what antibiotics he was given during his childhood.

   B. refer to allergy and immunology for further evaluation.

   C. inform the patient to start an antihistamine whenever he is given an antibiotic.

   D. provide a prescription for a systemic corticosteroid to take if he develops a reaction to his next antimicrobial course.

93. Serious allergic reactions caused by the use of TMP-SMX include all of the following except:

   A. anaphylaxis.

   B. Stevens-Johnson syndrome.

   C. toxic epidermal necrolysis.

   D. fixed drug eruptions.

94. A 37-year-old man presents with acute bacterial rhinosinusitis (ABRS) that has failed to respond to 5 days of treatment with amoxicillin. He reports that he experienced an allergic reaction to ciprofloxacin a few years ago that caused a rash as well as swelling of the lips and tongue. In deciding on a new antimicrobial, you consider avoiding the use of:

A. amoxicillin-clavulanate.

B. azithromycin.

C. moxifloxacin.

D. cefpodoxime.

95. You prescribe a regimen of oral doxycycline to treat an acute exacerbation of chronic obstructive pulmonary disease for a 56-year-old man. This is his first exposure to this antimicrobial. You advise that:

A. he should not experience an allergic reaction because he has no reported penicillin allergy.

B. if he experiences any allergic reaction, he should stop taking the antibiotic and seek appropriate health care.

C. if he experiences an allergic reaction, he should continue taking the medication until he meets with a health-care provider to avoid resistance development.

D. any allergic reaction will eventually resolve once the regimen is complete.

For answers and rationales, see end of chapter.

Acute Bacterial Rhinosinusitis

Overview

ABRS is a clinical condition resulting from inflammation of the lining of the membranes of the paranasal sinuses caused by bacterial infection. Risk factors include any condition that alters the normal cleansing and drainage mechanisms of the sinuses, including viral infection, poorly controlled allergic rhinitis, tobacco use, and abnormalities in sinus structure.

Clinical Presentation

Because viral infections typically improve after 5 to 10 days, the diagnosis of ABRS is considered only in patients with URI-like symptoms with persistent or worsening symptoms for 10 or more days who continue to have:

1. maxillary/facial pain and

2. purulent nasal discharge.

In addition, the patient with a report of "double sickening," that is, approximtately 3 to 4 days or more of URI-like symptoms that gradually improve and then suddenly worsen, is suggestive of superimposed bacterial sinus infection. Alternatively, patients can present with severe illness (pain and fever), 3 to 4 days after onset of symptoms (Table 5-8). The physical examination during ABRS, including sinuses tender to palpation, is often quite similar to what is seen during viral URI and therefore contributes little to the diagnosis.

Diagnostic Testing

ABRS is a clinical diagnosis with history of present illness being more sensitive and specific for the condition when compared to physical examination. Nearly all patients with ABRS do not require radiographic (x-ray or CT) imaging because it is nonspecific and cannot distinguish between viral or bacterial infection. Advanced imaging such as CT or MRI can be helpful for recurrent or complicated situations, with treatment failure, or when suppurative complications are suspected.

Treatment

Empiric antimicrobial therapy in ABRS should be aimed at choosing an agent with significant activity against gram-positive (*S pneumoniae*) and gram-negative organisms (*H influenzae*, *M catarrhalis*), with consideration for drug-resistant *S pneumoniae* risk and possible need for stability in the presence of

TABLE 5-8 Causative Pathogens in Acute Otitis Media (AOM)/Acute Bacterial Rhinosinusitis (ABRS) and Algorithm for ABRS Management

ORGANISM	DESCRIPTION	RESISTANCE
S pneumoniae	Gram-positive diplococci Most common ABRS and AOM bacterial pathogen	Approximately 25% drug-resistant S pneumoniae via altered protein-binding sites that limit antibiotic's ability to bind to the pathogen
H influenzae	Gram-negative bacillus Second most common ABRS and AOM bacterial pathogen	Approximately 30% to 40% penicillin-resistant via production of beta-lactamase that cleaves the beta-lactam ring
M catarrhalis	Gram-negative coccus A distant third most common ABRS and AOM pathogen	Approximately 90% penicillin-resistant via beta-lactamase production

Algorithm for the Management of Acute Bacterial Rhinosinusitis

Abbreviations
CT: computed tomography
MRI: magnetic resonance imaging

Signs and symptoms either:
a) Persistent and not improving (≥10 days);
b) Severe (≥3–4 days); or
c) Worsening or "double-sickening" (≥3–4 days)

Risk for antibiotic resistance
• Age <2 or >65, day care
• Prior antibiotics within the past month
• Prior hospitalization past 5 days
• Comorbidities
• Immunocompromised

Risk for Resistance

No → Initiate first-line antimicrobial therapy

Yes → Initiate second-line antimicrobial therapy

Symptomatic management

Improvement after 3–5 days → Complete 5–7 days of antimicrobial therapy

Worsening or no improvement after 3–5 days

Improvement after 3–5 days → Complete 7–10 days of antimicrobial therapy

Improvement → Complete 5–7 days of antimicrobial therapy

Broaden coverage or switch to different antimicrobial class

Improvement → Complete 7–10 days of antimicrobial therapy

Worsening or no improvement after 3–5 days

Refer to specialist

• CT or MRI to investigate noninfectious causes or suppurative complications
• Sinus or meatal cultures for pathogen-specific therapy

Source: Clinical Infectious Diseases Advance Access, http://cid.oxfordjournals.org

Source: Chow AW, Benninger MS, Brook I, et al. IDSA clinical practice guideline for acute bacterial rhinosinusitis in children and adults. Clin Infect Dis. 2012;54:e72–e112.

beta-lactamase. If there is treatment failure, the choice of a new antimicrobial depends on the initial medication that failed to eradicate the infection and patterns of recent antimicrobial use (Table 5-9). The use of the macrolide antimicrobials (erythromycin, clarithromycin, azithromycin) is not recommended in ABRS therapy due to relatively poor *S pneumoniae* coverage and higher risk of treatment failure. Intervention in underlying contributory causes, such as treating allergic rhinitis and encouraging the cessation of tobacco use, is crucial to treatment success.

Treatments should also be considered to reduce the symptoms associated with ABRS. Saline via nasal spray or neti pot can be used to rinse nasal passages, whereas a nasal corticosteroid (fluticasone [Flonase], budesonide [Rhinocort Aqua], or triamcinolone [Nasacort], others) can be used to reduce inflammation; nasal corticosteroid use is most effective in ABRS when allergic rhinitis is a contributor. According to evidence-based practice recommendations, the use of decongestants, either oral or nasal sprays, is not recommended as adjunctive treatment for patients with ABRS as their use has little to no influence on patient outcomes. However, an individual patient can find a degree of symptom relief with these adjunctive therapies. OTC pain relievers (acetaminophen or ibuprofen) can help alleviate pain. (See Table 5-8 and the algorithm on the management of ABRS.)

Discussion Source

Chow AW, Benninger MS, Brook I, et al. IDSA clinical practice guideline for acute bacterial rhinosinusitis in children and adults. *Clin Infect Dis.* 2012;54:e72–e112.

TABLE 5-9 Antimicrobial Regimens for Acute Bacterial Rhinosinusitis (ABRS) in Adults

INDICATION	DOSE	COMMENTS
Initial empiric therapy	**First-line therapy** ■ Amoxicillin-clavulanate 2,000 mg/125 mg PO BID **Second-line therapy** ■ Doxycycline 100 mg PO BID or 200 mg PO daily	■ High dose (HD, 3 to 4 g/d) amoxicillin needed against DRSP, increasing advocated as first-line therapy due to higher rate of efficacy ■ Clavulanate as a beta-lactamase inhibitor, allows amoxicillin to have activity against beta-lactamase producing organisms such as *H influenzae, M catarrhalis* ■ Doxycycline: DRSP treatment failure risk, activity against gram-negative organisms, stable in presence of beta-lactamase, pregnancy risk category D
Beta-lactam allergy (allergy to antimicrobials with beta-lactam ring such as penicillins, cephalosporins)	One of the following: ■ Doxycycline 100 mg PO BID or 200 mg PO daily ■ Levofloxacin 750 mg PO daily ■ Moxifloxacin 400 mg PO daily	■ Respiratory fluoroquinolones (FQs): Activity against DRSP, gram-negative organisms, stable in presence of beta-lactamase, not to be used as first-line ABRS therapy
Risk for antibiotic resistance or failed initial therapy	Mild-to-moderate disease; one of the following: ■ Amoxicillin-clavulanate 2,000 mg/125 mg PO BID ■ Cefpodoxime 200 mg po bid ■ Cefprozil 250 to 500 mg po bid ■ Cefdinir 300 mg PO q12h or 600 mg PO q24h Severe disease: ■ Levofloxacin 750 mg PO daily ■ Moxifloxacin 400 mg PO daily	■ All options with activity against gram-positive and gram-negative organisms, stable in presence of and/or active against beta-lactamase

Sources: Chow AW, Benninger MS, Brook I, et al. IDSA clinical practice guideline for acute bacterial rhinosinusitis in children and adults. Clin Infect Dis. 2012;54:e72–e112; Gilbert DN, Chambers HF, Eliopoulos GM, Saag MS, Pavia AT. The Sanford Guide to Antimicrobial Therapy. 50th ed. Sperryville, VA: Antimicrobial Therapy, Inc.; 2020:51.

QUESTIONS

96. A 45-year-old otherwise well woman presents with a chief complaint of a "sinus infection." In evaluating her for this problem, which of the following findings is most supportive of the diagnosis of ABRS?

    A. upper respiratory tract infection-like symptoms persisting beyond 7 to 10 days

    B. mild midfacial fullness and tenderness

    C. bilateral cervical lymphadenopathy

    D. purulent nasal discharge for the past 4 days

97. The most common causative bacterial pathogen in ABRS in a 40-year-old adult with type 2 diabetes mellitus and A1C of 8.2% is:

    A. *M pneumoniae*.

    B. *S pneumoniae*.

    C. *M catarrhalis*.

    D. *E coli*.

98. Which of the following patients is least likely to develop ABRS?

    A. a 22-year-old with a 2-week history of viral URI symptoms

    B. a 35-year-old with allergic rhinitis who is currently not using controller or rescue medications

    C. a 38-year-old who has a 40 pack-year cigarette smoking history, currently smoking 2 packs per day

    D. an 18-year-old with a history of recurrent epistaxis

99. Which of the following is a first-line therapy for the treatment of ABRS in a 32-year-old adult with hypertension, taking an ACE inhibitor and thiazide diuretic, who has no allergies and last took an antimicrobial approximately 2 years ago?

    A. amoxicillin-clavulanate

    B. TMP-SMX

    C. clarithromycin

    D. moxifloxacin

100. Which of the following represents an oral therapeutic option for ABRS in a 25-year-old woman with well-controlled asthma, using an inhaled corticosteroid daily and a beta-2 agonist as needed, with no recent antimicrobial use and with treatment failure after 72 hours of appropriate-dose oral doxycycline therapy?

    A. clindamycin

    B. clarithromycin

    C. TMP-SMX

    D. high-dose amoxicillin with clavulanate

101. A 34-year-old man with penicillin allergy with a history of hive-form reaction and difficulty breathing presents with ABRS. Three weeks ago, he was treated with doxycycline for "bronchitis." You now prescribe:

    A. standard-dose clarithromycin.

    B. standard-dose moxifloxacin.

    C. standard-dose cephalexin.

    D. high-dose amoxicillin.

102. A 45-year-old man with ABRS has shown no clinical improvement after a total of 10 days of oral antimicrobial therapy. Initially treated with doxycycline for 5 days, he was then switched to levofloxacin for the past 5 days. This is his third episode of ABRS in the past 12 months. You consider:

    A. initiating a course of oral corticosteroid.

    B. switching treatment to oral moxifloxacin.

  C. prompt referral for sinus imaging with a CT scan.

  D. discontinuing antimicrobial therapy, performing a nasal swab for culture and sensitivity, and treatment dependent on these results.

103. All of the following have demonstrated efficacy in relieving symptoms of ABRS except:

  A. saline nasal spray.

  B. nasal corticosteroid.

  C. oral decongestant.

  D. oral acetaminophen.

For answers and rationales, see end of chapter.

Oral Cancer

Overview

The most common form of oral cancer is squamous cell carcinoma (SCC), which accounts for 95% of cases. Tobacco use, whether from chewing tobacco, dipping or smokeless tobacco, or cigarette or pipe smoking, is likely the most common lifestyle oral cancer risk factor, with risk increasing according to duration of use. Other risk factors for oral cancer include male gender, advancing age (two-thirds of individuals are older than 55 years at time of diagnosis), and alcohol abuse. More recently, chronic infection with human papillomavirus (HPV) type 16 is recognized as a potent HPV risk factor.

Clinical Presentation

Most commonly SCC, an oral cancer, is characterized by a relatively painless, firm ulceration, or raised lesion; the oral lesion is typically present for a number of months prior to patient presentation for evaluation and diagnosis.

Diagnostic Testing/Screening Recommendations

When oral cancer is suspected, referral to otolaryngology or oral surgery for a lesion biopsy is recommended. Additional treatment is based on these results.

Oral cancer screening should be part of regularly scheduled dental checkups that include an examination of the entire mouth. The American Cancer Society also recommends that health-care providers examine the mouth and throat as part of a routine cancer-related checkup, while the U.S. Preventive Services Task Force (USPSTF) concludes that the current evidence is insufficient to assess the balance of benefits and harms of screening for oral cancer in asymptomatic adults.

> **CLINICAL CONCEPT**
>
> Given that oral cancer is unfortunately often diagnosed after it has spread beyond the oral cavity, the lymphadenopathy associated with oral cancer consists of immobile nodes usually greater than 1 cm in diameter that are nontender when palpated.

Oral Lesions: Differential Diagnosis

The differential diagnosis of oral lesions is broad. Nonmalignant, often infectious, oral lesions, such as herpes simplex, oral candidiasis, and aphthous stomatitis, differ from oral SCC in that these conditions usually cause considerable oral discomfort. With these infectious causes, the associated lymphadenopathy, if present, follows drainage tracts and is characterized by tenderness and mobility. In addition, these conditions usually resolve within weeks, often with or without treatment. In contrast, the lesion associated with SCC persists.

Discussion Sources

Oral Cancer Foundation. Oral cancer facts. http://www.oralcancerfoundation.org/facts

Schiff BA. Oral squamous cell carcinoma. Merck Manual online. http://www.merckmanuals.com/professional/ear_nose_and _throat_disorders/tumors_of_the_head_and_neck/oral_squamous_cell_carcinoma.html

QUESTIONS

104. You inspect the oral cavity of a 72-year-old man who has an 80 pack-year cigarette smoking history as well as a history of alcohol abuse for 20 years, currently with 10 years of sobriety. You find an oral lesion suspicious for malignancy and describe it as:

  A. a raised, red, painful shallow ulcer.

  B. a denuded patch with a removable white coating.

    C. an ulcerated lesion with indurated margins.

    D. a painful vesicular-form lesion with macerated margins.

105. Firm, painless, relatively fixed anterior cervical nodes would most likely be seen in the diagnosis of:

    A. herpes simplex.

    B. AOM.

    C. bacterial pharyngitis.

    D. oral cancer.

106. Which of the following is the most common form of oral cancer?

    A. adenocarcinoma

    B. sarcoma

    C. SCC

    D. basal cell carcinoma

107. One of the risk factors of oral cancer is infection with:

    A. human herpes virus type 1.

    B. HPV16.

    C. adenovirus type 16.

    D. EBV.

108 to 114. See the following image and match the nodes with their respective letters.

_____ **108.** Preauricular nodes

_____ **109.** Posterior cervical nodes

_____ **110.** Anterior cervical nodes

_____ **111.** Supraclavicular nodes

_____ **112.** Submandibular nodes

_____ **113.** Submental nodes

_____ **114.** Tonsillar nodes

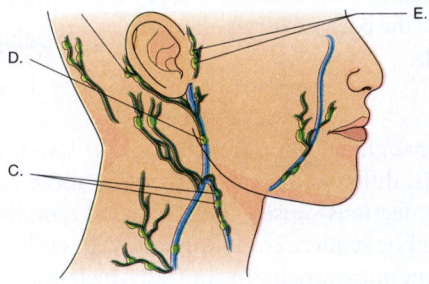

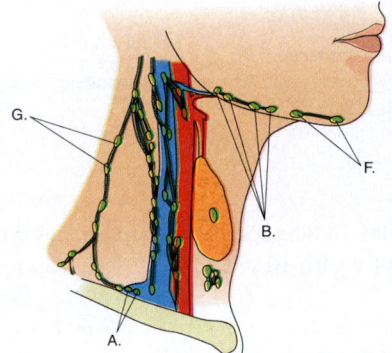

For answers and rationales, see end of chapter.

Acute Bacterial Pharyngitis

Overview

Streptococcus pyogenes, also known as group A beta-hemolytic streptococcus (GABHS), also known as "strep throat," is the causative pathogen in 15% to 40% of sore throats in school-aged children but is less common in children younger than 3 years and in teenagers and adults. The organism is transmitted primarily via saliva and droplet contact. The incubation period lasts an average of 3 to 5 days but can be up to 3 months.

Clinical Presentation

Clinical presentation of exudative pharyngitis caused by *S pyogenes* includes complaints of sore throat and fever, and evidence of large, beefy tonsils usually covered with exudate, pharyngeal erythema, palatal petechiae, and bilateral anterior cervical lymphadenopathy. Signs and symptoms such as cough, nasal discharge, conjunctivitis, and/or hoarseness are usually absent with GABHS pharyngitis and are more indicative of viral infection. In viral pharyngitis, the degree of pharyngeal erythema does not correlate with the degree of discomfort.

Scarlet fever associated with bacterial pharyngitis is the clinical condition seen when a scarlatiniform rash with a fine sandpaper-like texture, usually without significant pruritus, erupts during streptococcal pharyngitis, usually on the second day of illness. The rash starts on the trunk and spreads widely, usually sparing the palms and soles, and usually peels during recovery.

Diagnostic Testing

A rapid antigen detection test, or rapid strep test (RST), is performed by swabbing the tonsils or posterior pharynx, avoiding the teeth, gums, and tongue, to detect the presence of the group A streptococcus carbohydrate antigen; it can be completed in minutes. If a rapid streptococcal test result is positive, antimicrobial treatment should be initiated immediately; prompt antimicrobial treatment provides more rapid symptom relief and helps prevent suppurative and nonsuppurative complications. Owing to the test's high sensitivity and specificity, with a negative RST in the teen and adult, no further diagnostic testing is needed.

Treatment

In the treatment of bacterial pharyngitis caused by *S pyogenes*, penicillin formulations remain highly effective. When the total daily dosage is given in equally divided twice-daily doses, treatment outcomes are equivalent to regimens of three or four times daily with significantly improved adherence. A single dose of injectable penicillin given intramuscularly offers a one-time treatment option. Limitations to using intramuscular penicillin include increased risk of serious reaction with penicillin allergy and a treatment failure rate similar to that of a completed course of oral therapy. For patients with a penicillin allergy without immediate reaction, an oral cephalosporin can be prescribed. With immediate reaction in penicillin allergy, azithromycin and clindamycin are alternatives (see Table 5-6). Of group A beta-hemolytic streptococcus isolates, 35% are resistant to macrolides such as azithromycin or clarithromycin or to clindamycin; these drugs should be used only when a patient has severe penicillin allergy. While the use of all antimicrobials is associated with the development of *Clostridium difficile* colitis, clindamycin use poses particular risk. Advice on the use of symptomatic treatment with saltwater gargles, throat lozenges, and analgesics such as ibuprofen or acetaminophen should also be given. Treatment of scarlet fever is identical to treatment of streptococcal pharyngitis and carries no increased risk of complications or sequelae.

Patients with bacterial pharyngitis are no longer contagious within 24 hours of initiation of appropriate systemic antimicrobial therapy and when without fever. Hence, the child, teen, or adult can return to school and/or work at that time. Communicability gradually decreases over several weeks in untreated patients.

Asymptomatic nasopharyngeal carriage is common. Groups C and G streptococci cause pharyngitis but without rheumatic fever risk. These organisms are not detected on rapid strep screen but can be revealed on standard throat culture. The infection and its resulting symptoms clear without antimicrobial therapy, but taking an appropriate antimicrobial helps minimize symptoms.

Bacterial Pharyngitis Complications

Complications of bacterial pharyngitis include peritonsillar abscess, acute glomerulonephritis, and, as mentioned, rheumatic fever. Peritonsillar abscess is most commonly caused by *Fusobacterium necrophorum* GABHS or groups C and G streptococcus. Clinical presentation of peritonsillar abscess includes progressively worsening sore throat, often worse on one side; trismus (inability or difficulty in opening the mouth); drooling; a muffled, "hot potato" voice with an erythematous, swollen tonsil with contralateral uvular deviation; and cervical lymphadenopathy. Because airway compromise is a potentially life-threatening consequence of peritonsillar abscess, ultrasonography or CT of the affected region should be promptly obtained to confirm the diagnosis. Referral to emergency and specialty ENT care and treatment with appropriate antimicrobial therapy, needle aspiration, and airway maintenance must be initiated promptly. Antimicrobial therapy initiated early in the course of acute pharyngitis minimizes peritonsillar abscess risk. (See Chapter 18 for additional information on the role of bacterial pharyngitis treatment and its role in rheumatic fever prevention.)

Discussion Sources

Gerber MA, Baltimore RS, Eaton CB, et al. Prevention of rheumatic fever and diagnosis and treatment of acute streptococcal pharyngitis (American Heart Association guidelines). *Circulation.* 2009;119:1541–1551.

Gilbert DN, Chambers HF, Eliopoulos GM, Saag MS, Pavia AT. *The Sanford Guide to Antimicrobial Therapy.* 50th ed. Sperryville, VA: Antimicrobial Therapy, Inc.; 2020:49.

University of Michigan Health System. Pharyngitis guideline, May 2013. Ann Arbor, MI. http://www.med.umich.edu/1info/FHP /practiceguides/pharyngitis/pharyn.pdf

QUESTIONS

115. An 18-year-old woman has a chief complaint of a "sore throat and swollen glands" for the past 3 days. Her physical examination includes a temperature of 101°F (38.3°C), exudative pharyngitis, and tender anterior cervical lymphadenopathy. Right and left upper quadrant abdominal tenderness is absent. The most likely diagnosis is:

A. *S pyogenes* pharyngitis.

B. infectious mononucleosis.

C. viral pharyngitis.

D. Vincent angina.

116. Treatment options for streptococcal pharyngitis for a patient with severe penicillin allergy include all of the following except:

A. azithromycin.

B. TMP-SMX.

C. clarithromycin.

D. clindamycin.

117. *S pyogenes* is transmitted primarily through:

A. sexual contact.

B. skin-to-skin contact.

C. saliva and droplet contact.

D. contaminated surfaces.

118. You are seeing a 25-year-old man with *S pyogenes* pharyngitis. He asks whether he can get a "shot of penicillin" for therapy. He has no history of drug allergy. You consider the following when counseling about the use of intramuscular penicillin:

A. Injectable penicillin formulation is stable in the presence of beta-lactamase.

B. This is a treatment option when nonadherence to oral therapy is a possibility.

C. This is the preferred agent in treating group G streptococcal infection.

D. Injectable penicillin has a superior spectrum of antimicrobial coverage compared with the oral version of the drug.

119. The incubation period for infection with *S pyogenes* is usually:

A. 1 to 3 days.

B. 3 to 5 days.

C. 6 to 9 days.

D. 10 to 13 days.

120. You see a patient with a positive rapid strep screen. Antimicrobial therapy has been initiated. This person can be cleared to return to work or school after _____ hours of antimicrobial therapy.

A. 12

B. 24

C. 36

D. 48

121. A 21-year-old man presents with a 4-day history of sore throat, without nasal discharge, cough, or other viral illness signs and symptoms. On examination, he has pharyngeal erythema and slightly tender bilateral anterior cervical lymphadenopathy. His rapid strep screen is negative. When considering pharyngitis caused by group C or G streptococci as a possible cause of this illness, the NP considers that:

A. potential complications include glomerulonephritis.

B. appropriate antimicrobial therapy helps to facilitate more rapid resolution of symptoms.

C. infection with these organisms carries a significant risk of subsequent rheumatic fever.

D. acute infectious hepatitis can occur if not treated with an appropriate antimicrobial.

122. When advising a patient with scarlet fever, the NP considers that:

A. there is increased risk for poststreptococcal glomerulonephritis.

B. the rash often peels during recovery.

C. an injectable cephalosporin is the preferred treatment option.

D. throat culture is usually negative for group A streptococci.

123. The rash associated with scarlet fever typically occurs how long after the start of the symptomatic infection?

A. 2 days

B. 4 days

C. 7 to 10 days

D. 2 to 3 weeks

124. Treatment of scarlet fever in a 19-year-old woman with no allergy to penicillin can include all of the following except:

A. penicillin.

B. cefdinir.

C. TMP-SMX.

D. cefpodoxime.

125 to 126. Match the patient with the likely causative pathogen for pharyngitis.

_____ 125. *S pyogenes*

_____ 126. Respiratory virus

   A. a 34-year-old with cough, nasal discharge, hoarseness, conjunctival inflammation, and diarrhea

   B. a 26-year-old woman with sore throat and fever, swollen tonsils covered with exudate, palatal petechiae, and anterior cervical lymphadenopathy

127. All of the following are common causes of penicillin treatment failure in streptococcal pharyngitis except:

A. infection with a strain of *Streptococcus* producing beta-lactamase.

B. failure to initiate or complete the antimicrobial course.

    C. concomitant infection or carriage with an organism producing beta-lactamase.

    D. inadequate penicillin dosage.

128. A 24-year-old woman presents with a 1-week history of progressively worsening sore throat with dysphagia, trismus, and unilateral otalgia. Her voice is muffled, and examination reveals an erythematous, swollen tonsil with contralateral uvular deviation. The most likely diagnosis is:

    A. infectious mononucleosis.

    B. viral pharyngitis.

    C. peritonsillar abscess.

    D. early stage scarlet fever.

129. Common causative organisms of peritonsillar abscess include all of the following except:

    A. *F necrophorum*.

    B. *Candida albicans*.

    C. group C or G streptococcus.

    D. GABHS.

130. The most appropriate next step for a patient diagnosed with peritonsillar abscess is:

    A. intramuscular penicillin with follow-up in 24 hours.

    B. emergent referral to emergency department and specialty ENT consult.

    C. pharyngeal x-ray.

    D. to obtain throat culture prior to initiation of antimicrobial therapy.

For answers and rationales, see end of chapter.

Infectious Mononucleosis

Overview

Infectious mononucleosis is an acute systemic viral illness usually caused by EBV, a DNA herpes virus that typically enters the body via oropharyngeal secretions and infects B lymphocytes. Nearly all cases occur in people younger than 35 years of age. EBV has an incubation period of 30 to 50 days.

Clinical Presentation

The usual course of infectious mononucleosis includes a 3- to 5-day prodrome of headache, malaise, myalgia, and anorexia, followed by acute symptoms that last about 5 to 15 days with fatigue, exudative pharyngitis and tonsillar enlargement, fever, and headache. Marked anterior and posterior cervical lymphadenopathy is usually noted. Splenomegaly develops in more than 50% of patients, and hepatomegaly develops in about 10%; these organs are also tender to palpation. Additional findings include jaundice, periorbital edema, soft palatal petechiae, generalized adenopathy, maculopapular rash, and a 30% incidence of concurrent streptococcal pharyngitis. Full recovery time varies but is usually about 4 to 6 weeks.

Diagnostic Testing

Diagnostic testing for patients with infectious mononucleosis usually includes obtaining a heterophile antibody test (Monospot), which has a sensitivity of 85% and specificity of 100%. The test does have limitations, however. Positivity increases during the first 6 weeks of illness, with only 60% of patients positive by the second week of illness. Furthermore, false negatives occur in 10% of adults and 50% of children. To complicate this issue further, acute infection with cytomegalovirus, adenovirus, *Toxoplasma gondii,* HIV, and other agents can cause an infectious mononucleosis-like illness with a risk of heterophile antibody cross-reactivity and a resulting infectious mononucleosis false-positive rate of 5% to 15%. Leukopenia with lymphocytosis is present. The presence of atypical lymphocytes is not unique to infectious mononucleosis and is commonly found in systemic viral infection. Mild thrombocytopenia is seen in 50% of patients; 85%

of infected individuals develop a twofold to threefold elevation in hepatic enzymes (aspartate and alanine aminotransferases) by the second and third weeks of the illness.

Treatment

Treatment of infectious mononucleosis is usually supportive, with recovery slow but complete. There is a potential, however, for upper pharyngeal obstruction and respiratory distress when enlarged tonsils and lymphoid tissue impinge on the upper airway.

Use of a systemic corticosteroid such as prednisone, 40 to 60 mg/day PO for 3 days, is the treatment of choice when upper pharyngeal obstruction is present, although little evidence exists to support this practice. However, the use of prednisone in a person with infectious mononucleosis who is having difficulty swallowing because of pharyngeal edema often provides symptomatic relief. In uncomplicated infectious mononucleosis, neither the use of antiviral agents such as acyclovir nor routine prescribing of systemic corticosteroid agents is indicated.

If there is evidence of a concomitant condition such as AOM where antimicrobial therapy is indicated, the use of amoxicillin or ampicillin should be avoided as this can cause a cutaneous reaction (rash) in patients with EBV infection. This rash is thought to be the result of altered immune status during the infection and not indicative of penicillin allergy.

Infectious Mononucleosis Complications

In a person who participates in contact or collision sports or other similar activities, the risk of splenic rupture in response to even modest abdominal trauma, the most common cause of mortality and morbidity in patients with infectious mononucleosis, needs to be considered during acute and convalescent stages.

When the spleen is easily palpated, its size is usually increased by two or more times normal. The physical examination is a relatively insensitive measure of splenic size, however. Obtaining an ultrasound examination is considered a prudent measure to ensure splenic regression before approving return to sports play. All persons with infectious mononucleosis are at risk of splenic rupture, however, regardless of spleen size. In addition, the person with infectious mononucleosis should return to his or her baseline state of health, without pharyngeal symptoms, prior to returning to sports or other physically active pursuits.

Discussion Source

Dunmire SK, Hogquist KA, Balfour Jr HH. Infectious mononucleosis. *Curr Top Microbiol Immunol.* 2015;390:211–240. https://www.ncbi.nlm.nih.gov/pmc/articles/PMC4670567/

> **CLINICAL CONCEPT**
> With infectious mononucleosis, the risk for splenic rupture is greatest in the second and third weeks of illness—hence the mandate of abstaining from collision or contact sports for at least 1 month. The risk of rupture is greatest in the enlarged spleen; the size of the normal spleen can be recalled by the "rules of odds": $1 \times 3 \times 5$ inches in size, weighing 7 oz (about 200 g), and lying between ribs 9 and 11.

QUESTIONS

131. A 21-year-old woman presents with a chief complaint of a 3-day history of "sore throat and swollen glands," fatigue, and intermittent fever. Her physical examination includes exudative pharyngitis, minimally tender anterior and posterior cervical lymphadenopathy, and maculopapular rash. She is diagnosed with infectious mononucleosis and was likely infected with the causative organism how many days ago?

A. 5 to 10

B. 20 to 30

C. 30 to 50

D. more than 100

132. EBV, the most common causative organism of infectious mononucleosis, is primarily transmitted via:

A. skin-to-skin contact.

B. contact with blood.

C. oropharyngeal secretions.

D. genital contact.

133. Which of the following is most likely to be found in the laboratory data of a person with infectious mononucleosis?

A. neutrophilia with reactive forms

B. lymphocytosis with atypical lymphocytes

C. thrombocytosis

D. macrocytosis

134. You examine a 20-year-old college student who has infectious mononucleosis with tonsillar hypertrophy; exudative pharyngitis; poor fluid intake due to painful, difficult swallowing; and a patent airway. You prescribe which of the following oral medications?

A. amoxicillin

B. prednisone

C. ibuprofen

D. acyclovir

135. In patients with infectious mononucleosis, which medication should be avoided because of a risk of rash development?

A. acetaminophen

B. sulfamethoxazole

C. erythromycin

D. amoxicillin

136. What percentage of patients with infectious mononucleosis have splenomegaly during the acute phase of the illness?

A. at least 10%

B. about 25%

C. at least 50%

D. nearly 100%

137. The size of a normal spleen is approximately:

A. $1'' \times 1'' \times 3''$.

B. $1'' \times 3'' \times 5''$.

C. $2'' \times 4'' \times 6''$.

D. $3'' \times 5'' \times 7''$.

138. A 16-year-old ice hockey player was recently diagnosed with infectious mononucleosis. Because of a risk for splenic rupture, she should be advised to wait how long before participating back on the ice with her team?

A. at least 2 weeks

B. at least 1 month

C. at least 3 months

D. at least 6 months

For answers and rationales, see end of chapter.

QUESTION ANSWERS AND RATIONALES

Conjunctivitis

1. Correct: A. suppurative or bacterial conjunctivitis.
Suppurative conjunctivitis is the most likely diagnosis due to the unilateral nature of the condition and the presence of purulent eye discharge.
Incorrect:
Viral conjunctivitis (B) and allergic conjunctivitis (C) are typically bilateral conditions. Additionally, viral conjunctivitis is associated with clear, watery discharge. There is no mention of injury in the patient history in order to consider a mechanical injury diagnosis (D).

2. Correct: C. an allergen
Bilateral, itchy eyes on an intermittent basis throughout the year points to allergic conjunctivitis.
Incorrect:
Bacterial (suppurative) conjunctivitis (A) is typically associated with unilateral involvement, while viral infection (B) is associated with a clear, watery discharge; neither of which would occur on an intermittent basis throughout the year. There is no mention of injury in the patient history to consider this diagnosis (D).

3. Correct: D. *Pseudomonas aeruginosa.*
In outpatient infections, *P aeruginosa* is an uncommon cause of infection, including bacterial conjunctivitis.
Incorrect:
Bacterial or suppurative conjunctivitis is caused by select gram-positive (*S pneumoniae* [C] or *S aureus* [A]) or gram-negative (*H influenzae* [B]) organisms. Knowledge of the most likely causative organisms in infectious diseases is critical in selecting appropriate initial empirical antimicrobial therapy.

4. Correct: B. levofloxacin.
Ocular solutions of fluoroquinolones (e.g., levofloxacin, moxifloxacin) are considered first-line therapy as they remain highly effective against the most common causative organisms.
Incorrect:
Empirical treatment of suppurative conjunctivitis should provide coverage against common gram-positive (*S pneumoniae* or *S aureus*) and gram-negative (*H influenzae*) organisms. Macrolides (e.g., azithromycin) (D), tobramycin (A), or gentamicin (C) are not preferred due to high rates of resistance exhibited by *S pneumoniae*.

5. Correct: D. corticosteroid ophthalmic drops.
The use of ophthalmic corticosteroid solution increases the risk of eye infection, particularly among patients wearing contact lenses. Other adverse effects with the use of corticosteroid eye drops include increased risk of cataracts and a rise in intraocular pressure that can lead to optic disk and visual field damage similar to open-angle glaucoma.
Incorrect:
Treatment of allergic disorders includes the use of medications to reduce production of inflammatory mediators, such as the mast cell stabilizer cromolyn (A), and medications that block the action of inflammatory mediators, such as antihistamines (B, C).

6. Correct: B. adenovirus.
Adenovirus is the most common virological cause of conjunctivitis.
Incorrect:
Coronavirus (A), rhinovirus (C), and human papillomavirus (D) are not typical causes of conjunctivitis. In viral conjunctivitis, the patient often exhibits signs and symptoms of a viral upper respiratory tract infection. Transmission of virus to the eye can occur through accidental inoculation of viral particles from the patient's hands or by contact with infected upper respiratory droplets.

7. Correct: D. cool artificial tear solution.
Treatment should focus on relieving irritative symptoms, such as with the use of cold artificial tear solution.
Incorrect:
Viral conjunctivitis is most often self-limiting and will resolve without the use of antibiotics over days to weeks. The use of antibacterials, such as moxifloxacin (A) or polymyxin (B), or antivirals such as acyclovir (C) are not warranted. The development of a secondary bacterial ophthalmological infection after viral conjunctivitis is rare.

Ophthalmological Emergencies

8. Correct: B. nausea and vomiting.
Nausea, vomiting, and even headache can occur in select emergency conditions, such as angle-closure glaucoma, but are not considered the classic symptoms for an ophthalmological emergency.
Incorrect:
Severe eye pain (A), red eye (C), and new-onset change in visual acuity (D) are the major classic signs/symptoms of ophthalmological emergency. In more limiting eye problems, such as viral or bacterial conjunctivitis, there are no visual changes (once eye discharge is wiped away), and the eye can be irritated but not painful and can have a slightly red "pink eye" appearance.

9. Correct: C. angle-closure glaucoma.
This patient has multiple risk factors for angle-closure glaucoma (i.e., female gender, systemic anticholinergic use), plus the classic presentation for this diagnosis including unilateral headache, visual changes, firm eyeball, and poorly reactive pupil.
Incorrect:
OAG (B) is associated with painless, slowly progressive peripheral vision loss. Anterior uveitis (D) is

characterized by a constricted, irregularly shaped pupil and no change in IOP. Herpetic conjunctivitis (A) is characterized by itching and redness of the eye, eye pain and inflammation of the eyelids, and continuous watery discharge.

10. **Correct: A. prompt referral to an ophthalmologist.**
For a patient diagnosed with angle-closure glaucoma, prompt referral to ophthalmology is needed to confirm diagnosis and initiate therapy to preserve vision. If the IOP is not lowered within a few hours (with IOP-lowering medications and/or laser or incisional surgical therapy), permanent vision loss is possible.
Incorrect:
As such, treating the symptoms, such as with an analgesic (B), and delaying treatment (D) to reduce IOP are not appropriate. The use of a topical corticosteroid (C) is not warranted for angle-closure glaucoma.

11. **Correct: D. anterior uveitis.**
This patient presents the classic signs and symptoms of anterior uveitis, particularly dully painful red eye with vision changes and a pupil that is constricted, nonreactive, and irregularly shaped. Furthermore, anterior uveitis occurs in a large percentage of patients with spondyloarthropathy, particularly in persons with the HLA-B27 allele.
Incorrect:
Angle-closure glaucoma (C) is characterized by eye pain, a firm eyeball, visual changes, and dilated and unreactive pupil. OAG (B) is associated with painless, slowly progressive vision loss. Herpetic conjunctivitis (A) is characterized by itching and redness of the eye, eye pain and inflammation of the eyelids, and continuous watery discharge.

12. **Correct: D. retinal detachment.**
This patient presents with the typical symptoms of retinal detachment, including an increasing number of floaters and decreased visual acuity. She is also at higher risk of retinal detachment due to her older age and history of cataract surgery.
Incorrect:
OAG (A) is associated with painless, slowly progressive vision loss associated with elevated IOP. Anterior uveitis (C) is characterized by a dully painful red eye and a constricted, irregularly shaped pupil. Central renal artery occlusion (B) is associated with sudden, severe vision loss.

13. **Correct: D. immediate referral to an ophthalmologist.**
In primary care, a high index of suspicion is needed for vision-threatening conditions. For retinal detachment, early diagnosis and treatment by an ophthalmologist are needed to prevent permanent vision loss.
Incorrect:
There is no sign of infection or localized inflammation; thus, treatment with an antimicrobial (B) or topical corticosteroid (C) is not necessary. Delaying treatment

with the use of an eye shield (A) causes pupillary dilation that can worsen IOP and lead to permanent vision loss.

14. **Correct: B. immediately removing any protruding foreign body from the eye.**
In primary care, it is best not to attempt removal of a foreign body from the eye globe. The patient should be referred immediately to an ophthalmologist.
Incorrect:
The patient should be referred immediately to an ophthalmologist (D). Fluorescein staining (C) can be helpful in identifying corneal injury including corneal abrasion and small foreign body fragments. Primary prevention through patient education on appropriate eye protection (A) can help prevent future eye trauma events.

Primary Open-Angle Glaucoma

15. **Correct: A. peripheral vision loss**
Although all of these changes can be seen in patients with advanced POAG, peripheral vision loss is specific to POAG.
Incorrect:
New onset of difficulty with distance vision (C) can be found in patients with cataracts or with age-related ocular changes. Changes in near vision (B) are a common part of the aging process because of hardening of the lens (i.e., presbyopia) and the need for increased illumination (D).

16. **Correct: B. elevated intraocular pressure.**
All forms of glaucoma are caused by elevated IOP.
Incorrect:
Knowledge of the pathophysiology of disease is key to appreciating its clinical presentation and rationale for treatment. Hardening of the lens (A) is an age-related process, while degeneration of the optic nerve (C) and hypotension in the anterior maxillary artery (D) are not causes of POAG.

17. **Correct: A. excessive cupping of the optic disk**
Excessive IOP results in an optic disk and cup that are "pushed in," creating a classic finding called glaucomatous cupping.
Incorrect:
Papilledema (C), in which the optic disk bulges and the margins are blurred, is seen when there is excessive pressure behind the eye, as in increased intracranial pressure (Fig. 5-6). Flame-shaped hemorrhage (D) and arteriovenous nicking (B), which is an indentation of retinal veins by stiff retinal arteries, are most commonly seen in the presence of chronic hypertension.

18. **Correct: D. blue eye color.**
The presence of one or more risk factors for a given disease increases the likelihood of a condition being present. However, the absence of risk factors does not necessarily eliminate disease risk. Blue eye color is not a known risk factor for POAG.

Incorrect:

Risk factors for POAG include African ancestry (A), diabetes mellitus (B), family history of POAG, history of certain eye trauma or uveitis, and advancing age (C). Therefore, patients with one or more of these factors should be prioritized for screening for POAG.

19. **Correct: A. intraocular pressure greater than 25 mm Hg**

All forms of glaucoma are caused by elevated IOP (greater than 25 mm Hg). As a result of the increased IOP, the optic disk and cup are "pushed in" and create a cup-to-disk ratio typically greater than 0.3.

Incorrect:

Papilledema (B), in which the optic disk bulges and the margins are blurred, is seen when there is excessive pressure behind the eye, as in increased intracranial pressure. Change in pupillary response (D) is not a key diagnostic finding for POAG and can be indicative of other ophthalmological conditions. In POAG, the optic disk and cup are "pushed in" and create a cup-to-disk ratio typically greater than 0.3 (C).

20. **Correct: C. a 68-year-old man of African ancestry with type 2 diabetes mellitus**

Knowing risk factors for a given disease can help guide clinicians in making a differential diagnosis. Risk factors for POAG include African ancestry, diabetes mellitus, family history of POAG, history of certain eye trauma or uveitis, and advancing age. Therefore, among the choices given, the elderly man of African ancestry and type 2 diabetes is likely to be at greatest risk of POAG.

Incorrect:

Knowing risk factors for a given disease can help guide clinicians in making a differential diagnosis. Risk factors for POAG include African ancestry, diabetes mellitus, family history of POAG, history of certain eye trauma or uveitis, and advancing age. The 22-year-old (A) has one major risk factor for POAG (diabetes), bilateral cataracts are not a risk factor for POAG (B), and being of Native American ancestry or having asthma are not risk factors for POAG (D).

21. **Correct: D. mast cell stabilizers.**

Treatment of POAG is aimed at reducing IOP to normal levels. Mast cell stabilizers halt the degradation or mast cells and the subsequent release of histamine and other inflammatory mediators. These agents are typically used to treat allergic conjunctivitis but have no role in the treatment of POAG.

Incorrect:

Treatment of POAG is aimed at reducing IOP to normal levels. Topical beta-adrenergic antagonists (A) and α_2-agonists (B) can be used to reduce the production of intraocular fluid. Topical prostaglandin analogues (C) increase the outflow of intraocular fluid.

Eyelid Disorders

22. **Correct: B. a hordeolum.**

A pustule is a small, raised lesion filled with purulent fluid. This is most consistent with a hordeolum or stye, which is an acute, localized swelling of the eyelid (internal or external) usually caused by infection.

Incorrect:

A chalazion (A) is an inflammatory condition characterized by a hard, nontender swelling of the upper or lower eyelid. Blepharitis (C) is an inflammatory condition associated with lid redness, crusting, and flaking. Cellulitis (D), when noted in the ocular region, is typically caused by an acute bacterial infection and is characterized by a warm, red, edematous area with sharply demarcated borders. This is a rare complication of hordeolum.

23. **Correct: A. a chalazion.**

A chalazion is an inflammatory condition characterized by a hard, nontender swelling of the upper or lower eyelid.

Incorrect:

A hordeolum (B) is acute, localized swelling of the eyelid (internal or external) usually caused by infection forming a pustule or abscess. Blepharitis (C) is an inflammatory condition associated with lid redness, crusting, and flaking. When noted in the ocular region, cellulitis (D) is typically caused by an acute bacterial infection and is characterized by a warm, red, edematous area with sharply demarcated borders.

24. **Correct: B. warm compresses multiple times a day to the affected area.**

Warm compresses are effective in treating hordeolum as this lesion usually opens spontaneously due to a thin pustular wall and then heals rapidly.

Incorrect:

Risk of secondary infection is low; therefore, antimicrobial therapy (D) (topical/ocular or systemic) is not warranted. Incision and drainage (C) are rarely indicated. Topical corticosteroid (A) is not recommended for hordeolum and can increase the risk of secondary infection.

25. **Correct: B. cellulitis of the eyelid.**

On rare occasions, hordeolum will progress to cellulitis of the eyelid. If cellulitis occurs, ENT consultation is warranted. *S aureus* is the most common causative organism.

Incorrect:

Hordeolum or stye is localized and does not result in insult to the conjunctiva (A) or cornea (C). On rare occasions, hordeolum will progress to cellulitis of the eyelid but will not cause sinusitis (D).

26. **Correct: C. warm compresses of the affected area.**

Initial treatment for a chalazion includes frequent warm soaks of the area.

Incorrect:

Since chalazion is an inflammatory condition and not infectious, antimicrobial therapy (A) is not warranted. If the condition fails to resolve with warm soaks, then referral to an ophthalmologist for intralesional corticosteroid injection or excision (D) is recommended, particularly if the chalazion impairs lid closure or presses on the cornea. Topical corticosteroid (B) is not recommended and can increase the risk of secondary infection.

27. **Correct: C. blepharitis.**
Blepharitis is an inflammatory condition associated with lid redness, crusting, and flaking and is often accompanied by burning, itching, or a grainy sensation. The condition is caused by bacteria and inflammation due to congested oil glands at the base of each eyelash.
Incorrect:
A chalazion (A) is an inflammatory condition characterized by a hard, nontender swelling of the upper or lower eyelid. A hordeolum (B) is acute, localized swelling of the eyelid usually caused by infection forming a pustule or abscess. Cellulitis (D), typically caused by an acute bacterial infection, is characterized by a warm, red, edematous area with sharply demarcated borders.

28. **Correct: B. intralesional corticosteroid injection.**
Intralesional corticosteroid injection is not warranted for blepharitis.
Incorrect:
Treatment of blepharitis includes warm compresses (C) several times per day and gentle cleansing with diluted baby shampoo (D) to remove any crust and flakes in the area. This can be followed with application of a topical antimicrobial (A). Blepharitis is frequently a recurring condition that requires chronic treatment. Poorly controlled blepharitis can lead to lid deformity.

Otitis Externa

29. **Correct: D. *Moraxella catarrhalis***
Though *M catarrhalis* is a common pathogen for AOM, it is not a common pathogen for OE.
Incorrect:
It is important for health-care providers to recognize the most likely causative organisms in order to select appropriate initial empirical therapy. The most common pathogens for OE include gram-positive bacteria (*S epidermidis* [B] [46%] and *S aureus* [C] [11%]) as well as gram-negative *Pseudomonas* species (A) (11%).

30. **Correct: A. a 22-year-old who travels frequently by airplane**
Risk factors for OE include a history of recent ear canal trauma, vigorous use of a cotton swab or other device to clean the ear canal, conditions in which moisture is frequently held in the ear canal (such as with cerumen impaction), and frequent swimming. Frequent air travel is not a risk factor for OE but can be a risk factor for AOM.
Incorrect:
Risk factors for OE include a history of recent ear canal trauma, vigorous use of a cotton swab or other device to clean the ear canal (B), conditions in which moisture is frequently held in the ear canal (such as with cerumen impaction) (D), and frequent swimming (C).

31. **Correct: C. fluoroquinolone otic drops.**
Antimicrobial otic drops are the preferred treatment choice for OE as these provide highly effective localized therapy. Fluoroquinolones are the preferred first-line agent.
Incorrect:
Systemic antimicrobial therapy (A, B) can be considered in OE if the ear canal is sufficiently swollen to prevent proper distribution of the otic drops, or in complicated cases such as malignant/necrotizing OE. Aminoglycoside otic drops (D) are not the preferred first-line agent due to spectrum of activity and should not be used in the presence of a ruptured tympanic membrane.

32. **Correct: B. increased ear pain with tragus pull.**
The clinical presentation of OE includes the hallmark findings of pain on tragus palpation or with the application of traction to the pinna.
Incorrect:
Tympanic membrane immobility (A), erythema (C), and bullae (D) are all consistent with AOM, and recognizing these differences is an important aspect of making the differential diagnosis.

33. **Correct: A. the presence of an immunocompromised condition.**
Those at risk for malignant or necrotizing OE include patients who are immunocompromised or who have received radiotherapy to the skull base.
Incorrect:
Malignant/necrotizing OE can occur at any age though it is more common in older adults (B). A history of URI (C) or a complicated course of OME (D) are risk factors for AOM.

34. **Correct: B. pain disproportionate to the clinical presentation.**
The clinical presentation of malignant or necrotizing OE includes the usual features of OE with the addition of pain disproportionate to clinical findings.
Incorrect:
The usual features of OE include purulent or serous discharge (A), pain on application of traction to the pinna (C), and marked ear canal edema (D). The presence of these findings would not necessarily indicate malignant or necrotizing OE.

35. **Correct: D. use of analgesic otic drops.**
While management of pain through the use of analgesic otic drops is an important part of malignant OE therapy, choosing this option does not set the priorities of care, including ENT consult, appropriate systemic antimicrobial therapy, and imaging to detect complications. In addition, topical analgesia will likely be inadequate to control the severe pain usually noted with this condition.
Incorrect:
Setting the priorities of care for the person with malignant OE would include performing imaging studies (C), initiating systemic antimicrobial therapy (B), and making prompt referral to a specialist (A).

Acute Otitis Media in Teens and Adults

36 to 39. Yes or No

36. **Correct: Yes**

37. **Correct: No**

38. **Correct: Yes**

39. **Correct: Yes**

Understanding the likely causative pathogens of infection is important in safe practice and guiding management decisions. Common viral pathogens in AOM include RSV, influenza virus, and rhinovirus. Herpes simplex virus 2 is not a common cause of AOM. Viral AOM typically presents with milder symptoms compared to bacterial infections and usually resolves within 7 to 10 days with supportive care alone (antimicrobials not needed).

40 to 43. Yes or No

40. **Correct: Yes**

41. **Correct: Yes**

42. **Correct: No**

43. **Correct: Yes**

Common bacterial pathogens that cause AOM include *S pneumoniae* (gram-positive pathogen) and the gram-negative pathogens *H influenzae* and *M catarrhalis*. These are also the leading pathogens of ABRS. *E coli*, a gram-negative bacterium, is not typically implicated in AOM.

44. **Correct: D. aggressive ear canal hygiene.**

Eustachian tube dysfunction contributes to the development of AOM. As such, upper respiratory infection, allergic rhinitis, and tobacco use are risk factors for AOM. Aggressive ear canal hygiene can increase the risk of OE but not AOM.

Incorrect:

Eustachian tube dysfunction contributes to the development of AOM. As such, URI (A), allergic rhinitis (B), and tobacco use (C) are risk factors for AOM.

45. **Correct: B. tympanic membrane immobility.**

In AOM, the tympanic membrane may be retracted or bulging and is typically reddened with loss of translucency and immobility on insufflation.

Incorrect:

Prominent tympanic membrane bony landmarks (A) are usually not visual in AOM as the middle ear is filled with purulent discharge. Crackling and itchiness in the affected ear (C) are often reported following AOM, during OME that is usually noted for a number of weeks after acute infection. Lymphadenopathy of the anterior cervical nodes on the ipsilateral side are often noted in AOM, but the submental node (D) is not part of the middle ear's drainage tract and, thus, will not be involved in AOM findings.

46. **Correct: C. high-dose amoxicillin.**

This patient is at risk of infection with drug-resistant *S pneumoniae* due to recent use of an antimicrobial. As such, high-dose amoxicillin will be an appropriate choice.

Incorrect:

Azithromycin (A) is not recommended due to high rates of resistance by *S pneumoniae*, and high-dose amoxicillin provides better coverage compared to cephalexin (B) (first-generation cephalosporin) and TMP-SMX (D).

47. **Correct: A. cefpodoxime.**

With milder forms of penicillin allergy, a second- or third-generation cephalosporin (e.g., cefpodoxime) can be considered due to a lower risk of cross-reactivity compared to first-generation agents (e.g., cephalexin) and robust coverage.

Incorrect:

There is higher risk of cross-reactivity between penicillins and first-generation cephalosporins (C) compared to second-generation cephalosporins. Erythromycin (B) offers poor coverage against *S pneumoniae*, a leading cause of AOM. Cefpodoxime also provides more robust *S pneumoniae* coverage compared to TMP-SMX (D).

48. **Correct: D. respiratory fluoroquinolones such as levofloxacin**

Among the answer choices, the respiratory fluoroquinolones provide the best coverage against *S pneumoniae* with relatively low rates of resistance. These agents are recommended for the treatment of infection when DRSP is suspected.

Incorrect:

S pneumoniae exhibits higher rates of resistance to the macrolides (A), doxycycline (B), and first-generation cephalosporins (C) compared to the respiratory fluoroquinolones.

49. **Correct: C. fever**

Since OME marks the resolution of acute infection, fever is not an anticipated finding.

Incorrect:

With resolution of AOM, tympanic membrane mobility returns to normal within 1 to 2 weeks, but fluid in the middle ear (A) remains for several weeks. This can result in a sensation of ear fullness (B) and itching (D) or crackling in the ear.

50. **Correct: A. advising that this condition self-resolves.**

With resolution of AOM, the tympanic membrane mobility returns to normal within 1 to 2 weeks, but fluid in the middle ear remains for several weeks. Thus, time is the best intervention for the resolution of OME.

Incorrect:

Repeating a course of antimicrobial therapy (B) or the use of antihistamines (C) or a mucolytic agent (D) will not be effective in hastening symptom resolution and, thus, is not recommended.

Ménière's Disease, Ménière's Syndrome

51 to 53. Matching Questions

51. **Correct: Syndrome (S)**

52. **Correct: Syndrome (S)**

53. **Correct: Syndrome (S)**

Ménière's disease is idiopathic in origin without a clearly identifiable underlying cause. Ménière's syndrome presents with identical signs as Ménière's disease but with an identified underlying cause. Ménière's syndrome is usually secondary to various processes that interfere with normal production or resorption of endolymph, and can include endocrine dysfunction, trauma, electrolyte imbalance, autoimmune dysfunction, medications, infection, or hyperlipidemia. For each of the examples, an underlying cause is present that can contribute to the condition (i.e., trauma, osteoarthritis, and rheumatoid arthritis).

54. **Correct: C. This is largely a diagnosis of exclusion.**
Ménière's disease is idiopathic in origin without a clearly identifiable underlying cause; thus, it is largely a diagnosis of exclusion. The tetrad of symptoms includes fluctuating hearing loss, episodic vertigo, tinnitus, and aural fullness.
Incorrect:
Neuroimaging (A) is not warranted, and hearing loss (B) is usually in the low-frequency range. Tinnitus (D), or ringing in the ears, is usually present and is part of the four components of the disease.

55 to 59. Yes or No

55. **Correct: No**
The Weber tuning test evaluates the nature of hearing loss. A vibrating tuning fork is placed in the middle of the patient's forehead, and the patient is asked to identify in which ear the sound is louder. A normal Weber test has the patient reporting the sound is heard equally on both sides. During Ménière's disease, the Weber tuning test usually lateralizes to the unaffected ear.

56. **Correct: Yes**
The Rinne test is performed by placing a vibrating tuning fork against the patient's mastoid bone and asking the patient to indicate when the sound is no longer audible (bone conduction). Once the patient reports the sound is no longer heard, then the fork is quickly moved 1 to 2 cm from the auditory canal and the patient is again asked if he or she can hear it (air conduction). A normal finding shows that air conduction exceeds bone conduction, which is what is observed with Ménière's disease.

57. **Correct: Yes**
During pneumatic otoscopy, an otoscope is fitted snugly on the patient's external auditory canal to produce an airtight chamber. Gently squeezing a rubber bulb in rapid succession allows observation of the eardrum mobility. Performing this on the affected ear of a patient with Ménière's disease can elicit symptoms and/or cause nystagmus (repetitive, uncontrolled movements of the eyes).

58. **Correct: No**
The Romberg test evaluates a patient's ability to maintain balance by having the patient stand erect with feet together and eyes closed and observing movement for a minute. A positive sign is observed with swaying, irregular swaying, or toppling over. This test is usually positive in patients with Ménière's disease.

59. **Correct: Yes**
The Fukuda marching step test has the patient perform a march step with the eyes closed. Patients with Ménière's disease generally have a positive result where there is directional drift, usually toward the affected ear.

60. **Correct: B. Dix-Hallpike test.**
The Dix-Hallpike test evaluates the ability to elicit nystagmus while moving the patient from sitting to supine with the head angled 45° to one side and then the other.
Incorrect:
The Romberg test (A) evaluates a patient's ability to maintain balance by having the patient stand erect with feet together and eyes closed and observing movement for a minute. The Fukuda marching step test (D) has the patient perform a march step with the eyes closed. The Rinne test (C) uses a tuning fork to determine if air conductance exceeds bone conductance.

61. **Correct: D. restricting fluid intake.**
Measures to decrease fluid pressure load in the inner ear can help prevent symptoms. However, these measures do not include fluid restriction.
Incorrect:
Risk factors for Ménière's disease include the use of ototoxic drugs (A), long-term high-dose salicylate use, certain cancer chemotherapeutics, and exposure to loud noise (B). Triggers of attacks can include certain foods and drinks, mental and physical stress, and variations in the menstrual cycle. Measures to decrease fluid pressure load in the inner ear can also help prevent symptoms, such as the use of thiazide diuretics or limiting sodium intake (C).

62 to 65. Matching Questions

62. **Correct: B. subjective perception of altered equilibrium**

63. **Correct: A. perception that the person or the environment is moving**

64. **Correct: C. rhythmic oscillations of the eyes**

65. **Correct: D. perception of abnormal hearing or head noises**
Dizziness can include the perception of an altered equilibrium that can include unsteadiness, lightheadedness, or a feeling of impending fainting (B). Possible causes of dizziness can include hypotension or postural hypotension as well as hyperventilation and anxiety. Vertigo is a sense of spinning or whirling when the person is not actually moving (A) and is usually caused by a disorder of the vestibular system (structures of the inner ear, vestibular nerve, brainstem, and cerebellum). Nystagmus is characterized by rhythmic, uncontrolled oscillations of the eye (C), often found in persons with Ménière's disease. Movements can be side to side, up and down, or circular in motion and can affect vision, depth

perception, balance, and coordination. Tinnitus is the perception of noise or ringing in the ears (D). Tinnitus is typically a symptom of an underlying condition, such as age-related hearing loss or injury to the ear.

Anterior Epistaxis

66. **Correct: C. a 42-year-old man who works outdoors during the months of December to March in the northeastern United States**
Anterior epistaxis is most commonly the result of localized nasal mucosa dryness or trauma. Nosebleeds tend to increase in the winter months due to lower humidity.
Incorrect:
Hypertension (A) and coagulation disorders (B) are uncommon reasons for nosebleeds in the outpatient setting, while the presence of nasal polyps is not a risk factor for epistaxis (D).

67. **Correct: C. firm pressure in an "entire nose pinched" position for a minimum of 10 minutes.**
Most episodes of anterior epistaxis can be easily managed with simple pressure as first-line therapy, either with firm pressure to the area superior to the nasal alar cartilage or an "entire nose pinched closed" approach for at least 10 minutes; often up to 30 minutes of pressure is needed.
Incorrect:
If simple pressure is ineffective, second-line approaches can include nasal packing (A) and cautery (D). Topical antifibrinolytic agents can be used when other methods are unsuccessful (B).

68. **Correct: B. accelerated hypertension.**
Though hypertension is not a common reason for acute anterior epistaxis, poorly controlled hypertension is among the more common reasons for epistaxis that is refractory to first-line therapies.
Incorrect:
Diabetes mellitus (A), acute bacterial sinusitis (C), and thrombocytopenia (D) are not commonly associated with protracted nasal bleeding.

69. **Correct: A. initiating systemic prothrombotic therapy.**
The use of systemic prothrombotic therapy is not recommended for recurrent epistaxis.
Incorrect:
Epistaxis is nearly always treated with localized therapy, including pressure, nasal packing (B), cautery (C), and/or topical antifibrinolytic agents (D). For refractory cases, arterial embolization or surgical therapy can be considered.

Allergic Rhinitis

70. **Correct: C. "After a rain shower."**
Pollens are major triggers in seasonal AR and allergic conjunctivitis and are likely at the lowest levels after a rain shower.
Incorrect:
Pollen counts are generally the highest early in the morning (A) as they are released shortly after dawn.

Pollen travels best on warm, dry, breezy days (B) and lowest during chilly, wet periods. Overcast skies (D) have no effect on pollen counts in the absence of precipitation.

71 to 74. Matching Questions

71. **Correct: B. most common seasonal allergen**

72. **Correct: C. common indoor allergen**

73. **Correct: A. most common perennial allergen**

74. **Correct: C. common indoor allergen**
Pollens are major triggers in seasonal AR and allergic conjunctivitis and achieve highest levels early in the morning. Dust mites are the most common trigger for perennial allergy symptoms. Pet dander, cockroaches, and mold spores are other indoor allergens found to cause nasal and ocular allergy symptoms. Some outdoor mold spores can also cause allergy symptoms.

75. **Correct: C. in a few days to a week.**
Unlike a topical nasal decongestant that can provide an immediate effect, the use of a nasal corticosteroid can take a few days to a week before symptom relief is achieved.
Incorrect:
When prescribing these agents, patient education is needed to ensure consistent use to achieve the desired effect. Patients initiating nasal corticosteroid therapy should be advised that effects will not be immediate (A) or even within 1 to 2 days (B). If no effects are observed after 1 to 2 weeks (D), treatment approaches should be reevaluated.

76. **Correct: D. oral loratadine**
Due to this patient's symptoms and occupation, he requires a rapid reliever that is nonsedating. Loratadine, a second-generation antihistamine, is recommended as first-line therapy due to its effectiveness in providing rapid relief and nonsedating quality.
Incorrect:
Nasal cromolyn (A) is not recommended as first-line treatment, and diphenhydramine (B), a first-generation antihistamine, is sedating. Nasal corticosteroids, such as flunisolide (C), can be used as controller medications but will not provide immediate relief.

77. **Correct: B. action on the histamine-1 (H_1) receptor sites.**
Antihistamines work by blocking the H_1 receptor sites and preventing the action of histamines, a potent inflammatory mediator. These agents can be used to treat acute allergy symptoms. Second-generation products such as loratadine (Claritin®) can be given as first-line treatment. First-generation products, such as diphenhydramine, should be avoided due to their sedative and anticholinergic effects.
Incorrect:
Antihistamines work by blocking the H_1 receptor sites and prevent the action of histamines. This action prevents inflammatory mediation (C) and has no clinically significant impact on vasoconstriction (A) or peripheral vasodilation (D).

78. Correct: A. vasoconstriction.

Decongestants act as vasoconstrictors, opening edematous nasal passages and relieving congestion. These agents only provide relief of nasal congestion. Topical decongestants should be limited to use for less than 5 days, and use should be avoided in preschoolers. Regular use of oral decongestants should be avoided due to potential adverse effects, including tachycardia, hypertension, dizziness, and sedation.

Incorrect:

Decongestants act as vasoconstrictors rather than vasodilators (D) and have no impact on H_1 receptor sites (B) or inflammatory mediation (C).

79. Correct: D. oral antihistamine

An oral second-generation antihistamine can be used as first-line therapy to treat acute symptoms of AR, including nasal itch.

Incorrect:

The use of an anticholinergic nasal spray (A) should be limited to the relief of refractory rhinorrhea. Oral decongestants (B) should be avoided in AR, while corticosteroid nasal spray (C) can be used as a controller agent, though its effect may not be achieved until consistent use for several days to a week.

80. Correct: C. nasal decongestant

A nasal decongestant can be used for rescue therapy and symptom relief of nasal congestion. However, these agents should not be used for prolonged periods of time (less than 5 days).

Incorrect:

Leukotriene modifiers (B), such as montelukast, can be considered for treatment of AR. However, these agents are generally not preferred as they tend to be more expensive with similar or less effectiveness compared with other products. The use of anticholinergic nasal spray (A) should be limited to the relief of refractory rhinorrhea. An oral first-generation antihistamine (D) is not recommended as treatment for AR because of sedation effects, though a nasal antihistamine has first-line benefits for seasonal AR associated with nasal congestion.

81. Correct: B. oral antihistamine

The American Academy of Otolaryngology-Head and Neck Surgery (AAO-HNS) recommends the use of an oral antihistamine to treat rhinorrhea associated with AR.

Incorrect:

Leukotriene modifiers (D), such as montelukast, can be considered for treatment of AR. However, these agents are generally not preferred as they tend to be more expensive with similar or less effectiveness compared with other products. The use of anticholinergic nasal spray (A) should be limited to the relief of refractory rhinorrhea. Corticosteroid nasal spray (C) can be used as controller therapy, though relief can take several days of consistent use.

82. Correct: B. anticholinergic effect.

Ipratropium bromide is an anticholinergic that can be useful as part of rescue therapy for patients with bothersome nasal discharge. These agents work by inhibiting the parasympathetic transmission to submucosal glands.

Incorrect:

Ipratropium bromide works as an anticholinergic with no or minimal vasodilation (C), vasoconstriction (D), or antihistaminic (A) action.

83. Correct: C. cardiovascular disease.

Oral decongestants have the potential for vasoconstriction and increased blood pressure and heart rate. These agents should be avoided in patients with hypertension and cardiovascular disease. As decongestants are a common ingredient in many OTC medications, patient education is important to raise awareness of the possible risks when considering these medications.

Incorrect:

In general, regular use of oral decongestants should be avoided due to potential adverse effects, including tachycardia, hypertension, dizziness, and sedation. There are no warnings or precautions with their use associated with AR (A), migraine headache (B), or chronic bronchitis (D).

84. Correct: C. a mast cell stabilizer.

Cromolyn is a mast cell stabilizer used as a nasal spray to treat AR. Mast cells are involved in the inflammatory process through the release of mediators, including histamines. Cromolyn stabilizes the mast cells and prevents the release of inflammatory mediators and can be used as controller therapy for AR.

Incorrect:

Cromolyn is a mast cell stabilizer and thus does not work as an anti-immunoglobulin E antibody (A), vasoconstrictor (B), or leukotriene modifier (D).

85. Correct: B. an inflammatory inhibitor.

Leukotrienes are inflammatory chemicals that are released upon exposure to an allergen. Upon release, these chemicals cause airway constriction and mucus production. Leukotriene modifiers work by blocking the action of leukotriene that can cause nasal congestion and rhinorrhea. These agents are typically used as controller therapy in AR by blocking the inflammatory process.

Incorrect:

Leukotriene modifiers are typically used as controller therapy in AR and thus would not be used as a rescue drug (C) or to treat acute inflammation (D) or acute nasal itch (A).

86. Correct: A. when allergy symptoms are controlled with environmental management.

Allergen immunotherapy can be helpful in managing persistent AR and conjunctivitis and should be considered in patients with multiorgan symptoms of IgE-mediated allergic sensitization (e.g., asthma). Allergen immunotherapy would not be appropriate for patients whose allergy symptoms can be controlled with simple environmental management.

Incorrect:
Allergen immunotherapy can be helpful in managing persistent AR and conjunctivitis and should be considered in patients with multiorgan symptoms of IgE-mediated allergic sensitization (e.g., asthma) (D). This method can be highly effective in select patients and should be considered when other treatments fail (B) or if the patient desires to reduce the use of allergy medications (C).

87. **Correct: A. initiation of daily oral corticosteroids.**
A short course of oral corticosteroids is recommended in moderate-to-severe AR and conjunctivitis when symptoms are not controlled with current therapy.

Incorrect:
Daily intranasal corticosteroids (C) as well as mast cell stabilizers (D) can be used as controller therapy once symptoms are managed. Parenteral or intramuscular corticosteroids (B) are not preferred over oral corticosteroids, and repeated doses are needed for full effect.

Antibiotic Allergy

88. **Correct: D. imipenem**
Safe practice involves recognizing the properties and characteristics of drug classes and knowing to which class each medication belongs. Imipenem belongs in the carbapenem drug class, which typically has a "penem" suffix.

Incorrect:
The prefix or suffix of generic drug names can be helpful in recognizing the drug class. Agents in the penicillin drug class typically have the "cillin" suffix and include ampicillin (B), amoxicillin (A), and dicloxacillin (C).

89. **Correct: D. Epstein-Barr virus (EBV).**
EBV is the leading causative organism in mononucleosis. When certain penicillin forms, such as ampicillin and amoxicillin, are administered to a person with EBV infection, a cutaneous reaction (rash) nearly always occurs. Though the mechanism is not entirely known, the rash is thought to be the result of altered immune status during the infection and not indicative of penicillin allergy.

Incorrect:
Other than the reaction between certain penicillins and EBV infection, there are no other known reactions between antibiotic use and other select pathogens, including infections caused by human herpes virus type 1 (A), human papilloma virus type 11 (B), and adenovirus type 20 (C).

90. **Correct: A. cephalexin**
The greatest rate of cross-reactivity to the penicillins appears to arise from use of the first-generation cephalosporins (e.g., cephalexin and cefadroxil).

Incorrect:
There is less cross-reactivity with second-generation (e.g., cefprozil [B]), third-generation (e.g. cefpodoxime [D]), and fourth-generation (e.g., cefuroxime [C]) agents, with a cross-reactivity rate of less than 1%.

91. **Correct: B. the beta-lactams**
The beta-lactam class (e.g., penicillin, amoxicillin, cephalosporins) is associated with the highest rate of allergic reactions, with about 10% of the population reporting a penicillin allergy. However, the rate is likely not as high as reported in the past.

Incorrect:
Approximately 3% to 6% report an allergy to sulfonamides (D) (e.g., TMP-SMX). Allergic reaction to the macrolides (A) (e.g., azithromycin, clarithromycin) is relatively uncommon (0.4% to 3%), as well as immediate allergic reactions to fluoroquinolones (C) (e.g., ciprofloxacin, levofloxacin), with rates ranging from 0.4% to 2%.

92. **Correct: B. refer to allergy and immunology for further evaluation.**
Safe practice dictates that the exact nature of this patient's allergy, if any, be determined by a specialist. This information will be essential if antimicrobial therapy is needed for this patient in the future.

Incorrect:
The use of antihistamines (C) or corticosteroids (D) as a measure to help avoid an allergic reaction is not appropriate. It is also important to note that family reports (A) of allergies can often be inaccurate. Antimicrobial allergy does not appear to have a strong genetic or familial tendency.

93. **Correct: D. fixed drug eruptions.**
Fixed drug eruptions are the development of one or more erythematous patches. The condition associated with the use of TMP-SMX is usually mild and self-limiting.

Incorrect:
Use of TMP-SMX can on occasion lead to serious reactions including anaphylaxis (A) (overreaction of the immune system) that can lead to hypotension, vomiting, syncope, and upper airway edema. Stevens-Johnson syndrome (B) and toxic epidermal necrolysis (C) are severe skin reactions that eventually cause the skin to blister and peel, leaving raw areas.

94. **Correct: C. moxifloxacin.**
Though a respiratory fluoroquinolone, such as moxifloxacin or levofloxacin, would be appropriate due to the likely presence of a beta-lactamase-producing organism or drug-resistant *S pneumoniae*, a history of facial edema with ciprofloxacin is problematic given the risk for potential respiratory distress. Thus, the use of another fluoroquinolone should be avoided for this patient.

Incorrect:
Given the report of facial edema with prior use of a fluoroquinolone, an antimicrobial from another class would

be most appropriate, including beta-lactams (D), macrolides (A), and cephalosporins (B).

95. **Correct: B. if he experiences any allergic reaction, he should stop taking the antibiotic and seek appropriate health care.**

When taking an antimicrobial for the first time, the patient should be instructed that if an allergic reaction occurs, he should stop taking the medication and immediately contact a health-care provider. This is generally true for all medications as the allergic reaction can worsen with continued use.

Incorrect:

The absence of a penicillin allergy (A) does not necessarily predict the absence of a reaction to doxycycline since they belong to different drug classes. With the development of an allergic reaction, the patient should not continue taking the medication (C) as the reaction can worsen rather than resolve with continued use (D).

Acute Bacterial Rhinosinusitis

96. **Correct: A. upper respiratory tract infection-like symptoms persisting beyond 7 to 10 days**

Patient history of present illness, especially the length of symptoms, is more sensitive and specific for ABRS than is physical examination. Symptoms that persist beyond 7 to 10 days, especially with a report of double sickening, is most indicative of ABRS.

Incorrect:

ABRS can include symptoms of facial fullness and tenderness (B), cervical lymphadenopathy (C), and nasal discharge (D). However, these conditions can also occur in the presence of a viral upper respiratory infection, allergic rhinitis, and a variety of other conditions. Having symptoms that persist beyond 7 to 10 days, especially with a report of double sickening, is most indicative of ABRS.

97. **Correct: B. S pneumoniae.**

Understanding the common pathogens of infection is helpful in deciding appropriate initial empiric therapy. The gram-positive bacteria *S pneumoniae* is the most common causative pathogen of ABRS and is most likely to cause the most significant symptoms.

Incorrect:

H influenzae and *M catarrhalis* (C) are common gram-negative organisms that cause ABRS. *M pneumoniae* (A) and *E coli* (D) are not typically found in ABRS.

98. **Correct: D. an 18-year-old with a history of recurrent epistaxis**

Risk factors for ABRS include any condition that alters the normal cleansing mechanism of the sinuses. Recurrent epistaxis is not a risk factor for ABRS.

Incorrect:

Risk factors for ABRS include any condition that alters the normal cleansing mechanism of the sinuses. These can include viral URI (A), poorly controlled allergic rhinitis (B), cigarette smoking (C), and abnormalities of sinus structure.

99. **Correct: A. amoxicillin-clavulanate**

The most common pathogens for ABRS include *S pneumoniae* (gram-positive), *H influenzae* (gram-negative), and *M catarrhalis* (gram-negative). Amoxicillin-clavulanate exhibits activity against these pathogens and is considered an appropriate first-line agent.

Incorrect:

A respiratory fluoroquinolone (D) can be considered in the presence of risk factors for DRSP; however, hypertension is not a comorbid condition associated with DRSP risk, and there has been no recent use of antimicrobials for this patient. TMP-SMX (B) and clarithromycin (C) are not preferred due to elevated rates of *S pneumoniae* resistance to these agents.

100. **Correct: D. high-dose amoxicillin with clavulanate**

Doxycycline exhibits effective activity against certain gram-positive and gram-negative pathogens but is not effective against DRSP, which is the likely pathogen in this patient. Among the choices, high-dose amoxicillin with clavulanate represents the best option to overcome resistance.

Incorrect:

TMP-SMX (C) and the macrolides (B) are not recommended for DRSP, and clindamycin (A) is not recommended for ABRS. A respiratory fluoroquinolone would be another appropriate option for this patient.

101. **Correct: B. standard-dose moxifloxacin.**

Because of a recent history of antimicrobial use, this patient is at risk of infection by DRSP. A respiratory fluoroquinolone (i.e., moxifloxacin) is the preferred choice when DRSP is suspected.

Incorrect:

The macrolides (i.e., clarithromycin [A]) and first-generation cephalosporins (i.e., cephalexin [C]) are not recommended for the treatment of DRSP. High-dose amoxicillin (D) should be avoided in this patient due to penicillin allergy.

102. **Correct: C. prompt referral for sinus imaging with a CT scan.**

For the patient who has experienced treatment failure with antimicrobials that should have been effective, imaging will likely help with rethinking the original diagnosis. A CT scan can help identify a sinus structural abnormality or possibly a complication such as extension of infection beyond the sinus space. ENT consultation should also be considered.

Incorrect:

With treatment failure with moxifloxacin, prescribing a second fluoroquinolone (B) would not be appropriate as it would likely result in the same clinical response. A nasal swab (D) can be useful in identifying the causative organism, but appropriate management should not be delayed for culture results, which can take 1 to 2 days. An oral corticosteroid (A) is not warranted, particularly when a definitive diagnosis with imaging studies has not been made.

103. Correct: C. oral decongestant

Adjunctive treatments should be considered to reduce the symptoms associated with ABRS. Decongestants, either oral or nasal, are not recommended as adjunctive therapy in patients with ABRS as they do not substantially impact outcomes.

Incorrect:

Saline nasal spray (A) or neti pot can be used to rinse nasal passages. Nasal corticosteroids (B) can be effective in reducing inflammation. Analgesics such as acetaminophen (D) or ibuprofen can help alleviate pain.

Oral Cancer

104. Correct: C. an ulcerated lesion with indurated margins.

An ulcerated lesion with indurated margin is the classic presentation of oral SCC. Oral cancer is typically painless, while other self-limiting conditions can be at minimum uncomfortable (candidiasis) with an irritated feeling to painful (herpetic lesion, aphthous stomatitis).

Incorrect:

A raised, red, painful shallow ulcer (A) best describes a self-limiting aphthous stomatitis. A denuded patch with a removable white coating best (B) describes oral candidiasis. A painful vesicular-form lesion (D) is likely due to herpes infection.

105. Correct: D. oral cancer.

Lymphadenopathy associated with oral cancer consists of immobile nodes that are nontender when palpated.

Incorrect:

In infection (herpes simplex [A], AOM [B], bacterial pharyngitis [C]), the associated lymphadenopathy follows drainage tracks and is characterized by tenderness and mobility.

106. Correct: C. SCC

SCC is by far the most common cause of oral cancer, accounting for over 90% of cancers in the oral cavity and oropharynx.

Incorrect:

Other types of oral cancer include verrucous carcinoma, adenocarcinoma (A), sarcoma (B), basal cell carcinoma (D), minor salivary gland carcinoma, and lymphomas, which occur much less frequently than SCC.

107. Correct: B. HPV16.

There is a growing body of evidence supporting the increasing role of HPV16 in oral cancers, particularly among young, nonsmoking oral cancer patients. Among people under the age of 50 years, HPV16 will likely replace tobacco as the leading cause of initiation of the cancer process. With the availability and growing utilization of the HPV vaccine that protects against HPV16, it is hoped that the incidence of oral cancers will decrease in the future.

Incorrect:

Other virus types, including human herpes virus type 1 (or the "cold sore" virus) (A) and EBV (common cause of mononucleosis) (D) are not typically associated with oral cancer formation. Though adenovirus has been implicated in certain cancers, adenovirus type 16 (C) has not been identified as a risk factor for oral cancer.

108 to 114. Matching Questions

108. Correct: E

109. Correct: G

110. Correct: C

111. Correct: A

112. Correct: B

113. Correct: F

114. Correct: D

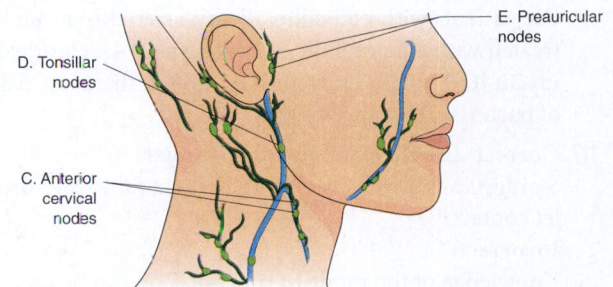

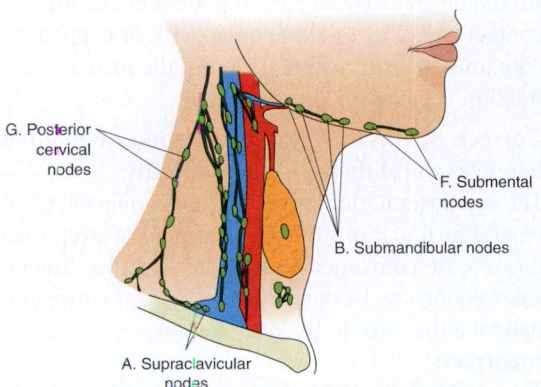

The preauricular nodes are located just anterior to the ears and drain lymph fluid from the eyes, cheeks, and scalp. The posterior cervical nodes are located along the back of the neck, while the anterior cervical nodes are located along the front part of the neck, in front of the sternocleidomastoid muscle. Supraclavicular nodes are located on either side of the hollow of the clavicle near the sternoclavicular joint. The submandibular nodes are located between the submandibular salivary glands and along the underside of the jaw. The submental nodes are located under the chin and drain the anterior mandible and associated structures. The tonsillar nodes are located just below the angle of the mandible.

Acute Bacterial Pharyngitis

115. Correct: A. *S pyogenes* pharyngitis.

Classic symptoms of *S pyogenes* pharyngitis or strep throat include sore throat, fever, enlarged tonsils that are usually covered with exudate, and anterior cervical lymphadenopathy.

Incorrect:

Viral pharyngitis (C) is accompanied by cough, nasal discharge, hoarseness, and pharyngeal ulcerations. The presentation of infectious mononucleosis (B) includes fatigue, exudative pharyngitis with tonsillar enlargement, fever, headache, and anterior and posterior cervical lymphadenopathy. Vincent angina (D) is associated with infection of the gums and tooth margins.

116. **Correct: B. TMP-SMX.**

TMP-SMX is not typically used for the treatment of strep throat but can be considered for other infections caused by a susceptible organism.

Incorrect:

For patients with penicillin allergy, strep throat can be treated with a macrolide (azithromycin [A], clarithromycin [C]) or clindamycin [D], though there is a risk of bacterial resistance to these agents.

117. **Correct: C. saliva and droplet contact.**

S pyogenes is primarily transmitted via saliva and droplet contact.

Incorrect:

Knowledge of the mode of transmission can be an important step in minimizing risk of transmission and should be an essential part of patient education. Sexual contact (A), skin-to-skin contact (B), or exposure to contaminated surfaces (D) are not the primary transmission vehicles for this pathogen.

118. **Correct: B. This is a treatment option when nonadherence to oral therapy is a possibility.**

The oral formulation of penicillin is preferred over parenteral formulations for the treatment of strep throat due to cost, convenience, and safety factors. The injectable version can be considered if there is concern with patient adherence to the oral therapy.

Incorrect:

The oral and injectable forms of penicillin exhibit an identical spectrum of activity (D), including group G streptococci (C), and both are susceptible to beta-lactamase (A). However, the disadvantages of the intramuscular formulation include a greater risk of severe allergic reaction, higher cost, and injection site pain.

119. **Correct: B. 3 to 5 days.**

The incubation period of *S pyogenes* lasts an average of 3 to 5 days but can be up to 3 months. Knowledge of the incubation period of an organism is important in helping identify exposure and pre-illness onset and also to let patients know when they could have passed on the organism to others. This is particularly helpful when the patient is a member of a household or in other situations where individuals are in close physical contact.

Incorrect:

The incubation period of *S pyogenes* lasts an average of 3 to 5 days but can be up to 3 months.

120. **Correct: B. 24**

Patients are no longer contagious within 24 hours of initiation of antimicrobial therapy and without fever. Patients should be educated on when they are no longer contagious as this will dictate when they can return to work or school. A premature return to work or school can increase contagion risk through droplet transmission.

Incorrect:

Patients are no longer contagious within 24 hours of initiation of antimicrobial therapy and without fever. Patients should be educated on when they are no longer contagious as this will dictate when they can return to work or school.

121. **Correct: B. appropriate antimicrobial therapy helps to facilitate more rapid resolution of symptoms.**

Infections caused by groups C and G streptococci typically clear without antimicrobial therapy. However, resolution of symptoms is quicker with appropriate antimicrobial treatment. It is important to note that the RST will not detect these organisms; a throat culture is needed.

Incorrect:

Groups C and G streptococci can cause pharyngitis but carry minimal risk for rheumatic fever (C) or glomerulonephritis (A). Though infection with group C or G streptococci can cause peritonsillar abscess, this is a rare complication. These organisms are not associated with acute infectious hepatitis (D).

122. **Correct: B. the rash often peels during recovery.**

Scarlet fever is characterized by the formation of a scarlatiniform rash during streptococcal pharyngitis. The rash can peel during recovery, typically without any great discomfort.

Incorrect:

Treatment is similar to strep throat treatment (C) (i.e., oral penicillin), and there is no increased risk for sequelae, including glomerulonephritis (A). Throat culture of the patient with scarlet fever would often reveal the presence of GABHS (D).

123. **Correct: A. 2 days**

Scarlet fever is characterized by the formation of a scarlatiniform rash with a fine sandpaper-like texture. The rash usually appears on the second day of illness.

Incorrect:

The rash associated with scarlet fever usually appears on the second day of illness.

124. **Correct: C. TMP-SMX.**

Treatment of scarlet fever is identical to treatment of streptococcal pharyngitis. TMP-SMX is not recommended for the treatment of bacterial pharyngitis.

Incorrect:

Treatment of scarlet fever is identical to treatment of streptococcal pharyngitis. Penicillin (A) remains highly effective and is the treatment of choice. Cephalosporins (e.g., cefdinir [B], cefpodoxime [D]) can be useful in the presence of concomitant infection or carriage of an organism that produces beta-lactamase.

125 to 126. Matching Questions

125. **Correct: B. a 26-year-old woman with sore throat and fever, swollen tonsils covered with exudate, palatal petechiae, and anterior cervical lymphadenopathy**

126. **Correct: A. a 34-year-old with cough, nasal discharge, hoarseness, conjunctival inflammation, and diarrhea**

Understanding the differences in signs and symptoms of a bacterial and viral infection is important in making a differential diagnosis and selecting appropriate management options. Classic symptoms of *S pyogenes* pharyngitis or strep throat include sore throat, fever, enlarged tonsils that are usually covered with exudate, and anterior cervical lymphadenopathy (B). Viral pharyngitis is accompanied with cough, nasal discharge, hoarseness, and pharyngeal ulcerations (A).

127. **Correct: A. infection with a strain of *Streptococcus* producing beta-lactamase.**

GABHS do not produce beta-lactamase and remain susceptible to penicillin.

Incorrect:

A concomitant infection or carriage with an organism, such as *H influenzae*, that produces beta-lactamase can lead to treatment failure (C). Inadequate dosage (D) as well as nonadherence to therapy (B) can also contribute to treatment failure as an insufficient concentration of antimicrobial is attained and maintained at the site of infection to eradicate the pathogen.

128. **Correct: C. peritonsillar abscess.**

The patient presents with symptoms most consistent with peritonsillar abscess, including progressively worsening sore throat, often worse on one side, a muffled "hot potato" voice, and swollen tonsils with contralateral uvular deviation.

Incorrect:

Scarlet fever (D) has a similar presentation as strep throat with the addition of a scarlatiniform rash on the second day of illness. Viral pharyngitis (B) typically has more mild symptoms and is accompanied with cough, nasal discharge, hoarseness, and pharyngeal ulcerations. The presentation of mononucleosis (A) includes fatigue, exudative pharyngitis with tonsillar enlargement, fever, headache, and anterior and posterior cervical lymphadenopathy.

129. **Correct: B. *Candida albicans*.**

Understanding the most common etiology of infection is important when deciding on initial empiric antimicrobial therapy. *C albicans* is a yeast implicated in candidiasis but does not cause peritonsillar abscess.

Incorrect:

Understanding the most common etiology of infection is important when deciding on initial empiric antimicrobial therapy. Peritonsillar abscess is most commonly

caused by *F necrophorum* (A), GABHS (D), and group C or G streptococcus (C).

130. **Correct: B. emergent referral to emergency department and specialty ENT consult.**

Because airway compromise is a potentially life-threatening complication of peritonsillar abscess, an immediate referral to the emergency department with an ENT specialty consult is needed.

Incorrect:

Appropriate antimicrobial treatment, needle aspiration, and airway maintenance should be promptly initiated. Confirmation of a peritonsillar abscess diagnosis can be performed via ultrasonography or CT of the affected region, rather than a pharyngeal x-ray (C). Due to the life-threatening nature of this condition, there should be no delay in antimicrobial therapy (D) or specialty care (A).

Infectious Mononucleosis

131. **Correct: C. 30 to 50**

Knowledge of the incubation period of an organism is important in helping identify exposure pre-illness onset and also to let patients know when they could have passed on the organism. Infectious mononucleosis is most commonly caused by EBV, which has a 30- to 50-day incubation period. This is followed by an intense T cell–mediated immune response that coincides with the development of symptoms.

Incorrect:

Knowledge of the incubation period of an organism is important in helping identify exposure pre-illness onset and also to let patients know when they could have passed on the organism. Infectious mononucleosis has a 30- to 50-day incubation period.

132. **Correct: C. oropharyngeal secretions.**

Recognizing the mechanism of transmission in infectious diseases is important in minimizing further transmission of contagion and should be part of patient education. Infectious mononucleosis is primarily transmitted through oropharyngeal secretions, hence why this infection is commonly referred to as the "kissing disease."

Incorrect:

Recognizing the mechanism of transmission in infectious diseases is important in minimizing further transmission of contagion. Skin-to-skin, blood exposure, and genital contacts (A, B, D) are not methods of transmitting the EBV that is the causative organism in the majority of cases of mononucleosis.

133. **Correct: B. lymphocytosis with atypical lymphocytes**

Lymphocytosis with atypical lymphocytes is a common white blood cell (WBC) finding in many significant viral infections such as infective mononucleosis.

Incorrect:

Neutrophilia with reactive forms (A) is associated with bacterial infection. Thrombocytosis (C), an increase in platelets, is not noted in mononucleosis, though a transient modest thrombocytopenia (a platelet count reduction) is found in about 50% of patients with mononucleosis. Macrocytosis (D) refers to increased red blood cell (RBC) size, which is not found in mononucleosis.

134. Correct: B. prednisone

Prednisone has long been used to help relieve symptoms of pharyngeal edema associated with infectious mononucleosis. A 3-day regimen is usually sufficient.

Incorrect:

Antivirals, such as acyclovir (D), are not helpful in this infection. Ibuprofen (C) can help alleviate some discomfort caused by the infection but will likely not be effective for severe pharyngitis. Amoxicillin (A) should be avoided during infectious mononucleosis as it can cause a rash in patients with EBV infection.

135. Correct: D. amoxicillin

Amoxicillin should be avoided during infectious mononucleosis as it can cause a rash in patients with EBV infection. The exact mechanism that causes the reaction is unclear and could involve a true allergic drug reaction, a virus-dependent rash, or a transient loss of drug tolerance due to the virus that is responsible for the symptoms. The condition is more common in children than in adults with mononucleosis.

Incorrect:

Acetaminophen (A), sulfamethoxazole (B), and erythromycin (C) have not been associated with development of a rash in patients with infectious mononucleosis.

136. Correct: C. at least 50%

Splenomegaly develops in at least 50% of patients. In a person who participates in contact or collision sports or other activities, the risk of splenic rupture in response to even modest abdominal trauma needs to be considered during acute and convalescent stages. The risk for splenic rupture is greatest in the second and third weeks of illness—hence the mandate of

abstaining from collision or contact sports for at least 1 month.

Incorrect:

Knowing the percentage of patients who will develop this risk factor for splenic rupture is critical to safe practice.

137. Correct: B. 1″ × 3″ × 5″.

The size of the normal spleen can be recalled by the "rules of odds": 1 × 3 × 5 inches in size, weighing 7 oz (about 200 g), and lying between ribs 9 and 11. When the spleen is easily palpated, its size is usually increased by two or more times normal. However, physical examination is a relatively insensitive measure of splenic size.

Incorrect:

Knowledge of splenic size is critical to safe practice.

138. Correct: B. at least 1 month

Splenic rupture is a rare occurrence in infectious mononucleosis (0.1% to 0.5% of patients) but is the leading cause of mortality among these patients. All persons with infectious mononucleosis are at risk of splenic rupture regardless of spleen size, with the highest risk occurring during the second and third weeks of illness. Because of this, patients should abstain from collision or contact sports for at least 1 month. Though there are no specific guidelines, sports teams may require a left upper quadrant abdominal ultrasound to ensure splenic regression prior to allowing a return to play. Physical examination provides a relatively insensitive measure of spleen size. In addition, the person with infectious mononucleosis should return to his or her baseline state of health, without pharyngeal symptoms, prior to returning to sports or other physically active pursuits.

Incorrect:

All persons with infectious mononucleosis are at risk of splenic rupture regardless of spleen size, with the highest risk occurring during the second and third weeks of illness. Because of this, patients should abstain from contact or collision sports for at least 1 month.

Cardiac Disorders

6

Cardiovascular Disease Risk Assessment and Reduction

Overview

In the United States, coronary heart disease (CHD), most often caused by atherosclerosis, is the leading cause of death in both men and women. Guidelines from the American College of Cardiology (ACC) and American Heart Association (AHA) recommend routine evaluation of atherosclerotic cardiovascular disease (ASCVD) risk in asymptomatic adults, with ASCVD being broadly defined as acute coronary syndrome (ACS), myocardial infarction (MI), angina (stable or unstable), arterial revascularization, stroke/transient ischemic attacks (TIA), peripheral arterial disease (PAD), heart failure (HF), and/or atrial fibrillation (AF).

ASCVD risk is based on nonmodifiable factors (e.g., age, gender, or ethnicity) and modifiable factors (e.g., cholesterol level or blood pressure [BP]). All patients should be counseled on healthy lifestyle habits and encouraged to adopt lifestyle modifications to reduce cardiovascular disease (CVD) risk when necessary. These can involve a change in diet, weight loss for those who are overweight or obese, and increased physical activity (Table 6-1). For those at higher risk of CVD, lifestyle modifications should be combined with appropriate pharmacotherapy, typically to reduce cholesterol level or BP (also refer to the "Dyslipidemia" section in Chapter 12).

> **HYPERTENSION: A MODIFIABLE ATHEROSCLEROTIC CARDIOVASCULAR DISEASE RISK FACTOR**

Overview

Hypertension (HTN), a major modifiable ASCVD risk factor, is a complex disease with a core defect of vascular dysfunction that leads to select target organ damage (TOD); the target organs include the brain, eye, heart, and kidneys (Table 6-2). Appropriate HTN treatment significantly reduces TOD risk, including ASCVD. When a BP reading of 115/75 mm Hg is used as a starting point, ASCVD disease risk doubles with each increment of 20/10 mm Hg. HTN control leads to a reduction of stroke incidence by 35% to 40%, reduction of MI by 20% to 25%, and reduction of HF by 50%. Long-standing poorly controlled HTN is the leading cause of new-onset HF.

Making the Hypertension Diagnosis

Accurate clinical assessment depends on proper measurement of BP. The patient should be seated in a chair with feet flat on the floor, without crossed legs, with arm supported at heart level, for at least 5 minutes before taking the BP measurement, not on an examination table with feet dangling. Failure to perform these measures can lead to an artificially elevated reading and lack of standardization from visit to visit. The BP cuff should be wide enough to cover more than 80% of the upper arm, and the cuff's bladder should be approximately 40% of the arm circumference. The use of a cuff that does not meet these qualifications can lead to a falsely elevated BP reading (Box 6-1). Two or more measurements should be performed at least 1 to 2 minutes apart at the visit. In the absence of HTN TOD, when BP is elevated, BP readings should be performed at a subsequent visit 1 to 4 weeks later to confirm an HTN diagnosis. In the presence of HTN TOD, the diagnosis of HTN can be made with a single office visit.

Clinical Presentation

HTN is known as "the silent killer," referring to the fact that most people with elevated BP, including individuals with markedly high BP, are often without symptoms. As a result, HTN can go unnoticed for many years without a BP measurement, causing considerable and often irreversible TOD. However, damage to blood vessels and the heart can occur in asymptomatic patients. For those with HTN who present with symptoms, usually with hypertensive emergency, these can include headache, shortness of breath, epistaxis, flushing, dizziness, chest pain, and hematuria. (See the section "Hypertension Emergency Versus Hypertension Urgency" later in this chapter.)

"White coat" HTN refers to the condition where consistently elevated BP is observed in the health-care office or when a health-care provider (HCP) is present, but BP is normal in other, more comfortable environments. This is likely caused by patient anxiety in the health setting. The HCP and team should certainly work to ensure the patient is as

TABLE 6-1 Lifestyle Modifications in Hypertension

MODIFICATION	RECOMMENDATION	AVERAGE SYSTOLIC BLOOD PRESSURE REDUCTION RATE	
		Hypertension	*Normotension*
Weight reduction in overweight/obesity	Maintain normal body weight (BMI = 18.5 to 24.9 kg/m²) or at least 1-kg (2.2-lb) reduction in overweight (~1 mm Hg reduction for each 1-kg loss)	–5 mm Hg	–2/3 mm Hg
DASH eating plan	Diet rich in fruits, vegetables, whole grains, and low-fat dairy products with reduced content of saturated and total fat	–11 mm Hg	–3 mm Hg
Dietary sodium reduction	Optimal = less than 1,500 mg/day Alternative = At least 1,000 mg/day reduction	–5/6 mm Hg	–2/3 mm Hg
Enhanced intake of dietary potassium	Aim for 3,500 to 5,000 mg/day, preferably by consumption of a diet rich in potassium	–4/5 mm Hg	–2 mm Hg
Physical activity	Aerobic (90 to 150 min/week)	–5/8 mm Hg	–2/4 mm Hg
	Dynamic resistance (90–150 min/week)	–4 mm Hg	–2 mm Hg
	Isometric resistance (4 × 2 min [hand grip], 1 min rest between exercises, 3 sessions/week)	–5 mm Hg	–4 mm Hg
Moderation in alcohol intake	In individuals who drink alcohol, reduce intake to: Men: ≤2 drinks daily* Women: ≤1 drink daily*	–4 mm Hg	–3 mm Hg

*One drink = 12 oz (0.35 L) of beer, 5 oz (0.15 L) of wine, 1.5 oz (0.04 L) of 80-proof liquor.

Source: Data from Whelton PK, Carey RM, Aronow WS, et al. 2017 ACC/AHA guideline for the prevention, detection, evaluation, and management of high blood pressure in adults. J Am Coll Cardiol. 2017;71:e127–e248. http://www.onlinejacc.org/content/71/19/e127?_ga=2.35459041.138023780.1570631377-352956434.1570631377

TABLE 6-2 Hypertension: A Complex Disease Potentially Leading to Select Target Organ Damage

TARGET ORGAN	POTENTIAL DAMAGE OUTCOME WITH KNOWN MODERATION AS A RESULT OF EFFECTIVE ANTIHYPERTENSION THERAPY
Brain	Stroke, vascular (multi-infarct) dementia
Cardiovascular system	Atherosclerosis, myocardial infarction, left ventricular hypertrophy, heart failure
Kidney	Hypertensive nephropathy, renal failure
Eye	Hypertensive retinopathy with risk for blindness

BOX 6-1 Keys to an Accurate Blood Pressure Measurement

■ Take two or more measurements per visit (auscultatory method preferred)
■ Have patient be seated comfortably for ≥5 minutes with back supported, feet on floor, and arm supported in horizontal position
■ Blood pressure cuff placed at heart level

To detect postural hypotension or hypertension:

■ Take blood pressure measurement with patient standing for 1 to 3 minutes

TABLE 6-3 Hypertensive Retinopathy Grades

GRADE	COMMON FINDINGS
1	Common in long-standing, poorly controlled hypertension
	Narrowing of arteriolar branches; usually reversible when hypertension is treated
	No vision changes or permanent findings
2	Common in long-standing, poorly controlled hypertension
	Narrowing of arterioles with severe local constriction; usually reversible when hypertension is treated
	No vision changes or permanent findings
3	Usually with diastolic blood pressure ≥110 mm Hg (implies hypertensive emergency)
	Preceding signs with flame-shaped hemorrhages
	Potential for visual change and permanent findings
4	Usually with diastolic blood pressure ≥130 mm Hg (implied hypertensive emergency)
	Preceding signs with papilledema
	Potential for visual change and permanent findings

comfortable as possible during the clinical encounter to minimize this risk. At the same time, studies reveal that ASCVD risk is increased in the presence of white coat HTN. Ongoing BP evaluation is important in white coat HTN due to the higher risk of developing chronically elevated HTN.

Eye examination should be performed to detect signs of hypertensive retinopathy and to grade the extent of this condition with long-standing, poorly controlled HTN (Table 6-3).

Diagnostic Testing

With an HTN diagnosis, laboratory testing should be performed to establish a baseline for medication use and screen for secondary causes of HTN. These tests include fasting blood glucose, complete blood count (CBC) and lipid profile, serum creatinine and estimated glomerular filtration rate (eGFR), serum sodium, potassium and calcium, thyrotropin (TSH), urinalysis, and electrocardiogram (ECG). Additional testing is dictated by patient presentation and risk factors.

Treatment

Recommendations on the management of HTN are largely based on guidelines released from the Eighth Joint National Committee (JNC-8) and ACC/AHA. Though there are minor differences in BP goals and treatment recommendations, clinicians should focus on the general agreement, or overlap, between the

CLINICAL CONCEPT

The ACC/AHA provide a convenient online heart risk calculator that provides a 10-year risk ASCVD estimate that can be used to help guide management decisions.

CLINICAL CONCEPT
For any individual with
HTN or elevated BP,
lifestyle modification
should be considered as
part of first-line treatment,
as these can yield
significant improvement
in BP measurements
(see Table 6-1).

two guidelines. When determining BP goal, the JNC-8 generally recommends less than or equal to 140/90 mm Hg for nearly all patient populations, including those with diabetes mellitus and chronic kidney disease. ACC/AHA generally recommends a goal of less than or equal to 130/80 mm Hg.

According to both sets of HTN guidelines, the preferred first-line and later-line medications are generally confined to four classes: thiazide-type diuretics, calcium channel blockers (CCBs), angiotensin-converting enzyme inhibitors (ACEIs), and angiotensin receptor blockers (ARBs). Certain patient factors should be taken into consideration when deciding on an initial agent. People of African ancestry show reduced BP responses to monotherapy with ACEIs and ARBs compared with diuretics or CCBs. Although complete explanations for these racial differences are unknown, what is known is that HTN is the most common cause of renal failure in African Americans. In those with chronic kidney disease (CKD) and greater than or equal to 18 years of age (regardless of race or diabetes status), initial or add-on therapy should include an ACEI or ARB to improve kidney outcomes. The American Diabetes Association advocates for ACEI or ARB in diabetes with HTN, also related to improved renal outcomes.

Patients should take their medication for 1 month before assessing response to treatment and considering adjustment to the medication regimen. When intensification of therapy is needed, treatment can be adjusted to include higher doses or combinations of agents in these four classes (Table 6-4). In more than two-thirds of individuals with HTN, their HTN cannot be controlled on one drug, and two or more antihypertensive agents selected from different drug classes will be required. Prior to using beta blockers, aldosterone antagonists, or other classes of agents, patients should first receive a dose adjustment and combination of the four first-line agents. Triple therapy with an ACEI/ARB, CCB, and thiazide-type diuretic would precede use of a beta blocker, aldosterone antagonist, or other alternative agent. ACEIs and ARBs should not be used in combination.

■ ACE inhibitors and ARBs work by attenuating the activity of angiotensin II, a potent vasoconstrictor. These agents should not be used in combination as well as with a direct renin inhibitor. Dosing should be adjusted for renal insufficiency, and there is a modest hyperkalemia risk with their use, particularly in those with CKD or taking potassium supplements or potassium-sparing medications. These agents should not be used in the presence of severe bilateral renal artery stenosis due to risk of acute renal failure, and these agents should be avoided in pregnancy.

■ Nondihydropyridine calcium channel blockers (CCBs) (e.g., diltiazem) are particularly helpful for BP control and renal protection. However, these drugs are inhibitors of cytochrome P450 3A4 isoenzyme and should be used with caution with other medications that are substrates of this isoenzyme, such as select statins. Nondihydropyridines also reduce the heart rate as they induce bradycardic and negatively inotropic effects and thus should be limited to patients with normal left ventricular function. These agents are contraindicated in patients with severe left ventricular dysfunction and in those with second- or third-degree atrioventricular (AV) block in the absence of a pacemaker.

■ Dihydropyridine (DHP) calcium channel blockers (e.g., amlodipine) tend to be more potent vasodilators than non-DHP CCBs and are generally used for patients with difficult-to-treat HTN. The agents are associated with dose-related lower extremity and pedal edema and should not be used in patients with heart failure with reduced ejection fraction (HFrEF).

■ Thiazide diuretics result in low-volume sodium depletion that leads to a reduction in peripheral vascular resistance, thus decreasing BP. Chlorthalidone is preferred over hydrochlorothiazide (HCTZ) based on its prolonged half-life and superior efficacy. These agents are calcium sparing, but patients should be monitored for sodium, potassium, and magnesium depletion. They are less effective in patients with advanced renal impairment.

Along with the traditional risks, microalbuminuria (MA) or glomerular filtration rate of less than 60 mL/min is identified as a cardiovascular risk factor. When adjusted for other risk factors, the relative risk of ischemic heart disease associated with MA is increased twofold. An interaction between MA and cigarette smoking has been noted, and the presence of MA more than doubled the predictive effect of the conventional atherosclerotic risk factors for development of ischemic heart disease. MA not only is an independent predictor of ischemic heart disease, but it also substantially increases the risk associated with other established risk factors. Because the person with MA has significant CVD risk, recommendations for

TABLE 6-4 Comparison of Hypertension Guideline Recommendations

	JNC-8	ACC/AHA
HTN stages (SBP/DBP, mm Hg)	Less than 120 and less than 80 (Normal) 120 to 139 or 80 to 89 (Prehypertension) 140 to 159 or 90 to 99 (HTN stage 1) ≥160 or ≥100 (HTN stage 2)	Less than 120 and less than 80 (Normal) 120 to 129 and less than 80 (Elevated) 130 to 139 or 80 to 89 (HTN stage 1) ≥140 or ≥90 (HTN stage 2)
BP Goals (SBP/DBP, mm Hg)		
Clinical CVD or 10-year ASCVD risk ≥10%	NS	Less than 130/80
No clinical CVD and 10-year ASCVD risk less than 10%	NS	Less than 130/80
Age less than 60 years	Less than 140/90	NS
Age ≥60 years	Less than 150/90	NS
Age ≥65 years	NS	Less than 130 (SBP)
Diabetes mellitus (no CKD)	Less than 140/90	Less than 130/80
CKD	Less than 140/90	Less than 130/80
CKD after renal transplant	NS	Less than 130/80
HF	NS	Less than 130/80
Stable ischemic heart disease	NS	Less than 130/80
Secondary stroke prevention	NS	Less than 130/80
Secondary stroke prevention (lacunar)	NS	Less than 130/80
Peripheral arterial disease	NS	Less than 130/80
First-line antihypertensive agents	Thiazide diuretic CCB ACEI or ARB African ancestry: Thiazide diuretic or CCB Non-African ancestry: Thiazide diuretic, CCB, ACEI, or ARB With CKD: Include ACEI or ARB	Thiazide diuretic CCB ACEI or ARB In adults with African ancestry without CKD, HF, thiazide diuretics, CCB priority initial medications

*Avoid combining ACEI with ARB. Combined use of these agents can increase risk of serious adverse events, including hyperkalemia, hypotension, and worsening kidney function.

ACEI, angiotensin-converting enzyme inhibitor; ARB, angiotensin II receptor blocker; CCB, calcium channel blocker; CKD, chronic kidney disease; DBP, diastolic blood pressure; HF, heart failure; HTN, hypertension; SBP, systolic blood pressure.

Sources: James PA, Oparil S, Carter BL, et al. 2014 evidence-based guideline for the management of high blood pressure in adults: report from the panel members appointed to the Eighth Joint National Committee (JNC 8). JAMA. 2014;311(5):507–520; Whelton PK, Carey RM, Aronow WS, et al. 2017 ACC/AHA guideline for the prevention, detection, evaluation, and management of high blood pressure in adults. J Am Coll Cardiol. 2017;71:e127–248. http://www.onlinejacc.org/content/71/19/e127?_ga=2.35459041.138023780.1570631377-352956434.1570631377

HTN treatment include thiazide diuretics, beta blockers, ACEIs, and CCBs, particularly non-DHP. In the presence of chronic renal disease, as manifested by MA, recommendations also include the use of an ACEI or, alternatively, an ARB if an ACEI is not tolerated.

HYPERTENSION IN THE OLDER ADULT

The prevalence of HTN increases in older populations. According to the National Health Interview Survey (NHIS, United States, 2018), the prevalence of HTN increases from about 9% among those 18 to 44 years old, to 55% among those 65 to 74 years old, and 61% for those 75 years old and older. In the elderly, HTN is characterized by an elevated systolic BP with normal or low diastolic BP, which is a consequence of age-associated stiffening of the large arteries.

The clinical presentation of and diagnostic testing for HTN in the older adult is unchanged from that of the younger adult. The therapeutic target BP goal in the elderly is less than 150/90 mm Hg in persons 60 years and older (JNC-8) or less than 130 mm Hg systolic BP in adults 65 years old and older (ACC/AHA). According to ACC/AHA, the intensity of BP lowering and choice of antihypertensive medications in the elderly should take into consideration various factors, including burden of comorbidity, life expectancy, clinical judgment, and patient preference.

Some major concerns with the use of BP medications include electrolyte disturbances, renal dysfunction, and excessive orthostatic BP decline. Postural hypotension, defined as a fall in BP of less than or equal to 20 mm Hg systolic, less than or equal to 10 mm Hg diastolic, or both within 3 minutes of standing upright, increases the risk of falls, syncope, and cardiovascular events in the elderly. Similar to younger adults, a combination of medications is often needed to control HTN in the elderly, and initiation with combination therapy should be considered if BP is greater than 20/10 mm Hg above goal. Many conditions provide compelling indications to use certain drugs in the elderly (Table 6-5).

CLINICAL CONCEPT

When considering BP medications, HCPs must be vigilant about treatment-related adverse effects in the older adult because of a high prevalence of cardiovascular and noncardiovascular comorbidities.

TABLE 6-5 Compelling Indications for Individual Drug Classes in Elderly Patients

	THIAZIDE DIURETIC	BETA-ADRENERGIC RECEPTOR ANTAGONIST (BETA BLOCKER)	ANGIOTENSIN-CONVERTING ENZYME INHIBITOR (ACEI)	ANGIOTENSIN RECEPTOR BLOCKER (ARB)	CALCIUM ANTAGONIST (CALCIUM CHANNEL BLOCKER)	ALDOSTERONE ANTAGONIST
Heart failure	√	√	√	√	√	√
Postmyocardial infarction		√	√	√		√
Coronary artery disease or high cardiovascular disease risk	√	√	√		√	
Diabetes	√	√	√	√	√	
Angina pectoris		√			√	
Aortopathy/aortic aneurysm	√	√	√		√	
Recurrent stroke prevention	√		√	√	√	

Source: Aronow WS, Fleg JL, Pepine CJ, et al. ACCF/AHA 2011 expert consensus document on hypertension in the elderly. J Am Coll Cardiol. 2011;57:2037–2114. http://www.medpage today.com/upload/2011/4/25/j.jacc.2011.01.008v1.pdf

HYPERTENSION EMERGENCY VERSUS HYPERTENSION URGENCY

A hypertensive emergency is characterized by a severe elevation in BP, exceeding 180/120 mm Hg, that is also associated with new or worsening TOD. These patients require immediate reduction in BP to prevent further TOD, including hypertensive encephalopathy, intracranial hemorrhage, acute ischemic stroke, acute MI, and acute renal failure, among others. In addition to BP measurement, physical examination should include an eye examination to identify the presence of new retinal hemorrhages or papilledema. The presence of jugular distension, crackles on auscultation, and peripheral edema can indicate HF. Electrolyte levels, blood urea nitrogen (BUN), and creatinine can be used to identify renal impairment, while a dipstick urinalysis can be used to detect hematuria and proteinuria. With evidence of new or worsening TOD, patients should be immediately admitted to the intensive care unit (ICU) and administered intravenous antihypertensive medication to reduce BP, though not necessarily to normal levels. The goal of treatment is to reduce mean arterial BP by no more than 25% within the first few minutes to an hour, then if stable, to attain a BP of 160/100 mm Hg within the next 2 to 6 hours, with a normal BP achieved within 24 to 48 hours.

Hypertensive urgency is defined as a severe BP elevation in a patient who is otherwise stable and without acute or impending change in TOD. Typically, these patients have a history of HTN and have discontinued or are nonadherent to antihypertensive medication. These patients do not need to be referred to emergency care or for hospitalization, but they should reinstitute or intensify their antihypertensive medications and schedule a follow-up visit. No in-office BP-lowering medications should be given.

Discussion Sources

Aronow WS, Fleg JL, Pepine CJ, et al. ACCF/AHA 2011 expert consensus document on hypertension in the elderly. *J Am Coll Cardiol.* 2011;57:2037–2114. http://www.medpagetoday.com/upload/2011/4/25/j.jacc.2011.01.008v1.pdf

Eckel RH, Jakicic JM, Ard JD, et al. 2013 AHA/ACC guideline on lifestyle management to reduce cardiovascular risk: a report of the American College of Cardiology/American Heart Association Task Force on Practice Guidelines. *Circulation.* 2014;63 (25 pt B):2960–2984.

Graham TP. Hypertension. In: Kellerman RD, Rakel DP, eds. *Conn's Current Therapy 2019.* Philadelphia, PA: Saunders Elsevier; 2019:118–124.

James PA, Oparil S, Carter BL, et al. 2014 Evidence-based guideline for the management of high blood pressure in adults: report from the panel members appointed to the Eighth Joint National Committee (JNC 8). *JAMA.* 2014;311(5):507–520. http://jama.jamanetwork.com/article.aspx?articleid=1791497

Recarti C, Unger T. Prevention of coronary artery disease: recent advances in the management of hypertension. *Curr Atheroscler Rep.* 2013;15:311.

Whelton PK, Carey RM, Aronow WS, et al. 2017 ACC/AHA guideline for the prevention, detection, evaluation, and management of high blood pressure in adults. *J Am Coll Cardiol.* 2017;71:e127–248. http://www.onlinejacc.org/content/71/19/e127?_ga=2.35459041.138023780.1570631377-352956434.1570631377

QUESTIONS

1. Which of the following would be expected to result in the greatest reduction in systolic BP (SBP) in a middle-aged man with HTN?

    A. initiating a DASH eating plan

    B. starting an exercise regimen involving 100 min/week of dynamic resistance

    C. weight reduction of 4 kg in an overweight individual

    D. limiting alcohol consumption to two drinks or less

2. Enhanced intake of which of the following is recommended to decrease BP?

    A. sodium

    B. iron

    C. calcium

    D. potassium

3. You examine a 38-year-old woman who has presented for an initial examination and Papanicolaou test. She has no complaint. Her BP is 154/98 mm Hg bilaterally, and her body mass index (BMI) is 31 kg/m². The rest of her physical examination is unremarkable. Your next best action is to:

    A. initiate antihypertensive therapy.

    B. arrange for at least two additional BP measurements during the next 2 weeks.

C. order blood urea nitrogen, creatinine, and potassium measurements and urinalysis.

D. advise her to reduce her sodium intake.

4. You see a 68-year-old woman as a patient who is transferring care into your practice. She has a 10-year history of HTN, diabetes mellitus, and hyperlipidemia. Current medications include HCTZ, glipizide, metformin, simvastatin, and daily low-dose aspirin. Today's BP reading is 158/92 mm Hg, and the rest of her history, examination, and laboratory testing are unremarkable. Documentation from her former HCP indicates that her BP has been consistently near this value for the past 12 months. Your next best action is to:

A. prescribe an ACEI.

B. have her return for a BP check in 1 week.

C. advise that her current therapy is adequate.

D. add therapy with an aldosterone antagonist.

5. You examine a 78-year-old woman with long-standing, poorly controlled HTN. When evaluating her for hypertensive TOD, you look for evidence of:

A. lipid abnormalities.

B. insulin resistance.

C. left ventricular hypertrophy.

D. clotting disorders.

6. Diagnostic testing for a patient with newly diagnosed primary HTN should include all of the following except:

A. fasting blood glucose.

B. uric acid.

C. creatinine.

D. potassium.

7. In the person with HTN, the nurse practitioner (NP) recommends all of the following to potentially reduce BP in a patient with a BMI of 30 kg/m² except:

A. 10-kg (22-lb) weight loss.

B. dietary sodium restriction to less than 1,500 mg per day.

C. regular aerobic physical activity, such as 30 to 40 minutes of brisk walking most days of the week.

D. consuming at least one to two servings of alcohol daily.

8 to 12. Match the anti-HTN medication with its appropriate class.

_____ 8. Amlodipine

_____ 9. Diltiazem

_____ 10. Trandolapril

_____ 11. Telmisartan

_____ 12. Pindolol

A. beta-adrenergic receptor antagonist

B. nondihydropyridine calcium channel blocker

C. dihydropyridine calcium channel blocker

D. angiotensin receptor antagonist

E. ACEI

13. You see a 38-year-old man of African ancestry with HTN who is currently being treated with thiazide-type diuretic. His current BP reading is 156/94 mm Hg, and he has no history of diabetes mellitus or CKD. Following current best evidence, you consider adding which of the following medications?

A. ACEI

B. ARB

C. beta-adrenergic receptor antagonist

D. CCB

14. Non-DHP CCBs are contraindicated in patients with:
   A. type 1 diabetes mellitus.
   B. a history of venous thromboembolism.
   C. severe left ventricular dysfunction.
   D. concomitant treatment with an ACEI.

15. In obtaining an office BP measurement, which of the following is most reflective of the best practice?
   A. The patient should sit in a chair with feet flat on the floor for at least 5 minutes before obtaining the reading.
   B. The BP cuff should not cover more than 50% of the upper arm.
   C. The patient should sit on the edge of the examination table without arm support to enhance reading accuracy.
   D. Obtaining the BP reading immediately after the patient walks into the examination room is recommended.

16. A BP elevation noted only at an office visit is commonly known as _____ HTN.
   A. provider-induced
   B. clinical
   C. white coat
   D. pseudo

17. The most important long-term goal of treating HTN is to:
   A. strive to reach recommended numeric BP measurement.
   B. avoid disease-related TOD.
   C. develop a plan of care with minimal adverse effects.
   D. treat concomitant health problems often noted in the person with this condition.

18. You initiate spironolactone therapy for a patient with HTN who is already receiving an ACEI as well as two other HTN medications. You advise the patient to return in 4 weeks to check which of the following laboratory parameters?
   A. sodium
   B. calcium
   C. potassium
   D. chloride

19. A 68-year-old woman presents with HTN and BP of 152 to 158/92 to 96 mm Hg documented over 2 months on three different occasions. ECG and creatinine are normal, and she has no proteinuria. Clinical findings include the following: BMI 26.4 kg/m^2; no S_3, S_4, or murmur; and point of maximal impulse at fifth intercostal space, midclavicular line. Which of the following represents the best intervention?
   A. Initiate therapy with metoprolol.
   B. Initiate therapy with chlorthalidone.
   C. Initiate therapy with methyldopa.
   D. Continue to monitor BP, and start drug therapy if evidence of TOD.

20. Which of the following can have a favorable effect on a comorbid condition in a person with HTN?
   A. chlorthalidone in gout
   B. propranolol with lower airway disease

C. aldosterone antagonist in HF

D. methyldopa in an older adult

21. According to JNC-8 and ACC/AHA guidelines, all of the following medications are first-line agents for use in a middle-aged white man without diabetes mellitus except:

A. lisinopril.

B. chlorthalidone.

C. metoprolol.

D. amlodipine.

22. You see a 59-year-old man with poorly controlled HTN. On physical examination, you note grade 1 hypertensive retinopathy. You anticipate all of the following will be present except:

A. patient report of acute visual change.

B. narrowing of the terminal retinal arterioles.

C. sharp optic disc borders.

D. absence of retinal hemorrhage.

23. According to JNC-8 and ACC/AHA, a 52-year-old well woman with a healthy BMI whose BP is consistently 114 to 118/72 to 76 mm Hg is considered to have:

A. normal BP.

B. HTN requiring therapy with a CCB.

C. HTN requiring therapy with a beta blocker.

D. HTN requiring therapy with a thiazide-type diuretic.

24. Which of the following is associated with the highest risk of ischemic heart disease?

A. presence of MA plus heavy alcohol intake

B. absence of MA plus use of a thiazolidinedione

C. absence of MA plus chronic physical inactivity

D. presence of MA plus cigarette smoking

25. When compared with patients of European ancestry, patients of African ancestry tend to have a reduced effect with monotherapy with all of the following BP medications except:

A. ACEIs.

B. ARBs.

C. CCBs.

D. beta blockers.

26. You see a 62-year-old man with HTN and asthma, currently being treated with low-dose HCTZ and low-dose losartan. His BP has been in the 162/88 mm Hg range, noted in office and in his home BP log. All of the following are appropriate next courses of action except:

A. increasing the dose of losartan.

B. adding a beta-adrenergic receptor antagonist.

C. adding a CCB.

D. increasing the dose of HCTZ.

27. Which of the following statements concerning postural hypotension in the elderly is false?

A. It increases the risk of falls and syncope.

B. It is characterized by a drop in BP when going from a standing to a sitting position.

C. It increases the risk of cardiovascular events.

D. It is associated with the use of vasodilating medications.

28 to 33. According to the American College of Cardiology Foundation/American Heart Association (ACCF/AHA) guidelines, when treating elderly patients with HTN, which of the following medications have a compelling indication for use in the following patient conditions? *(The medications listed can be used more than once. A given condition can have more than one medication indicated.)*

_____ **28.** HF

_____ **29.** Diabetes mellitus

_____ **30.** Angina pectoris

_____ **31.** Coronary artery disease

_____ **32.** Aortic aneurysm

_____ **33.** Recurrent stroke prevention

    A. thiazide diuretic

    B. beta blocker

    C. ACEI

    D. ARB

    E. aldosterone antagonist

    F. CCB

For answers and rationales, see end of chapter.

Acute Coronary Syndrome

Overview

ACS and angina pectoris, most often caused by atherosclerosis, result from an imbalance in the ability to supply the myocardium with sufficient oxygen to meet its metabolic demands. ACS includes an umbrella of cardiovascular conditions that include ST-segment elevation myocardial infarction (STEMI), non–ST-segment elevation myocardial infarction (NSTEMI), and unstable angina. Typically, STEMI is associated with transmural MI (full-thickness necrosis of the myocardium in the region of the MI), subsequent development of Q waves on the ECG, and total occlusion of a coronary artery. NSTEMI involves nontransmural MI, no Q-wave evolution of the ECG, and subtotal occlusion of the vessel. Certain clinical characteristics increase or decrease the likelihood of ACS (Table 6-6).

MI/ACS most commonly occurs when an atherosclerotic plaque ruptures, leading to the formation of an occlusive thrombus. Coronary artery spasm can also occur, adding to the vessel obstruction. A patient with suspected ACS needs to be assessed promptly and accurately because therapy to reinstitute vessel patency (e.g., thrombolysis, percutaneous angioplasty, stent placement, or coronary artery bypass grafting) should be initiated early in the process to limit myocardial damage.

Clinical Presentation

Men often have their first manifestation of CHD in the form of MI, whereas women initially present first with angina pectoris, which often leads to MI. Women younger than 60 years often have a presentation similar to that of men, however. Chest pain associated with ACS is typically associated with myocardial ischemia or MI and commonly described as substernal compression or crush; pressure; tightness; heaviness; cramping; aching sensation; unexplained indigestion; belching; epigastric pain; radiating pain to neck, jaw, shoulders, back, or one or both arms; and/or dyspnea, nausea/vomiting, and diaphoresis.

Women usually have onset of CHD at significantly older ages and are likely to present differently than men. Dyspnea is often an anginal equivalent in older women. In a study of 515 women with ACS, 95% reported new or different symptoms in weeks before the event, including unusual fatigue (70%), sleep disturbance (48%), shortness of breath (42%), indigestion (39%), and anxiety (35%). Symptoms experienced by the women during ACS included shortness of breath (58%), weakness (55%), unusual fatigue (43%), diaphoresis (39%), dizziness (39%), and chest pain or pressure (30%); 43% of the woman had no chest discomfort during the event.

CLINICAL CONCEPT

Atypical ACS presentation is often noted in both sexes when patients are older than 80 years, which can include confusion, dyspnea, and cognitive impairment, and less often, with the classic symptoms such as chest pain.

TABLE 6-6 Likelihood That Signs and Symptoms Represent Acute Coronary Syndrome

FEATURES	HIGH LIKELIHOOD: ANY OF THE FOLLOWING PRESENT	INTERMEDIATE LIKELIHOOD: ABSENCE OF HIGH-LIKELIHOOD FEATURES AND PRESENCE OF ANY OF THE FOLLOWING	LOW LIKELIHOOD: ABSENCE OF HIGH- OR INTERMEDIATE-LIKELIHOOD FEATURES BUT MANY HAVE THE FOLLOWING
History	Chest or left arm pain or discomfort as chief symptom producing documented angina	Chest or left arm pain or discomfort as chief symptom Age older than 70 years at onset Male sex Diabetes mellitus	Probable ischemic symptoms in absence of any intermediate-likelihood characteristics Recent cocaine use
Examination	Pulmonary edema New rales or crackles Transient mitral regurgitation murmur Hypotension	Extracardiac vascular disease	Chest discomfort reproduced by palpation
ECG findings	New or presumably new transient ST segment deviation (≥0.05 mV) or T wave inversion (≥0.2 mV) with symptoms	Fixed Q waves Abnormal ST segments or E waves not documented as new	T-wave flattening or inversion in leads with dominant R waves ECG
Cardiac markers	Elevated cTnT, cTnI, or CPK-MB	Normal	Normal

Source: McConaghy JR, Oza RS. Outpatient diagnosis of acute chest pain in adults. Am Fam Physician. 2013;87(3):177–182. https://www.aafp.org/afp/2013/0201/p177.html

The discomfort associated with an anginal episode is described with many terms—*pressure, pain, tightness, heaviness,* and *suffocation*. In stable angina, patterns of symptom provocation are usually predictable, with exertion often causing discomfort that is promptly relieved with rest, use of sublingual (tablet or spray) nitroglycerin, or both. Unstable angina is defined as a new onset of symptoms at rest or worsening symptoms with activities that did not previously provoke symptoms. The clinical presentation of unstable angina represents an emergency and should be handled accordingly.

S_4 is often heard with myocardial ischemia and poorly controlled angina pectoris or recurrent myocardial ischemia. This sound of poor myocardial relaxation (compliance) and diastolic dysfunction may potentially cause decreased cardiac output. The third heart sound (S_3) is that of poor myocardial contractility and systolic dysfunction and usually leads to decreased cardiac output; this abnormal heart sound is often heard in the presence of HF.

Diagnostic Testing

In approximately 75% of patients admitted to the hospital for MI/ACS, this condition is ruled out. At least 25% of all MIs are clinically silent, however, with few if any symptoms. To reduce unneeded hospitalization and to detect asymptomatic MI/ACS, diagnostic tests that are highly sensitive and specific for myocardial damage are needed. An ECG is typically the first test done to diagnose MI and is often performed by an emergency medical technician (EMT) while the patient is en route to the hospital in order to activate the cardiac team. This can be critical in reducing the arrival-to-catheterization time. Other tests may be used to determine the extent of heart damage caused by an MI or to determine whether symptoms are due to another cause. These tests include a chest x-ray, echocardiogram, nuclear scan, computed tomography (CT) angiogram, or coronary angiogram.

Select blood tests are also used to detect specific substances noted in the presence of heart damage induced by myocardial damage. Troponin is a regulatory protein of the myofibril with three major subtypes: C, I, and T. Subtypes I (cTnI) and T (cTnT) are released in the presence of myocardial damage. Both increase rapidly within the first 12 hours after MI; cTnT typically remains elevated for about 168 hours, and cTnI remains elevated for about 192 hours. cTnI is the more cardiac-specific measure and is sensitive for small-volume myocardial damage. cTnT levels can be elevated in chronic renal failure, muscle trauma, and rhabdomyolysis. cTnI is more sensitive and specific than ECG and creatine kinase myocardial band (CK-MB) in diagnosing unstable angina and non-Q-wave MI. In addition, cTnI results are available quickly through a rapid assay. Protracted elevation of cTnI after MI or unstable angina is a predictor of increased mortality. People with angina without documented MI have a significantly higher risk of death within 42 days if cTnI is persistently elevated. Newer, more sensitive troponin assays, such as high-sensitivity cardiac troponin T (hs-cTnT) allow identification of up to 80% of patients with acute MI within 2 to 3 hours of arrival to the emergency department (ED). The use of these tests is generally preferred over older assays, such as myoglobin or CK-MB. Other markers being studied to diagnose ACS and stratify patients for risk of MI or death include B-type (brain) natriuretic peptide (BNP) and N-terminal pro-BNP (NT-pro-BNP). A combination of these tests can be useful in predicting patient outcomes following ACS, though more research is needed.

Testing to support the angina diagnosis includes a resting 12-lead ECG (although this is normal in about 50% of individuals with the disease) and exercise tolerance or other form of stress testing, often with myocardial nuclear imaging. CT to document coronary artery calcification is another noninvasive test.

Treatment

Initial Therapy in Acute Coronary Syndrome

A patient who presents with ACS in the primary care setting represents a 911 emergency and should be immediately referred to the ED and transported by emergency medical services when available. The AHA periodically publishes guidelines for the management of patients with ST-segment elevation MI, unstable angina, and NSTEMI developed from consensus of nursing and medical experts and evidence-based health care. The AHA recommends the following therapy:

- Nitroglycerin via sublingual spray or tablet should be given, followed by parenteral nitroglycerin.
- Supplemental oxygen should be administered to patients with cyanosis or respiratory distress, and pulse oximetry or arterial blood gas determination should be done to confirm adequate arterial SaO_2 (greater than 90%).
- Adequate analgesia should be provided with intravenous morphine sulfate when symptoms are not immediately relieved by nitroglycerin or when pulmonary congestion or severe agitation or both are present.
- A beta blocker should be given if there are no contraindications. The first dose should be administered intravenously. An ACEI should be given if no contraindications exist.
- Aspirin (162 to 325 mg orally in a chewable, nonenteric form) should be given as soon as possible after hospital presentation or in the field and continued indefinitely in patients who can tolerate it, and a maintenance dose (81 mg) should be continued indefinitely. Other antiplatelet agents (i.e., $P2Y_{12}$ inhibitors such as clopidogrel [Plavix®]) can be used if aspirin allergy or intolerance is present or as adjunctive therapy.
- A history should be taken and a physical examination, 12-lead ECG, and cardiac marker tests should be performed promptly.

Reperfusion Therapy

With a diagnosis of ACS and ST-segment elevation, the patient should be evaluated for reperfusion; the examiner should look for ST-segment elevation greater than 1 mm in contiguous leads. The presence of these changes usually indicates acute coronary artery occlusion, usually from thrombosis.

These therapies have the best effect on clinical outcomes if used within 6 hours after onset of chest pain but may be helpful 7 to 12 hours or more after MI symptoms begin.

- Percutaneous coronary intervention (PCI) is recommended in the presence of STEMI and ischemic symptoms of less than 12 hours' duration. If fibrinolytic therapy is contraindicated, PCI should be performed in patients with STEMI and ischemic symptoms of less than 12 hours' duration, irrespective of any time delay in first medical contact. Following PCI, dual antiplatelet therapy (aspirin plus clopidogrel, prasugrel, or ticagrelor) should be given for at least 12 months.
- Thrombolysis usually involves heparin given for at least 48 hours to ensure continued vessel patency. Before giving a thrombolytic agent such as tissue plasminogen

CLINICAL CONCEPT

Clinically significant ST-segment elevation largely dictates reperfusion therapy with the use of thrombolytic therapy, primary percutaneous transluminal coronary angioplasty, or other revascularization options.

activator or streptokinase, the prescriber must be aware of absolute and relative contraindications to thrombolytic therapy. Absolute contraindications include any prior intracranial hemorrhage, known structural cerebral vascular lesion (e.g., arteriovenous malformation), known malignant intracranial neoplasm (primary or metastatic), ischemic stroke within 3 months *except* acute ischemic stroke within 4.5 hours, suspected aortic dissection, active bleeding or bleeding diathesis (excluding menses), significant closed-head or facial trauma within 3 months, intracranial or intraspinal surgery within 2 months, severe uncontrolled HTN (unresponsive to emergency therapy), and for streptokinase, prior treatment within the previous 6 months.

If left bundle branch block is evident on ECG and the clinical scenario is consistent with acute MI, standard acute MI care should be offered. Patients with a presentation suggestive of MI but without ST-segment changes should not receive thrombolysis. These patients should be hospitalized and placed on continuous ECG monitoring for rhythm disturbances; disturbances that are noted should be appropriately treated. Serial 12-lead ECGs should be obtained, and results should be correlated with clinical measures of myocardial necrosis, such as troponin. Aspirin therapy should be continued, and heparin use should be considered, particularly in the presence of a large anterior MI or left ventricular mural thrombus because of increased risk of embolic stroke.

Evaluation and Treatment After Acute Coronary Syndrome

Drug therapy after ACS includes beta blockers and aspirin. Beta blockers reduce myocardial workload through lowering heart rate, lowering stroke volume, and blunting catecholamine response. Most patients with ACS also have an indication for ACEI use. A CCB is often added if anginal symptoms occur two or more times per week and no contraindications to CCB use exist. A CCB can be useful to relieve ischemia, lower BP, or control the ventricular response rate to AF in patients who are intolerant of beta blockers. Caution, however, is advised for use in patients with left ventricular systolic dysfunction. Dihydropyridine CCBs (e.g., nifedipine, amlodipine) tend to be more potent vasodilators than nondihydropyridines (e.g., verapamil, diltiazem), whereas the latter tend to have more marked inotropic effects. Sustained-effect nitroglycerin via the oral or topical route (patch or ointment) can be added, particularly if nocturnal symptoms are present. Nitroglycerin via sublingual tablet or spray should be prescribed with advice on its use for acute symptoms and education to monitor frequency of use to detect patterns of anginal triggers and disease instability. Use of nitrates enhances myocardial perfusion through peripheral and central vasodilation.

> **CLINICAL CONCEPT**
>
> An exercise tolerance test can be routinely performed for patients at high risk to check the effectiveness of procedures done to improve coronary circulation and can predict the risk of future cardiovascular events, such as an MI.

Before hospital discharge, ACS patients should undergo standard exercise testing to assess functional capacity, efficacy of current medical regimen, and risk stratification for subsequent cardiac events. Beta blocker and ACEI therapy should be continued indefinitely. Dual antiplatelet therapy (DAPT) with low-dose aspirin plus a $P2Y_{12}$ inhibitor (e.g., clopidogrel) should be considered for up to 12 months for patients treated initially with either early invasive or ischemia-guided therapy. For those treated with a stent implantation, DAPT should be continued for at least 12 months. Pharmacological intervention (i.e., statin therapy) is likely to be needed in patients with considerable cardiovascular risk, including those with HTN, diabetes mellitus, and vascular disease. This ongoing care is in keeping with an overall plan to reduce or eliminate all cardiac risk factors, including inactivity, smoking, and obesity.

Coronary angiography should be considered if exercise tolerance is poor, significant abnormality is noted on resting or exercise ECG or myocardial imaging, or symptoms become less stable.

Discussion Sources

American College of Cardiology/American Heart Association (ACC/AHA) Task Force on Practice Guidelines. 2014 ACC/AHA/AATS/PCNA/SCAI/STS Focused Update of the Guideline for the Diagnosis and Management of Patients with Stable Ischemic Heart Disease. *J Am Coll Cardiol.* 2014;64(18). doi:10.1016/j.jacc.2014.07.017. http://www.onlinejacc.org/content/64/18/1929

American College of Cardiology/American Heart Association (ACC/AHA) Task Force on Practice Guidelines. 2012 ACCF/AHA Focused Update of the Guideline for the Management of Patients with Unstable Angina/Non–ST-Elevation Myocardial Infarction (Updating the 2007 Guideline and Replacing the 2011 Focused Update). *Circulation.* 2012;126:875–910. http://content.onlinejacc.org/article.aspx?articleid=1217906

American College of Cardiology/American Heart Association (ACC/AHA) Task Force on Practice Guidelines. 2013 ACCF/AHA Guideline for the Management of ST-Elevation Myocardial Infarction. *J Am Coll Cardiol.* 2013;61:e78–e140. http://content.onlinejacc.org/article.aspx?articleid=1486115

American College of Cardiology/American Heart Association (ACC/AHA) Task Force on Practice Guidelines. 2014 AHA/ ACC Guideline for the Management of Patients with Non-ST-Elevation Acute Coronary Syndromes. *J Am Coll Cardiol.* 2014;64:e139–e228. http://www.onlinejacc.org/content/accj/64/24/e139.full.pdf?_ga=2.195787308.1257041792.1571236610 -471937103.1571236610

American College of Cardiology/American Heart Association (ACC/AHA) Task Force on Practice Guidelines. 2016 ACC/AHA Guideline Focused Update on Duration of Dual Antiplatelet Therapy in Patients with Coronary Artery Disease. *J Am Coll Cardiol.* 2016;68:1082–1115. http://www.onlinejacc.org/content/68/10/1082?_ga=2.233904670.1257041792.1571236610 -471937103.1571236610

Held EP, Chugh SS. Warning signs of impending acute cardiac events. *Circulation.* 2018;138:1617–1619.

McSweeney J, Cody M, O'Sullivan P, Elberson K, Moser D, Garvin B. Women's early warning symptoms of acute myocardial infarction. *Circulation.* 2003;108:2619–2623.

QUESTIONS

34. Causes of unstable angina include all of the following except:

A. left ventricular hypertrophy.

B. vasoconstriction.

C. nonocclusive thrombus.

D. inflammation or infection.

35. Which of the following is most consistent with a person presenting with unstable angina?

A. a 5-minute episode of chest tightness brought on by stair climbing and relieved by rest

B. a severe, searing pain that penetrates the chest and lasts about 30 seconds

C. chest pressure lasting 20 minutes that occurs at rest

D. "heartburn" relieved by position change

36. The initial manifestation of CHD in men is most commonly:

A. unstable angina.

B. MI.

C. intracranial hemorrhage.

D. stable angina.

37. In assessing a 62-year-old woman with or at risk for ACS, the NP considers that the patient will likely present:

A. in a manner similar to that of a man with equivalent disease.

B. at the same age as a man with similar health problems.

C. more commonly with angina and less commonly with acute MI.

D. with confusion and cognitive impairment.

38. Rank the following signs and symptoms in the order of most common to least common in a 60-year-old woman in the time preceding an ACS event.

A. dyspnea

B. indigestion

C. sleep disturbance

D. unusual fatigue

39. The cardiac finding most commonly associated with unstable angina is:

A. physiological split S_2.

B. S_4.

C. opening snap.

D. summation gallop.

40. Which of the following changes on the 12-lead ECG do you expect to find in a patient with ACS?

A. flattened T wave

B. R wave larger than 25 mm

C. ST-segment deviation (greater than 0.05 mV)

D. fixed Q wave

41. Beta-adrenergic antagonists are used in ACS therapy because of their ability to:

A. reverse obstruction-fixed vessel lesions.

B. reduce myocardial oxygen demand.

C. enhance myocardial vessel tone.

D. stabilize arterial volume.

42. Nitrates are used in ACS therapy because of their ability to:

A. reverse fixed vessel obstruction.

B. reduce myocardial oxygen demand.

C. cause vasodilation.

D. stabilize cardiac rhythm.

43. Which of the following is most consistent with a 50-year-old man presenting with acute MI?

A. a 2-minute episode of chest tightness brought on by stair climbing

B. a severe, localized pain that penetrates the chest and lasts about 3 hours

C. chest pressure lasting 20 minutes that occurs at rest

D. retrosternal diffuse pain for 30 minutes accompanied by diaphoresis

44 to 47. Match the clinical syndrome with its pathophysiological characteristic.

_____ **44.** Unstable angina

_____ **45.** Stable angina

_____ **46.** NSTEMI

_____ **47.** STEMI

A. new onset of chest pain and discomfort at rest or worsening of symptoms with activities that previously did not provoke symptoms

B. predictable onset of chest pain or discomfort, usually with physical exertion

C. results from full-thickness (transmural) necrosis of the myocardium and total occlusion of coronary artery

D. results from severe coronary artery narrowing, transient occlusion, or microembolization of thrombus and/or atheromatous material

48. Which of the following changes on the 12-lead ECG would you expect to find in a patient with history of acute transmural MI 6 months ago?

A. 2-mm ST-segment elevation

B. R wave larger than 25 mm

C. T-wave inversion

D. deep Q waves

49. Which of the following changes on the 12-lead ECG would you expect to find in a patient with myocardial ischemia?

A. 2-mm ST-segment elevation

B. S wave larger than 10 mm

C. T-wave inversion

D. deep Q waves

50. The ECG of a 57-year-old man who presents in the ED complaining of chest pain and shortness of breath lasting over 20 minutes is shown.

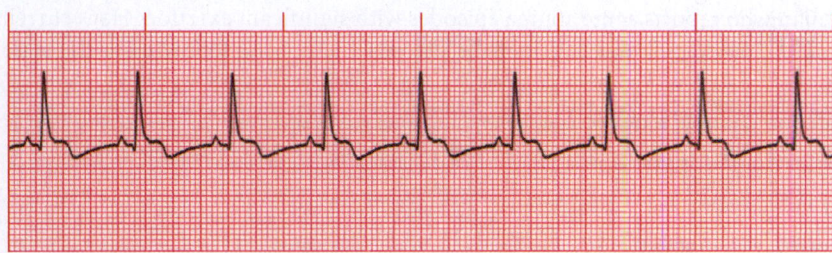

Jones SA. *ECG Notes: Interpretation and Management Guide.* 3rd ed. Philadelphia, PA: F.A. Davis; 2016.

This most likely demonstrates:

A. a normal ECG reading.

B. NSTEMI.

C. STEMI.

D. AF.

51. The ECG of a 72-year-old woman with a history of MI is shown.

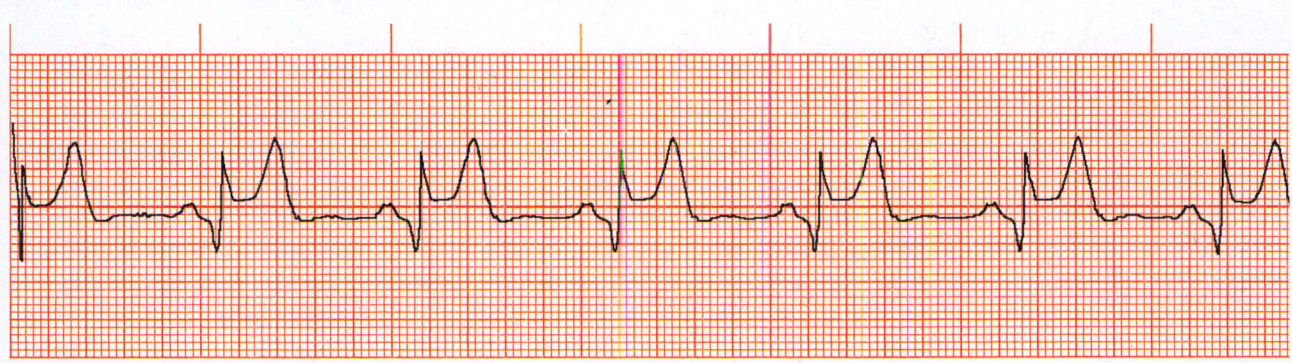

Geiter HB Jr. *E-Z ECG Rhythm Interpretation.* Philadelphia, PA: F.A. Davis; 2007.

Transmural injury in this patient is best demonstrated by the presence of:

A. U waves.

B. pathological Q waves.

C. low QRS voltage.

D. ST-segment depression.

52. Thrombolytic therapy is indicated in patients with chest pain and ECG changes such as:

A. 1-mm ST-segment depression in leads V1 and V3.

B. physiological Q waves in leads aVF, V5, and V6.

C. 3-mm ST-segment elevation in leads V1 to V4.

D. T-wave inversion in leads aVL and aVR.

53. An abnormality of which of the following is the most sensitive marker for myocardial damage?

A. aspartate aminotransferase

B. creatine phosphokinase (CPK)

C. troponin I (cTnI)

D. lactate dehydrogenase

54. All of the following should be prescribed as part of therapy in ACS except:

A. aspirin.

B. metoprolol.

    C. lisinopril.

    D. nisoldipine.

55. You see a 54-year-old man who reports acute angina episodes with significant exertion. He is currently taking a beta blocker and clopidogrel. You consider the use of which of the following at the start of anginal symptoms?

    A. an oral dose of a calcium channel blocker

    B. a dose of nitroglycerin via oral spray

    C. an extra dose of the beta blocker

    D. a sustained-effect nitroglycerin patch

56. Which of the following is an absolute contraindication to the use of thrombolytic therapy?

    A. history of hemorrhagic stroke

    B. BP of 160/100 mm Hg or greater at presentation

    C. current use of warfarin

    D. active peptic ulcer disease

57. For a patient with a history of MI and who demonstrates intolerance to aspirin, an acceptable alternative antiplatelet medication is:

    A. ibuprofen.

    B. clopidogrel.

    C. warfarin.

    D. rivaroxaban.

58. Routine use of the treadmill exercise tolerance test is most appropriate for:

    A. a healthy 34-year-old woman.

    B. a 56-year-old man following two-vessel stenting to establish activity tolerance.

    C. an 84-year-old man with stable angina who uses a walker.

    D. a 52-year-old woman with dyslipidemia and no history of ACS.

59. According to the recommendations of the ACC/AHA, the recommended first-line lipid-lowering therapy for a patient with elevated ASCVD risk is:

    A. niacin.

    B. statin.

    C. fish oil.

    D. fibrate.

60. Which of the following is least likely to be reported in ACS?

    A. newly noted pulmonary crackles

    B. transient mitral regurgitation murmur

    C. hypotension

    D. pain reproduced with palpation

For answers and rationales, see end of chapter.

Heart Failure

Overview

HF occurs as a result of altered cardiac function that leads to inadequate cardiac output and a resulting inability to meet the oxygen and metabolic demands of the body. This can be a consequence of any structural or functional impairment of ventricular filling or ejection of blood.

Hypertensive heart disease and atherosclerosis are the leading causes of HF. Less common HF triggers in the adult at risk for the condition include pneumonia (as a result of increased right-sided heart workload), anemia (because of the resulting decreased oxygen-carrying capability of the blood), and increased sodium intake (because of the resultant increase in circulating volume).

Patients with HF can be divided into those with reduced left ventricular ejection fraction (HFrEF) and those with preserved ejection fraction (HFpEF). HFrEF is generally defined as a diagnosis of HF with an ejection fraction 40% or less (healthy individuals typically have a left ventricular ejection fraction of 50% to 75%). The most common cause of HFrEF is ACS with antecedent MI, though several other risk factors can contribute to the condition. About half of patients with HF have preserved ejection fraction (typically defined as greater than 50%, with those in the 40% to 50% range belonging to an intermediate group). HTN is the most common cause of HFpEF, though other risk factors can include obesity, coronary artery disease, diabetes mellitus, AF, and hyperlipidemia. HFpEF is more common in women and with increasing age.

> **CLINICAL CONCEPT**
> The trajectory of HF is characterized by the baseline problems with periods of HF exacerbation, with worsening signs and symptoms.

Clinical Presentation

A careful patient history and physical examination are the cornerstones in the assessment of a patient with HF. A patient history can provide clues as to the cause of HF, while the physical examination can assess the severity of disease.

Clinical presentation of stable HF typically includes dyspnea on exertion, unexplained fatigue, and lower extremity edema. The clinical presentation of acute exacerbation of HF, one of the most common reasons for acute care hospital admission, includes unexplained weight gain and worsening dyspnea from baseline. The degree of dyspnea can occur in a wide spectrum range, increasing in severity from exertional dyspnea (shortness of breath with exercise), to orthopnea (shortness of breath that typically develops quickly when the individual is recumbent and is relieved with elevation of the head), paroxysmal nocturnal dyspnea (shortness of breath that occurs at night, characterized by a sudden awakening after a couple of hours of sleep, with a feeling of severe anxiety, breathlessness, and suffocation), and dyspnea at rest to eventual acute pulmonary edema. Additional reported history in HF often includes nocturia, worsening fatigue, and weakness. Except for the mildest cases, crackles heard over the lung bases are characteristic; in severe cases, there is wheezing and expectoration of frothy, blood-tinged sputum. S_3 is usually noted, typically disappearing on resolution of the acute event. Additional findings usually include tachycardia, diaphoresis, pallor, and peripheral cyanosis with pallor. Although edema is considered a classic finding in HF, a substantial gain of extracellular fluid volume (i.e., a minimum of 5 L in adults) must occur before peripheral edema is manifested. As a result of liver engorgement from elevated right-sided heart pressures, hepatojugular reflux, hepatic engorgement, and tenderness are typically noted. The point of maximal impulse (PMI) is normally at the fifth intercostal space, midclavicular line. This shifts laterally and perhaps over more than one intercostal space in the presence of dilated cardiomyopathy and its resultant increase in cardiac size.

Patient history and symptom presentation are usually not sufficient to differentiate between HFrEF and HFpEF, as both can present similarly and will depend on the severity of disease. Patients with HF are often assigned a classification of heart disease from either the ACCF/AHA (stages A through D) or the New York Heart Association (NYHA I to IV). The ACCF/AHA stages of HF emphasize development and progression of disease, whereas the NYHA classes focus on exercise capacity and symptomatic status of the disease (Table 6-7). In treating an acute HF exacerbation, a patient often is initially consistent with a higher classification category (NYHA III or IV). After treatment, the assignment of a lower category (NYHA I or II) is likely noted and should be a clinical goal. In the primary care setting, patients in ACCF/AHA stage A or B are generally managed by treating underlying risk factors and comorbidities along with guideline-directed medical therapy. The goal is to cease or slow progression of disease. Patients who reach stage B HF require expert consultation with cardiology, while those at stage C or D are co-managed with cardiology specialists.

Diagnostic Testing

Laboratory testing in HF usually includes evaluation to rule in or rule out potential underlying causes (e.g., anemia, infection, renal insufficiency, or others) and should include CBC, urinalysis, serum electrolytes, BUN, serum creatinine, glucose, fasting lipid profile, liver function tests, and TSH. BNP is an amino acid structure common to all natriuretic peptides. The cardiac ventricles are the major source of plasma BNP; the amount in circulation is in proportion to ventricular volume expansion and pressure overload.

TABLE 6-7 Comparison of Heart Failure Classification Criteria for ACCF/AHA and NYHA

ACCF/AHA STAGES OF HEART FAILURE (HF)	NYHA FUNCTIONAL CLASSIFICATION
A At high risk for HF but without structural heart disease or symptoms of HF	I. No limitation of physical activity. Ordinary physical activity does not cause symptoms of HF.
B Structural heart disease but without signs or symptoms of HF	II. Slight limitation of physical activity. Comfortable at rest, but ordinary physical activity results in symptoms of HF.
C Structural heart disease with prior or current symptoms of HF	III. Marked limitation of physical activity. Comfortable at rest, but less than ordinary activity causes symptoms of HF.
D Refractory HF requiring specialized interventions	IV. Unable to carry on any physical activity without symptoms of HF, or symptoms of HF at rest.

Source: Yancy CW, Jessup M, Bozkurt B, et al. 2013 ACCF/AHA guideline for the management of heart failure: a report of the American College of Cardiology Foundation/American Heart Association Task Force on Practice Guidelines. Circulation. 2013;128:e240–e327. http://circ.ahajournals.org/content/128/16/e240.extract

As part of the evaluation of a patient with dyspnea and suspected HF, an elevated BNP or N-terminal pro-BNP level helps to support the diagnosis. The increased circulating volume found in HF can occasionally lead to evidence of hemodilution on hemogram; this corrects as circulating volume is normalized.

ECG helps to identify the presence of left atrial enlargement, left ventricular hypertrophy, and dysrhythmias often noted in HF but not specific to the diagnosis. ECG changes consistent with acute myocardial ischemia or MI as the cause of HF can also be revealed.

Findings on chest radiograph in HF include cardiomegaly and alveolar edema with pleural effusions and bilateral infiltrates in a butterfly pattern. Additional findings are loss of sharp definition of pulmonary vasculature; haziness of hilar shadows; and thickening of interlobular septa, also known as Kerley B lines. As part of the evaluation of heart valve function and competency, an echocardiogram is usually obtained. Radionuclide evaluation of left ventricular function provides helpful information on global heart function. Angiography and further studies should be directed by clinical presentation and other health risks.

Treatment

In the primary care setting, management goals in HF include stopping or slowing the progression of disease by addressing risk factors.

For those with stage B HF (structural heart disease but without symptoms), risk reduction along with pharmacotherapy should be initiated. In some cases, surgical intervention such as revascularization or valvular surgery or an implantable cardioverter-defibrillator may be considered. It is important to note that clinical trials have primarily focused on treatment of HFrEF, and so little is known about optimal management of HFpEF. In general, patients with HFpEF are treated for underlying risk factors and comorbidities as well as pharmacotherapy similar to HFrEF. Lifestyle modifications are also an important part of HFpEF treatment, including low-sodium diet, restricted fluid intake, daily weight measurement, exercise, and weight loss when appropriate.

The goal of HF pharmacotherapy is threefold: reduction of preload, reduction of systemic vascular resistance (afterload reduction), and inhibition of the renin and sympathetic nervous system. Because ACEIs and ARBs cause central and peripheral vasodilation, these medications result in a reduction in cardiac workload and improvement in cardiac output. Although ACEIs and ARBs are the cornerstone of HF therapy, their use can be associated with adverse effects. Most common is hypotension, particularly when one of these agents is prescribed for a person who is currently taking a diuretic or vasodilator. To avoid hypotension, ACEI or ARB therapy should

CLINICAL CONCEPT

For those with stage A HF (high risk of HF but without structural heart disease or symptoms), interventions include treating HTN and hyperlipidemia, encouraging smoking cessation and regular exercise, and discouraging alcohol intake or illicit drug use.

be started at low dosages and increased slowly to achieve a therapeutic response. Renal insufficiency can be precipitated by ACEI or ARB therapy; this usually occurs only in the presence of renal artery stenosis or underlying renal disease. Hyperkalemia with ACEI or ARB use is usually seen only with concurrent use of a potassium-sparing diuretic/aldosterone antagonist, such as spironolactone (Aldactone®); in advancing renal disease; or in a poor hydration state, including overly aggressive diuretic use.

Beta-adrenergic blockers are used to inhibit chronotropic and inotropic responses to beta-adrenergic stimulation; the use of an alpha/beta blocker such as carvedilol (Coreg®) can provide the additional benefit of a vasodilating effect through its action blockade at the alpha receptors. Long-term beta-adrenergic antagonist (beta blocker) use has been shown to improve cardiac function, to reduce myocardial ischemia, to decrease myocardial oxygen consumption, and possibly to reduce the incidence of sudden cardiac death. This drug class is underused in HF therapy.

Additional medications are used to treat HF symptoms, such as diuretics, angiotensin receptor-neprilysin inhibitors (ARNIs), and/or a sinoatrial node modulator (ivabradine). Diuretics assist with circulating volume and preload reduction, with the goal of a careful balance. Unless contraindicated, a potassium-sparing diuretic such as spironolactone should be used because of its neurohumoral effects, allowing sodium excretion and enhanced vasodilation. These effects are achieved by the drug's ability to bind competitively at receptors found in aldosterone-dependent sodium-potassium exchange sites in the renal tubule. The use of ivabradine in addition to recommended therapy in patients with stage C HF has been shown to reduce hospitalization. For those with refractory HF (stage D), in addition to previously mentioned interventions, other options can include heart transplantation, placement of a left ventricular assist device, or pulmonary catheterization.

> **CLINICAL CONCEPT**
>
> Because digoxin is a medication with narrow therapeutic index and with significant drug-drug interactions and a potential proarrhythmic effect, clinical vigilance is needed with its use.

Digoxin, an older medication less frequently used in HF therapy, has a positive inotropic effect and slows conduction through the atrioventricular node. A prolongation of the PR interval and cupping of the ST segment are typically seen in ECGs of patients taking a therapeutic dose of digoxin.

Drugs that interact with digoxin include amiodarone, diltiazem, select macrolides (clarithromycin and erythromycin), oral (but not topical) azole antifungals, cyclosporine, and verapamil. Drugs that can cause potassium depletion, such as many diuretics, can also increase the risk of digoxin toxicity. In digoxin toxicity, numerous cardiac effects can be seen; atrioventricular block is the most common, whereas anorexia is the most commonly reported by patients. Visual changes are rarely reported. Digoxin use is associated with reduced hospital admissions along with improved symptoms of HF, quality of life, and exercise tolerance in patients with mild to moderate HF. Long-term use of digoxin in patients with more severe HF (NYHA II or III) has been shown to have no effect on mortality but can reduce hospitalizations.

For those with AF, an antithrombotic is recommended to reduce the risk of thromboembolic events including stroke. Warfarin (Coumadin®) remains commonly used, though this agent has a narrow therapeutic index. Regular monitoring of the international normalized ratio level is needed to ensure a safe and effective dose is utilized (see Table 11-5 for warfarin dosing strategies). Patients should also be well informed of potential drug-drug and drug-food interactions. Additional antithrombotics include direct factor Xa inhibitors (e.g., rivaroxaban [Xarelto®], apixaban [Eliquis®]) and direct thrombin inhibitors (e.g., dabigatran [Pradaxa®]). These agents provide more convenient dosing compared with warfarin and do not require regular monitoring, though these are costlier options and associated with adverse effects, namely increased bleeding risk. Dabigatran in particular should be used with caution in patients greater than or equal to 75 years because of increased risk of bleeding. The availability of reversal agents should also be considered when initiating long-term therapy with antithrombotics.

Discussion Sources

Dumitru I. Heart failure. Medscape. http://emedicine.medscape.com/article/163062-overview

Yancy CW, Jessup M, Bozkurt B, et al. 2017 ACC/AHA/HFSA focused update of the 2013 ACCF/AHA guideline for management of heart failure. *J Am Coll Cardiol.* 2017;70:776–803. http://www.onlinejacc.org/content/accj/70/6/776.full.pdf?_ga=2.149459766 .1255144026.1571407591-2136470166.1571407591

QUESTIONS

61. HF pathophysiology is characterized by:

    A. impaired atrial filling and ejection of blood.

    B. incomplete closure of tricuspid valve.

    C. near normal ventricular function.

    D. inadequate cardiac output to meet oxygen and metabolic demands of the body.

62. A leading cause of HF is:

    A. hypertensive heart disease.

    B. AF.

    C. pulmonary embolism.

    D. type 2 diabetes.

63 to 65. Match each of the following conditions with its mechanism for contributing to HF exacerbation:

_____ **63.** Pneumonia

_____ **64.** Anemia

_____ **65.** High sodium intake

    A. increase in circulating volume of blood

    B. increased right-sided heart workload

    C. decreased oxygen-carrying capacity of blood

66. The condition of a sudden shortness of breath that usually occurs after 2 to 3 hours of sleep and leads to sudden awakening followed by a feeling of severe anxiety and breathlessness is known as:

    A. dyspnea.

    B. orthopnea.

    C. resting dyspnea.

    D. paroxysmal nocturnal dyspnea.

67. You examine an 82-year-old woman who has a history of HF. She is in the office because of increasing shortness of breath in the last 2 days. When auscultating her heart, you note tachycardia with a rate of 104 beats per minute and a single extra heart sound early in diastole. This sound most likely represents:

    A. summation gallop.

    B. S_3.

    C. opening snap.

    D. S_4.

68. You examine a 65-year-old man with dilated cardiomyopathy and HF. On examination, you expect to find all of the following except:

    A. jugular venous distention.

    B. tenderness on right upper-abdominal quadrant palpation.

    C. point of maximal impulse at the fifth intercostal space, midclavicular line.

    D. peripheral edema.

69. In patients with HF, the point of maximum impulse usually:

    A. remains unchanged near the fourth intercostal space.

    B. remains unchanged near the fifth intercostal space.

    C. shifts lower on the midclavicular line.

    D. shifts laterally by one or more intercostal spaces.

70 to 72. Match the term with the correct impact on the heart.

_____ **70.** Inotropic

_____ **71.** Chronotropic

_____ 72. Dromotropic

    A. cardiac rate

    B. cardiac conduction

    C. force of the cardiac contraction

73. The rationale for using beta blocker therapy in treating a patient with HF is to:

    A. increase myocardial contractility.

    B. reduce the effects of circulating catecholamines.

    C. relieve concomitant angina.

    D. stabilize cardiac rhythm.

74. An ECG finding in a patient who is taking digoxin in a therapeutic dose typically includes:

    A. shortened PR interval.

    B. slightly depressed, cupped ST segments.

    C. widened QRS complex.

    D. tall T waves.

75. A potential adverse effect of ACEI when used with spironolactone therapy is:

    A. HTN.

    B. hyperkalemia.

    C. renal insufficiency.

    D. proteinuria.

76. ECG findings in a patient with digoxin toxicity would most likely include:

    A. atrioventricular heart block.

    B. T-wave inversion.

    C. sinus tachycardia.

    D. pointed P waves.

77. Symptoms of digoxin toxicity as reported by patients are most likely to include:

    A. anorexia.

    B. disturbance in color perception.

    C. blurred vision.

    D. constipation.

78. Which of the following medications is an aldosterone antagonist?

    A. clonidine

    B. spironolactone

    C. hydrochlorothiazide

    D. furosemide

79. Which of the following best describes orthopnea?

    A. shortness of breath with exercise

    B. dyspnea that develops when the individual is recumbent and is relieved with elevation of the head

    C. shortness of breath that occurs at night, characterized by a sudden awakening after a couple of hours of sleep, with a feeling of severe anxiety, breathlessness, and suffocation

    D. dyspnea at rest

80. Which of the following is unlikely to be noted in the person experiencing HF?

    A. elevated serum BNP

    B. Kerley B lines noted on chest x-ray

    C. left ventricular hypertrophy on ECG

    D. evidence of hemoconcentration on hemogram

81. Which of the following medications is an alpha-/beta-adrenergic antagonist?

    A. atenolol

    B. metoprolol

    C. propranolol

    D. carvedilol

82. The risk for digoxin toxicity increases with concomitant use of all of the following medications except:

    A. amiodarone.

    B. clarithromycin.

    C. cyclosporine.

    D. levofloxacin.

83. During a routine physical for a 64-year-old man, the following ECG is revealed:

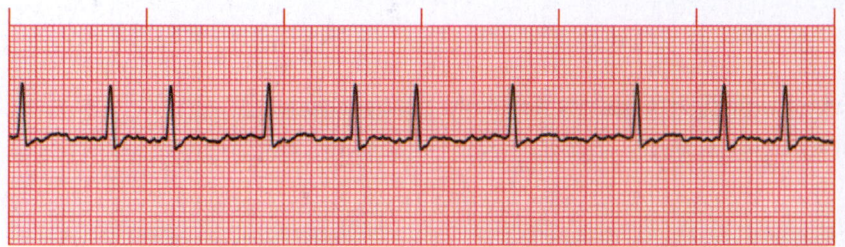

Jones, SA. *ECG Notes: Interpretation and Management Guide.* 3rd ed. Philadelphia, PA: F.A. Davis; 2016.

He has no complaints of dyspnea, syncope, or chest pain, and has no history of HTN. The most likely diagnosis is:

    A. TIA.

    B. dilated cardiomyopathy.

    C. NSTEMI.

    D. AF.

84. Agents used for the prevention of thromboembolic events in a patient with atrial fibrillation include all of the following except:

    A. dabigatran.

    B. prasugrel.

    C. rivaroxaban.

    D. apixaban.

85. A risk factor for HFrEF can include:

    A. female gender.

    B. history of intracranial hemorrhage.

    C. prior MI.

    D. history of postural hypotension.

86. Risk factors for HFpEF include all of the following except:

    A. female gender.

    B. HTN.

    C. long-term corticosteroid use.

    D. older age.

87. Which of the following statements is false regarding presentation of HFrEF and HFpEF?

    A. Both conditions commonly present with dyspnea and fatigue.

    B. Among patients with stage B HF, those with HFpEF present with more severe symptoms compared to those with HFrEF.

    C. Differentiation between HFrEF and HFpEF requires further evaluation beyond patient history and physical examination.

    D. Patients with HFrEF and HFpEF will commonly have a history of HTN.

88. A key component in the initial management of HFpEF is:

    A. CCBs.

    B. thiazide diuretics.

    C. an implantable cardioverter-defibrillator.

    D. addressing risk factors and comorbidities.

89. First-line pharmacotherapy for HFrEF can include any of the following except:

    A. ACEI.

    B. ARB.

    C. aldosterone antagonist.

    D. beta blocker.

For answers and rationales, see end of chapter.

Disorders Revealed by the Cardiac Examination

Overview

A careful clinical examination, including assessment for abnormal heart sounds and murmurs, remains the mainstay of diagnosing many cardiac conditions. Indeed, the cardiac examination is the first step, as the clinician needs to provide information from this evaluation to guide the ordering of confirmatory diagnostic tests or whether such testing is not needed.

MURMURS AND ABNORMAL HEART SOUNDS

Overview

Heart murmurs are caused by the sounds produced from turbulent blood flow. Blood traveling through the chambers and great vessels is usually silent. When the flow is sufficient to generate turbulence in the wall of the heart or great vessel, a murmur occurs.

Murmurs are often benign; the examiner simply hears the blood flowing through the heart, but no cardiac structural abnormality exists. Certain cardiac structural problems, such as valvular and myocardial disorders, however, can contribute to the development of a murmur (Table 6-8).

Normal heart valves allow one-way, unimpeded, forward blood flow through the heart. The entire stroke output is able to pass freely during one phase of the cardiac cycle (diastole with the atrioventricular valves, systole with the others), and there is no backflow of blood. When a heart valve fails to open to its normal orifice, it is stenotic.

> **CLINICAL CONCEPT**
>
> When a heart valve fails to close appropriately, the valve is incompetent, causing regurgitation of blood to the previous chamber or vessel. Both of these events place a patient at significant risk for embolic disease.

TABLE 6-8 Assessment of Common Systolic Heart Murmurs in Adults

MURMUR	IMPORTANT CARDIAC EXAMINATION FINDINGS	ADDITIONAL FINDINGS	COMMENTS
Physiological (also known as innocent, functional)	Grade 1 to 3/6 early to midsystolic murmur heard best at left sternal border, but usually audible over precordium	No radiation beyond precordium. Softens or disappears with standing, increases in intensity with activity, fever, anemia; S_1, S_2 intact, normal PMI*	Etiology probably flows over aortic valve. May be heard in ~80% of thin adults if examined in soundproof room. Asymptomatic with no report of chest pain, heart failure symptoms, palpitations, syncope, activity intolerance
Aortic stenosis	Grade 1 to 4/6 harsh systolic murmur, usually crescendo-decrescendo pattern, heard best at second right intercostal space, apex, softens with standing	Radiates to carotids, may have diminished S_2, slow filling carotid pulse, narrow pulse pressure, loud S_4, heaving PMI. The greater the degree of stenosis, the later the peak of murmur	In younger adults, usually congenital bicuspid valve. In older adults, usually calcific, rheumatic in nature. Dizziness and syncope ominous signs, pointing to severely decreased cardiac output
Mitral regurgitation	Grade 1 to 4/6 high-pitched blowing systolic murmur, often extending beyond S_2. Sounds like long "haaa," "hooo." Heard best at right lower scapular border	Radiates to axilla, often with laterally displaced PMI. Decreased with standing, Valsalva maneuver. Increased by squat, hand grip	Found in ischemic heart disease, endocarditis, RHD. With RHD, often with other valve abnormalities (aortic stenosis, mitral stenosis, aortic regurgitation)
Mitral valve prolapse	Grade 1 to 3/6 late-systolic crescendo murmur with honking quality heard best at apex. Murmur follows midsystolic click	With Valsalva or standing, click moves forward into earlier systole, resulting in a longer sounding murmur. With hand grasp, squat, click moves back further into systole, resulting in a shorter murmur	Often seen with minor thoracic deformities such as pectus excavatum, straight back, and shallow anterior-posterior diameter. Chest pain is sometimes present, but there is a question as to whether mitral valve prolapse itself is cause

*PMI, point of maximal impulse; RHD, rheumatic heart disease.

During auscultation, the bell of the stethoscope is most helpful for detecting lower-pitched sounds, whereas the diaphragm is most helpful for higher-pitched sounds (Table 6-9). Systolic murmurs are graded on a 1 to 6 scale, from barely audible to audible with stethoscope off the chest. Grade 3 murmur is about as loud as S_1 or S_2, whereas grade 2 murmur is slightly softer; grade 1 murmur is difficult to hear. Grade 4 murmurs are usually accompanied by a thrill, or the feel of turbulent blood flow. Diastolic murmurs are usually graded on the same scale but abbreviated to grades 1 through 4 because these murmurs are not loud enough to reach grades 5 and 6.

Clinical Presentation

Any patient where an abnormality is revealed on cardiac examination should undergo a focused health history. The patient should be asked about major symptoms of heart disease including chest pain, HF symptoms, palpitations, syncope, and activity intolerance.

Physiological Murmurs

Physiological murmurs are heard in the absence of cardiac pathology. The term *physiological* implies that the reason for the murmur is something other than obstruction to flow and that the murmur is present with a normal gradient across the valve. This murmur is heard in 80% of thin adults or children if the cardiac examination is performed in a soundproof booth, and it is best heard at the left sternal border.

A physiological murmur occurs in early to midsystole, usually with a crescendo-decrescendo (louder then softer) quality, leaving the S_1 and S_2 heart sounds intact. In addition, an individual with a benign

TABLE 6-9 Heart Sounds

HEART SOUND	SIGNIFICANCE	COMMENT	HEARD BEST
S_1	Marks beginning of systole. Produced by events surrounding closure of mitral and tricuspid valve	Best heard at apex with the diaphragm	"**Lub** dub" heard nearly simultaneous with carotid upstroke
S_2	Marks end of systole. Produced by events surrounding closure of aortic and pulmonic valves	Best heard at base with diaphragm	"Lub **dub**" heard
Physiological split S_2	Widening of normal interval between aortic and pulmonic components of S_2. Caused by delay in pulmonic component	Heard best in pulmonic region	The split *in*creases on patient *in*spiration Found in most adults younger than 30 years old, fewer beyond this age Benign finding
Pathological split S_2	Fixed split—no change with inspiration Paradoxical split—narrows or closes with inspiration	Heard best in pulmonic region	Fixed split often found in uncorrected septal defect Paradoxical split often found in conditions that delay aortic closure, such as left bundle branch block Finding can resolve with treatment of underlying condition
Pathological S_3	Marker of ventricular overload, systolic dysfunction, or both	Heard in early diastole, can sound like it is "hooked on" to the back of S_2 Low pitch, best heard with bell, might miss with diaphragm	For diagnosis of heart failure, correlate with additional findings such as dyspnea, tachycardia, crackles Finding can resolve with treatment of underlying condition
S_4	Marker of poor diastolic function, most often found in poorly controlled hypertension or recurrent myocardial ischemia	Heard late in diastole, can sound like it is "hooked on" to the front of S_1 Sometimes called a presystolic sound Soft, low pitch (higher pitch than S_3), best heard with bell	Finding can resolve with treatment of underlying condition

systolic ejection murmur denies having cardiac symptoms and has an otherwise normal cardiac examination, including an appropriately located point of maximum impulse and full pulses.

Aortic Stenosis

Aortic stenosis (AS) is the inability of the aortic valves to open to an optimal orifice. The aortic valve normally opens to 3 cm²; AS usually does not cause significant symptoms until the valvular orifice is limited to 0.8 cm². The disease is characterized by a long symptom-free period with rapid clinical deterioration at the onset of symptoms, including dyspnea, syncope, chest pain, and HF. Low pulse pressure, the difference between the systolic and diastolic BP, is a characteristic of severe AS.

When AS is present in adults who are middle-aged and older, it is most often the acquired form. Risk factors for acquired AS include older age and previous rheumatic fever. In an older adult, the problem is usually calcification, leading to the inability of the valve to open to its normal orifice. Valvular changes in middle-aged adults without congenital AS are usually the sequelae of rheumatic fever and represent about 30% of valvular dysfunction seen in rheumatic heart disease.

AS is occasionally noted in children and younger adults and is usually caused by a congenital bicuspid (rather than tricuspid) valve or by a three-cusp valve with leaflet fusion. This congenital heart problem is most often found in boys and young men and is commonly accompanied by a history of excellent exercise tolerance. With higher-grade congenital AS, the health history can include becoming excessively short of breath with increased activity such as running. The physical examination is usually normal except for the associated cardiac findings.

Mitral Regurgitation

The heart murmur of mitral regurgitation (MR) arises from mitral valve incompetency or the inability of the mitral valve to close properly. This incompetency allows a retrograde flow from a high-pressure area (left ventricle) to an area of lower pressure (left atrium). MR is most often caused by the degeneration of the mitral valve, commonly by rheumatic fever, endocarditis, calcific annulus, rheumatic heart disease, ruptured chordae, or papillary muscle dysfunction. In MR resulting from rheumatic heart disease, there is usually some degree of mitral stenosis. After the person becomes symptomatic, the disease progresses in a downhill course leading to HF over the next 10 years.

Mitral Valve Prolapse

Mitral valve prolapse (MVP) is likely the most common valvular heart problem; it is present in perhaps 10% of the population. The degree of distress (chest pain, dyspnea) may depend in part on the degree of MR, although some studies have failed to reveal any difference in the rates of chest pain in patients with or without MVP. Potentially the greatest threat is the rupture of chordae, usually seen only in those with connective tissue disease, especially Marfan syndrome.

Most patients with MVP have a benign condition in which one of the valve leaflets is unusually long and buckles or prolapses into the left atrium, usually in midsystole. At that time, a click occurs that is followed by a short murmur caused by regurgitation of blood into the atrium. Cardiac output is usually uncompromised, and the event goes unnoticed by the patient; however, the clinician could detect this on examination.

One way of describing MVP variation from the norm is to inform the patient that one leaflet of the mitral valve is a bit longer than usual. The "holder" (valve orifice) is of average size, however. This discrepancy causes the valve to buckle a bit, just as a person's foot would if forced into a shoe that is one or two sizes too small. As a result, the heart makes an extra set of sounds (click and murmur) but is not diseased or damaged. MVP is often found in patients with minor thoracic deformities such as pectus excavatum, a dish-shaped concave area at T1, and scoliosis. The exact nature of this correlation of findings is not understood.

The second and much smaller group of patients with MVP has systolic displacement of one or both of the mitral leaflets into the left atrium alone with valve thickening and redundancy, usually accompanied by mild to moderate MR. This group typically has additional health problems, such as Marfan syndrome or other connective tissue disease. There is a risk of bacterial endocarditis in this group because structural cardiac abnormality is present.

Murmur of Hypertrophic Cardiomyopathy

Hypertrophic cardiomyopathy is a disease of the cardiac muscle. The ventricular septum is thick and asymmetrical, leading to potential blockage of the outflow tract. Patients often exhibit symptoms of cardiac outflow tract blockage with activity because the hypertrophic ventricular walls better approximate with the increased force of myocardial contraction associated with exercise. The presentation of hypertrophic cardiomyopathy can be sudden cardiac death. Idiopathic hypertrophic subaortic stenosis is a type of cardiomyopathy. A mutation in one of several genes can cause the condition. The mutation is inherited in an autosomal-dominant pattern, thus requiring only one copy of the mutant gene to cause the disorder. In most cases, an affected person has one parent with the condition. Patients with this disorder are usually young adults with a history of dyspnea with activity, but they are often asymptomatic. Chest pain and postexertion syncope are occasionally reported. Physical examination typically reveals a systolic murmur that gets louder with position change from supine to standing along with a loud S_4 heart sound.

Diagnostic Testing

Once a potentially pathological heart murmur is detected, an ECG is used to detect heart rhythm and structural problems including chamber hypertrophy. A transthoracic or transesophageal echocardiogram is used to create moving images of the heart to identify abnormal heart valves, such as those that are calcified or leaking, as well as other heart defects. A cardiac CT scan or magnetic resonance imaging (MRI) can also be used to visualize heart defects that cause the murmur; its use is typically limited to clinical situations in which the echocardiogram results require clarification. In hypertrophic cardiomyopathy, genetic testing is usually warranted. Specialty evaluation is usually required to confirm diagnosis of pathological cardiac murmurs and contribute to the treatment plan.

Treatment

Because no cardiac pathology is present with a physiological murmur, no endocarditis prophylaxis is needed, and there is no particular treatment required.

For mild AS in the asymptomatic child or young adult, treatment is not necessary, but ongoing monitoring is important to detect any change toward a moderate to severe level. This usually involves ECG, echocardiogram, exercise stress test, CT scan, and/or MRI, in consultation with cardiology referral. Surgical correction or replacement of the valve is often needed for moderate-to-severe AS.

Benign MVP is characterized by echocardiography findings that fail to reveal any abnormality, simply noting the valve buckling followed by a small-volume MR. If there are no cardiac complaints and the rest of the cardiac examination, including the ECG, is normal, no further evaluation is needed.

> **CLINICAL CONCEPT**
> Barring other health problems, patients with MVP usually have normal cardiac output and tolerate a program of aerobic activity.

This activity should be encouraged to promote health and well-being. When circulating volume is low, the degree of MVP is increased, which increases the intensity of the murmur. Maintaining a high level of fluid intake should be encouraged for patients with MVP. Treatment with a beta-adrenergic antagonist (beta blocker) is indicated only when symptomatic recurrent tachycardia or palpitations are an issue.

The murmur of MR is usually noted in the presence of significant cardiac disease. While there is no specific MR therapy, treatment is directed at management of the underlying condition.

Hypertrophic cardiomyopathy therapy includes efforts to minimize the risk of cardiac outflow track and sudden cardiac death. Beta blocker therapy helps lower heart rate and has a mild negative inotropic and antiarrhythmic effect. Surgical intervention includes septum myomectomy, where the hypertrophic septum is surgically minimized; septal ablation is also an option. An implantable cardioverter-defibrillator is often recommended to minimize dysrhythmic death risk.

The AHA has developed guidelines for the evaluation of infectious endocarditis risk. Although in the past, infectious endocarditis prophylaxis was used liberally for most individuals with a past or current history of heart murmur or structural cardiac abnormality, the AHA has long advocated for restraint in this practice, recognizing that infectious endocarditis is much more likely to result from frequent exposure to random bacteremias associated with daily activities than from bacteremia caused by a dental, gastrointestinal (GI) tract, or genitourinary tract procedure; maintenance of optimal oral health and hygiene is likely more important than prophylactic antibiotics for a dental procedure in reducing infectious endocarditis risk. Infectious endocarditis prophylaxis is considered a reasonable option, however, for people at highest risk, including individuals with an infectious endocarditis history or a prosthetic heart valve (Table 6-10).

PREPARTICIPATION SPORTS SCREENING EXAMINATION

A preparticipation sports screening examination is an important step toward safe involvement in organized sports. The purpose of the screening examination is to maintain the health and safety of the athlete, not simply to disqualify or exclude athletes from participating in sports. Cardiovascular evaluation is one of the most important components of the sports participation evaluation. Reducing the risk of exercise-induced sudden cardiac death and the progression or deterioration of cardiovascular function caused by exercise are the primary goals of preparticipation evaluation. The precise conditions responsible for athletic field deaths differ considerably according to age. In victims younger than 35 years, most sudden cardiac deaths are caused by cardiac malformations. Hypertrophic cardiomyopathy is the predominant abnormality in about one-third of cases, and congenital coronary anomalies rank as the second most common etiology. Most of these deaths occur while the victims are playing team sports. In athletes 35 years or older, most deaths are caused by atherosclerotic coronary artery disease, usually while the victims are participating in an individual endeavour such as long-distance running.

The preparticipation cardiovascular history should include questions about the following:

■ Prior occurrence of exertional chest pain/discomfort or syncope/near syncope
■ Excessive, unexpected, and unexplained shortness of breath or fatigue associated with exercise
■ Past detection of a heart murmur or high BP

TABLE 6-10 Prevention of Endocarditis: Guidelines from the American Heart Association

PRIMARY REASONS FOR REVISIONS OF INFECTIOUS ENDOCARDITIS (IE) PROPHYLAXIS GUIDELINES

IE is much more likely to result from frequent exposure to random bacteremias associated with daily activities than from bacteremia caused by a dental, gastrointestinal (GI) tract, or genitourinary (GU) tract procedure.

Prophylaxis may prevent very few, if any, cases of IE in individuals who undergo a dental, GI tract, or GU tract procedure.

The risk of antibiotic-associated adverse events exceeds the benefit, if any, from prophylactic antibiotic therapy.

Maintenance of optimal oral health and hygiene may reduce incidence of bacteremia from daily activities and is more important than prophylactic antibiotics for a dental procedure to reduce the risk of IE.

CARDIAC CONDITIONS ASSOCIATED WITH HIGHEST RISK OF ADVERSE OUTCOME FROM ENDOCARDITIS FOR WHICH PROPHYLAXIS WITH DENTAL PROCEDURES IS REASONABLE

Prosthetic cardiac valve or prosthetic material used for cardiac valve repair

Previous IE

Congenital heart disease (CHD)*

■ Unrepaired cyanotic CHD, including palliative shunts and conduits

■ Completely repaired congenital heart defect with prosthetic material or device, whether placed by surgery or by catheter intervention, during the first 6 months after the procedure[†]

■ Repaired congenital heart disease with residual defects at the site or adjacent to the site of a prosthetic patch or prosthetic device (which inhibits endothelialization)

■ Cardiac transplantation recipients who develop cardiac valvulopathy

DENTAL, ORAL, OR RESPIRATORY TRACT OR ESOPHAGEAL PROCEDURES: GIVE 30 TO 60 MINUTES BEFORE PROCEDURE

Adults	*Children*
Amoxicillin 2 g PO	Amoxicillin 50 mg/kg PO

IF UNABLE TO TAKE ORAL MEDICATION

Ampicillin 2 g IM or IV Cefazolin or ceftriaxone 1 g IM or IV	Ampicillin 50 mg/kg IM or IV
	Cefazolin or ceftriaxone 50 mg/kg IM or IV

ORAL, IF PENICILLIN OR AMPICILLIN ALLERGIC

Clindamycin 600 mg	Clindamycin 20 mg/kg
Cephalexin[‡,§] 2 g	Cephalexin[§] 50 mg/kg
Azithromycin or clarithromycin 500 mg	Azithromycin or clarithromycin 15 mg/kg

IF PENICILLIN OR AMPICILLIN ALLERGIC AND UNABLE TO TAKE ORAL MEDICATION

Cefazolin[§] or ceftriaxone[§] 1 g IM or IV	Cefazolin[§] or ceftriaxone[§] 50 mg/kg IM or IV
Clindamycin 600 mg IM or IV	Clindamycin 20 mg/kg IM or IV

*Except for the conditions listed, antibiotic prophylaxis is no longer recommended for any other form of CHD.

[†]Prophylaxis is reasonable because endothelialization of prosthetic material occurs within 6 months after the procedure.

[‡]Or other first- or second-generation oral cephalosporin in equivalent adult or pediatric dosage.

[§]Cephalosporins should not be used in an individual with a history of anaphylaxis, angioedema, or urticaria with penicillins or ampicillin.

Source: Wilson W, Taubert KA, Gewitz M, et al. Prevention of infective endocarditis: guidelines from the American Heart Association. Circulation. 2007;116:1736–1754. http://circ.ahajournals.org/content/116/15/1736.full.pdf

- Family history of the following: premature death (sudden or otherwise), significant disability from cardiovascular disease in one or more close relatives younger than age 50 years, or specific knowledge of the occurrence of certain conditions (hypertrophic cardiomyopathy, dilated cardiomyopathy, long QT syndrome, Marfan syndrome, or clinically important dysrhythmias)

The cardiovascular physical examination should include the following:

- Precordial auscultation in the supine and standing positions to identify heart murmurs consistent with dynamic left ventricular outflow obstruction
- Assessment of the femoral artery pulses to exclude coarctation of the aorta
- Recognition of the physical stigmata of Marfan syndrome
- BP measurement in the sitting and standing positions

When abnormalities on the cardiac examination are noted during the preparticipation sports physical examination, the patient should undergo appropriate diagnostics as well as specialty consultation. Clearance to play the sport should be held until evaluation is complete.

INFECTIVE ENDOCARDITIS

Overview

Infective endocarditis is an infection of the inner lining of the heart, most commonly occurring in persons with damaged heart valves, prosthetic heart valves, or other heart defects. Risk factors also include a history of endocarditis or intravenous drug use.

The infection can develop slowly or rapidly, depending on the causative pathogen, and signs and symptoms can vary accordingly.

> **CLINICAL CONCEPT**
>
> Endocarditis rates due to methicillin-resistant *Staphylococcus aureus* have been increasing, likely because of the opioid epidemic.

Clinical Presentation

The most common symptoms include fever, chills, a new or altered heart murmur, fatigue, aching joints and muscles, shortness of breath, edema, persistent cough, unexplained weight loss, hematuria, tenderness of the spleen, Osler's nodes, and petechiae. Petechiae are best described as flat, pinpoint purple, red, or brown spots on the skin that can appear as clusters.

Diagnostic Testing

Endocarditis diagnosis involves a blood culture to detect the infection and a transesophageal echocardiogram to identify vegetation formation or infected tissue in the heart. An ECG can be used to detect alteration to heart function, whereas a chest x-ray, CT scan, or MRI are often used to detect spread of the infection to other sites.

Treatment

Endocarditis is treated with high doses of intravenous antibiotics that should be tailored to the causative pathogen and susceptibility profile, as well as the patient's risk factor for the disease's development. Treatment lasts at least 4 to 6 weeks to eradicate the infection. Surgery is occasionally required to repair or replace a damaged valve caused by infective endocarditis.

Discussion Sources

Baddour LM, Wilson WR, Bayer AS, et al. Infective endocarditis in adults: diagnosis, antimicrobial therapy, and management of complications: a scientific statement for healthcare professionals from the American Heart Association. *Circulation.* 2015;132:1435–1486.

Goolsby MJ, Grubbs L. *Advanced Assessment: Interpreting Findings and Formulating Differential Diagnoses.* 4th ed. Philadelphia, PA: F.A. Davis; 2019.

Wilson W, Taubert KA, Gewitz M, et al. Prevention of infective endocarditis: guidelines from the American Heart Association. *Circulation.* 2007;116:1736–1754. http://circ.ahajournals.org/content/116/15/1736.full.pdf

QUESTIONS

90. You examine a 24-year-old woman with MVP. Her physical examination findings may also include:

A. pectus excavatum.

B. obesity.

C. petite stature.

D. hyperextensible joints.

91. Among individuals younger than 35 years, the most common cause of sudden cardiac death is:

A. non-ST-segment MI.

B. ST-segment MI.

C. a congenital cardiac malformation.

D. AS.

92. During a preparticipation cardiovascular history, all of the following questions should be included except:

A. past detection of a heart murmur.

B. excessive, unexplained, and unexpected shortness of breath.

C. prior occurrence of exertional chest pain/discomfort.

D. prior use of NSAIDs.

93. During a preparticipation sports examination, you hear a grade 2/6 early to midsystolic ejection murmur, heard best at the second intercostal space of the left sternal border, in an asymptomatic young adult. The murmur disappears with position change from supine to standing position. This most likely represents:

A. an innocent flow murmur.

B. mitral valve incompetency.

C. aortic regurgitation.

D. MVP.

94. In performing a cardiac examination in a person with MVP, you expect to find:

A. an early to midsystolic, crescendo-decrescendo murmur.

B. a pansystolic murmur.

C. a low-pitched, diastolic rumble.

D. a mid- to late-systolic murmur.

95. A risk factor for MVP includes a history of:

A. rheumatic fever.

B. rheumatoid arthritis.

C. Kawasaki disease.

D. Marfan syndrome.

96. Aside from heart murmur, additional findings in MVP include:

A. an opening snap.

B. a midsystolic click.

C. a paradoxical splitting of the second heart sound (S_2).

D. a fourth heart sound (S_4).

97. Intervention for patients with MVP often includes advice about which of the following?

A. restricted activity because of low cardiac output

B. control of fluid intake to minimize risk of volume overload

C. routine use of beta-adrenergic antagonists to control palpitations

D. encouragement of a regular program of aerobic activity

98. When a heart valve fails to open to its normal orifice size, it is said to be:
   A. stenotic.
   B. incompetent.
   C. sclerotic.
   D. regurgitant.

99. When a heart valve fails to close properly, it is said to be:
   A. stenotic.
   B. incompetent.
   C. sclerotic.
   D. regurgitant.

100. Upon detection of a suspected pathological cardiac murmur, the next step in obtaining a diagnostic procedure usually includes a(n):
   A. ventilation perfusion scan.
   B. echocardiogram.
   C. pulmonary artery angiography.
   D. cardiac CT scan.

101. You are evaluating a 45-year-old woman who has a history of rheumatic heart disease. When assessing her for mitral stenosis, you auscultate the heart, anticipating finding the following murmur:
   A. systolic with wide radiation over the precordium.
   B. localized diastolic with little radiation.
   C. systolic with radiation to the neck.
   D. systolic with radiation to the axilla.

102. In evaluating mitral valve incompetency, you expect to find the following murmur:
   A. systolic with radiation to the axilla.
   B. diastolic with little radiation.
   C. late diastolic with opening snap.
   D. localized systolic.

103. In evaluating an 88-year-old man with a 10-year history of AS, the NP anticipates finding 12-lead ECG changes consistent with:
   A. right bundle branch block.
   B. extreme axis deviation.
   C. right atrial enlargement.
   D. left ventricular hypertrophy.

104. Signs and symptoms consistent with endocarditis include all of the following except:
   A. bradycardia.
   B. Osler's nodes.
   C. hematuria.
   D. petechiae.

105. From the following list, the most helpful test in suspected bacterial endocarditis includes:
   A. urine culture.
   B. blood culture.

C. chest x-ray.

D. myocardial biopsy.

106. Of the following patients, who is in greatest need of endocarditis prophylaxis when planning dental work?

   A. a 22-year-old woman with MVP with trace MR noted on echocardiogram

   B. a 54-year-old woman with a prosthetic aortic valve

   C. a 66-year-old man with cardiomyopathy

   D. a 58-year-old woman who had a three-vessel coronary artery bypass graft with drug-eluting stents 1 year ago

107. Of the following people, who has no significant increased risk for developing bacterial endocarditis?

   A. a 43-year-old woman with a bicuspid aortic valve

   B. a 55-year-old man who was diagnosed with a physiological murmur during childhood

   C. a 45-year-old woman with a history of endocarditis

   D. a 24-year-old man with a history of injection drug use

108. You are examining an 85-year-old woman and find a grade 3/6 crescendo-decrescendo systolic murmur with radiation to the neck. She states she sometimes gets "lightheaded when I walk up a flight of stairs." This is most likely caused by:

   A. AS.

   B. aortic regurgitation.

   C. anemia.

   D. mitral stenosis.

109. AS in a 15-year-old asymptomatic male during a sports-clearance physical examination is most likely:

   A. a sequela of rheumatic fever.

   B. a result of a congenital defect.

   C. calcific in nature.

   D. found with atrial septal defect.

110. A risk factor for acquired AS is:

   A. history of pulmonary embolism.

   B. chronic obstructive pulmonary disease (COPD).

   C. type 2 diabetes.

   D. prior rheumatic fever.

111. Management of mild AS with normal limit cardiac output and excellent exercise tolerance in a 12-year-old boy usually includes:

   A. periodic monitoring with ECG and echocardiogram.

   B. use of a balloon catheter to separate fused valve leaflets.

   C. valve replacement.

   D. use of an anticoagulant/antiplatelet therapy to minimize stroke risk.

112. A physiological murmur has which of the following characteristics?

   A. occurs late in systole

   B. is noted in a localized area of auscultation

    C. becomes softer when the patient moves from supine to standing

    D. frequently obliterates S₂

113. You are examining a 19-year-old man who is diagnosed with a murmur of MR. When he asks about participation in sports activities, you counsel that:

    A. participation in sports activities should not be affected by his condition.

    B. he should refrain from any activities requiring physical exertion.

    C. participation will depend on the degree of atrial atrophy.

    D. participation will depend on the degree of ventricular enlargement.

114. You are examining an 18-year-old man who is seeking a sports clearance physical examination. You note a midsystolic murmur that gets louder when he stands. This could represent:

    A. AS.

    B. hypertrophic cardiomyopathy.

    C. a physiological murmur.

    D. a Still's murmur.

115. According to recommendations of the AHA, which of the following antibiotics should be used for endocarditis prophylaxis in patients who are allergic to penicillin?

    A. erythromycin

    B. dicloxacillin

    C. azithromycin

    D. ofloxacin

116. A grade 3 systolic heart murmur is usually:

    A. softer than the S₂ heart sound.

    B. about as loud as the S₁ heart sound.

    C. accompanied by a thrill.

    D. heard across the precordium but without radiation.

117. The S₃ heart sound has all of the following characteristics except:

    A. it is heard in early diastole.

    B. it is a presystolic sound.

    C. it is noted in the presence of ventricular overload.

    D. it is heard best with the bell of the stethoscope.

118. The S₄ heart sound has which of the following characteristics?

    A. After it is initially noted, it is a permanent finding.

    B. It is noted in the presence of poorly controlled HTN.

    C. It is heard best in early diastole.

    D. It is a high-pitched sound best heard with the diaphragm of the stethoscope.

119. Which of the following is most consistent with the presentation of hypertrophic cardiomyopathy?

    A. a 52-year-old who reports angina and chest tightness with exercise

    B. a 29-year-old who reports a gradual and steady decrease in exercise tolerance

    C. a 21-year-old athlete who reported postexertional syncope

    D. a 25-year-old injection drug user who reports fatigue and shortness of breath

For answers and rationales, see end of chapter.

QUESTION ANSWERS AND RATIONALES

Cardiovascular Disease Risk Assessment and Reduction

1. Correct: A. initiating a DASH eating plan

Lifestyle modifications are an important component in reducing the risk of CVD. Among the items listed, the adoption of a DASH eating plan will result in the greatest reduction in SBP (about 11 mm Hg on average) in an individual with HTN (A). A DASH eating plan is rich in fruits, vegetables, whole grains, and low-fat dairy with reduced content of saturated and total fat.

Incorrect:

Other lifestyle modifications that can be beneficial in reducing SBP include starting an exercise regimen of aerobic exercise (~5/8 mm Hg with 90 to 150 minutes per week) or dynamic resistance (~4 mm Hg with 90 to 150 minutes per week) (B), limiting alcohol consumption in individuals who drink alcohol (~4 mm Hg) (D), and weight reduction in overweight or obese individuals (~1 mm Hg reduction for each kilogram loss) (C).

2. Correct: D. potassium

Consumption of a diet rich in potassium has been identified as an important component in reducing BP (D). Individuals should aim for 3,500 to 5,000 mg per day. High potassium foods include bananas, oranges, cantaloupe, grapefruit, prunes, raisins, and certain legumes (e.g., lima beans, pinto beans, lentils).

Incorrect:

A reduction in sodium is generally recommended to reduce HTN, aiming for a goal of less than 1,500 mg per day or a reduction of at least 1,000 mg per day (A). Enhanced intake of iron (B) or calcium (C) is not anticipated to help reduce BP.

3. Correct: B. arrange for at least two additional BP measurements during the next 2 weeks.

In the absence of hypertensive symptoms or any indication of TOD, the best approach to confirm a diagnosis of HTN would be to schedule repeat BP measurements during the following 2 weeks (B). If the readings continue to indicate HTN, then consultation on lifestyle modification and/or pharmacotherapy can be done.

Incorrect:

A diagnosis of HTN in an otherwise healthy individual with an elevated BP measurement should be confirmed with a repeated BP measurement 1 to 4 weeks later. If the elevated BP reading is confirmed, then additional laboratory testing should be performed (C) as well as counseling on lifestyle modifications, such as reducing sodium intake (D). The initiation and selection of antihypertensive medication will depend on the degree of HTN and patient preference (A).

4. Correct: A. prescribe an ACEI.

This patient with a long history of HTN is not meeting her BP goal of at least less than 140/90 mm Hg with her current regimen. Escalation of therapy is warranted and can include the addition of an ACEI or ARB (A), which will also provide renal protection in the presence of diabetes mellitus.

Incorrect:

There is no need for the patient to return for another BP reading in 1 week as she has been in an elevated range for the past 12 months (B). She is not meeting her BP goal and requires escalation of therapy (C). An aldosterone antagonist is not preferred over an ACEI or ARB due to lack of renal protection (D).

5. Correct: C. left ventricular hypertrophy.

Long-standing, poorly controlled HTN can result in specific TOD. Cardiovascular effects of HTN include atherosclerosis, MI, left ventricular hypertrophy (C), and HF.

Incorrect:

Lipid abnormalities are not a consequence of poorly controlled HTN but can contribute to CVD (A). Insulin resistance is associated with type 2 diabetes mellitus and is not a consequence of HTN (B). Clotting disorders are not associated with the presence of long-standing HTN (D).

6. Correct: B. uric acid.

With a diagnosis of HTN, laboratory analysis should be performed to establish a baseline for medication use and screen for secondary causes of HTN. Uric acid level, typically measured in patients with symptoms of gout, is not warranted in patients with newly diagnosed HTN (B).

Incorrect:

Laboratory analyses performed in newly diagnosed patients with HTN can include fasting blood glucose (check for diabetes) (A), CBC and lipid profile, serum creatinine (C) and eGFR (check for renal impairment), serum sodium, potassium (D), and calcium.

7. Correct: D. consuming at least one to two servings of alcohol.

Lifestyle modifications can be an important aspect in comprehensive management of HTN. For individuals who consume alcohol, it is recommended to limit the number of alcoholic drinks to two per day for men and one per day for women. Consumption of at least one to two servings is not recommended to help manage HTN (D).

Incorrect:

Weight loss in individuals who are overweight or obese (A) as well as regular aerobic exercise (C) can be effective in reducing BP. Dietary sodium restriction to less than 1,500 mg per day (or a reduction of at least 1,000 mg per day) can also be beneficial in reducing BP (B).

8 to 12. Matching Questions

8. Correct: C. dihydropyridine calcium channel blocker

9. Correct: B. nondihydropyridine calcium channel blocker

10. Correct: E. ACEI

11. Correct: D. angiotensin receptor antagonist

12. Correct: A. beta-adrenergic receptor antagonist
First-line treatments of HTN include thiazide diuretics, CCBs, ACEIs, and ARBs. ACEIs, such as trandolapril (10), and ARBs, such as telmisartan (11) work by attenuating angiotensin II, a potent vasoconstrictor. CCBs cause vasodilatation. Nondihydropyridine CCBs, such as diltiazem (9), are helpful for BP control and renal protection but can reduce heart rate and so should be limited to patients with normal left ventricular function. Dihydropyridine CCBs, such as amlodipine (8), are more potent vasodilators than non-DHP CCBs and are generally reserved for those with difficult-to-treat HTN. Beta-adrenergic receptor antagonists, or beta blockers such as pindolol (12), block adrenergic B1-receptor sites and blunt catecholamine response, leading to decreased heart rate and stroke volume.

13. Correct: D. CCB
People of African ancestry have demonstrated a better response with CCBs and thiazide diuretics compared to other antihypertensive classes (D). JNC-8 guidelines prefer the use of these agents among African Americans in the absence of diabetes mellitus or CKD.
Incorrect:
Among patients of African ancestry without diabetes mellitus or CKD, CCBs and thiazide diuretics are preferred over ACEIs (A), ARBs (B), and beta blockers (C), as evidence demonstrates a better response with thiazide diuretics and CCBs.

14. Correct: C. severe left ventricular dysfunction.
CCBs are associated with a negative inotropic effect and bradycardia, and so their use should be limited to patients with normal left ventricular function. The use of these agents is contraindicated in patients with severe left ventricular dysfunction (C) and in those with second- or third-degree AV block in the absence of a pacemaker.
Incorrect:
There are no specific warnings with the use of CCBs in patients with type 1 diabetes mellitus (A) or who have a history of venous thromboembolism (B). They can be safely used in combination with an ACEI (D).

15. Correct: A. The patient should sit in a chair with feet flat on the floor for at least 5 minutes before obtaining the reading.
Obtaining an accurate BP measurement requires following proper procedures. A BP reading should be performed with the patient sitting in a chair with feet flat on the floor for at least 5 minutes prior to the reading (A).
Incorrect:
The BP cuff should be wide enough to cover more than 80% of the upper arm (B). The arm should be supported at heart level during the reading (C). Patients should be seated for at least 5 minutes prior to the reading (D).

16. Correct: C. white coat
White coat HTN refers to the patient condition where consistently elevated BP is observed in the medical office or when a physician is present, but BP is normal in other, more comfortable environments (e.g., home) (C). This is likely caused by patient anxiety in the medical setting. This condition does not necessarily need to be treated with pharmacotherapy. Rather, an improved patient-provider interaction through improved communication, empathy, and trust can help to alleviate anxiety and reduce the impact of white coat HTN.
Incorrect:
Elevated BP observed only in the medical office setting refers to white coat HTN and not provider-induced (A), clinical (B), or pseudo (D) HTN.

17. Correct: B. avoid disease-related TOD.
When managing a patient with HTN, it is important to recognize that an important goal is to prevent or minimize the risk of disease-related TOD (B). Serious and life-threatening conditions can result from TOD including stroke, MI, HF, and renal failure, among others.
Incorrect:
Management of HTN should aim to achieve BP goals recommended in evidence-based guidelines (A) while minimizing adverse effects of pharmacotherapy (C). However, the main goal of HTN management is to avoid TOD that can lead to serious and life-threatening conditions. Treatment of concomitant conditions should be part of the comprehensive health plan to avoid TOD (D).

18. Correct: C. potassium
The use of an ACEI is associated with a modest hyperkalemia risk, particularly when used concomitantly with an aldosterone antagonist, such as spironolactone. Therefore, potassium levels should be routinely monitored to identify elevated levels (C) and addressed accordingly.
Incorrect:
The use of an ACEI with spironolactone is not associated with substantial clinical effect with regard to sodium (A), calcium (B), or chloride (D) levels.

19. Correct: B. Initiate therapy with chlorthalidone.
The recommended BP goal for this patient is at least less than 140/90 mm Hg, which has not been observed on multiple readings over 2 months. First-line treatment can include a thiazide diuretic, such as chlorthalidone (B), ACEI, ARB, or CCB.
Incorrect:
This patient has consistently elevated BP, and treatment should be initiated prior to the development of TOD (D). Beta blockers, such as metoprolol (A), and centrally acting agents, such as methyldopa (C), are not recommended first-line treatment options.

20. Correct: C. aldosterone antagonist in HF
Aldosterone antagonists, such as spironolactone, can offer benefits in patients with HF, as these agents can

help regulate sodium and water homeostasis and maintenance of intravascular volume. These agents have been shown to improve morbidity and mortality among patients with HF (C).

Incorrect:
Thiazide diuretics, such as chlorthalidone, are not recommended in patients with a history of gout, as these agents can trigger an acute gouty attack (A). The use of beta blockers, such as propranolol, can worsen bronchospasm in a patient with lower airway disease and will inhibit the activity of beta-2 agonist medications (B). Methyldopa is not recommended in older adults as this can lead to cognitive alterations (D).

21. **Correct: C. metoprolol.**
The JNC-8 and ACC/AHA guidelines recommend the use of ACE inhibitors, ARBs, CCBs, or a thiazide diuretic as first-line treatment of HTN without diabetes mellitus or CKD. Metoprolol, a beta blocker, is not recommended as first-line treatment (C).

Incorrect:
First-line treatment for this patient can include an ACEI (e.g., lisinopril [A]), a thiazide diuretic (e.g., chlorthalidone [B]), a calcium channel blocker (e.g., amlodipine [D]), or an ARB.

22. **Correct: A. patient report of acute visual change.**
Patients with grade 1 or grade 2 hypertensive retinopathy will not report changes in vision (A). These typically occur at the higher grades (grade 3 or grade 4).

Incorrect:
Grade 1 is the mildest form of hypertensive retinopathy and is not associated with the presence of retinal hemorrhages (D) but should have a normal finding of sharp optic disc borders (C). The characteristic finding in grade 1 hypertensive retinopathy is a narrowing of the terminal retinal arterioles (B).

23. **Correct: A. normal BP.**
There are slight differences in the categories of HTN when comparing the JNC-8 and ACC/AHA guidelines. In both guidelines, a normal HTN is considered less than 120/80 mm Hg (A).

Incorrect:
HTN requiring pharmacotherapy is generally considered 140/90 mm Hg or higher in JNC-8 guidelines, and 130/80 mm Hg or higher in ACC/AHA guidelines. Thus, this patient does not have HTN and does not require treatment with antihypertensive medications (B, C, D). When treatment is needed, first-line agents can include an ACEI, ARB, CCB, or thiazide diuretic.

24. **Correct: D. presence of MA plus cigarette smoking.**
MA has been identified as a risk factor for CVD and ischemic heart disease. The presence of cigarette smoking further increases the risk of ischemic heart disease (D). HTN in a patient with MA should include the use of a thiazide diuretic, beta blocker, ACEIs, and CCBs.

Incorrect:
The presence rather than absence of MA increases the risk of ischemic heart disease (B, C). The addition of cigarette smoking has been identified to further increase this risk. A link between MA and heavy alcohol intake on ischemic heart disease has not been established (A).

25. **Correct: C. CCBs.**
People of African ancestry have demonstrated a better response with CCBs (C) and thiazide diuretics compared to other antihypertensive classes. JNC-8 guidelines prefer the use of these agents among African Americans in the absence of diabetes mellitus or CKD.

Incorrect:
Among patients of African ancestry, CCBs and thiazide diuretics tend to result in greater BP-lowering effects when compared to ACEIs (A), ARBs (B), and beta blockers (D).

26. **Correct: B. adding a beta-adrenergic receptor antagonist.**
For a patient who does not meet BP goal with current therapy, escalation of therapy can include increasing the dose of the current regimen or adding a new class of agent. However, for a patient with asthma or other lower airway disease, a beta-adrenergic receptor antagonist should be avoided, as this can exacerbate bronchospasm and minimize the effect of beta-2 agonist therapy (B).

Incorrect:
Acceptable treatment options for this patient can include increasing the dose of losartan (A) or HCTZ (D) as well as adding a new class of agents, such as a CCB (C).

27. **Correct: B. It is characterized by a drop in BP when going from a standing to a sitting position.**
When managing the elderly, the risk of postural hypotension should be assessed as this can increase the risk of falls and serious injury. Postural hypotension is defined as a drop in BP when going from a sitting to a standing position, not from a standing to a sitting position (B).

Incorrect:
Postural hypotension in the elderly can increase the risk of falls (A) as well as cardiovascular events (C). The condition is associated with the use of vasodilating medications (D), such as CCBs.

28 to 33. Matching Questions

28. **Correct: A. thiazide diuretic; B. beta blocker; C. ACEI; D. ARB; E. aldosterone antagonist; F. CCB**

29. **Correct: A. thiazide diuretic; B. beta blocker; C. ACEI; D. ARB; F. CCB**

30. **Correct: B. beta blocker; F. CCB**

31. **Correct: A. thiazide diuretic; B. beta blocker; C. ACEI; F. CCB**

32. **Correct: A. thiazide diuretic; C. ACEI; D. ARB; F. CCB**

33. **Correct: A. thiazide diuretic; C. ACEI; D. ARB; F. CCB**
ACC/AHA provide guidance on the selection of appropriate antihypertensive medications in the elderly

depending on the compelling indication. For those with HF, any of the listed medications is acceptable for lowering BP (28). For those with diabetes, preferred agents include thiazide diuretics, beta blockers, ACEIs, ARBs, or CCBs (29). In patients who experience angina pectoris, a beta blocker or CCB is preferred (30). For those with coronary artery disease or aortic aneurysm, selection can include a thiazide diuretic, beta blocker, ACEI, or CCB (31, 32). In considering recurrent stroke prevention, preferred agents include a thiazide diuretic, ACEI, ARB, or CCB (33).

Acute Coronary Syndrome

34. Correct: A. left ventricular hypertrophy.
Unstable angina is predominantly caused by CHD or another condition that can diminish the flow of blood in the coronary arteries to adequately supply the heart with oxygen. Left ventricular hypertrophy is often caused by long-standing, poorly controlled HTN but would not impact blood flow to the heart (A).
Incorrect:
Vasoconstriction (B) or a nonocclusive thrombus (C) present in the coronary artery can lead to diminished blood flow to the heart and result in unstable angina. Inflammation and infection, such as acute endocarditis, can also trigger unstable angina, particularly with the development of embolisms from vegetative growth (D).

35. Correct: C. chest pressure lasting 20 minutes that occurs at rest
Unstable angina presents with chest pain that is typically described as pressure, tightness, heaviness, or aching sensation. The pain can occur at rest or with exercise or stress and can last several minutes (C).
Incorrect:
Chest tightness that results from exercise and is relieved by stress best describes stable angina rather than unstable angina (A). Chest pain associated with unstable angina is described as pressure, tightness, or heaviness rather than severe or searing pain, and the pain will last for several minutes in duration rather than only 30 seconds (B). A feeling of "heartburn" that is relieved by a positional change would more likely be GI in nature and not unstable angina (D).

36. Correct: B. MI.
The most common initial manifestation of CHD in men is MI (B).
Incorrect:
In women, the most common initial manifestation of CHD is angina (A, D), which often leads to MI. In men, MI is more common than intracranial hemorrhage (C) or angina as the initial manifestation of CHD.

37. Correct: C. more commonly with angina and less commonly with acute MI.
The most common initial presentation of ACS in women is angina, while the most common initial manifestation in men is MI (C).

Incorrect:
Women usually have disease onset at an older age compared to men and will present differently (B). However, women younger than 60 years will often present in a similar manner as men (A). Atypical presentation of ACS can occur in both men and women 80 years and older and can include symptoms of confusion and cognitive impairment (D).

38. Correct: D. unusual fatigue; C. sleep disturbance; A. dyspnea; B. indigestion
A study of 515 women with ACS identified new or different symptoms preceding their ACS episode. The most common symptom was unusual fatigue (70%), followed by sleep disturbance (48%), shortness of breath (42%), and indigestion (39%).

39. Correct: B. S_4.
The fourth heart sound, also known as S_4 or atrial gallop, is frequently heard with myocardial ischemia and poorly controlled angina pectoris (B). The sound occurs just before S_1 and can be a sign of poor myocardial relaxation and diastolic dysfunction that can cause diminished cardiac output.
Incorrect:
A physiological split S_2 occurs when closure of the aortic valve and closure of the pulmonary valve are not aligned (A) and is usually a benign finding. An opening snap can occur early in diastole and is caused by thickened valve leaflets, which produce a snapping sound when they open, as observed with mitral stenosis (C). A summation gallop is more likely associated with tachycardia and not angina pectoris (D).

40. Correct: C. ST-segment deviation (greater than 0.05 mV)
The characteristic finding on ECG for ACS is a new or presumably new transient ST-segment deviation or a T-wave inversion along with symptoms (C).
Incorrect:
T-wave flattening (A) or inversion in leads with dominant R waves (B) usually indicates a low likelihood of ACS. A finding of fixed Q waves typically indicates an intermediate likelihood of ACS (D).

41. Correct: B. reduce myocardial oxygen demand.
Beta-adrenergic antagonists, or beta blockers, are typically used first-line during ACS due to their ability to reduce myocardial workload and oxygen demand by lowering heart rate, lowering stroke volume, and blunting catecholamine response (B).
Incorrect:
Beta blockers are not able to reverse vessel lesions (A), enhance myocardial vessel tone (C), or stabilize arterial volume (D).

42. Correct: C. cause vasodilation.
Nitrates primarily work by causing vasodilation and improving blood flow (C). Nitroglycerin can be administered as soon as possible either via sublingual spray or tablet followed by parenteral administration.

Incorrect:

Beta blockers are used to reduce myocardial oxygen demand (B). Nitrates are not involved in reversing fixed vessel obstruction (A) or stabilizing cardiac rhythm (D), such as with an antiarrhythmic drug (e.g., amiodarone, flecainide).

43. **Correct: D. retrosternal diffuse pain for 30 minutes accompanied by diaphoresis**

In a younger patient presenting with acute MI, a classic presentation would be expected. This would include chest pain lasting several minutes that is described as pressure, tightness, heaviness, or aching and can be accompanied by dyspnea, nausea/vomiting, or diaphoresis (D).

Incorrect:

Chest tightness that occurs with exercise, such as stair climbing, is more likely due to stable or unstable angina (A). Meanwhile, chest pressure that lasts 20 minutes and occurs at rest is likely to be due to unstable angina (C). Severe, localized chest pain that lasts 3 hours is not a typical presentation of MI, but other causes should be investigated, possibly related to the GI system (B).

44 to 47. Matching questions.

44. **Correct: A. new onset of chest pain and discomfort at rest or worsening of symptoms with activities that previously did not provoke symptoms**

45. **Correct: B. predictable onset of chest pain or discomfort, usually with physical exertion**

46. **Correct: D. results from severe coronary artery narrowing, transient occlusion, or microembolization of thrombus and/or atheromatous material**

47. **Correct: C. results from full-thickness (transmural) necrosis of the myocardium and total occlusion of coronary artery**

Stable angina is characterized by symptoms that occur in a predictable manner, usually with exertion and relieved with rest (45). Unstable angina is associated with the appearance of symptoms either at rest or with activities that previously did not provoke symptoms (44). STEMI is associated with transmural MI (full-thickness necrosis) and total occlusion of the coronary artery (47). NSTEMI involves nontransmural MI and subtotal occlusion of the coronary vessel (46).

48. **Correct: D. deep Q waves**

Long-term ECG findings in a person who experienced a past acute transmural MI will include the presence of deep Q waves, which are indicative of preexisting structural or ischemic heart disease (D).

Incorrect:

An acute transmural MI, or STEMI, is characterized by ST deviation on ECG. However, this deviation is transient and will resolve when symptoms abate (A). A T-wave inversion is also an early indication of STEMI but will likely resolve soon after the episode (C). R waves are not a typical indication for acute transmural MI (B).

49. **Correct: C. T-wave inversion**

Myocardial ischemia occurs with inadequate blood flow to the heart leading to oxygen deficiency. The reduced blood flow could be the result of a complete or partial blockage of a coronary artery. The classic ECG finding of myocardial ischemia is a T-wave inversion (C).

Incorrect:

ST elevation indicates cardiac injury and is transiently found during STEMI (A). Q waves indicate necrosis of myocardial tissue and persist following MI (D). S waves in excess of 1 mV (10 mm) can be considered a normal finding, depending on the lead (B).

50. **Correct: C. STEMI.**

The ECG shows a clear elevation in the ST segment following the QRS complex. This is a characteristic finding in individuals who have experienced a STEMI (C).

Incorrect:

A normal ST segment will not have an elevation or depression, of which a clear elevation is demonstrated in this example (A). An NSTEMI will not produce ST-segment elevation by its definition (B). AF is characterized by a very rapid atrial rate (up to 400 to 600 beats per minute) so that the action potential is very low, resulting in an absence of P waves, which are evident in this example (D).

51. **Correct: B. pathologic Q waves.**

This ECG demonstrates a broadening of the QRS complex that is consistent with a pathological Q wave (B). The pathological Q waves are an indication of cardiac tissue damage from a prior MI.

Incorrect:

A U wave is not evident in this ECG, which would come after the T wave and possibly represent repolarization of the Purkinje fibers (A). There is no indication of low QRS voltage as evident by the peak of the QRS complex (C). There is no ST-segment depression or elevation indicated in this example (D).

52. **Correct: C. 3-mm ST-segment elevation in leads V1 to V4.**

Clinically significant ST-segment elevation largely determines the use of reperfusion therapy with thrombolytic therapy. Among the answer choices, the patient with an ST-segment elevation of 3 mm will be the best candidate for thrombolytic therapy (C), though the presence of absolute and relative contraindications must be considered.

53. **Correct: C. troponin I (cTnI)**

The presence of several biomarkers can be used to detect myocardial tissue damage and provide an early indication for MI. Troponin subtypes cTnI and cThT are released in the presence of myocardial damage. Both biomarkers increase rapidly during the first 12 hours after MI. However, cTnI is more cardiac specific and is sensitive to small-volume cardiac damage (C).

Incorrect:

Aspartate aminotransferase is a liver enzyme used to detect for liver damage, such as due to hepatitis or cirrhosis (A). CPK is released in the presence of muscle damage and is not specific to myocardial damage (B). Creatine kinase myocardial band (CK-MB) is more specific to cardiac damage. However, its utility in detecting MI is being replaced with other more sensitive and specific tests, such as troponin subtypes. Lactate dehydrogenase is used to detect tissue and organ damage but is not specific for myocardial damage (D).

54. **Correct: D. nisoldipine.**

Nisoldipine is an NHP calcium channel blocker that can provide potent vasodilation. These agents can be a useful option when the patient is intolerant of beta blockers, which is considered a first-line treatment option during ACS (D).

Incorrect:

During ACS, a beta blocker (e.g., metoprolol) should be given if there are no contraindications in order to decrease myocardial workload and oxygen demand (B). An ACEI (e.g., lisinopril) is also recommended in the absence of contraindications (C). Aspirin is recommended at the first sign of ACS due to its antiplatelet effect (A).

55. **Correct: B. a dose of nitroglycerin via oral spray**

At the first signs of an anginal episode, nitroglycerin is recommended due to its powerful vasodilation effects. A rapid-acting formulation is preferred, either as an oral spray or quick-dissolving tablet.

Incorrect:

Immediate administration of rapid-acting nitroglycerin is the preferred treatment at the start of an anginal episode rather than a sustained-effect patch (D). An extra dose of a beta blocker (C) or a dose of a calcium channel blocker (A) will not have an immediate impact to alleviate anginal symptoms and can be associated with adverse effects depending on patient factors.

56. **Correct: A. history of hemorrhagic stroke**

For patients with ACS due to coronary artery occlusion, treatment options can include fibrinolysis, stenting, or revascularization procedures (e.g., percutaneous coronary intervention). When fibrinolytic therapy is selected, it is important to recognize contraindications to ensure patient safety. A history of intracranial hemorrhage is an absolute contraindication for this treatment (A).

Incorrect:

Relative contraindications include the use of oral anticoagulant therapy, such as warfarin (C), and active peptic ulcer disease (D). Significant HTN of greater than 180/110 mm Hg is also a relative contraindication (B).

57. **Correct: B. clopidogrel.**

The P2Y$_{12}$ inhibitors can be used as an alternative to aspirin in the situation of aspirin intolerance. Members of this class include clopidogrel (B), ticagrelor, and prasugrel.

Incorrect:

Warfarin (C) and rivaroxaban (D) are oral anticoagulant therapies and not antiplatelet medications. Ibuprofen and other NSAIDs provide only a transient antiplatelet effect and are not considered an acceptable alternative to aspirin (A).

58. **Correct: B. a 56-year-old man following two-vessel stenting to establish activity tolerance.**

For patients with a history of ACS and who underwent a reperfusion intervention, routine use of the treadmill exercise test should be performed to assess restoration or change in functional capacity as well as the efficacy of the current medication regimen (B). Routine testing can also be useful in stratifying patient risk for future ACS events.

Incorrect:

Routine use of the treadmill exercise test is not warranted in healthy individuals (A) as well as individuals with dyslipidemia and no history of ACS (D). Due to safety concerns, the treadmill exercise test should be avoided in elderly individuals who have difficulty walking without assistance (C).

59. **Correct: B. statin.**

The latest recommendations for ACC/AHA recommend statin therapy as the preferential first-line treatment for dyslipidemia (B). The use of moderate- or high-intensity statin therapy should be determined based on current low-density lipoprotein (LDL) cholesterol level and patient factors.

Incorrect:

Statin therapy is the preferred first-line agent to reduce LDL levels. If intensification is needed beyond optimized statin dosing, ezetimibe or a PCSK9 inhibitor can be added to statin therapy. Dietary supplements of fish oil are not recommended to reduce LDL (C). Fibrates (D) and niacin (A) are not recommended due to lack of evidence demonstrating cardiovascular benefits with use of these agents.

60. **Correct: D. pain reproduced with palpation**

Patient signs and symptoms can provide an early indication if they are experiencing an actual ACS event or some other condition. The presence of chest discomfort or pain that is reproduced by palpation would suggest a low likelihood of an ACS event (D).

Incorrect:

Signs and symptoms associated with a high likelihood of an ACS event include hypotension (C), pulmonary edema, new rales or crackles (A), and a transient MR murmur (B).

Heart Failure

61. **Correct: D. inadequate cardiac output to meet oxygen and metabolic demands of the body.**

HF can be due to a number of structural or functional impairments of cardiac function. The condition manifests when there is inadequate cardiac output to meet the oxygen and metabolic demands of the body, leading to its associated symptoms (D).

Incorrect:
There are many causes of HF. Approximately half of patients have reduced ventricular ejection fraction (C), while atrial filling and ejection is not a typical cause of HF (A). Valvular disease can contribute to HF but is not essential in its pathophysiology (B).

62. **Correct: A. hypertensive heart disease.**
HTN is a significant risk factor for both HFrEF and HFpEF (A). Initial management approaches of HF are often focused on controlling HTN to slow or stop progression of disease, typically with lifestyle modifications and antihypertensive medications.

Incorrect:
Type 2 diabetes mellitus is a risk factor for HF but is not as strongly associated to the condition as HTN (D). AF is often seen in later stages of HF but is not frequently a cause of the condition (B). Pulmonary embolism is a serious medical condition that is not usually related to the development of HF (C).

63 to 65. Matching Questions

63. **Correct: B. increased right-sided heart workload.**

64. **Correct: C. decreased oxygen-carrying capacity of blood**

65. **Correct: A. increase in circulating volume of blood**
For adults at risk of HF, other conditions can trigger symptoms associated with HF. Pneumonia can result in increased right-sided heart workload as inflammation in the lungs can inhibit blood flow through the pulmonary arteries (63). Anemia results in decreased hemoglobin content in the blood, thus decreased oxygen-carrying capacity, resulting in increased cardiac workload (64). High sodium intake will result in increased circulating volume, thus increasing workload demand by the heart (65).

66. **Correct: D. paroxysmal nocturnal dyspnea.**
Dyspnea, or shortness of breath, is the classic symptom of HF or exacerbation of HF. Paroxysmal nocturnal dyspnea is characterized by sudden shortness of breath that usually occurs after 2 to 3 hours of sleep and leads to sudden awakening (D).

Incorrect:
Dyspnea is the general term for shortness of breath (A). Dyspnea typically occurs with exertion, though in severe cases, it can occur when the individual is at rest, though the term *resting dyspnea* is not defined (C). Orthopnea is defined as shortness of breath that develops when the individual is recumbent and is relieved with elevation of the head (B).

67. **Correct: B. S_3.**
The third heart sound known as S_3 is an extra sound heard early in diastole following the normal "lub-dub"

heart sound and is typically associated with HF (B). The sound is produced when the mitral valve opens and blood strikes a compliant left ventricle.

Incorrect:
The fourth heart sound, also known as S_4 or atrial gallop, is frequently heard with myocardial ischemia and poorly controlled angina pectoris (D). The sound occurs just before S_1 and can be a sign of poor myocardial relaxation and diastolic dysfunction that can cause diminished cardiac output. An opening snap can occur early in diastole and is caused by thickened valve leaflets, which produce a snapping sound when they open (C). A summation gallop is a finding with tachycardia and occurs when S_3 and S_4 are superimposed and appear as one sound (A).

68. **Correct: C. point of maximal impulse at the fifth intercostal space, midclavicular line.**
In healthy individuals, the normal position of the PMI is the fifth intercostal space and midclavicular line. In the presence of dilated cardiomyopathy and associated increase in cardiac size, the PMI will shift laterally by as much as one or more intercostal spaces (C).

Incorrect:
Expected findings in the patient with dilated cardiomyopathy and HF include jugular venous extension (A), tenderness on the right upper-abdominal quadrant upon palpation (B), and peripheral edema (D).

69. **Correct: D. shifts laterally by one or more intercostal spaces.**
In healthy individuals, the normal position of the PMI is the fifth intercostal space and midclavicular line. In the presence of HF, the PMI can shift laterally by as much one or more intercostal spaces (D).

Incorrect:
The normal PMI position is the fifth intercostal space and not the fourth intercostal space (A), and is along the midclavicular line. HF can cause the PMI to shift laterally from this position (B), rather than lower on the midclavicular line (C).

70 to 72. Matching Questions

70. **Correct: C. force of the cardiac contraction**

71. **Correct: A. cardiac rate**

72. **Correct: B. cardiac conduction**
Proper care of cardiac conditions requires a thorough understanding of the terms used. Inotropic drugs are used to modify the force or speed of contractions and can include positive inotropic medications (such as digoxin, epinephrine, or norepinephrine), and negative inotropic drugs such as calcium channel blockers (70). Chronotropic drugs are used to alter heart rate and rhythm and can include atropine, dopamine, and beta blockers (71). Dromotropic drugs affect cardiac conduction and can include phenytoin or verapamil (72).

73. Correct: B. reduce the effects of circulating catecholamines.

Beta blockers are an important aspect in HF management, and long-term use of these agents has been shown to improve cardiac function, reduce myocardial ischemia, and decrease myocardial oxygen consumption. These drugs inhibit chronotropic and inotropic responses by reducing the effects of circulating catecholamines (B).

Incorrect:

A positive inotropic medication, such as digoxin, can be used to increase myocardial contractility (A). Beta blockers are useful in managing HF regardless of the presence of angina, which is typically treated with nitroglycerin (C). An antiarrhythmic medication is used to stabilize cardiac rhythm, such as amiodarone (D).

74. Correct: B. slightly depressed, cupped ST segments.

Digoxin has a positive inotropic effect and slows tissue conduction. An expected ECG finding among individuals who are taking a therapeutic dose of the medication is prolongation of the PR interval and cupping of the ST segment (B).

Incorrect:

Digoxin can result in prolonging the PR interval rather than shortening this interval (A). The medication is not associated with a widened QRS complex (C) or tall T waves (D).

75. Correct: B. hyperkalemia.

The use of an ACEI or ARB is associated with a moderate risk of hyperkalemia, which increases with inadequate fluid intake or with concomitant use of an aldosterone antagonist, such as spironolactone (B).

Incorrect:

ACEI use with spironolactone is not associated with renal insufficiency (C) or proteinuria (D). These agents are used to treat HTN and will not cause HTN (A).

76. Correct: A. atrioventricular heart block.

Digoxin has a positive inotropic effect and slows conduction through the atrioventricular node. Digoxin toxicity can be identified on ECG findings by the presence of atrioventricular heart block (A).

Incorrect:

The most likely finding of digoxin toxicity is AV heart block rather than a T-wave inversion (B), sinus tachycardia (C), or pointed P waves (D).

77. Correct: A. anorexia.

Anorexia is the most common adverse effect associated with digoxin toxicity, as well as a variety of cardiac effects such as AV block (A). Use of digoxin with potassium-depleting medications can increase the risk of digoxin toxicity.

Incorrect:

Visual changes are rarely reported with digoxin toxicity, such as disturbance in color perception (B) or blurred vision (C). Other signs of digoxin toxicity can include lethargy, confusion, and GI symptoms such as anorexia, nausea, vomiting, diarrhea, and abdominal pain. Constipation is not typically associated with digoxin toxicity (D).

78. Correct: B. spironolactone

Aldosterone antagonists can include spironolactone and eplerenone (B). These agents are used to regulate sodium and water homeostasis and maintenance of intravascular volume. The use of these agents is associated with hyperkalemia risk, particularly when combined with an ACEI or ARB.

Incorrect:

Hydrochlorothiazide belongs to the class of thiazide diuretics (C), while furosemide is a loop diuretic (D). Clonidine is an α_2-agonist used in the treatment of HTN (A).

79. Correct: B. dyspnea that develops when the individual is recumbent and is relieved with elevation of the head

One sign of HF is the development of orthopnea, which is shortness of breath that develops when the individual is recumbent and is relieved with elevation of the head (B).

Incorrect:

Dyspnea is shortness of breath that can occur with exercise or exertion (A) or in severe cases at rest (D). Paroxysmal nocturnal dyspnea is best described as shortness of breath that occurs at night, characterized by a sudden awakening after a couple of hours of sleep, with a feeling of severe anxiety, breathlessness, and suffocation (C).

80. Correct: D. evidence of hemoconcentration on hemogram

Hemoconcentration is a decrease in plasma volume, which subsequently causes an increase in the concentration of RBCs and other components of blood. This is unlikely to occur in HF as there is usually excessive extracellular fluid volume resulting in hemodilution on hemogram (D).

Incorrect:

Biomarkers for HF can include elevated levels of BNP and N-terminal pro-BNP (A). Signs from chest x-ray can include thickening of interlobular septa, known as Kerley B lines (B), and a loss of sharp definition of pulmonary vasculature. An expected finding on ECG would include left ventricular hypertrophy (C).

81. Correct: D. carvedilol

An alpha-/beta-adrenergic antagonist, such as carvedilol, can add the benefits of a beta blocker with the additional vasodilating effects seen with blockade at the alpha receptors (D).

Incorrect:

Atenolol (A), metoprolol (B), and propranolol (C) all belong to the beta blocker class and can be used to blunt catecholamine response.

82. Correct: D. levofloxacin.

The use of digoxin is limited due to its narrow therapeutic index and potential for drug-drug interactions.

However, the agent does not have a substantial interaction with the fluoroquinolones, such as levofloxacin (D).
Incorrect:
Medications known to have a substantial interaction with digoxin include amiodarone (A), diltiazem, clarithromycin (B), erythromycin, azole antifungals, and cyclosporine (C).

83. **Correct: D. AF.**
The ECG reveals irregular QRS complexes and an absence of discrete P waves. These findings, together with abnormally conducted beats after long and short R-R cycles are most indicative of AF (D).
Incorrect:
A TIA, characterized by brief neurological dysfunction caused by reduced blood flow to the brain, spinal cord, or retina without tissue death, does not typically result in changes in ECG (A) but can be triggered by cardiac conditions, such as AF, that can be identified on ECG. ECG findings of dilated cardiomyopathy can include reduced voltage QRS complexes as well as abnormal Q waves, which are not evident in this example (B). NSTEMI can be identified with a depressed ST wave or T wave inversion. In the absence of symptoms, NSTEMI is unlikely given the ECG example (C).

84. **Correct: B. prasugrel.**
Anticoagulant medications are recommended for patients with AF for the prevention of thromboembolic events. Prasugrel is a $P2Y_{12}$ inhibitor that has antiplatelet effect but is not an anticoagulant (B).
Incorrect:
Anticoagulants used to prevent thromboembolic events can include dabigatran (A), rivaroxaban (C), or apixaban (D).

85. **Correct: C. prior MI.**
Patients with HFrEF typically have structural changes that cause reduced left ventricular ejection fraction. This can be caused by heart tissue damage following MI (C).
Incorrect:
Female gender is a risk factor for HFpEF rather than HFrEF (A). A history of intracranial hemorrhage (B) or postural hypotension (D) are not linked to the development of HFrEF.

86. **Correct: C. long-term corticosteroid use.**
About half of patients with clinical HF can be categorized in HFpEF. The diagnosis of HFpEF is more difficult than that of HFrEF as it is a diagnosis of exclusion. Certain risk factors have been identified for HFpEF; however, long-term corticosteroid use is not among those risk factors (C).
Incorrect:
HFpEF is more commonly found among women (A) and older adults (D). The condition is also associated with the presence of comorbidities, such as HTN (B) and diabetes mellitus.

87. **Correct: B. Among patients with stage B HF, those with HFpEF present with more severe symptoms compared to those with HFrEF.**
Patients with HFrEF and HFpEF can present similarly and will require evaluation beyond patient history and clinical presentation to differentiate between the two conditions. For those with stage B HF, individuals typically have structural heart disease but without any signs or symptoms, regardless of HFrEF or HFpEF (B).
Incorrect:
Patients with HFrEF and HFpEF can present similarly and will require evaluation beyond patient history and clinical presentation to differentiate between the two conditions (C). Common findings in patients with HFpEF and HFrEF include dyspnea and fatigue (A), and HTN is a frequent finding in both conditions (D).

88. **Correct: D. addressing risk factors and comorbidities.**
Clinical trials on HF have primarily focused on HFrEF, and so optimal management of HFpEF is largely unknown. A key focus in these patients should include proper management of risk factors and comorbidities, such as HTN, hyperlipidemia, and diabetes mellitus (D).
Incorrect:
Addressing risk factors and comorbidities is a key component in the management of HFpEF. These patients are commonly treated with similar pharmacotherapy as HFrEF, which would include the use of ACEIs or ARBs, as well as a beta blocker as first-line treatment. CCBs (A), thiazide diuretics (B), and an implantable cardioverter-defibrillator (C) would not normally be considered in the initial treatment of HFpEF but can be considered in later disease.

89. **Correct: C. aldosterone antagonist.**
Aldosterone antagonists, such as spironolactone, can be considered to help manage HTN in patients with HF. However, these agents would not normally be used in first-line selection and should be used with caution in patients already taking an ACEI or ARB due to risk of hyperkalemia (C).
Incorrect:
Initial pharmacological approaches in the treatment of HFrEF can include an ACEI (A) or ARB (B) along with a beta blocker (D).

Disorders Revealed by the Cardiac Examination

90. **Correct: A. pectus excavatum.**
MVP is often seen in individuals with minor thoracic deformities such as pectus excavatum, straight back, or a shallow anterior-posterior diameter (A). Pectus excavatum is characterized by a deformity of the anterior thoracic wall in which the sternum and rib cage are shaped abnormally, which can produce a caved or sunken chest appearance.
Incorrect:
MVP is more commonly found with thoracic structural deformities rather than in individuals with obesity (B),

petite stature (C), or hyperextensible joints (D), such as those with Marfan syndrome.

91. Correct: C. a congenital cardiac malformation.
Among younger individuals (35 years and younger), the most common cause of sudden cardiac death is due to a congenital cardiac malformation (C). The most common reason is hypertrophic cardiomyopathy, while congenital coronary anomalies are also frequently found in these cases.
Incorrect:
Sudden cardiac death in individuals older than 35 years is most frequently caused by atherosclerotic coronary artery disease, which can include MI (A, B). AS is not a frequent cause of sudden cardiac death, and individuals can still participate in select activities in mild-to-moderate AS (D), though no participation in sports is recommended in severe AS.

92. Correct: D. prior use of NSAIDs.
A preparticipation sports evaluation should include a thorough patient history and cardiac evaluation. However, prior use of NSAIDs is not a critical component of the cardiovascular history, as these agents do not have a substantial impact on cardiac function (D). However, chronic use of NSAIDs should be further investigated to determine the reason for NSAID use and assess risk of adverse effects, such as GI conditions.
Incorrect:
A thorough cardiovascular history should include questions related to prior detection of a heart murmur (A); any instances of excessive, unexpected, or unexplained dyspnea (B); or reports of chest pain or discomfort with exertion (C). A thorough family history of cardiac events should also be evaluated.

93. Correct: A. an innocent flow murmur.
A physiological or innocent flow murmur is best characterized by a grade 1 to 3/6 early to midsystolic murmur that is heard best at the left sternal murmur that softens or disappears when changing from supine or sitting to a standing position (A). These murmurs are associated with no symptoms, and individuals can participate fully in sports.
Incorrect:
Mitral valve incompetence or regurgitation is characterized by a grade 1 to 4/6 high-pitched blowing systolic murmur that often extends beyond S$_2$ (B). Aortic regurgitation is characterized as a grade 1 to 3/4 high-pitched blowing diastolic murmur (C). MVP is best described as a grade 1 to 3/6 late systolic crescendo murmur with a honking quality (D).

94. Correct: D. a mid- to late-systolic murmur.
MVP is best described as a grade 1 to 3/6 late systolic crescendo murmur with a honking quality that is best heard at apex (D). The murmur usually follows a midsystolic click (D). With standing, the click moves forward earlier into systole.

Incorrect:
An early to midsystolic, crescendo-decrescendo murmur most likely describes a physiological murmur (A). A pansystolic murmur is most likely due to MR and is described as a high-pitched blowing murmur often extending beyond S$_2$ (B). A low-pitched, diastolic rumble best describes mitral stenosis (C).

95. Correct: D. Marfan syndrome.
Marfan syndrome is a rare connective tissue disorder that is associated with a higher risk for MVP (D). This can be due to valve leaflets that become floppy and do not close tightly, allowing blood to leak backward across the valve.
Incorrect:
Rheumatic fever is more likely to be associated with the development of MR with also a possibility of mitral stenosis (A). Though Kawasaki disease can have cardiac effects, this does not usually lead to the development of MVP (C). Rheumatoid arthritis is not typically associated with the development of heart defects (B).

96. Correct: B. a midsystolic click.
MVP is characterized by a grade 1 to 3/6 late-systolic crescendo murmur with a honking quality. The murmur typically follows a midsystolic click (B). The click will move forward into earlier systole upon standing from the sitting or supine position.
Incorrect:
An opening snap is often found with mitral stenosis (A). A paradoxical splitting of the second heart sound can be due to a condition that delays aortic closure, such as left bundle branch block (C). A fourth heart sound can be heard during diastolic dysfunction (D), such as AS.

97. Correct: D. encouragement of a regular program of aerobic activity
Those who present with MVP alone can be managed with standard of care with no restriction on physical activities and require no pharmacotherapy (D).
Incorrect:
With MVP alone, standard of care with encouragement for regular aerobic exercise is the usual course of management. Beta blockers are not warranted to control palpitations (C), and there is no need for fluid restriction (B). Activity restriction can be considered when MVP presents with other conditions, such as moderate regurgitation or dysrhythmias (A).

98. Correct: A. stenotic.
A stenotic heart valve will fail to open to its normal orifice (A).
Incorrect:
When a heart valve fails to close appropriately, it is called incompetent (B), and will lead to regurgitation of blood to the previous chamber or blood vessel (D). A sclerotic heart valve will have a benign thickening or calcification of the leaflets that can prevent proper closure of the valve (C).

99. Correct: B. incompetent.
When a heart valve fails to close appropriately, it is called incompetent (B) and will lead to regurgitation of blood to the previous chamber or blood vessel.
Incorrect:
An incompetent heart valve can result in blood regurgitation (D). A stenotic heart valve will fail to open to its normal orifice (A). A sclerotic heart valve will have a benign thickening or calcification of the leaflets that can prevent proper closure of the valve (C).

100. Correct: B. echocardiogram.
An echocardiogram is typically the initial diagnostic test once a potentially pathological murmur is detected (B). This procedure can allow visualization of the heart and its structures while pumping, as well as evaluate blood flow through the valves and into each chamber and blood vessel. Depending on what needs to be observed, several types of echocardiogram can be used, including a transthoracic echocardiogram or transesophageal echocardiogram.
Incorrect:
An echocardiogram is typically the first diagnostic procedure as it is low cost and noninvasive. A CT scan would not be considered at initial evaluation due to its high cost but can be considered when additional visualization is needed beyond the echocardiogram (B). A pulmonary artery angiography would not be an initial diagnostic procedure due to its highly invasive nature (C). A ventilated perfusion scan is typically used to evaluate blood flow in the lungs and not for cardiac anomalies (A).

101. Correct: B. localized diastolic with little radiation.
Mitral stenosis is characterized by a grade 1 to 3/4 low-pitched late diastolic murmur that is localized and heard best at the apex (B). This type of murmur is nearly always rheumatic in origin.
Incorrect:
MR is characterized as a high-pitched blowing systolic murmur that radiates to the axilla (D). AS is characterized by a harsh systolic murmur that radiates to the carotids (C). A physiological murmur is best described as early to midsystolic and is audible over the precordium, but there is no radiation beyond the precordium (A).

102. Correct: A. systolic with radiation to the axilla.
Mitral valve incompetency, or MR, is best described as a grade 1 to 4/6 high-pitched blowing systolic murmur that radiates to the axilla (A). The murmur is decreased with standing.
Incorrect:
A diastolic murmur with little radiation best describes mitral stenosis (B). A ventricular septal defect can lead to a regurgitant systolic murmur that is occasionally holosystolic and usually localized (D). Mitral stenosis can result in a low-pitched late diastolic murmur, often with an opening snap (C).

103. Correct: D. left ventricular hypertrophy.
Individuals with a prolonged history of AS are at greater risk of left ventricular hypertrophy due to the extra effort needed by the left ventricle to maintain cardiac output while working against the defective stenotic valve (D).
Incorrect:
AS is not associated with the development of right bundle branch block (A) or extreme axis deviation (B). Right atrial enlargement can result from a defect in the tricuspid valve, such as tricuspid regurgitation or stenosis (C).

104. Correct: A. bradycardia.
Signs and symptoms of endocarditis can include a broad range of findings. However, bradycardia, or a slow heart rate, is not considered a common finding with this condition (A).
Incorrect:
Common signs and symptoms of endocarditis include fever, chills, new or altered heart murmur, fatigue, Osler's nodes (i.e., painful raised red lesions commonly found on the hands and feet) (B), hematuria (C), and petechiae (D).

105. Correct: B. blood culture.
For a patient suspected of endocarditis, the initial test should include a blood culture to detect and identify the organism (B).
Incorrect:
A chest x-ray will offer little help in the diagnosis of bacterial endocarditis but can be used to rule out other conditions that have similar symptoms, such as pneumonia (C). Myocardial biopsy would not be warranted during the initial workup for suspected endocarditis (D). Positive or negative findings on urine culture will not be helpful in helping to confirm a diagnosis of bacterial endocarditis (A).

106. Correct: B. a 54-year-old woman with a prosthetic aortic valve
Antimicrobial prophylaxis should be limited only to those at highest risk of infective endocarditis. These would include individuals with a prior history of bacterial endocarditis, those with prosthetic cardiac valves or prosthetic material used for cardiac valve repair, and certain congenital heart diseases. Among the patients listed, the 54-year-old with a prosthetic heart valve would be the only individual who should receive antimicrobial prophylaxis (B).
Incorrect:
Antibacterial prophylaxis should only be considered for those at highest risk of infective endocarditis and is not routinely recommended for individuals undergoing a genitourinary, GI, or dental procedures. Prophylaxis is also not warranted for individuals with MVP (A), cardiomyopathy (C), or a history of coronary artery bypass graft (D).

107. Correct: B. a 55-year-old man who was diagnosed with a physiological murmur during childhood

A physiological murmur during childhood is associated with no increased risk for the development of infective endocarditis (B).

Incorrect:

Those at highest risk include individuals with a prior history of bacterial endocarditis (C), those with prosthetic cardiac valves or prosthetic material used for cardiac valve repair, and certain congenital heart diseases (A). Injection drug use also increases the risk of infective endocarditis, possibly due to repeated episodes of bacteremia (D).

108. Correct: A. AS.

The patient's symptoms are consistent with low cardiac output. The presence of a grade 3/6 crescendo-decrescendo systolic murmur is most consistent with AS (A).

Incorrect:

Aortic regurgitation is characterized by a grade 1 to 3/4 high-pitched blowing diastolic murmur (B). Anemia can sometimes be associated with an innocent murmur, which is characterized by a grade 1 to 3/6 early to midsystolic murmur that softens or disappears when standing (C). Mitral stenosis is identified by a grade 1 to 3/4 low-pitched late diastolic murmur that is localized (D).

109. Correct: B. a result of a congenital defect.

AS found in younger adults is most frequently caused by a congenital defect, such as bicuspid valve (B). The impact of AS on sports participation will depend on the degree of stenosis, with full participation allowed with mild stenosis.

Incorrect:

In older adults found with AS, there is a greater likelihood that the condition is caused by an acquired form such as by calcification (C) or a result of rheumatic fever (A). AS is not typically related to an atrial septal defect (D).

110. Correct: D. prior rheumatic fever.

Acquired AS is typically found in older adults and can be the result of a number of conditions, including calcification or rheumatic disease (D). For younger patients, AS is more likely caused by congenital bicuspid valve.

Incorrect:

Acquired AS is not associated with a history of pulmonary embolism (A), COPD (B), or type 2 diabetes (C).

111. Correct: A. periodic monitoring with ECG and echocardiogram.

Active management is typically not needed in patients with mild AS who have normal cardiac output and excellent exercise tolerance. Periodic monitoring of the condition should be performed to detect any changes in the condition and whether further intervention is needed (A).

Incorrect:

For the AS patient with no symptoms and normal cardiac output, surgical (B, C) or pharmacological management (D) is not warranted.

112. Correct: C. becomes softer when the patient moves from supine to standing

A physiological or innocent murmur is best characterized as a grade 1 to 3/6 early to midsystolic murmur with no radiation beyond the precordium. The murmur typically softens or disappears with standing (C).

Incorrect:

A physiological murmur occurs early to midsystole and not late in systole (A). It is noted over the entire precordium but not beyond that (B). S_1 and S_2 are normally intact with this type of murmur (D).

113. Correct: D. participation will depend on the degree of ventricular enlargement.

For patients with MR, the level of sports participation will depend on the size and function of the left ventricle (D). With normal size and function, full participation can be done. With mild left ventricle enlargement but normal function at rest, selected participation is recommended. No sports participation should be allowed in the presence of enlarged left ventricle or any left ventricle dysfunction observed at rest.

Incorrect:

Participation in sports will depend on the size and function of the left ventricle (A). Sports participation should be avoided only when the left ventricle is enlarged or if there is left ventricle dysfunction at rest (B). MR should not lead to atrial atrophy (C).

114. Correct: B. hypertrophic cardiomyopathy.

Hypertrophic cardiomyopathy is characterized by a harsh midsystolic crescendo-decrescendo murmur that can increase when moving from a sitting to standing position (B). The condition is a leading cause of sudden cardiac death among younger participants in sports, and participation should be determined on an individual basis according to the degree of ventricular function and symptoms.

Incorrect:

A physiological murmur (C) and AS (A) will soften or disappear upon standing rather than get louder. Similarly, a Still's murmur will soften or disappear when going from supine to sitting or standing (D).

115. Correct: C. azithromycin

For those at high risk of bacterial endocarditis and antimicrobial prophylaxis is warranted, several agents can be considered. In the presence of penicillin allergy, choices can include clindamycin, cephalexin, azithromycin (C), or clarithromycin.

Incorrect:

Dicloxacillin would not be recommended due to cross-allergy with penicillin (B). Erythromycin (A) and the fluoroquinolones (i.e., ofloxacin) (D) are not recommended agents for prophylaxis.

116. Correct: B. about as loud as the S_1 heart sound.
Systolic murmurs are graded from 1 (barely audible) to 6 (audible with stethoscope off the chest). A grade 3 heart murmur is about as loud as S_1 or S_2 (B).
Incorrect:
Grade 2 systolic murmur is softer than the S_2 heart sound (A). A grade of 4 or higher is usually accompanied by a thrill (C). The grade does not take into account localization or radiation of the sound (D).

117. Correct: B. it is a presystolic sound.
The S_3 heart sound is a marker of ventricular overload, systolic dysfunction, or both. The heart sound is typically heard in early diastole but can also hook onto the back of S_2 and is not heard in presystole (B).
Incorrect:
S_3 is typically heard in early diastole (A) and noted in the presence of ventricular overload (C) and/or systolic dysfunction. It produces a low pitch that is heard best with the bell of the stethoscope (D).

118. Correct: B. It is noted in the presence of poorly controlled HTN.
The S_4 heart sound is a marker of poor diastolic function and is most often found in poorly controlled HTN or recurrent myocardial ischemia (B). Treatment of the underlying condition can resolve the S_4 heart sound.

Incorrect:
The S_4 heart sound can develop with poorly controlled HTN. S_4 is not a permanent finding as treatment of the underlying condition can resolve it (A). The sound is typically heard late in diastole (C) and is described as a soft, low-pitched sound heard best with the bell of the stethoscope (D).

119. Correct: C. a 21-year-old athlete who reported postexertional syncope
Hypertrophic cardiomyopathy is a leading cause of sudden cardiac death in younger athletes. Common signs include dyspnea, chest pain, and postexertional syncope. The 21-year-old most likely fits this description (C).
Incorrect:
Angina and chest tightness reported by an older adult is less likely to be due to hypertrophic cardiomyopathy, but another cause should be investigated. This can include ACS as well as AS, likely from calcification of the leaflets (A). Individuals with mitral stenosis typically undergo a protracted latency period followed by a gradual decrease in exercise tolerance, reflecting a decrease in cardiac output (B). Injection drug users are at high risk of bacterial endocarditis that can present with signs of fever, chills, fatigue, shortness of breath, and aching joints and muscles (D).

Respiratory Disorders 7

Asthma

Overview

Asthma is a common chronic disorder of the lower airways that is complex and characterized by variable and recurring symptoms, airflow obstruction, bronchial hyperresponsiveness, and underlying inflammation. Risk factors contributing to the development of asthma include atopy, genetic-environmental interactions, and viral respiratory tract infections.

Clinical Presentation

In well-controlled asthma (the goal of therapy), cough and wheeze are noted infrequently, and activity tolerance is normal. Signs and symptoms consistent with asthma, especially with poor asthma control and flare, include recurrent cough, wheeze, shortness of breath and/or chest tightness, and evidence of air trapping (Table 7-1). This is due to variable airflow obstruction and bronchial hyperresponsiveness triggered by underlying airway inflammation and subsequent air trapping. Symptoms often occur or worsen at night or with exercise, during viral respiratory infections, or with exposure to aeroallergens and/or pulmonary irritants (such as first- or secondhand smoke). The history and measurement of lung function, such as forced expiratory volume at 1 second (FEV_1) or peak expiratory flow rate (PEFR) are essential and more reliable than the physical examination.

Diagnostic Testing

Spirometry is needed to make the diagnosis of asthma; the anticipated results consistent with asthma include an increase in FEV_1 12% or greater from baseline post short-acting beta-2 agonist (SABA) use. A peak flow meter should be used for monitoring, not for diagnosing, asthma. Objective evaluation for airflow obstruction should be conducted with every asthma-related visit. Other conditions to consider when making the differential diagnosis can include alpha-1 antitrypsin deficiency, upper respiratory tract infection, gastroesophageal reflux, bronchiolitis, chronic obstructive pulmonary disease (COPD), chronic sinusitis, cystic fibrosis, heart failure, pulmonary embolism, and sarcoidosis (Box 7-1).

Treatment

Upon initial diagnosis of asthma, the level of asthma severity is assessed to guide decisions regarding therapeutic interventions. Asthma severity is classified as intermittent or persistent and is determined by the level of impairment and level of risk. Persistent asthma is subdivided as mild, moderate, and severe. Follow-up visits are essential for the assessment of asthma control. Use of the Asthma Control Test (ACT) can provide a simple and convenient way for the health-care provider to evaluate how well asthma symptoms were controlled in the past 4 weeks; the ACT is available online. This questionnaire includes five questions that are rated from 0 to 5, with total scores ranging from 0 to 25. A score of less than 20 indicates asthma is not well controlled. The level of control (well controlled, not well controlled, or very poorly controlled) determines whether to maintain therapy, step up therapy, or step down therapy (Figs. 7-1 to 7-3).

One of the major goals of asthma therapy is to reduce impairment, including prevention of chronic asthma symptoms, require infrequent use of SABAs, and maintain normal or near-normal lung function and be able to participate in normal activity levels. Well-controlled asthma will allow full participation in sports, exercise, and recreational activities as well as result in minimal impact on normal activities of daily living (ADLs).

Another major goal is to reduce risk, including the likelihood of future asthma attacks, progressive decline in lung function (or, for children, reduced lung growth), and death rates from poor asthma control.

This is achieved with a variety of therapies where the patient and family are actively engaged in the treatment plan, including drug therapy, environmental control, reducing asthma comorbidity, and appropriate immunization.

Medications are typically divided into two groups in asthma care: controller medications are used for regular maintenance treatment to reduce airway inflammation, control symptoms, and prevent exacerbations; reliever (rescue) medications are provided for as-needed relief of breakthrough symptoms including worsening asthma or exacerbations. Reduction of impairment and asthma exacerbation is achieved by the prevention of symptoms, use of a SABA limited to 2 or fewer days/week (unless for prevention of exercise-induced bronchospasm), maintenance of normal pulmonary function and normal activity levels, and meeting patients' and families' expectations of and satisfaction with asthma care.

Because of the wide range of asthma medications currently available, the nurse practitioner (NP), patient, and family can work together to find a lifestyle and treatment regimen that provide optimal care with minimal to no adverse medication effects. Inhalers are an integral part of asthma treatment, and the correct use of these medications is essential in optimizing patient outcomes. Unfortunately, up to 70% to 80% of patients do not use their inhalers correctly, thus emphasizing the need to educate patients on the proper administration of these medications.

Reliever Medications

Relievers consist of SABAs, short-acting muscarinic agents (SAMAs), and oral corticosteroids (OCSs). SABAs include albuterol (Proventil®, Ventolin®, ProAir®), levalbuterol (Xopenex®), and pirbuterol (Maxair®). SABAs are the drug of choice for all age groups to relieve acute asthma symptoms including bronchoconstriction and to prevent exercise-induced bronchoconstriction. SABA use more than 2 days/week (unless for prevention of exercise-induced bronchospasm) indicates a need for better

TABLE 7-1 Clinical Findings in Asthma or Chronic Obstructive Pulmonary Disease Flare

CONDITION	PHYSICAL EXAMINATION FINDINGS
Lower airway disease with resulting air trapping as found in asthma or chronic obstructive pulmonary disease flare or poor disease control	■ Hyperresonance on thoracic percussion ■ Decreased tactile fremitus wheeze (expiratory first, inspiratory later) ■ Prolonged expiratory phase of forced exhalation ■ Low diaphragms ■ Increased anterior-posterior diameter ■ Reduction in forced expiratory volume at 1 second (FEV_1) or peak expiratory flow rate (early finding) ■ Reduction in arterial oxygen saturation (Sao_2) (later finding)

Source: Mangione S. *Physical Diagnosis Secrets*. 3rd ed. Philadelphia, PA: Mosby Elsevier; 2012.

BOX 7-1 Making the Diagnosis: Is It Asthma?

■ Symptoms consistent with asthma
  ■ Recurrent cough, wheeze, shortness of breath, and/or chest tightness
  ■ Symptoms occur or worsen at night, exercise, viral respiratory infections, aeroallergens, and/or pulmonary irritants (such as secondhand smoke)
■ Airflow obstruction is at least partially reversible
  ■ Increase in FEV_1 ≥12% from baseline
  ■ Increase in FEV_1 ≥12% post short-acting beta-2 agonist
■ Consider the diagnosis of asthma and perform spirometry if any of these indicators are present. These indicators are not diagnostic by themselves, but the presence of multiple key indicators increases the probability of the diagnosis of asthma.
■ Spirometry is needed to make the diagnosis of asthma.
  ■ A peak flow meter is used for monitoring, not for diagnosing, asthma.

Sources: National Heart, Lung, and Blood Institute. Expert Panel Report 4 (EPR-4) Working Group: National Asthma Education and Prevention Program Coordinating Committee. https://www.nhlbi.nih.gov/about/advisory-and-peer-review-committees/national-asthma-education-and-prevention-program-coordinating/EPR4-working-group

Global Initiative for Asthma. Global Strategy for Asthma Management and Prevention, 2018. https://ginasthma.org

	Intermittent Asthma	Management of Persistent Asthma in Individuals Ages 12+ Years				
Treatment	STEP 1	STEP 2	STEP 3	STEP 4	STEP 5	STEP 6 ■
Preferred	PRN SABA	Daily low-dose ICS and PRN SABA or PRN concomitant ICS and SABA▲	Daily and PRN combination low-dose ICS-formoterol▲	Daily and PRN combination medium-dose ICS-formoterol▲	Daily medium-high dose ICS-LABA + LAMA and PRN SABA▲	Daily high-dose ICS-LABA + oral systemic corticosteroids + PRN SABA
Alternative		Daily LTRA* and PRN SABA or Cromolyn,* or Nedocromil,* or Zileuton,* or Theophylline,* and PRN SABA	**Daily medium-dose ICS and PRN SABA** or **Daily low-dose ICS-LABA, or daily low-dose ICS + LAMA,▲ or daily low-dose ICS + LTRA,* and PRN SABA** or **Daily low-dose ICS + Theophylline* or Zileuton,* and PRN SABA**	Daily medium-dose ICS-LABA or daily medium-dose ICS + LAMA, and PRN SABA▲ or Daily medium-dose ICS + LTRA,* or daily medium-dose ICS + Theophylline,* or daily medium-dose ICS + Zileuton,* and PRN SABA	Daily medium-high dose ICS-LABA or daily high-dose ICS + LTRA,* and PRN SABA	
		Steps 2–4: Conditionally recommend the use of subcutaneous immunotherapy as an adjunct treatment to standard pharmacotherapy in individuals ≥ 5 years of age whose asthma is controlled at the initiation, build up, and maintenance phases of immunotherapy▲			Consider adding Asthma Biologics (e.g., anti-IgE, anti-IL5, anti-IL5R, anti-IL4/IL13)**	

Assess Control

- First check adherence, inhaler technique, environmental factors,▲ and comorbid conditions.
- **Step up** if needed; reassess in 2–6 weeks
- **Step down** if possible (if asthma is well controlled for at least 3 consecutive months)

Consult with asthma specialist if Step 4 or higher is required. Consider consultation at Step 3.

Control assessment is a key element of asthma care. This involves both impairment and risk. Use of objective measures, self-reported control, and health care utilization are complementary and should be employed on an ongoing basis, depending on the individual's clinical situation.

Abbreviations: ICS, inhaled corticosteroid; LABA, long-acting beta$_2$-agonist; LAMA, long-acting muscarinic antagonist; LTRA, leukotriene receptor antagonist; SABA, inhaled short-acting beta$_2$-agonist

▲ Updated based on the 2020 guidelines.

* Cromolyn, Nedocromil, LTRAs including Zileuton and montelukast, and Theophylline were not considered for this update, and/or have limited availability for use in the United States, and/or have an increased risk of adverse consequences and need for monitoring that make their use less desirable. The FDA issued a Boxed Warning for montelukast in March 2020.

** The AHRQ systematic reviews that informed this report did not include studies that examined the role of asthma biologics (e.g. anti-IgE, anti-IL5, anti-IL5R, anti-IL4/IL13). Thus, this report does not contain specific recommendations for the use of biologics in asthma in Steps 5 and 6.

■ Data on the use of LAMA therapy in individuals with severe persistent asthma (Step 6) were not included in the AHRQ systematic review and thus no recommendation is made.

FIGURE 7-1 Stepwise approach for managing asthma in patients 12 years of age and older.

National Heart, Lung, and Blood Institute; National Institutes of Health; U.S. Department of Health and Human Services. 2020 Focused Updates to the Asthma Management Guidelines: A Report from the National Asthma Education and Prevention Program Coordinating Committee Expert Panel Working Group.

Components of Severity		Classification of Asthma Severity (Youths ≥12 years of age or adults)			
		Intermittent	Persistent		
			Mild	Moderate	Severe
Impairment **Normal FEV₁/FVC:** 8–19 yr 85% 20–39 yr 80% 40–59 yr 75% 60–80 yr 70%	Symptoms	≤2 days/week	>2 days/week but not daily	Daily	Throughout the day
	Nighttime awakenings	≤2x/month	3–4x/month	>1x/week but not nightly	Often 7x/week
	Short-acting beta₂-agonist use for symptom control (not prevention of EIB)	≤2 days/week	>2 days/week but not daily and no more than 1x on any day	Daily	Several times per day
	Interference with normal activity	None	Minor limitation	Some limitation	Extremely limited
	Lung function	• Normal FEV₁ between exacerbations • FEV₁ >80% predicted • FEV₁/FVC normal	• FEV₁ ≥80% predicted • FEV₁/FVC normal	• FEV₁ = >60% but <80% predicted • FEV₁/FVC reduced 5%	• FEV₁ <60% predicted • FEV₁/FVC reduced 5%
Risk	Exacerbations requiring oral systemic corticosteroids	0–1/year (see note)	≥2/year (see note) ⟶		
		Consider severity and interval since last exacerbation. Frequency and severity may fluctuate over time for patients in any severity category. Relative annual risk of exacerbations may be related to FEV₁.			
Recommended Step for Initiating Therapy		Step 1	Step 2	Step 3	Step 4
				and consider short course of oral systemic corticosteroids	
		In 2–6 weeks, evaluate level of asthma control that is achieved, and adjust therapy accordingly.			

Key: FEV₁, forced expiratory volume in 1 second; FVC, forced vital capacity; ICU, intensive care unit.

Notes:

- The stepwise approach is meant to assist, not replace, the clinical decision making required to meet individual patient needs.
- Level of severity is determined by assessment of both impairment and risk. Assess impairment domain by patient's/caregiver's recall of previous 2–4 weeks and spirometry. Assign severity to the most severe category in which any feature occurs.
- At present, there are inadequate data to correspond frequencies of exacerbations with different levels of asthma severity. In general, more frequent and intense exacerbations (e.g., requiring urgent, unscheduled care, hospitalization, or ICU admission) indicate greater underlying disease severity. For treatment purposes, patients who had ≥2 exacerbations requiring oral systemic corticosteroids in the past year may be considered the same as patients who have persistent asthma, even in the absence of impairment levels consistent with persistent asthma.

FIGURE 7-2 Classifying asthma severity in youths ≥12 years of age and adults.
Expert Panel Report 3: Guidelines for the Diagnosis and Management of Asthma. https://www.nhlbi.nih.gov/guidelines/asthma/asthgdln.pdf.

CLINICAL CONCEPT

A poor perception of symptoms, use of two or more canisters of SABA per month, and prior severe exacerbations are important risk factors for death from asthma and should influence decisions regarding asthma management (Box 7-2).

asthma control via improvement of airway inflammation. Frequent use of asthma rescue medications is a surrogate marker for poorly controlled airway inflammation. SABAs work by binding to the β₂-adrenergic receptor, causing smooth muscle relaxation and bronchodilation. This effect occurs within 3 to 5 minutes. Compared with albuterol and pirbuterol, levalbuterol, a single isomer of the racemic albuterol, is often reported as better tolerated than the other SABAs, because of greater bronchodilation at a reduced dose.

Ipratropium bromide (Atrovent®) is a SAMA, also known as an anticholinergic, indicated for the treatment of moderate or severe asthma exacerbations to provide additional bronchodilation to albuterol. This inhaled agent inhibits muscarinic cholinergic receptors, reducing vagal tone in the airway, decreasing mucus secretion, and blocking reflex bronchoconstriction because of reflex esophagitis.

Systemic corticosteroids are considered reliever medications and are indicated in moderate to severe asthma exacerbations and when there is partial response to initial SABA use in exacerbations. Oral prednisone is preferred over a parenteral corticosteroid form. These medication forms are equally effective, and there is less risk

Components of Control		Classification of Asthma Control (Youths ≥12 years of age or adults)		
		Well Controlled	**Not Well Controlled**	**Very Poorly Controlled**
Impairment	Symptoms	≤2 days/week	>2 days/week	Throughout the day
	Nighttime awakenings	≤2x/month	1–3x/week	≥4x/week
	Interference with normal activity	None	Some limitation	Extremely limited
	Short-acting beta₂-agonist use for symptom control (not prevention of EIB)	≤2 days/week	>2 days/week	Several times per day
	FEV₁ or peak flow	>80% predicted/ personal best	60%–80% predicted/ personal best	<60% predicted/ personal best
	Validated Questionnaires			
	ATAQ	0	1–2	3–4
	ACQ	≤0.75*	≥1.5	N/A
	ACT	≥20	16–19	≤15
Risk	Exacerbations	0–1/year	≥2/year (see note)	
		Consider severity and interval since last exacerbation.		
	Progressive loss of lung function	Evaluation requires long-term follow-up care.		
	Treatment-related adverse effects	Medication side effects can vary in intensity from none to very troublesome and worrisome. The level of intensity does not correlate to specific levels of control but should be considered in the overall assessment of risk.		
Recommended Action for Treatment		• Maintain current step • Regular follow-ups every 1–6 months to maintain control • Consider step down if well-controlled for at least 3 months	• Step up 1 step and reevaluate in 2–6 weeks • For side effects, consider alternative treatment options	• Consider short course of oral systemic corticosteroids • Step up 1–2 steps and reevaluate in 2 weeks • For side effects, consider alternative treatment options

FEV_1 or peak flow

*ACQ values 0.76-1.4 are indeterminant regarding well-controlled asthma.
Key: EIB, exercise–induced bronchospasm; FEV_1, forced expiratory volume in 1 second.

Notes:

- The stepwise approach is meant to assist, not replace, the clinical decision making required to meet individual patient needs.

- The level of control is based on the most severe impairment or risk category. Assess impairment domain by patient's recall of previous 2-4 weeks and by spirometry/or peak flow measures. Symptom assessment for longer periods should reflect a global assessment, such as inquiring whether the patient's asthma is better or worse since the last visit.

- At present, there are inadequate data to correspond frequencies of exacerbations with different levels of asthma control. In general, more frequent and intense exacerbations (e.g., requiring urgent, unscheduled care, hospitalization, or ICU admission) indicate poorer disease control. For treatment purposes, patients who had ≥2 exacerbations requiring oral systemic corticosteroids in the past year may be considered the same as patients who have not-well-controlled asthma, even in the absence of impairment levels consistent with not-well-controlled asthma.

- Validated Questionnaires for the impairment domain (the questionnaires do not assess lung function or the risk domain)
  ATAQ = Asthma Therapy Assessment Questionnaire© (See sample in "Component 1: Measures of Asthma Assessment and Monitoring.")
  ACQ = Asthma Control Questionnaire© (user package may be obtained at www.qoltech.co.uk or juniper@qoltech.co.uk)
  ACT = Asthma Control Test™ (See sample in "Component 1: Measures of Asthma Assessment and Monitoring.")
  Minimal Important Difference: 1.0 for the ATAQ; 0.5 for the ACQ; not determined for the ACT.

- Before step up in therapy:
  – Review adherence to medication, inhaler technique, environmental control, and comorbid conditions.
  – If an alternative treatment option was used in a step, discontinue and use the preferred treatment for that step.

FIGURE 7-3 Assessing asthma control in youths ≥12 years of age and adults.
Expert Panel Report 3: Guidelines for the Diagnosis and Management of Asthma. 2007. https://www.nhlbi.nih.gov/guidelines/asthma/asthgdln.pdf.

of serious adverse reaction with OCSs. The duration of OCSs for asthma is usually 5 to 10 days. There is no need to taper the dose for a 5- to 7-day course and usually no need to taper for a 10-day course, particularly if a patient is on an inhaled corticosteroid (ICS) (Table 7-2). A taper should be considered for patients taking systemic corticosteroids for 14 days or longer to avoid recurrence of inflammation and prevent cortisol deficiency, as the gradual dose reduction allows recovery from corticosteroid-induced adrenal suppression.

Controller Medications

The backbone of persistent asthma therapy is medications that prevent and/or reduce airway inflammation to gain and maintain asthma control. Asthma controllers consist of ICSs, leukotriene modifiers (LTMs), ICSs combined with long-acting beta-2 agonists (ICSs/LABAs), and the long-acting muscarinic antagonists (LAMAs). ICSs (i.e., fluticasone [Flovent®], mometasone [Asmanex®], budesonide [Pulmicort®], others) have proved to be most effective in preventing airway inflammation and are the preferred controller treatment for all levels of persistent asthma. Risks of asthma exacerbations are reduced with routine use of ICSs. Improvement in asthma control is seen within 2 to 8 days of starting an ICS. Local adverse effects include sore throat, oral candidiasis, and hoarseness. Rinsing the mouth after ICS use and use of a spacer can help reduce these effects. Primary care providers are often poorly informed as to the relative potency of a given ICS and prescribe too low a dose for the asthma severity; this is a major issue and impacts the attainment of asthma control (Table 7-3). Systemic absorption varies among the ICS agents but is usually quite modest and not clinically significant. Use the lowest ICS dose possible, and implement corticosteroid-sparing strategies.

For children taking ICSs, there is a potential but small risk of delayed growth as well as a potential for a small reduction (0.2 cm) in final adult height in select children, such as those at highest risk for asthma

---

BOX 7-2 Risk Factors for Death From Asthma

■ Infants less than 1 year old
■ Previous severe exacerbations
■ ≥Two hospitalizations in past year
■ ≥Three emergency department visits in past year
■ Hospitalization/emergency department visit in past month
■ More than two canisters SABA (200 puffs per canister) use per month
■ Poor patient perception of symptoms
■ Lack of written asthma care plan
■ Sensitivity to *Alternaria*
■ Low socioeconomic status
■ Recreational drug use
■ Major psychosocial problems
■ Comorbidities (cardiovascular disease, other chronic lung disease)
■ Urban residence
■ Major psychological disease
■ Current or recent withdrawal from systemic corticosteroids

Sources: *National Heart, Lung, and Blood Institute.* Expert Panel Report 3: Guidelines for the Diagnosis and Management of Asthma. *Washington, DC: U.S. Department of Health and Human Services. http://www.nhlbi.nih.gov/health-pro/guidelines/current/asthma-guidelines*

Global Initiative for Asthma. Global Strategy for Asthma Management and Prevention, 2018. https://ginasthma.org

---

TABLE 7-2 Relative Potency of Systemic Corticosteroids

Higher potency corticosteroids (equipotent doses)	Betamethasone, 0.6–0.75 mg Dexamethasone, 0.75 mg	Half-life 36 to 54 hours
Medium potency corticosteroids (equipotent doses)	Methylprednisolone, 4 mg Triamcinolone, 4 mg Prednisolone, 5 mg Prednisone, 5 mg	Half-life 18 to 36 hours
Lower potency (equipotent doses) corticosteroids	Hydrocortisone, 20 mg Cortisone, 25 mg	Half-life 8 to 12 hours

Source: *Facts & Comparisons. Philadelphia, PA: Wolters Kluwer Health. http://www.wolterskluwercdi.com/facts-comparisons-online/*

TABLE 7-3 Estimated Comparative Daily Doses for Inhaled Corticosteroid (ICS) Therapy in Patients 12 Years and Older

	LOW DAILY DOSE	MEDIUM DAILY DOSE	HIGH DAILY DOSE
Beclomethasone HFA	100 to 200 mcg	Greater than 200 to 400 mcg	Greater than 400 mcg
Budesonide DPI	200 to 400 mcg	Greater than 400 to 800 mcg	Greater than 800 mcg
Fluticasone propionate HFA	100 to 250 mcg	Greater than 250 to 500 mcg	Greater than 500 mcg
Fluticasone propionate DPI	100 to 250 mcg	Greater than 250 to 500 mcg	Greater than 500 mcg
Mometasone furoate	110 to 220 mcg	Greater than 220 to 440 mcg	Greater than 440 mcg
Triamcinolone acetonide	400 to 1000 mcg	Greater than 1000 to 2000 mcg	Greater than 2000 mcg

Source: Global Initiative for Asthma. Global Strategy for Asthma Management and Prevention, 2018. https://ginasthma.org

adverse effects. However, this potential risk is well balanced by the effectiveness of these medications. Interpretations of study results evaluating linear growth in childhood asthma are difficult because of the unknown influence from the uncontrolled disease itself versus the treatment.

An LTM (less commonly called a leukotriene receptor antagonist [LTRA]), such as montelukast (Singulair®), is used to control asthma by inhibiting the inflammatory actions of leukotrienes. This medication class is indicated as an alternative to ICS in mild persistent asthma and as an add-on therapy to ICS in moderate and severe persistent asthma. However, LTM use results in only about 50% of the anti-inflammatory effect of an ICS. This drug class is most often used as an add-on therapy when asthma is not well controlled with an ICS only.

LABAs, including salmeterol (Serevent®) and formoterol (Foradil®), have a pharmacodynamic profile identical to SABAs, but with a significantly different pharmacokinetic profile. LABAs improve symptoms, improve lung function, reduce exacerbations, and enhance the anti-inflammatory action of corticosteroids. Adding a LABA to an ICS is the preferred treatment for moderate and severe asthma when disease control cannot be achieved with the use of an ICS alone; a LABA should not be used without an ICS in asthma treatment.

LAMAs, such as tiotropium, can be used as an add-on therapy for individuals with a history of asthma flares. These agents are generally well tolerated and can improve lung function while increasing the time between flares despite use of ICS with LABA.

Mast cell stabilizers (cromolyn and nedocromil) are mentioned in some asthma guidelines; however, these agents are no longer available in the United States because of superior agents on the market. These are older inhalation agents that are safe, but inferior in potency to ICS and require multiple dosing daily. Theophylline is also mentioned; however, it is rarely used because there are superior agents now available and because of its significant drug-drug interaction potential, narrow therapeutic index, and requirement for periodic serological drug-level monitoring (Table 7-4).

Once asthma control is achieved and maintained, assess the patient at regular intervals and consider stepping down asthma therapy. Step-down asthma therapy should only be considered when asthma symptoms are well controlled and lung function has plateaued, demonstrated by an objective measure such as FEV_1 or PEFR, for at least 3 months. In addition, the step-down therapy is not advised during pregnancy, when traveling, and/or during active respiratory tract infection; these are all risks for worsening asthma control and flare. The patient and/or caregiver and family must agree to proceed with step-down therapy and be actively engaged in the process. At each step, the patient should be carefully evaluated for worsening asthma control; if this occurs, therapy should be intensified. Common examples of step-down therapy include lowering ICS dose and/or discontinuing use of LAMA.

Certain drug-drug interactions should be considered in patients with asthma. For those with hypertension, the use of beta blockers should be avoided, as these agents can mitigate the effects of LABAs or

CLINICAL CONCEPT

The LABA class previously received a boxed warning from the U.S. Food and Drug Administration (FDA) about increased death risk with LABA use in asthma, but that warning has been removed.

TABLE 7-4 Medications Used for Treating Patients With Asthma and Chronic Obstructive Pulmonary Disease (COPD)

MEDICATION	MECHANISM OF ACTION	INDICATION	COMMENT
Inhaled short-acting beta-2 agonists (SABAs) Albuterol (Proventil®, Ventolin®, ProAir®), pirbuterol (Maxair®)	SABA: Bronchodilation via activation of beta-2 receptor site	SABA: Reliever drug; treatment of acute asthma and COPD symptoms.	Onset of action = 15 minutes. *Used prn.*
Inhaled levalbuterol (Xopenex®) (SABA) Inhaled short-acting muscarinic agents (SAMAs) ipratropium (Atrovent®)	SAMA: Muscarinic antagonist; yielding bronchodilation	SAMA: Reliever drug for COPD; add-on for asthma exacerbation.	Onset of action = 30 minutes. Duration 4 to 6 hours. *Used prn.*
Inhaled long-acting bronchodilators Long-acting beta-2 agonists (LABAs) Salmeterol (Serevent®), formoterol (Foradil®), indacaterol (Onbrez®), others	LABA: Bronchodilation through stimulation of receptor site beta-2	LABA: Controller drug; treatment and prevention of bronchospasm in asthma and COPD.	LABA: Onset of action 1 hour (15 to 30 minutes for formoterol). Duration of action 12 hours. Not to be used as monotherapy in asthma. *Used on a set schedule, not prn.*
Inhaled long-acting muscarinic agents (LAMAs) Tiotropium (Spiriva®), aclidium (Pressair®), others	LAMA: Muscarinic antagonist; yielding bronchodilation	LAMA: In asthma and COPD, prevention of bronchospasm and minimizing airway inflammation.	Consistent use minimizes risk of asthma flare, COPD exacerbation. *Used on a set schedule, not prn.*
Inhaled corticosteroids (ICSs) Mometasone (Asmanex®), fluticasone (Flovent®), budesonide (Pulmicort®), beclomethasone (Qvar®), ciclesonide (Alvesco®), others	Block late-phase activation to allergen, inhibit inflammatory cell migration and activation	Controller drug, preferred treatment for persistent asthma to prevent and control inflammation. In COPD, routine use recommended with FEV_1 less than 50% predicted and/or with recurrent exacerbations, albeit with a modestly increased pneumonia risk.	Need consistent use to be helpful. Cornerstone medication of most asthma levels. *Used on a set schedule, not prn.*
Oral leukotriene modifier (LTM) (montelukast [Singulair®])	Inhibit action of inflammatory mediator (leukotriene) by blocking select receptor sites	Controller drug, prevention of inflammation in asthma.	Less effective than inhaled corticosteroids. Particularly effective add-on medication with ICS use and with allergic rhinitis. In mild persistent asthma, an alternative, although not preferred. *Used on a set schedule, not prn.*

Continued

TABLE 7-4 Medications Used for Treating Patients With Asthma and Chronic Obstructive Pulmonary Disease (COPD)—cont'd

MEDICATION	MECHANISM OF ACTION	INDICATION	COMMENT
Systemic corticosteroids, orally or parenterally Prednisone, prednisolone, dexamethasone, others	Inhibit eosinophilic action and other inflammatory mediators	Treatment of acute inflammation such as in asthma flare or COPD exacerbation.	Oral route preferred whenever possible. Indicated in treatment of acute asthma flare or COPD exacerbated to reduce inflammation. In higher dose and with longer therapy (more than 2 weeks), adrenal suppression may occur. No taper needed if use is short term (less than 10 days) and at lower dose (prednisone, 40 to 60 mg/day or less).
Inhaled mast cell stabilizers Cromolyn sodium (Intal®), nedocromil (Tilade®)	Halts degradation of mast cells and release of histamine and other inflammatory mediators	Controller drug, prevention of inflammation in asthma.	No longer available in United States due to poor sales, not safety issues. Need consistent use to be helpful. Less effective than other controller therapies.
Oral theophylline	Mild bronchodilator via nonphosphodiesterase inhibitor. Possible mild anti-inflammatory effect	Prevention of bronchospasm in asthma and COPD.	Narrow therapeutic index drug with numerous potential drug interactions. Monitor carefully for toxicity by checking drug levels and clinical presentation.
Oral phosphodiesterase-4 inhibitors Roflumilast (Daliresp®)	Not well defined; thought to be because of the effects of increased intracellular cAMP in lung cells	Indicated as a treatment to reduce the risk of COPD exacerbations in patients with severe COPD associated with chronic bronchitis and a history of exacerbations. Not recommended for use in asthma.	Is not a bronchodilator and is not indicated for the relief of acute bronchospasm. *Used on a set schedule, not prn.*

Sources: *Global Initiative for Asthma. Global Strategy for Asthma Management and Prevention, 2018. https://ginasthma.org*
Global Initiative for Chronic Obstructive Lung Disease (GOLD). 2020 Global Strategy for Prevention, Diagnosis and Management of COPD. https://goldcopd.org/gold-reports/

SABAs. Beta blockers can also exacerbate bronchial symptoms via increased bronchial obstruction and airway reactivity.

Asthma Medications Requiring Specialty Referral

Several monoclonal antibodies are available for the treatment of allergic asthma that is not controlled by recommended treatment regimens (e.g., high-dose ICS/LABA with or without LAMA). Omalizumab (Xolair®) is a humanized monoclonal antibody indicated for moderate to severe persistent allergic asthma uncontrolled on ICS. The patient usually has poorly controlled asthma with recurrent exacerbations and quality of life limitations, despite optimal asthma treatment. Mepolizumab (Nucala®) and reslizumab (Cinquair®) are both interleukin-5 (IL-5) antagonist monoclonal antibodies indicated as add-on therapy for severe asthma with an eosinophilic phenotype. Omalizumab and mepolizumab are given as subcutaneous injection every

2 to 4 weeks, while reslizumab is administered as an IV infusion every 4 weeks. The use of these medications requires specialized evaluation prior to initiation and ongoing monitoring during their use.

Allergic immunotherapy is another recommendation for asthma treatment in multiple treatment guidelines. Numerous well-documented studies have shown it to be an effective treatment for asthma, improving lung function, where there is an allergic contribution that triggers asthma episodes.

ASSESSMENT AND TREATMENT OF ASTHMA FLARE

Overview

An asthma exacerbation can occur in individuals with a preexisting diagnosis of asthma or as the initial presentation of asthma. Common causes for asthma flares or exacerbations are aeroallergen exposure, viral respiratory tract infections, and nonadherence to controller medications. It is important to identify triggers and develop a plan for avoiding or minimizing them. The patient should have an individualized asthma action plan to guide care during an exacerbation. Severe exacerbations can occur at all asthma severity levels.

Clinical Presentation

An asthma flare is characterized by a progressive increase in symptoms that can include dyspnea, cough, wheezing, or chest tightness and is associated with decreased lung function. In asthma exacerbations, breath sounds are often reduced, and hyperinflation is present because of significant air trapping.

> **CLINICAL CONCEPT**
> A chest x-ray is not required when evaluating a person with an asthma flare unless there is a suspicion of pneumonia.

Diagnostic Testing

Diagnostic testing should evaluate any change in lung function, either with FEV_1 or PEFR, and compare with values from the patient's previous lung function or predicted values. The frequency of symptoms can also be an important measure to determine the onset of a flare, though in some patients, symptoms can be perceived poorly, and patients can experience a substantial decline in lung function without a change in symptoms. The physical examination can be relatively normal during asthma and does not correlate well with asthma severity. Routine measurement of arterial blood gas is not needed.

Treatment

A severe exacerbation can be life-threatening, and patients who deteriorate rapidly should be advised to promptly see their health-care provider or a facility that provides emergency access for patients with acute asthma. When a patient presents with an asthma flare in primary care, the goals are to rapidly relieve airflow obstruction and hypoxemia, address the underlying inflammatory condition, and prevent relapse. Approaches to treat an acute exacerbation in primary care include the following (GINA guidelines):

■ For mild to moderate exacerbations, repeated administration of inhaled SABA up to 4 to 10 puffs every 20 minutes for the first hour. Depending on response after the first hour, SABA dosing can then be adjusted from 4 to 10 puffs every 3 to 4 hours to 6 to 10 puffs every 1 to 2 hours. There is no difference in effectiveness when SABA is administered via metered dose inhaler (MDI) and spacer, a dry powder inhaler (DPI), or a nebulizer. However, the most cost-effective approach is the use of albuterol with an MDI and spacer.

■ Controlled or titrated oxygen therapy should be used to maintain oxygen saturation at 93% to 95% (94% to 98% for children 6 to 11 years old).

■ OCSs should be given promptly at a dose of prednisolone 1 mg/kg/day (usually with a maximum dose of 50 mg/day) in adults and 1 to 2 mg/kg/day (maximum dose of 40 mg/day) in children 6 to 11 years old. OCSs should be continued for 5 to 7 days. Oral administration is preferred over IV administration as it is as effective, quicker to administer, less invasive, and less expensive.

■ Controller medication dosage (e.g., ICS with or without LABA) should be increased for the next 2 to 4 weeks. If not on a controller medication, an ICS-containing therapy should be initiated. In adults with acute deterioration, high-dose ICS for 7 to 14 days can be equally effective as a short course of OCS therapy.

■ Antibiotics are not recommended without evidence of bacterial lung infection.

■ Sedation should be avoided during an acute asthma flare as anxiolytic and hypnotic drugs can cause respiratory depression, increasing the risk of asthma-related death.

A severe asthma episode is characterized by talking in single words (rather than phrases); sitting hunched forward; having respiratory rate greater than 30/minute, pulse rate greater than 120 bpm, oxygen saturation less than 90%, and PEF 50% or less than predicted or best. These patients should be immediately transferred to an acute care facility while promptly administering SABA, oxygen therapy, and OCS.

Discussion Sources

Cloutier MM, Dixon AE, Krishnan JA, et al. Managing asthma in adolescents and adults: 2020 asthma guideline update from the National Asthma Education and Prevention Program. *JAMA.* 2020;324:2301–17. https://jamanetwork.com/journals/jama/article-abstract/2773482

Cox L, Nelson H, Lockey R, et al. Allergen immunotherapy: a practice parameter third update. *J Allergy Clin Immunol.* 2011;127(1):S1–S55. https://www.aaaai.org/Aaaai/media/MediaLibrary/PDF%20Documents/Practice%20and%20Parameters/Allergen-immunotherapy-Jan-2011.pdf

Global Initiative for Asthma. Global Strategy for Asthma Management and Prevention, 2018. https://ginasthma.org

Guilbert TW, Mauger DT, Allen, DB, et al. Growth of preschool children at high risk for asthma 2 years after discontinuation of fluticasone. *J Allergy Clin Immunol.* 2011;128:956–963.

National Heart, Lung, and Blood Institute. *Expert Panel Report 3: Guidelines for the Diagnosis and Management of Asthma.* Washington, DC: U.S. Department of Health and Human Services. http://www.nhlbi.nih.gov/health-pro/guidelines/current/asthma-guidelines

Thomas A, Lemanske RF Jr, Jackson DJ. Approaches to stepping up and stepping down care in asthmatic patients. *J Allergy Clin Immunol.* 2011;128(5):915–924.

QUESTIONS

1. Which of the following best describes asthma?

   A. intermittent airway inflammation with occasional bronchospasm

   B. a disease of bronchospasm that leads to airway inflammation

   C. chronic airway inflammation with superimposed bronchospasm

   D. relatively fixed airway constriction

2. The patient you are evaluating is having an asthma flare. You have assessed that his condition is appropriate for office treatment. You expect to find the following on physical examination:

   A. tripod posture.

   B. inspiratory crackles.

   C. increased vocal fremitus.

   D. hyperresonance on thoracic percussion.

3. A 44-year-old man has a long-standing history of moderate persistent asthma that is normally well controlled by fluticasone with salmeterol (Advair®) via metered-dose inhaler, one puff twice a day, and the use of albuterol one to two times a week as needed for wheezing. Three days ago, he developed a sore throat, clear nasal discharge, body aches, and a cough with a small amount of white sputum production. In the past 24 hours, he has had intermittent wheezing that necessitated the use of albuterol, two puffs every 3 hours, which produced partial relief. Your next most appropriate action is to obtain a:

   A. chest radiograph.

   B. measurement of oxygen saturation (SaO_2).

   C. spirometry measurement.

   D. sputum smear for white blood cells (WBCs).

4. You examine Jane, a 24-year-old woman who has an acute asthma flare following a 3-day history of upper respiratory tract symptoms (clear nasal discharge, dry cough, no fever). She has a history of moderate persistent asthma that is in good control and an acceptable peak expiratory flow (PEF). She is using budesonide (Pulmicort®) and albuterol as directed and continues to have difficulty with coughing and wheezing. At home, her PEF is 55% of personal best. In the office, her forced expiratory volume at 1 second (FEV_1) is 65% of predicted. Her medication regimen should be adjusted to include:

   A. oral theophylline.

   B. inhale salmeterol (Serevent®) via MDI.

   C. oral prednisone.

   D. oral montelukast (Singulair®).

5. For Jane in question 4, the NP also considers prescribing:

   A. a 10-day course of oral amoxicillin.

   B. a 5-day course of oral azithromycin.

   C. a 14-day course of levofloxacin.

   D. no antimicrobial therapy.

6. Which of the following describes a PEF meter?

   A. should only be used in the presence of a medical professional

   B. provides a convenient method to check expiratory air flow at home

   C. is as accurate as spirometry

   D. should not be used more than once daily

7. Which of the following is most accurate regarding the use of a chest x-ray during an acute asthma flare?

   A. Chest radiograph should be performed with each asthma flare.

   B. Chest radiograph should be performed during and following resolution of the flare.

   C. Chest radiograph should be avoided as it can further exacerbate a flare.

   D. Chest radiograph should be limited to those with signs of respiratory tract infection (e.g., fever, congested cough).

8. A 36-year-old man with asthma also needs antihypertensive therapy. Which of the following products should you avoid prescribing?

   A. hydrochlorothiazide

   B. propranolol

   C. amlodipine

   D. enalapril

9 to 12. Which of the following is consistent with the presentation of asthma that is not well controlled? (Yes or No)

   _____ **9.** A troublesome nocturnal cough more than two nights per week

   _____ **10.** Need for albuterol to relieve shortness of breath more than twice a week

   _____ **11.** Evidence of consolidation on chest x-ray

   _____ **12.** Two or more exacerbations/year requiring OCSs

13. The cornerstone of moderate persistent asthma controller drug therapy is the use of:

   A. oral theophylline.

   B. inhaled mast cell stabilizers.

   C. inhaled SABAs.

   D. ICSs.

14. Sharon is a 29-year-old woman with moderate persistent asthma. She has a prescription for an ICS that she does not use, stating, "I'm finding that the albuterol works better." Currently she uses about two albuterol metered-dose inhalers per month, "that keeps my cough and wheeze under control." She is requesting a prescription refill. You consider that:

   A. her asthma is well controlled, and albuterol use can continue.

   B. excessive albuterol use is a risk factor for asthma death.

   C. her asthma is not well controlled, and salmeterol (Serevent®) should be added to relieve broncho-spasm and reduce her albuterol use.

   D. her asthma has better control with albuterol than ICSs.

15. In the treatment of asthma, an LTM should be used as a:

A. controller to prevent bronchospasm.

B. controller to inhibit inflammatory responses.

C. reliever to treat acute bronchospasm.

D. reliever to treat inflammation.

16. Which of the following is not a risk for asthma death?

A. hospitalization or an emergency department visit for asthma in the past month

B. current use of systemic corticosteroids or recent withdrawal from systemic corticosteroids

C. difficulty perceiving airflow obstruction or its severity

D. rural residence

17. An 18-year-old high school senior presents, asking for a letter stating that he should not participate in gym class because he has asthma. The most appropriate action is to:

A. write the note because gym class participation could trigger asthma symptoms.

B. excuse him from outdoor activities only to avoid pollen exposure.

C. assess his level of asthma control and make changes in his treatment plan if needed so he can participate.

D. write a note excusing him from gym until his follow-up examination in 2 months.

18. You see a 34-year-old man with moderate persistent asthma who has an asthma flare, and a regimen of oral prednisone is prescribed for 7 days. Which of the following is true?

A. A taper is needed for prednisone therapy lasting longer than 4 days.

B. A taper is not needed if the prednisone regimen is usually for 14 days or less.

C. A taper is not needed regardless of duration of prednisone therapy.

D. A taper is needed if the patient is taking concomitant ICSs.

19. After ICS is initiated, improvement in control is usually seen:

A. on the first day of use.

B. within 2 to 8 days.

C. in about 3 to 4 weeks.

D. in about 1 to 2 months.

20. Compared with albuterol, levalbuterol (Xopenex®) has:

A. a different mechanism of action.

B. the potential ability to provide greater bronchodilation with a lower dose.

C. an anti-inflammatory effect similar to that of an ICS.

D. a contraindication to use in elderly patients.

21. Which of the following is consistent with the use of ICSs for a child with asthma?

A. The potential but small risk of delayed growth with ICSs is well balanced by their effectiveness.

B. ICSs should be used only if an LTM fails to control asthma.

C. Permanent growth stunting is consistently noted in children using ICSs.

D. An LTM is equal in therapeutic effect to the use of a LABA.

22. A potential adverse effect from ICS use is:

A. oral candidiasis.

B. tachycardia.

C. gastrointestinal upset.

D. insomnia.

23. Clinical findings characteristic of poorly controlled asthma include all of the following except:
    A. a recurrent spasmodic cough that is worse at night.
    B. recurrent shortness of breath and chest tightness with exercise.
    C. a congested cough that is worse during the day.
    D. wheezing with and without associated respiratory infections.

24. Which of the following best describes the mechanism of action of SABAs?
    A. reducer of inflammation
    B. inhibition of secretions
    C. modification of leukotriene action
    D. smooth muscle relaxation

25. Regarding the use of LABAs, which of the following is false?
    A. LABAs enhance the anti-inflammatory action of corticosteroids.
    B. Use of LABAs is associated with an increase in the risk of asthma death.
    C. Adding a LABA to an ICS can be considered to enhance asthma control.
    D. LABAs should not be used as monotherapy to relieve bronchospasms in asthma.

26. Which of the following is the therapeutic objective of using inhaled SAMA?
    A. as an anti-inflammatory
    B. to increase vagal tone in the airway
    C. as a bronchodilator
    D. as a mucolytic

27. Which of the following is true regarding the use of systemic corticosteroids in the treatment of asthma?
    A. Frequent short bursts are preferred over daily ICSs.
    B. The OCS should be started at days 3 to 4 of the asthma flare for optimal effect.
    C. The oral route is preferred over parenteral therapy in most patients.
    D. The adult dose to treat an asthma flare should not exceed the equivalent of prednisone 40 mg daily.

28. Concerning LABA use, the NP realizes that LABAs:
    A. are recommended as a first-line therapy in mild intermittent asthma.
    B. have a significantly different pharmacodynamic profile when compared to SABAs.
    C. have the most rapid onset of action across the drug class.
    D. should be added to therapy only when ICS use does not provide adequate asthma control.

29. Which of the following statements is false regarding the use of biologics in the management of asthma?
    A. Their use is recommended for patients with mild persistent asthma to prevent asthma flares.
    B. The medications are administered via injection or IV infusion.
    C. Labeled indications are generally for patients with asthma that is poorly controlled despite active standard treatment.
    D. Special evaluation is required prior to its use, and ongoing monitoring is needed during use.

30. Immunotherapy is recommended for use in patients:
    A. with well-controlled asthma and infrequent exacerbations.
    B. with allergic-based asthma.
    C. with moderate persistent asthma who are intolerant of ICSs.
    D. with poorly controlled asthma demonstrated by SABA use multiple times per day.

31 to 35. Answer the following questions True or False.

_____ **31.** Most prescribers are well-versed in the relative potency of ICSs and prescribe an appropriate dose for the patient's clinical presentation.

_____ **32.** Approximately 80% of the dose of an ICS is systemically absorbed.

_____ **33.** An LTM and an ICS are interchangeable clinically because both groups of medications have equivalent anti-inflammatory effects.

_____ **34.** LAMAs can be used to reduce the risk of asthma flares.

_____ **35.** Due to safety concerns, mast cell stabilizers are no longer available.

36. Common findings during an asthma flare can include all of the following except:

A. increased dyspnea.

B. increased chest tightness.

C. increased sputum production.

D. increased cough.

37 to 39. Answer the following questions True or False regarding treatment of an asthma exacerbation for an adult in the primary care setting.

_____ **37.** A SABA given via a nebulizer is more effective compared to an MDI.

_____ **38.** During a severe asthma flare, OCSs should be given once the patient is transferred to an acute care facility.

_____ **39.** Oxygen therapy should be titrated to maintain oxygen saturation greater than 96%.

40. During an acute asthma exacerbation, the dose of controller therapy should be increased:

A. for 7 days.

B. for 2 to 4 weeks.

C. for 3 months.

D. indefinitely.

41. For a patient presenting with an acute exacerbation, the goals of treatment include all of the following except:

A. restore lung function to baseline.

B. relieve airflow obstruction.

C. address underlying inflammation.

D. relieve hypoxemia.

For answers and rationales, see end of chapter.

Chronic Obstructive Pulmonary Disease

Overview

COPD is a preventable and treatable disease with significant extrapulmonary effects that can contribute to the severity in individual patients. The pulmonary component is characterized by airflow limitation that is not fully reversible; this differs from asthma. The airflow limitation is usually progressive and associated with an abnormal inflammatory response of the lung to noxious particles or gases. Continued inhalation of the problematic substance worsens airway changes and contributes to COPD's progression.

Genetic factors are likely contributors as well, given that not everyone who has a significant smoking history develops COPD. Patients with the disease typically present for care in the fifth and sixth decades of life, usually after having symptoms for more than a decade. The majority of patients with COPD have significant concurrent disease, including cardiovascular disease, that contributes to mortality and morbidity.

CLINICAL CONCEPT

The major COPD risk factor is tobacco smoking; however, chronic exposure to air pollution and biomass fuel exposure through burning of wood, coal, and kerosene are major contributors to the disease's development in select populations.

The pathophysiology of COPD involves inflammation and narrowing of the peripheral airways that lead to the characteristic decrease in lung function, typically measured by FEV_1. Emphysema, or destruction of alveoli, is a common finding in COPD and contributes to airflow limitation and decreased gas transfer. The loss of small airways in addition to airway narrowing is a significant contributor to airflow limitation and air trapping.

Clinical Presentation

The clinical presentation of COPD typically includes symptoms of recurrent dyspnea, chronic cough, and persistent sputum production as a result of airway inflammation, smooth muscle constriction, and altered lung mechanics. Historically, the hallmark symptom of chronic bronchitis is a chronic productive cough, whereas for emphysema it is shortness of breath. However, these terms are not used as part of the Global Initiative for Obstructive Lung Disease (GOLD) guidelines for the diagnosis and management of COPD, in favor of recognition of the concurrence of the two conditions in most patients with a COPD diagnosis.

COPD diagnosis should be considered in any patient with progressive dyspnea, chronic cough or sputum production, and/or a history of risk factors, such as tobacco use. Dyspnea is typically persistent and progressive and is worse with exercise and exacerbations. Cough can be intermittent and is often unproductive. However, the cough is often productive and chronic. Spirometry should then be performed and is required to make the clinical diagnosis of COPD.

Diagnostic Testing

COPD is characterized by a decrease in the ratio of forced expiratory volume at 1 second (FEV_1) to forced vital capacity (FVC). The FEV_1:FVC ratio is considered the most sensitive indicator of early airflow limitation. The presence of a postbronchodilator FEV_1:FVC less than 70% confirms persistent airflow obstruction. The degree of spirometric abnormality generally reflects the severity of COPD. However, symptoms often do not correlate well with objective measurements and/or patients may deny symptoms and meet diagnostic criteria for COPD. The COPD Assessment Test (CAT) is a useful adjunct to symptoms, spirometry abnormality, and identification of risk for exacerbations for the assessment of the level of COPD severity and for choosing pharmacological therapy (Tables 7-5 to 7-8). This questionnaire includes eight simple questions that are rated from 0 to 5, with total scores ranging from 0 to 40 (http://www.catestonline.org/). A score of less than 10 indicates a low impact of COPD on an individual's well-being and daily life. Other conditions to consider when making the differential diagnosis include alpha-1 antitrypsin deficiency, bronchitis, chronic cough, congestive heart failure, emphysema, and pulmonary embolism.

Treatment

Nonpharmacological Therapy

The goals of treating COPD are to reduce COPD symptoms, reduce frequency and severity of COPD exacerbations, and improve exercise tolerance and health status. Nonpharmacological achievement of these goals includes smoking cessation and avoidance of other pulmonary irritants. Because 80% of all cases of COPD can be attributed directly to tobacco use, encouraging the patient to stop smoking is an important clinical goal.

TABLE 7-5 Classification of Severity of Airflow Limitation in Chronic Obstructive Pulmonary Disease Based on Postbronchodilator FEV_1

IN PATIENTS WITH FEV_1/FVC LESS THAN 0.70:

GOLD 1	Mild	$FEV_1 \geq 80\%$ predicted
GOLD 2	Moderate	$50\% \leq FEV_1 < 80\%$ predicted
GOLD 3	Severe	$30\% \leq FEV_1 < 50\%$ predicted
GOLD 4	Very severe	$FEV_1 < 30\%$ predicted

Source: *Global Initiative for Chronic Obstructive Lung Disease (GOLD)*. 2020 Global Strategy for Prevention, Diagnosis and Management of COPD. *https://goldcopd.org/gold-reports/*

TABLE 7-6 Global Initiative for Chronic Obstructive Pulmonary Disease (GOLD) Pharmacological Therapy for Stable COPD*

PATIENT GROUP	INITIAL THERAPY	COMMENTS
A Low risk for exacerbation Less symptoms One or fewer moderate exacerbations per year mMRC 0 to 1; CAT less than 10	Short-acting or long-acting bronchodilator such as SA beta-2 agonist (albuterol [Ventolin® HFA] SABA) *or* LA muscarinic antagonist (tiotropium [Spiriva®]) *or* LA beta$_2$-agonist (salmeterol [Serevent®] LABA)	After initial evaluation, continue, stop, or try alternative class of bronchodilator, dependent on patient response.
B Low risk for exacerbation More symptoms One or fewer moderate exacerbations per year mMRC greater than or equal to 2; CAT greater than or equal to 10	Long-acting bronchodilator *And/or* LA muscarinic antagonist (LAMA; tiotropium [Spiriva®]) *or* LA beta-2 agonist (LABA; salmeterol [Serevent®])	For patients with severe breathlessness, initial therapy with two bronchodilators from different drug classes (LABA and LAMA) can be considered.
C High risk for exacerbation Less symptoms Two or more exacerbations per year (one or more leading to hospitalization) mMRC 0 to 1; CAT less than 10	LA muscarinic antagonist (LAMA; tiotropium [Spiriva®])	Patients with persistent exacerbations may benefit from adding a second long-acting bronchodilator or a combination of LABA and ICS.
D High risk for exacerbation More symptoms Two or more exacerbations per year (one or more leading to hospitalization) mMRC greater than or equal to 2; CAT greater than or equal to 10	LA muscarinic antagonist (LAMA; tiotropium [Spiriva®])	LAMA/LABA can be used as initial therapy in patients with greater dyspnea and/or exercise limitation. LABAs/ICSs can also be considered in patients with history of asthma or with eosinophil count greater than or equal to 300 cells/mm^3. In patients with exacerbations despite LABA/ICS or LABA/LAMA/ICS, chronic bronchitis, and severe to very severe airflow limitation, the addition of PDE-4 inhibitor can be considered.**

CAT, COPD Assessment Test; COPD, chronic obstructive pulmonary disease; ICS, inhaled corticosteroid; LA, long acting; mMRC, modified Medical Research Council dyspnea score; SA, short acting.

*Medications mentioned are representative of drug class, not priority medications.

**Roflumilast (Daliresp®) (phosphodiesterase 4 [PDE4] inhibitor), therapeutic option to reduce the risk of COPD exacerbations in patients with severe and very severe COPD associated with chronic bronchitis who have a history of exacerbations. Not a bronchodilator and not indicated for relief of acute bronchospasm. Adverse effects include unintended weight loss and changes in mood, thinking, and behavior. Not to be used with theophylline.

Source: Global Initiative for Chronic Obstructive Lung Disease (GOLD). 2020 Global Strategy for Prevention, Diagnosis and Management of COPD. https://goldcopd.org/gold-reports/

TABLE 7-7 Global Initiative for Chronic Obstructive Pulmonary Disease (GOLD) Pharmacological Therapy for Follow-up Treatment

ADDRESSING DYSPNEA (PERSISTENT BREATHLESSNESS OR EXERCISE LIMITATION):

■ If on long-acting bronchodilator monotherapy:	■ Addition of second bronchodilator (or switch inhaler device or treatment)
■ If on long-acting beta-2 agonist (LABA)/inhaled corticosteroid (ICS):	■ Addition of long-acting muscarinic antagonist (LAMA) for triple therapy, or switch to LABA/LAMA (if original indication for ICS was inappropriate)

ADDRESSING PERSISTENT EXACERBATIONS:

■ If on long-acting bronchodilator monotherapy:	■ Escalate to LABA/LAMA or LABA/ICS
■ If on LABA/LAMA therapy:	■ Escalate to LABA/LAMA/ICS (if eosinophil count greater than 100 cells/mm^3) or add roflumilast or azithromycin (if blood eosinophil count less than 100 cells/mm^3)
■ If on LABA/ICS:	■ Add a LAMA for triple therapy or switch to LABA/LAMA
■ If on LABA/LAMA/ICS:	■ Add roflumilast (especially if FEV$_1$ less than 50% predicted and chronic bronchitis), or add a macrolide, or consider stopping ICS

Source: Global Initiative for Chronic Obstructive Lung Disease (GOLD). 2020 Global Strategy for Prevention, Diagnosis and Management of COPD. https://goldcopd.org/gold-reports/

TABLE 7-8 Combined Assessment of Chronic Obstructive Pulmonary Disease

PATIENT GROUP	CHARACTERISTIC	SPIROMETRIC CLASSIFICATION	EXACERBATIONS PER YEAR	CAT
A	Low risk fewer symptoms	GOLD 1–2	Less than or equal to 1	Less than 10
B	Low risk more symptoms	GOLD 1–2	Less than or equal to 1	≥10
C	High risk fewer symptoms	GOLD 3–4	≥2	Less than 10
D	High risk more symptoms	GOLD 3–4	≥2	≥10

Source: Global Initiative for Chronic Obstructive Lung Disease (GOLD). 2020 Global Strategy for Prevention, Diagnosis and Management of COPD. https://goldcopd.org/gold-reports/

Despite symptoms, many patients continue to smoke. Raising the issue of smoking cessation at every visit and offering assistance with this is an important part of the ongoing care of the person with COPD. Counseling about general hygiene should also be provided, including information on minimizing exposure to passive smoking, allergens, and air pollution, and advice on hydration, nutrition, and avoiding respiratory tract infection.

Patients at all severity levels of COPD benefit from exercise training and pulmonary rehabilitation. The goal of this intervention is to improve quality of life, decrease symptoms, and increase physical participation in ADLs. Pulmonary rehabilitation can also reduce the symptoms of anxiety and depression among patients with COPD. Components of a pulmonary rehabilitation program include reversing the effects of physical deconditioning, social isolation, weight loss, muscle wasting, and altered mood often noted with COPD. Improvements in exercise tolerance and symptoms of dyspnea and fatigue can be sustained even after a single pulmonary rehabilitation program. Issues of funding, access, and lack of provider and patient knowledge about this helpful intervention make pulmonary rehabilitation an underused, although helpful, intervention in patients with COPD.

Immunizations

Patients with COPD are at higher risk of a number of vaccine-preventable diseases, and immunization should be encouraged. Routine seasonal influenza vaccination is recommended to be given annually for patients with COPD. A variety of influenza vaccines can be used, but the live-attenuated influenza vaccine (LAIV) administered via a nasal spray should not be used in individuals with airway disease. Pneumococcal vaccination is currently recommended for all adults 65 years and older as well as younger adults considered at higher risk of disease, including cigarette smokers, people with asthma, and anyone with COPD. (See Chapter 2 for further information on influenza and pneumococcal immunization.)

Pharmacology in Chronic Obstructive Pulmonary Disease Treatment

Pharmacological therapy can be helpful in minimizing COPD symptoms and preventing exacerbations. Unfortunately, there is no definitive evidence that any available COPD medication will alter the long-term decline in lung function.

> **CLINICAL CONCEPT**
> The backbone of pharmacological therapy for COPD is a variety of inhaled bronchodilators.

Patients at all levels of COPD severity should be prescribed a SABA for acute relief of symptoms such as cough and bronchospasm. Routine use of daily long-acting bronchodilators is begun at the moderate severity stage COPD (group B) and continued throughout very severe COPD (group D). Options include a LAMA (tiotropium [Spiriva®], aclidium bromide [Tudorza Pressair®]), a LABA (salmeterol [Serevent®], formoterol [Foradil®], arformoterol [Brovana®], indacaterol [Onbrez®]), or a SAMA agent dosed several times daily (ipratropium [Atrovent®]). With COPD therapy, the long-acting bronchodilators are preferred over the multidosed, short-acting agents because of superior effectiveness and convenience. The choice between the long-acting bronchodilators depends on availability of the drug, the patient's individual response in terms of symptom relief, and adverse effects. Combining bronchodilators of different pharmacological classes can improve therapeutic efficacy. In addition, LAMA use in COPD offers a complementary method of bronchodilation to the LABAs as well as reduces the risk of COPD exacerbation.

Routine use of ICSs in COPD patients with FEV_1 less than 60% predicted improves symptoms and lung function and reduces the frequency of exacerbations. Combination ICS/long-acting bronchodilator is more effective in improving symptoms and lung function and reducing exacerbations in patients with moderate to very severe COPD than either individual component. ICS use can increase the risk of certain adverse effects, such as pneumonia; initiating ICS therapy in COPD should occur only after careful consideration of benefits versus risks.

Long-term treatment with OCSs is not recommended due to the well-recognized risk, including negative impact on bone density, increase in blood pressure and glucose, and gastropathy risk. Theophylline is less effective and less well tolerated than other bronchodilators. There is a risk for drug–drug interactions, and it has a narrow therapeutic index. Roflumilast (Daliresp®) is a phosphodiesterase-4 inhibitor indicated for the reduction of exacerbations in severe and very severe COPD.

Long-term oxygen therapy for patients with COPD should be considered, particularly as the disease progresses, or when a patient presents with advanced disease (Table 7-9). The goal of therapy is to ensure

---

TABLE 7-9 Long-Term Oxygen Therapy in Chronic Obstructive Pulmonary Disease

Goal	To ensure adequate oxygen delivery to vital organs by increasing baseline Pao_2 at rest to ≥60 mm Hg at sea level or producing SaO_2 ≥90%, or both
Indications to initiate long-term (>15 hr/day) oxygen therapy	Pao_2 less than 55 mm Hg *or* SaO_2 less than 88% with or without hypercapnia Pao_2 55 to 69 mm Hg *or* SaO_2 89% in the presence of cor pulmonale, right heart failure, or polycythemia (hematocrit greater than 56%)

Source: Global Initiative for Chronic Obstructive Lung Disease (GOLD). 2020 Global Strategy for Prevention, Diagnosis and Management of COPD. https://goldcopd.org/gold-reports/

adequate oxygen delivery to the vital organs by increasing the baseline PaO_2 at rest to 60 mm Hg or greater at sea level, or producing SaO_2 equal to or greater than 90%, or both. In patients with chronic respiratory failure, oxygen therapy administered more than 15 hours per day has been shown to increase survival. Many patients wait until they are breathless, then attempt to correct this with as-needed oxygen use and fail to achieve maximum benefit; these benefits include not only improved overall well-being but also increased survival.

ASSESSMENT AND TREATMENT OF CHRONIC OBSTRUCTIVE PULMONARY DISEASE EXACERBATION

Overview

Exacerbations of respiratory symptoms that necessitate intensified therapy are important clinical events in COPD. The most common causes of an exacerbation are infection, usually viral and less commonly bacterial in origin, of the tracheobronchial tree and air pollution, but the cause of at least one-third of severe exacerbations cannot be identified. COPD exacerbations contribute to disease progression, with many patients unable to return lung function to the preexacerbation state.

Clinical Presentation

An exacerbation is characterized by acute worsening of respiratory symptoms that requires additional therapy. An exacerbation typically lasts 7 to 10 days but can last considerably longer with a prolonged time to recovery. Patients present with evidence of increased airway inflammation, mucus production, and air trapping, resulting in increased dyspnea. Other symptoms can include increased sputum purulence and volume along with increased cough and wheeze.

Diagnostic Testing

For a patient with a prior diagnosis of COPD, an exacerbation diagnosis can be suspected based on patient presentation, history of symptoms, and objective measure of airflow obstruction. However, respiratory symptoms can also worsen due to other conditions that are common among COPD patients, and clinical assessment should be performed to rule these out as a possible cause of symptoms. These conditions can include pneumonia, pneumothorax, pleural effusion, pulmonary embolism, and cardiac arrythmias. Because of the possibility of a concomitant pneumonia, a chest x-ray should be obtained when the patient presents with fever or unusually low SaO_2 or both; in the absence of these findings, a chest x-ray is not usually needed.

Treatment

Inhaled bronchodilators (beta-2 agonists or muscarinic antagonists or both) are effective for the treatment of COPD exacerbation. A SABA with or without a SAMA is the recommended first-line bronchodilator to treat an exacerbation, with a focus on limiting acute bronchospasm. Consideration should be given to adding a long-acting bronchodilator, such as a LABA or a LAMA or combined LABA/LAMA therapy, if the patient is not currently using one and adding an ICS to reduce the risk of future exacerbations. A systemic corticosteroid, with oral route preferred, such as prednisone 40 mg daily for 5 to 7 days, should be added; knowledge of the relative potency of these drugs is important for safe and effective clinical practice (see Table 7-3). Although a 10-day course of systemic corticosteroid therapy has been advised, recent study supports the efficacy and safety of a shorter 5-day course. Oxygen therapy can be considered for patients with hypoxemia and should be titrated to achieve a target saturation of 88% to 92%.

Antimicrobial therapy is not always needed as part of treatment of a COPD exacerbation because the cause can be nonbacterial in origin, such as an environmental problem or viral infection. Use of an antibiotic is likely indicated when symptoms of breathlessness and cough are accompanied by altered sputum characteristics that suggest bacterial infection, such as increased purulence or change in volume. Appropriate use of antimicrobials can shorten recovery time and reduce the risk of early relapse, treatment failure, and hospitalization duration. The duration of therapy should be 5 to 7 days, and the therapeutic choice should be dictated by antimicrobial coverage for the major bacterial pathogens involved in COPD exacerbation, while taking into account local patterns of bacterial resistance (Table 7-10).

Discussion Sources

Gilbert DN, Chambers HF, Eliopoulos GM, Saag MS, Pavia AT. *The Sanford Guide to Antimicrobial Therapy*. 50th ed. Sperryville, VA: Antimicrobial Therapy, Inc.; 2020.

Global Initiative for Chronic Obstructive Lung Disease (GOLD). *2020 Global Strategy for Prevention, Diagnosis and Management of COPD*. https://goldcopd.org/gold-reports/

TABLE 7-10 Etiology and Recommendations for Antimicrobial Therapy in Chronic Obstructive Pulmonary Disease (COPD) Exacerbations

ETIOLOGY	Viruses (20% to 50%) ■ Aside from infection, tobacco use, air pollution, and viruses common contributing factors Bacteria: ■ Causative bacterial pathogens (30% to 50%) include *Haemophilus influenzae, Haemophilus parainfluenzae, Streptococcus pneumoniae, Moraxella catarrhalis* ■ Less common pathogens include atypical pathogens, other gram-positive and gram-negative organisms
MILD TO MODERATE DISEASE	*Antimicrobial therapy usually not indicated.* If prescribed, consider using one of the following agents: ■ Amoxicillin ■ Doxycycline ■ Trimethoprim-sulfamethoxazole ■ Cephalosporin
SEVERE DISEASE (INCREASED DYSPNEA, INCREASED SPUTUM VISCOSITY/PURULENCE, AND INCREASED SPUTUM VOLUME) *Role of antimicrobial therapy debated even for severe disease*	Use one of the following agents: ■ Amoxicillin-clavulanate ■ Cephalosporin ■ Azithromycin ■ Clarithromycin ■ Fluoroquinolone with activity against drug-resistant *S pneumoniae* such as moxifloxacin, levofloxacin, others

Source: Gilbert DN, Chambers HF, Eliopoulos GM, Saag MS, Pavia AT. The Sanford Guide to Antimicrobial Therapy. 50th ed. Sperryville, VA: Antimicrobial Therapy, Inc.; 2020:37.

QUESTIONS

42. When discussing immunizations with a 67-year-old woman with COPD, you advise that she:

A. receive live attenuated influenza virus vaccine.

B. avoid immunization against influenza because of the risk associated with the vaccine.

C. receive inactivated influenza virus vaccine.

D. take an antiviral for the duration of the influenza season.

43 to 46. Indicate whether each statement is True or False.

_____ **43.** Seasonal influenza vaccination is recommended for household members of people with COPD.

_____ **44.** A 66-year-old woman with COPD ideally should receive an influenza vaccine specifically developed for use in older adults.

_____ **45.** People with COPD should not receive the pneumococcal vaccine until 65 years of age.

_____ **46.** A 52-year-old immunocompetent patient with COPD who receives the pneumococcal polysaccharide 23 vaccine (PPSV 23, Pneumovax) should get revaccinated in 5 years.

47. When used in treating COPD, ipratropium bromide (Atrovent®) is prescribed to achieve which of the following therapeutic effects?

A. increase mucociliary clearance

B. reduce alveolar volume

    C. bronchodilation

    D. mucolytic action

48. What is the desired therapeutic action of ICSs and LAMA therapy when used to treat COPD?

    A. reversal of fixed airway obstruction

    B. improvement of central respiratory drive

    C. reduction of airway inflammation

    D. mucolytic activity

49. A potential adverse effect of ICS therapy in COPD is:

    A. potential development of concomitant asthma.

    B. more rapid lung function decline.

    C. increased risk of pneumonia.

    D. more severe exacerbations.

50. Which is most consistent with the diagnosis of COPD?

    A. FEV_1:FVC ratio equal to or less than 0.70 after properly timed SABA use

    B. dyspnea on exhalation

    C. elevated diaphragms noted on x-ray

    D. polycythemia noted on complete blood cell count

51. The most effective nonpharmacological method to prevent exacerbations in patients with COPD is:

    A. weight loss for those with a body mass index (BMI) greater than 25 kg/m².

    B. to avoid exposure to children or day-care centers.

    C. brisk walking for at least 5 minutes three to five times a day as tolerated.

    D. to avoid exposure to pulmonary irritants, including active or passive exposure to cigarette smoke.

52. When managing patients with COPD who continue to smoke cigarettes, a discussion on the importance of smoking cessation should occur:

    A. at the initial diagnosis visit.

    B. with each COPD exacerbation.

    C. once ICS therapy is initiated.

    D. at every office visit.

53. According to the GOLD COPD guidelines, which of the following medications is indicated for use in all COPD stages?

    A. short-acting inhaled beta-2 agonist

    B. ICS

    C. phosphodiesterase-4 (PDE-4) inhibitor

    D. mucolytic

54. According to the GOLD COPD guidelines, the goal of ICS use in severe COPD is to:

    A. minimize the risk of repeated exacerbations.

    B. improve cough function.

    C. reverse alveolar hypertrophy.

    D. help mobilize secretions.

55. What is the recommended duration of OCS therapy during a COPD exacerbation?

    A. 5 to 7 days

    B. at least 10 days

C. 14 days

D. 28 days

56. Which of the following pathogens is among the most commonly implicated in a COPD exacerbation caused by respiratory tract infection?

A. *Legionella* species

B. *Streptococcus pyogenes*

C. respiratory tract viruses

D. *Staphylococcus aureus*

57. Which is the most appropriate choice of therapy in the treatment of an acute exacerbation in a 55-year-old man who has moderate COPD and who presents without fever or evidence of consolidation?

A. a 5-day course of oral levofloxacin

B. a 7-day course of oral amoxicillin

C. a 10-day course of oral doxycycline

D. antimicrobial therapy usually not indicated

58. Which is the most appropriate statement about therapy for a severe COPD exacerbation in a 52-year-old man?

A. A 5-day course of azithromycin should be prescribed.

B. A 10-day course of amoxicillin/clavulanate is advisable.

C. A 7-day course of trimethoprim-sulfamethoxazole (TMP-SMX) is recommended.

D. The role of antimicrobial therapy is debated, even for a severe exacerbation.

59. You see a 67-year-old man with very severe (GOLD 4) COPD who asks, "When should I use my home oxygen?" You respond:

A. "As needed when short of breath."

B. "Primarily during sleep hours."

C. "Preferably during waking hours."

D. "For at least 15 hours a day."

60. With a COPD exacerbation, a chest x-ray should be obtained:

A. routinely in all patients.

B. when attempting to rule out a concomitant pneumonia.

C. if sputum volume is increased.

D. when work of breathing is increased.

61. Which of the following best describes the role of theophylline in COPD treatment?

A. routinely indicated in moderate to very severe COPD

B. use limited by narrow therapeutic profile and drug–drug interaction potential

C. a potent bronchodilator

D. available only in parenteral form

62. All of the following are consistent with the GOLD COPD recommendation for pulmonary rehabilitation except:

A. it is reserved for very severe COPD.

B. its goals include improvement in overall well-being.

C. it is an underused therapeutic option.

D. it can lead to a reduction in symptoms of anxiety and depression.

63. All of the following are consistent findings during COPD exacerbation except:

   A. increased FEV_1.

   B. increased cough.

   C. increased sputum purulence.

   D. increased sputum production.

For answers and rationales, see end of chapter.

Tuberculosis

Overview

Pulmonary tuberculosis (TB) is a bacterial infection caused by *Mycobacterium tuberculosis* and transmitted through aerosolized droplets. With an estimated 20% to 43% of the world's population chronically infected, the disease occurs disproportionately in disadvantaged populations, such as in individuals who are unhoused, in those who are malnourished, and among people living in overcrowded and substandard housing.

> **CLINICAL CONCEPT**
>
> Public health measures to ensure adequate shelter, hygiene, and nutrition for the vulnerable public are an important primary prevention measure against the spread of TB infection.

About 30% of individuals exposed to the causative organism become infected. In an immunocompetent host, when the organism is acquired, an immune reaction ensues to help contain the infection within granulomas. This stage, known as primary TB, is usually symptom free. Viable organisms can lie dormant within the granulomas for years, however; this stage is known as latent TB infection (LTBI). A person with LTBI does not have active disease and is not contagious.

Without treatment, individuals with LTBI have a 10% lifetime risk of reactivation of the disease, known as postprimary TB, with 50% of the reactivations occurring within the first 2 years of primary infection. This increases to a risk of 10% per year in the presence of HIV infection; increased rates of reactivation are also noted with other forms of immunocompromise (systemic corticosteroid or other immunosuppressive drug used for many chronic illnesses) or diabetes mellitus. After primary infection, about 5% of patients do not mount an adequate immune response and develop progressive primary TB.

Clinical Presentation

Symptoms of an active pulmonary TB infection include cough, unexplained weight loss or anorexia, fever, night sweats, and fatigue; the duration of these findings is often variable, and these symptoms often have occurred intermittently over a protracted period of time. Atypical presentation can occur in immunocompromised individuals. Although hemoptysis (coughing up blood or bloody sputum) is occasionally reported, the cough associated with TB is often dry; frank hemoptysis is rarely reported. The chest examination is usually normal, with dyspnea seldom reported unless disease is extensive. TB can also infect extrapulmonary tissues that can result in nonspecific signs and symptoms. Acute TB pericarditis can result in chest pain, while tuberculous meningitis can present with a chronic, intermittent headache and subtle mental status changes. Other common areas of infection can include the skeletal, genitourinary, and gastrointestinal systems.

Diagnostic Testing

Tuberculin skin test (TST) is one method of identifying individuals infected with *M tuberculosis*. This test, when performed on an asymptomatic patient, is an example of secondary prevention or health screening. (See Chapter 2.) The test is performed by injecting 0.1 mL of purified protein derivative (PPD) transdermally. The results should be checked within 48 to 72 hours, with the transverse measurement of any change in the test site measured in millimeters of induration, not simply redness. A positive TST result is usually noted within 2 to 10 weeks of acquiring the organism. Thresholds for a positive TST result vary in different clinical conditions (Table 7-11). The interpretation of the test is the same in the presence or absence of bacille Calmette-Guérin (BCG) vaccination history. In certain circumstances, two-step testing and anergy testing should be considered.

The TST has limitations, including the need for multiple visits, one to inject the PPD and then a return visit to read or interpret the test, and a low sensitivity in people with immunosuppression, a group at high risk for reactivation. In addition, test results can be compromised by poor injection technique or the use of an inferior PPD product. As a result, alternative testing has been developed and is gaining increased acceptance. A blood test, known by its trade name QuantiFERON®-TB, detects interferon-γ, which is released by T lymphocytes in response to *M tuberculosis*–specific antigens. This test can be performed from a blood sample obtained on a single provider visit, with results available within 24 hours. In addition, its sensitivity is greater in patients with immunocompromise or with a history of receiving BCG vaccine.

TABLE 7-11 Classification of Tuberculin Skin Test Reaction

An induration of ≥5 mm is considered positive in:

- People living with HIV or AIDS
- A recent contact of a person with tuberculosis (TB) disease
- Persons with fibrotic changes on chest radiograph consistent with prior TB
- Patients with organ transplants
- Persons who are immunosuppressed for other reasons (e.g., taking the equivalent of more than 15 mg/day of prednisone for ≥1 month, taking TNF-α antagonists)

An induration of ≥10 mm is considered positive in:

- Recent immigrants (less than 5 years) from high-prevalence countries
- Injection drug users
- Residents and employees of high-risk congregate settings
- Mycobacteriology laboratory personnel
- Persons with clinical conditions that place them at high risk
- Children younger than 4 year old
- Infants, children, and adolescents exposed to adults in high-risk categories

An induration of ≥15 mm is considered positive in any person, including persons with no known risk factors for TB. Targeted skin testing programs should be conducted only in high-risk groups, however

Sources: Centers for Disease Control and Prevention (CDC). Targeted tuberculosis testing and interpreting tuberculin skin test results. https://www.cdc.gov/tb/publications/factsheets/testing/skintestresults.htm

Lewinsohn DM, Leonard MK, LoBue PA, et al. Official ATS/IDSA/CDC clinical practice guidelines: diagnosis of tuberculosis in adults and children. Clin Infect Dis. 2017;64:111–115. https://academic.oup.com/cid/article/64/2/111/2811357

Any patient with a positive TST or QuantiFERON®-TB test result should have a chest x-ray to help exclude the diagnosis of active pulmonary TB. In addition, a careful evaluation for clinical evidence of active disease, including malaise, weight loss, fever, night sweats, and chronic cough, should be carried out; these findings often evolve over 4 to 6 weeks in a person with active TB, and atypical presentation is common in immunocompromised individuals. In active TB, consolidations, infiltrates, and/or cavitation are usually noted on chest x-ray, usually involving the upper lobes. Mediastinal or hilar lymphadenopathy is often present. For those suspected of active TB disease, the presence of acid-fast bacilli from sputum should be performed via acid-fast microscopy. A culture for *M tuberculosis* will confirm the diagnosis, and susceptibility testing should be performed to help guide treatment. When managing a patient with suspected or confirmed active TB disease, the use of respiratory protective equipment is recommended to reduce risk of exposure of health-care personnel to infectious droplets expelled in the air by the patient. Patients should be educated on respiratory hygiene and the importance of cough etiquette procedures to minimize the spread of infection to others.

Treatment

Chemoprophylaxis therapy with isoniazid and other agents to prevent the development of active pulmonary TB should be considered for patients with latent TB—that is, positive tuberculin test results but negative chest radiograph results and no suspicion of disease revealed by health history or physical examination. The duration of isoniazid therapy is 6 to 9 months, depending on the dosing regimen. Rifampin is an alternative choice if isoniazid cannot be taken or is poorly tolerated. Although the risk of liver toxicity with anti-TB drug use increases with age, age alone is not a contraindication to its use, particularly in individuals at higher risk.

In the presence of active pulmonary TB, multiple antimicrobial therapies are administered that are aimed not only at eradicating the infection but also at minimizing the risk of developing a resistant pathogen. With latent and active disease, public health involvement is critical to maximize patient outcome and minimize risk to the general population.

> **CLINICAL CONCEPT**
>
> In this era of multidrug-resistant TB, it is prudent to consult with local TB experts to ascertain the local patterns of susceptibility.

Discussion Sources

Lewinsohn DM, Leonard MK, LoBue PA, et al. Official ATS/IDSA/CDC clinical practice guidelines: diagnosis of tuberculosis in adults and children. *Clin Infect Dis.* 2017;64:111–115. https://academic.oup.com/cid/article/64/2/111/2811357

Nahid P, Dorman SE, Alipanah N, et al. Official ATS/CDC/IDSA clinical practice guidelines: treatment of drug-susceptible tuberculosis. *Clin Infect Dis.* 2016;63:e147–e195. https://academic.oup.com/cid/article/63/7/e147/2196792

Pasipanodya J, Hall R, Gumbo T. Tuberculosis and other mycobacterial diseases. In: Kellerman RD, Rakel DP, eds. *Conn's Current Therapy 2019.* Philadelphia, PA: Saunders Elsevier; 2018:851–857.

QUESTIONS

64. You examine a 22-year-old woman who has been living in the United States for 4 years and grew up in a country where TB is endemic. She has documentation of receiving BCG vaccine as a child. With this information, you consider that:

    A. she will always have a positive TST result.

    B. biannual chest radiographs are needed to assess her health status accurately.

    C. a TST finding of 10 mm or more induration should be considered a positive result.

    D. isoniazid therapy should be given for 6 months before TST is undertaken.

65. A 33-year-old woman works in a small office with a man recently diagnosed with active pulmonary TB. Which of the following would be the best plan of care for this woman?

    A. She should receive TB chemoprophylaxis if her TST result is 5 mm or more in induration.

    B. Because of her age, TB chemoprophylaxis is contraindicated even in the presence of a positive TST result.

    C. If the TST result is positive but the chest radiograph is normal, no further evaluation or treatment is needed.

    D. Further evaluation is needed only if the TST result is 15 mm or more in induration.

66. Compared with TST, potential advantages of the QuantiFERON®-TB Gold test (QTF-G) include all of the following except:

    A. the ability to have the entire testing process complete with one clinical visit.

    B. the results are available within 24 hours.

    C. the interpretation of the test is not subject to reader bias.

    D. it is able to predict who is at greatest risk for active disease development.

67 to 71. For the following individuals, answer Yes or No in response to the question, "Does this patient have a reactive TST?"

    _____ **67.** a 45-year-old woman who works in a mycobacteriology laboratory and a 7-mm induration

    _____ **68.** a 21-year-old man with no identifiable TB risk factors and a 10-mm induration

    _____ **69.** a 31-year-old man living with HIV and a 6-mm induration

    _____ **70.** a 45-year-old woman from a country in which TB is endemic who has an 11-mm induration

    _____ **71.** a 42-year-old woman with rheumatoid arthritis who is taking etanercept (Enbrel®) who has a 7-mm induration

72. Risk factors for development of infection reactivation in patients with latent TB infection include all of the following except:

    A. diabetes mellitus.

    B. immunocompromise.

    C. long-term OCS therapy.

    D. male gender.

73. Clinical presentation of progressive primary TB most commonly includes all of the following except:

    A. malaise.

    B. fever.

    C. dry cough.

    D. frank hemoptysis.

74. For a patient suspected of active pulmonary TB disease, which of the following approaches is least helpful in confirming the diagnosis?

A. chest radiograph

B. Gram stain from blood sample

C. acid-fast microscopy from sputum sample

D. culture and susceptibility from sputum sample

For answers and rationales, see end of chapter.

Community-Acquired Pneumonia

Overview

Pneumonia is the most common cause of death from infectious disease and is the eighth-leading cause of overall mortality in the United States. Although pneumonia is often considered a disease primarily of older adults and persons with chronic illness, most episodes occur in immunocompetent community-dwelling individuals; about 20% of children develop pneumonia by age 5 years.

The term *community-acquired pneumonia* (CAP) is used to refer to an acute infection that was acquired outside of a health-care setting, as opposed to health-care–associated pneumonia or hospital-acquired pneumonia, which can be acquired in an acute care facility, long-term care or nursing facility, or other health-care settings.

Although numerous organisms are capable of causing pneumonia, relatively few are seen with frequency. *Streptococcus pneumoniae,* also known as the pneumococcal organism, is a gram-positive diplococcus, the most common CAP pathogen in adults, and is found in most deaths caused by CAP. *Haemophilus influenzae* is a predominant pathogen in CAP patients with COPD. *Mycoplasma pneumoniae* and *Chlamydophila* (formerly *Chlamydia*) *pneumoniae* are common causative pathogens of CAP. These organisms are transmitted by coughing and are often found among people living in closed communities, such as households, college dormitories, military barracks, and residential centers, including long-term care facilities. *M pneumoniae, C pneumoniae, Legionella* species, and respiratory viruses are often referred to as atypical pathogens (causing atypical pneumonia) because these organisms are not detectable via Gram stain, cannot be cultured on standard bacterial media, and clinically do not have a classic pneumonia presentation. Usually contracted by inhaling mist or aspirating liquid that comes from a water source contaminated with the organisms, pulmonary infection with *Legionella* species can result in pneumonia ranging from mild to severe disease; there is no evidence for person-to-person spread of the disease. Risk factors for severe disease with *Legionella* species, capable of causing the most serious illness of the atypical pathogens, include tobacco use, airway disease, and diabetes mellitus. Aspiration likely increases the risk of pneumonia caused by anaerobic organisms, though more research is needed to fully understand the role of these organisms in the pathological process.

> **CLINICAL CONCEPT**
> Most often caused by bacteria or virus, pneumonia is an acute lower respiratory tract infection involving lung parenchyma, interstitial tissues, and alveolar spaces.

Clinical Presentation

Patients with pneumonia usually present with cough (more than 90%), dyspnea (66%), sputum production (66%), and pleuritic chest pain (50%), although nonrespiratory symptoms, including fatigue and gastrointestinal upset, are also commonly reported. As with other infectious diseases, elderly patients often report fewer symptoms and often present with an elevated resting respiratory rate and generally feeling ill; altered mental status is often noted in the older adult with pneumonia.

Diagnostic Testing

Chest x-ray is helpful in the assessment of the person with CAP. Characteristic infiltrate patterns are typically seen with certain pathogens, such as interstitial infiltrates with atypical pathogens or viruses and areas of consolidation with *S pneumoniae.* Therapy should be based on patient characteristics and risk factors, however, rather than the pattern of the radiographic abnormality. According to the recommendations of the Infectious Diseases Society of America (IDSA)/American Thoracic Society (ATS) Consensus Guidelines, an abnormal chest radiograph and clinical findings are required to confirm the diagnosis of pneumonia. Complete blood count (CBC) with WBC differential, blood urea nitrogen (BUN), and creatinine should also be obtained.

For patients with nonsevere CAP being treated in the community, a sputum Gram stain and culture are not needed as there is often a poor yield of organisms in sputum and the results are not likely to impact management decisions or patient outcomes. Similarly, blood cultures are not needed as the yield in nonsevere CAP is very low and would rarely result in an appropriate change in therapy. The use of *Legionella* and pneumococcal urinary antigen testing is also not needed for nonsevere CAP. Testing for the presence of sepsis markers, such as procalcitonin or lactate, is not recommended for patients treated in the outpatient setting.

Treatment

Successful community-based care of a person with pneumonia depends on many factors. The patient must have intact gastrointestinal function and be able to take and tolerate oral medications and adequate amounts of fluids. A competent caregiver must be available, in part to ensure that the patient is able to seek help if the clinical condition worsens. Also, the patient should be able to return for follow-up examination and evaluation.

Certain patient characteristics increase the likelihood of death from pneumonia and should alert the NP to consider hospitalization. These include age older than 65 years and severe electrolyte or hematological disorder, such as serum sodium concentration of less than 130 mEq/L, hematocrit less than 30%, or absolute neutrophil count of less than 1,000/mm³. The CURB-65 criteria can provide a convenient approach to assist the clinician in determining whether a patient should be hospitalized. CURB-65 allocates one point for each of the following five criteria: confusion, BUN greater than 19 mg/dL, respiratory rate greater than 30/minutes, blood pressure less than 90/60 mm Hg, and 65 years of age and older. A score of 1 or less indicates that the patient can be treated as an outpatient, whereas a score greater than 1 indicates hospitalization is needed. The presence of a comorbid disease—such as impaired renal function, diabetes mellitus, heart failure, immunosuppression, and airway dysfunction—poses increased risk, as do abnormalities in vital signs, such as fever, tachycardia, tachypnea, and hypotension.

The pathogen responsible for pneumonia must also be considered because pneumonia death risk is increased when *S aureus,* often seen in postinfluenza pneumonia, or gram-negative rods such as *Klebsiella pneumoniae* or *Pseudomonas aeruginosa,* cause infection. Risk factors for pneumonia caused by gram-negative bacilli include alcoholism, underlying chronic bronchiectasis (e.g., cystic fibrosis), chronic tracheostomy and/or mechanical ventilation, and febrile neutropenia. Sputum analysis for Gram stain or culture is not recommended for the majority of patients with CAP, although it is commonly obtained during the evaluation of a person with pneumonia who is treated in the hospital.

Because definitive identification of the organism is unlikely, the choice of antimicrobial agent to treat pneumonia is largely empirical, directed at the most likely causative organism in view of patient characteristics, such as age and comorbidity. Because pneumococcal pneumonia, caused by *S pneumoniae,* carries a significant risk for mortality, the chosen antimicrobial should always be effective against this pathogen, regardless of patient presentation. Choosing an antimicrobial with activity against atypical organisms (*M pneumoniae, C pneumoniae, Legionella* species) and gram-positive and gram-negative organisms (*S pneumoniae, H influenzae* if patient risk is present) helps ensure optimal outcome.

An additional consideration is antimicrobial resistance. Factors that facilitate the development of resistant microbes include repeated exposure to a given agent, underdosing (eradicating more sensitive organisms, leaving more resistant pathogens untouched), and an unnecessarily prolonged period of treatment. Shorter course high-dose antimicrobial therapy in pneumonia treatment maximizes and exploits concentration-dependent killing by achieving higher maximum concentration and area under the concentration-time curve/minimal inhibitory concentration (AUC/MIC) values. This allows for effective treatment of difficult pathogens by increasing tissue penetration, and likely improves patient adherence to the regimen, thus minimizing the development of resistant pathogens. Patients with CAP should be treated for a minimum of 5 days, should be afebrile for 48 to 72 hours, and should have no more than one CAP-associated sign of clinical instability (e.g., elevated heart rate and respiratory rate, hypotension) before discontinuing therapy. A longer duration is occasionally needed if the initial therapy was not effective against the identified pathogen or if an extrapulmonary complication is present (e.g., meningitis).

The ATS and the IDSA offer guidelines for CAP assessment and intervention. Factors influencing the choice of antimicrobial agent include patient comorbidity and risk for infection by a difficult pathogen (e.g., *S aureus* or *P aeruginosa*).

CLINICAL CONCEPT

All first-line recommended CAP treatment options offer activity against *S pneumoniae, H influenzae,* and/or atypical pathogens, the most common organisms implicated in CAP (Tables 7-12 and 7-13).

TABLE 7-12 Community-Acquired Pneumonia: Likely Causative Pathogens, Characteristics, and Effective Antimicrobials

PATHOGEN	DESCRIPTION	MECHANISM OF ANTIMICROBIAL RESISTANCE	COMMENT
Streptococcus pneumoniae	Gram-positive diplococci	Via altered protein binding sites in bacterial cell (approximately 25% nationwide). Risk factors that increase likelihood of infection with drug-resistant *S pneumoniae* (DRSP) include recent systemic (oral or parenteral) antimicrobial use (within past 3 months), age ≥65 years, exposure to a child in day care, alcohol abuse, medical comorbidities, immunosuppressive therapy or illness. Effective antimicrobials for nonresistant *S pneumoniae*, keeping in mind regional variations in resistance rates: Macrolides (azithromycin, clarithromycin, erythromycin), standard amoxicillin, select cephalosporins, tetracyclines including doxycycline. Preferred antimicrobials with risk: combination therapy with amoxicillin-clavulanate or cephalosporin plus macrolide or doxycycline; or monotherapy with a respiratory fluoroquinolone (moxifloxacin, levofloxacin, others).	Most common cause of fatal community-acquired pneumonia.
Mycoplasma pneumoniae *Chlamydophila pneumoniae*	Not revealed by Gram stain	Due to naturally occurring resistance, effective antimicrobials: Macrolides, respiratory fluoroquinolones, tetracyclines including doxycycline. Ineffective antimicrobials: Beta-lactams (cephalosporins, penicillins).	Largely transmitted by cough, often seen in people who have recently spent extended time in close proximity (closed communities such as correctional facilities, college dormitories, long-term care facilities). "Atypical pneumonia" or "walking pneumonia" pathogens, usually characterized by dry cough, less severe signs and symptoms.
Haemophilus influenzae	Gram-negative bacillus	Beta-lactamase production (approximately 30% nationwide). Effective antimicrobials: Agents with activity against gram-negative organisms and stable in presence of or active against beta-lactamase—macrolides, cephalosporins, amoxicillin-clavulanate, respiratory fluoroquinolones, tetracyclines including doxycycline.	Common respiratory pathogen with tobacco-related lung disease.
Legionella spp.	Not revealed by Gram stain	Due to naturally occurring resistance, effective antimicrobials: Macrolides, respiratory fluoroquinolones, tetracyclines, including doxycycline. Ineffective antimicrobials: Beta-lactams (cephalosporins, penicillins).	Usually contracted by inhaling mist or aspirating liquid that comes from a water source contaminated with *Legionella*. No evidence for person-to-person spread of the disease. Major risk factors for severe *Legionella* disease: older age, male, smoking, diabetes mellitus, especially with poor glycemic control.

DRSP, drug-resistant Streptococcus pneumoniae.

Source: Gilbert DN, Chambers HF, Eliopoulos GM, Saag MS, Pavia AT. The Sanford Guide to Antimicrobial Therapy. *50th ed. Sperryville, VA: Antimicrobial Therapy, Inc.; 2020.*

TABLE 7-13 Infectious Diseases Society of America/American Thoracic Society (IDSA/ATS) Classification for Outpatient Treatment of Community-Acquired Pneumonia

Minimum diagnostic evaluation in CAP: CBC with WBC differential, BUN/Cr, chest x-ray. Additional testing based on patient presentation, comorbidity.

Recommended length of CAP therapy: Minimum of 5 days with evidence of increasing stability, afebrile for 48 to 72 hours prior to antimicrobial discontinuation (average 5 to 7 days).

(Therapies not listed in order of priority.)

IDSA/ATS CLASSIFICATION	IDSA/ATS TREATMENT OPTIONS
No significant comorbidities (including COPD, diabetes, renal or heart failure, asplenia, alcoholism) or risk factors for MRSA or *P aeruginosa**	Oral doxycycline *Or* Oral azithromycin, clarithromycin, or erythromycin, taking into consideration local *S pneumoniae* macrolide resistance rates (do not use if greater than 20% rate of resistance) *Or* Oral amoxicillin (high dose)
Likely causative pathogens *S pneumoniae* (gram-positive) *M pneumoniae* (atypical pathogen) *C pneumoniae* (atypical pathogen) Respiratory viruses, including influenza A/B, respiratory syncytial virus (RSV), others	
Significant comorbidities including COPD, diabetes, renal or heart failure, asplenia, alcoholism	Respiratory fluoroquinolone PO (moxi-, levofloxacin, others) *Or* Doxycycline, azithromycin or clarithromycin (macrolide) PO **plus** beta-lactam, such as amoxicillin-clavulanate (up to amox 4 g/d), cefpodoxime (Vantin®), cefuroxime (Ceftin®), all given PO
Likely causative pathogens *S pneumoniae* (gram-positive) *H influenzae* (gram-negative) *M pneumoniae* (atypical pathogen) *C pneumoniae* (atypical pathogen) *Legionella* spp. (atypical pathogen) Respiratory viruses as above Greater risk for resistant pathogens	

**Risk factors include respiratory isolation of MRSA or* P aeruginosa *or recent hospitalization and use of parenteral antibiotics in the last 90 days.*

Sources: Metlay JP, Waterer GW, Long AC, et al; Infectious Diseases Society of America, American Thoracic Society. Diagnosis and treatment of adults with community-acquired pneumonia. Am J Respir Crit Care Med. 2019;200:e45–e67. https://www.atsjournals.org/doi/full/10.1164/rccm.201908-1581ST. Gilbert DN, Chambers HF, Eliopoulos GM, Saag MS, Pavia AT. The Sanford Guide to Antimicrobial Therapy. 50th ed. Sperryville, VA: Antimicrobial Therapy, Inc.; 2020:40–43.

Consideration should be given to the possibility of resistant pathogens, whether naturally occurring or acquired resistance. To maximize the likelihood of a positive clinical outcome and minimize the risk of resistant pathogen development, higher-dose, shorter-course antimicrobial therapy should be prescribed.

NPs are ideally positioned to help minimize risk for pneumonia through immunization and hygienic measures. Nearly two-thirds of all fatal cases of pneumonia are caused by *S pneumoniae,* the pneumococcal organism. Although available for decades, pneumococcal vaccines (e.g., Pneumovax®, Prevnar®) continue to be underused. Remaining up to date on the latest immunization recommendations is critical to safe practice; see Chapter 2. The use of the influenza vaccine can help minimize the risk of postinfluenza pneumonia, an often debilitating and potentially fatal condition. Both vaccines can be given together and in the presence of moderately severe illness. Ensuring adequate ventilation, reinforcing cough hygiene, and proper hand washing can help minimize pneumonia risk.

Discussion Sources

Gilbert DN, Chambers HF, Eliopoulos GM, Saag MS, Pavia AT. *The Sanford Guide to Antimicrobial Therapy.* 50th ed. Sperryville, VA: Antimicrobial Therapy, Inc.; 2020:40–43.

Metlay JP, Waterer GW, Long AC, et al; Infectious Diseases Society of America, American Thoracic Society. Diagnosis and treatment of adults with community-acquired pneumonia. *Am J Respir Crit Care Med.* 2019;200:e45–e67. https://www.atsjournals.org/doi/full/10.1164/rccm.201908-1581ST

QUESTIONS

75 to 80. According to the American Thoracic Society/Infectious Diseases Society of America (ATS/IDSA) Consensus Guidelines on the Management of Community-Acquired Pneumonia in Adults, which of the following is the most appropriate antimicrobial for treatment of CAP in:

75. a 42-year-old man with no comorbidity, no reported drug allergy, and no recent antimicrobial use?

    A. oral doxycycline

    B. oral cefpodoxime

    C. oral TMP-SMX

    D. oral ciprofloxacin

76. a 46-year-old well woman with a history of a bilateral tubal ligation who is macrolide intolerant?

    A. oral clarithromycin

    B. oral cephalexin

    C. oral doxycycline

    D. oral fosfomycin

77. a 78-year-old woman with a history of COPD, hypertension, and dyslipidemia who is taking lovastatin and a dihydropyridine calcium channel blocker?

    A. oral clindamycin

    B. oral amoxicillin-clavulanate with oral doxycycline

    C. oral clarithromycin

    D. IM ceftriaxone

78. a 69-year-old man with heart failure, prior myocardial infarction, and type 2 diabetes?

    A. oral respiratory fluoroquinolone

    B. oral amoxicillin with clavulanate

    C. oral cephalosporin

    D. oral TMP-SMX

79. a 28-year-old woman with a severe beta-lactam allergy who has a dry cough, headache, malaise, and no comorbidity who takes no medication?

    A. oral clarithromycin

    B. oral amoxicillin

    C. IV levofloxacin

    D. IM ceftriaxone

80. a 47-year-old woman who was recently hospitalized and given parenteral antimicrobials for diverticulitis?

    A. oral amoxicillin-clavulanate

    B. high-dose oral amoxicillin

    C. oral clarithromycin

    D. oral moxifloxacin

81. Criteria to distinguish whether pneumonia is community acquired include all of the following except that the person:

    A. lives in the community.

    B. is not a resident of a long-term care facility.

    C. had no prior antimicrobial use in the previous 3 months.

    D. had no recent hospitalization.

82. Common symptoms of CAP in otherwise well adults include all of the following except:

    A. cough.

    B. altered mental status.

    C. dyspnea.

    D. pleuritic chest pain.

83. A clinically suspected diagnosis of pneumonia is typically confirmed by:

    A. sputum culture.

    B. sputum Gram stain.

    C. bronchoalveolar lavage.

    D. chest radiograph.

84. Which of the following is a quality of respiratory fluoroquinolones?

    A. activity against drug-resistant *S pneumoniae* (DRSP)

    B. poor activity against atypical pathogens

    C. predominantly hepatic route of elimination

    D. poor activity against beta-lactamase–producing organisms.

85. The mechanism of resistance of DRSP is through the cell's:

    A. beta-lactamase production.

    B. hypertrophy of cell membrane.

    C. alteration in protein-binding sites.

    D. failure of DNA gyrase reversal.

86. The primary mechanism of antimicrobial resistance of *H influenzae* is through the organism's:

    A. beta-lactamase production.

    B. hypertrophy of cell membrane.

    C. alteration in protein-binding sites.

    D. failure of DNA gyrase reversal.

87. Which of the following characteristics applies to macrolides?

    A. consistent activity against DRSP

    B. contraindicated for use during penicillin allergy

    C. effective against atypical pathogens

    D. unstable in the presence of beta-lactamase

88. According to the ATS/IDSA guidelines, what is the usual length of antimicrobial therapy for the treatment of CAP for outpatients?

    A. fewer than 5 days

    B. 5 to 7 days

    C. 7 to 10 days

    D. 10 to 14 days

89 to 91. Based on the CURB-65 criteria, indicate which patients should be treated as an inpatient (I) or outpatient (O).

_____ 89. a 47-year-old man with no confusion, BUN = 18 mg/dL, respiratory rate = 32/minutes, and blood pressure = 110/72 mm Hg

_____ 90. a 56-year-old woman with no confusion, BUN = 22 mg/dL, respiratory rate = 27/minutes, blood pressure = 88/56 mm Hg

_____ 91. a 72-year-old man with confusion, BUN = 18 mg/dL, respiratory rate = 35/minutes, blood pressure = 102/66 mm Hg

92. Risk factors for pneumonia caused by methicillin-resistant *S aureus* (MRSA) or *P aeruginosa* include all of the following except:

A. living in a rural setting.

B. recent hospitalization.

C. recent receipt of parenteral antimicrobial.

D. prior respiratory isolation of MRSA or *P aeruginosa*.

93. Which of the following most accurately describes sputum analysis in the evaluation of the person with CAP?

A. Gram stain is routinely advised.

B. Antimicrobial therapy should not be initiated until sputum specimen for culture has been obtained.

C. Sputum analysis is not recommended in the majority of patients with CAP.

D. If required, chest physical therapy can be used to facilitate sputum production.

94. Which of the following best describes the mechanism of transmission in an atypical pneumonia pathogen?

A. microaspiration

B. respiratory droplet

C. surface contamination

D. aerosolized contaminated water

95. Risk factors for death resulting from pneumonia include:

A. viral origin.

B. history of allergic reaction to multiple antimicrobials.

C. renal insufficiency.

D. polycythemia.

96. All of the following antimicrobial strategies help facilitate the development of resistant pathogens except:

A. longer course of therapy.

B. lower antimicrobial dosage.

C. higher antimicrobial dosage.

D. prescribing a broader-spectrum agent.

97. Findings of increased tactile fremitus and dullness to percussion at the right lung base in the person with CAP likely indicate an area of:

A. atelectasis.

B. pneumothorax.

C. consolidation.

D. cavitation.

98. You are caring for a 52-year-old man who is currently smoking 1.5 packs per day (PPD), has a 40 pack-year cigarette smoking history, and has CAP. It is the third day of his antimicrobial therapy, and he is without fever, is well hydrated, and is feeling less short of breath. His initial chest x-ray revealed a right lower lobe infiltrate. Physical examination today reveals peak inspiratory crackles with increased tactile fremitus in the right posterior thorax. Which of the following represents the most appropriate next step in this patient's care?

A. His current plan of care should continue because he is improving by clinical assessment.

B. A chest radiograph should be taken today to confirm resolution of pneumonia.

C. Given the persistence of abnormal thoracic findings, his antimicrobial therapy should be changed.

D. A computed tomography (CT) scan of the thorax is needed today to image any potential thoracic abnormalities.

99. While seeing a 66-year-old who was recently hospitalized with CAP, clinically improved, and is now being seen for a posthospitalization visit, the NP notes the patient is not up to date with certain immunizations. The NP appreciates that:

    A. pneumococcal vaccine should be given when antimicrobial therapy has been completed.

    B. pneumococcal vaccine can be given today, and influenza vaccine can be given in 2 weeks.

    C. influenza vaccine can be given today, and pneumococcal vaccine can be given in 2 weeks.

    D. influenza and pneumococcal vaccines should be given today.

100. The mechanism of transmission of *Legionella* species is primarily via:

    A. respiratory droplet.

    B. inhalation of aerosolized contaminated water.

    C. contact with a contaminated surface.

    D. hematogenous spread.

101 to 107. Identify the following organisms as a gram-positive, gram-negative, or atypical pathogen.

_____ **101.** *S pneumoniae*

_____ **102.** *H influenzae*

_____ **103.** *Legionella* species

_____ **104.** *C pneumoniae*

_____ **105.** *M pneumoniae*

_____ **106.** *S aureus*

_____ **107.** *P aeruginosa*

108 to 111. Indicate (*Yes or No*) whether the following diagnostic studies should be routinely performed for a patient suspected of CAP and managed in the outpatient setting.

_____ **108.** Procalcitonin

_____ **109.** Lactate

_____ **110.** *Legionella* urinary antigen

_____ **111.** Pneumococcal urinary antigen

For answers and rationales, see end of chapter.

COVID-19

Overview

COVID-19 (coronavirus disease 2019) is caused by the severe acute respiratory syndrome coronavirus 2 (SARS-CoV-2) that likely originated in Wuhan, China, in late 2019. Several factors have helped to spread the virus into a worldwide pandemic. First, the virus is a novel organism with little to no existing immunity within the population. The virus can efficiently replicate in humans and cause serious disease. Additionally, the virus is easily transmitted person-to-person, predominantly via respiratory droplets.

Though infection can cause serious and life-threatening disease, majority of infected individuals are asymptomatic or only present with mild symptoms. Risk factors for severe infection include age 65 years and older, resident in a nursing home or long-term care facility, and presence of one or more comorbidities (e.g., pulmonary disease, cardiac disease, immunocompromised, BMI greater than 40 kg/m², renal failure, liver disease, and diabetes). Male gender and certain ethnicities (i.e., Latino, African American, and Native American) have also been identified as risk factors for severe disease.

Clinical Presentation

Symptomatic adults will typically present with flu-like symptoms that can include fever, cough, fatigue, sputum production, and dyspnea. Less common symptoms can include myalgia/arthralgia, sore throat, chills, and GI upset. Anecdotal reports also suggest that loss of sense of smell and taste can be an early indication of infection, though further study is needed. Older adults and those in LTCFs are more likely to report loss of appetite, altered mental status, and diarrhea, as well as experience O_2 desaturation (which can be sudden, severe, and with minimal cough).

Diagnostic Testing

Individuals experiencing COVID-19 symptoms should first contact their health-care provider to determine if testing and/or in-person evaluation is needed. COVID-19 testing is the most accurate method to identify someone with active infection. However, the types of tests available and recommendations on who should be tested are evolving rapidly as more tests become available and as we learn more about the disease. Testing recommendations vary from state to state and often depend on the availability of tests. When testing availability is limited, the CDC offers a hierarchy for those who should receive higher priority for testing (refer to the CDC Web site for their latest recommendations).

It is important to note that there are a number of types of tests for COVID-19. A viral test will identify patients who have a current infection by detecting the presence of viral nucleic acid or antigen. This involves testing a respiratory sample (e.g., nasal swab) to identify the presence of the virus. A serological antibody test can determine if an individual has been previously infected with the virus. Antibodies are typically produced 1 to 3 weeks after infection, and so a negative result can occur in individuals who have been recently exposed to the virus. Awareness of emerging test options is critical.

Treatment

Certain treatments have been identified that improve outcomes and survival among hospitalized patients with severe disease, including the use of the antiviral remdesivir, as well as dexamethasone in those requiring oxygen therapy or ventilation. However, outpatient management of mild-to-moderate COVID-19 largely involves supportive care. Home care of COVID-19 is appropriate for individuals who meet certain criteria, such as the patient is stable, appropriate caregivers are available, a separate bedroom is available for the patient to recover, and the patient and other household members are able to adhere to precautions for home care or isolation. Individuals should be cautioned that some patients can deteriorate rapidly one week after illness onset and should seek emergency care with onset of severe symptoms (e.g., shortness of breath, respiratory rate greater than or equal to 30/minute, chest pain or pressure, and/or loss of speech or movement). Acute respiratory distress syndrome occurs a median of 8 to 12 days after disease onset.

For symptomatic individuals with suspected or confirmed COVID-19, home isolation should continue until the following three criteria are met: at least 3 days without fever, improvement in respiratory symptoms (e.g., cough, dyspnea), and at least 10 days since onset of symptoms. For asymptomatic individuals who tested positive for COVID-19, home isolation should continue until at least 10 days have passed since the first positive test and there have been no subsequent symptoms.

Interventions in the treatment and prevention of COVID-19 are likely to evolve as more becomes known about the disease and new interventions become available. Health-care providers are encouraged to stay up-to-date with validated resources, such as the CDC and WHO, on the latest approaches in the management of the infection.

Discussion Sources

Centers for Disease Control and Prevention. Coronavirus (COVID-19). https://www.cdc.gov/coronavirus/2019-ncov/index.html
National Institutes of Health. Coronavirus (COVID-19). https://www.nih.gov/coronavirus
World Health Organization. Coronavirus disease (COVID-19) pandemic. https://www.who.int/emergencies/diseases/novel
   -coronavirus-2019

Acute Bronchitis

Overview

Acute bronchitis is a condition of lower airway, self-limited inflammation, usually caused by viral infection, that can persist for approximately 3 weeks, though occasionally persists as long as 4 to 6 weeks. The diagnosis is usually limited to those without chronic airway disease (e.g., asthma or COPD). Acute bronchitis can be differentiated from the common cold (which lasts approximately 7 to 10 days, frequently with nasal congestion and rhinorrhea) or pneumonia (presence of fever, tachypnea, tachycardia, and clinical lung findings).

Though rarely identified in clinical practice, the causative pathogen for acute bronchitis is viral in more than 95% of cases. These include adenovirus, coronavirus,

CLINICAL CONCEPT

Persistent cough is one of the most common reasons for health-care provider office visits, and acute bronchitis is usually the diagnosis for these patients.

influenza A or B, respiratory syncytial virus, and rhinovirus. When a bacterial infection is implicated in acute bronchitis, which is quite rare and usually resolves without antimicrobials, the most common species are *Bordetella pertussis*, *C pneumoniae*, and *M pneumoniae*.

Clinical Presentation

Acute bronchitis is a clinical diagnosis made by taking an appropriate history of present illness and physical examination. As mentioned, problematic cough is the prominent sign, while disordered sleep and fatigue, caused by recurrent cough, are commonly reported symptoms. Typically, the cough developed during a viral upper respiratory track infection (URI) but persisted beyond the average 7 to 10 days for this condition. Sputum production is usually scant to absent; with sputum production, the color can range from clear to yellow or green. Contrary to common belief, colored sputum, reported by up to 50% of patients with acute bronchitis, is not a marker of bacterial infection but rather evidence of the presence of leukocytes, mobilized by the body to counter the infecting agents. Fever is rare and, when present, should direct the diagnosis toward influenza or pneumonia.

Examination of the lungs in acute bronchitis is usually normal, without use of accessory muscles or other signs of respiratory distress. Crackles are absent as is evidence of consolidation. If these findings are present, a diagnosis other than acute bronchitis, such as pneumonia or heart failure, should be considered. In acute bronchitis, occasionally expiratory wheezes are present.

When making a differential diagnosis, other conditions to consider beyond influenza and pneumonia can include exercise-induced asthma or bronchospasm, cystic fibrosis, bacterial tracheitis, and hyperreactive airway disease. Exercise-induced asthma should be considered for individuals complaining of exercise-related respiratory symptoms, including chest tightness, cough, dyspnea, wheezing, fatigue, and prolonged recovery time. A diagnosis of persistent asthma can also be considered for individuals who report "acute bronchitis" symptoms multiple times each year, particularly when cold outside or following viral URIs, along with nighttime awakenings due to symptoms several times each month.

Diagnostic Testing

The diagnosis of acute bronchitis is made clinically, by history and physical examination. Sputum culture is not recommended given the high prevalence of viral infections and the low yield of viral cultures. However, testing for select organisms may be helpful during outbreaks of acute bronchitis in select scenarios, especially when a bacterial pathogen is suspected (e.g., pertussis outbreak). Chest x-ray is not required or advised in acute bronchitis, unless there is a question of pneumonia where the patient has cough plus fever and/or evidence of consolidation. Spirometry to measure FEV_1 or PEFR can be useful for patients with significant bronchospasm and can help support a decision to use a rescue medication (i.e., SABA or SAMA). SaO_2 measurement is not usually warranted as this is a late marker for respiratory distress.

Treatment

Treatment of acute bronchitis should focus on symptom management. Practice guidelines suggest that the use of antitussives (e.g., dextromethorphan) is a reasonable choice despite a lack of consistent evidence supporting their use. However, antitussives should not be used in children younger than 8 years because of a lack of effectiveness and risk of adverse effects. Inhaler medications such as bronchodilators (SABA, SAMA) are not recommended for routine use in patients with acute bronchitis as there is a lack of evidence showing benefit with the use of these agents when there is no underlying history of lung disease or evidence of wheeze or airway obstruction. However, patients with wheezing have shown some response to the use of beta-2 agonist inhalers, particularly if there is evidence of impaired airflow as demonstrated by a low FEV_1 or PEFR. For severe, persistent cough, a short course of a systemic corticosteroid such as prednisone 40 mg daily for 3 to 5 days can offer significant symptom relief. For patients with sputum production, the use of a mucolytic can be considered, though proper hydration, helping to facilitate the production of thinner sputum, is the most effective method to mobilize secretions. The expectorant guaifenesin can be helpful in decreasing mucus viscosity, particularly in the person who is well hydrated, and has been shown to offer some benefit in decreasing cough frequency and intensity.

Routine use of antimicrobial therapy is not recommended for the treatment of acute bronchitis. Historically, the overuse of antimicrobials to treat viral infections has contributed to the rising prevalence of antimicrobial resistance in the community and, potentially, the growing number of cases of community-associated *Clostridium difficile* infection. Clinical studies demonstrate that antimicrobial therapy does not significantly change the course of acute bronchitis and only provides minimal benefit compared with the risks associated with their use. Current guidelines do not recommend the routine use of antimicrobials for acute bronchitis and suggest that health-care providers take the time to explain the reasoning to patients who are typically expecting a prescription. Antimicrobials can be considered in certain situations, such as if pertussis is suspected, which can be treated with a macrolide; with suspected pertussis, appropriate testing and health authority notification should take place. Antiviral medications can also be considered during influenza season for high-risk patients who present within 36 hours of symptom onset.

Discussion Sources

Braman SS. Chronic cough due to acute bronchitis: ACCP evidence-based clinical practice guidelines. *Chest.* 2006;129(suppl 1):95S–103S.

Gilbert DN, Chambers HF, Eliopoulos GM, Saag MS, Pavia AT. *The Sanford Guide to Antimicrobial Therapy.* 50th ed. Sperryville, VA: Antimicrobial Therapy, Inc.; 2020:37–38.

Kincade S, Long NA. Acute bronchitis. *Am Fam Physician.* 2016;94:560–565.

QUESTIONS

112. Cough associated with acute bronchitis can typically last approximately:

A. 1 week.

B. 2 weeks.

C. 3 weeks.

D. 3 months.

113. Approximately _____ of acute bronchitis cases are caused by a viral infection.

A. 15%

B. 30%

C. 65%

D. 95% or more

114. Bacterial pathogens implicated in causing acute bronchitis include all of the following except:

A. *S pneumoniae.*

B. *M pneumoniae.*

C. *C pneumoniae.*

D. *B pertussis.*

115. A 34-year-old woman presents with a 7-day history of cough with no fever or difficulty breathing. She is otherwise healthy. She is producing small amounts of yellow-tinged sputum. As part of her treatment, you recommend:

A. an antitussive.

B. an antihistamine.

C. a macrolide antimicrobial.

D. a beta-lactam antimicrobial.

116. Which of the following would most likely be noted upon chest examination of a normally healthy person who presents with acute bronchitis?

A. normal findings

B. evidence of consolidation

C. inspiratory wheeze

D. crackles

117. Which one of the following statements is most accurate regarding the use of chest x-ray in diagnosing acute bronchitis?

A. generally required to confirm a diagnosis

B. should be routinely performed at initial presentation and upon resolution of symptoms

C. will typically reveal multilobar infiltrates

D. usually not needed unless there is suspicion of pneumonia

118. A 28-year-old man with no history of tobacco use and who is normally healthy reports coughing episodes that last a few weeks multiple times during the year. The episodes become more evident during the winter months or following a "cold." He also reports coughing that disrupts his sleep a few times each month throughout the year, regardless of illness. The most likely diagnosis is:

A. acute bronchitis.

B. active TB.

C. persistent asthma.

D. walking pneumonia.

For answers and rationales, see end of chapter.

Lung Cancer

Overview

Nearly a quarter of a million Americans are diagnosed with lung cancer annually; this malignancy is the second most diagnosed cancer in men and woman annually and the most common cause of cancer death in either gender. The 5-year survival rate for localized stage lung cancer is 56% versus 19% for all stages combined. Currently, however, only 16% of lung cancers are diagnosed at the localized stage. As a result, efforts need to be focused on prevention or early detection of lung cancer.

While cigarette smoking is the leading lung cancer risk factor, approximately 20% will occur in nonsmokers. The highest-risk patients include current smokers aged 55 to 74 years with a smoking history of at least 30 pack-years as well as former smokers of the same age who have quit within the past 15 years but have the same smoking history. Other modifiable risk factors include exposure to secondhand smoke; exposure to radon or asbestos; exposure to cancer-causing agents in the workplace; routine use of certain dietary supplements including vitamin B, beta carotene, and vitamin E; and arsenic in the drinking water. Homes or buildings in any part of the United States can have high indoor radon levels, especially buildings with basements. To avoid radon exposure, homes should be tested and properly treated when necessary. To avoid secondhand smoke, homes and cars should be designated as smoke-free, places of employment that are smoke-free should be selected when possible, and restaurants and businesses that are smoke-free should be chosen. Nonmodifiable risk factors include previous radiation therapy to the lungs, air pollution, and personal or family history of lung cancer. Primary prevention of lung cancer includes helping patients avoid tobacco smoking or lending support and assistance in quitting.

Clinical Presentation

Typically, early lung cancer has no identifiable signs or symptoms. More commonly, in the absence of a screening program, lung cancer presentation occurs at late-stage disease when patients become symptomatic. Patients usually present with nonspecific systemic symptoms of fatigue, anorexia, and unexplained weight loss. The presence of a primary tumor, particularly with partial airway obstruction, can be associated with chest discomfort, cough, dyspnea, and hemoptysis. Upward of 40% of patients diagnosed with lung cancer initially present with signs and symptoms of intrathoracic spread. This can be associated with hoarseness (from laryngeal nerve paralysis), phrenic nerve paralysis, a superior pulmonary sulcus tumor (Pancoast tumor) with Horner's syndrome, and/or chest wall invasion with persistent, pleuritic pain. Nearly one-third of patients present with signs and symptoms of extrathoracic disease including spread to the bones, liver, adrenal glands, lymph nodes, brain, and spinal cord.

Diagnostic Testing

Early detection is essential, because early stage lung cancers are more likely to respond to treatment, such as surgery, radiation, and chemotherapy. Guidelines from the American College of Chest Physicians (ACCP) recommend that patients at significant risk for lung cancer be offered annual screening with low-dose computed tomography (LDCT), including current smokers aged 55 to 77 years with at least a 30 pack-years history as well as former smokers of the same age who have quit within the past 15 years but have the same smoking history. Guidelines from the U.S. Preventive Services Task Force (USPSTF) are similar to those from ACCP with the exception of extending the age for LDCT screening for those up to 80 years. The NCCN (National Comprehensive Cancer Network) recommends annual LDCT screening for patients

55 to 74 years with a 30 or more pack-year history of smoking, as well as younger patients (50 years or older) with a less extensive smoking history (at least 20 pack-years) who have one additional risk factor, such as a history of cancer or lung disease, family history of lung cancer, radon exposure, or occupational exposure. Screening of high-risk smokers is predicted to prevent one death from lung cancer for every 320 individuals screened. In comparison, breast cancer screening with mammograms prevents one death for every 780 screened.

Although screening certain high-risk patients offers the potential to reduce lung cancer mortality, the decision-making process concerning whether to offer screening must take into consideration its associated risks. These include relatively high false-positive rates, radiation exposure from multiple CT scans, patient anxiety, and unnecessary invasive procedures. Clinicians can mitigate these risks by offering screening only to those patients who fall within the parameters outlined in the ACCP, USPSTF, or NCCN guidelines.

Treatment

The first step in lung cancer treatment is, as mentioned, early detection. In the presence of a positive lung cancer screening test or with an incidental finding of imaging done for another reason, consultation with radiology and oncology is warranted. Next steps include biopsy to confirm the diagnosis. Once all pertinent information has been gathered, treatment options are presented and therapy proceeds, keeping in mind overall patient health and comorbidity.

Discussion Sources

American Cancer Society. *Cancer Facts and Figures 2019*. Atlanta, GA: American Cancer Society; 2019. http://www.cancer.org /research/cancer-facts-statistics/all-cancer-facts-figures/cancer-facts-figures-2019.html

Mazzone PJ, Silvestri GA, Patel S, et al. Screening for lung cancer: CHEST guideline and expert panel report. *Chest*. 2018;153:954–985.

National Lung Screening Trial Research Team, Aberle DR, Adams AM, Berg CD, et al. Reduced lung-cancer mortality with low-dose computed tomographic screening. *N Engl J Med*. 2011;365(5):395–409.

QUESTIONS

119. Lung cancer ranks number _____ as a cause of cancer-related death in men and women.

    A. 1

    B. 2

    C. 3

    D. 4

120. Symptoms of lung cancer caused by a primary tumor include all of the following except:

    A. chest discomfort.

    B. dyspnea.

    C. stridor.

    D. hemoptysis.

121. According to ACCP guidelines, annual screening with LDCT for lung cancer should occur in 55- to 77-year-old smokers with a smoking history of at least _____ pack-years.

    A. 15

    B. 30

    C. 50

    D. 70

122. Guidelines from the NCCN recommend screening high-risk smokers beginning at age:

    A. 40 years.

    B. 45 years.

    C. 50 years.

    D. 55 years.

123. Current limitations of screening smokers with LDCT include all of the following except:
    A. a high false-positive rate.
    B. low sensitivity.
    C. radiation exposure from multiple CT scans.
    D. patient anxiety.

124. Risk factors for lung cancer include all of the following except:
    A. high chlorine levels in drinking water.
    B. asbestos exposure.
    C. air pollution.
    D. radiation therapy to the lungs.

125. Other than smoking cessation or avoiding exposure to secondhand smoke, prevention of lung cancer can include:
    A. avoiding outdoor exercise.
    B. use of air purifiers.
    C. detection and treatment of radon in the home.
    D. ICS use.

For answers and rationales, see end of chapter.

QUESTION ANSWERS AND RATIONALES

Asthma

1. **Correct: C. chronic airway inflammation with super-imposed bronchospasm**
   Asthma is best described as a disease involving chronic airway inflammation that is associated with a history of respiratory symptoms that can include wheeze, dyspnea, chest tightness, and cough that can vary over time in intensity (C). Bronchospasm often results as a consequence of airway inflammation.
   Incorrect:
   Asthma is associated with chronic rather than intermittent airway inflammation (A). Bronchospasm is often the result of airway inflammation and not the other way around (B). Airway constriction varies over time and depends on disease progression, exacerbation, as well as adherence to medical treatment (D).

2. **Correct: D. hyperresonance on thoracic percussion.**
   Mild to moderate asthma exacerbation episodes are appropriate for treatment in the office setting. A typical finding during an asthma flare is hyperresonance upon thoracic percussion, which is a louder and lower-pitched sound than normal and can indicate the presence of air trapping (D).
   Incorrect:
   Vocal fremitus is a vibration felt on the chest wall and detected during auscultation when the patient speaks. Crackles are a clicking or rattling noise heard upon auscultation of the lungs, usually arising from airway secretions. Crackles (B) and vocal fremitus (C) are not typical findings of asthma but are more common with

pneumonia. The tripod posture would be an indication of severe respiratory distress, and a patient presenting with this would not be appropriately treated in the office setting but should be immediately transferred to acute care (A).

3. **Correct: C. spirometry measurement.**
   During an asthma flare, an objective measure of airflow obstruction is needed to assess severity of the episode and help guide treatment. Spirometry is the most common lung function test used to monitor asthma and provides a rapid method to evaluate changes to the airways (C).
   Incorrect:
   A chest radiograph is not needed during an asthma flare unless there is a suspicion for pneumonia (such as fever and/or evidence of consolidation) (A). Oxygen saturation will fall late during an asthma flare and will not be useful during the early stage of a flare (B). A sputum smear for WBC or culture and susceptibility testing is not needed for an asthma flare (D).

4. **Correct: C. oral prednisone.**
   During an asthma flare, OCS can be helpful to relieve airway inflammation, which is quite evident in this patient with FEV_1 of 65% predicted (C).
   Incorrect:
   Theophylline is not recommended during an asthma flare (A). The LABA, salmeterol, does not have a role in treating an asthma flare but is used in combination with ICS to prevent bronchospasm (B). Similarly, montelukast is used as a controller agent and not a rescue medication during an asthma flare (D).

5. Correct: D. no antimicrobial therapy.

The use of antimicrobials during an asthma flare should be avoided unless there is evidence of a bacterial infection. This patient presents with clear nasal discharge and an absence of fever, which would suggest a possible viral infection. Thus, antimicrobials would not be needed (D).

Incorrect:

Antimicrobials are not needed for this patient as she likely has a viral infection. Thus, the use of amoxicillin (A), azithromycin (B), or levofloxacin (C) is not warranted.

6. Correct: B. provides a convenient method to check expiratory air flow at home

A peak flow meter can provide a helpful measure of lung function with proper patient education on how to use the device. Though the result is not as accurate as spirometry, it provides a convenient, portable, and inexpensive way to monitor lung function (B).

Incorrect:

Unlike spirometry, a peak flow meter is a portable device that can be used outside of the office setting (A). Patients should be educated on its proper use, though these devices are not as accurate as spirometry (C). Peak flow meters can be used multiple times per day to monitor lung function (D).

7. Correct: D. Chest radiograph should be limited to those with signs of respiratory tract infection (e.g., fever, congested cough).

During an acute asthma exacerbation, a chest radiograph is not warranted unless there is a suspicion of pneumonia (D). Signs of pneumonia can include the presence of fever, elevated WBC count, purulent sputum, and congested cough.

Incorrect:

A chest radiograph has limited usefulness during an asthma flare (A) or to measure resolution of the flare (B). Chest x-ray will not contribute to the severity of the asthma flare (C).

8. Correct: B. propranolol

The use of beta blockers, particularly noncardioselectives, such as propranolol, to treat hypertension should be avoided in patients with asthma, as this can interfere with asthma treatment, particularly the LABAs or SABAs (B). These agents can also cause increased bronchial obstruction and airway reactivity.

Incorrect:

Antihypertensive medications that are preferred for patients with asthma can include thiazide diuretics, such as hydrochlorothiazide (A), or calcium channel blockers, such as amlodipine (C). Angiotensin-converting enzyme (ACE) inhibitors, such as enalapril, are also useful to treat hypertension in asthma patients, though this class is associated with medication-induced cough that can be confused with symptoms of asthma (D).

9 to 12. Yes or No

9. Correct: Yes

10. Correct: Yes

11. Correct: No

12. Correct: Yes

Control of asthma symptoms should be evaluated at every health-care visit to help determine whether medications need adjustment. A convenient and simple way to measure asthma control is through the use of the ACT. Signs of asthma that is not well-controlled include nighttime awakenings that occur more than twice per week (9), a need for SABA use more than twice per week (10), or having two or more exacerbations per year (12). The presence of consolidation on chest x-ray is likely not related to asthma but is a typical finding with pneumonia (11).

13. Correct: D. ICSs.

The use of ICSs is the first-line controller medication for moderate persistent asthma as this is the most effective approach to control airway inflammation (D). Depending on the severity of asthma symptoms, ICS can also be used in combination with a LABA.

Incorrect:

Oral theophylline can be used as a bronchodilator but is not preferred as first-line therapy due to the availability of more effective alternatives (i.e., ICS), a narrow therapeutic index, and potential for drug-drug interactions (A). Mast cell stabilizers are no longer available in the United States due to the availability of more effective treatment options, such as ICSs (B). SABAs are used as rescue medications and not as a controller agent (C).

14. Correct: B. excessive albuterol use is a risk factor for asthma death.

Excessive use of SABA (i.e., more than two canisters per month) suggests that asthma is not well controlled and is a risk factor for asthma-related death (B), as overuse of SABAs is a surrogate marker for poor control of airway inflammation. The best approach for this patient is to initiate an ICS along with a short course of OCS therapy to control airway inflammation.

Incorrect:

Excessive use of SABA indicated that her asthma is not well controlled (A). An ICS would be the preferred approach to reduce airway inflammation, rather than continuing with the SABA (D) or initiating treatment with a LABA (C). LABAs should not generally be used as monotherapy but in combination with ICS.

15. Correct: B. controller to inhibit inflammatory responses.

LTMs, such as montelukast, are used as controller medications that inhibit the inflammatory actions of leukotrienes (B). These agents are generally used as add-on therapy to ICS in moderate or severe persistent asthma.

Incorrect:

LTMs are not used as reliever medications to treat acute inflammation (D) or acute bronchospasm (C). They are used as controller medications to reduce inflammation rather than to prevent bronchospasm (A).

16. Correct: D. rural residence

Several risk factors have been identified for asthma-related death. Among these are urban residence, not rural residence (D).

Incorrect:

Recognizing risk factors for asthma-related death can help guide management decisions. Risk factors include previous severe exacerbations, hospitalization or emergency department visit for asthma in the past month (A), more than two canisters SABA use per month, current or recent withdrawal from systemic corticosteroids (B), poor patient perception of asthma symptoms (C), illicit drug use, low socioeconomic status, and certain comorbidities.

17. Correct: C. assess his level of asthma control and make changes in his treatment plan if needed so he can participate.

The goal for patients with asthma is to have symptoms well controlled that will allow full participation in sports and activities as well as have minimal impact on normal ADLs. At this visit, the patient's asthma control should be evaluated, such as with the ACT, and his medications adjusted to ensure full participation in sports (C).

Incorrect:

Patients with asthma should not be routinely excused from sports participation but should be managed to attain the goal of well-controlled asthma. The patient should be evaluated for asthma control and the medications adjusted accordingly (D). Exercise will not typically trigger symptoms with well-controlled asthma (A). Allergic asthma is more commonly caused by indoor allergens, such as dust mites, rather than pollen exposure (B). For those with allergic asthma, referral to a specialist can be considered for evaluation and potential treatment with immunotherapy.

18. Correct: B. A taper is not needed if the prednisone regimen is usually for 14 days or less.

OCS therapy can be effective in controlling airway inflammation, and a short course can be considered. Typically, systemic corticosteroid use for 14 days or less will not require a tapering regimen (B). Longer durations of corticosteroid use should be tapered to avoid recurrence of inflammation as well as prevent possible cortisol deficiency and its complications.

Incorrect:

Typically, systemic corticosteroid therapy lasting over 14 days will require a tapering regimen to avoid adverse effects (A, C). The use of concomitant ICSs is not a significant factor in determining whether a taper is needed due to low systemic absorption of ICSs (D).

19. Correct: B. within 2 to 8 days.

There is often a delay of several days between the initiation of ICS and improvement in asthma symptoms (B). For those with evidence of inflammation due to asthma, an improved outcome can be achieved with a short course of OCSs at the time of initiating ICSs.

20. Correct: B. the potential ability to provide greater bronchodilation with a lower dose.

Albuterol and levalbuterol are both SABAs used as rescue medications in asthma. Levalbuterol is a single isomer of the racemic mixture found in albuterol. Levalbuterol can provide greater bronchodilation at a reduced dose, thus potentially improving its tolerability (B).

Incorrect:

Albuterol and levalbuterol are both SABAs with the same mechanism of action (A). These agents cause bronchodilation and not anti-inflammatory effects as seen with ICS (C). Levalbuterol is not contraindicated in the elderly (D).

21. Correct: A. The potential but small risk of delayed growth with ICSs is well balanced by their effectiveness.

For children taking ICSs, there is a potential but small risk of delayed growth as well as a potential for a small reduction (0.2 cm) in final adult height in select children (A). However, interpretations of these studies can be difficult because it is difficult to separate any unknown influence from uncontrolled asthma itself versus the treatment.

Incorrect:

ICSs remain the first-line treatment for asthma in children and are preferred over LTMs (B). Though there is a small potential risk for growth stunting in children, this is not a consistent finding and can be a result of other factors, such as uncontrolled asthma (C). The therapeutic effect of LTMs (i.e., anti-inflammatory) is different than that of LABAs (i.e., bronchodilation) (D).

22. Correct: A. oral candidiasis.

The anti-inflammatory action of an ICS can increase the risk of certain adverse effects, such as sore throat, oral candidiasis (A), and hoarseness. Adverse effects can be minimized by rinsing the mouth after each use as well as using a spacer.

Incorrect:

ICS use is not associated with tachycardia (B), gastrointestinal upset (C), or insomnia (D).

23. Correct: C. a congested cough that is worse during the day.

In addition to documented airflow obstruction as measured by FEV_1, several symptoms are consistent with the diagnosis of asthma. However, a congested cough that is worse during the day is more likely to be associated with a respiratory tract infection than asthma (C).

Incorrect:

Characteristic symptoms for asthma include recurrent cough, wheeze (D), shortness of breath, and/or chest tightness (B). Symptoms such as cough are often worse at night (A) or with exercise.

24. Correct: D. smooth muscle relaxation

The mechanism of action of SABAs as well as LABAs is through smooth muscle relaxation that leads to bronchodilation, thus improving airflow in the lungs (D).

Incorrect:

Anti-inflammatory action is observed with the use of ICSs or LTMs (A). LTMs inhibit inflammation by modifying leukotriene action (C). SABAs are not involved in inhibiting the production of secretions (B).

25. Correct: B. Use of LABAs is associated with an increase in the risk of asthma death.

LABAs can be an important part of asthma controller therapy due to their bronchodilation effect. Though the LABA class once had an FDA warning regarding an increased risk of asthma death if used as monotherapy, the warning has since been removed with subsequent research findings (B).

Incorrect:

LABAs used as controller therapy can help improve asthma symptoms, enhance the anti-inflammatory effect of corticosteroids (A), and enhance asthma control when combined with an ICS (C). LABAs in general should not be used as monotherapy to reduce exacerbations and relieve bronchospasm but should be combined with an ICS (D).

26. Correct: C. as a bronchodilator

SAMAs can be used as a rescue medication for the relief of acute asthma symptoms. This class has anticholinergic activity and works as a muscarinic antagonist to yield bronchodilation (C).

Incorrect:

SAMAs generally work as a bronchodilator and not as an anti-inflammatory agent (such as ICSs) (A) or as a mucolytic (D). Use of SAMAs does not result in an increase in the vagal tone of the airway (B).

27. Correct: C. The oral route is preferred over parenteral therapy in most patients.

Systemic corticosteroids can be an effective treatment option to establish control of inflammation in asthma or during an asthma flare. Oral administration is generally preferred as the effectiveness is nearly identical, and there is less risk for serious adverse reactions with oral dosing (C).

Incorrect:

A short course of systemic corticosteroids can be used concomitantly with ICSs to establish control of inflammation. ICS therapy should then continue on a set schedule as the controller medication (A). During an asthma flare, OCSs should be initiated immediately to control inflammation rather than waiting 3 to 4 days, particularly as there can be a delay of several days if ICS therapy is initiated (B). During an asthma flare, the maximum dose in adults generally should not exceed 50 mg/day (D).

28. Correct: D. should be added to therapy only when ICS use does not provide adequate asthma control.

LABAs offer an effective bronchodilation effect that is useful as an asthma controller medication. This class is generally added to an ICS when the ICS does not provide adequate control of symptoms, as LABAs can enhance the anti-inflammatory effect and improve asthma control when used in combination (D). LABAs are not typically used as monotherapy.

Incorrect:

For mild intermittent asthma, the preferred first-line agent is an ICS rather than a LABA (A). LABAs have a similar pharmacodynamic profile as SABAs, though they differ in pharmacokinetics (B). SABAs, used as rescue medications, have a more rapid onset of action compared to LABAs (C).

29. Correct: A. Their use is recommended for patients with mild persistent asthma to prevent asthma flares.

There are a growing number of biological agents available for the management of asthma. These agents are generally reserved for patients with asthma that is not well controlled despite active treatment with recommended agents. Their use would not be considered for patients with mild persistent asthma (A).

Incorrect:

Biological agents available for the treatment of asthma include omalizumab (Xolair®), mepolizumab (Nucala), and reslizumab (Cinquair®). These agents are generally reserved for patients with poorly controlled asthma despite active treatment (C). These monoclonal antibodies are administered via injection or, in the case of reslizumab, IV infusion (B). The use of these medications requires specialized evaluation prior to initiation and ongoing monitoring during its use (D).

30. Correct: B. with allergic-based asthma.

The use of immunotherapy can be considered for patients diagnosed with allergic asthma (B). Treatment can involve subcutaneous immunotherapy or sublingual immunotherapy, and clinical studies demonstrate some improvement in symptom scores and medication requirements with immunotherapy. This approach is generally used as add-on therapy for asthma control.

Incorrect:

Immunotherapy can be considered if allergy plays a prominent role in asthma, such as for those who experience asthma with allergic rhinoconjunctivitis. This approach should not be considered in patients with well-controlled asthma (A) or in other patients with persistent or poorly controlled asthma without a demonstrated component of allergy in their disease process (C, D).

31 to 35. True or False

31. Correct: False

32. Correct: False

33. Correct: False

34. Correct: True

35. Correct: False

In general, primary care providers are not well versed on the relative potency of a given ICS and tend to prescribe too low of a dose for the asthma severity, which can be a barrier to adequate asthma control (31). Systemic absorption of ICSs can vary among the various types of molecules but is usually low and not clinically significant (32). LTMs act as anti-inflammatory agents similar to ICSs but are generally less effective (33). LAMAs can be used as add-on therapy to improve symptom control and have been shown to reduce the risk of asthma exacerbations (34). Mast cell stabilizers are no longer available in the United States due to the availability of more effective options to treat asthma, such as ICSs, rather than any safety concerns (35).

36. Correct: C. increased sputum production.
An asthma flare is characterized by a progressive increase in asthma symptoms. This is not typically associated with an increase in sputum production, which would more likely indicate a respiratory tract infection (C).
Incorrect:
Characteristic findings of an asthma flare include a progressive increase in shortness of breath (A), cough (D), wheezing or chest tightness (B), all associated with decreased lung function. In asthma exacerbations, breath sounds are often reduced, and hyperinflation is present because of significant air trapping.

37 to 39. True or False

37. Correct: False

38. Correct: False

39. Correct: False
During an asthma flare, a SABA should be administered about 4 to 10 puffs every 20 minutes for the first hour and then adjusted afterward. There is no difference in improvement whether the SABA is administered via an MDI with spacer, a DPI, or a nebulizer (37). OCSs should be administered as soon as possible for all patients experiencing a flare; there should not be a wait until symptoms become severe or after transfer to an acute care facility (38). Oxygen therapy should be given to maintain oxygen saturation between 93% and 95% in adults (39).

40. Correct: B. for 2 to 4 weeks.
For patients experiencing an asthma flare, controller therapy should be prescribed to reduce the risk of further exacerbations. For those already on controller medication, increased doses should be maintained for 2 to 4 weeks (B).

41. Correct: A. restore lung function to baseline.
Patients who present with an acute asthma flare require immediate medical attention as this is a potentially life-threatening event. Interventions should aim to relieve airflow obstruction and hypoxemia. However, depending on the severity of the exacerbation and progression of disease, restoration of lung function to baseline may not be achievable (A).
Incorrect:
The goals of treatment of an asthma flare are to rapidly relieve airflow obstruction (B) and hypoxemia (D), address the underlying inflammatory condition (C), and prevent relapse.

Chronic Obstructive Pulmonary Disease

42. Correct: C. receive inactivated influenza virus vaccine.
Patients with COPD are advised to remain up to date with recommended vaccinations, including the pneumococcal vaccine and annual seasonal influenza vaccine. The trivalent or quadrivalent inactivated influenza vaccine administered via injection is recommended for all persons 6 months of age or older (C).
Incorrect:
Annual seasonal influenza vaccination is recommended for all adults with COPD, as there is little risk associated with the inactivated viral vaccine (B). The LAIV vaccine is not recommended for individuals with airway disease (A). Antiviral prophylaxis throughout the flu season is not a recommended approach for prevention of influenza (D).

43 to 46. True or False

43. Correct: True

44. Correct: True

45. Correct: False

46. Correct: False
Annual influenza vaccination is generally recommended for all individuals 6 months and older. Vaccination is especially important for those with close contact with people with comorbidities, such as COPD, as infection can cause serious and life-threatening complications (43). For older adults, high-dose and adjuvanted influenza vaccines are available to help elicit a productive immune response and should be preferred when available (44). If these vaccines are not available, other age-appropriate vaccines are also acceptable. The Centers for Disease Control and Prevention (CDC) recommend administering one dose of the pneumococcal polysaccharide vaccine (PPSV23) to individuals younger than 65 years who have a chronic respiratory disease, such as COPD (45). A second dose of PPSV23 should be given once the individual reaches 65 years (or at least 5 years after the first dose), and a dose of the pneumococcal conjugate vaccine (PCV13) should be considered (46).

47. Correct: C. bronchodilation
Ipratropium bromide is a short-acting anticholinergic agent that has a similar effect as beta-2 agonists in achieving bronchodilation (C). Ipratropium bromide must be dosed several times per day to achieve the desired effect, and long-acting bronchodilators are generally preferred over this agent because of its better effectiveness and convenience.
Incorrect:
Ipratropium bromide works as a bronchodilator and is not involved in mucociliary clearance (A) and does not provide mucolytic activity (D). This agent does not reduce alveolar volume (B), which would be a negative outcome in the treatment of COPD.

48. **Correct: C. reduction of airway inflammation**

ICS and LAMA therapy can be an important part of the management of COPD, as these agents reduce airway inflammation (C), therefore reducing the risk of COPD exacerbation.

Incorrect:

ICS or LAMA use does not impact the central respiratory drive (B), and they do not exhibit mucolytic activity (D). Fixed airway obstruction can be a consequence of chronic airway inflammation resulting in airway remodeling, but ICS or LAMA use will not reverse these effects (A).

49. **Correct: C. increased risk of pneumonia.**

ICSs can be used to reduce airway inflammation found in COPD. However, use of these agents is associated with certain adverse effects, such as a small increased risk of the development of pneumonia (C).

Incorrect:

The use of ICSs is not associated with the development of concomitant asthma (A), nor will it lead to more severe exacerbations in COPD (D). ICSs can help to prevent exacerbations, which are events that can hasten lung function decline (B).

50. **Correct: A. FEV$_1$:FVC ratio equal to or less than 0.70 after properly timed SABA use**

Though most individuals with COPD will be symptomatic at the time of diagnosis, symptoms are not needed. Objective measures of lung function are used to confirm the diagnosis of COPD since many in the early stages of disease will be asymptomatic. The accepted diagnostic measure is a FEV$_1$:FVC ratio of 0.70 or less (A).

Incorrect:

Though dyspnea is a common symptom of COPD, this is not needed to make a diagnosis (B). Spirometry is used to evaluate lung function and confirm the diagnosis. A chest radiograph is not needed unless the physician is trying to rule out another condition, such as pneumonia (C). Polycythemia, or elevated levels of red blood cells, is occasionally noted in advanced disease but is not an essential finding in a COPD diagnosis (D).

51. **Correct: D. to avoid exposure to pulmonary irritants, including active or passive exposure to cigarette smoke.**

Several nonpharmacological approaches can be used to prevent COPD exacerbations. However, the most effective approach is to limit exposure to pulmonary irritants, especially tobacco smoke (D). For patients who continue to smoke despite a COPD diagnosis, the issue of smoking cessation should be raised at every office visit along with offering resources and assistance as part of the ongoing care.

Incorrect:

Weight loss in individuals who are overweight or obese can help to alleviate respiratory restriction (A). Avoiding or limiting exposure to children who attend day-care centers can help to prevent respiratory tract infections that can trigger an exacerbation (B). Increasing physical activity can be helpful in increasing fitness and help with respiratory function (C).

52. **Correct: D. at every office visit.**

The most effective approach to prevent COPD exacerbations and slow disease progression is to limit exposure to pulmonary irritants, especially tobacco smoke. For patients who continue to smoke despite a COPD diagnosis, the issue of smoking cessation should be raised at every visit along with offering resources and assistance as part of ongoing care (D).

Incorrect:

Raising the issue of smoking cessation and offering assistance should be done at every visit as part of ongoing care (A). Consistent and persistent discussions will help the patient recognize the consequences of tobacco use. The issue should not be limited to only when there is an exacerbation (B) or when ICS therapy is initiated (C), as the delay will cause irreversible progression of lung function decline.

53. **Correct: A. short-acting inhaled beta-2 agonist**

According to the GOLD COPD guidelines, a SABA is appropriate at all stages of COPD as a bronchodilator and rescue medication (A).

Incorrect:

An ICS is usually reserved for COPD patients with more severe disease (group C or D) as an add-on to long-acting bronchodilator therapy (B). A PDE-4 inhibitor can be considered in patients with severe or very severe airflow limitation (group D), despite combination therapy with a LABA, LAMA, and/or ICS (C). The regular use of a mucolytic can be considered in patients who are not currently taking an ICS, though these agents would not generally be needed for patients with mild disease (D).

54. **Correct: A. minimize the risk of repeated exacerbations.**

According to the GOLD COPD guidelines, the use of an ICS can be considered as add-on therapy for patients with persistent exacerbations (group C or D). These agents provide an anti-inflammatory effect and can reduce the frequency of exacerbations when combined with a LABA (A).

Incorrect:

ICSs provide anti-inflammatory activity and are not used to improve cough function (B) or reverse alveolar hypertrophy (C). Mucolytics can be used to help mobilize secretions in the airways (D).

55. **Correct: A. 5 to 7 days**

When OCS therapy is warranted to reduce airway inflammation during a COPD exacerbation, a regimen of 5 to 7 days is generally recommended (A). Clinical evidence demonstrates that a 5-day course is just as effective as a 10-day course and will reduce the risk of adverse effects. Tapering doses are not typically needed for regimens lasting 14 days or less.

56. **Correct: C. respiratory tract viruses**

Respiratory tract infection is a common cause of COPD exacerbation. Respiratory tract viruses are often overlooked as the causative pathogen, though they are implicated in up to 50% of exacerbations (C).

Incorrect:

The most common bacterial causes of COPD exacerbations include *H influenzae*, *H parainfluenzae*, *S pneumoniae*, and *M catarrhalis*. Atypical pathogens, such as *Legionella*, are less commonly identified (A). *S pyogenes* (B) and *S aureus* (D) are not typically associated with COPD exacerbations.

57. **Correct: D. antimicrobial therapy usually not indicated**

The role of antimicrobial therapy during COPD exacerbation is debated even for severe disease. Antimicrobials should be limited to those individuals who present with signs and symptoms of bacterial infection, such as fever and consolidation, as therapy can help to prevent early relapse or treatment failure and hasten recovery. However, in the absence of any indication of a bacterial infection, antimicrobial therapy is not indicated (D).

Incorrect:

For this patient with no evidence of a bacterial infection, antimicrobial therapy is not warranted. Amoxicillin (B) and doxycycline (C) can be used when bacterial infection is suspected in mild to moderate disease. A respiratory fluoroquinolone can be used in severe disease when a bacterial infection is suspected or confirmed (A).

58. **Correct: D. The role of antimicrobial therapy is debated, even for a severe exacerbation.**

The role of antimicrobial therapy during COPD exacerbation is debated even for severe disease (D). Antimicrobials should be limited to those individuals who present with signs and symptoms of bacterial infection, such as fever and consolidation, as therapy can help to prevent early relapse or treatment failure and hasten recovery.

Incorrect:

When a bacterial infection is suspected or confirmed during a COPD exacerbation, antimicrobial therapy can be considered to prevent early relapse or treatment failure and hasten recovery. When prescribed, antimicrobial treatment duration should be limited to 5 to 7 days, and severe disease can be treated with oral forms of amoxicillin-clavulanate (B), azithromycin (A), clarithromycin, a respiratory fluoroquinolone, or cephalosporin. TMP-SMX is not recommended for treatment of COPD exacerbation (C).

59. **Correct: D. "For at least 15 hours a day."**

When oxygen therapy is prescribed for severe COPD, it is recommended to be used for at least 15 hours each day, as this prolonged duration is needed to correct hypoxemia and reduce heart workload (D). The long-term administration of oxygen therapy has been shown to increase survival in patients with severe resting hypoxemia.

Incorrect:

Maximum effects of oxygen therapy require prolonged use (more than 15 hours) during the day. Oxygen therapy can be used during waking or sleeping hours (B, C) and should not be limited to only when the individual is short of breath (A). Many patients who wait until they are breathless before starting oxygen therapy and/or only use oxygen therapy on an as-needed basis will fail to achieve the maximum benefits of this therapy.

60. **Correct: B. when attempting to rule out a concomitant pneumonia.**

Chest radiograph has limited usefulness in diagnosing a COPD exacerbation but can be used to rule out concomitant conditions that can cause respiratory symptoms. These include pneumonia (B), pneumothorax, or pleural effusion.

Incorrect:

Routine use of chest radiography has limited utility during a COPD exacerbation unless there is a need to rule out other conditions (A). An increase in sputum volume (C) and shortness of breath/labored breathing (D) are common features during an exacerbation and do not warrant chest radiography.

61. **Correct: B. use limited by narrow therapeutic profile and drug–drug interaction potential**

The use of theophylline as a bronchodilator is limited in the management of COPD as other bronchodilators are more effective and better tolerated. Theophylline is also associated with a narrow therapeutic index that requires regular monitoring for levels and has the potential for numerous drug-drug interactions (B).

Incorrect:

Theophylline acts as a bronchodilator but is not as potent as other available agents (C). Theophylline is available in oral and IV formulations (D). Due to its narrow therapeutic index and drug–drug interaction potential, it is not a preferred treatment option in COPD (A) and would not be effective in moderate to severe disease due to its mild bronchodilator effect.

62. **Correct: A. it is reserved for very severe COPD.**

The goals of pulmonary rehabilitation are to improve quality of life, decrease symptoms, and increase physical participation in ADLs. Patients at all severity levels of COPD can benefit from pulmonary rehabilitation (A).

Incorrect:

Pulmonary rehabilitation can be helpful in reducing anxiety and depression among patients with COPD (D). The goals of pulmonary rehabilitation are to improve quality of life, decrease symptoms, and increase physical participation in ADLs (B). Pulmonary rehabilitation is often underused because of issues of funding, access, and lack of provider and patient knowledge (C).

63. **Correct: A. increased FEV_1.**

A COPD exacerbation is associated with an increase in COPD symptoms as well as decreased lung function that could be at least partially irreversible. This would lead to a decrease, rather than increase, in FEV_1 values as determined by spirometry (A).

Incorrect:
Characteristic findings during COPD exacerbation are typically an increase in symptoms, including increased cough (B) and wheezing, sputum production (D), and shortness of breath. Sputum can also have increased purulence (C), suggesting the presence of a bacterial infection and/or higher levels of white blood cells.

Tuberculosis

64. Correct: C. a TST finding of 10 mm or more induration should be considered a positive result.
Individuals who have a higher risk of being infected, such as those who emigrated from high-prevalence countries, are considered to have a positive result from the TST with an induration of 10 mm (C). Receipt of the BCG vaccine as a child does not impact the interpretation of the TST result.

Incorrect:
Individuals from areas with high prevalence of TB will not always have a positive TST result, thus emphasizing the need to test individuals at higher risk of TB exposure to identify those who may require treatment (A). Chest radiographs are not required unless there is a positive TST result to exclude active pulmonary TB (B). Prophylaxis with isoniazid should only be initiated with evidence of a latent infection that is detected with a positive TST or other test result but a negative finding on chest radiograph for active infection (D).

65. Correct: A. She should receive TB chemoprophylaxis if her TST result is 5 mm or more in induration.
For an individual with recent contact with a person with documented TB disease, a TST result of 5 mm or more is considered positive. To prevent active TB, chemoprophylaxis should be considered with a positive TST result (A).

Incorrect:
Though there is a greater risk of drug-induced adverse effects with increasing age, older age by itself is not a contraindication for chemoprophylaxis (B). A positive TST test with normal chest radiograph would suggest a latent TB infection, and treatment should be considered to prevent future active TB infection (C). For patients with recent close contact of a person with TB disease, a positive result on the TST is 5 mm or more in induration (D).

66. Correct: D. it is able to predict who is at greatest risk for active disease development.
The QuantiFERON®-TB Gold test does offer several advantages compared to the TST. However, neither of these tests is able to predict which individuals with latent TB infection will progress to active TB disease (D).

Incorrect:
The QuantiFERON®-TB Gold test is a blood test that detects interferon-γ that is released in response to *M tuberculosis*–specific antigens. The test can be performed with a blood sample taken during a single clinical visit (A), and the results are available within 24 hours compared with the 2 to 3 days needed for the TST (B). This test also provides a quantitative result that is not subject to reader bias (C).

67 to 71. Yes or No

67. Correct: No

68. Correct: No

69. Correct: Yes

70. Correct: Yes

71. Correct: Yes
When evaluating a TST reaction, health-care providers should consider several criteria when determining whether a result is positive or negative. An induration of 5 mm or greater can be considered positive for TB among individuals with HIV (69) or other immunosuppressed individuals, such as those taking a TNF-α antagonist (71). Individuals who emigrated from high-endemic countries will be considered positive with a TST result of 10 mm or greater induration (70). In healthy individuals with no risk factor for TB, a TST result of 15 mm or greater induration is needed for a positive result (68). For those who work in a mycobacteriology laboratory, an induration of 10 mm or higher is needed for a positive result (67).

72. Correct: D. male gender.
Without treatment, individuals with latent TB infection have a 10% lifetime risk of reactivation to develop postprimary TB. Certain individuals are at higher risk, though male gender is not considered a risk factor for reactivation (D).

Incorrect:
Risk factors for reactivation of TB include HIV or other forms of immunocompromise (B), including the use of systemic corticosteroids (C). Several chronic conditions can also increase risk, such as diabetes mellitus (A).

73. Correct: D. frank hemoptysis.
Blood-tinged sputum is occasionally reported in patients with active TB infection. However, frank hemoptysis is rarely found in patients with TB disease (D).

Incorrect:
Common signs and symptoms of progressive primary TB include a dry cough (C), fever (B), malaise (A), weight loss or anorexia, and night sweats.

74. Correct: B. Gram stain from blood sample
Though *M tuberculosis* can infect extrapulmonary tissues, a Gram stain of blood sample is not sensitive or specific to detect active pulmonary TB disease (B).

Incorrect:
Findings from a chest radiograph can be used to detect signs of active TB disease (typically a patchy or nodular infiltrate) or exclude the diagnosis (A). Acid-fast microscopy can provide a rapid approach to detect for acid-fast bacilli in sputum suggesting the presence of *M tuberculosis* (C). Confirmation of active TB disease requires culture for the presence of the infecting organism, while susceptibility testing can help guide treatment decisions (D).

Community-Acquired Pneumonia

75. Correct: A. oral doxycycline

For adults with CAP and no risk factors for antimicrobial resistance, preferred treatment choices can include oral formulations of amoxicillin, doxycycline, or the macrolides (A).

Incorrect:

For individuals with risk factors for antimicrobial-resistant infection, including comorbidities, asplenia, and alcoholism, treatment can include monotherapy with an oral respiratory fluoroquinolone or combination therapy with oral formulations of doxycycline, azithromycin, or clarithromycin plus a beta-lactam (amoxicillin-clavulanate or a cephalosporin [B]). Ciprofloxacin is not considered a respiratory fluoroquinolone and would not be used in the treatment of CAP (D). TMP-SMX is not recommended for the treatment of CAP (C).

76. Correct: C. oral doxycycline

For adults with CAP and no risk factors for antimicrobial resistance, preferred treatment choices can include oral formulations of amoxicillin, doxycycline (C), or the macrolides.

Incorrect:

In the presence of macrolide intolerance, the use of clarithromycin should be avoided in this patient (A). Cephalexin (B) and fosfomycin (D) are not recommended agents for the treatment of CAP. Fosfomycin is typically used for the treatment of urinary tract infections.

77. Correct: B. oral amoxicillin-clavulanate with oral doxycycline

For individuals with risk factors for antimicrobial-resistant infection, including the presence of significant comorbidities such as COPD, treatment can include monotherapy with an oral respiratory fluoroquinolone or combination therapy with oral formulations of doxycycline, azithromycin, or clarithromycin plus a beta-lactam (amoxicillin-clavulanate or a cephalosporin). A combination of amoxicillin-clavulanate plus doxycycline would be appropriate (B).

Incorrect:

Clindamycin is not a recommended treatment option for CAP (A). Clarithromycin monotherapy would be appropriate for a patient with no risk factor for antimicrobial resistance but would need to be combined with a beta-lactam in higher-risk patients (C). Similarly, a cephalosporin such as ceftriaxone should be combined with a macrolide or doxycycline for patients with significant comorbidities (D).

78. Correct: A. oral respiratory fluoroquinolone

For individuals with risk factors for antimicrobial-resistant infection, including the presence of significant comorbidities such as heart failure and type 2 diabetes, treatment can include monotherapy with an oral respiratory fluoroquinolone (A) or combination therapy with oral formulations of doxycycline, azithromycin,

or clarithromycin plus a beta-lactam (amoxicillin-clavulanate or a cephalosporin).

Incorrect:

For this patient with significant comorbidities, beta-lactam therapy with amoxicillin-clavulanate (B) or a cephalosporin (C) should be combined with a macrolide or doxycycline to ensure adequate coverage of the causative pathogen. TMP-SMX is not a preferred antimicrobial for the treatment of CAP (D).

79. Correct: A. oral clarithromycin

For a patient presenting with a dry cough and mild signs and symptoms, this would suggest infection with an atypical pathogen. In the absence of comorbidities or other risk factors for antimicrobial resistance, treatment with an oral macrolide would be appropriate (A).

Incorrect:

In the presence of severe beta-lactam allergy, the use of amoxicillin (B) and cephalosporins (D) should be avoided. A respiratory fluoroquinolone is not warranted in the absence of risk factors for resistance (C).

80. Correct: D. oral moxifloxacin

For patients with risk factors for resistant pathogens infection caused by monotherapy with a respiratory fluoroquinolone is appropriate (D). Risk factors can include hospitalization and administration of parenteral antimicrobials.

Incorrect:

This patient is at higher risk of infection with MRSA or *P aeruginosa* and so should receive either monotherapy with a respiratory fluoroquinolone or combination therapy with oral formulations of doxycycline, azithromycin, or clarithromycin plus a beta-lactam. Monotherapy with amoxicillin-clavulanate (A), amoxicillin (B), or a macrolide (C) would not be preferred.

81. Correct: C. had no prior antimicrobial use in the previous 3 months.

Criteria for CAP are primarily focused on the setting of where the infection originated. Recent use of an antimicrobial is not part of the criteria, though this could increase the risk of an antimicrobial-resistant infection (C).

Incorrect:

Criteria for CAP include onset of disease that occurs in the community (A) and should not be associated with living in a nursing home or other long-term care facility (B) as well as not be due to recent hospitalization (D).

82. Correct: B. altered mental status.

Respiratory symptoms are the most common among those with CAP. Altered mental status is not a common finding among CAP patients who are otherwise well (B). However, this can be part of an atypical presentation in older adults with CAP.

Incorrect:

Common signs and symptoms of CAP include cough (A), dyspnea (C), sputum production, and pleuritic chest pain (D). Some nonrespiratory symptoms can also be evident, including fatigue and gastrointestinal upset.

83. Correct: D. chest radiograph.

Chest radiographs should be obtained in all patients suspected of CAP to confirm the diagnosis with the presence of pulmonary infiltrates or to exclude other conditions that may mimic CAP (D).

Incorrect:

In the outpatient setting, a sputum Gram stain (B) and sputum culture (A) are not recommended, as these frequently have low yield of organisms in nonsevere disease, and the results will not likely affect management decisions or clinical outcomes. Bronchoalveolar lavage is typically only performed in severe disease that requires hospitalization (C).

84. Correct: A. activity against drug-resistant *S pneumoniae* (DRSP)

The respiratory fluoroquinolones retain activity against *S pneumoniae* that exhibit resistance to other classes of antimicrobials, such as beta-lactams and macrolides (A). However, the use of these agents should be reserved, when necessary, due to increasing rates of resistance and certain safety concerns.

Incorrect:

The respiratory fluoroquinolones exhibit potent activity against *S pneumoniae*, usually including DRSP, as well as atypical pathogens (B) and beta-lactamase–producing organisms (D). Levofloxacin is predominantly excreted as an unchanged drug in the urine and is not hepatically metabolized (C).

85. Correct: C. alteration in protein-binding sites.

The predominant mechanism of resistance exhibited by *S pneumoniae* is an alteration in protein-binding sites (e.g., penicillin-binding protein) that makes antimicrobials ineffective (C).

Incorrect:

Beta-lactamase production is the most common mechanism utilized by *H influenzae* and *M catarrhalis* that provides resistance against beta-lactam agents, such as penicillin, ampicillin, and amoxicillin (A). Mutations in DNA gyrase and topoisomerase can result in resistance against fluoroquinolones, but this is not a common mechanism in *S pneumoniae* (D). Hypertrophy of the cell membrane is not a common mechanism of resistance by *S pneumoniae* (B).

86. Correct: A. beta-lactamase production.

Beta-lactamase production is the most common mechanism utilized by *H influenzae* and *M catarrhalis* that provides resistance against beta-lactam agents, such as penicillin, ampicillin, and amoxicillin (A).

Incorrect:

The predominant mechanism of resistance exhibited by *S pneumoniae* is an alteration in protein-binding sites (e.g., penicillin-binding protein) that makes antimicrobials ineffective (C). Mutations in DNA gyrase and topoisomerase can result in resistance against fluoroquinolones, but this is not a common mechanism in *H influenzae* (D). Hypertrophy of the cell membrane is not a common mechanism of resistance for *H influenzae* (B).

87. Correct: C. effective against atypical pathogens

The macrolides, such as clarithromycin and azithromycin, can be used for the treatment of CAP caused by atypical pathogens, such as *M pneumoniae*, *C pneumoniae*, and *Legionella* species (C).

Incorrect:

The macrolides are not recommended for use against infections suspected or confirmed by drug-resistant *S pneumoniae* due to high rates of resistance to this class of agents (A). Macrolides are generally safe to use in patients with penicillin allergy as there is no cross-reactivity (B). Macrolides do not possess a beta-lactam ring and so are stable in the presence of beta-lactamase (D).

88. Correct: B. 5 to 7 days

Guidelines recommend duration of antimicrobial therapy of at least 5 days, with evidence of increasing clinical stability and absence of fever for 48 to 72 hours before discontinuing therapy. On average, treatment should last 5 to 7 days (B).

Incorrect:

Treatment should last at least 5 days (A) with the average duration of 5 to 7 days, depending on evidence of clinical stability and absence of fever. Longer duration of treatment should be avoided as this can increase the risk of resistance development and drug-induced adverse effects without improving clinical outcomes (C, D).

89 to 91. Indicate inpatient (I) or outpatient (O)

89. Correct: Outpatient

90. Correct: Inpatient

91. Correct: Inpatient

The CURB-65 criteria are a simple method to determine whether a patient with CAP should be treated in the inpatient or outpatient setting. CURB-65 allocates one point for each of the following five criteria: confusion, BUN greater than 19 mg/dL, respiratory rate greater than 30/minutes, blood pressure less than 90/60 mm Hg, and 65 years of age and older. A score of 1 or less indicates that the patient can be treated as an outpatient, whereas a score greater than 1 indicates hospitalization is needed. The 47-year-old would have a score of 1, indicating outpatient management is appropriate (89). The 56-year-old will have a score of 2, suggesting inpatient management is needed (90). The 72-year-old has a score of 3 supporting the need for inpatient management, possibly in the intensive care unit (ICU) (91).

92. Correct: A. living in a rural setting.

According to the ATS/IDSA guidelines, empiric antimicrobial selection should be based on risk factors for infection caused by MRSA or *P aeruginosa*. However, living in a rural setting is not identified as a risk factor for infection by these pathogens (A).

Incorrect:

Risk factors for CAP caused by MRSA or *P aeruginosa* include prior respiratory isolation of these pathogens (D), recent hospitalization (B), and recent receipt of parenteral antimicrobials (within the past 90 days) (C).

93. **Correct: C. Sputum analysis is not recommended in the majority of patients with CAP.**

For patients with nonsevere CAP who will be treated in the outpatient setting, sputum Gram stain and/or culture is not recommended as the yield of organisms is typically low from sputum samples, and findings will unlikely impact management decisions and clinical outcomes (C). For severe CAP requiring hospitalization, a culture should be considered to identify the pathogen and resistance profile to help guide antimicrobial selection.

Incorrect:

Routine Gram stain from a sputum sample is not recommended as part of the diagnostic process in nonsevere CAP (A). Once a CAP diagnosis is made, typically following a chest radiograph, antimicrobial therapy should not be delayed until culture results, which can take 2 to 3 days (B). Sputum analysis is not required or recommended in most patients with CAP, and thus chest physical therapy is not warranted (D).

94. **Correct: B. respiratory droplet**

Atypical pneumonia is most commonly caused by *C pneumoniae* or *M pneumoniae*. These organisms are largely transmitted by respiratory droplets resulting from cough (B), and atypical pneumonia is often seen in individuals who spend extended time in close proximity to others, such as correctional facilities, college dormitories, or long-term care facilities.

Incorrect:

Microaspiration is a common mechanism of transmission of *S pneumoniae* and *H influenzae* (A). Aerosolized contaminated water is the usual mechanisms of transmission of *Legionella* (D). Surface contamination is not a typical route of transmission for pneumonia pathogens (C).

95. **Correct: C. renal insufficiency.**

ATS/IDSA guidelines provide criteria for determining severe pneumonia that would warrant hospitalization due to a higher risk of death. Major criteria include the presence of septic shock or respiratory failure, while minor criteria include elevated respiratory rate, leukopenia, thrombocytopenia, uremia (indicating renal insufficiency [C]), hypothermia, and hypotension, among others.

Incorrect:

S pneumoniae is the most common cause of fatal CAP, while viral infection is not a risk factor for mortality (A). Leukopenia and thrombocytopenia, rather than polycythemia, are associated with higher mortality risk (D). History of allergic reaction to multiple antimicrobials is not identified as a risk factor for death (B).

96. **Correct: C. higher antimicrobial dosage.**

The use of higher antimicrobial doses for shorter periods of time optimizes the pharmacokinetic/pharmacodynamic properties of the antimicrobial to eradicate the infection and reduce the risk of resistance development (C). This strategy is particularly true for concentration-dependent antimicrobials, such as the fluoroquinolones, where a regimen of levofloxacin 750 mg for 5 days is preferred over the 500 mg for 7 to 10 days.

Incorrect:

Using a longer course of therapy (A), lower antimicrobial dose (B), and broad-spectrum agent (D) will encourage resistance development, as these strategies will eradicate susceptible pathogens but encourage growth of intermediate or resistant pathogens.

97. **Correct: C. consolidation.**

Consolidation describes an area of the lung that has filled with liquid instead of air. Consolidation can be identified by findings of increased tactile fremitus and dullness to percussion (C).

Incorrect:

Atelectasis describes a collapse of lung tissue with loss of volume and is indicated by an absence of breath sounds (A). Pneumothorax is characterized by a decrease, rather than an increase, in tactile fremitus (B). Cavitation refers to a gas-filled space in the lung and usually cannot be detected by physical examination but would require chest radiography (D).

98. **Correct: A. His current plan of care should continue because he is improving by clinical assessment.**

The patient is showing clinical improvement with the current management strategy and so the current antimicrobial regimen should be continued for at least a total of 5 days and discontinued when clinical stability and absence of fever are sustained for 48 to 72 hours (A).

Incorrect:

A chest radiograph is not needed to confirm improvement of CAP, especially since pulmonary findings will not typically resolve for up to 1 month or longer following disease (B). The patient is improving and so a change in antimicrobial therapy is not needed (C), and there is no need for additional imaging studies (D).

99. **Correct: D. influenza and pneumococcal vaccines should be given today.**

Annual seasonal influenza vaccination is recommended for nearly all individuals 6 months and older, while pneumococcal vaccine is recommended for all immunocompetent adults at age 65 years who have not yet received a pneumococcal vaccine. The vaccines can be administered at the same office visit. Vaccines of any kind can be given to individuals in the absence of moderate to severe illness, with or without fever. For this patient who has resolved the CAP episode and is now back in the community, immunization with both vaccines is appropriate (D).

Incorrect:

Vaccines can be administered to individuals who are taking antimicrobial therapy and who are absent of moderate to severe illness (A). The influenza and pneumococcal vaccines can be administered at the same office visit without the need for an interval between vaccinations (B, C).

100. Correct: B. inhalation of aerosolized contaminated water.

Aerosolized contaminated water is the usual mechanism of transmission of *Legionella* (D).

Incorrect:

C pneumoniae or *M pneumoniae* are largely transmitted by respiratory droplets resulting from cough (A). Hematogenous spread (D) or surface contamination (C) are not typical routes of transmission for pneumonia pathogens.

101 to 107. Indicate gram-positive, gram-negative, or atypical

101. Correct: gram-positive

102. Correct: gram-negative

103. Correct: atypical

104. Correct: atypical

105. Correct: atypical

106. Correct: gram-positive

107. Correct: gram-negative

Understanding the characteristics of bacterial pathogens can be important in guiding management decisions. Among CAP pathogens, gram-positive bacteria include *S pneumoniae* (101) and *S aureus* (106). Gram-negative pathogens include *H influenzae* (102) and *P aeruginosa* (107). Atypical pathogens, which cannot be identified by Gram stain, include *C pneumoniae*, *M pneumoniae*, and *Legionella* species (104, 105, 103).

108 to 111. Yes or No

108. Correct: No

109. Correct: No

110. Correct: No

111. Correct: No

The latest CAP guidelines from ATS/IDSA do not recommend routine use of the pneumococcal urinary antigen (111) or *Legionella* urinary antigen test (110) except in cases of severe CAP. Evidence has demonstrated that the use of these tests does not provide any benefit. Procalcitonin (108) and lactate (109) are used as markers for the presence of sepsis, which is a serious and life-threatening condition that would not be treated in the outpatient setting but would require hospitalization and possibly ICU care.

Acute Bronchitis

112. Correct: C. 3 weeks

Acute bronchitis is characterized as a self-limited infection that can last for approximately 3 weeks but sometimes will persist for up to 4 to 6 weeks (C). Chronic bronchitis is defined as respiratory symptoms, including cough, that last for at least 3 months of the year for 2 consecutive years.

113. Correct: D. 95% or more

The predominant cause of acute bronchitis is viral infection, which causes at least 95% of episodes.

Because of this, the use of antimicrobial therapy is not recommended, as acute bronchitis will typically resolve on its own.

114. Correct: A. *S pneumoniae*.

The predominant pathogen in acute bronchitis is typically a viral organism. On the rare occasion a bacterial pathogen is identified, *S pneumoniae* is not implicated in these infections, though it is a common pathogen in CAP and upper respiratory tract infections.

Incorrect:

Bacterial causes of acute bronchitis can include the atypical pathogens *M pneumoniae* (B) and *C pneumoniae* (C) as well as *B pertussis* (D) that is implicated in pertussis and whooping cough (in children).

115. Correct: A. an antitussive.

In the absence of any evidence for a bacterial infection, such as pneumonia, patients with symptoms of acute bronchitis should receive symptomatic therapy only. This can include an antitussive (A), mucolytic, or expectorant to help relieve frequency and severity of cough.

Incorrect:

Antimicrobial therapy with a macrolide (C) or beta-lactam agent (D) is not routinely recommended for the treatment of acute bronchitis in the absence of signs or symptoms of bacterial infection. An antihistamine is also not warranted, as these agents are used to treat an allergic reaction rather than a likely viral infection (B).

116. Correct: A. normal findings

Acute bronchitis is typically a clinical diagnosis made by patient history and physical examination. Examination of the lungs in acute bronchitis is usually normal (A) in the absence of a more serious infection, such as influenza or pneumonia.

Incorrect:

During acute bronchitis, crackles are absent (D) as is evidence of consolidation (B). If these findings are present, a diagnosis other than acute bronchitis, such as pneumonia or heart failure, should be considered. Wheezing is not a common finding in acute bronchitis, though occasionally expiratory wheeze rather than inspiratory wheeze can be present (C).

117. Correct: D. usually not needed unless there is suspicion of pneumonia

A chest x-ray is not needed and is not recommended for the diagnosis of acute bronchitis as it will offer little information about the clinical condition (D). A chest x-ray can be considered when there is concern about pneumonia for a patient who presents with cough plus fever and/or consolidation.

Incorrect:

Acute bronchitis is usually a clinical diagnosis that does not require a chest x-ray for confirmation (A). Multilobar infiltrates would not be observed with acute bronchitis but would more likely indicate pneumonia or other serious infection (C). Routine chest x-ray at presentation and upon resolution of symptoms is not needed and is not recommended (B).

118. Correct: C. persistent asthma.

When considering acute bronchitis, it is important to recognize other clinical conditions that can present similarly when making the differential diagnosis. For this patient who experiences coughing episodes several times each year as well as frequent nighttime awakening due to respiratory symptoms, a likely diagnosis would be persistent asthma (C). Spirometry can be used to measure lung function and help confirm an asthma diagnosis.

Incorrect:

Acute bronchitis is defined as a persistent cough that lasts approximately 3 weeks and then typically resolves rather than persistent symptoms throughout the year (A). Walking pneumonia is caused by infection with an atypical pathogen and is characterized by a dry cough that would persist until resolution rather than undergo repeated periods of resolution followed by symptoms throughout the year (D). Active TB is characterized by chronic cough, malaise, night sweats, fever, and weight loss, which were not reported for this patient (B).

Lung Cancer

119. Correct: A. 1

Lung cancer is the leading cause of cancer death in both men and women, accounting for approximately 142,000 deaths each year (A). Lung cancer is the second leading cause of new cancer cases in each gender, trailing only prostate cancer in men and breast cancer in women.

120. Correct: C. stridor.

Stridor is caused by obstructed airflow in the lungs and results in a high-pitched, wheezing sound. The airflow blockage is typically in the upper respiratory system, such as near the trachea or larynx, and is not typically associated with lung cancer (C).

Incorrect:

Early stages of lung cancer are typically asymptomatic with symptoms manifesting in later disease. The most common signs of lung cancer can include nonspecific symptoms of fatigue, anorexia, or weight loss. Signs of a primary tumor can include chest discomfort (A), cough, dyspnea (B), and hemoptysis (D).

121. Correct: B. 30

The ACCP guidelines recommend annual LDCT screening for high-risk individuals, which can include current smokers aged 55 to 77 years with a smoking history of at least 30 pack-years (B) as well as former smokers of the same age who have quit within the past 15 years but have the same smoking history. Guidelines from the USPSTF are similar to those of ACCP with the exception of extending the age for LDCT screening up to 80 years.

122. Correct: C. 50 years.

The NCCN recommends annual LDCT screening for patients 55 to 74 years with a 30 or more pack-year history of smoking, as well as younger patients (50 years or older) with a less extensive smoking history (at least 20 pack-years) who have one additional risk factor (C). Additional risk factors can include a history of cancer or lung disease, family history of lung cancer, radon exposure, or occupational exposure.

123. Correct: B. low sensitivity.

LDCT can be an important tool in screening high-risk patients for lung cancer. However, there are a number of limitations with this approach. LDCT has a high sensitivity in detecting abnormalities that can be related to lung cancer (B).

Incorrect:

Limitations of LDCT screening include a high false-positive rate (A), radiation exposure from repeated CT scans over the years (C), as well as patient anxiety during the process (D). As such, LDCT should only be used for individuals who meet the criteria outlined in current guidelines.

124. Correct: A. high chlorine levels in drinking water.

Smoking and exposure to secondhand smoke are major risk factors for lung cancer. However, other factors have been identified beyond tobacco smoke that can increase risk. Though not typically a concern in the United States, asbestos in drinking water can increase the risk of lung cancer. However, high levels of chlorine have not been implicated in this disease (A).

Incorrect:

Modifiable risk factors for lung cancer include exposure to radon or asbestos (B), exposure to cancer-causing agents in the workplace, certain dietary supplements, and arsenic in the drinking water. Non-modifiable risk factors include previous radiation therapy to the lungs (D), air pollution (C), and personal or family history of lung cancer.

125. Correct: C. detection and treatment of radon in the home.

Exposure to radon is a risk factor for lung cancer. Radon gas can be found in any home or building throughout the United States, and radon testing and appropriate treatment should be performed to minimize this risk (C).

Incorrect:

Though air pollution can be a risk factor for lung cancer, the benefits of outdoor exercise far outweigh the risk under most circumstances (A). Air purifiers can be effective in reducing the level of allergens but are unlikely to be effective in removing pollutants and smoke that can cause lung cancer (B). ICS use, such as in asthma or COPD treatment, has not been shown to decrease lung cancer risk (D).

Gastrointestinal Disorders

8

Anal Fissure

Overview

In anal fissure, there is an ulcer or tear of the margin of the anus; most fissures occur posteriorly. Anal fissure risk factors include a history of recent or recurrent constipation (most potent risk factor), recurrent or recent severe diarrhea, recent childbirth, and anal intercourse or other anal insertion practices.

Clinical Presentation

The most common patient report is one of severe anal pain during a bowel movement, with the pain lasting several minutes to hours afterward. The pain recurs with every bowel movement, and the patient commonly becomes afraid or unwilling to have a bowel movement, leading to a cycle of worsening constipation, harder stools, and more anal pain. If rectal bleeding is noted with anal fissure, this is usually limited to drops of blood noted when wiping, not protracted bleeding. If the fissure is off the midline, transverse across the anal mucosa, or irregular, an alternative diagnosis should be considered.

Other conditions to consider when evaluating a patient with suspected anal fissure can include hemorrhoids, Crohn's disease, anal fistula, anal squamous cell carcinoma, and anal condyloma acuminata. Anal fissure can sometimes be mistaken for hemorrhoids, which can have a similar bleeding pattern but are typically not associated with the degree of pain attributed to anal fissure.

Diagnostic Testing

The diagnosis of anal fissure is usually made clinically, through history of present illness coupled with physical examination. Digital rectal examination with anal fissure is quite painful and should not be done. Additional testing including anoscopy or colonoscopy is typically undertaken with severe symptoms, complications, or when the diagnosis is in question. In particular, the diagnosis should be questioned if standard anal fissure therapy does not result in clinical improvement.

Treatment

Given that constipation is the most common anal fissure risk factor, the primary treatment goal is to prevent constipation and, therefore, break the cycle that contributes to the condition. First-line therapies include increased dietary fluid and fiber intake as well as fiber supplementation and stool softener; prescribing a stool softener as a solo intervention is seldom effective. Osmotic laxatives (e.g., magnesium citrate, magnesium hydroxide [Milk of Magnesia], and polyethylene glycol [MiraLAX®]) will help pull water into the intestines to soften stools to help relieve constipation. However, long-term use of magnesium salts is not recommended due to the risk of magnesium toxicity, particularly in patients with renal failure. These interventions alone are often not sufficient to facilitate stool passing, and an additional measure may need to be added. Mineral oil, given orally or via small-volume enema, helps lubricate the stool, renders defecation more comfortable, and minimizes anal mucosal damage; long-term use is discouraged owing to its potential to attenuate the absorption of the fat-soluble vitamins A, D, E, and K and essential fatty acids when used consistently in large amounts. Local measures such as sitz baths and cool compresses can provide additional relief. With this approach, the majority of anal fissures will heal within a few weeks. Relapse is common and is usually noted when recommended therapy is abandoned and constipation recurs.

If symptoms persist despite treatment with the above-mentioned therapies or symptoms are particularly severe, intra-anal application of 0.4% nitroglycerin (NTG) or a dihydropyridine (DHP) calcium channel blocker, such as nifedipine ointment, can be applied directly to the internal sphincter. These products are believed to relax the internal sphincter and increase blood flow to the anal mucosa. This offers pain relief and hastens the healing process. Adverse effects are identical to what is reported with other forms of these medications and include headache and dizziness, though nifedipine is associated with fewer adverse effects compared with NTG. An additional option, available through specialty consultation, is botulinum toxin injection (Botox®) into the anal sphincter; spasm at this point is thought to be the cause of particularly painful anal fissure. Botulinum injections provide relief for approximately 3 months, during which time the hope is that the fissure will heal. Surgical sphincterotomy is an option in the most recalcitrant of cases.

Discussion Sources

Poritz LS. Anal fissure. Medscape. http://emedicine.medscape.com/article/196297

Wald A, Bharucha AE, Cosman BC, Whitehead WE. ACG clinical guidelines: management of benign anorectal disorders. *Am J Gastroenterol.* 2014;109:1141–1157. https://www.ncbi.nlm.nih.gov/pubmed/25022811

QUESTIONS

1. The most common anal fissure location is:

   A. posterior midline of the anus.

   B. anterior anal midline.

   C. anterior and posterior anal midline.

   D. transversely across the anal mucosa.

2. Rectal bleeding associated with anal fissure is usually described by the patient as:

   A. drops of blood noticed when wiping.

   B. dark brown to black in color and mixed in with normal-appearing stool.

   C. a large amount of brisk red bleeding.

   D. significant blood clots and mucus mixed with stool.

3. A 62-year-old woman who reports frequent constipation is diagnosed with an anal fissure. First-line therapy includes all of the following except:

   A. stool-bulking supplements.

   B. high-fiber diet.

   C. intra-anal corticosteroids.

   D. the periodic use of oral mineral oil.

4. A 54-year-old man with an anal fissure responds inadequately to dietary intervention and standard therapy during the past 2 weeks. Additional treatment options include all of the following except:

   A. intra-anal nitroglycerin ointment.

   B. botulinum toxin injection to the internal anal sphincter.

   C. surgical sphincterotomy.

   D. rubber band ligation of the lesion.

5 to 8. In a patient who presents with a history consistent with anal fissure but with notation of an atypical anal lesion, alternative diagnoses to consider can include which of the following? (Yes or No)

   _____ 5. Condyloma acuminata

   _____ 6. Crohn's disease

   _____ 7. Anal squamous cell carcinoma

   _____ 8. *Clostridium difficile* colitis

9. Which of the following is the most likely patient report with anal fissure?

   A. "I have anal pain that is relieved with having a bowel movement."

   B. "Even after having a bowel movement, I feel like I still need to 'go' more."

   C. "I have anal pain for up to 1 to 2 hours after I have a bowel movement."

   D. "I itch down there almost all the time."

10. Long-term, recurrent, high-dose, oral use of mineral oil can lead to deficiency in:

   A. iron.

   B. vitamin A.

   C. vitamin C.

   D. vitamin B_{12}.

For answers and rationales, see end of chapter.

Hemorrhoids

Overview

The superior hemorrhoidal veins form internal hemorrhoids, whereas the inferior hemorrhoidal veins form external hemorrhoids. Both forms are normal anatomical findings but cause discomfort when there is an increase in the venous pressure and resulting dilation and inflammation. Contrary to common thought, hemorrhoids do not represent varicosities.

In many cases, the cause for hemorrhoids is unknown. At the same time, a number of clinical conditions and activities increase the risk for development of hemorrhoids, including excessive alcohol use, chronic diarrhea or constipation, obesity, high-fat/low-fiber diet, prolonged sitting, sedentary lifestyle, being a receptive partner in anal intercourse, and loss of pelvic floor muscle tone. Over time, tissue and vessel redundancy develop, resulting in rectal protrusion and increased risk for bleeding.

Clinical Presentation

Internal hemorrhoids are graded on a scale of I to IV as follows:

■ Grade I—the hemorrhoids do not prolapse.

■ Grade II—the hemorrhoids prolapse upon defecation but reduce spontaneously.

■ Grade III—the hemorrhoids prolapse upon defecation and must be reduced manually.

■ Grade IV—the hemorrhoids are prolapsed and cannot be reduced manually.

External hemorrhoids are not graded.

The rectal bleeding associated with hemorrhoids is usually minor and typically described as a red streak on the stool.

With chronically protruding or prolapsing hemorrhoids, the patient often reports itch, mucus leaking, and staining of undergarments with streaks of stool. Manual reduction of the protruding hemorrhoid after evacuation can be helpful. Other conditions to consider when evaluating a patient with suspected hemorrhoids can include acute proctitis, anal fissure, condyloma acuminata, and rectal prolapse.

> **CLINICAL CONCEPT**
>
> Reports of persistent bleeding, dark blood mixed with stool, or development of anemia related to rectal bleeding warrant prompt referral for colonoscopy for evaluation for colorectal cancer or alternative diagnosis.

Diagnostic Testing

The diagnosis of hemorrhoids is made clinically, through history of present illness coupled with physical examination. Additional testing including anoscopy or colonoscopy is typically only undertaken with severe symptoms or complications, or when the diagnosis is in question.

Treatment

As with anal fissure, prevention of hemorrhoidal engorgement and inflammation is the best treatment. Strategies include weight control, high-fiber diet, fiber supplements, regular aerobic physical activity, and increased fluid intake. The average adult should strive for a minimum of 20 to 30 grams of fiber per day, preferably through eating high-fiber foods. Examples of high-fiber foods include dry beans, peas, oat products such as oatmeal and oat bran, and most, but not all, whole fruits and vegetables.

Treatment for acute hemorrhoid flare-ups includes the use of astringents and topical corticosteroids, sitz baths, and analgesics. Though not well studied in the treatment of hemorrhoids, the use of topical corticosteroids can ease the symptoms of pruritis and inflammation. However, steroid-containing creams, particularly higher-potency agents, should not be used for prolonged periods because of their potential to cause permanent atrophic skin and tissue effects.

Surgical intervention is warranted when more conservative therapy fails to yield clinical improvement:

■ Rubber band ligation is often the surgical intervention of choice for lower grade (I and II) internal hemorrhoids and a single grade III or IV hemorrhoid; this procedure is done in an office, usually in a surgical practice.

■ Surgical hemorrhoidectomy is recommended with multiple hemorrhoid columns, especially grades III and IV, as well as extensive external and internal hemorrhoids.

Thrombosed external hemorrhoids can cause sudden-onset excruciating anal pain; the patient with this condition often reports for emergency care. On physical examination, a deep purple-blue, exquisitely tender anal lesion is visible. Surgical excision of the skin overlying the thrombosed hemorrhoid provides rapid symptomatic relief. If this intervention is not available or is declined by the patient, conservative therapy with cool compresses, sitz baths, stool softener, and analgesics can be used. The thrombus will resolve in 1 to 2 weeks without surgical intervention.

Discussion Sources

Thornton SC. Hemorrhoids. Medscape. https://emedicine.medscape.com/article/775407-overview

Wald A, Bharucha AE, Cosman BC, Whitehead WE. ACG clinical guidelines: management of benign anorectal disorders. *Am J Gastroenterol*. 2014;109:1141–1157. https://www.ncbi.nlm.nih.gov/pubmed/25022811

QUESTIONS

11. Rectal bleeding associated with hemorrhoids is usually described as:

    A. streaks of bright red blood on the stool.

    B. dark brown to black in color and mixed in with normal-appearing stool.

    C. a large amount of brisk red bleeding.

    D. significant blood clots and mucus mixed with stool.

12. Therapy for hemorrhoids includes all of the following except:

    A. weight control.

    B. low-fat diet.

    C. topical corticosteroids.

    D. the use of a stool softener.

13. The nurse practitioner (NP) is advising a 58-year-old woman about the benefits of a high-fiber diet. Which of the following foods provides the highest fiber content?

    A. a small banana

    B. 1 cup of cooked oatmeal

    C. a half-cup serving of brown rice

    D. a medium-sized blueberry muffin

14. A 62-year-old man presents with a 2-month history of noting a "bit of dark blood mixed in with my stool most days." Physical examination reveals external hemorrhoids, no rectal mass, and a small amount of dark brown stool on the examining digit. In-office fecal occult blood test is positive, and hemogram reveals a microcytic hypochromic anemia. The next best step in his care is to:

    A. perform in-office anoscopy.

    B. advise the patient to use sitz baths post–bowel movement.

    C. refer to gastroenterology practice for colonoscopy.

    D. order a double-contrast barium enema.

15. Risk factors for the development of hemorrhoidal symptoms include all of the following except:

    A. prolonged sitting.

    B. insertive partner in anal intercourse.

    C. chronic diarrhea.

    D. excessive alcohol use.

16. Which of the following best describes grade III internal hemorrhoids?

   A. The hemorrhoids do not prolapse.

   B. The hemorrhoids prolapse upon defecation but reduce spontaneously.

   C. The hemorrhoids prolapse upon defecation and must be reduced manually.

   D. The hemorrhoids are prolapsed and cannot be reduced manually.

17. Which of the following patients should be evaluated for possible surgical intervention for hemorrhoids?

   A. a 28-year-old woman with symptomatic external hemorrhoids who gave birth 6 days ago

   B. a 48-year-old man with grade II internal hemorrhoids and improvement with standard medical therapy

   C. a 44-year-old woman who has internal and external hemorrhoids with recurrent prolapse

   D. a 58-year-old man who has grade I internal hemorrhoids and improvement with psyllium supplements

For answers and rationales, see end of chapter.

Acute Appendicitis

Overview

Acute appendicitis is an inflammatory disease of the vermiform appendix caused by infection or obstruction. The peak age of patients with acute appendicitis is 10 to 30 years; this condition is uncommon in infants and elderly adults. At either end of the life span, a delay in diagnosis of appendicitis commonly occurs because providers do not consider appendicitis a possibility.

Clinical Presentation

There is no true classic presentation of acute appendicitis. Vague epigastric or periumbilical pain often heralds its beginning, with the discomfort shifting to the right lower quadrant over the next 12 hours. Pain is often aggravated by walking or coughing. Nausea and vomiting are late symptoms that invariably occur a number of hours after the onset of pain; this late onset helps to differentiate appendicitis from gastroenteritis, in which vomiting usually precedes abdominal cramping. The presentation of appendicitis also differs significantly according to the anatomical position of the appendix, with pain being reported in the epigastrium, flank, or groin. The obturator and psoas signs indicate inflammation of the respective muscles and strongly suggest peritoneal irritation and the diagnosis of appendicitis; these signs are also known as obturator muscle and iliopsoas muscle signs (Figs. 8-1 and 8-2). Rebound tenderness, which is abdominal pain that worsens with release of deep palpation, indicates the likelihood of peritoneal irritation and helps with the diagnosis of acute appendicitis. The presence of rebound tenderness is also known as a positive Blumberg's sign. Other common conditions to consider when evaluating a patient with suspected acute appendicitis can include constipation, cholecystitis, Crohn's disease, diverticulitis, ectopic pregnancy, pelvic inflammatory disease, and endometriosis, among others.

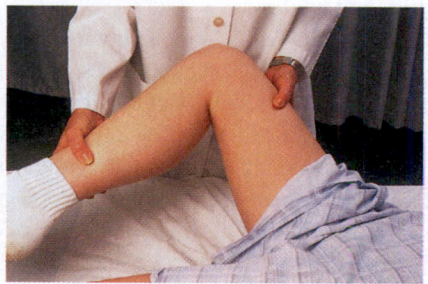

FIGURE 8-1 Obturator muscle sign.
Dillion PM. Nursing Health Assessment: The Foundation of Clinical Practice, 3rd ed. Philadelphia, PA: F.A. Davis; 2016.

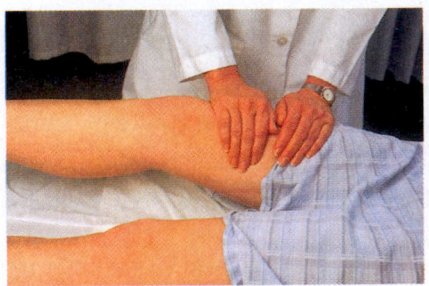

FIGURE 8-2 Iliopsoas muscle sign.
Dillion PM. Nursing Health Assessment: The Foundation of Clinical Practice, 3rd ed. Philadelphia, PA: F.A. Davis; 2016.

Diagnostic Testing

A total white blood cell (WBC) count and differential are obtained as part of the evaluation of patients with suspected appendicitis. The most typical WBC count pattern found in this situation is the "left shift."
The following are typically noted in the "left shift":

■ Leukocytosis: An elevation in the total WBC.
■ Neutrophilia: An elevation in the number of neutrophils in circulation. Neutrophilia is defined as an absolute neutrophil count (ANC) of greater than 7,000 neutrophils/mm³. The ANC is calculated by multiplying the percentage of neutrophils by the total WBC in cubic millimeters (mm³). A total WBC (TWBC) of 12,000/mm³ × 70% neutrophils yields an ANC of 8,300 neutrophils/mm³. Neutrophils are also known as "polys" or "segs," both referring to the polymorph shape of the segment nucleus of this WBC.
■ Bandemia: An elevation in the number of bands or young neutrophils in circulation. Usually less than 4% of the total WBCs in circulation are bands. When this percentage is exceeded, and the absolute band count (ABC) is greater than 500/mm³, bandemia is present. A TWBC of 12,000/mm³ with 8% bands yields an ABC of 860/mm³. The presence of bandemia indicates that the body has called up as many mature neutrophils as were available in the storage pool and is now accessing less mature forms. The presence of bandemia further reinforces the seriousness of the infection. An increase in circulating bands also occurs in pneumonia, meningitis, septicemia, pyelonephritis, and tonsillitis when caused by bacterial infection.

Given that appendicitis is an inflammatory disease, adding a test to detect inflammation, such as the C-reactive protein (CRP), is also an option. An elevated CRP provides a degree of support for the diagnosis, whereas a normal value helps to rule out the condition. For women of childbearing age, pregnancy should be ruled out via urinary beta-human chorionic gonadotropin (beta-hCG); the presentations of acute appendicitis and early ectopic pregnancy have many features in common.

Computed tomography (CT) of the abdomen, usually with oral or rectal contrast, is generally considered the imaging of choice in suspected appendicitis; its ability to define the anatomical abnormality associated with appendicitis is superior to other imaging options. Abdominal CT is the preferred diagnostic procedure when there is a suspicion of appendiceal perforation, because this study reveals periappendiceal abscess formation, or when an atypical presentation raises the issue of another possible diagnosis. Because of concerns about patient exposure to radiation during a CT scan, abdominal or pelvic ultrasonography (US) is considered a diagnostic modality for appendicitis, particularly in children, teens with body mass index (BMI) within a healthy range, and adults.

With abnormality noted on ultrasound, including an inability to clearly visualize the appendix, CT is then used to further help with the diagnostic process. In particular, this is an appealing option to minimize radiation exposure in children and women of reproductive age. Magnetic resonance imaging (MRI) has limited use in the evaluation of suspected appendicitis. Because of its lack of ionizing radiation, this is an option when evaluating a pregnant woman with suspected appendicitis; unfortunately, the normative changes noted during pregnancy render abdominal ultrasound of limited use for evaluation of a pregnant woman with abdominal pain.

Given the variety of imaging modalities available and the frequency of their use, the ionizing radiation burden of a study should be considered prior to ordering. (See Table 8-1.) The long-term risk of excessive ionizing radiation is presumed to include carcinogenesis; children and women of reproductive age are particularly vulnerable.

Appendiceal perforation, commonly referred to as a ruptured or burst appendix, is usually associated with a marked leukocytosis with total WBC count often exceeding 20,000/mm³ to 30,000/mm³, fever

TABLE 8-1 Radiation Doses From Common Imaging Studies*

TEST	DOSE (mSv)	EQUIVALENT PERIOD OF BACKGROUND RADIATION
Chest x-ray (standard two views)	0.06 to 0.1	8 to 12 days
Abdomen x-ray	0.5 to 0.7	62 to 88 days
Abdomen and pelvis CT*	10.0	3 years
Virtual colonoscopy	10.2	3 years
Whole-body positron emission tomography (PET)/low-dose CT	8.5 to 10.3	3 years
Whole-body PET/full-dose CT	23.7 to 26.4	8 to 9 years
Abdominal ultrasound	No ionizing radiation exposure	Not applicable
Abdominal MRI	No ionizing radiation exposure	Not applicable

*The ionizing radiation doses mentioned here represent an average for the study.

Source: Coakley F, Gould R, Yeh B, Arenson R. CT radiation dose: what can you do right now in your practice? AJR. 2011;196:619–625. https://www.ajronline.org/content/196/3/619.full.pdf+html

greater than 102°F (greater than 38.8°C), peritoneal inflammation findings, and symptoms lasting longer than 48 hours. An ill-defined right lower quadrant abdominal mass, usually dull to percussion with or without a degree of rebound tenderness, in a person with a presentation consistent with appendiceal perforation is suggestive of abscess formation.

Treatment

Surgical removal of an inflamed appendix via laparoscopy or laparotomy is usually indicated. If there is evidence of rupture with localized abscess and peritonitis, CT-directed abscess aspiration can be indicated first, with an appendectomy performed after appropriate antimicrobial therapy. Occasionally, with an intact appendix, antimicrobial therapy and close follow-up is an option.

Discussion Sources

Craig S. Appendicitis. Medscape. https://emedicine.medscape.com/article/773895-overview

Ferri F. Appendicitis. In: Ferri F. *Ferri's Best Test: A Practical Guide to Clinical Laboratory Medicine and Diagnostic Imaging.* 4th ed. Philadelphia, PA: Elsevier Saunders; 2017;254.

QUESTIONS

18. All of the following are typically noted in a young adult with the diagnosis of acute appendicitis except:

    A. periumbilical pain.

    B. positive obturator sign.

    C. rebound tenderness.

    D. marked febrile response.

19. A 26-year-old man presents with acute abdominal pain. As part of the evaluation for acute appendicitis, you order a WBC count with differential and anticipate the following results:

    A. total WBCs, 4,500/mm³; neutrophils, 35%; bands, 2%; lymphocytes, 45%.

    B. total WBCs, 14,000/mm³; neutrophils, 55%; bands, 3%; lymphocytes, 38%.

    C. total WBCs, 16,500/mm³; neutrophils, 66%; bands, 8%; lymphocytes, 22%.

    D. total WBCs, 18,100/mm³; neutrophils, 55%; bands, 3%; lymphocytes, 28%.

20. You see a 72-year-old woman who reports nausea and abdominal pain occurring over the past 24 hours. In evaluating a patient with suspected appendicitis, the clinician considers that:

    A. the presentation can differ according to the anatomical location of the appendix.

    B. this is a common reason for acute abdominal pain in elderly patients.

    C. vomiting before onset of abdominal pain is often seen.

    D. the presentation is markedly different from the presentation of pelvic inflammatory disease.

21. The psoas sign can be best described as abdominal pain elicited by:

    A. passive extension of the hip.

    B. passive flexion and internal rotation of the hip.

    C. deep palpation.

    D. asking the patient to cough.

22. The obturator sign can be best described as abdominal pain elicited by:

    A. passive extension of the hip.

    B. passive flexion and internal rotation of the hip.

    C. deep palpation.

    D. asking the patient to cough.

23. An 18-year-old man with a BMI = 40 kg/m² presents with periumbilical pain, vomiting, and abdominal cramping over the past 48 hours. Physical examination reveals rebound tenderness, and laboratory analysis shows the presence of bandemia and a total WBC of 28,000/mm³. To support the diagnosis of acute appendicitis with suspected appendiceal rupture, you consider obtaining the following abdominal imaging study:

    A. MRI.

    B. CT scan.

    C. ultrasound.

    D. flat plate.

24. Appropriate management of acute appendicitis without evidence of appendiceal perforation is:

    A. appendectomy.

    B. IV antimicrobial therapy.

    C. appendectomy with IV antimicrobial therapy.

    D. oral antimicrobial therapy plus systemic corticosteroids.

25. Which of the following best represents the peak ages for occurrence of acute appendicitis?

    A. 1 to 20 years

    B. 20 to 40 years

    C. 10 to 30 years

    D. 30 to 50 years

26. Clinical findings most consistent with appendiceal rupture include all of the following except:

    A. abdominal discomfort less than 48 hours in duration.

    B. fever greater than 102°F (greater than 38°C).

    C. palpable abdominal mass.

    D. marked leukocytosis with total WBC greater than 20,000/mm³.

27. Which of the following imaging studies potentially exposes the patient being evaluated for abdominal pain to the lowest ionizing radiation burden?

A. ultrasound

B. barium enema

C. CT scan

D. abdominal flat plate

28. Commonly encountered diagnoses other than acute appendicitis can include which of the following in a 28-year-old woman with a 2-day history of lower abdominal pain and with right-sided pain slightly worse than left? *(More than one can apply.)*

A. constipation

B. PID

C. ectopic pregnancy

D. splenic infarct

29. Rebound tenderness is best described as abdominal pain that worsens with:

A. light palpation at the site of the discomfort.

B. release of deep palpation at the site of the discomfort.

C. palpation on the contralateral side of the abdomen.

D. deep palpation at the site of the discomfort.

30 to 32. Match each sign used in the diagnosis of acute appendicitis with its appropriate description.

_____ 30. Markle sign

_____ 31. Dunphy sign

_____ 32. Blumberg sign

A. a sharp pain in the right lower quadrant of the abdomen that is elicited by cough

B. abdominal palpation yields rebound tenderness

C. pain in the right lower quadrant of the abdomen when dropping from standing on toes to heels with a jarring landing

33. Which of the following findings would you expect to encounter in a 33-year-old man with appendiceal abscess?

A. leukopenia with lymphocytosis

B. positive Cullen's sign

C. diffuse maculopapular rash

D. dullness to percussion in the abdominal right lower quadrant

For answers and rationales, see end of chapter.

Gallbladder Disease

Overview

Gallstone formation occurs when substances in bile are present in high concentrations; the bile becomes supersaturated, and the substance precipitates out into a microscopic crystal. The crystals are trapped in the gallbladder mucosa, with resulting formation of sludge. Over time, more substance precipitates out and the crystals grow, forming macroscopic stones. Duct occlusion by stones or sludge causes the majority of symptoms and clinical problems with gallstone disease. The most common form of stones is cholesterol or is cholesterol dominant (80% to 85%). Gallstones cause the most common form of gallbladder disease.

Major risk factors for gallstone formation include age older than 50 years, female gender, obesity, hyperlipidemia, rapid weight loss (including patients who have undergone bariatric surgery), pregnancy, genetic factors, European or Native American ancestry, and chronic ingestion of a [...] glycemic index.

Cholelithiasis is defined as a condition in which there is the formation of calculi or gallst[...] out the presence of gallbladder or associated structure. About 75% of all patients with chole[...] symptoms and become aware of the condition only when it is found during evaluation for a[...] problem. About 10% to 25% of individuals initially without symptoms become symptoma[...] decade. In the absence of symptoms, prophylactic cholecystectomy is not usually indicated[...]

Clinical Presentation

Many patients with gallstones have intermittent discomfort as a result of this condition[...] described as being of sudden onset, usually postprandial, particularly within 1 hour [...] abdominal right upper quadrant or epigastrium, occasionally radiating to the tip of th[...] the presence of radiating pain is known as Collins' sign. Episodes of discomfort typical[...] with a pattern of increasing then decreasing discomfort as the gallbladder contracts a[...] shifts. Nausea and vomiting are common during painful episodes. Indeed, vomiting ofte[...] cant pain relief. *Biliary colic* is a term used to describe the acutely painful paroxysms d[...] called, colloquially, a "gallbladder attack."

Acute cholecystitis results from an acute inflammation of the gallbladder, nearly al[...] stones. Right upper quadrant or epigastric pain and tenderness are present along wit[...] more) and occasional fever (33%); vomiting often affords temporary symptom relief[...] pating the right upper quadrant of the abdomen significant enough to cause inspirator[...] sign) is nearly always present. A palpable gallbladder is rarely noted. Approximately [...] affected have some degree of jaundice. Other conditions to consider in the differential[...] appendicitis, acute pyelonephritis, peptic ulcer disease (PUD), and cholelithiasis.

Diagnostic Testing

Combined with the health history, physical examination findings, and laborator[...] results help to support the diagnosis of cholecystitis. Right upper quadrant abdom[...] ally reveals stones and is considered the diagnostic test of choice; given the lack [...] with ultrasound, this is also a test that can be used during pregnancy. Abdominal [...] the diagnosis when compared with US but can assist in ruling out other gastroint[...] ogy. A hepatoiminodiacetic acid (HIDA) scan is more sensitive and specific at reveal[...] cystic duct.

Most gallstones are radiolucent—that is, unable to be visualized on standard [...] an abdominal flat plate is of limited value. Abdominal MRI seldom plays a role i[...] stone disease. A variety of percutaneous and endoscopic diagnostic procedures are [...] cated or uncertain scenarios. With acute cholecystitis, leukocytosis is usually pr[...] total WBC count of 12,000/mm³ to 20,000/mm³, coupled with elevated levels of t[...] (Table 8-2).

Treatment

Acute cholecystitis symptoms usually subside with conservative therapy, such as a l[...] liquids and analgesics. Antimicrobial therapy is occasionally indicated with evidence [...] cystectomy, typically performed via laparoscope, should be considered[...] likelihood of recurrence.

In a person who is seriously ill with other health problems an[...] high a risk to undergo cholecystectomy, US-guided gallbladder asp[...] cutaneous cholecystectomy can delay or occasionally eliminate the[...] surgical intervention. Stone-dissolving medications, such as urso[...] are available but can take 2 years to dissolve stones. Approximately [...] treated with stone-dissolving medications have a return of stones with[...] sequently, the use of this therapy has largely fallen out of favor.

Discussion Source

Heuman DM. Gallstones (cholecystitis). Medscape. https://emedicine.medscape.com[...]

CLINICAL CONCEPT

Complications of gallstone disease include pancreatitis and sepsis; both are most common in the older adult who develops the condition.

TABLE 8-2 Hepatic Enzyme Elevations and Their Significance

ENZYME ELEVATION	CLINICAL SIGNIFICANCE	EXAMPLE
Alanine aminotransferase (ALT, formerly known as SGPT) Highly liver specific	Measure of hepatic cellular enzymes. Elevated with hepatocellular damage. With hepatitis A, B, C, D, or E, or drug-induced or industrial chemical-associated hepatitis, ALT greater than AST with enzyme increases ≥10 × ULN. In nonalcoholic fatty liver steatohepatitis (NASH, AKA nonalcoholic fatty liver disease [NAFLD]) ALT>AST, within 3 × ULN.	A 22-year-old woman with acute hepatitis A AST 678 U/L (normal 0 to 31 U/L) ALT 828 U/L (normal 0 to 31 U/L) ALT:AST ratio ≥1 A 66-year-old woman with obesity, type 2 diabetes mellitus, and nonalcoholic fatty liver disease AST 44 U/L ALT 78 U/L ALT:AST ratio >1
Aspartate aminotransferase (AST, formerly known as SGOT) Found in liver, myocardium, skeletal muscle	Measure of hepatic cellular enzymes. Elevated with hepatocellular damage In alcohol-related hepatic injury, AST often greater than ALT, usually within 3 × ULN. In acetaminophen overdose, AST and ALT elevation ≥20 times × ULN	A 38-year-old man with a 10-year history of increasingly heavy alcohol use AST 83 U/L (normal 0 to 31 U/L) ALT 50 U/L (normal 0 to 31 U/L) AST:ALT ratio ≥1 A 26-year-old man with intentional acetaminophen overdose AST 15,083 U/L (normal 0 to 31 U/L) ALT 10,347 U/L (normal 0 to 31 U/L)
Alkaline phosphatase (ALP)	Levels increase in response to biliary obstruction, intrahepatic or extrahepatic cholestasis Enzyme found in rapidly dividing or metabolically active tissue, such as liver, bone, intestines, placenta	A 40-year-old woman with acute cholecystitis AST 45 U/L (0 to 31) ALT 55 U/L (0 to 31) ALP 225 U/L (0 to 125)
Gamma glutamyl transferase (GGT)	In hepatic disease, rise parallels increase in ALP Marked elevation often noted in obstructive jaundice, hepatic metastasis, intrahepatic cholestasis	A 40-year-old woman with acute cholecystitis AST 45 U/L (0 to 31) ALT 55 U/L (0 to 31) ALP 225 U/L (0 to 125) GGT 245 U/L (0 to 45)

ULN, upper limit of normal.

Source: Ferri FF. Ferri's Best Test: A Practical Guide to Clinical Laboratory Medicine and Diagnostic Imaging. 4th ed. Philadelphia, PA: Elsevier Saunders; 2017.

QUESTIONS

34. A 43-year-old woman has a 12-hour history of sudden onset of right upper quadrant abdominal pain with radiation to the shoulder, fever, and chills. She has had similar, milder episodes in the past, especially after eating fatty foods. Examination reveals marked tenderness to right upper quadrant abdominal palpation. Her most likely diagnosis is:

A. hepatoma.

B. acute cholecystitis.

C. acute hepatitis.

D. cholelithiasis.

35. Which of the following is usually not seen in the diagnosis of acute cholecystitis?
    A. elevated serum creatinine
    B. increased alkaline phosphatase level
    C. leukocytosis
    D. elevated aspartate aminotransferase (AST) level

36. Murphy's sign can be best described as abdominal pain elicited by:
    A. right upper quadrant abdominal palpation.
    B. asking the patient to stand on tiptoes and then letting body weight fall quickly onto the heels.
    C. asking the patient to cough.
    D. percussion.

37. Which of the following is the most common serious complication of cholecystitis?
    A. adenocarcinoma of the gallbladder
    B. gallbladder empyema
    C. hepatic failure
    D. pancreatitis

38. A 58-year-old man reports intermittent right upper quadrant abdominal pain. He has obesity and being actively treated for hyperlipidemia. Imaging in a patient with suspected symptomatic cholelithiasis usually includes obtaining an abdominal:
    A. MRI.
    B. CT scan.
    C. ultrasound of the right upper quadrant.
    D. flat plate.

39. Which of the following is most likely to be found in a person with acute cholecystitis?
    A. fever
    B. vomiting
    C. jaundice
    D. palpable gallbladder

40. Risk factors for the development of cholelithiasis include all of the following except:
    A. rapid weight loss.
    B. male gender.
    C. obesity.
    D. Native American ancestry.

41. A gallstone that is not visualized on standard x-ray is said to be:
    A. radiopaque.
    B. radiolucent.
    C. calcified.
    D. unclassified.

For answers and rationales, see end of chapter.

Colorectal Cancer

Overview

Colorectal cancer is the third leading cause of cancer death in both genders in the United States, with approximately 5% of the population developing the disease. Only lung cancer (both genders), prostate cancer (men), and breast cancer (women) exceed this disease in cancer-related mortality. Most colorectal malignancies prove to be adenocarcinomas, with about 70% found in the colon and 30% found in the rectum. Risk factors include a history of inflammatory bowel disease (ulcerative colitis [UC] and Crohn's disease), personal history of neoplasia, age older than 50 years, a family history of colorectal cancer, and familial polyposis syndrome. In addition, an autosomal dominant condition known as hereditary non-polyposis colorectal cancer (HNPCC) has been identified. Although HNPCC is the likely cause for only about 3% of all colorectal cancers, persons with this risk factor tend to develop disease earlier and have a 70% likelihood of colon cancer by age 65 years. A thorough family history is important in assessing an individual's risk of colorectal cancer. A diet high in fat, high in red meat, and low in calcium has also been implicated as a contributing factor. The use of antioxidants, calcium supplements, and low-dose aspirin has been shown in limited study to reduce colorectal cancer rates.

Clinical Presentation

A person presenting with colorectal cancer is usually asymptomatic until the disease is quite advanced. At that time, vague abdominal complaints coupled with iron-deficiency anemia (as a result of chronic low-volume blood loss) often are noted. The mass is most often beyond the examining digit. As a result, digital rectal examination is an ineffective method of colorectal cancer screening. Bowel obstruction, including sudden onset of vomiting, abdominal pain, and distension, is a late, not early, manifestation of colorectal cancer.

Screening and Diagnostic Testing

Given that this condition does not present clinically until the disease is advanced, colorectal cancer screening is recommended (Box 8-1). Colorectal cancer screening is recommended for individuals at average risk starting at age 45 or 50 years and should continue until age 75 years while in good health (i.e., life expectancy >10 years). The decision to screen between the ages of 76 and 85 years should be based on individual patient factors and preferences, while individuals over 85 years should no longer undergo colorectal cancer screening. Screening can involve stool-based tests or examination that allows visualization of the colon. The most commonly recommended colorectal cancer screening method in adults is visual examination via colonoscopy at 10-year intervals. Alternative visual testing methods and schedules include flexible sigmoidoscopy or CT colonography (virtual colonoscopy) performed every 5 years. A CT scan can also be useful in detecting the presence of partial or complete bowel obstruction. With an abnormal finding from flexible sigmoidoscopy or CT colonography, the patient should then undergo a colonoscopy in order to allow biopsy of suspicious lesions.

> **CLINICAL CONCEPT**
> Toilet-bowl fecal occult blood tests (FOBTs) as well as the FOBT obtained via the digital rectal examination in the provider's office are not recommended as colorectal cancer screening.

Stool-based tests include highly sensitive fecal immunochemical test (FIT; annually), highly sensitive guaiac-based fecal occult blood test (gFOBT; annually), or the multitargeted stool DNA test (MT-sDNA; every 3 years). Compared with guaiac-based tests for the detection of occult blood, immunochemical tests are more patient-friendly and are likely to be equal or better in sensitivity and specificity. The MT-sDNA test (Cologuard®) is a highly sensitive test that detects the presence of blood in the stool as well as DNA mutations from colorectal cancer or polyp cells. With a positive finding from stool tests, repeat testing is not justified, as a colonoscopy should be performed.

Alternative screening schedules, usually including more frequent testing or earlier testing or both, are considered when colorectal cancer risk factors are present. These risk factors include a personal history of colorectal cancer or certain types of polyps, Crohn's disease or UC, a strong family history (first-degree relative [parent, sibling, or child]) of colorectal cancer or polyps, a known family history of hereditary colorectal cancer syndromes such as familial adenomatous polyposis (FAP) or HNPCC, or a personal history of radiation to the abdomen or pelvic area to treat a prior cancer. These alternative schedules should be pursued in conjunction with expert consultation.

As mentioned, colorectal cancer typically presents clinically when quite advanced, usually with new-onset iron-deficiency anemia coupled with GI symptoms. Initial diagnostic testing includes FOBT testing and, if positive, referral for colonoscopy. With signs and symptoms of acute large bowel obstruction, an uncommon presentation of colorectal cancer, GI imaging includes abdominal flat plate and/or abdominal CT. Subsequent care and referral are dependent on the outcome of these studies.

BOX 8-1 Colorectal Screening Tests: Pros and Cons

- Fecal immunochemical test (FIT)—checks for blood in stool
  - Pros: No direct risk to colon, no bowel preparation, sampling done at home, inexpensive
  - Cons: annual test, can miss some cancers/polyps, false positives
- Guaiac-based fecal occult blood test (gFOBT)—checks for blood in stool
  - Pros: No direct risk to colon, no bowel prep, sampling done at home, inexpensive
  - Cons: Annual test, can miss some cancers/polyps, false positives, pretest diet changes needed
- Stool DNA test (Cologuard®)—tests for DNA mutations and blood in stool
  - Pros: No direct risk to colon, no bowel preparation, sampling done at home, done every 3 years
  - Cons: Can miss some cancers/polyps, false positives
- Colonoscopy—visual examination of the colon and rectum
  - Pros: Views the entire colon, can biopsy and remove polyps, every 10 years
  - Cons: Full bowel preparation needed, can miss small polyps, expensive, sedation needed
- CT colonography—two-dimensional and three-dimensional views of colon and rectum
  - Pros: Fairly quick and safe, can view the entire colon, done every 5 years, no sedation needed
  - Cons: Full bowel preparation needed, can miss small polyps, some false positives, radiation exposure, cost
- Flexible sigmoidoscopy—visual examination of rectum and lower part of colon
  - Pros: Fairly quick and safe, full bowel preparation and sedation not usually needed, done every 5 years
  - Cons: Views only part of the colon, can miss small polyps, discomfort, risk of bleeding or bowel tear

Treatment

Treatment of colorectal cancer requires expert consultation and usually includes surgery combined with chemotherapy and radiation. In the presence of large bowel obstruction, surgery is usually needed to remove the obstruction as well as part of the affected intestines. Long-term survival depends on many factors, including the size and depth of the tumor, the presence of positive nodes, and the overall health of the patient. If iron-deficiency anemia is present as a result of colorectal cancer and resulting chronic, low-volume blood loss, this should also be treated with iron supplementation.

Discussion Sources

American Cancer Society. Guideline for Colorectal Cancer Screening. https://www.cancer.org/cancer/colon-rectal-cancer/detection-diagnosis-staging/acs-recommendations.html

Maxwell PJ, Isenberg GA. Tumors of the colon and rectum. In: Bope ET, Kellerman RD, eds. *Conn's Current Therapy*. Philadelphia, PA: Saunders Elsevier; 2017:248–251.

QUESTIONS

42. Which of the following is true concerning colorectal cancer?

    A. The majority of colorectal cancers are found during rectal examination.

    B. Anal carcinoma is more common than cancers involving the colon.

    C. Early manifestations include abdominal pain and cramping.

    D. Later disease presentation often includes iron-deficiency anemia.

43. According to current recommendations, which of the following is the preferred method for annual colorectal cancer screening in a 51-year-old man?

    A. digital rectal examination

    B. gFOBT

    C. colonoscopy

    D. FIT-DNA test (Cologuard®)

44. Which of the following is most likely to be noted in a person with early stage colorectal cancer?

    A. gross rectal bleeding

    B. unintended weight loss

C. ...y symptoms

D. ...and vomiting

45. ...following does not increase a patient's risk of developing colorectal cancer?

A. ...sion of colorectal cancer

B. ...dysosis

C. ...history of neoplasm

D. ...aspirin therapy

46. ...current data, colorectal cancer is the number _____ cause of cancer death in men and

A.

B.

C.

D.

47. ...following types of anemia is most likely to be found in an individual with advanced
...cancer?

A. ...chronic disease

B. ...anemia

C. ...ency anemia

D. ...ency anemia

...onales, see end of chapter.

Colonic Diverticular Disease: Diverticulosis/Diverticulitis

Overview

...osis, bulging pockets are present in the intestinal wall, most commonly in the wall of ...though the abnormality can occur in any part of the large intestine. In North America, ...third of the population will develop diverticulosis by age 50 years and approximately ...years. Inflammation is not present, however, and the patient is usually asymptomatic. ...major risk factor for the condition was thought to be a long-term ...because the condition is more common in developed countries in ...high levels of processed foods is the normal. However, addi- ...support this as a cause. Major risk factors are considered to be ...history of the disease, and select connective tissue disorders, including ...in diverticulitis, the diverticular pouches become inflamed. The ...inflammation is usually unclear but could be triggered from fecal par- ...the colonic outpouching, causing obstruction and diverticular dis- ...tension can result in colonic microtears, alteration in gut flora, and ...and inflammation. Uncomplicated diverticulitis refers to localized ...Complicated disease is inflammation associated with abscess, fistula, ...bleeding, and/or perforation.

> **CLINICAL CONCEPT**
>
> Diverticulosis is often found during studies done for other reasons, such as colonoscopy for colorectal cancer screening.

Clinical Presentation

...culosis, where there is colonic outpouching but no inflammation, no symptoms are usually ...symptomatic diverticulosis, mild left-sided abdominal cramping, increased flatus, and a ...constipation alternating with diarrhea are reported. In acute colonic diverticulitis, the diver- ...inflamed, usually resulting in fever, leukocytosis, diarrhea, and left lower quadrant abdominal ...perforation is the likely origin of the condition, with the perforation ranging from pinpoint ...majority, which cause local infection and respond to conservative management, to major ...necessitate surgical repair and are often complicated by intra-abdominal abscess or peritonitis. ...often obtained to support the diagnosis and assess disease severity or complications.

Diagnostic Testing

As mentioned, given that most individuals with diverticulosis are without specific symptoms, this condition is most often found as an incidental finding during another study. Most often, diverticulosis is found during routine colonoscopy done for colorectal cancer screening.

In diverticulitis, an abdominal CT scan with contrast is helpful in confirming the diagnosis. The abdominal CT in acute diverticulitis usually reveals bowel wall thickening; complications including abscess and fistulas can also be identified with this diagnostic modality. A plain abdominal film can identify free air, indicating diverticular perforation, or altered bowel air patterns consistent with obstruction; this study is usually normal in milder disease. Because of the potential risk of complication, a barium enema should not be obtained during an acute episode of diverticular disease. Abdominal ultrasound is not helpful in this condition.

Colonoscopy evaluation is contraindicated in acute diverticulitis, as insufflation of air can result in or exacerbate free perforation and peritonitis. At the same time, colonoscopy is advised about 4 to 6 weeks after an episode of acute diverticulitis in patients who had or are at risk for complication and/or to update colorectal cancer screening.

Treatment

In asymptomatic or mildly symptomatic diverticulosis without evidence of diverticulitis or intestinal obstruction, intervention can include a high-fiber diet, along with the use of fiber supplements such as bran, psyllium, and methylcellulose. The goal of treatment is to minimize the risk of complications such as diverticulitis. Although avoidance of seeds and other similar food products has been recommended in the past as a way to avoid acute diverticulitis, few studies exist to support this dietary change.

In mild cases of diverticulitis, conservative management is adequate, including a liquid diet to ensure gut rest, with an emphasis on adequate hydration, for the duration of the illness. In mild, uncomplicated diverticulitis, antimicrobial therapy has been shown to provide no added benefit. Antimicrobial therapy should be considered in more severe cases and complicated diverticulitis disease. Metronidazole is the antibiotic of choice because of its strong activity against anaerobic organisms implicated in the conditions. Because the infection is often polymicrobial, a second agent should be added that exhibits activity against the gram-negative organisms that are implicated, such as *Escherichia coli*. These antimicrobials include ciprofloxacin, levofloxacin, moxifloxacin, amoxicillin-clavulanate, or trimethoprim-sulfamethoxazole (TMP-SMX) (Table 8-3). If the patient fails to respond within 2 to 3 days or becomes significantly worse during that time, particularly if peritoneal signs develop, an abdominal CT scan and specialty surgical consultation should be obtained. Approximately 4 to 6 weeks following resolution of acute diverticulitis, patients should undergo colonoscopy to rule out colorectal cancer, particularly if the patient is not up to date with colorectal cancer screening.

Measures to prevent colonic diverticulosis and diverticulitis include regular aerobic exercise, adequate hydration, and a high-fiber diet. All of these measures help increase bowel motility and tone.

> **CLINICAL CONCEPT**
>
> With recurrent diverticulitis episodes, particularly with a complicated course, surgical intervention with partial colectomy is an option to remove the problematic portion of the intestines.

TABLE 8-3 Antimicrobial Treatment Options in Acute Diverticulitis

CAUSATIVE ORGANISMS	PRIMARY ORAL TREATMENT REGIMEN WHEN SUITABLE FOR OUTPATIENT THERAPY	ALTERNATIVE ORAL TREATMENT REGIMEN WHEN SUITABLE FOR OUTPATIENT THERAPY
Enterobacteriaceae, *Pseudomonas aeruginosa*, *Bacteroides* spp., enterococci	TMP-SMX-DS bid *or* ciprofloxacin 750 mg bid or levofloxacin 750 mg daily plus metronidazole 500 mg q6h, all for 7 to 10 days	Amoxicillin-clavulanate ER 1,000/62.5 mg 2 tabs bid for 7 to 10 days *or* Moxifloxacin 400 mg q24h for 7 to 10 days

TMP-SMX, trimethoprim-sulfamethoxazole.

Source: Gilbert DN, Chambers HF, Eliopoulos GM, Saag MS, Pavia AT. *The Sanford Guide to Antimicrobial Therapy. 50th ed.* Sperryville, VA: Antimicrobial Therapy, Inc.; 2020:22.

Discussion Sources

Gilbert DN, Chambers HF, Eliopoulos GM, Saag MS, Pavia AT. *The Sanford Guide to Antimicrobial Therapy.* 50th ed. Sperryville, VA: Antimicrobial Therapy, Inc.; 2020.

Wilkins T, Embry K, George R. Diagnosis and management of acute diverticulitis. *Am Fam Physician.* 2013;87:612–620.

QUESTIONS

48. Colonic diverticulosis most commonly occurs in the walls of the:

  A. ascending colon.

  B. descending colon.

  C. transverse colon.

  D. sigmoid colon.

49. Approximately what percentage of the population will develop diverticulosis by the time they reach 50 years of age?

  A. 10%

  B. 20%

  C. 33%

  D. 50%

50. Which of the following is most consistent with the presentation of a patient with colonic diverticulosis?

  A. diarrhea and leukocytosis

  B. constipation and fever

  C. few or no symptoms

  D. frank blood in the stool with reduced stool caliber

51. Which of the following is most consistent with the presentation of a patient with acute colonic diverticulitis?

  A. cramping, diarrhea, and leukocytosis

  B. constipation and fever

  C. right-sided abdominal pain

  D. frank blood in the stool with reduced stool caliber

52. Major risk factors for diverticulosis include all of the following except:

  A. low-fiber diet.

  B. family history of the condition.

  C. older age.

  D. select connective tissue disorders (e.g., Marfan syndrome).

53. To avoid the development of acute diverticulitis, treatment of diverticulosis can include:

  A. avoiding foods with seeds.

  B. the use of fiber supplements.

  C. ceasing cigarette smoking.

  D. limiting alcohol intake.

54. The location of discomfort with acute diverticulitis is usually in which of the following areas of the abdomen?

  A. epigastrium

  B. left lower quadrant

    C. right lower quadrant

    D. suprapubic

55. Which of the following best describes colonic diverticulosis?

    A. bulging pockets in the intestinal wall

    B. poorly contracting intestinal walls

    C. strictures of the intestinal lumen

    D. flaccidity of the small intestine

56. You are seeing Mr. Lopez, a 68-year-old man with suspected acute colonic diverticulitis. In choosing an appropriate imaging study to support this diagnosis, which of the following abdominal imaging studies is most appropriate?

    A. flat plate

    B. ultrasound

    C. CT scan with contrast

    D. barium enema

57. In the evaluation of acute diverticulitis, the most appropriate diagnostic approach to rule out free air in the abdomen includes:

    A. barium enema.

    B. plain abdominal film.

    C. abdominal ultrasound.

    D. lower endoscopy.

58. A 56-year-old woman is diagnosed with moderate diverticulitis. This is her second episode in the past 6 weeks. In addition to counseling her about increased fluid intake and adequate rest, you recommend antimicrobial treatment with:

    A. amoxicillin with clarithromycin.

    B. linezolid with daptomycin.

    C. ciprofloxacin with metronidazole.

    D. nitrofurantoin with doxycycline.

59. A complication of colonic diverticulitis can include:

    A. Crohn's disease.

    B. diverticular hemorrhage.

    C. colorectal cancer.

    D. intussusception.

For answers and rationales, see end of chapter.

Peptic Ulcer Disease

Overview

GI irritation and ulcer occur when there is an imbalance between gastric protective mechanisms and irritating factors such as hydrochloric acid and other digestive juices. Gastric parietal cells secrete hydrochloric acid, mediated by histamine$_2$-receptor sites.

    Clinically, the description of the resulting disease includes a notation of where the ulcer is—for example, duodenal ulcer, gastric (stomach) ulcer, or esophageal ulcer. PUD usually includes loss of mucosal surface, extending to muscularis mucosae, that is at least 5 mm in diameter, with most losses two to five times this size.

    In the past, the adage "no stress, no extra acid, no ulcer" was often quoted. PUD treatment often included the use of psychotropic medications for relief of stress,

> **CLINICAL CONCEPT**
>
> PUD is located in areas, such as the duodenum, stomach, esophagus, and small intestine, that are exposed to peptic juices such as acid and pepsin.

according to the hypothesis that this would reduce the acid production. In reality, only 30% to 40% of persons with PUD have higher than average acid secretion rates. In addition, coffee drinking and occasional alcohol use are not PUD risk factors. Alcohol abuse with cirrhosis remains a risk factor, however.

Besides the use of NSAIDs and systemic corticosteroid use, major risk factors for gastric ulcer include age older than 60 years, history of PUD (especially gastric ulcer), and previous use of histamine$_2$-receptor antagonists (H$_2$RA), proton pump inhibitors (PPIs), or antacids for the treatment of GI symptoms. Additional, less potent risk factors include cigarette smoking, cardiac disease, and alcohol use; taking more than one NSAID; the concurrent use of NSAIDs, direct oral anticoagulants (DOACs), and other anticoagulant/antiplatelet products such as warfarin and clopidogrel; and also pose bleeding risk.

Duodenal ulcer (DU) is more common than gastric ulcer. The most potent risk DU factor is infection with *Helicobacter pylori*. *H pylori* is a gram-negative, spiral-shaped organism with sheathed flagella found in at least 90% of patients with duodenal ulcer. The pathogen is also found in about 40% to 70% of individuals with gastric ulcer. Infection with *H pylori* is transmitted via the oral-fecal and oral-oral routes, and rates of infection approach 100% in developing nations with impure water supplies. In developed nations with pure water supplies, at least 75% of the population older than 50 years has been infected at some time. Eradication of the organism dramatically alters the risk of relapse. Numerous antimicrobial combinations are effective in treating symptomatic *H pylori* infection (Table 8-4). *H pylori* is also found in individuals with asymptomatic gastritis and dyspepsia without ulceration; eradication of the organism does not appear to make a difference in symptoms in patients with these conditions.

Clinical Presentation

The clinical presentation of PUD differs according to the location of the lesion. Symptoms associated with acute gastritis and gastric ulcer often become worse with eating because of the increase in irritating stomach acid production that happens with food ingestion. The symptoms often lessen within an hour as food buffers the acid. In contrast, DU symptoms often worsen as the stomach pH decreases when emptying after a meal, resulting in a sensation of stomach burning about 2 hours after a meal. However, significant variation in clinical presentation is common, and the exact diagnosis of PUD location cannot be made by history and presentation alone. A variety of other conditions, including acute coronary syndrome, gastroesophageal reflux, cholecystitis, and others, can mimic PUD.

Diagnostic Testing

Diagnostic testing in PUD differs according to whether gastric ulcer, gastritis, or DU is suspected. When DU is suspected, stool antigen testing is the most cost-effective method of diagnosing *H pylori* infection, particularly when coupled with a clinical presentation consistent with PUD. The organism produces urease, which breaks down urea into ammonia and CO_2; this allows the organism to control pH in its local environment in the stomach by neutralizing H^+ ions in gastric acid. As a result, urea breath testing is also a helpful diagnostic procedure when attempting to establish the presence of *H pylori* infection, although it is usually more expensive than the stool antigen test. In fecal and urea breath *H pylori* testing,

TABLE 8-4 Treatment Options in *Helicobacter pylori* Infection Associated With Duodenal/Gastric Ulcer

ANTIMICROBIALS AND ACID-SUPPRESSING MEDICATION	USUAL DURATION OF THERAPY	COMMENTS
Bismuth subsalicylate 2 tabs qid plus metronidazole 500 mg tid plus tetracycline 500 mg qid plus PPI	14 days total	Repeat stool antigen and/or urea breath test more than 8 weeks posttreatment
PPI + amoxicillin 1,000 mg bid + metronidazole 500 mg bid + clarithromycin 500 mg bid	14 days	Prevalence of pretreatment resistance increasing, especially clarithromycin About 20% failure rates with previously recommended triple therapy (PPI + amoxicillin + clarithromycin)

Source: Gilbert DN, Chambers HF, Eliopoulos GM, Saag MS, Pavia AT. The Sanford Guide to Antimicrobial Therapy. 50th ed. Sperryville, VA: Antimicrobial Therapy, Inc.; 2020:21.

current PPI use could result in a false negative. Ideally, the patient should not take a PPI for 2 weeks prior to these tests. Serological testing for *H pylori* is also available, with the limitation that titers can take years to decline after effective treatment; however, 50% of patients have undetectable titers 12 to 18 months after therapy.

A significant amount of PUD, particularly gastric ulcer, acute gastritis, and NSAID-induced gastropathy, is caused by use of NSAIDs and the use of systemic corticosteroids. This is partly because the action of these products inhibits cyclooxygenase-1 (COX-1), an enzyme found in gastric mucosa, small and large intestine mucosa, kidneys, platelets, and vascular epithelium. COX-1 contributes to the health of these organs through numerous mechanisms, including the maintenance of the protective gastric mucosal layer and proper renal perfusion. In suspected NSAID-induced gastropathy, upper GI endoscopy with biopsy is critical to differentiate between an ulcer and gastric malignancy. Upper GI imaging (e.g., CT scan, UGI series) is limited in being able to make this distinction.

A variety of diagnostic measures are available when confirmation of the lesion(s)'s location is required. An upper GI series identifies more than 80% of all ulcers larger than 0.5 cm, whereas upper GI endoscopy identifies nearly all such ulcers. In particular, upper endoscopy should be considered as a first-line diagnostic test in adults older than 50 years of age who present with new-onset PUD symptoms, as this modality also allows for ruling out gastric ulcer or gastric cancer. (See Table 8-5 for further information on diagnostic testing in PUD.) The presence of PUD alarm findings can also warrant immediate endoscopy

TABLE 8-5 Assessing a Patient With Peptic Ulcer Disease

LOCATION AND TYPE OF PEPTIC ULCER DISEASE	RISK AND CONTRIBUTING FACTORS	PRESENTING SIGNS AND SYMPTOMS	DIAGNOSTIC TESTING
Duodenal ulcer	*Helicobacter pylori* infection (most common), NSAID use, systemic corticosteroid use (much less common)	Epigastric burning, gnawing pain about 2 to 3 hours after meals; relief with foods, antacids Clusters of symptoms with periods of feeling well; awakening at 1 to 2 a.m. with symptoms common, morning waking pain rare Tender at the epigastrium, left upper quadrant abdomen; slightly hyperactive bowel sounds	Stool antigen testing ≥90% sensitive and specific If *H pylori* stool antigen test is positive and PUD history, assume active infection and treat because cost of treatment less than that of confirmatory endoscopy. Repeat stool antigen test ≥8 weeks posttreatment. Urea breath test used to establish presence of acute infection. PPI use should be avoided for 2 weeks prior to stool or urea breath testing. *H pylori* testing; serological testing for anti–*H pylori* antibodies positive with acute infection but can take decades postinfection to decline. Use of serological testing for *H pylori* not recommended.
Gastric ulcer	NSAID and corticosteroid use (potent risk factor) Cigarette smoking Male:female ratio equal Peak incidence in fifth and sixth decades of life; nearly all found in patients without *H pylori* infection Are a result of chronic NSAID or long-term systemic corticosteroid use	Pain often reported with or immediately after meals Nausea, vomiting, weight loss common	Difficulty distinguishing gastric ulcer from stomach cancer through UGI imaging UGI endoscopy with biopsy vital to rule out gastric malignancy Need confirmation of presence of *H pylori* before treatment, as is present in some cases

Continued

TABLE 8-5 Assessing a Patient With Peptic Ulcer Disease—cont'd

LOCATION AND TYPE OF PEPTIC ULCER DISEASE	RISK AND CONTRIBUTING FACTORS	PRESENTING SIGNS AND SYMPTOMS	DIAGNOSTIC TESTING
Nonerosive gastritis, chronic type B (antral) gastritis	Most likely caused by *H pylori* infection	Nausea Burning and pain limited to upper abdomen without reflux symptoms	Upper GI endoscopy helpful diagnostic test, likely with *H pylori* testing
Erosive gastritis	Usually secondary to alcohol and NSAID use, ASA use, stress *H pylori* infection usually not a factor	Nausea Burning and pain limited to upper abdomen without reflux symptoms; bleeding common	Upper GI endoscopy is helpful diagnostic test, likely with *H pylori* testing

ASA, acetylsalicylic acid; PUD, peptic ulcer disease; UGI, upper gastrointestinal.

and gastroenterology referral. The findings include bleeding or anemia, unexplained weight loss, progressive dysphagia or odynophagia, recurrent vomiting, and family history of GI cancer.

Treatment

In documented *H pylori* infection, treatment is aimed at the eradication of the causative organism. A variety of antimicrobial regimens are available. (See Table 8-4.) In NSAID- or corticosteroid-induced gastropathy, first-line therapy is discontinuation of the offending medication.

Suppression or neutralization of gastric acid is a critical part of PUD therapy. H2RAs (whose names have the -*tidine* suffix, such as ranitidine [Zantac®] and famotidine [Pepcid®]) competitively block the binding of histamine to the H2-receptor site, reducing the secretion of gastric acid. Cimetidine should be avoided due to its CYP 450 inhibition and resulting drug interaction potential that is not found in the other H2RAs. These products are generally well tolerated. H2RAs likely offer protection against NSAID-induced duodenal ulcer and perhaps gastritis, but not against gastric ulcer. PPIs afford better protection against PUD. A prostaglandin analogue, misoprostol (Cytotec®), is a drug specifically designed for gastric protection with NSAIDs; the use of this medication is possibly helpful in minimizing renal injury secondary to NSAID use.

PPIs include omeprazole (Prilosec®), esomeprazole (Nexium®), and lansoprazole (Prevacid®). These drugs inhibit gastric acid secretion by inhibiting the final step in acid secretion by altering the activity of the "proton pump" (H^+, K^+-ATPase). As a result, there is a virtual cessation of stomach hydrochloric acid production, particularly owing to its significant action against the postprandial acid surge. With many of the PPIs, clinical efficacy is improved when the medication is taken on an empty stomach one-half hour prior to breakfast.

> **CLINICAL CONCEPT**
> Protracted PPI use has been associated with reduced absorption of iron, vitamin B_{12}, and other micronutrients.

An increase in fracture risk of the hip, spine, wrist, and forearm as well as *C difficile* colitis has also been noted with long-term PPI use. As a result, PPI use should not extend beyond 2 months, if possible.

Often, patients report an increase in upper GI distress when discontinuing long-term PPI use. The likely cause is rebound gastric hyperacidity; this problem can be minimized by gradually tapering the PPI dose (if possible) or trying every-other-day dosing with a supplemental dose of an antacid when symptoms flare. An alternative is to try low-dose H2RA therapy with supplemental antacid use as needed. This gap therapy is usually continued for approximately 1 month.

Discussion Sources

Abraham N. Proton pump inhibitors: potential adverse effects. *Curr Opin Gastroenterol.* 2012;28(6):615–620.

Gilbert DN, Chambers HF, Eliopoulos GM, Saag MS, Pavia AT. *The Sanford Guide to Antimicrobial Therapy.* 50th ed. Sperryville, VA: Antimicrobial Therapy, Inc.; 2020:21.

Vincent K. Gastritis and peptic ulcer disease. In: Bope ET, Kellerman RD, eds. *Conn's Current Therapy.* Philadelphia, PA: Saunders Elsevier; 2018:204–206.

QUESTIONS

60. Long-term effects of PPI use include all of the following except:
    A. increased risk of hip fracture.
    B. increased risk of inflammatory bowel disease (IBD).
    C. increased risk of *C difficile* colitis.
    D. decreased absorption of iron.

61. Antiprostaglandin drugs such as systemic corticosteroids and NSAIDS cause stomach mucosal injury primarily by:
    A. a direct irritative effect.
    B. altering the thickness of the protective mucosal layer.
    C. decreasing peristalsis.
    D. modifying stomach pH level.

62. A 24-year-old man presents with a 3-month history of upper abdominal pain. He describes it as an intermittent, centrally located "burning" feeling in his upper abdomen, most often occurring 2 to 3 hours after meals. He denies taking NSAIDs, aspirin, or systemic corticosteroids and drinks approximately one to two 12-oz beers a week. His presentation is most consistent with the clinical presentation of:
    A. acute gastritis.
    B. gastric ulcer.
    C. duodenal ulcer.
    D. cholecystitis.

63. When choosing pharmacological intervention to prevent recurrence of duodenal ulcer in a middle-aged man, you prescribe:
    A. omeprazole (Prilosec®).
    B. bismuth subsalicylate (Pepto-Bismol™).
    C. tetracycline plus metronidazole.
    D. ranitidine (Zantac®).

64. The H$_2$RA most likely to cause drug interactions with phenytoin and theophylline is:
    A. cimetidine.
    B. famotidine.
    C. nizatidine.
    D. ranitidine.

65. Which of the following is least likely to be found in a patient with gastric ulcer?
    A. history of long-term naproxen use
    B. age younger than 50 years
    C. previous use of H$_2$RA or antacids
    D. cigarette smoking

66. NSAID-induced PUD can be best limited by the use of:
    A. timed antacid doses.
    B. taking the medication with food.
    C. an appropriate antimicrobial.
    D. PPI use.

67. A 64-year-old woman presents with a 3-month history of upper abdominal pain. She describes the discomfort as an intermittent, centrally located "burning" feeling in the upper abdomen, most often with meals and often accompanied by mild nausea. Use of an over-the-counter H_2RA affords partial symptom relief. She also uses diclofenac on a regular basis for the control of osteoarthritis pain. Her clinical presentation is most consistent with:

A. acute gastroenteritis.

B. gastric ulcer.

C. duodenal ulcer.

D. chronic cholecystitis.

68. To minimize the risk of adverse effects, PPI use should be limited to no longer than:

A. 2 weeks.

B. 4 weeks.

C. 2 months.

D. 6 months.

69. PUD can occur in any of the following locations except:

A. duodenum.

B. stomach.

C. esophagus.

D. large intestine.

70. An ulcer that is noted to be located in the region below the lower esophageal sphincter and before the pylorus is usually referred to as a(n) _____ ulcer.

A. duodenal

B. esophageal

C. gastric

D. stomach

71. A 56-year-old man with a 60 pack-year cigarette smoking history, recent 5-lb unintended weight loss, and a 3-month history of new-onset symptoms of peptic disease presents for care. He is taking no medications on a regular basis and reports drinking approximately six 12-oz beers per week with no more than three beers per day. Physical examination is unremarkable except for mild pharyngeal erythema and moderate epigastric tenderness without rebound. The most helpful diagnostic test at this point in his evaluation is:

A. an upper endoscopy.

B. a barium swallow.

C. an evaluation of *H pylori* status.

D. esophageal pH monitoring.

72. Which of the following can be considered as an alternative to PPI for protection against NSAID-induced gastropathy?

A. sucralfate

B. misoprostol

C. esomeprazole

D. metoclopramide

73. *H pylori* is least likely to cause which of the following PUDs?

A. duodenal ulcer

B. gastric ulcer

    C. nonerosive (antral) gastritis

    D. erosive gastritis

74. To avoid rebound gastric hyperacidity following discontinuation of long-term PPI use, all of the following methods can be used except:

    A. gradually tapering the PPI dose with supplemental antacid.

    B. switching to every-other-day dosing of PPI with supplemental antacid.

    C. switching to a low-dose H₂RA therapy with supplemental antacid.

    D. initiating empiric *H pylori* therapy.

For answers and rationales, see end of chapter.

Gastroesophageal Reflux Disease

Overview

Gastroesophageal reflux disease (GERD) is a common but troublesome condition. Reflux of stomach contents into the esophagus occurs regularly. Most reflux is asymptomatic with no resulting esophageal injury. GERD is present when there are symptoms or evidence of tissue damage. Decreased lower esophageal sphincter tone and the resulting reflux of gastric contents cause GERD. Esophageal mucosal irritation results from exposure to hydrochloric acid and pepsin. The use of certain medications and consuming certain foods can worsen GERD symptoms. (See Treatment section.)

> **CLINICAL CONCEPT**
>
> Non-GI GERD symptoms, including chronic hoarseness, sore throat, nocturnal cough, and wheezing, are often reported, occasionally in the absence of more classic GERD symptoms, and particularly when the condition is chronic.

Clinical Presentation

The most common GERD presentation includes dyspepsia, chest pain at rest, and postprandial fullness. Other conditions to consider when making the differential diagnosis include acute and chronic gastritis, esophagitis, cholelithiasis, PUD, *H pylori* infection, and irritable bowel syndrome (IBS).

Diagnostic Testing

In patients with classic GI symptoms, the diagnosis of GERD is usually made clinically with no specific diagnostic testing performed, particularly when clinical response is noted with standard therapy.

Treatment

Behavioral intervention in GERD includes avoiding or minimizing conditions or situations that encourage esophageal reflux: remaining upright and avoiding assuming the supine position within 3 hours of a meal, eating smaller meals, and eliminating occasions of overeating. Because abdominal obesity contributes to GERD, weight loss can also be helpful. Elevation of the head of the bed on 4-inch blocks can also offer some relief; propping the head and upper thorax on pillows is not effective.

The use of certain medications, including estrogen, progesterone/progestins, theophylline, calcium channel blockers, and nicotine, can result in a decrease in lower esophageal sphincter pressure and worsen GERD. These medications should be discontinued if clinically possible. Initial therapy for patients with GERD includes identifying triggers and reducing their intake. The most commonly mentioned include alcohol, tomato-based products, chocolate, peppermint, colas, citrus juices, and food high in fat.

The use of antacids after meals and at bedtime is often sufficient to control milder, particularly intermittent, GERD symptoms. Antacids neutralize secreted acids and inactivate pepsin and bile salts. These medications are most effective when used 1 to 3 hours after meals and at bedtime. Antacids interact with many other medications and should be used at least 2 hours apart; with the use of a fluoroquinolone such as ciprofloxacin, antacid use should be 2 to 4 hours before or 4 to 6 hours after the fluoroquinolone.

If the use of antacids and lifestyle modification are inadequate to control milder, intermittent GERD symptoms, an H₂RA at full prescription strength should be added. H₂RAs are effective in healing only mild esophagitis in a majority of cases and can be considered for maintenance therapy to prevent relapse. If there is no improvement in 6 weeks, longer-term H₂RA therapy is unlikely to be helpful. With moderate-to-severe symptoms that do not respond to a prescription dosage of H$_2$RA, a PPI such as omeprazole (Prilosec®) or lansoprazole (Prevacid®) should be prescribed; an alternative is to simply start therapy for a confirmed diagnosis with a PPI. Compared with H$_2$RAs, PPIs have superior postprandial and nocturnal acid suppression. An 8-week course of PPI therapy is usually adequate to heal acute esophageal inflammation noted with ongoing GERD. If GERD symptoms do not resolve with this PPI course, referral to gastroenterology for further evaluation, including upper GI endoscopy, is warranted.

In the past, sucralfate and prokinetic agents were considered to be treatment options for GERD; little evidence supports the use of these medications, and these medications are no longer considered therapeutic options in this condition.

The clinical course of GERD is usually straightforward; however, "alarm" symptoms in GERD that warrant further evaluation include:

■ Dysphagia (difficulty swallowing)
■ Odynophagia (painful swallowing)
■ GI bleeding
■ Unexplained weight loss
■ Persistent chest pain

The development of iron-deficiency anemia as a result of chronic low-volume GI blood loss in the presence of GERD symptoms is a rare but worrisome finding. A component of the additional evaluation is referral to gastroenterology for upper endoscopy. These alarm findings can be indicative of erosive esophagitis or esophageal cancer; upper endoscopy can clarify the diagnosis and provide, if required, a vehicle of esophageal biopsy.

> **CLINICAL CONCEPT**
> Reflux-induced esophageal injury, also known as reflux esophagitis, is present in 40% of patients with GERD.

Surgical intervention in GERD is a treatment option usually limited to patients with the most severe symptoms that are not improved by the use of standard treatment. In obesity, weight loss, with a consideration for bariatric surgery, should be discussed prior to GERD surgery. Symptoms are likely to continue even with GERD surgery if there is no weight loss.

Erosions and ulcerations in squamous epithelium of the esophagus are present and are most common in elderly patients and individuals with long-standing GERD history.

Complications of reflux esophagitis include esophageal stricture and columnar epithelial metaplasia, also known as Barrett's esophagus (BE), which typically involves the distal esophagus. In patients at risk for BE, an upper GI endoscopy should be performed and appropriate biopsy specimens taken. Although BE has long been mentioned as a potent risk factor for esophageal adenocarcinoma, this risk is not thought to be as significant as it was in the past. Risk factors for BE include GERD of long duration, certain ethnicity (i.e., white, Latino), male gender, advancing age (older than 50 years of age), tobacco use, alcohol use, and obesity. Intervention in BE is similar to GERD treatment and is based on aggressive acid suppression, with the anticipated end product of minimizing further esophageal damage. For patients with established BE of any length and with no dysplasia, endoscopic surveillance should occur at 3- to 5-year intervals. The clinician and patient should remain aware of the latest recommendations on BE intervention and surveillance.

Discussion Sources

Katz PO, Gerson LB, Vela MF. Diagnosis and management of gastroesophageal reflux disease. *Am J Gastroenterol*. 2013;108(3): 308–328. http://gi.org/guideline/diagnosis-and-managemen-of-gastroesophageal-reflux-disease/

Shaheen NJ, Falk GW, Iyer PG, Gerson L. Diagnosis and management of Barrett's esophagus. *Am J Gastroenterol*. 2016;111:30–50. https://gi.org/guideline/diagnosis-and-management-of-barretts-esophagus/

QUESTIONS

75. A 35-year-old woman complains of a 6-month history of periodic "heartburn" primarily after eating tomato-based sauces. Her weight is unchanged, and examination reveals a single altered finding of epigastric tenderness without rebound. As first-line therapy, you advise:

   A. avoiding trigger foods.

   B. the use of an oral prokinetic medication.

   C. addition of oral sucralfate with meals.

   D. increased fluid intake with food intake.

76. You see a 62-year-old man diagnosed with esophageal columnar epithelial metaplasia. You realize he is at increased risk for:

    A. duodenal ulcer.

    B. esophageal adenocarcinoma.

    C. gastroesophageal reflux.

    D. *H pylori* colonization.

77. In caring for a patient with symptomatic gastroesophageal reflux, you prescribe a PPI to:

    A. enhance motility.

    B. increase the pH of the stomach.

    C. reduce esophageal pressure.

    D. help limit *H pylori* growth.

78. A 38-year-old nonsmoking man presents with signs and symptoms consistent of GERD. He has self-treated with over-the-counter antacids and acid suppression therapy with effect. His weight is stable, and he denies nausea, vomiting, diarrhea, or melena. Which of the following represents the most appropriate diagnostic plan for this patient?

    A. fecal testing for *H pylori* antigen

    B. upper GI endoscopy

    C. barium swallow

    D. no specific diagnostic testing is needed

79. Which of the following is most likely to be found in a 40-year-old woman with new-onset reflux esophagitis?

    A. recent initiation of estrogen-progestin hormonal therapy

    B. recent weight loss

    C. report of melena

    D. evidence of *H pylori* infection

80. Which of the following is likely to be reported in a patient with persistent GERD?

    A. hematemesis

    B. chronic sore throat

    C. diarrhea

    D. melena

81. A 58-year-old man recently began taking an antihypertensive medication and reports that his "heartburn" has become much worse. He is most likely taking:

    A. atenolol.

    B. trandolapril.

    C. amlodipine.

    D. losartan.

82. You prescribe a fluoroquinolone antibiotic to treat pyelonephritis in a 54-year-old woman who has occasional GERD symptoms that she treats with a prn antacid. When discussing appropriate medication use, you advise that she should take the antimicrobial:

    A. with the antacid.

    B. separated from the antacid use by 2 to 4 hours before or 4 to 6 hours after taking the fluoroquinolone.

    C. without regard to antacid use.

    D. apart from the antacid by about 1 hour on either side of the fluoroquinolone dose.

83. A 43-year-old man with obesity and a 1-year history of classic GERD symptoms has been on consistent use of a therapeutic dose of a PPI for the past 6 months. He states he is "really no better with the medicine and I have cut out most of the food that bothers my stomach. I even cut out all alcohol and soda." Physical examination reveals stable weight, mildly erythematous pharynx, and epigastric tenderness without rebound. Next-step options include:

   A. obtaining an upper GI series.

   B. referral for GERD surgery.

   C. further evaluation with upper GI endoscopy.

   D. obtaining FOBT testing.

84. Which of the following is not an "alarm" finding in the person with GERD symptoms?

   A. weight gain

   B. dysphagia

   C. odynophagia

   D. iron-deficiency anemia

85. Risk factors for BE include all of the following except:

   A. a history of cigarette smoking.

   B. being older than 50 years of age.

   C. male gender.

   D. African American ethnicity.

86. A 57-year-old male is in need of evaluation for BE. You recommend:

   A. *H pylori* testing.

   B. thoracic CT scan with contrast.

   C. upper GI endoscopy with biopsy.

   D. barium swallow.

87. A 64-year-old male with diagnosed BE has shown no sign of dysplasia in two consecutive evaluations within the past year. You recommend additional surveillance testing should be conducted every:

   A. 6 to 12 months.

   B. 12 to 18 months.

   C. 2 years.

   D. 3 to 5 years.

For answers and rationales, see end of chapter.

Esophageal Cancer

Overview

Esophageal cancer can be found in a variety of forms and is the sixth most common cause of cancer deaths worldwide. Until the 1970s, squamous cell carcinoma (SCC), usually found in the upper part of the esophagus, represented approximately 90% to 95% of all esophageal cancers in the United States and was most frequently found in African American men with a long history of smoking and alcohol consumption. Rates of esophageal adenocarcinoma, usually located at the junction of the esophagus and stomach, have been increasing over the past few decades, particularly among whites. The incidence of adenocarcinoma now exceeds SCC in white men and women. As with BE, esophageal cancer is more common in men, with a male-to-female ratio of approximately 3:1. The disease is most often diagnosed in the sixth and seventh decades of life. Human papillomavirus (HPV) is recognized as a potential contributing factor in the development of esophageal cancer. However, recent research suggests HPV infection is not an important risk factor, though certain HPV types might play a role in a small subset of esophageal cancers. The HPV vaccine, now approved for adults up to 45 years of age, can offer protection against certain types of HPV types that cause genital cancers; its effectiveness in preventing oral, throat, or esophageal cancer is currently unknown with further study ongoing.

Clinical Presentation

In early esophageal cancer, regardless of etiology, the patient is usually without symptoms.

Less commonly reported symptoms are epigastric or retrosternal pain, persistent hoarseness, and cough, though these are also common to GERD. Because of chronic low-volume bleeding from the cancerous esophageal tumor, iron-deficiency anemia often develops.

Diagnostic Testing and Treatment

Often, esophageal cancer is not detected until it has become advanced. Prognosis is dependent on the extent of the disease. When esophageal cancer is suspected, esophagogastroduodenoscopy (EGD, upper GI endoscopy) with appropriate biopsies is the preferred method of initial diagnostic testing. Additional testing is based on initial findings.

Discussion Source

Masab M, Espat J. Esophageal cancer. Medscape. http://emedicine.medscape.com/article/277930

QUESTIONS

88. Among white men and women in the United States, the most common form of esophageal cancer is:
    A. squamous cell cancer.
    B. adenocarcinoma.
    C. basal cell carcinoma.
    D. HPV induced.

89. Risk factors for esophageal cancer include all of the following except:
    A. female gender.
    B. HPV infection.
    C. older age.
    D. BE.

90. From the following, who is at greatest risk of esophageal cancer?
    A. a 34-year-old male who eats a high-fat diet
    B. a 76-year-old male who stopped smoking 15 years ago
    C. a 45-year-old woman with a history of six full-term pregnancies
    D. a 58-year-old woman who follows a plant-based diet

91. The presence of more advanced esophageal cancer is commonly associated with:
    A. renal impairment.
    B. chronic bronchitis.
    C. iron-deficiency anemia.
    D. unexplained weight gain.

For answers and rationales, see end of chapter.

Viral Hepatitis

Overview

Numerous infective agents cause viral hepatitis (Table 8-6). The most common hepatic-specific viral agents in the United States are those that result in hepatitis A (hepatitis A virus, referred to as HAV), hepatitis B (hepatitis B virus, referred to as HBV), hepatitis C (hepatitis C virus, referred to as HCV), and hepatitis D (hepatitis D virus, referred to as HDV). These viral hepatitis forms have specific routes of transmission, risk factors for acquisition, diagnostic testing, and treatment.

TABLE 8-6 Infectious Hepatitis: Key Features to Transmission and Diagnosis

TYPE	ROUTE OF TRANSMISSION	IZ AVAILABLE? POSTEXPOSURE PROPHYLAXIS?	SEQUELAE	DISEASE MARKER
Hepatitis A	Fecal-oral	IZ = Yes Postexposure prophylaxis with IZ and/or IG for close contacts	None, survive or die (low mortality rate)	Acute disease marker ■ HAV IgM (M = miserable) ■ Elevated hepatic enzymes ≥10 × ULN Chronic disease marker ■ None, as chronic hepatitis A does not exist Disease in past, Hx IZ = ■ Anti-HAV (total of HAV IgM and HAV IgG [G = gone]) present ■ Hepatic enzymes normalize Still susceptible to hepatitis A infection ■ Anti-HAV negative (Negative = "Never had")
Hepatitis B	Blood, body fluids	IZ = Yes Postexposure prophylaxis with IZ and/or HBIG for blood, body fluid contacts	Chronic hepatitis B, hepatocellular carcinoma (HCC, primary liver cancer, hepatoma), hepatic failure	Acute disease markers ■ HBsAg = Always growing ■ HBeAg = Extra contagious, extra growing ■ Elevated hepatic enzymes ≥10 × ULN Chronic disease marker ■ Patient without symptoms ■ NL or slightly elevated hepatic enzymes ■ HBsAg (Ag = Always growing) ■ Only present if HBV on board ■ Surrogate marker for HBV Hepatitis B in past, Hx IZ (in most) ■ HBsAb (Anti-HBs) ■ B = Bye, as no HBV on board ■ A protective antibody, unable to get HBV in the future ■ Hepatic enzyme normalized Still susceptible to hepatitis B infection ■ HBsAg negative ■ Anti-HBc negative ■ HBsAb (Anti-HBs) negative

Continued

TABLE 8-6 Infectious Hepatitis: Key Features to Transmission and Diagnosis—cont'd

TYPE	ROUTE OF TRANSMISSION	IZ AVAILABLE? POSTEXPOSURE PROPHYLAXIS?	SEQUELAE	DISEASE MARKER
Hepatitis C	Blood, body fluids	No No	Chronic hepatitis C, hepatocellular carcinoma (HCC, primary liver cancer, hepatoma), hepatic failure	Acute disease marker ■ Anti-HCV present ■ HCV viral RNA ■ Elevated hepatic enzymes Chronic disease marker ■ Anti-HCV present ■ HCV viral RNA ■ Normal to slightly elevated hepatic enzymes Disease in the past ■ Anti-HCV present (nonprotective antibody) ■ HCV RNA absent ■ Normalized hepatic enzymes
Hepatitis D	Blood, body fluids	No, but prevent B and you can prevent D	Severe infection, hepatic failure, death	Acute or chronic hepatitis B (HBsAg) markers *plus* hepatitis D IgM. Usually with markedly elevated hepatic enzymes.

NB: The content of this table is not meant to be a comprehensive guide for the diagnosis of infectious hepatitis but rather an overview. For additional information, see Ferri F. Ferri's Best Test: A Practical Guide to Clinical Laboratory Medicine and Diagnostic Imaging. 4th ed. St. Louis, MO: Elsevier Saunders; 2017; and Desai S. Clinician's Guide to Laboratory Medicine: Pocket. 3rd ed. Houston, TX: MD2B; 2009; CDC. Viral hepatitis–hepatitis A information, hepatitis B information, hepatitis C information. https://www.cdc.gov/hepatitis/hav

---

CLINICAL CONCEPT

Laboratory findings in infectious hepatitis include elevated serum aminotransferase (hepatic enzyme) levels, most often 20 or more times the upper limit of normal (ULN).

Clinical Presentation

The presentation of viral hepatitis usually includes malaise, myalgia, fatigue, nausea, and anorexia. Aversion to cigarette smoke exposure is often reported. Clay-colored stools, arthritis-like symptoms, and skin rash are also noted, though not universally. Mild fever occasionally occurs. Hepatomegaly with usually mild right upper quadrant abdominal tenderness without rebound is found in about 50% of patients, with splenomegaly in about 15%. Jaundice, when present, occurs about 1 week after the onset of symptoms; jaundice is not found in most cases, however. The course of the illness is typically 2 to 3 weeks. During this period, a gradual increase in energy, appetite, and well-being is reported. Onset of symptoms after viral acquisition differs by the organism's incubation period. In general, patients with hepatitis A, B, and D are more symptomatic than patients presenting with hepatitis C. Indeed, most patients with acute HCV infection have minimal to no symptoms.

Diagnostic Testing

Virus-specific testing differs with different hepatitis forms and is outlined in the corresponding section.

Laboratory findings common to all forms of viral hepatitis include leukopenia with lymphocytosis. Atypical lymphocytes are often found. Excess bilirubin, reflected in the urine, is usually found in the absence of icterus. Knowledge of measures to prevent hepatitis or minimize its acquisition after exposure is important to safe, effective practice (see Table 8-6).

HEPATITIS A

Overview

Hepatitis A infection is caused by HAV, a small RNA virus. Transmitted primarily by the fecal/oral route, hepatitis A is typically a self-limiting infection with a low mortality rate unless there is underlying preexisting hepatic disease.

Fecal-contaminated water supplies are the most common source of infection, although eating raw shell-fish that grew in impure water can be problematic. In areas with limited safe water supply, most children contract this disease by school age; the majority (more than 70%) of children younger than age 6 years will have few or no symptoms during HAV infection.

In North America, adults 20 to 39 years old account for nearly 50% of the reported cases. Because of the risk to a given population, the local public health department should be consulted for advice when an outbreak of hepatitis A infection occurs.

Unlike hepatitis B and C, there are no long-term known sequelae of HAV infection, no chronic infection state, and a history of hepatitis A infection does not carry risk for hepatocellular carcinoma or cirrhosis. The onset of symptoms in hepatitis A usually occurs about 15 to 50 days after the organism is contracted; the average incubation period for the virus is about 28 days, with a range of 15 to 50 days.

Prevention

HAV is a heat-sensitive virus that can be killed by heating food to higher than 185°F (higher than 85°C) for 1 minute. Adequate chlorination and purification of municipal water, as recommended in the United States, kills HAV before it enters the water supply. The virus is capable of surviving on select surfaces for many weeks. Proper hand hygiene and cleaning environmental surfaces with a 1:100 bleach solution are measures that can help minimize the spread of this infection.

All children and any unimmunized adult who requests the HAV vaccine should be immunized. See Chapter 2 for details about immunizations, at-risk populations, and additional candidates for HAV vaccine. Hepatitis A vaccine, which does not contain live virus, is usually well tolerated without systemic reaction. Postvaccine HAV immunity typically lasts at least 20 years. Postexposure prophylaxis against hepatitis A is also available; immune globulin (IG) and HAV vaccine are used for this purpose. Refer to the latest immunization guidelines for further information on this important public health issue.

Diagnostic Testing

Because the clinical presentation of the various viral hepatitis forms is similar, the diagnosis must be confirmed by a positive serological test for the specific hepatitis viral infection. See Tables 8-2 and 8-6 for details.

Treatment

There is no specific treatment for HAV infection as the body will clear the virus on its own, with the liver typically healing itself within a month or two. HAV treatment primarily focuses on alleviating the signs and symptoms of the infection. Patients often feel tired and have decreased energy levels, and thus should rest when needed. To combat nausea, patients can try to eat small snacks rather than larger meals and choose higher-calorie foods over lower-calorie foods if having trouble ingesting enough calories. Finally, any insult to the liver should be avoided during HAV infection. If possible, any medications potentially toxic to the liver, including frequent, high-dose acetaminophen, should be stopped or changed, and alcohol consumption should be avoided while signs and symptoms persist.

HEPATITIS B AND D

Overview

Hepatitis B is caused by a small double-stranded DNA virus that contains an inner core protein of hepatitis B core antigen and an outer surface of HBsAg. HBV is usually transmitted through an exchange of blood and body fluids. The virus has a long incubation period, with symptoms occurring an average of 90 days after exposure but could range from 60 to 150 days.

The predominant modes of transmission of the HBV virus are through sexual activity and/or injection drug use. Risk factors for HBV infection include having multiple partners, men who have sexual contact with other men, sharing needles during injection drug use, having a job with exposure to human blood, or traveling to areas with high infection rates of HBV (such as Africa, central and Southeast Asia, and central Europe). HBV is also a major occupational hazard of health workers. HBV cannot be spread by contaminated food or water, nor can it be spread through casual contact in the workplace or other settings. Because of the risk to a given population, the local public health department should be notified whenever hepatitis B is diagnosed. See Chapter 2 for additional information about at-risk populations.

Acute hepatitis B is a serious illness that can lead to hepatic failure. Approximately 5% to 10% of individuals with acute hepatitis B go on to develop chronic hepatitis B; chronic hepatitis B is a potent risk factor for hematoma or primary hepatocellular carcinoma and hepatic cirrhosis. A person with chronic hepatitis B continues to be able to transmit the virus, although the person appears clinically well. A patient with hepatitis B and D acute co-infection has a course of illness similar to that in a patient with only acute hepatitis B infection. Because the hepatitis D virus is an RNA virus that can occur only concurrently in the presence of HBV, hepatitis D disease is found only in persons with acute or chronic hepatitis B. If a patient with chronic hepatitis B becomes superinfected with hepatitis D virus, a fulminant or severe acute hepatitis often results.

Prevention

Hepatitis B infection can be prevented by limiting exposure to blood and body fluids. HBV can be killed with a 1:10 dilution of bleach to clean up blood spills. Gloves and eye protection should be worn when cleaning up blood or body fluids spills. Condom use with sexual activity also dramatically reduces HBV acquisition.

Vaccination against HBV is widely available and recommended. Recombinant hepatitis B vaccine, which does not contain live virus, is well tolerated; one contraindication to receiving the vaccine is a personal history of anaphylaxis to baker's yeast. The vaccine should be offered to adults born before 1991 and to all who have not been immunized, particularly persons at highest risk for contracting the virus. Non-immunized individuals being treated for other sexually transmitted infections should be encouraged to receive protection against HBV. See Chapter 2 for detailed information about HPV vaccinations, including at-risk populations. Refer to the latest immunization guidelines from the Centers for Disease Control and Prevention for further information on this important public health issue. Unvaccinated persons should receive hepatitis B immune globulin (HBIG) and hepatitis B vaccine as soon as possible after HBV exposure, preferably within 24 hours.

Testing for HIV, other sexually transmitted infections, and hepatitis A and C should also be offered, and postexposure prophylaxis and immunization should be offered when applicable. Owing to the complexity of care, intervention for a person with occupational exposure should be done with expert consultation in this area.

Prevention of hepatitis B through immunization also prevents hepatitis D.

Diagnostic Testing

Because the clinical presentation of the various viral hepatitis forms is similar, the diagnosis must be confirmed by a positive serological test for the specific hepatitis viral infection. See Tables 8-2 and 8-6 for details.

Treatment

Treatment for acute hepatitis B is largely supportive. Treatment with interferon (interferon-α and pegylated interferon) or a nucleoside/nucleotide analog (i.e., telbivudine, adefovir, entecavir, tenofovir, and lamivudine) has shown clinical utility in inducing remission in some patients with chronic hepatitis B. Entecavir and tenofovir have potent antiviral activity and will lead to undetectable levels of HBV DNA in most patients. Because of the rapid advances being made in this area, the NP and patient must be aware of the most up-to-date treatment options.

HEPATITIS C

Overview

Hepatitis C infection is transmitted through the exchange of blood and body fluids. A single-strand RNA virus causes the infection. Prior to 1992, HCV was commonly spread through blood transfusions and organ transplants; however, since the advent of screening of the blood supply for HCV, the risk of transfusion-associated hepatitis C has decreased from 10% in the early 1980s to 1 in a million (0.0001%) per unit transfused today.

Other at-risk behaviors include tattooing, branding, piercing, or other similar practices when shared or poorly sanitized equipment is used. Transmission through sexual contact is possible, but this risk is relatively low. Maternal-fetal transmission is also uncommon and is usually limited to women with high circulating HCV levels. Transmission through breastfeeding has not been reported.

Clinical Presentation

The HCV incubation period is about 6 to 7 weeks, and the infection rarely causes a serious acute illness. At least 50% to 80% of individuals with hepatitis C go on to develop a chronic infection. As with chronic hepatitis B, the person with chronic hepatitis C usually appears well but is carrying an oncogenic virus and remains capable of transmitting HCV.

Progression to cirrhosis occurs in about 20% of people infected with chronic hepatitis C after 20 years of untreated disease. HCV-related cirrhosis risk in individuals with untreated HCV is increased in men, with disease acquisition after age 40 years, and in people who drink the equivalent of 50 g or more of alcohol per day (15 g alcohol = 12 oz beer, 5 oz wine, or 1.5 oz 80-proof whiskey).

> **CLINICAL CONCEPT**
> More than 50% of HCV infections are caused by injection drug use with needle sharing.

Diagnostic Testing

Because the clinical presentation of the various viral hepatitis forms is similar, the diagnosis must be confirmed by a positive serological test for the specific hepatitis viral infection. See Tables 8-2 and 8-6 for details.

Treatment

Due to the significant potential sequelae of chronic hepatitis C infection, expert consultation should be obtained so that the patient and primary care provider are well versed on the latest evaluation, monitoring, and treatment options. A number of highly effective oral HCV protease inhibitors are available that can achieve sustained virological response (SVR, defined as absence of detectable virus 12 weeks after completion of treatment) used as monotherapy or combination therapy. More than 90% of HCV-infected individuals can achieve SVR with 12 weeks or less of oral antiviral therapy. Because of the rapid advances being made in this area, the clinician and patient must be aware of the most up-to-date treatment options. There is a lack of evidence supporting surveillance for hepatocellular carcinoma (HCC) among individuals with chronic HCV or a past history of HCV infection. However, surveillance should be performed (either via serological testing such as with periodic α-fetoprotein measurement or imaging) for any adult with evidence of cirrhosis due to any etiology, as this can improve survival and early detection of HCC. This also applies to a patient with untreated chronic hepatitis B.

Discussion Sources

Centers for Disease Control and Prevention. Hepatitis A questions and answers for health professionals. https://www.cdc.gov/hepatitis/hav/havfaq.htm

Centers for Disease Control and Prevention. Viral hepatitis—hepatitis B information. https://www.cdc.gov/hepatitis/hbv

Centers for Disease Control and Prevention. Viral hepatitis—hepatitis C information. https://www.cdc.gov/hepatitis/hcv/index.htm

Centers for Disease Control and Prevention. Viral hepatitis—hepatitis D information. https://www.cdc.gov/hepatitis/hdv/index.htm

QUESTIONS

92. A 36-year-old man complains of a 3-day history of new-onset nausea, fever, malaise, and abdominal pain. He shows signs of jaundice and reports darkly colored urine. Diagnostic results show elevated serum aminotransferase in excess of 10 times the ULN. His most likely diagnosis is:

A. cholecystitis.

B. viral hepatitis.

C. pancreatitis.

D. BE.

93. The serological marker for acute HAV infection is:

A. HAV IgM.

B. HAV viral DNA.

C. HAV IgG.

D. alkaline phosphatase.

94. You are caring for a 45-year-old woman who was born and raised in a rural community in Central America. She reports that she had "yellow jaundice" as a young child. Her physical examination is unremarkable. Her laboratory studies are as follows:
AST, 22 U/L (normal, 0 to 31 U/L)
ALT, 25 U/L (normal, 0 to 40 U/L)
HAV IgG, positive.
Laboratory testing reveals:

    A. chronic hepatitis A.

    B. no evidence of prior or current hepatitis A infection.

    C. resolved hepatitis A infection.

    D. prodromal hepatitis A.

95. The most common source of hepatitis A infection is:

    A. sharing intravenous drug equipment.

    B. cooked seafood.

    C. contaminated water supplies.

    D. sexual contact.

96. A well 48-year-old man presents for routine health maintenance and has a normal abdominal examination. He denies use of alcohol or other liver toxins, has a modest hepatic enzyme elevation, and is hepatitis B surface antigen (HBsAg) positive. These findings are most consistent with:

    A. no evidence of hepatitis B infection.

    B. resolved hepatitis B infection.

    C. chronic hepatitis B.

    D. evidence of effective hepatitis B immunization.

97 to 100. Match each hepatitis virus with the correct incubation times (some answers may be used more than once).

_____ 97. Hepatitis A

_____ 98. Hepatitis B

_____ 99. Hepatitis C

_____ 100. Hepatitis D

    A. 15 to 45 days (average 28 days)

    B. 14 to 180 days (average 45 days)

    C. 45 to 160 days (average 120 days)

101. All of the following are effective methods to kill HAV except:

    A. heating food to more than 185°F (85°C) for at least 1 minute.

    B. adequately chlorinating or purifying water.

    C. cleaning surfaces with a 1:100 bleach solution.

    D. freezing food for at least 1 hour.

102. A 54-year-old man has been recently diagnosed with HAV infection. You recommend all of the following except:

    A. eating smaller, more frequent meals to help combat nausea.

    B. avoiding consumption of any alcohol.

    C. reviewing current medication use for consideration of discontinuation.

    D. prescribing a systemic antibacterial to prevent superinfection.

103. A 38-year-old man with a current history of injection drug use presents with malaise, nausea, fatigue, and "yellow eyes" for the past week. After ordering diagnostic tests, you confirm the diagnosis of acute hepatitis B. Anticipated laboratory results include:

A. the presence of hepatitis B surface antibody (HBsAb).

B. neutrophilia.

C. thrombocytopenia.

D. the presence of HBsAg.

104. Clinical findings in a 45-year-old woman with acute hepatitis B likely include all of the following except:

A. abdominal rebound tenderness.

B. scleral icterus.

C. a smooth, tender, palpable hepatic border.

D. report of myalgia.

105 to 108. Indicate (Yes or No) if each of the following is a risk factor for HBV infection.

_____ **105.** Having multiple sexual partners

_____ **106.** Having an occupation that potentially involves exposure to human blood

_____ **107.** Injection drug use

_____ **108.** Eating food prepared by a person with chronic HBV infection

109. You see a 50-year-old woman who has not received immunization against hepatitis B. She is sexually active without condom use with a man newly diagnosed with acute hepatitis B. You advise her to:

A. start hepatitis B immunization series.

B. limit the number of sexual partners.

C. be tested for HBsAb.

D. receive HBIG and start hepatitis B immunization series.

110. The HBV vaccine should not be offered to individuals who have a history of anaphylactic reaction to:

A. eggs.

B. baker's yeast.

C. peanuts.

D. shellfish.

111. You see a 22-year-old male who is an injection drug user who has recently been diagnosed with chronic HBV infection. You recommend additional testing for all of the following except:

A. Lyme disease.

B. HIV.

C. HAV.

D. HCV.

112. Which of the following statements is true concerning hepatitis C infection?

A. It usually manifests with jaundice, fever, and significant hepatomegaly.

B. Among health-care workers, it is most commonly found in nurses.

C. At least 50% of persons with acute hepatitis C go on to develop chronic infection.

D. Interferon therapy is consistently curative.

113. Which of the following characteristics is predictive of severity of chronic liver disease in a patient with chronic hepatitis C?

    A. female gender, age younger than 30 years

    B. co-infection with hepatitis B, daily alcohol use

    C. acquisition of virus through intravenous drug use, past history of hepatitis A infection

    D. frequent use of aspirin, nutritional status

114. To prevent an outbreak of hepatitis D infection, an NP plans to:

    A. promote a campaign for clean food supplies.

    B. immunize the at-risk population against hepatitis B.

    C. offer antiviral prophylaxis against the virus.

    D. encourage frequent hand washing.

115. Monitoring for hepatoma in a patient with chronic hepatitis B or C often includes periodic evaluation of:

    A. erythrocyte sedimentation rate (ESR).

    B. HBsAb.

    C. α-fetoprotein.

    D. bilirubin.

116. Which of the following is an expected laboratory result in a 38-year-old man with acute hepatitis A infection (normal values: AST, 0 to 31 U/L; ALT, 0 to 40 U/L)?

    A. AST, 55 U/L; ALT, 50 U/L

    B. AST, 320 U/L; ALT, 190 U/L

    C. AST, 320 U/L; ALT, 300 U/L

    D. AST, 640 U/L; ALT, 870 U/L

117. Which of the following is most likely to be reported in a patient on long-term use of atorvastatin therapy (normal values: AST, 0 to 31 U/L; ALT, 0 to 40 U/L)?

    A. AST, 22 U/L; ALT, 28 U/L

    B. AST, 320 U/L; ALT, 190 U/L

    C. AST, 32 U/L; ALT, 120 U/L

    D. AST, 440 U/L; ALT, 670 U/L

118. You see a 48-year-old woman with nonalcoholic fatty liver disease. Evaluation of infectious hepatitis includes the following:
    Anti-HAV IgG—negative
    Anti-HBs—negative
    Anti-HCV—negative
    When considering her overall health status, you advise receiving which of the following vaccines?

    A. immunization against hepatitis A and B as based on her lifestyle risk factors

    B. immunization against hepatitis B and C

    C. immunization against hepatitis A and B

    D. immunization against hepatitis A, B, and C

119. Which of the following hepatitis forms is least effectively transmitted from man to woman via heterosexual vaginal intercourse?

    A. hepatitis A

    B. hepatitis B

C. hepatitis C

D. hepatitis D

For answers and rationales, see end of chapter.

Irritable Bowel Syndrome and Irritable Bowel Disease

IRRITABLE BOWEL SYNDROME

Overview

IBS is a functional bowel disorder characterized by abdominal pain or discomfort and altered bowel habits in the absence of detectable structural abnormalities. This condition is sometimes called spastic colon, irritable colon, or nervous colon. Around the world, 10% to 20% of adults and adolescents have symptoms consistent with IBS, and most studies show a female predominance. IBS affects all ages, but most have their first symptoms before age 45 years.

Advances in research and science have demonstrated that the etiology of IBS is likely multifactorial, with proposed mechanisms involving abnormal gut motor/sensory activity, central neural dysfunction, psychological disturbances, mucosal inflammation, stress, and luminal factors. The risk of developing IBS increases after an episode of acute gastroenteritis. Although anxiety or depression has often been attributed to the resulting disease-induced suffering, in reality, mood disorders often predate IBS onset.

> **CLINICAL CONCEPT**
> Women are diagnosed with IBS two to three times as often as men and make up 80% of the population with severe IBS.

Clinical Presentation

IBS symptoms tend to come and go over time, usually presenting with a protracted history of intermittent diarrhea and constipation with accompanying abdominal pain.

Patients with IBS frequently complain of abdominal distension, increased belching, or flatulence, which they say contribute to increased gas, while most IBS patients have normal amounts of intestinal gas but have impaired transit and tolerance to the intestinal gas loads. Belching is explained by reflux gas from the distal to more proximal intestine. Approximately 25% to 50% of patients complain of upper GI symptoms, including dyspepsia, heartburn, and nausea, especially with the most severe symptoms. However, fever, vomiting, and involuntary weight loss are typically absent. Severity of symptoms varies and can significantly impact quality of life.

On physical examination, a person with IBS usually has tenderness in the sigmoid region; the remainder of the examination is usually normal.

Diagnostic Testing

Diagnosis of the condition is usually made via careful history and clinical presentation, with a focus on excluding other conditions as there are no clear diagnostic markers. Indeed, extensive diagnostic workup in IBS is not recommended in the absence of alarm findings in the adult younger than 45 years old. However, it is important to identify any alarm findings that could suggest more serious disease. IBS alarm findings include overt GI bleeding, iron-deficiency anemia, nocturnal passage of stool, unintentional weight loss, family history of IBD or colorectal cancer, recent changes in bowel habits, leukocytosis, and the presence of a palpable abdominal mass or lymphadenopathy.

Because of the nonspecific GI symptoms of IBS, several other diagnoses must be considered, including IBD, colonic neoplasia, celiac disease, lactase deficiency, endometriosis, depression and anxiety, sexual and physical abuse, and small bowel bacterial overgrowth.

The Rome IV criteria for the diagnosis of IBS require that patients must have recurrent abdominal pain on average at least 1 day/week in the past 3 months associated with two or more of the following: symptoms related to defecation, associated with a change in stool frequency, or associated with a change in stool form or appearance. Abdominal pain is highly variable in its intensity and location. Often it is episodic and crampy, from mild to capable of interfering with activities of daily living (ADLs).

> **CLINICAL CONCEPT**
> Additional IBS symptoms usually include altered stool frequency, form, or passage (or a combination of two or all three), usually accompanied by mucorrhea and abdominal bloating or the sensation of distention or both.

Sleep deprivation is infrequent except for those with severe IBS; nocturnal pain is a poor discriminator of organic versus functional bowel disease. Bleeding is not a feature of IBS unless hemorrhoids or another condition are present. Malnutrition and unintended weight loss do not occur.

People with IBS often present with one of three main subtypes based on bowel patterns:

- IBS, diarrhea prominent (IBS-D): small volumes of loose stools, volumes less than 200 mL without nocturnal diarrhea; is often aggravated by emotional stress or eating, with passage of large amounts of mucus
- IBS, constipation predominant (IBS-C): can be first episodic then become intractable to laxatives with hard, narrowed stool caliber and a sense of incomplete evacuation for weeks or months interrupted by brief periods of diarrhea
- IBS, mixed diarrhea and constipation (IBS-M)

Individuals who meet the diagnostic criteria for IBS but whose bowel habits do not fall into one of the three subtypes are categorized as IBS unclassified.

Gut dysfunction occurs along a continuum, with most patients moving from type to type. Usually the patient reports that these symptoms have been present for many years before care was sought.

Women are diagnosed with the condition more often than men. Most individuals with the condition have onset of symptoms before age 35 years, often reporting problems since childhood. Although IBS onset can occur after age 40 years, an alternative GI diagnosis, including malignancy, becomes more likely and should be carefully considered in an adult in this age group presenting with IBS-like symptoms.

Diagnostic testing is not required initially in patients whose history and symptoms are compatible with IBS. However, further tests are warranted in those who do not improve in 2 to 4 weeks of empiric therapy. Laboratory analysis is usually directed at ruling out another cause for the condition and typically reveals a normal hemogram, a normal ESR, and a negative test for fecal occult blood. Glucose or lactulose breath tests can be used to rule out small bowel bacterial overgrowth. Stool analysis for ova, parasite, enteric pathogens, leukocytes, and *C difficile* toxin are negative. If imaging studies, such as GI barium study, ultrasound, or abdominal CT or endoscopy, are indicated by clinical presentation, the results are usually normal. In refractory cases, referral to a gastroenterology specialist can be considered, particularly if the diagnosis is in question. A high prevalence of small intestinal bacterial overgrowth detected by positive lactulose hydrogen breath testing has been noted; testing is usually done in conjunction with GI consultation.

Treatment

Intervention in IBS involves patient support and education about the nature of the condition, including information that life expectancy is not affected, the condition is usually chronic with periodic exacerbations, and stress is a common trigger. Nutritional intervention can be helpful, with adequate hydration, addition of dietary fiber (at least 25 to 35 grams daily with at least four to six glasses of water), avoidance of trigger foods, and moderation of caffeine intake often reported as being helpful. Common triggers to aggravate IBS symptoms include coffee, disaccharides, legumes, cabbage, a high-carbohydrate diet, and excessive fructose and artificial sweeteners, such as sorbitol or mannitol. Fiber supplementation is often helpful with diarrhea and constipation; polycarbophil-based products, such as FiberCon®, offer a potential advantage over psyllium by causing less flatulence. Although some patients with IBS report improvement with avoidance of lactose, fructose, or gluten, others do not.

Intervention with medications is usually aimed at treating the predominant symptom (Table 8-7). A low-dose tricyclic antidepressant or selective serotonin reuptake inhibitor use can be helpful for IBS. For IBS-D, the antidiarrheal medication loperamide (Imodium®) is often used, though there is a general lack of evidence supporting its use in IBS. Eluxadoline (Viberzi®), a mixed-opioid receptor agonist, is approved for the treatment of IBS-D and offers an alternative to antidiarrheals or antispasmodics. Rifaximin (Xifaxan®) is an antibiotic that has also been shown to improve symptoms of IBS-D.

For IBS-C, prokinetic or promotility agents have traditionally been used. Because of safety issues, select prokinetics, such as metoclopramide (Reglan®), are not recommended for long-term use. Lubiprostone (Amitiza®), linaclotide (Linzess®), and plecanatide (Trulance®) are agents approved for the treatment of IBS-C and have been shown to be superior to placebo in clinical trials. Lubiprostone is a chloride channel activator, while linaclotide and plecanatide are guanylate cyclase-C agonists. Prudent practice dictates keeping up to date with the latest IBS treatment options.

The use of prebiotics and probiotics is an emerging treatment option that might help to normalize the possibly altered gut flora; however, current evidence does not support the use of these products for treatment of IBS.

TABLE 8-7 Treatment Medication Classifications for Irritable Bowel Syndrome

MEDICATION CLASS	EXAMPLES	MECHANISM OF ACTION
Antispasmodic (Anticholinergic) agents	Dicyclomine, hyoscyamine, methscopolamine	Reduces stool frequency, but can worsen constipation
Antidiarrheal agent	Loperamide	Decreases peristalsis and fluid secretion in the gut; evidence supporting use in IBS-D generally lacking; long-term use can lead to constipation
Osmotic laxatives	PEG 3350 (Miralax®); magnesium hydroxide (MOM, Milk of Magnesia)	Helps to retain water in the stool (PEG 3350) or draws fluid into the gut (MOM); helpful in IBS-C
Chloride channel activator	Lubiprostone (Amitiza®)	Promotes fluid secretion into the intestinal lumen; helpful in IBS-C
Guanylate cyclase-C agonists	Linaclotide (Linzess®), plecanatide (Trulance®)	Promotes fluid secretion in the gut; helpful in IBS-C
Mixed-opioid receptor agonist	Eluxadoline (Viberzi®)	Agonist of μ and κ opioid receptors to decrease motility and reduce visceral pain; antagonist of δ opioid receptor to modulate μ agonism to reduce risk of constipation; helpful in IBS-D
Antimicrobial	Rifaximin (Xifaxan®)	Antibacterial approved for treatment of IBS-D
Tricyclic and related antidepressants	Nortriptyline, desipramine, imipramine, amitriptyline	Alters gut pain threshold, resulting in less abdominal pain; the anticholinergic effects of TCAs can help with limiting stool frequency; helpful in IBS-D
Selective serotonin reuptake inhibitors	Sertraline, fluoxetine, citalopram, paroxetine	Alters gut pain threshold, resulting in less abdominal pain; helpful in IBS-C

INFLAMMATORY BOWEL DISEASE

Overview

IBD is a disease of unclear etiology but likely involves an autoimmune response in the GI tract. This condition has a genetic component; whether this is a predisposition or susceptibility is unclear.

In contrast to IBS, the male-to-female ratio is approximately equal for UC and Crohn's disease. Similar to IBS, IBD is most often diagnosed in late adolescence to early adulthood, with most individuals who develop the disease showing symptoms by their late 20s. Less commonly, new-onset IBD is diagnosed in a child or older adult.

Clinical Presentation

The diagnosis of IBD is usually made through a combination of careful health history, physical examination, and appropriate diagnostic investigations, including radiography, endoscopy, and biopsy. The manifestations of IBD generally depend on the area of the intestinal tract involved. Patients with UC or Crohn's disease frequently have bloody diarrhea, occasionally with tenesmus. Patients with Crohn's disease involving the small intestine frequently have abdominal pain, involuntary weight loss, and diarrhea, and occasionally they have symptoms of intestinal obstruction. The presence of anterior and posterior anal fissures should raise suspicion for Crohn's disease.

> **CLINICAL CONCEPT**
>
> The two major types of IBD are UC, in which the pathological changes are limited to the colon, and Crohn's disease, in which the changes can involve any part of the GI tract.

A cobblestone mucosal pattern is often identified on endoscopy or contrast radiography in Crohn's disease. "Skip lesions," areas of affected mucosal tissue alternating with normal tissue, are common; the rectum is often spared with the terminal ileum and right colon involved in most cases. In UC, inflammation is limited to the mucosa, whereas in Crohn's disease, the entire intestinal wall is involved. Additional extraintestinal manifestations in IBD include a nondestructive axial or peripheral arthritis in 15% of cases. Renal calculi are often found with Crohn's disease.

Diagnostic Testing

During an IBD flare, serological markers of inflammation, including CRP and ESR (or sed rate) are usually elevated. Leukocytosis is often present. In Crohn's disease, fistulas and perianal disease are often noted. Toxic colitis, characterized by nonobstructive colonic dilation with signs of systemic toxicity, can occur as a potentially life-threatening complication of either condition; this condition is usually infectious in origin, with *C difficile* often implicated.

Anemia is a common problem in IBD; its etiology is often from multiple causes. Iron-deficiency anemia, manifesting as a microcytic, hypochromic anemia, occurs as a result of chronic blood loss. Anemia of chronic disease, a normocytic, normochromic anemia, is a result of inflammation of IBD, whereas anemia associated with acute blood loss can occur as a result of GI hemorrhage during a flare. Vitamin B_{12} deficiency, manifesting as a macrocytic, normochromic anemia, can also result in Crohn's disease, usually in the presence of significant terminal ileum disease. Other conditions to consider for patients with suspected IBD can include celiac disease, IBS, ischemic colitis, diverticulitis, and colorectal malignancy.

Treatment

The health care for a person with IBD is usually a combination of lifestyle support, medication, and occasionally surgery. A person with IBD should be counseled to keep track of dietary triggers. Lactose intolerance is common in Crohn's disease but no more common than in the general population in people with UC. Tobacco use is associated with greater Crohn's disease, but not UC, flares. Smoking cessation should be encouraged for this and its numerous additional health benefits. Gut rest is often used during treatment of Crohn's disease, but not UC flares. Although IBD is likely genetic, not psychological, in origin, mental health and social support are important treatment components as the patient and family cope with this chronic, life-altering, and potentially life-threatening disease.

Medication therapy in IBD is usually initiated at the time of a flare, often the most common point of disease diagnosis. In Crohn's disease and UC, oral aminosalicylates, including sulfasalazine (Azulfidine®) and mesalamine (Apriso®), are usually the first-line therapy and are equally effective. Mesalamine is usually better tolerated and can be used in the presence of sulfa allergy. In UC, when disease is limited to the distal colon, mesalamine and corticosteroids can be administered rectally. Oral or parenteral corticosteroid use can provide rapid symptom relief because of potent anti-inflammatory effects. In Crohn's disease, metronidazole and ciprofloxacin are used when perineal disease or an inflammatory mass is noted; antibiotic use in UC is discouraged because of the increased risk of *C difficile* infection. Immune modulators including 6-mercaptopurine and azathioprine are often prescribed to provide long-term disease control. A monoclonal antibody against tumor necrosis factor (TNF)-α, infliximab (Remicade®), is also a potentially helpful, although costly, treatment option, assisting in remission in about 80% of individuals with Crohn's disease and about 50% of individuals with UC. Additional biologics approved for the treatment of IBD include other anti-TNF agents (adalimumab [Humira®], certolizumab [Cimzia®], and golimumab [Simponi®]), and monoclonal antibodies against α_4-integrin (natalizumab [Tysabri®] and vedolizumab [Entyvio®]). Given the increasing role of biologics in IBD therapy, the NP should stay abreast with clinical advances. Other immune modulators such as methotrexate and cyclosporine have been used with some success. More recent studies have demonstrated that elimination of inflammation, through the use of either biologics or immune modulators, can lead to deep mucosal healing and result in decreased rates of surgery, hospitalization, and local or systemic corticosteroid use among IBD patients. Therefore, an earlier introduction of these agents in disease management is being advocated. These medications are prescribed in consultation with gastroenterology.

No dietary or lifestyle changes have been shown to prevent IBD, though stress and dietary indiscretions can contribute to IBD flares. Probiotic therapy is an emerging option used to help normalize gut flora and minimize inflammation and IBD flare risk. Because of the difficulty with micronutrient absorption,

TABLE 8-8 Irritable Bowel Syndrome (IBS) Versus Inflammatory Bowel Disease (IBD)

What these have in common: history

Chronically recurring symptoms of abdominal pain, discomfort (urgency and bloating), and alterations in bowel habits

What are their differences?

IBS	IBD (ULCERATIVE COLITIS, CROHN'S DISEASE)
No detectable structural abnormalities	Intestinal ulceration, inflammation
Absence of rectal bleeding, fever, weight loss, elevated CRP, ESR	■ Crohn's: Mouth to anus
	■ UC: Colon only
	Rectal bleeding, diarrhea, fever, weight loss, elevated CRP, ESR, leukocytosis, especially during flares
Intervention	Intervention
■ Lifestyle modification such as diet, fiber, fluids, exercise	■ Aminosalicylates
■ Medications as indicated by symptoms (see Table 8-7)	■ Immune modulators
	■ Biologics (anti-TNF-α and anti-α_4-integrin)
	■ Anti-inflammatory medications (e.g., systemic corticosteroids) as indicated by clinical presentation and response
	■ Surgical intervention often needed and careful ongoing monitoring for gastrointestinal malignancy

CRP, C-reactive protein; ESR, erythrocyte sedimentation rate.

including iron and vitamin B_{12}, with Crohn's disease, parenteral replacement therapy is often preferred over the oral route.

The course of IBD is quite variable. A person with UC has approximately a 50% chance of having a flare in 2 years after achieving disease remission; this number is lower, about 40%, for a person with Crohn's disease. With UC, colorectal cancer risk is greatly increased after about a decade of disease; as a result, surveillance colonoscopy is recommended every 2 years after 8 to 10 years of disease. In contrast, with Crohn's disease, there is an increased risk for small bowel malignancy. At present, no effective screening is available for IBD. Given the complexities in diagnosis and treatment for a person with IBD, expert consultation should be sought. Table 8-8 compares IBS and IBD.

Discussion Sources

Ford AC, Moayyedi P, Lacy BE, et al. American College of Gastroenterology monograph on the management of irritable bowel syndrome and chronic idiopathic constipation. *Am J Gastroenterol.* 2014;109:S2-S26.

Kasper F, Fauci A, Longo D, Mauser S, Jameson JL, Loscalzo, J. *Harrison's Principles of Internal Medicine.* 20th ed. New York, NY: McGraw-Hill Education/Medical; 2018.

Lehrer J, Lichtenstein G. Irritable bowel syndrome. Medscape. http://emedicine.medscape.com/article/180389

Rowe W. Inflammatory bowel disease. Medscape. http://emedicine.medscape.com/article/179037

QUESTIONS

120. In a 28-year-old man who presents with a 6-month history of involuntary weight loss, recurrent abdominal cramping, loose stools, and anterior and posterior anal fissure, which of the following diagnoses should be considered?

    A. UC

    B. Crohn's disease

    C. *C difficile* colitis

    D. condyloma acuminata

121 to 124. Which of the following patient complaints should be evaluated further when making the differential diagnosis of IBS? (Yes or No)

_____ **121.** A 52-year-old female with a first-degree family history of colorectal cancer, recent constipation, and abdominal pain

_____ **122.** A 45-year-old man with low albumin and leukocytosis

_____ **123.** A 22-year-old with complaints of flatulence and abdominal pain that are usually relieved with defecation

_____ **124.** A 16-year-old female with chronic, alternating constipation and diarrhea when she is studying for high school exams and worrying about her parents' impending divorce

125. The pathophysiology of IBS can be best described as:

A. sharing the same pathophysiology as IBD.

B. a patchy inflammatory process in the small bowel that most adolescents will outgrow with vigorous exercise and a low-residue diet.

C. a condition that is the result of abnormal gut motor/sensory activity.

D. an overstimulation of pancreatic β-cell production.

126. Diagnostic criteria for IBS include abdominal pain that is associated with all of the following except:

A. improvement with defecation.

B. a change in frequency of stool.

C. a change of stool form.

D. unexplained weight loss.

127. When considering an IBS diagnosis, the NP should be aware that:

A. diagnosis is largely based on clinical presentation and application of the Rome IV criteria.

B. a colonoscopy should be done routinely when the diagnosis is suspected.

C. complete blood count (CBC), ESR, CRP, and serum albumin should be the initial laboratory tests for an IBS workup.

D. once an IBS diagnosis has been confirmed, you can assure the patient that treatment is generally curative.

128. Which of the following oral medications is approved for the treatment of diarrhea-predominant IBS?

A. vancomycin (Vancocin®)

B. linaclotide (Linzess®)

C. bismuth subsalicylate (Pepto-Bismol™)

D. eluxadoline (Viberzi®)

129. Tenesmus is defined as which of the following?

A. rectal burning with defecation

B. a sensation of incomplete bowel emptying that is distressing and sometimes painful

C. weight loss that accompanies many bowel diseases

D. appearance of frank blood in the stool

130. Concerning IBS, which of the following statements is most accurate?

A. Patients most often report chronic diarrhea as the most distressing part of the problem.

B. Weight gain is often reported.

C. Patients can present with bowel issues ranging from diarrhea to constipation.

D. The condition is associated with a strongly increased risk of colorectal cancer.

131. An example of a medication with prokinetic activity is:

  A. dicyclomine (Bentyl®).

  B. metoclopramide (Reglan®).

  C. loperamide (Imodium®).

  D. psyllium (Metamucil®).

132. Diagnostic testing in IBS often reveals:

  A. evidence of underlying inflammation.

  B. anemia of chronic disease.

  C. normal results on most testing.

  D. mucosal thickening on abdominal radiological imaging.

133 to 137. Which of the following can be helpful in the management of IBS? (Yes or No)

_____ **133.** Moderate protein, low-residue diet

_____ **134.** Fiber supplementation

_____ **135.** Stress modification and regular aerobic exercise

_____ **136.** Antispasmodics and loperamide for diarrhea predominance

_____ **137.** Tricyclic antidepressants for constipation predominance

138. Which of the following is the best candidate for the use of lubiprostone (Amitiza®)?

  A. a 32-year-old man with diarrhea-predominant IBS

  B. a 45-year-old woman with newly diagnosed IBD

  C. a 22-year-old woman with constipation-predominant IBS

  D. a 52-year-old man with an acute flare of IBD

139. IBS is characterized by all of the following except:

  A. weight loss and malnutrition.

  B. abdominal pain at least one time per week for a 3-month period.

  C. altered bowel pattern in the absence of detected structural abnormalities.

  D. occurs two to three times more often in women than men.

140. Diagnostic testing in IBD often reveals:

  A. evidence of underlying inflammation.

  B. notation of intestinal parasites.

  C. normal results on most testing.

  D. a characteristic intra-abdominal mass on radiological imaging.

141. Laboratory evaluation during an IBD flare will reveal elevated levels of all of the following except:

  A. CRP.

  B. serum Cr.

  C. ESR.

  D. WBC.

142. IBD is associated with all of the following types of anemia except:

  A. anemia of chronic disease.

  B. iron-deficiency anemia.

  C. megaloblastic anemia.

  D. hemolytic anemia.

143. IBD is a term usually used to describe:

    A. UC and IBS.

    B. *C difficile* colitis and Crohn's disease.

    C. Crohn's disease and UC.

    D. inflammatory colitis and ileitis.

144. "Skip lesions" are usually reported during colonoscopy in:

    A. IBS.

    B. UC.

    C. Crohn's disease.

    D. *C difficile* colitis.

145. Deep mucosal healing can be achieved in patients with IBD with the use of:

    A. oral aminosalicylates.

    B. parenteral corticosteroids.

    C. antibiotics.

    D. immune modulators.

146. After a decade of disease, a person with UC is at increased risk of malignancy involving which of the following sites? Choose all that apply.

    A. small bowel

    B. large intestine

    C. duodenum

    D. stomach

147. Crohn's disease is associated with increased risk of malignancy involving which of the following sites? Choose all that apply.

    A. small bowel

    B. large intestine

    C. duodenum

    D. stomach

148 to 158. Which of the following statements is most consistent with IBD, with IBS, or with both conditions?

_____ **148.** Onset of symptoms is before age 30 to 40 years in most cases.

_____ **149.** The patient population is predominately female.

_____ **150.** The condition is often referred to as spastic colon by the general population.

_____ **151.** Extraintestinal manifestations occasionally include nondestructive arthritis and renal calculi.

_____ **152.** This is a potentially life-threatening condition.

_____ **153.** The etiology likely involves an autoimmune response to the GI tract.

_____ **154.** Patients should be advised to avoid trigger foods.

_____ **155.** Involvement can be limited to intestinal mucosa only, or the full thickness of the intestinal wall can be involved.

_____ **156.** The etiology is considered to be an alteration in small and large bowel motility.

_____ **157.** Potential complications include fistula formation and perineal disease.

_____ **158.** Potential complications include increased risk for colonic malignancy.

For answers and rationales, see end of chapter.

Celiac Disease

Overview

Celiac disease (also called sprue, celiac sprue, and gluten enteropathy) is a chronic disorder caused by an immunological response to gluten, a storage protein found in certain grains that results in diffuse damage to the proximal small intestinal mucosa with malabsorption of nutrients. Although symptoms can manifest between 6 months and 24 months of age after the introduction of solid foods, the majority of cases of celiac disease present in childhood or adulthood. Population screening with serological testing suggests that the disease is present in 1:100 whites of northern European ancestry.

Although the precise pathogenesis is unclear, celiac disease arises in a small subset of genetically susceptible (HLA-DQ2 or HLA-DQ8) individuals when dietary gluten stimulates an inappropriate immunological response. Glutens are partially digested in the intestinal lumen into glutamine-rich peptides. Some of the glutamines are deamidated by the enzyme tTG, generating negatively charged glutamic acid residues. If these peptides are able to bind to HLA-DQ2 or HLA-DQ8 molecules on antigen-presenting cells, they may stimulate an inappropriate T cell–mediated activation in the intestinal submucosa that results in destruction of mucosal enterocytes as well as a humoral immune response that results in antibodies to gluten, tTG, and other autoantigens.

Clinical Presentation

Celiac disease's clinical presentation in adults is often confused with other diseases because of overlapping signs and symptoms. Symptoms of celiac disease are typically present for at least 10 years before a correct diagnosis is made and often depend on the patient's age and extent of small bowel disease. Other conditions that can be considered in a patient with suspected celiac disease include Crohn's disease, IBS, hypothyroidism, malabsorption syndrome, jejunoileitis, and bacterial overgrowth syndrome.

> **CLINICAL CONCEPT**
> Many patients with celiac disease who have chronic diarrhea and flatulence are misdiagnosed as having IBS.

Celiac sprue must be distinguished from other causes of malabsorption. Severe pan-malabsorption of multiple nutrients almost always implies mucosal disease.

Other causes such as tropical sprue, bacterial overgrowth, cow's milk intolerance, viral gastroenteritis, eosinophilic gastroenteritis, and acid hypersecretion from gastrinoma need to be ruled out.

Treatment

Celiac disease treatment is focused on a number of factors, including the following:

■ A gluten-free diet is essential (all wheat, rye, and barley must be eliminated). Examples of food that do not contain gluten are rice, corn, millet, potato, buckwheat, and soybeans. Refer to a knowledgeable dietician/nutritionist and encourage a lay support group.

■ Avoid dairy products temporarily or permanently if necessary until intestinal symptoms resolve. Dairy products should be reintroduced slowly, gauging symptom response.

■ Dietary supplements should provide micronutrient repletion until intestinal symptoms have resolved (folate, iron, calcium, and vitamins A, B_{12}, D, and E). Vitamin and mineral levels should be checked periodically to prevent deficiencies.

Discussion Sources

Celiac Disease Foundation. https://celiac.org.

Katz KD, Rashtak S, Lahr BD, et al. Screening for celiac disease in a North American population: sequential serology and gastrointestinal symptoms. *Am J Gastroenterol.* 2011;106(7):1333–1339.

Papdakis MA, McPhee SJ, Rabow MW. *Current Medical Diagnosis and Treatment 2019.* 58th ed. New York, NY: McGraw-Hill Medical; 2019.

Rubio-Tapia A, Hill ID, Kelly CP, et al. Diagnosis and management of celiac disease. *Am J Gastroenterol.* 2013;108:656–76. https://gi.org/guideline/diagnosis-and-management-of-celiac-disease/

QUESTIONS

159. Celiac disease is also called all of the following except:

A. gluten-induced enteropathy.

B. celiac sprue.

    C. sprue.

    D. small bowel malabsorption syndrome.

160. All of the following characterize celiac disease except that:

    A. it is a temporary immunological gluten disorder.

    B. it affects more often people of northern European ancestry.

    C. it causes diffuse damage to the proximal small intestinal mucosa with malabsorption of nutrients.

    D. it is often misdiagnosed as IBD.

161. Celiac disease's classic presentation can include which of the following? Choose all that apply.

    A. weight loss, chronic diarrhea, and muscle wasting

    B. flatulence and abdominal distension

    C. as growth restriction when diagnosed in children younger than 2 years old

    D. reported egg intolerance

162. The most accurate laboratory markers to diagnose celiac sprue are:

    A. ESR and CRP.

    B. IgA endomysial and IgA tTG antibodies.

    C. mucosal biopsies of the terminal ileum.

    D. *H pylori* IgG antibodies.

163. Patients with celiac disease present with similar signs and symptoms of all of the following conditions except:

    A. acute appendicitis.

    B. small bowel bacterial overgrowth.

    C. cow's milk intolerance.

    D. tropical sprue.

164. Which of the following would be an acceptable food choice, using standard products, for a person with celiac disease?

    A. beer and popcorn

    B. vegetarian pizza and grape juice

    C. steak with mashed potatoes

    D. chicken nuggets and green salad (no dressing)

165. An 8-year-old girl is diagnosed with celiac disease. When counseling her parents, you advise that the child should:

    A. consume whole grains, especially wheat, oats, and barley.

    B. carefully plan exercise to minimize symptoms.

    C. avoid intake of semolina, spelt, and rye.

    D. avoid birthday parties or other gatherings that could expose the child to offending foods.

For answers and rationales, see end of chapter.

Pancreatitis, Pancreatic Pseudocysts, and Pancreatic Cancer

PANCREATITIS

Overview

Pancreatitis, characterized by an acute or chronic inflammation of the organ, is a potentially life-threatening condition, characterized by autodigestion of pancreatic and peripancreatic tissues. This destruction occurs when pancreatic cells are damaged, releasing naturally occurring digestive enzymes including trypsin, amylase, and lipase.

Although alcohol abuse is commonly thought of as being one of the most common contributing factors for the disease, a small percentage of people who are problem drinkers develop the condition; likely the etiology of pancreatitis is multifactorial. Most alcohol-related cases of acute pancreatitis occur in people with a minimum of 5 to 7 years of heavy ethanol ingestion, with binge drinkers having much lower risk. Less common risk factors are use of opioids, use of select medications including systemic corticosteroids and the thiazide diuretics, viral infection, and blunt abdominal trauma.

Clinical Presentation

Guidelines from the American College of Gastroenterology state that at least two of the following three criteria should be present to diagnose acute pancreatitis: (1) characteristic (severe) abdominal pain, (2) serum amylase and/or lipase exceeding three times the upper limit of normal, and/or (3) characteristic abdominal imaging findings (see later).

The overall patient presentation in pancreatitis is a person who appears acutely ill. The pain that is characteristic with pancreatitis is typically described as a band-like pattern across the abdomen that bores through to the back. Nausea, vomiting, and anorexia often accompany the pain as does fever, dehydration, and diaphoresis. Physical examination usually reveals hypoactive bowel sounds and abdominal distention with epigastric tenderness with or without rebound. There is typically a history of significant alcohol ingestion and/or a heavy meal immediately preceding the attack. In addition, when the disease involves the head of the pancreas, jaundice is often present, but usually without localized right upper quadrant abdominal tenderness seen in hepatic and biliary disorders such as cholecystitis and acute hepatitis.

Rarely, two characteristic but ominous signs, associated with elevated mortality rates, are present in acute pancreatitis. Grey-Turner sign is present, revealed as ecchymosis around the flanks. Cullen's sign (Fig. 8-3) is characterized by periumbilical ecchymosis with superficial edema, usually found in pancreatic necrosis with intra-abdominal bleeding. Either sign is indicative of retroperitoneal or abdominal hemorrhage from the liberation of pancreatic enzymes and often signals pancreatic necrosis.

Diagnostic Testing

Abdominal CT scan usually provides a diagnostic view of the inflamed pancreas. Abdominal ultrasound can assist in diagnosing contributing gallbladder disease in acute pancreatitis; this study does not typically help with diagnosing acute or chronic pancreatitis because of limited views of the organ.

In a patient with acute pancreatitis, serum amylase level is typically elevated; however, this is also indicated in other conditions, such as perforated duodenal ulcer and other surgical abdominal emergencies. Because elevated amylase level is often found in many other conditions aside from acute pancreatitis, concurrently measuring serum lipase level increases diagnostic specificity (Table 8-9). If amylase and lipase levels are initially three times the upper limit of normal and gut perforation and infarction have been ruled out, these laboratory values clinch the diagnosis of pancreatitis. With expert consultation, additional studies are occasionally obtained if the diagnosis is unclear.

Treatment

Treatment of the underlying cause of pancreatitis, such as gallbladder disease or hypertriglyceridemia, or discontinuation of the causative agent, such as alcohol, corticosteroids, or thiazide diuretics, is the first-line therapy. Significant pain and volume constriction are common in patients with acute pancreatitis. Intervention includes parenteral hydration, analgesia, and gut rest. While patients with pancreatitis often present to primary care or other outpatient practices, often inpatient admission is needed. At the same time, the clinical course can range from a self-limiting condition to life-threatening illness. The Ranson criteria (Table 8-10) are usually used in assessing severity of pancreatitis. With a Ranson score of 3 to 5, there is a 10% to 20% mortality rate, and the patient should be admitted to the intensive care unit (ICU). With a score greater than 5, the mortality rate is more than 50%, and more systemic complications are likely.

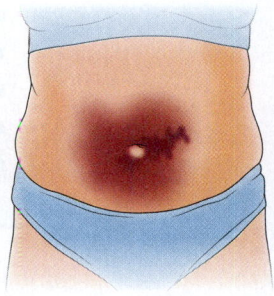

FIGURE 8-3 Cullen's sign.
Thompson J. Essential Health Assessment. Philadelphia, PA: F.A. Davis; 2017.

TABLE 8-9 Lipase and Amylase Evaluation in Acute Pancreatitis

AMYLASE

In pancreatitis

- Appears 2 to 12 hours after symptom onset
- Back to normal within 7 days of pancreatitis resolution

Amylase level greater than 1,000 U/L

- Seen in cholelithiasis as well as alcoholic pancreatitis diagnosis

Nonpancreatic amylase sources

- Salivary glands
- Ovarian cysts
- Ovarian tumors
- Tubo-ovarian abscess
- Ruptured ectopic pregnancy
- Lung cancer

LIPASE

In pancreatitis

- Appears 4 to 8 hours after symptom onset
- Peaks at 24 hours, decreases 8 to 14 days after pancreatitis resolution

Nonpancreatic reasons for elevated lipase

- Renal failure
- Perforated duodenal ulcer
- Bowel obstruction
- Bowel infarction

TABLE 8-10 Ranson Criteria of Severity of Acute Pancreatitis

AT TIME OF PATIENT PRESENTATION	DEVELOPMENT OF THE FOLLOWING WITHIN FIRST 48 HOURS INDICATIVE OF WORSENING PROGNOSIS
Age older than 55 years	Hematocrit decrease greater than 10%
WBC greater than 16,000/mm^3	Arterial P_{O_2} less than 60 mm Hg
Blood glucose greater than 200 mg/dL (greater than 11.1 mol/L)	Serum Ca^{++} less than 8 mg/dL
AST greater than 250 U/L	Base deficit greater than 4 mEq/L
LDH greater than 350 IU/L	Estimate fluid sequestration of greater than 6 L
	BUN increase greater than 8 mg/dL over admission value

NUMBER OF CRITERIA	MORTALITY RATE PER RANSON CRITERIA
0 to 2	1%
3 to 4	15%
5 to 6	40%
Greater than 6	100%

AST, aspartate aminotransferase; BUN, blood urea nitrogen; LDH, lactate dehydrogenase; WBC, white blood cell count.

Sources: Ranson JH, Rifkind KM, Roses DF, Fink SD, Eng K, Spencer FC. Prognostic signs and the role of operative management in acute pancreatitis. Surg Gynecol Obstet. 1974;139(1):69–81; Carroll JK, Herrick B, Gipson T, Lee SP. Acute pancreatitis: diagnosis, prognosis, and treatment. Am Fam Physician. 2007;75:1513–1520.

PANCREATIC PSEUDOCYSTS

Overview

Pancreatic pseudocysts consist of benign pockets of fluid lined with scar or inflammatory tissue. A pancreatic pseudocyst is most often a consequence of and occurs after an episode of pancreatitis, usually occurring several weeks after the acute illness. A high index of suspicion for the development of this condition should be maintained, particularly in the patient with recurrent or chronic pancreatitis.

Clinical Presentation

Though pseudocysts are most often asymptomatic, signs and symptoms can include persistent abdominal pain that radiates to the back, nausea, vomiting, as well as a palpable upper abdominal mass. A ruptured pseudocyst can be life-threatening as fluid released can damage nearby blood vessels and cause massive bleeding. In addition, infection can occur in the abdominal cavity.

Diagnostic Testing

Often, pancreatic pseudocysts are identified during abdominal scans for other health issues. CT can allow a determination of the wall thickness of the pseudocyst, which can help guide the therapeutic strategy. CT with contrast can provide greater detail, allowing a determination of any pancreatitis that might be present. MRI offers improved contrast compared to CT scans and can be used to better characterize fluid collections as well as any debris within the pseudocysts. Though MRI and CT scans can help differentiate a pseudocyst from cancer, additional testing is sometimes needed to arrive at a conclusive diagnosis. Fluid collected from the pseudocyst can be used to test for evidence of malignancy. Serological testing can also be used to differentiate pancreatic cancer from pseudocyst.

In pancreatic malignancy, levels of carcinoembryonic antigen (CEA) and carcinoembryonic antigen-125 (CEA-125) are elevated. Given that with pseudocyst, there is often no pancreatic inflammation or hepatic involvement, amylase, lipase, and liver enzymes are usually within normal limits. In cases of moderate-to-severe pancreatitis that included peripancreatic fluid collection, follow-up should include imaging to check for the presence of a pseudocyst.

> **CLINICAL CONCEPT**
>
> Abdominal CT scan is the preferred method to visualize pancreatic pseudocysts, with a sensitivity of 90% to 100%.

Treatment

The main goal of pancreatic pseudocyst treatment is to avoid complications, including infection and rupture that can lead to internal hemorrhage. The size of the cyst is a poor predictor of complications, and whether treatment is needed should depend on the presence of symptoms, risk for complications, and concern about possible malignancy. The management decision is typically made with consultation from a gastroenterologist, surgeon, and radiologist. Most pseudocysts resolve over time without any intervention beyond supportive care. A pseudocyst that is causing bothersome symptoms or growing larger must be drained. This is usually performed via endoscopic ultrasound-guided fine needle aspiration or placement of an endoscopically guided stent. Surgery is sometimes needed to remove an enlarged pseudocyst.

PANCREATIC CANCER

Overview

Risk factors for pancreatic cancer include a history of chronic pancreatitis, tobacco use, and diabetes mellitus (DM). About 5% of the time, a genetic factor contributes to the disease. About 40% of cases occur sporadically with no identifiable risk factors. Pancreatic cancer has high mortality rates because clinical presentation usually occurs with late disease with metastatic spread.

Clinical Presentation

Early pancreatic cancer signs and symptoms are nonspecific and include anorexia, nausea, fatigue, and epigastric or midback pain. In later disease, pancreatic cancer presentation usually includes significant unintended weight loss, worsening abdominal pain, especially at night, and painless jaundice. Other findings include thrombophlebitis or diffuse lymphadenopathy. A less common but significant finding is St. Mary Joseph's nodule, a palpable umbilical nodule, often with a vascular appearance, that is noted in an advanced intra-abdominal or pelvic cancer, including pancreatic, ovarian, or colonic cancer.

Diagnostic Testing

Abdominal CT scan is helpful in identifying pancreatic cancer, though other imaging techniques are often used, including endoscopic ultrasonography, MRI, and positron emission tomography (PET). The usefulness of abdominal ultrasound is limited by the presence of intestinal gas. Normochromic, normocytic anemia is a common finding, as is elevated total and direct bilirubin and alkaline phosphatase. An elevation in amylase is an uncommon finding in pancreatic cancer, unless concomitant pancreatitis is present.

CLINICAL CONCEPT

Unfortunately, given usual later stage presentation, pancreatic cancer continues to rank in the top five causes of cancer death in adults.

Treatment

Once detected, or suspected, further evaluation and treatment of pancreatic cancer require expert consultation. Prognosis is typically based on cancer staging and comorbidity.

Discussion Sources

Crockett SD, Wani S, Gardner TB, et al. American Gastroenterological Association Institute guideline on initial management of acute pancreatitis. *Gastroenterology*. 2018;154;1096–1101.

Dragovich T. Pancreatic cancer. Medscape. https://emedicine.medscape.com/article/280605

Gardner TB, Berk BS. Acute pancreatitis. Medscape. http://emedicine.medscape.com/article/181364-overview

Papadakis MA, McPhee SJ, Rabow MW. *Current Medical Diagnosis and Treatment 2019*. 58th ed. New York, NY: McGraw-Hill Medical; 2019.

Sawyer MAJ. Pancreatic pseudocyst imaging. Medscape. https://emedicine.medscape.com/article/373117-overview#a1

QUESTIONS

166. Risk factors for acute pancreatitis include all of the following except:

A. hypothyroidism.

B. dyslipidemia.

C. abdominal trauma.

D. thiazide diuretic use.

167. Ms. Lane, a 38-year-old woman with a long-standing history of alcohol abuse, presents with a 4-day history of a midabdominal ache that radiates through to the back, remains relatively constant, and has been accompanied by nausea and three episodes of vomiting. Her last vomiting episode was 15 minutes ago. She has tried taking antacids without relief. Her skin is cool and moist with a blood pressure of 90/72 mm Hg, pulse rate of 120 bpm, and respiratory rate of 24/min. Findings that would support a diagnosis of acute pancreatitis include all of the following except:

A. elevated serum amylase level.

B. elevated lipase level.

C. jaundice.

D. upper abdominal tenderness without localization or rebound.

168. Your next best action in caring for Ms. Lane in the previous question is to:

A. refer to the acute care hospital for admission.

B. attempt office hydration after administration of an analgesic agent.

C. initiate therapy with ranitidine (Zantac®) and an antacid.

D. obtain serum electrolyte levels.

169 to 172. Indicate whether each of the following conditions will lead to elevated levels of amylase, lipase, both, or neither.

_____ **169.** Lung cancer

_____ **170.** Renal failure

_____ **171.** Ovarian cyst

_____ **172.** Obesity

173. Which of the following statements is true when evaluating a patient with acute pancreatitis?

A. Diagnosis can be made by clinical assessment alone.

B. The pancreas can be clearly visualized by abdominal ultrasound.

C. Measuring serum lipase level along with amylase level increases diagnostic specificity in acute pancreatitis.

D. Hypocalcemia is a nearly universal finding.

174. When using the Ranson criteria to evaluate the severity of acute pancreatitis, what score would warrant consideration for ICU admission?

   A. less than 2

   B. 3 or greater

   C. 6 or greater

   D. 8 or greater

175. Common signs and symptoms of a pancreatic pseudocyst include all of the following except:

   A. abdominal pain that radiates to the back.

   B. nausea and vomiting.

   C. jaundice.

   D. a mass that can be palpated in the upper abdomen.

176. Which of the following diagnostic tests is most effective in determining whether a pancreatic pseudocyst is benign?

   A. CT scan

   B. MRI scan

   C. analysis of cyst fluid

   D. serum amylase and lipase levels

177. A 56-year-old man with a history of acute pancreatitis undergoes a follow-up abdominal MRI scan. A small mass is identified on the pancreas that is later diagnosed as a benign pseudocyst. The pseudocyst is not causing any symptoms and measures 8 mm in diameter. You consider:

   A. monitoring the pseudocyst for any change in size or resolution.

   B. draining the pseudocyst.

   C. surgical removal of the pseudocyst.

   D. initiating a regimen of anti-inflammatory medication to decrease the size of the pseudocyst.

178. Risk factors for pancreatic cancer include all of the following except:

   A. hypertension.

   B. history of chronic pancreatitis.

   C. tobacco use.

   D. diabetes mellitus.

179 to 185. Indicate (Yes or No) whether each of the following would be an anticipated finding in a patient with suspected pancreatic cancer.

_____ **179.** Involuntary weight loss

_____ **180.** Painless jaundice

_____ **181.** Presence of Cullen's sign

_____ **182.** Positive obturator and psoas signs

_____ **183.** Normochromic, normocytic anemia

_____ **184.** Hematuria

_____ **185.** Midepigastric pain that radiates to the midback or lower back region

186. All of the following laboratory findings are expected in a patient with pancreatic cancer except:

   A. elevated total bilirubin.

   B. diminished platelet count.

   C. elevated alkaline phosphatase.

   D. elevated direct bilirubin.

187. Which of the following imaging techniques would be least helpful in the diagnosis of pancreatic cancer?

    A. abdominal ultrasound

    B. abdominal CT

    C. endoscopic ultrasound

    D. MRI

For answers and rationales, see end of chapter.

Ionizing Radiation

The use of radiography can be an essential tool in clinical evaluation and diagnosis. However, rapid growth in the use of these procedures, such as CT scans, has led to concern about low-dose ionizing radiation doses.

> **CLINICAL CONCEPT**
>
> The primary concern with high-level radiation exposure is an increased risk for developing a malignancy.

Other adverse effects of exposure to low-dose ionizing radiation have also been suspected, such as an increased risk for the development of cataracts following repeated head CT scans that include the lens of the eye. Appropriate use of these techniques requires understanding the balance of long-term risks inherent with radiation exposure with the necessity of utilizing these imaging studies.

The amount of radiation exposure can vary significantly depending on the type of imaging study being conducted. It is important to remember that we are all exposed to radiation on a daily basis, mainly from the sun and soil. The entire body is exposed to this background radiation, compared with only certain parts of the body when conducting medical imaging studies. A comparison of the radiation doses from various types of imaging studies is shown in Table 8-1.

Minimizing exposure to radiation depends on sound methodology and quality control. Using the lowest possible dose should be desired, with consideration of first using nonionizing radiation examinations, such as MRI or ultrasound, if possible. Repeated radiological examinations, where the same test is completed more than once but results not communicated or shared, should be avoided.

Discussion Source

Coakley F, Gould R, Yeh B, Arenson R. CT radiation dose: what can you do right now in your practice? *AJR.* 2011;196:619–625. https://www.ajronline.org/content/196/3/619.full.pdf+html

QUESTIONS

188 to 191. Match the imaging study with the equivalent amount of background radiation. *(An answer can be used more than once.)*

_____ 188. Abdominal CT scan

_____ 189. Abdominal MRI

_____ 190. Abdominal ultrasound

_____ 191. Abdominal x-ray

    A. no radiation

    B. 62 to 88 days

    C. 3 years

For answers and rationales, see end of chapter.

QUESTION ANSWERS AND RATIONALES

Anal Fissure

1. Correct: A. posterior midline of the anus.
The most common site of anal fissure is posterior midline of the anus (A).

Incorrect:
Fissures occurring anterior midline of the anus (B) are less frequent than posterior. About 2% of patients have both posterior and anterior fissures (C). Fissures

occurring off the midline (D) should raise suspicion of another diagnosis, such as Crohn's disease, cancer, or infection.

2. **Answer: A. drops of blood noticed when wiping.**
Bleeding associated with anal fissures is best described as drops of blood noted when wiping (A) and not protracted bleeding.
Incorrect:
Significant amounts of blood clots and mucus in stool (D) can be associated with more serious GI conditions, such as cancer or Crohn's disease. Dark stools (melena) are typically attributed to digested blood originating from an upper GI bleeding event. Report of persistent bleeding (C) or dark brown to black in color mixed with stool (B) warrants further investigation by colonoscopy to possibly identify colorectal cancer or another diagnosis.

3. **Correct: C. intra-anal corticosteroids.**
The use of intra-anal, vasodilating ointments, such as nitroglycerin or nifedipine, can help to increase blood flow, reduce pain, and hasten healing of anal fissures. However, intra-anal corticosteroids (C) are not indicated for this condition.
Incorrect:
A primary management strategy to prevent and treat anal fissures is to prevent constipation and prevent the cycle that contributes to this condition. Treatments can include stool-bulking agents (A), osmotic laxatives and stool softeners, a high-fiber diet (B), and the occasional use of oral mineral oil (D).

4. **Correct: D. rubber band ligation of the lesion.**
Rubber band ligation is typically used as a management option for internal or external hemorrhoids when conservative treatment is inadequate. This is not a technique to manage anal fissures.
Incorrect:
Second-line treatment of anal fissures can include intra-anal administration of nitroglycerin (A) or nifedipine to increase blood flow, relieve pain, and improve the healing process. A botulinum toxin (B) injection can be considered to alleviate spasm that can contribute to anal fissure pain. For refractory cases, surgical management via sphincterotomy can be used (C).

5 to 8. Yes or No

5. **Correct: Yes**

6. **Correct: Yes**

7. **Correct: Yes**

8. **Correct: No**
Anal fissure is most commonly noted with a fissure on the posterior midline of the anus. An atypical anal lesion can be due to a number of other conditions including condyloma acuminata (i.e., genital warts via HPV infection), Crohn's disease, or anal squamous cell carcinoma. *C difficile* colitis is not typically associated with anal lesions and would present with other notable symptoms, including severe abdominal pain and/or cramping and frequent watery bowel movements.

9. **Correct: C. "I have anal pain for up to 1 to 2 hours after I have a bowel movement."**
Correct:
The most common complaint of anal fissure is severe anal pain during a bowel movement that can last minutes to hours afterward and recurs with each bowel movement (C).
Incorrect:
The report of anal pain that is relieved following a bowel movement is most likely due to IBS (A). The feeling on an incomplete evacuation of bowels (B) is typically associated with constipation, which is a major risk factor for anal fissure. Reports of constant itch in the anal region can be caused by hemorrhoids, infection, or skin irritation due to a number of causes (e.g., poor hygiene, aggressive wiping, psoriasis) (D).

10. **Correct: B. vitamin A.**
Chronic use of mineral oil will diminish the absorption of fat-soluble vitamins, such as vitamin A (B), D, E, and K.
Incorrect:
Mineral oil can hinder the absorption of fat-soluble vitamins. Its use will have less of an impact on the absorption of water-soluble vitamins and minerals, such as iron (A), vitamin C (C), and vitamin B_{12} (D).

Hemorrhoids

11. **Correct: A. streaks of bright red blood on the stool.**
Bleeding associated with hemorrhoids are best described as streaks of bright red blood on the stool (A) and not protracted bleeding.
Incorrect:
Significant amounts of blood clots and mucus in stools (D) can be associated with more serious GI conditions, such as cancer or Crohn's disease. Dark stools are typically attributed to digested blood originating from an upper GI bleeding event. Reports of persistent bleeding (C) or dark brown to black in color mixed with stool (B) warrants further investigation by colonoscopy to possibly identify colorectal cancer or another diagnosis.

12. **Correct: B. low-fat diet.**
Certain lifestyle changes can help prevent hemorrhoidal engorgement and inflammation and include weight control, high-fiber diet, regular aerobic exercise, and adequate fluid intake. A low-fat diet (B) is not necessarily a treatment for hemorrhoids, though this could be part of a weight control plan.
Incorrect:
Prevention and treatment of hemorrhoids can include lifestyle changes, such as weight control (A) and increased physical activity. Topical corticosteroids (C) can help reduce inflammation, though prolonged use is not recommended due to atrophic effects on the skin, particularly with higher-potency agents. Measures to reduce constipation, such as high-fiber diets and stool softeners (D), can help prevent hemorrhoidal engorgement.

13. Correct: B. 1 cup of cooked oatmeal

The average adult should strive to consume 20 to 30 grams of fiber per day, preferably through consuming high-fiber foods. High-fiber foods can include dry beans, peas, and oat products, such as oatmeal (B).

Incorrect:

It is important to note that most, but not all, whole fruits and vegetables are high in fiber. Oatmeal is a high-fiber food, and 1 cup would provide the greatest amount of fiber compared to a small banana (A), a half-cup of brown rice (C), or a small blueberry muffin (D).

14. Correct: C. refer to gastroenterology practice for colonoscopy.

The presence of a microcytic hypochromic anemia is indicative of iron-deficiency anemia, likely resulting from chronic low-volume GI blood loss. This is consistent with dark brown stool suggesting digested blood from an upper GI bleed. The most appropriate course of action is referral for colonoscopy to rule out colorectal cancer or other GI condition beyond hemorrhoids.

Incorrect:

The findings are consistent with an upper GI bleed that requires further evaluation via colonoscopy to rule out colorectal cancer. The use of anoscopy (A) and sitz baths (B) can be helpful in the evaluation and management of the patient's hemorrhoids, but these will not address the potentially more serious condition in the GI tract. Colonoscopy is the preferred method to screen and diagnose colorectal cancer, though double-contrast barium enema (D) can be considered for those who cannot undergo a colonoscopy.

15. Correct: B. insertive partner in anal intercourse.

Though the cause of hemorrhoids can be uncertain for many cases, several risk factors have been identified for the development of hemorrhoids, including being a receptive partner in anal intercourse. However, being the insertive partner (B) in anal intercourse is not a risk factor.

Incorrect:

Risk factors for the development of hemorrhoids include excessive alcohol use (D), chronic diarrhea (C) or constipation, obesity, high-fat/low-fiber diet, and prolonged sitting (A).

16. Correct: C. The hemorrhoids prolapse upon defecation and must be reduced manually.

A grade III classification best describes hemorrhoids that prolapse upon defecation and must be reduced manually (C).

Incorrect:

Grade I hemorrhoids do not prolapse (A), while grade II hemorrhoids prolapse upon defecation but reduce spontaneously (B). A grade IV hemorrhoid is prolapsed and cannot be reduced manually (D).

17. Correct: C. a 44-year-old woman who has internal and external hemorrhoids with recurrent prolapse

Surgical intervention should be considered when conservative approaches are unsuccessful in managing hemorrhoids. Recurrent external hemorrhoids described in the 44-year-old woman (C) can cause sudden-onset severe pain that can require emergency care. Surgical interventions can include rubber band ligation or surgical hemorrhoidectomy.

Incorrect:

Surgical interventions should not be considered when conservative treatments provide adequate relief, such as the 48-year-old man with grade II internal hemorrhoids (B) and the 58-year-old man with grade I internal hemorrhoids (D). For the 28-year-old woman following childbirth (A), her hemorrhoids should resolve with conservative treatments, such as sitz baths, astringents, or topical corticosteroid treatment.

Acute Appendicitis

18. Correct: D. marked febrile response.

Though there is no true classic presentation for acute appendicitis, certain signs and physical findings can occur frequently to aid in its diagnosis. However, the presence of fever (D) is not a frequent or reliable indication for this condition. Fever can be pronounced, however, during appendiceal rupture.

Incorrect:

The most common findings in acute appendicitis include a history of anorexia and periumbilical or epigastric pain (A) followed by nausea, right lower quadrant (RLQ) pain, and vomiting, occurring in 50% of cases. RLQ tenderness is present in approximately 96% of cases. Other common findings include rebound tenderness (C), Rovsing's sign, obturator sign (B), psoas sign, and pain on percussion.

19. Correct: C. total WBCs, 16,500/mm³; neutrophils, 66%; bands, 8%; lymphocytes, 22%.

A "left shift" in the WBC pattern is typically seen in acute appendicitis associated with severe bacterial infection. This is associated with an increase in total WBCs, elevation in neutrophils, and elevation in bands (bandemia) (C).

Incorrect:

In the case of mild leukopenia (total WBCs, 4,500/mm³; neutrophils, 35%; bands, 2%; lymphocytes, 45% [A]), this is not likely reflective of a bacterial infection but possibly a viral infection. Elevated WBCs and relatively normal WBC differentials (B, D) are often seen in acute pain or other physiological stressor as well as a response to exercise or environmental extremes such as hot or cold weather.

20. Correct: A. the presentation can differ according to the anatomical location of the appendix.

Making an appendicitis diagnosis can be challenging as there is no true classic presentation for this condition. Additionally, presentation can differ significantly depending on the anatomical position of the appendix (A), which can cause pain in the epigastrium, flank, or groin region.

Incorrect:

Acute appendicitis is uncommon in the elderly and can be associated with a less than typical presentation and can include signs and symptoms beyond acute abdominal pain (B). The signs can be similar to PID and are included in the differential diagnosis (D). Nausea and vomiting are typically late symptoms and occur hours after the onset of pain (C).

21. **Correct: A. passive extension of the hip.**

Psoas sign (A) is elicited by having the patient lie on his or her left side while the hip is extended. Pain can indicate inflammation of the psoas muscle as well as peritoneal irritation.

Incorrect:

Pain with flexion and internal rotation of the hip is the obturator sign (B). Rebound tenderness is abdominal pain that worsens with release of deep palpation (C). Asking the patient to cough (D) is not part of an evaluation of the patient with suspected acute appendicitis.

22. **Correct: B. passive flexion and internal rotation of the hip.**

Pain with flexion and internal rotation of the hip is the obturator sign (B). Pain can indicate inflammation of the obturator muscle as well as peritoneal irritation.

Incorrect:

Psoas sign is elicited by having the patient lie on his or her left side while the hip is extended (A). Rebound tenderness is abdominal pain that worsens with release of deep palpation (C). Asking the patient to cough (D) is not part of an evaluation of the patient with suspected acute appendicitis.

23. **Correct: B. CT scan.**

CT scan (B) is the imaging technique of choice in suspected appendicitis as it has superior ability to define anatomical abnormalities. The imaging technique is also preferred if appendiceal perforation is suspected and retains high-quality imaging for obese patients.

Incorrect:

MRI (A) has limited use in evaluating suspected appendicitis but is often used for pregnant women due to low ionizing radiation compared to CT scan. Ultrasound (C) can be considered as a safer primary diagnostic technique, particularly in children and lean adults. However, its usefulness in visualizing abnormalities in the gut is limited in overweight and obese patients. A flat plate (D) would not be useful in detecting anatomical abnormalities associated with appendicitis.

24. **Correct: C. appendectomy with IV antimicrobial therapy.**

Surgical intervention via appendectomy is the only curative approach for acute appendicitis. IV antimicrobial therapy also plays an important role and should be given as prophylaxis prior to surgery with coverage against both aerobic and anaerobic organisms (C).

Incorrect:

Antimicrobial therapy by itself is not consistently curative for acute appendicitis (B). Appendectomy is curative and will help prevent complications, though surgery should be accompanied with appropriate antimicrobial therapy (A). Systemic corticosteroids are not indicated for acute appendicitis (D).

25. **Correct: C. 10 to 30 years**

The peak age of patients with acute appendicitis is from 10 to 30 years (C).

Incorrect:

Acute appendicitis is less common in very young children and older and elderly adults. Given the infrequent nature of appendicitis among the very young and very old, a delay in diagnosis often occurs in these cases.

26. **Correct: A. abdominal discomfort less than 48 hours in duration.**

A key sign of abdominal rupture is duration of symptoms lasting longer than 48 hours, not less than 48 hours (A).

Incorrect:

Common findings of a ruptured or burst appendix include WBC exceeding 20,000/mm³ (D), fever greater than 102°F (greater than 38°C) (B), and peritoneal inflammation findings. A palpable ill-defined lower quadrant abdominal mass (C) is suggestive of abscess formation.

27. **Correct: A. ultrasound**

An ultrasound does not expose a patient to ionizing radiation and can be safely used to evaluate children and pregnant women.

Incorrect:

Among the imaging techniques listed, a CT scan (C) of the abdomen will expose a patient to the greatest amount of ionizing radiation (approximately 10 mSv), followed by barium enema (B) (7 mSv for a series of 10 images), and abdominal flat plate (D) (1.2 mSv).

28. **Correct: A. constipation; B. PID; and C. ectopic pregnancy**

Though the presentation of acute appendicitis can vary considerably, abdominal pain, typically right lower quadrant pain, is a frequent finding. The differential diagnosis can include several other conditions with similar pain symptoms, including constipation (A), PID (B), and ectopic pregnancy (C).

Incorrect:

The most common signs of splenic infarct (D) include left flank pain and left upper quadrant tenderness, which conflicts with typical findings associated with acute appendicitis (most frequently right lower quadrant pain).

29. **Correct: B. release of deep palpation at the site of the discomfort.**

Rebound tenderness describes abdominal pain that is greater with the release of deep palpation at the site of discomfort (B). This is also called Blumberg's sign.

Incorrect:

Light palpation (A) allows for determination of the areas of tenderness and abdominal wall resistance due to rigidity and guarding. Deep palpation (D) allows evaluation of the internal organs and intra-abdominal masses. Rovsing's sign describes when palpation of the left lower quadrant increases pain in the right lower quadrant (contralateral side [C]).

30 to 32. Matching Questions

30. **Correct: C. pain in the right lower quadrant of the abdomen when dropping from standing on toes to heels with a jarring landing**

31. **Correct: A. a sharp pain in the right lower quadrant of the abdomen that is elicited by cough**

32. **Correct: B. abdominal palpation yields rebound tenderness**

The Markle sign, or jar tenderness, will elicit pain in the right lower quadrant of the abdomen when dropping from standing on toes to heels with a jarring landing and is an indication of localized peritonitis due to acute appendicitis. This has a sensitivity of 74%. Rebound tenderness describes abdominal pain that is greater with the release of deep palpation at the site of discomfort and is called Blumberg's sign. This has a specificity of up to 75% in acute appendicitis. The Dunphy sign (cough test) is associated with increased pain during coughing, suggesting localized peritonitis, and can be present in a minority of patients with acute appendicitis.

33. **Correct: D. dullness to percussion in the abdominal right lower quadrant**

Dullness to percussion in the abdomen (D) would suggest either a solid mass or a collection of fluid beneath the region being examined, which would be expected in the presence of abscess formation.

Incorrect:

Appendiceal perforation and abscess would be associated with leukocytosis (elevated WBC) rather than leukopenia (diminished WBC) (A). Cullen's sign (B) is superficial edema and bruising in the tissue surrounding the umbilicus and is associated with pancreatitis, not appendiceal abscess. Appendiceal abscess is not associated with the formation of a maculopapular rash (C).

Gallbladder Disease

34. **Correct: B. acute cholecystitis.**

The classic symptoms of acute cholecystitis (B), or acute inflammation of the gallbladder, include right upper quadrant or epigastric pain along with vomiting and occasionally fever. Pain usually occurs soon after eating a meal, particularly one high in fat.

Incorrect:

Signs of acute hepatitis (C) can include nausea, anorexia, fever, malaise, abdominal pain, and jaundice. The timing of abdominal pain in acute hepatitis is not usually limited to the postprandial period. Hepatoma (A), or hepatocellular cancer, are usually asymptomatic until later stages of disease, when symptoms can include weight loss, abdominal pain and swelling, jaundice, anorexia, and nausea/vomiting. The majority of patients with cholelithiasis (D) are asymptomatic and become aware of the condition only when being evaluated for another health problem.

35. **Correct: A. elevated serum creatinine**

Acute cholecystitis is associated with inflammation and liver damage but should not substantially impact renal function. Thus, the condition will not result in elevated serum creatinine (A).

Incorrect:

Acute cholecystitis is associated with elevated WBC (leukocytosis [C]), as well as an increase in hepatic enzymes such as alkaline phosphatase (B) and aspartate aminotransferase (D).

36. **Correct: A. right upper quadrant abdominal palpation.**

Murphy's sign can be used to diagnose cholecystitis and is positive with the presence of pain during deep inspiration as the examiner palpates the right upper quadrant of the abdomen (A).

Incorrect:

The Markle sign, or jar tenderness, will elicit pain in the right lower quadrant of the abdomen when dropping from standing on toes to heels with a jarring landing (B) and is an indication of localized peritonitis due to acute appendicitis. Percussion (D) can be used to help determine whether there is gas, a solid mass, or a collection of fluid beneath the region being examined. A tympanic sound would indicate a gas-filled area, while dullness is associated with solid or fluid-filled compartment. Asking the patient to cough (C) is not a routine diagnostic tool in evaluating suspected cholecystitis.

37. **Correct: D. pancreatitis**

The most common serious complication of gallstone disease is pancreatitis (D). Approximately 40% of acute pancreatitis cases in developed countries are due to gallstones passing into the bile duct.

Incorrect:

Though the presence of gallstones is a risk factor for gallbladder cancer, only a very small percentage of individuals with gallstones will actually develop adenocarcinoma of the gallbladder (A). Gallbladder cancer is typically asymptomatic until later stages of disease. Gallbladder empyema (B), when the gallbladder fills with purulent material resulting from infected bile, can occur in 5% to 15% of patients with acute cholecystitis, which is nearly always caused by gallstones. Signs of gallbladder empyema include severe abdominal pain, high fever, chills, and sometimes rigors. Cirrhosis is a major risk factor for the development of gallstones, but hepatic failure (C) is not a common complication from the presence of gallstones.

38. **Correct: B. CT scan.**

Though an ultrasound is usually the preferred initial diagnostic test, ultrasound imaging is limited when used in overweight or obese patients. In this case, an abdominal CT scan (B) can be used to check for gallstones and also rule out other GI pathological conditions.

Incorrect:

Though an ultrasound (C) is the diagnostic test of choice for gallstones, its utility can be limited in obese patients.

Most gallstones are radiolucent and would not be visible on a standard flat plate (D). Abdominal MRI (A) is rarely used in the diagnosis of gallstone disease.

39. Correct: B. vomiting

Common signs of acute cholecystitis include right upper quadrant pain or epigastric pain along with vomiting (70% or more of cases) (B).

Incorrect:

Less frequent signs of acute cholecystitis include fever (33% of cases; A) and jaundice (25% to 50% of cases; C). A palpable gallbladder (D) is rarely noted for this condition.

40. Correct: B. male gender.

It is the female gender, rather than the male gender (B), that is at higher risk of developing cholelithiasis.

Incorrect:

In addition to female gender, other risk factors for cholelithiasis include age older than 50 years, obesity (C), hyperlipidemia, rapid weight loss (A), pregnancy, and European or Native American ancestry (D).

41. Correct: B. radiolucent.

Radiolucent (B) indicates an object or tissue that cannot be visualized on x-ray, as it does not block radiation but lets it pass.

Incorrect:

The opposite of radiolucent is radiopaque (A), which blocks radiation and is easily visualized on the x-ray. Calcified (C) refers to the accumulation of calcium salts. Calcified gallstones are more likely to be visualized on x-ray, though only 50% of pigment stones and 20% of cholesterol stones contain sufficient calcium to be visible on x-ray. Unclassified (D) is not a term typically used to describe the visualization of objects on x-ray.

Colorectal Cancer

42. Correct: D. Later disease presentation often includes iron-deficiency anemia.

Iron-deficiency anemia is a common finding in colorectal cancer (D) resulting from chronic low-volume blood loss. Iron supplementation should be included in treatment if iron-deficiency anemia is found.

Incorrect:

Colorectal cancer and polyps are usually located beyond an examining digit and so would not typically be found during rectal examination (A). Colorectal cancer is the third leading cause of cancer death and occurs more frequently than anal carcinomas (B). Colorectal cancer is typically asymptomatic during early stages of disease (C). The earliest signs and symptoms include vague abdominal pain along with iron-deficiency anemia.

43. Correct: B. gFOBT

The gFOBT is an acceptable screening test for colorectal cancer and can be performed annually in a patient at average cancer risk. With a positive result, a colonoscopy should be performed.

Incorrect:

Colonoscopy (C) is recommended every 10 years for screening of colorectal cancer, while Cologuard® can be performed every 3 years (D). Digital rectal examination (A) is not a recommended screening test for colorectal cancer as most cancers will be located beyond the examining digit.

44. Correct: C. few if any symptoms

Early stages of colorectal cancer are typically asymptomatic (C), which is why screening for the disease is important to detect the cancer before it progresses into later stages.

Incorrect:

Symptoms of colorectal cancer at later stages of disease can include gross rectal bleeding (A) and unintended weight loss (B). Nausea and vomiting (D) can also be present in later stages, particularly if there is a partial or complete obstruction of the bowel.

45. Correct: D. long-term aspirin therapy

The use of low-dose aspirin (D), as well as the use of antioxidants and calcium supplements, has been associated with a lower risk of colorectal cancer.

Incorrect:

A family history of colorectal cancer (A), the presence of familial polyposis (B), and having a personal history of neoplasm (C) are known risk factors for colorectal cancer.

46. Correct: B. 3

Colorectal cancer is the third leading cause of death from cancer (B). However, long-term outcomes are generally good when colorectal cancer is identified and treated during the early stages of disease.

Incorrect:

The types of cancer that cause greater cancer-related mortality than colorectal cancer are lung cancer (both genders), prostate cancer (men), and breast cancer (women).

47. Correct: C. iron-deficiency anemia

Chronic low-volume blood loss is frequently found in advanced colorectal cancer. As such, this will often lead to iron-deficiency anemia (C), which should be treated with iron supplementation.

Incorrect:

Folate-deficiency anemia (D; primarily caused by inadequate dietary intake of folate) and pernicious anemia (B; caused by malabsorption of vitamin B_{12}) are not associated with the development of advanced colorectal cancer. Anemia of chronic disease (A) is associated with certain chronic health problems, such as acute and chronic inflammatory conditions, renal insufficiency, and hypothyroidism.

Colonic Diverticular Disease: Diverticulosis/Diverticulitis

48. Correct: D. sigmoid colon.

Though colonic diverticulosis can occur in any part of the large intestines, it occurs most frequently in the sigmoid colon (D).

Incorrect:

The sigmoid colon is the most frequent site of colonic diverticulosis, and this location is consistent with a presentation of left lower quadrant abdominal pain without vomit (when symptoms of diverticulosis are present). The condition can occur less frequently in other parts of the colon, including the ascending colon (A), descending colon (B), and transverse colon (C).

49. **Correct: C. 33%**

In developed countries, approximately one-third (C) of individuals will develop diverticulosis by the time they reach age 50 years, and two-thirds will develop this condition by age 80 years.

Incorrect:

In addition to older age, other risk factors for diverticulosis include family history of disease and select connective tissue disorders, such as Marfan syndrome.

50. **Correct: C. few or no symptoms**

In colonic diverticulosis, inflammation is not present, and the patient is typically asymptomatic (C). The condition is often identified when diagnostic studies are performed for other reasons, such as colonoscopy screening for colorectal cancer.

Incorrect:

In the absence of inflammation, symptoms are usually not present during diverticulosis. When symptoms do occur, they typically consist of left-sided abdominal cramping, increased flatus, and a pattern of constipation alternating with diarrhea. Therefore, diarrhea with leukocytosis (A) or constipation and fever (B) are not typical findings for this condition. Frank blood in the stool with reduced stool quality (D) would be associated with a more severe condition (e.g., colorectal cancer) warranting immediate further evaluation.

51. **Correct: A. cramping, diarrhea, and leukocytosis**

Acute colonic diverticulitis is associated with inflammation that can cause left lower quadrant abdominal pain, fever, leukocytosis, and diarrhea (A).

Incorrect:

Diverticulitis is associated more frequently with diarrhea than constipation (B) as well as left-sided abdominal pain (C). Frank blood in the stool with reduced stool quality (D) is more likely a sign of colorectal cancer or possibly inflammatory bowel disease, warranting immediate further evaluation.

52. **Correct: A. low-fiber diet.**

A low-fiber diet has historically been identified as a risk factor for diverticulosis as this condition occurs more frequently in developed nations where the population consumes a greater quantity of processed foods. However, more recent research has failed to demonstrate a low-fiber diet as a risk factor.

Incorrect:

Risk factors for diverticulosis include older age (C), a family history of disease (B), and select connective tissue disorders, such as Marfan syndrome (D).

53. **Correct: B. the use of fiber supplements.**

Management of diverticulosis involves conservative approaches to reduce the risk of development of diverticulitis. This includes a high-fiber diet along with the use of fiber supplements.

Incorrect:

Though providing other health benefits, ceasing cigarette smoking (C) and limiting alcohol intake (D) are not part of the treatment plan for diverticulosis. Avoiding foods with seeds (A) was once recommended to avoid development of diverticulitis, but few studies support this practice. However, individuals might notice other dietary triggers that cause symptoms and should be encouraged to avoid those foods.

54. **Correct: B. left lower quadrant**

The most frequent location of diverticulitis is in the sigmoid colon, which would be associated with pain and discomfort in the left lower quadrant (B).

Incorrect:

Epigastric pain, located just below the ribs (A), can be caused by a number of GI disorders, including GERD, gastritis, PUD, or gallbladder disorder. Right lower quadrant (C) abdominal pain can be associated with appendicitis. Suprapubic (D) pain can be caused by cystitis, bladder stones, or prostatitis.

55. **Correct: A. bulging pockets in the intestinal wall**

The best description of colonic diverticulosis is the presence of bulging pockets in the intestinal wall, most commonly in the sigmoid colon.

Incorrect:

Diverticula are small pouches that bulge outward through the colon. When these pouches become inflamed, the condition is called diverticulitis. Diverticulosis is not related to poorly contracting intestinal walls (B), strictures of the intestinal lumen (C), or flaccidity of the small intestines (D).

56. **Correct: C. CT scan with contrast**

In suspected acute diverticulitis, a CT scan with contrast (C) would be most useful in identifying findings consistent with the condition. A CT scan can also visualize abscess and fistulas that might be present in complicated disease.

Incorrect:

A flat plate (A) would not be helpful in milder disease but can detect free air if an intestinal perforation is present or altered bowel air patterns are present in the case of bowel obstruction. Abdominal ultrasound (B) is not helpful for this condition, and a barium enema (D) should be avoided due to risk of complication during acute diverticular disease.

57. **Correct: B. plain abdominal film.**

A flat plate (B) would not be helpful in milder disease but can detect free air if an intestinal perforation is present or altered bowel air patterns are present in the case of bowel obstruction.

Incorrect:

Abdominal ultrasound (C) is not helpful for this condition, and a barium enema (A) should be avoided due to risk of complication during acute diverticular disease. Lower endoscopy (D) is contraindicated during acute diverticulitis as insufflation of air can result in or exacerbate free perforation and peritonitis.

58. Correct: C. ciprofloxacin with metronidazole.

Antimicrobial treatment for diverticulitis should include coverage against anaerobic bacteria as well as gram-negative bacteria. Metronidazole is effective against anaerobes, while the fluoroquinolones (e.g., ciprofloxacin, levofloxacin, and moxifloxacin) provide gram-negative coverage (C).

Incorrect:

Amoxicillin with clarithromycin (A) will offer some gram-negative coverage but will not be effective against anaerobes. Linezolid with daptomycin (B) are both effective against gram-positive bacteria. Nitrofurantoin (primarily used for urinary tract infections) and doxycycline (D) provide some gram-negative coverage but lack anaerobic coverage.

59. Correct: B. diverticular hemorrhage.

During acute diverticulitis, diverticular hemorrhage can occasionally occur with the erosion of a vessel contained within a diverticular sac. This can lead to painless lower GI bleeding, and surgical intervention is often needed.

Incorrect:

Crohn's disease (A) and colorectal cancer (C) are not complications resulting from acute diverticulitis. Intussusception (D) is a GI disorder found in newborns and not associated with diverticulitis.

Peptic Ulcer Disease

60. Correct: B. increased risk of inflammatory bowel disease (IBD).

The long-term use of PPIs is associated with various adverse effects, including reduced absorption of certain vitamins and minerals. However, an increased risk of IBD (B) is not one of them.

Incorrect:

Prolonged PPI use is associated with reduced absorption of iron (D), vitamin B_{12}, and other micronutrients. Absorption of calcium and magnesium might also be reduced, thus increasing the risk of bone fractures (A). Additionally, the use of PPIs has been attributed to an increased risk in developing *C difficile* colitis (C) among individuals already at higher risk of developing this infection. Thus, PPI use should not extend beyond 2 months if possible.

61. Correct: B. altering the thickness of the protective mucosal layer.

Endogenous prostaglandins help stimulate and thicken the protective mucosal layer of the stomach. The use of antiprostaglandin medications, such as systemic corticosteroids or NSAIDs, will inhibit this protective mechanism (B) and increase the risk of damage to the stomach lining.

Incorrect:

A substantial portion of PUD is caused by the use of antiprostaglandin medications. NSAIDS and systemic corticosteroids inhibit the action of cyclooxygenase (COX-1 and COX-2) that contributes to maintenance of the protective mucosal layer of the stomach. These agents do not have a direct irritative effect on the stomach lining (A), change the stomach pH level (D), or decrease peristalsis (C).

62. Correct: C. duodenal ulcer.

Epigastric burning and pain that occurs 2 to 3 hours after meals and is relieved with food is most consistent with a duodenal ulcer (C). These ulcers are most commonly associated with *H pylori* infection.

Incorrect:

Gastric ulcer (B) is typically characterized by epigastric pain occurring immediately after meals. Cholecystitis (D), or inflammation of the gallbladder, is characterized by upper right quadrant abdominal pain that often radiates to the right shoulder, usually following a fatty meal. Pain is often accompanied with nausea, vomiting, and fever. Symptoms of acute gastritis (A) include epigastric pain (that may improve or worsen with food), as well as nausea, vomiting, and loss of appetite.

63. Correct: C. tetracycline plus metronidazole.

Though several medications will help alleviate symptoms and promote healing of duodenal ulcer, only effective antimicrobial therapy that eradicates *H pylori* infection will prevent recurrence.

Incorrect:

Recommended treatment of duodenal ulcer includes quadruple therapy containing a PPI, bismuth subsalicylate, and tetracycline plus metronidazole. H_2RAs (e.g., ranitidine) (D) suppress hydrochloric acid production, while PPIs (e.g., omeprazole) (A) inhibit gastric acid secretion. These agents, as well as bismuth subsalicylate (i.e., Pepto-Bismol™) (B) can help reduce symptoms and promote healing but will not impact the presence of *H pylori*, which can lead to recurrence.

64. Correct: A. cimetidine.

Cimetidine is the only H_2RA that significantly inhibits cytochrome P450, which can slow the metabolism of many drugs, including phenytoin and theophylline.

Incorrect:

The H_2RAs act by reducing the secretion of gastric acid. They are generally well tolerated, and famotidine (B), nizatidine (C), and ranitidine (D) do not have a substantial impact on cytochrome P450.

65. Correct: B. age younger than 50 years

Older age is a key risk factor for gastric ulcer. Thus, among the answer choices, age younger than 50 years would not indicate a higher risk for this condition.

Incorrect:

In addition to older age, risk factors for gastric ulcer can include use of NSAIDs (A) or systemic corticosteroids, history of PUD, previous use of antacids or H_2RAs (C) for the treatment of GI symptoms, cigarette smoking (D), cardiac disease, and alcohol use.

66. Correct: D. PPI use.
NSAIDs have antiprostaglandin activity that reduces the protective mucosal layer in the stomach lining. Among the choices, a PPI would provide the best approach as these agents virtually cease production of hydrochloric acid production. However, long-term use of PPIs is associated with adverse effects, and treatment should be limited to no longer than 2 months.
Incorrect:
Antimicrobial therapy (C) would not be appropriate in this situation as NSAID-induced PUD is not caused by *H pylori* infection. Timed antacid doses (A) might provide some relief from symptoms but will not address the underlying mechanism of disease. As NSAIDs do not have a direct irritative effect on the stomach lining, but rather reduce the production of the protective mucosal layer via its antiprostaglandin effect, taking NSAIDs with food (B) will not have a substantial impact on the disease. The use of misoprostol can also be an effective alternative to provide protection against NSAID-induced PUD.

67. Correct: B. gastric ulcer.
Gastric ulcer (B) is typically characterized with epigastric pain occurring immediately after meals. She also presents with risk factors for gastric ulcer, including older age and chronic NSAID use.
Incorrect:
Duodenal ulcer is characterized by epigastric burning and pain that occurs 2 to 3 hours after meals and is relieved with food (C). Cholecystitis (D), or inflammation of the gallbladder, is characterized by upper right quadrant abdominal pain that often radiates to the right shoulder, usually following a fatty meal. Pain is often accompanied with nausea, vomiting, and fever. Gastroenteritis (A) is typically caused by an infection in the intestinal system and accompanied by watery diarrhea, abdominal cramps, nausea and vomiting, and sometimes fever.

68. Correct: C. 2 months.
Prolonged PPI use is associated with reduced absorption of iron, vitamin B_{12}, and other micronutrients. Absorption of calcium and magnesium might also be reduced, thus increasing the risk of bone fractures. Additionally, the use of PPIs has been attributed to an increased risk in developing *C difficile* colitis among individuals already at higher risk of developing this infection. Thus, PPI use should not extend beyond 2 months if possible.

69. Correct: D. large intestine.
PUD occurs when there is an imbalance between gastric protective mechanisms and irritation and damage caused by hydrochloric acid and other digestive juices produced in the stomach. The digestive juices would likely not impact the large intestines (D), as they are

normally neutralized before reaching that portion of the digestive system.
Incorrect:
Gastric acid can cause irritation and damage in the stomach (B) and surrounding segments of the digestive tract, including the esophagus (C) and duodenum (A) (segment of the small intestines immediately following the stomach).

70. Correct: C. gastric
The esophageal sphincter connects the esophagus with the stomach. The pyloric sphincter connects the stomach with the duodenum, which is the first segment of the small intestines. An ulcer occurring between these two sphincters is called a gastric ulcer (C).
Incorrect:
An esophageal ulcer (B) would occur in the esophagus prior to the stomach and esophageal sphincter. An ulcer occurring past the pyloric sphincter in the duodenum is called a duodenal ulcer (A). Ulcers occurring in the stomach (D) are known as gastric ulcers.

71. Correct: A. an upper endoscopy.
An upper endoscopy (A) is recommended in the presence of alarm findings. Alarm findings include bleeding or anemia, unexplained weight loss, progressive dysphagia or odynophagia, recurrent vomiting, and family history of GI cancer. In this patient, recent unintended weight loss would warrant further investigation with an upper endoscopy to check for gastric cancer.
Incorrect:
Upper endoscopy is the preferred diagnostic test in the presence of alarm findings. A barium swallow (B) can be used to identify abnormalities of the pharynx and esophagus but is less effective in identifying gastric abnormalities, such as gastric cancer. *H pylori* testing (C) might be useful in the absence of abnormal findings from upper endoscopy to identify a duodenal ulcer. Esophageal pH monitoring (D) is more helpful in the presence of GERD symptoms, albeit in select circumstances.

72. Correct: B. misoprostol
Misoprostol is a prostaglandin analogue that is specifically designed for gastric protection for patients taking NSAIDs. It might also help minimize renal injury secondary to NSAID use.
Incorrect:
Esomeprazole (C) belongs to the PPI class and so would not be an alternative. Sucralfate (A) can be used for treatment of duodenal ulcer but is inferior to misoprostol for protection against NSAID-induced gastropathy. Metoclopramide (D) is used to treat gastroparesis and can relieve symptoms of nausea, vomiting, heartburn, and loss of appetite. However, it does not provide protection against NSAID-induced gastropathy.

73. Correct: D. erosive gastritis
Erosive gastritis (D) usually occurs secondary to alcohol and NSAID use, aspirin use, and stress. *H pylori* infection is usually not a factor.

Incorrect:

H pylori infection is the most common risk factor for duodenal ulcer (A) and can also play an important role in gastric ulcer (B) and nonerosive (antral) gastritis (C). *H pylori* testing can be helpful in the diagnostic process for each of these conditions (typically in combination with upper endoscopy for the diagnosis of nonerosive and erosive gastritis).

74. Correct: D. initiating empiric *H pylori* therapy.

Patients often report upper GI distress when discontinuing long-term PPI use. This is likely caused by rebound gastric hyperacidity, which can be minimized by tapering the PPI dose. Providing empiric antimicrobial therapy against *H pylori* will not impact rebound gastric hyperacidity.

Incorrect:

Different strategies can be used to gradually reduce the PPI dose to prevent rebound gastric hyperacidity when trying to discontinue PPI therapy. These can include tapering the PPI dose with supplemental antacid (A) or switching to every-other-day dosing of PPI with supplemental antacid (B). Alternatively, a low-dose H_2RA can be used with supplemental antacid (C).

Gastroesophageal Reflux Disease

75. Correct: A. avoiding trigger foods.

Initial management approaches for GERD, particularly mild, intermittent cases, is to identify potential trigger foods (A) and avoid their consumption. The use of antacids after meals and at bedtime can also be considered in mild intermittent GERD.

Incorrect:

Though prokinetic (B) and sucralfate (C) were commonly used in the past for the treatment of GERD, these agents are no longer considered to be therapeutic options as clinical evidence does not support their use. Increasing fluid intake with meals (D) will not alleviate symptoms associated with GERD.

76. Correct: B. esophageal adenocarcinoma.

Esophageal columnar epithelial metaplasia, also known as BE, is a risk factor for esophageal adenocarcinoma. Patients with BE should undergo regular surveillance for the presence of dysplasia.

Incorrect:

The presence of esophageal columnar epithelial metaplasia, or BE, is typically a result of chronic GERD, and so would not be a risk factor for GERD (C). The condition is not related to colonization by *H pylori* (D) and does not increase the risk for the development of a duodenal ulcer (A).

77. Correct: B. increase the pH of the stomach.

PPIs inhibit gastric acid secretion by inhibiting the final step in acid secretion by altering the activity of the proton pump. As a result, the pH in the stomach remains higher.

Incorrect:

The mechanism of action of PPIs is to decrease gastric acid secretion and increase the pH in the stomach. This class of agents does not enhance GI motility (A), reduce esophageal pressure (C), or limit *H pylori* growth (D).

78. Correct: D. no specific diagnostic testing is needed

GERD is typically a presumptive diagnosis established by the presence of the usual symptoms of heartburn and regurgitation and response to standard therapy. Additional testing is not required, particularly in the absence of alarm findings.

Incorrect:

H pylori infection is typically not involved in GERD, and testing for this pathogen is not warranted (A). Upper GI endoscopy (B) would be appropriate in the presence of alarm symptoms and for patients at high risk for complications but is not required for routine diagnosis of GERD. Barium swallow (C) is not recommended for the diagnosis of GERD.

79. Correct: A. recent initiation of estrogen-progestin hormonal therapy

The use of certain medications can cause a decrease in lower esophageal sphincter pressure and cause or exacerbate GERD. These medications include estrogen, progesterone/progestins, theophylline, calcium channel blockers, and nicotine. These medications should be discontinued if clinically possible.

Incorrect:

Weight loss (B) can actually be helpful in relieving GERD and is strongly recommended for overweight or obese patients with GERD. Melena (C), or the presence of digested blood in stool, is a sign of GI bleeding and would not be an expected finding of new-onset GERD. *H pylori* infection is typically not involved in GERD, and testing for this pathogen is not warranted (D).

80. Correct: B. chronic sore throat

Common non-GI symptoms of GERD include chronic hoarseness, sore throat (B), nocturnal cough, and wheezing. These symptoms are occasionally found in the absence of classic symptoms of GERD, especially with chronic GERD.

Incorrect:

Hematemesis (A), or vomiting of blood, as well as melena (D) are indications of GI bleeding, suggesting a condition more serious than GERD that would require further evaluation. Diarrhea (C) is typically not a symptom of GERD.

81. Correct: C. amlodipine.

The use of certain medications can cause a decrease in lower esophageal sphincter pressure and cause or exacerbate GERD. These medications include estrogen, progesterone/progestins, theophylline, calcium channel blockers (e.g. amlodipine [C]), and nicotine. These medications should be discontinued if clinically possible.

Incorrect:

Among antihypertension medications, calcium channel blockers can exacerbate symptoms of GERD. Medications from other antihypertension drugs, such as beta blockers (e.g., atenolol [A]), angiotensin-converting enzyme inhibitors (e.g., trandolapril [B]), and angiotensin II receptor blockers (e.g., losartan [D]) have less impact on GERD.

82. **Correct: B. separated from the antacid use by 2 to 4 hours before or 4 to 6 hours after taking the fluoroquinolone.**

Antacids have a chelating effect with metals and can interact with several types of medications, including fluoroquinolones. Thus, when prescribing a fluoroquinolone for a patient who uses antacids, it is important to educate patients to separate antacid use by 2 to 4 hours before or 4 to 6 hours after taking the fluoroquinolone (B).

Incorrect:

Because of a potential for interaction, antacids should not be dosed concomitantly with fluoroquinolones (A, C) and should be separated by multiple hours either before or after the fluoroquinolone is taken (D).

83. **Correct: C. further evaluation with upper GI endoscopy.**

For patients who do not respond to PPI therapy and lifestyle modification for GERD, the most appropriate next step is further evaluation via upper GI endoscopy.

Incorrect:

An upper GI endoscopy is preferred over an upper GI series (A) when evaluating a patient for refractory GERD. Endoscopy will be helpful in confirming GERD or identifying an alternative cause of symptoms. The upper GI series would not be helpful in confirming a GERD diagnosis. Surgical intervention is typically reserved for the most severe cases (B). For obese patients, gastric bypass surgery can be considered as an approach to improve GERD symptoms. Screening for colorectal cancer via FOBT testing is not warranted in this patient (D).

84. **Correct: A. weight gain**

Unintended weight loss, rather than weight gain, is an alarm finding in a person presenting with GERD symptoms.

Incorrect:

In addition to unintended weight loss, other alarm findings include dysphagia (B), odynophagia (C), GI bleeding that can result in iron-deficiency anemia (D), and persistent chest pain.

85. **Correct: D. African American ethnicity.**

Among ethnic groups, whites and Hispanics are at higher risk of NE, and not African Americans (D).

Incorrect:

BE, or esophageal columnar epithelial metaplasia, is most commonly found in older patients (B) and those with a long-standing history of GERD. Other risk factors include male gender (C), tobacco use (A), and obesity.

86. **Correct: C. upper GI endoscopy with biopsy.**

Upper endoscopy (C) is the preferred method for initial diagnosis and surveillance of BE. This approach also allows the clinician to take biopsy samples for early detection of esophageal cancer.

Incorrect:

Screening for *H pylori* infection (A) is not recommended for GERD patients or those with BE as this organism does not typically play a role in pathogenesis. A CT scan (B) will likely not reveal any abnormalities in BE unless there is the presence of a Barrett ulcer or mass lesion, in which case follow-up evaluation with endoscopy and biopsy will be needed. An upper GI series or barium swallow (D) would not reliably establish a diagnosis of BE.

87. **Correct: D. 3 to 5 years.**

Current guidelines from the American College of Gastroenterology recommend endoscopic evaluation of BE every 3 to 5 years in the absence of dysplasia. The use of additional biomarkers is not recommended for risk stratification.

Incorrect:

ACG guidelines recommend endoscopic surveillance every 3 to 5 years for BE patients without dysplasia. More frequent surveillance is not necessary nor is it recommended as it can increase the risk of procedural adverse events and there is a low risk of progression from BE to esophageal adenocarcinoma (A, B, C).

Esophageal Cancer

88. **Correct: B. adenocarcinoma.**

Though squamous cell carcinoma has historically been the most common type of esophageal cancer in the United States, there has been a steady rise in the number of adenocarcinomas, particularly among white men and women. The number of esophageal adenocarcinomas (B) now outnumbers SCCs in this population.

Incorrect:

The two predominant types of esophageal cancer are adenocarcinoma and SCC. The frequency of adenocarcinomas has increased dramatically over the past four decades and now outnumbers SCC (A) among white men and women. Basal cell carcinoma occurs rarely in the esophagus (C). HPV infection has been implicated as a risk factor for esophageal cancer, but recent evidence suggested a more limited role in causing esophageal cancer (D).

89. **Correct: A. female gender.**

Esophageal cancer is more common in men than women (A), occurring at a ratio of approximately 3:1 male:female.

Incorrect:

The presence of a BE diagnosis is a strong risk factor for esophageal cancer (D), and patients should undergo routine endoscopy to check for the presence of dysplasias. Esophageal cancer is more common among older adults, with the diagnosis most frequently made among individuals in their 60s and 70s (C). HPV infection has been implicated as a risk factor for esophageal cancer, though more recent evidence is suggesting that HPV plays a more limited role in these types of cancers (B).

90. Correct: B. a 76-year-old male who stopped smoking 15 years ago

Risk factors for esophageal cancer include male gender and older age as well as tobacco use. Among the individuals listed, the 76-year-old man with a history of tobacco (B) use presents with the greatest risk for this condition.

Incorrect:

A diet low in fruits and vegetables might increase the risk of esophageal cancer. A high-fat (A) or plant-based diet (D) would not increase the risk of this type of cancer. Pregnancy is not a known risk factor for esophageal cancer (C).

91. Correct: C. iron-deficiency anemia

Advanced esophageal cancer is frequently associated with chronic low-volume blood loss. This can lead to the development of iron-deficiency anemia (C).

Incorrect:

Unexplained weight loss, not weight gain (D), can be an alarm finding of esophageal cancer. Though GERD can be associated with symptoms of sore throat, cough, and wheezing, findings consistent with chronic bronchitis are not typically related to esophageal cancer (B). Renal impairment is not associated with esophageal cancer (A).

Viral Hepatitis

92. Correct: B. viral hepatitis.

The most telling signs for this patient are the presence of jaundice and elevated liver enzymes suggesting clinically significant liver damage. The presence of fever also suggests an active infection is present. Among the answer choices, acute viral hepatitis (B) is the most likely diagnosis.

Incorrect:

BE (D) is associated with GERD that can present with abdominal pain but would not explain signs of liver damage or fever. Cholecystitis (A), or inflammation of the gallbladder, can be associated with constant, acute abdominal pain, often radiating to the right shoulder, as well as nausea, vomiting, and fever. Jaundice and elevated liver enzymes can be present in a proportion of these patients, though not usually to the high degree presented with this patient. Pancreatitis (C) is associated with abdominal pain and elevated levels of amylase and/or lipase. Jaundice is not a usual finding with pancreatitis.

93. Correct: A. HAV IgM.

During an acute hepatitis A infection, immunoglobulin M (IgM) antibody to the hepatitis A virus (A) develops, and this is the key serological marker for an acute HAV infection.

Incorrect:

HAV is an RNA virus, and so detection of viral DNA (B) is not possible. HAV RNA can be detected through the use of reverse transcription and PCR, which can offer earlier detection of HAV infection compared to testing the presence of IgM antibodies. HAV IgG (C) is present following resolution of HAV infection. Alkaline phosphatase (D) can be used to detect liver damage but would not be specific for HAV infection.

94. Correct: C. resolved hepatitis A infection.

The presence of normal liver enzyme levels and HAV IgG suggests a resolved hepatitis A virus infection (C). This is also supported by prior history of living in an area with endemic hepatitis A (rural Central America) and a history of jaundice.

Incorrect:

There is no chronic hepatitis A disease state (A). The presence of HAV IgG suggests prior exposure to HAV (B) that is now resolved, rather than an early stage of infection (D).

95. Correct: C. contaminated water supplies.

HAV is primarily transmitted by fecal-contaminated drinking water and food supplies (C). Raw shellfish that grew in impure water can also be a source of HAV infection.

Incorrect:

HAV is not transmitted via exposure to blood or body fluids, such as can happen with sharing intravenous drug equipment (A) or sexual contact (D). Properly cooking food, including contaminated seafood (B), will kill the HAV.

96. Correct: C. chronic hepatitis B.

HBsAg is a surrogate marker for the presence of HBV, either as an acute or chronic infection. This patient likely has a chronic infection as he presents with no symptoms and only mildly elevated hepatic enzymes (C).

Incorrect:

The presence of HBsAg suggests that HBV is currently present (A) and that the infection is not resolved (B). The presence of HBsAb (Anti-HBs) would indicate a resolved infection or successful immunization (D), and the patient is no longer susceptible to HBV infection.

97 to 100. Matching Questions

97. Correct: A. 15 to 45 days (average 28 days)

98. Correct: C. 45 to 160 days (average 120 days)

99. Correct: B. 14 to 180 days (average 45 days)

100. Correct: C. 45 to 160 days (average 120 days)

The incubation period spans the time from when a person becomes infected with the virus to the time that symptoms develop. Knowing the incubation period of a virus can be important in helping to identify the source of infection for public health efforts, as well as identifying other individuals who were possibly exposed to the virus. The incubation period for hepatitis D is identical to hepatitis B, as the hepatitis D virus requires co-infection with HBV.

101. Correct: D. freezing food for at least 1 hour.
Freezing food (D) will not kill HAV; thus, other methods must be used to kill the virus.
Incorrect:
HAV is heat sensitive and can be killed by heating food to ≥185°F (85°C) for at least 1 minute (A). Adequate chlorination of the water supply (B), as recommended in the United States, will kill the virus. A 1:100 bleach solution (C) is effective in killing the virus from surfaces.

102. Correct: D. prescribing a systemic antibacterial to prevent superinfection.
Antimicrobial therapy (D) is not warranted during hepatitis A infection. The infection typically resolves over time, and bacterial superinfection is not a common cause for concern.
Incorrect:
During acute hepatitis A infection, steps can be taken to combat nausea and prevent further liver damage. Eating smaller, more frequent meals (A) can help with nausea, while choosing high-calorie foods can also help maintain body weight during the illness. Alcohol should be avoided (B) and any medications should be reviewed (C) for hepatoxicity potential and discontinued if possible.

103. Correct: D. the presence of HBsAg.
Signs of acute HBV infection include HBsAg (D), HBeAg, as well as elevated hepatic enzymes ≥10 × ULN.
Incorrect:
The presence of HBsAb (A) would suggest HBV infection in the past that resolved or the patient was immunized against the virus. Neutrophilia (B) is an elevation of neutrophils, typically in response to a bacterial infection. Thrombocytopenia (C) is a decrease in the number of platelets, which is not a typical finding for acute HBV infection. Secondary thrombocytosis, an elevation in platelets, can occur during periods of infection.

104. Correct: A. abdominal rebound tenderness.
Abdominal rebound tenderness (A), characterized by pain upon removal of pressure to the abdomen, is not a usual finding with hepatitis but is more commonly found with peritonitis and appendicitis.
Incorrect:
Scleral icterus (B), or yellowing of the eyes, is a sign of jaundice, which is a typical sign of acute hepatitis. Myalgia (D), or muscle pain, is another expected finding with acute hepatitis infection, as well as a tender, palpable hepatic border (C) upon physical examination of the abdomen. Other common findings of all forms of acute viral hepatitis include nausea, anorexia, fever, malaise, abdominal pain, clay-colored stools, and dark-colored urine.

105 to 108. Yes or No
105. Yes
106. Yes
107. Yes
108. No
HBV is usually transmitted through an exchange of blood or body fluids. Thus, risk factors include having sex with multiple partners, men who have sex with men, sharing needles during injection drug use, having a job with exposure to human blood, or traveling to areas endemic for HBV infection. HAV is transmitted through contaminated food or water.

109. Correct: D. receive HBIG and start hepatitis B immunization series.
Postexposure prophylaxis can be effective in preventing HBV infection. For unvaccinated individuals, HBIG and the HBV vaccine should be administered (D) as soon as possible, preferably within 24 hours after exposure.
Incorrect:
Postexposure prophylaxis should include HBIG in addition to starting the HBV immunization series (A). The presence of HBsAb would indicate immunity to HBV, which would occur with prior exposure to HBV or through prior vaccination (C). Limiting the number of sexual partners would generally decrease her risk of HBV infection but is not pertinent in this situation where her only partner has HBV infection (B).

110. Correct: B. baker's yeast.
Though serious allergic reactions to vaccines are very rare overall, the HBV vaccine is contraindicated for individuals who experience life-threatening anaphylactic reaction to baker's yeast (B).
Incorrect:
Though individuals who have a history of severe allergic reaction to baker's yeast should not receive the HBV vaccine, there are no warnings or contraindications for vaccination among individuals with known allergies to eggs (A), peanuts (C), or shellfish (D).

111. Correct: A. Lyme disease.
For individuals diagnosed with HBV infection, testing for other sexually transmitted infections should be offered. Lyme disease (A) is not a sexually transmitted infection, and testing would not be warranted among individuals with HBV.
Incorrect:
For individuals diagnosed with HBV infection, testing for other sexually transmitted infections, including HIV (B), hepatitis A (C), and hepatitis C (D) should also be offered, and postexposure prophylaxis and immunization should be offered when applicable.

112. Correct: C. At least 50% of persons with acute hepatitis C go on to develop chronic infection.
Though HCV rarely causes severe acute illness, at least 50% to 80% of individuals will go on to develop

chronic infection (C). Progression to cirrhosis will develop in 20% of those with chronic HCV infection after 20 years of disease.

Incorrect:
Hepatitis C infection rarely causes acute symptoms (A) but remains asymptomatic. HCV is transmitted through an exchange of blood or body fluids; there is no evidence indicating a higher preponderance of HCV among nurses compared to other health-care workers (B). Treatment with pegylated interferon (D) has limited clinical efficacy, though the use of newer oral antiviral agents can achieve greater than 90% cure rates with 8 to 12 weeks of therapy.

113. Correct: B. co-infection with hepatitis B, daily alcohol use
For a patient with chronic hepatitis C infection, co-infection with hepatitis B can lead to rapid deterioration in hepatic function and contribute to the severity of disease; daily use of alcohol will also contribute to liver damage and cirrhosis (B).

Incorrect:
Co-infection with another hepatitis virus as well as alcohol use will contribute to the severity of liver damage in a patient with chronic HCV infection. Female gender, younger age (A), method of viral acquisition (C), and aspirin use (D) will not substantially impact progression of disease. Use of certain medications with hepatotoxicity can also contribute to liver damage, including high daily doses of acetaminophen (greater than 4 g per day).

114. Correct: B. immunize the at-risk population against hepatitis B.
The hepatitis D virus can only be found concurrently in the presence of hepatitis B. Thus, prevention of hepatitis B through immunization also protects the individual from hepatitis D (B).

Incorrect:
Hepatitis D is transmitted via exposure to infected blood or body fluids, so a campaign for clean food supplies (A) or improved hand washing (D) will have a limited impact on minimizing the spread of this virus. Antiviral prophylaxis (C) is not warranted for the prevention of any viral hepatitis.

115. Correct: C. α-fetoprotein.
Chronic hepatitis B and C are potent risk factors for hepatoma or primary hepatocellular carcinoma. Periodic monitoring for α-fetoprotein (C) can be used for surveillance of hepatic tumor growth, often coupled with imaging such as ultrasound or CT.

Incorrect:
α-Fetoprotein is the marker used to indicate hepatic tumor growth. ESR (A) is used to check for inflammation in the body, while bilirubin (D) can check for the presence of jaundice. HBsAb (B) is the marker for immunity against HBV infection.

116. Correct: D. AST, 640 U/L; ALT, 870 U/L
During acute hepatitis infection, AST and ALT values increase ≥10-fold than normal values, with ALT typically increasing greater than AST. Among the answer choices, choice D is most representative of acute HAV infection.

Incorrect:
All forms of acute viral hepatitis can lead to elevated levels of AST and ALT of >10-fold the upper limit of normal (ULN for AST=31 U/L; ULN for ALT=40 U/L), though often will reach levels of 20-fold or higher the ULN. Small increases in AST/ALT are not indicative of acute hepatitis (A). Additionally, ALT will increase to a greater degree than AST during these acute infections (B, C).

117. A. AST, 22 U/L; ALT, 28 U/L
With chronic use of statin therapy, there is a low likelihood of hepatic enzyme elevation. Choice A reflects normal values that are most likely to be found for this patient.

Incorrect:
Long-term statin use is not typically associated with elevated liver enzymes. Moderate elevations of one or both liver enzymes would suggest another cause of liver damage or dysfunction (B, C). Substantial elevations (≥10× ULN) of both liver enzymes can be caused by acute viral hepatitis (D).

118. Correct: C. immunization against hepatitis A and B
For the patient with nonalcoholic fatty liver disease, proactive steps should be taken to prevent further damage to the liver, including immunization against hepatitis A and B without regard to lifestyle risk factors.

Incorrect:
Vaccination against HAV and HBV should be given without regard to lifestyle risk factors (A) to prevent further damage to the liver caused by viral hepatitis. There is currently no vaccine available against HCV (B, D).

119. Correct: A. hepatitis A
Hepatitis A (A) is primarily transmitted via fecal-contaminated food or water and is not spread through an exchange of blood or body fluids as with the other hepatitis viruses.

Incorrect:
Hepatitis B (B), C (C), and D (D) are transmitted through an exchange of blood or body fluids and can be spread via heterosexual vaginal intercourse.

Irritable Bowel Syndrome and Irritable Bowel Disease

120. Correct: B. Crohn's disease
The presence of involuntary weight loss, recurrent abdominal cramping, and loose stools is consistent with IBD, either UC or Crohn's disease. Unlike UC where inflammation is limited to the mucosal lining, Crohn's disease (B) can involve the entire intestinal wall and frequently results in the development of anterior and posterior anal fissures.

Incorrect:

Condyloma acuminata (D) are caused by HPV infection and cause anogenital warts but would not be associated with the GI symptoms of this patient. *C difficile* colitis (C) is characterized by abdominal pain and frequent (often more than 8 to 12 times per day), watery bowel movements. UC (A) has similar symptoms as this patient but typically lacks the presence of anal fissures.

121 to 124. Yes or No

121. Correct: Yes

122. Correct: Yes

123. Correct: No

124. Correct: No

IBS is typically diagnosed through a careful patient history and clinical presentation. However, in the presence of alarm findings, further evaluation is warranted to rule out a more serious condition. Alarm findings include GI bleeding, iron-deficiency anemia, nocturnal passage of stool, unintentional weight loss, family history of IBD or colorectal cancer (121), recent changes in bowel habits, leukocytosis (122), and the presence of a palpable abdominal mass or lymphadenopathy. Patients in questions 123 and 124 are presenting with typical findings for IBS without alarm findings and, thus, would not need further evaluation.

125. Correct: C. a condition that is the result of abnormal gut motor/sensory activity.

IBS is characterized by abdominal pain and altered bowel habits in the absence of detectable structural abnormalities. The mechanism of disease is likely multifactorial and involves abnormal gut motor or sensory activity (C), as well as central neural dysfunction, psychological disturbances, mucosal inflammation, stress, and luminal factors.

Incorrect:

IBD (A) differs from IBS in that it involves an autoimmune response to the GI tract. IBS is not necessarily limited to the small bowel (B) but typically involves the colon, and symptoms extend into adulthood. There is no obvious role of the pancreas (D) in the pathophysiology of IBS.

126. Correct: D. unexplained weight loss.

Unexplained weight loss (D) is not part of the criteria for diagnosing IBS but is considered an alarm finding that would warrant further evaluation.

Incorrect:

The Rome IV criteria for the diagnosis of IBS require that patients must have recurrent abdominal pain on average at least 1 day/week in the past 3 months associated with two or more of the following: symptoms related to defecation (A), associated with a change in stool frequency (B), or associated with a change in stool form or appearance (C).

127. Correct: A. diagnosis is largely based on clinical presentation and application of the Rome IV criteria.

IBS is typically diagnosed through a careful patient history and clinical presentation as well as application of the Rome IV criteria. Further evaluation is usually not needed in the absence of alarm findings.

Incorrect:

A colonoscopy (B) is not warranted in the diagnosis of IBS, though it can be considered in the presence of alarm findings that warrant further evaluation. IBS is not typically associated with active infection or inflammation, and so laboratory testing (C) to detect these processes would not be helpful in confirming the diagnosis. IBS is a chronic condition with treatment available to address the symptoms but not cure the disease (D).

128. Correct: D. eluxadoline (Viberzi®)

Eluxadoline (Viberzi®) is a mixed-opioid receptor agonist that has been approved for the treatment of IBS-D and offers an alternative to antidiarrheals or antispasmodics (D). Additionally, the antibiotic rifaximin (Xifaxan®) has been shown to improve symptoms of IBS-D.

Incorrect:

Oral vancomycin (A) is used for the treatment of *C difficile* colitis but is not approved for IBS-D. Linaclotide (B) is approved for the treatment of constipation-predominant IBS. Pepto-Bismol™ (C) is commonly used for upset stomach, but evidence is lacking on its effectiveness in reducing symptoms associated with IBS-D.

129. Correct: B. a sensation of incomplete bowel emptying that is distressing and sometimes painful

Tenesmus is a common complaint among individuals with chronic constipation and IBS-C and is characterized by a sensation of incomplete bowel emptying that is distressing and sometimes painful (B).

Incorrect:

Rectal burning with defecation (A) can be due to a number of conditions, including hemorrhoids or anal fissure. Unexplained weight loss (C) and the appearance of frank blood in stool (hematochezia) (D) are alarm findings that would warrant further evaluation.

130. Correct: C. Patients can present with bowel issues ranging from diarrhea to constipation.

There are three major subtypes of IBS: constipation predominant, diarrhea predominant, and mixed etiology (C). Severity of symptoms can vary significantly and include abdominal pain, constipation, and diarrhea.

Incorrect:

Individuals with diarrhea-predominant IBS make up a subset of those with IBS, and diarrhea is typically episodic, often alternating between constipation and diarrhea rather than chronic diarrhea (A). Unlike IBD, IBS is not associated with an increased risk of colorectal cancer (D). Malabsorption and weight change (either gain or loss) are not usual findings with IBS (B).

131. Correct: B. metoclopramide (Reglan®).
Metoclopramide is a prokinetic agent that was traditionally used to treat IBS-C. However, due to safety concerns, long-term use of this agent is not recommended.

Incorrect:
Dicyclomine (A) is an anticholinergic/antispasmodic agent that has traditionally been used to treat IBS-D. Loperamide (C) is an antidiarrheal agent that is often used to treat IBS-D though clinical evidence supporting this practice is lacking. Psyllium (D) is a bulking agent that can be used to help alleviate symptoms associated with IBS-C.

132. Correct: C. normal results on most testing.
There are no specific tests used to diagnose IBS, as the diagnosis is usually made via detailed patient history, clinical presentation, and application of the Rome IV criteria. Laboratory tests and imaging typically reveal normal results (C).

Incorrect:
IBS is not a condition involving underlying inflammation (A), mucosal thickening of the GI tract (D), or any type of anemia (B). These findings are more typical of patients with IBD.

133 to 137. Yes or No

133. Correct: No

134. Correct: Yes

135. Correct: Yes

136. Correct: Yes

137. Correct: No
Nutritional intervention can be helpful in reducing the frequency of exacerbations and can include adequate hydration and fiber supplementation (134). However, a moderate-protein, low-residue diet would not substantially affect IBS (133). Avoiding stress, a common trigger, as well as regular aerobic exercise have been shown to be helpful in reducing IBS exacerbations (135). Antispasmodics and loperamide might offer some relief for IBS-D (136), though excessive use of loperamide can cause constipation. TCAs and antidepressants can be considered for IBS-D but are generally not recommended for IBS-C (137).

138. Correct: C. a 22-year-old woman with constipation-predominant IBS
Lubiprostone is a chloride channel activator that is approved for the treatment of IBS-C as well as chronic idiopathic constipation. The agent elicits fluid secretion into the intestinal lumen that promotes bowel movements.

Incorrect:
Lubiprostone is not indicated for patients with inflammatory bowel disease (B, D) or for individuals with diarrhea-predominant IBS (A).

139. Correct: A. weight loss and malnutrition.
IBS is typically not associated with weight loss or malnutrition (A). Unintended weight loss would be an alarm finding and warrant further evaluation in an individual suspected of IBS.

Incorrect:
The Rome IV criteria for diagnosing IBS include abdominal pain occurring at least once per week in the past 3 months (B). IBS is found more frequently in women (D) and is characterized by altered bowel pattern in the absence of structural abnormalities (C).

140. Correct: A. evidence of underlying inflammation.
IBD is associated with widespread inflammation (A), and diagnostic test results should confirm this, usually with elevated CRP and ESR.

Incorrect:
Inflammation associated with IBD will be noted on laboratory analysis (C). The condition is not related to the presence of intestinal parasites (B), and early diagnostic testing (D) will not reveal an intra-abdominal mass, though UC patients are at higher risk of colorectal cancer after many years of disease.

141. Correct: B. serum Cr.
An IBD flare is associated with widespread inflammation that can be detected by positive findings on a number of laboratory test results. However, serum Cr is used as a measure of renal function and would not be significantly impacted by inflammation associated with an IBD flare (B).

Incorrect:
IBD is associated with widespread inflammation, and diagnostic test results should confirm this, usually with elevated CRP (A) and ESR (C). Leukocytosis, or an elevation in WBCs, is also frequently present during an IBD flare (D).

142. Correct: D. hemolytic anemia.
Hemolytic anemia (D) occurs when red blood cells are destroyed and removed from circulation faster than the normal life span of the RBC. Though this can be due to an autoimmune reaction, this condition is not normally associated with IBD.

Incorrect:
Various types of anemia can result from IBD. Iron-deficiency anemia (B) can result from chronic blood loss from the GI tract. Widespread inflammation can contribute to the development of anemia of chronic disease, a normocytic, normochromic anemia (A). Malabsorption of vitamin B_{12} can result in megaloblastic (macrocytic) anemia (C).

143. Correct: C. Crohn's disease and UC.
Patients with IBD can be categorized into those with Crohn's disease and UC (C). In UC, the pathological changes are limited to the colon, and inflammation is limited to the mucosa. In Crohn's disease, the pathological changes can occur in any part of the GI tract,

and inflammation can involve the entire wall of the GI tract.

144. **Correct: C. Crohn's disease.**
"Skip lesions" refer to areas of affected tissue in the GI tract that alternates with normal tissue that is visualized during imaging studies. This is a common finding in the patient with Crohn's disease (C), with the terminal ileum and right colon most frequently involved.
Incorrect:
"Skip lesions" are a finding in Crohn's disease but not UC (B) or *C difficile* colitis (D). Colonoscopy of a patient with IBS will generally reveal normal findings (A).

145. **Correct: D. immune modulators.**
The elimination of inflammation, either through the use of biologics or immune modulators (D), can lead to deep mucosal healing and result in decreased rates of surgery, hospitalization, and corticosteroid use. Therefore, an earlier introduction of these agents in disease management is being advocated.
Incorrect:
The use of immune modulators (6-mercaptopurine and azathioprine) and biologics (anti-TNF and anti-α4-integrin agents) can eliminate inflammation and result in deep mucosal healing. Oral aminosalicylates (e.g., sulfasalazine and mesalamine) have traditionally been used as first-line agents for IBD (A) and remain effective in treating mild-to-moderate IBD. However, these agents are less likely to result in deep mucosal healing in UC or Crohn's disease. Oral or parenteral corticosteroids (B) can provide rapid symptom relief due to potent anti-inflammatory effect but are not recommended for long-term use, as these agents will not heal the damage to the mucosal lining. Antibiotics (C) are not generally recommended in IBD in the absence of infection, as these agents can increase the risk of *C difficile* colitis.

146. **Correct: B. large intestine.**
In UC, the pathological changes are limited to the colon (B). The risk of colorectal cancer is greatly increased in these patients after 10 years of disease duration.
Incorrect:
The pathological changes in UC are limited to the colon and would not impact the small bowel (A), duodenum (C), or stomach (D).

147. **Correct: A. small bowel**
In contrast to UC, Crohn's disease can impact any segment of the GI tract. However, an increased risk of malignancy is focused on the small bowel (A) among these patients.
Incorrect:
Crohn's disease is associated with increased malignancy of the small bowel, and not the large intestines (B), duodenum (C), or stomach (D). In contrast,

those with long-term ulcerative colitis (i.e., 10 years or longer) are at increased risk of colorectal cancer.

148 to 158. Indicate IBD, IBS, or both.

148. **Correct: Both**
IBS can affect persons of all ages, but onset of symptoms most often occurs before 45 years of age. IBD is most often diagnosed in late adolescence or early adulthood.

149. **Correct: IBS**
IBS is predominantly found in females. In IBD, the male-to-female ratio is close to 1.

150. **Correct: IBS**
IBS is also known as spastic colon, irritable colon, or nervous colon, and it is characterized by abdominal pain, discomfort, and/or altered bowel habits in the absence of detectable structural abnormalities.

151. **Correct: IBD**
For patients with IBD, approximately 15% will develop nondestructive axial or peripheral arthritis. Renal calculi are often found in those with Crohn's disease. IBS is not typically associated with extraintestinal manifestations.

152. **Correct: IBD**
IBD flares can be associated with the development of toxic colitis, a life-threatening condition characterized by nonobstructive colonic dilation with signs of systemic toxicity. Though IBS can negatively impact quality of life, the condition is not life-threatening.

153. **Correct: IBD**
IBD often has an unclear etiology but likely involves an autoimmune response to the GI tract. The etiology of IBS is likely multifactorial but does not involve an autoimmune response.

154. **Correct: Both**
Both IBS and IBD can be exacerbated with trigger foods. Common triggers of IBS include coffee, disaccharides, legumes, cabbage, and a high-carbohydrate diet. IBD patients should keep a diet diary to help identify food triggers. Lactose intolerance is more common among those with Crohn's disease.

155. **Correct: IBD**
In IBD, inflammation can be limited to the mucosa (UC) or can involve the entire intestinal wall (Crohn's disease). In IBS, physiological changes to the GI tract are typically not noted with imaging studies.

156. **Correct: IBS**
The etiology of IBS is multifactorial, often involving abnormal gut motor/sensory activity along with central neural dysfunction, psychological disturbances, mucosal inflammation, and stress. IBD typically involve an autoimmune response to the GI tract.

157. **Correct: IBD**
Fistulas and perianal abscess are often noted among those with Crohn's disease. Serious complications are not common among those with IBS.

158. Correct: IBD

Individuals with UC are at higher risk of colorectal cancer, particularly after 8 to 10 years of disease. Surveillance colonoscopy is recommended every 2 years for these patients. Crohn's disease is associated with a higher risk of small bowel malignancy. Increased colonic malignancy is not noted among those with IBS.

Celiac Disease

159. Correct: D. small bowel malabsorption syndrome.

Small bowel malabsorption syndrome (D) is not a term used to denote celiac disease.

Incorrect:

Celiac disease is a permanent dietary disorder caused by an immunological reaction to gluten. The condition is also known as gluten-induced enteropathy (A), celiac sprue (B), and sprue (C).

160. Correct: A. it is a temporary immunological gluten disorder.

Celiac disease is a permanent, not temporary (A), immunological disorder.

Incorrect:

Celiac disease occurs most frequently among whites of northern European ancestry (B), found in about 1% of this population. Its symptoms can include chronic diarrhea and flatulence, which can often lead to a misdiagnosis of IBS (D). The condition is characterized by diffuse damage to the proximal small intestinal mucosa with malabsorption of nutrients (C).

161. Correct: A. weight loss, chronic diarrhea, and muscle wasting; B. flatulence and abdominal distension; and C. as growth restriction when diagnosed in children younger than 2 years old

Celiac disease can cause weight loss, chronic diarrhea, and muscle wasting (A), as well as flatulence and abdominal distension (B). A sign of the condition in young children is growth restriction (C).

Incorrect:

Egg intolerance (D) is not a typical finding among individuals with celiac disease, though intolerance to cow's milk can contribute to symptoms. Dairy products should be avoided at least temporarily until intestinal symptoms resolve.

162. Correct: B. IgA endomysial and IgA tTG antibodies.

In celiac disease, glutamine-rich peptides derived from partially digested gluten bind to HLA-DQ2 or HLA-DQ8 molecules on antigen-presenting cells. This stimulates an inappropriate T cell–mediated activation in the intestinal submucosa that results in destruction of mucosal enterocytes as well as a humoral immune response that results in antibodies to gluten, tTG, and other autoantigens (B), which can be used as specific markers for the condition.

Incorrect:

ESR and CRP (A) are markers of inflammation, but they are not specific for celiac disease. A biopsy is a histological test, not serological (C). Duodenal biopsies can be used as part of the diagnostic process for celiac disease. The presence of *H pylori* IgG antibodies (D) can be used for the diagnosis of PUD, but *H pylori* is not involved in the pathogenesis of celiac disease.

163. Correct: A. acute appendicitis.

Symptoms of acute appendicitis (A) include abdominal pain, fever, rebound tenderness, as well as positive obturator and psoas signs. These are not consistent with typical findings in celiac disease.

Incorrect:

Celiac disease can be mistaken for other conditions because of overlapping signs and symptoms, such as weight loss, chronic diarrhea, flatulence, and abdominal distension. Other conditions to consider in the differential diagnosis can include small bowel bacterial overgrowth (B), cow's milk intolerance (C), and tropical sprue (D).

164. Correct: C. steak with mashed potatoes

Gluten is found in food products that contain wheat, rye, and barley. Substitutes for gluten-containing foods can include rice, corn, millet, potato, buckwheat, and soybeans. Among the answer choices, the steak and mashed potatoes (C) will not contain gluten.

Incorrect:

Beer (A) is not appropriate as it is derived from barley, while the crust of the pizza (B) and the breading of the chicken nuggets (D) will contain gluten from wheat.

165. Correct: C. avoid intake of semolina, spelt, and rye.

Individuals with celiac disease should avoid any food products that contain gluten, including all wheat, rye, and barley (C).

Incorrect:

Individuals with celiac disease should avoid consuming whole grains as these contain gluten (A). Though adequate exercise is important for maintaining overall health, exercise will not impact symptoms of celiac disease (B). Parents should be counseled about not avoiding normal childhood activities, such as birthday parties, because of celiac disease (D). The child should be made aware of appropriate food choices as early as possible, as this will be a lifelong process. With a proper understanding of the condition and dietary restrictions, celiac disease can be well managed.

Pancreatitis, Pancreatic Pseudocysts, and Pancreatic Cancer

166. Correct: A. hypothyroidism.

Several risk factors for acute pancreatitis have been identified. However, hypothyroidism (A) is not a recognized risk factor for this condition.

Incorrect:

Risk factors for acute pancreatitis are biliary tract disease including gallstones, excessive alcohol use, elevated triglyceride levels (B), viral infection, and blunt abdominal trauma (C). The use of certain medications, including opioids, thiazide diuretics (D), and systemic corticosteroids, can also increase the risk of acute pancreatitis.

167. Correct: C. jaundice.

Jaundice (C) is not a typical finding of acute pancreatitis but can be present if the condition involves the head of the pancreas. Unlike acute hepatic and biliary disorders (e.g., cholecystitis), jaundice caused by acute pancreatitis is not associated with localized right upper quadrant tenderness.

Incorrect:

Acute pancreatitis is typically characterized by elevations in serum amylase (A) and lipase (B). When serum amylase and serum lipase levels are both greater than threefold higher than the upper limit of normal and gut perforation and infarction have been ruled out, an acute pancreatitis diagnosis is virtually assured. Physical examination will reveal diffuse abdominal tenderness without rebound (D).

168. Correct: A. refer to the acute care hospital for admission.

In this patient, the presence of a narrow pulse pressure suggests poor circulating volume. This, combined with repeated acute vomiting episodes, would indicate that this patient should be admitted to an acute care setting for evaluation (A).

Incorrect:

Though it is important to maintain and assess hydration status in a patient with multiple episodes of vomiting (B, D), this patient presents with more urgent needs that should be evaluated in the acute care setting. The symptoms and patient history are not consistent with GERD, and so an H_2-receptor antagonist and antacids would not be warranted (C).

169 to 172. Indicate amylase, lipase, both, or neither.

169. Correct: amylase

170. Correct: lipase

171. Correct: amylase

172. Correct: neither

Though elevated levels of amylase and lipase are a key finding during acute pancreatitis, these laboratory findings are not specific for pancreatitis as there are several other sources of amylase and lipase. Nonpancreatic sources of amylase include salivary glands, ovarian cysts (171), ovarian tumors, tubo-ovarian abscess, ruptured ectopic pregnancy, and lung cancer (169). Elevated levels of lipase can occur in renal failure (170). However, amylase and lipase are not produced in adipose (fat) tissue, and so elevated levels would not be expected in obesity (172).

173. Correct: C. Measuring serum lipase level along with amylase level increases diagnostic specificity in acute pancreatitis.

Acute pancreatitis is typically characterized by elevations in serum amylase and lipase (C). When serum amylase and serum lipase levels are both more than

threefold higher than ULN and gut perforation and infarction have been ruled out, an acute pancreatitis diagnosis is virtually assured.

Incorrect:

Due to the nonspecific nature of symptoms and clinical findings associated with acute pancreatitis, confirmation of diagnosis typically involves laboratory analysis along with imaging studies (A). Ultrasound offers limited views of the pancreas (B), and so a CT scan is the preferred method to visualize abnormalities in the organ. Elevated serum amylase and lipase are universal findings in acute pancreatitis, not hypocalcemia (D).

174. Correct: B. 3 or greater

The Ranson criteria are usually used in assessing severity of pancreatitis. With a Ranson score of 0 to 2, the mortality rate is 1% and ICU admission would not normally be needed. With a Ranson score of 3 to 5, there is a 10% to 20% mortality rate, and the patient should be admitted to the ICU (B). With a score greater than 5, the mortality rate is greater than 50%, and more systemic complications are likely.

175. Correct: C. jaundice.

Jaundice (C) is not a typical sign associated with pancreatic pseudocyst. Jaundice can result in cases of acute pancreatitis where the head of the pancreas is affected.

Incorrect:

Pancreatic pseudocysts are often asymptomatic. However, when symptoms do occur, they most commonly include persistent abdominal pain that radiates to the back (A), a mass that can be felt in the upper abdomen (D), and nausea and vomiting (B).

176. Correct: C. analysis of cyst fluid

Though MRI and CT scans can help differentiate a pseudocyst from cancer, additional testing is usually needed to arise at a conclusive diagnosis. Fluid collected from the pseudocyst (C) can be used to test for signs of cancer. Serological testing with CEA and CEA-125 can also be used to differentiate pancreatic cancer from a pseudocyst.

Incorrect:

Though MRI and CT scans (A, B) can help differentiate a pseudocyst from cancer, additional testing is usually needed to arise at a conclusive diagnosis. Though serum amylase can be higher in pseudocysts and lower in tumors, the use of serum amylase and lipase levels (D) will not provide definitive evidence in differentiating between a pseudocyst and malignancy.

177. Correct: A. monitoring the pseudocyst for any change in size or resolution.

Most pseudocysts are self-limiting and resolve over time without any intervention other than supportive care. Intervention is usually not needed for pseudocysts that are asymptomatic and at low risk for complications and malignancy. A follow-up MRI should be scheduled to monitor any changes in pseudocyst morphology or check for resolution (A).

Incorrect:

Treatment goals are aimed at reducing the risk of complications including infection, hemorrhage, or rupture. However, conservative approaches might only be needed in cases of small pseudocysts that are asymptomatic and show no signs of growth. When an intervention is needed, treatment can include endoscopic drainage of fluid (B) or surgical removal (C) of the pseudocyst. No medications are available that will decrease the size of pseudocysts, including the use of anti-inflammatory agents (D).

178. **Correct: A. hypertension.**

Several risk factors have been identified for the development of pancreatic cancer. However, hypertension (A) is not among them.

Incorrect:

Risk factors for pancreatic cancer include a history of chronic pancreatitis (B), tobacco use (C), and diabetes mellitus (D). A genetic factor contributes to development of the disease in 5% of cases, though no identifiable risk factors are present in 40% of pancreatic cancer cases.

179 to 185. Yes or No

179. **Correct: Yes**

180. **Correct: Yes**

181. **Correct: No**

182. **Correct: No**

183. **Correct: Yes**

184. **Correct: No**

185. **Correct: Yes**

Typical signs of pancreatic cancer can include involuntary weight loss (179) and midepigastric pain that radiates to the back (185). Laboratory findings can include elevated alkaline phosphatase as well as elevated total and direct bilirubin (with involvement of the head of the pancreas). This can lead to painless jaundice (180). Anemia of chronic disease, a normochromic,

normocytic anemia, can also be present (183). Cullen's sign, or a bluish discoloration of the periumbilical region, is often found in acute pancreatitis but not pancreatic cancer (181). The obturator and psoas signs are typically noted in appendicitis (182). Hematuria, or blood in the urine, is not typically noted (184).

186. **Correct: B. diminished platelet count.**

Thrombocytopenia, or diminished platelet count (B), is not a typical finding in the patient with pancreatic cancer.

Incorrect:

For patients with pancreatic cancer, laboratory findings can include elevated alkaline phosphatase (C) as well as elevated total (A) and direct (D) bilirubin (with involvement of the head of the pancreas).

187. **Correct: A. abdominal ultrasound**

Several imaging techniques can be used to help with the diagnosis of pancreatic cancer. However, the usefulness of an abdominal ultrasound would be limited by the presence of intestinal gas (A).

Incorrect:

CT scan (B) is often the first imaging modality used in the diagnosis of pancreatic cancer. Other techniques that can help confirm the diagnosis include endoscopic ultrasound (C), MRI (D), and PET.

Ionizing Radiation

188 to 191. Matching Questions

188. **Correct: C. 3 years**

189. **Correct: A. no radiation**

190. **Correct: A. no radiation**

191. **Correct: B. 62 to 88 days**

When selecting a type of imaging study, the procedure with the lowest possible radiation exposure should be considered. Ultrasound and MRI do not expose the patient to any radiation. CT scans use the highest amount of radiation exposure, while x-rays are associated with moderate levels of exposure.

Genitourinary System, Reproductive System, and Gender-Related Health Care

9

Family Planning

Overview

Even with the availability of numerous methods of highly reliable contraception, nearly half of all pregnancies in the United States are unplanned. Rates of continued contraception use vary greatly according to the method. Helping adults choose an acceptable form of family planning is an important part of providing health care.

CONTRACEPTIVE OPTIONS FOR WOMEN

The U.S. Medical Eligibility Criteria for Contraceptive Use (U.S. MEC) was created to decrease the number of unintended pregnancies by removing unnecessary barriers in accessing and using contraceptives. The U.S. MEC includes recommendations for the use of specific contraceptive methods by women who have certain characteristics or health issues. When counseling women, men, and couples about contraceptive method choice, the U.S. MEC can be used to identify safe and effective contraceptive choices, above and beyond barrier methods, for nearly all women. U.S. MEC categories are as follows:

- Category 1: No restrictions on the use of the contraceptive method
- Category 2: Advantages outweigh risk
- Category 3: Exercise caution: Theoretical or proven risks usually outweigh benefit
- Category 4: Use represents unacceptable health risk

Combined Hormonal Contraceptives

Combined hormonal contraceptives (CHCs) have been available for more than five decades and used by millions of women worldwide. Examples include the standard combined oral contraceptive (COC), the patch (e.g., Ortho Evra®, Xulane®), and the vaginal ring (NuvaRing®).

CHCs achieve contraceptive effect via the progestin and estrogenic components. Progestin effects help to inhibit ovulation by suppressing luteinizing hormone (LH), thickening the endocervical mucus, and thinning the endometrium. Through estrogenic effects, ovulation is inhibited by suppression of follicle-stimulating hormone (FSH) and LH and alteration of endometrial cellular structure.

When the COC, ring, or patch is discontinued, fertility usually returns promptly. Contrary to common belief, there is no need to delay conception after discontinuing these contraceptive forms; prolonged CHC use is not associated with future infertility or other health problems.

Noncontraceptive benefits of CHCs include lower rates of benign breast tumors and dysmenorrhea. Menstrual volume is reduced by about 60%, resulting in decreased rates of iron-deficiency anemia. Decreased rates of endometrial, ovarian, and colon cancers are particularly noted among long-term users (more than 5 years). Decreased rates of acne, hirsutism, and ovarian cyst, as well as reduction in premenstrual syndrome and improvement in rheumatoid arthritis symptoms are also noted among CHC users. Improvement in acne is usually noted after about 3 months of use, whereas improvement in hirsutism usually takes about 6 months. This is likely associated with a reduction in free androgens and increase in the level of sex hormone-binding globulin (SHBG) with CHC use. These improvements persist while the woman is taking the CHC and are usually reversible when the CHC is discontinued. CHCs are also a highly effective family planning option for a wide variety of women with chronic health problems (Table 9-1).

In part because of the endometrial thinning, COCs can be safely used for an extended time (e.g., 91-day extended cycle) with withdrawal bleeding occurring every 3 months, which is an attractive option for a woman who does not wish to menstruate or who has a health problem that is exacerbated by menstruation, such as premenstrual syndrome, menstrual migraine, and dysmenorrhea. Similarly, continuous use of the patch or ring (rather than removal during week 4) will eliminate monthly withdrawal bleeding. Although CHCs are not protective against sexually transmitted infections (STIs), CHC users have a decreased frequency of pelvic

TABLE 9-1 Summary of the U.S. Medical Eligibility Criteria (U.S. MEC) for Contraception Use: Precautions for Use of Combined Hormonal Contraceptives*

Combined hormonal contraceptives (CHCs) include low-dose (less than 35 mg ethinyl estradiol [EE]) combined oral contraceptives (COCs), combined hormonal patch (Xulane®, Ortho Evra®, CombiPatch®), and combined vaginal ring (NuvaRing®, Annovera™): summary of U.S. MEC for contraceptive use

CATEGORY 4: USE REPRESENTS UNACCEPTABLE HEALTH RISK

- Breast cancer (current)
- Postpartum less than 21 days (with or without breastfeeding)
- Acute hepatitis
- Hepatic adenoma
- Migraine with aura
- Major surgery with prolonged immobilization
- Age ≥35 and smoking ≥15 cigarettes per day
- Hypertension (≥160/≥100 mm Hg or with vascular disease)
- History of DVT/PE and ≥one risk factor for recurrent DVT/PE
- Known thrombotic mutations (factor V Leiden, prothrombin mutations, protein S, C, or antithrombin deficiency)
- History of ischemic heart disease or stroke
- Moderate or severely impaired cardiac function (NYHA Functional Class III or IV)

CATEGORY 3: EXERCISE CAUTION: THEORETICAL OR PROVEN RISKS USUALLY OUTWEIGH BENEFIT

- 21 to 42 days postpartum (with or without breastfeeding), with other risk factors for VTE (such as age ≥35 years, previous VTE, thrombophilia, immobility, transfusion at delivery, BMI ≥30 mg/kg², postpartum hemorrhage, postcesarean delivery, preeclampsia, or smoking)
- Breastfeeding and 21 to 30 days without other risk factors for VTE
- Multiple risk factors for atherosclerotic CV disease (e.g., older age, smoking, diabetes, hypertension, low HDL, high LDL, or high triglyceride level)
- History of DVT/PE and no risk factor for recurrent DVT/PE
- Age ≥35 and smoking less than 15 cigarettes per day
- History breast cancer but no recurrence in past 5 years
- Interacting drugs (select antiepileptics such as phenytoin, carbamazepine, topiramate)
- Gallbladder disease (current or medically treated, but not after cholecystectomy
- DM type 1 or type 2 >20 years' duration or with vascular disease
- Hypertension adequately controlled without vascular disease
- Hypertension (systolic 140 to 159 mm Hg or diastolic 90 to 99 mm Hg)
- Bariatric surgery with malabsorptive procedures (i.e., gastric bypass) for COC only
- Rifampin or rifabutin therapy

CATEGORY 2: ADVANTAGES OUTWEIGH RISK

- Age ≤40
- Breastfeeding and 30 to 42 days postpartum, without risk factors for VTE
- Greater than 42 days postpartum with breastfeeding
- 21 to 42 days postpartum without breastfeeding and without other risk factors for VTE
- Cigarette smoking and age less than 35 years
- DM type 1 or type 2 without vascular disease
- Major surgery without prolonged immobilization
- Sickle cell disease
- History of high blood pressure during pregnancy
- Unexplained vaginal bleeding
- Undiagnosed breast mass
- Cervical cancer
- BMI ≥30 kg/m²
- Menarche to younger than 18 years and BMI ≥30 kg/m²
- Migraine without aura
- Asymptomatic gallbladder disease

CATEGORY 1: NO RESTRICTION

- Age menarche up to age 40 years
- Nulliparous or parous
- Postpartum greater than 42 days without breastfeeding
- Postabortion (first or second trimester, immediate postseptic abortion)
- Past ectopic pregnancy
- History of pelvic surgery
- Varicose veins
- Nonmigraine headache (mild or severe)
- PID, STI history
- HIV
- Benign breast disease
- Family history breast cancer
- Cervical ectropion
- Uterine fibroids
- Thyroid disease
- Depressive disorders
- Minor surgery without immobilization
- Heavy or prolonged menses
- Irregular menses
- History gestational DM
- Ovarian or endometrial cancer
- Bariatric surgery with restrictive procedure (i.e., laparoscopic band or gastric sleeve procedure)
- Broad-spectrum antimicrobial and antifungal use

BMI, body mass index; CHC, combined hormonal contraceptives; COC, combined oral contraceptive; DM, diabetes mellitus; DVT, deep vein thrombosis; HDL, high-density lipoprotein; LDL, low-density lipoprotein; PE, pulmonary embolism; PID, pelvic inflammatory disease; STI, sexually transmitted infection.

*Not a complete list.

Source: Centers for Disease Control and Prevention. United States Medical Eligibility Criteria (USMEC) for contraception use, 2016. MMWR. 2016;65(3):1–103. http://www.cdc.gov /reproductivehealth/contraception/usmec.htm

inflammatory disease (PID), which results from thickened endocervical mucus; this results in a lower rate of future ectopic pregnancy.

Combined Hormonal Contraceptive Adverse Effects

The highest dropout rates with CHCs are in the first 3 months of use. The most frequently mentioned reasons are breakthrough bleeding (BTB); with COC, inconvenience of use is often mentioned as well. Although BTB is bothersome, it is not harmful and does not indicate lesser contraceptive benefit. Compared with COC use, BTB rates with the use of the contraceptive ring and patch are usually lower after the first few weeks. This difference is largely due to the fact that the patch and ring do not require a daily action on the user's part, and adherence is significantly better. Therefore, the patch and ring can be preferable for women who are not as diligent in taking a pill every day. The patch and ring also provide a more consistent hormone dose than COCs, which can result in fewer systemic adverse effects (e.g., headaches, breast tenderness). With COC use, BTB can be minimized by taking the medication within the same 4-hour period every day. Cigarette smoking increases the likelihood of BTB and should be discouraged. The BTB rate increases dramatically with missed doses of the pill. Advice about what to do in the event of missed pills is an important part of providing contraceptive care (Table 9-2).

Nausea with COC, patch, ring, and hormone therapy (HT) is a commonly reported adverse effect. Nausea is usually a transient problem noted in the first months of use and can be minimized by taking the medication with food or at bedtime. If vomiting occurs within 2 hours of taking COC, the dose should be retaken.

CHC hormones interact with a few drugs. Interaction is noted, however, with many antiepileptic drugs (AEDs), including phenytoin, carbamazepine, topiramate, and primidone, as well as herbal products containing St. John's wort, potentially causing a reduction in the effectiveness of CHCs. Alternative methods should be encouraged, or if a COC is chosen, a preparation containing a minimum of 30 mcg ethinyl estradiol should be used. The BTB rate is greater in women using COC, patch, and ring concomitantly with an AED partly because of more rapid metabolism of estrogen.

> **CLINICAL CONCEPT**
>
> With appropriate use, CHC use usually results in fewer than 1 pregnancy per 100 women with perfect use during the first year, and 9 pregnancies per 100 women with typical use in the first year.

TABLE 9-2 Missed Combined Oral Contraceptive Pill Advice

MISSED PILL SITUATION	REQUIRED ACTION	COMMENT
If pill missed within 12 hours of the time that should have been taken	Take today's pills immediately.	No additional or emergency contraception needed; continue with the rest of the pack
If one pill missed for more than 12 hours but only one pill missed in a day	Take today's pills immediately.	No additional or emergency contraception needed; continue with the rest of the pack
If more than one pill missed	Take today's pill and the last forgotten pill today (two tablets in 1 day). If she has at least seven active pills in the pack, she has two options: 1. Take the rest of the active pills, skip the placebo pills, and start the next pack of pills without interruption, and use condoms or abstain for 7 days. *or* 2. Take the pills as in the pack and use condoms or abstinence until she has taken seven of the pills in the pack.	Encourage use of emergency contraception if she has had unprotected heterosexual intercourse in the prior 7 days

Source: Nelson AL, Cwiak C. Combined oral contraceptives (COCs). In: Hatcher RA, Trussell J, Nelson AL, Cates W, Kowal D, Policar MS, eds. Contraceptive Technology. 21st ed. Atlanta, GA: Managing Contraception; 2018.

COCs should also be used with caution in patients who have undergone certain types of bariatric surgery for weight loss. Restrictive-malabsorptive procedures, such as the Roux-en-Y gastric bypass, surgically limits the size of the stomach as well as bypasses a significant portion of the duodenum, thus intentionally creating a malabsorptive state. This will decrease the ability of the gut to absorb hormones from COCs, which can decrease contraceptive effectiveness. Restrictive procedures, such as gastric sleeve and gastric band surgery, do not interfere with the absorptive capacity of the gut and will not decrease the effectiveness of COCs.

The progestins used in most COC, patch, and ring formulations are testosterone derivatives. Drospirenone, found in the COC products Yasmin® and Yaz®, is an analogue of an aldosterone antagonist and has potassium-sparing qualities. Drospirenone should be used with caution in those with hepatic or renal dysfunction or with concomitant use of angiotensin receptor blocker, angiotensin-converting enzyme inhibitor, salt substitute, or a potassium-sparing diuretic.

Progestin-Only Pills, DMPA (Depo-Provera)

Progestin-only pills (POPs)/DMPA use offers certain advantages when compared with CHCs. These methods can provide an option for women who cannot take an estrogen-containing contraceptive because of chronic medical conditions, such as women with multiple risk factors for atherosclerotic cardiovascular disease, vascular disease, prolonged history of diabetes (greater than 20 years), or history of migraine with aura.

> **CLINICAL CONCEPT**
>
> POPs/DMPA do not alter the quality or quantity of breast milk and so can be a helpful option for nursing mothers.

One disadvantage with POP use is bleeding irregularity, ranging from prolonged flow to amenorrhea. With failure rates of up to 13% when used in a woman who is not breastfeeding, the POP is a less effective contraceptive than COC, but the nausea rate with its use is significantly lower than with COC use because of the lack of estrogen. POPs are taken daily, a schedule many women find more convenient than the typical 3-weeks-on/1-week-off schedule that is the classic way of taking COCs. As POP use inconsistently suppresses ovulation, this form of contraception likely works through thickening of the endocervical mucus and through the alteration of the endometrium.

DMPA (Depo-Provera®), given every 90 days by injection, is a highly reliable form of contraception (99.7% efficacy). DMPA is best suited for women who do not wish a pregnancy for at least 18 months, because resumption of fertility is frequently delayed 6 to 12 months after its discontinuation. When the injection is given within the first few days of menses, the contraceptive effect is immediate. When it is started 5 days after the onset of menses, a backup method of contraception should be used for 1 week. After 1 year of DMPA use, 30% to 50% of women have amenorrhea. DMPA is associated with weight gain, with an average of about 11 pounds (5 kg) over 3 years of use. According to observations from limited study, bone density is occasionally noted to be reduced in women using DMPA. This condition is largely reversible, however, when the medication is discontinued. The U.S. Food and Drug Administration (FDA) has assigned a boxed warning to DMPA, highlighting that prolonged use can result in the loss of bone density and recommending that the medication not be used for more than 2 years unless other methods cannot be used; bone density seems to normalize quickly with discontinuation of the medication. Calcium supplementation, at 1,000 to 1,500 mg/day, weight-bearing exercise, and vitamin D supplementation should be recommended; this advice is helpful for general bone health. Irregular bleeding is a common problem during the first few months of DMPA injection use but can be managed with a prostaglandin inhibitor or estrogen supplement (Table 9-3).

A self-injected formulation of DMPA (Depo-subQ Provera 104®) allows home-based administration of DMPA via a subcutaneous injection every 3 months using a prefilled, single-use syringe. Though this formulation contains only 70% of the active ingredient compared with the intramuscular (IM) formulation, effectiveness is unchanged.

Long-Acting Reversible Contraception

Long-acting reversible contraception (LARC), which includes intrauterine devices (IUDs) and progestin implants, is safe and effective for use in most women and provides highly effective contraception that does not depend, once inserted, on patient action. LARC forms are considered a preferred contraceptive option for many women, including adolescents, who are typically not considering pregnancy in the near future, given their protracted duration of activity, ranging from 3 to 10 or more years.

An etonogestrel-containing subdermal implant (Nexplanon®) is a LARC form that consists of a single rod inserted in the upper arm by a qualified health-care provider. The progestin released from the rod provides effective contraception (greater than 99%) for up to 3 years, thus making this a convenient

TABLE 9-3 Resolution of Common Adverse Effects of Hormonal Contraceptives

ADVERSE EFFECT (TYPE OF CONTRACEPTION)	COMMENTS/MANAGEMENT APPROACHES
Nausea (COCs)	Usually transient and resolves in the first months; consider taking COC with food or at bedtime.
Irregular bleeding (DMPA, LNG-IUD, Nexplanon®)	More common during the first few months of use. Minimized by the use of a prostaglandin inhibitor such as ibuprofen, 400 mg tid, or naproxen sodium, 375 to 540 mg bid, for 3 to 5 days. Estrogen supplements, such as a 0.1-mg estrogen patch used for 7 to 10 days, can also be helpful but are seldom needed.
Breakthrough bleeding (COCs, POPs)	Bothersome but not harmful. Minimized by taking pill within same 4-hour period each day; discourage cigarette smoking.
Loss of bone density (DMPA)	Possible with prolonged use (greater than 2 years). Calcium supplementation, at 1,000 to 1,500 mg/day, weight-bearing exercise, and vitamin D supplementation recommended.

COC, combined oral contraceptive; LNG-IUD, levonorgestrel-releasing intrauterine device; POP, progestin-only pill.

option for women who seek long-term contraception without a need for daily pills. Ovulation returns soon after removal of the rod (within 7 days). Nexplanon® is radiopaque and visible on x-ray, which can facilitate rod removal. Common adverse effects include irregular bleeding patterns and headache (see Table 9-3). As with the other progestin-based hormonal contraceptive option, the implant is acceptable (U.S. MEC 1 or 2) for use in women with a variety of health problems, including known thrombophilia (U.S. MEC 2).

IUDs offer a highly effective contraceptive form. Unfortunately, there are occasionally incorrect perceptions among patients and health-care providers that relatively few women can safely use these methods (Table 9-4). In reality, IUDs are U.S. MEC 1 or 2 for most women.

The Cu-IUD ParaGard® (Copper T 380A) is an effective LARC form with a failure rate of 0.5% to 2.2%. The mechanism of this contraceptive action is not entirely understood, but it is unlikely that its action is as an abortifacient. With a copper-containing IUD (Cu-IUD), there is often an increase in menstrual bleeding and upper reproductive tract infection. A Cu-IUD can be left in place for up to 10 years.

Mirena®, Skyla®, and Liletta® are examples of levonorgestrel-releasing IUDs (LNG-IUDs). LNG is a progestin form that helps produce marked reversible endometrial thinning. About 50% of LNG-IUD users are amenorrheic at the end of 2 years of use. Thickened endocervical mucus is also noted, which limits the ascent of infection into the upper reproductive tract and minimizes PID risk. Skyla® is effective for 3 years, Liletta® can be used for 4 years, and Mirena® is effective for 5 years.

CLINICAL CONCEPT
LNG-IUD is a particularly helpful method of contraception for women with menorrhagia.

NONHORMONAL CONTRACEPTIVE METHODS

For those who prefer to avoid hormonal contraceptives or cannot use hormonal contraception for health conditions, several nonhormonal options are available. Some of these approaches can also be effective in preventing STI acquisition and transmission. The effectiveness of these approaches typically depends on adherence by the user and, thus, is generally lower than that of hormonal contraceptives. Fortunately, nonhormonal contraceptives are easily accessible, with many sold over the counter (OTC), and there is virtually no limitation on use.

TABLE 9-4 Summary of the U.S. Medical Eligibility Criteria (U.S. MEC) for Contraception Use: Precautions for the Use of Intrauterine Devices

Summary of classification for use of intrauterine devices, including levonorgestrel-releasing intrauterine device (LNG-IUD; Mirena®, Skyla®, others) and copper-containing intrauterine device (Cu-IUD; Paragard®)*

CATEGORY 4: USE REPRESENTS UNACCEPTABLE HEALTH RISK	CATEGORY 3: EXERCISE CAUTION: THEORETICAL OR PROVEN RISK USUALLY OUTWEIGH BENEFIT	CATEGORY 2: ADVANTAGES OUTWEIGH RISK	CATEGORY 1: NO RESTRICTION
■ Pregnancy	■ Cirrhosis with severe decompensation (LNG-IUD)	■ Immediately after second-trimester therapeutic abortion	■ Age ≥20 years
■ Current PID	■ Severe thrombocytopenia (Cu-IUD)	■ High risk for HIV	■ Immediately after first-trimester therapeutic abortion
■ Current purulent cervicitis or chlamydia infection or gonorrhea	■ Positive antiphospholipids (LNG-IUS)	■ HIV infection (not clinically well or not receiving ARV therapy)	■ Parous
■ Unexplained vaginal bleeding		■ Age less than 20 years	■ Smoking (any age, any amount)
■ Cervical cancer, awaiting treatment		■ Nulliparous	■ Hypertension
■ Distorted uterine cavity		■ Vascular disease (LNG-IUD)	■ Vascular disease (Cu-IUD)
		■ Severe dysmenorrhea (Cu-IUD)	■ Uncomplicated or complicated valvular heart disease
		■ Cervical intraepithelial neoplasia (LNG-IUD)	■ Headaches (nonmigraine or migraine)
		■ Uterine fibroids	■ Cervical intraepithelial neoplasia (Cu-IUD)
		■ Severe thrombocytopenia (LNG-IUD)	■ Postpartum greater than 4 weeks

*Not a complete list.

Source: Centers for Disease Control and Prevention. United States Medical Eligibility Criteria (US MEC) for contraception use, 2016. 2016;MMWR 65(3):1–103. https://www.cdc.gov/reproductivehealth/contraception/usmec.htm.

The diaphragm (KoroFlex®), a barrier method of contraception, is placed in the vagina before intercourse. This device, which has an effectiveness rate of 88% to 94%, should be used in conjunction with a spermicide and removed no sooner than 6 hours after coitus. When properly fitted and in the appropriate position, the diaphragm should rest snugly in the vagina but without tension against the vaginal walls. When properly fitted, the woman and her partner should be unaware of the diaphragm's presence. If either partner can feel the diaphragm, the device is either the wrong size or not properly inserted. The failure rate of the diaphragm is about 20% and does not protect against STIs. Because a diaphragm should always be used with a spermicide, a woman with a history of recurrent urinary tract infection (UTI) is not an ideal candidate for diaphragm use. Although the thought behind this long-held advice is that the diaphragm increases UTI risk as a result of potential pressure on the woman's lower urinary tract, the risk more likely arises from the concurrent use of a spermicide.

Spermicides are available in various forms, including creams, jellies, foams, films, and vaginal suppositories. A woman who is exposed to the spermicide nonoxynol-9, either through vaginal use or with a male partner who uses condoms with this spermicide, is likely at increased risk of UTI. The proposed mechanism of this risk is the antibacterial effect of the spermicide, which reduces lactobacilli, a normal component of the periurethral flora. Lactobacilli produce hydrogen peroxide and lactic acid, providing the periurethral area and vagina with a pH that inhibits bacterial growth and blocks potential sites of attachment and is toxic to uropathogens. Spermicides do not protect against STIs and have a high failure rate when used alone (up to 30%).

Similar to a diaphragm, the cervical cap (FemCap) is a barrier method in which a flexible cap is placed over the cervix. The cap must be fitted and prescribed by a trained health-care provider. The cap is inserted prior to intercourse and should remain in place for at least 6 hours with a spermicide but no longer than 48 hours. The cap should not be used during menstruation due to a risk of toxic shock syndrome. There is a 20% to 40% failure rate, and this method does not protect against STIs.

A contraceptive sponge (Today® Sponge) is a barrier method to prevent conception but does not protect against STIs. These are available OTC without a prescription and consist of a foam-like insert embedded with spermicide that is inserted up to 24 hours prior to intercourse. These should remain in place for at least 6 hours after intercourse but be removed no longer than 30 hours after coitus. The sponge should not be used during menstruation due to risk of toxic shock syndrome. The failure rate can range from 20% to 40%.

Male and female condoms can offer an effective barrier method for contraception as well as protection against STIs if used correctly. Male condoms are generally inexpensive and easy to obtain, though there is a 15% to 20% contraceptive failure rate. A female condom, which consists of a thin lining that goes in the vagina to protect the uterus from sperm, can be placed up to 8 hours prior to intercourse. Female condoms (FC2® Female Condom) are available OTC. These are associated with a 20% failure rate and should not be used together with a male condom as this can cause tearing. A spermicide can be used to increase effectiveness with male and female condoms.

Discussion Sources

Bartz D, Goldberg AB. Injectable contraceptives. In: Hatcher RA, Trussell J, Nelson AL, Cates W, Kowal D, Policar MS, eds. *Contraceptive Technology*. 21st ed. Atlanta, GA: Managing Contraception; 2018.

Cates W, Harwood B. Vaginal barriers and spermicides. In: Hatcher RA, Trussell J, Nelson AL, Cates W, Kowal D, Policar MS, eds. *Contraceptive Technology*. 21st ed. Atlanta, GA: Managing Contraception; 2018.

Centers for Disease Control and Prevention. U.S. Medical Eligibility Criteria (U.S. MEC) for contraception use, 2016. *MMWR*. 2016;65(3):1–103. http://www.cdc.gov/reproductivehealth/contraception/usmec.htm

Dean G, Bimla Schwarz E. Intrauterine contraceptives (IUCs). In: Hatcher RA, Trussell J, Nelson AL, Cates W, Kowal D, Policar MS, eds. *Contraceptive Technology*. 21st ed. Atlanta, GA: Managing Contraception; 2018.

Nelson AL, Cwiak C. Combined oral contraceptives (COCs). In: Hatcher RA, Trussell J, Nelson AL, Cates Jr W, Kowal D, Policar MS, eds. *Contraceptive Technology*. 21st ed. Atlanta, GA: Managing Contraception; 2018.

Raymond EG. Progestin-only pills. In: Hatcher RA, Trussell J, Nelson AL, Cates W, Kowal D, Policar MS, eds. *Contraceptive Technology*. 21st ed. Atlanta, GA: Managing Contraception; 2018.

Trussell J, Guthrie KA. Choosing a contraceptive: efficacy, safety, and personal considerations. In: Hatcher RA, Trussell J, Nelson AL, Cates W, Kowal D, Policar MS, eds. *Contraceptive Technology*. 21st ed. Atlanta, GA: Managing Contraception; 2018.

QUESTIONS

1. Which of the following is a U.S. MEC category 4 (use represents unacceptable health risk) to the use of a CHC method (COC, patch [Ortho Evra®, Xulane®], or ring [NuvaRing®])?

   A. mother with a history of breast cancer

   B. personal history of hepatitis A at age 10 years

   C. presence of factor V Leiden mutation

   D. cigarette smoking one pack per day in a 22-year-old

2. A 22-year-old woman taking a 35-mcg ethinyl estradiol COC calls after forgetting to take her pills for 2 consecutive days. She is 2 weeks into the pack. You advise her to:

   A. take the last pill missed immediately and continue taking the remaining pills at the usual time, even if this means taking two pills today.

   B. discard two pills and take two pills today.

   C. discard the rest of the pack and start a new pack with the first day of her next menses.

   D. continue taking one pill daily for the rest of the cycle.

3. When counseling a woman about CHC use, you advise that:

   A. long-term use of any CHC is discouraged because the body needs a "rest" from CHC from time to time.

   B. fertility is often delayed for many months after CHC discontinuation.

   C. there is an increase in the rate of breast cancer after 3 years of CHC use.

   D. premenstrual syndrome symptoms are often improved with use of CHCs.

4. Noncontraceptive benefits of CHC use include a decrease in all of the following except:

   A. iron-deficiency anemia.

   B. PID.

    C. cervicitis.

    D. ovarian cancer.

5. Which of the following women is the best candidate for POP use?

    A. an 18-year-old woman who frequently forgets to take prescribed medications

    B. a 28-year-old woman with multiple sexual partners who does not use condoms

    C. a 32-year-old woman with adequately controlled hypertension

    D. a 26-year-old woman who wants to use the pill to help "regulate" her menstrual cycle

6. The most common reasons for discontinuing COC use is BTB and:

    A. nausea/vomiting.

    B. inconvenience of use.

    C. cost.

    D. high failure rate.

7. A 38-year-old nulliparous woman who smokes two and a half packs a day is in an "on-and-off" relationship. The woman presents seeking contraception. Which of the following represents the most appropriate method?

    A. contraceptive ring (NuvaRing®)

    B. COC (Ortho Tri-Cyclen®)

    C. contraceptive patch (Xulane®)

    D. vaginal diaphragm with spermicide

8. An alternative to the contraceptive ring (NuvaRing®) or patch (Xulane®) should be considered in all of the following women due to an increased venous thromboembolism (VTE) risk except:

    A. a 42-year-old nulliparous woman with type 2 diabetes mellitus and high low-density lipoprotein (LDL).

    B. a 31-year-old woman with a history of naturally occurring multiple gestation pregnancy.

    C. a 33-year-old who smokes more than 15 cigarettes per day.

    D. a 33-year-old with a family history of venous thrombosis.

9. According to the U.S. MEC, which of the following is a clinical condition in which the use of a Cu-IUD should be approached with caution?

    A. uncomplicated valvular heart disease

    B. current PID

    C. hypertension

    D. dysmenorrhea

10. Which of the following is the most appropriate response to a 27-year-old woman who is taking phenytoin (Dilantin®) for the treatment of a seizure disorder and is requesting hormonal contraception?

    A. "A barrier method would be the preferable choice."

    B. "COC is the best option."

    C. "Depo-Provera® (medroxyprogesterone acetate in a depot injection [DMPA]) use will likely not interact with your seizure medication."

    D. "LNG-IUD use is contraindicated."

11. Which of the following is commonly found after 1 year of using DMPA (Depo-Provera®)?

    A. weight gain

    B. hypermenorrhea

C. acne

D. rapid return of fertility when discontinued

12 to 16. According to the U.S. MEC, indicate the appropriate U.S. MEC category (1, 2, 3, or 4) for each candidate for CHCs (i.e., COC, patch, or vaginal ring).

_____ **12.** a 37-year-old woman who smokes 10 cigarettes per day

_____ **13.** a 29-year-old woman with PID

_____ **14.** a 45-year-old woman with history of migraine with aura

_____ **15.** a 32-year-old woman breastfeeding a 6-month-old infant

_____ **16.** a 28-year-old woman with type 1 diabetes mellitus without vascular disease

17 to 20. According to the U.S. MEC, indicate the appropriate category (1, 2, 3, or 4) for each candidate for a Cu-IUD or LNG-IUD.

_____ **17.** a 45-year-old woman with fibroids with uterine cavity distortion

_____ **18.** a 33-year-old woman who smokes two packs per day

_____ **19.** a 25-year-old woman with adequately controlled hypertension

_____ **20.** a 33-year-old woman with family history of breast cancer in a second-degree relative

21. As you prescribe a COC containing the progestin drospirenone (Loryna™, Ocella®, Vestura®, Yasmin®, Yaz®), you offer the following advice:

A. "Always take this pill on a full stomach."

B. "You should not take acetaminophen when using this birth control pill."

C. "Avoid using potassium-containing salt substitutes."

D. "You will likely notice that premenstrual syndrome symptoms might become worse."

22. A 26-year-old mother who breastfeeds her 4-month-old child queries about hormonal contraceptives. In counseling her on the use of the POP, you mention all of the following except:

A. the pill is taken every day.

B. the POP is a more effective contraceptive than COC.

C. the POP does not alter the quality or quantity of breast milk.

D. the POP is associated with bleeding irregularity, ranging from prolonged flow to amenorrhea.

23. With the use of a LNG-IUD (Mirena®, Skyla®), a form of LARC, which one of the following is normally noted?

A. endometrial hyperplasia

B. hypermenorrhea

C. increase in PID rates

D. reduction in menstrual flow

24. The reduction in free androgens noted in a woman using a COC can yield an improvement in:

A. cycle control.

B. acne vulgaris.

C. breast tenderness.

D. rheumatoid arthritis.

25. With DMPA in depot injection (Depo-Provera®), the recommended length of use in younger women is usually:

A. less than 1 year.

B. no more than 2 years.

C. as long as the woman desires this form of contraception.

D. as determined by her lipid response to the medication.

26. Irregular bleeding associated with DMPA (Depo-Provera®) can be minimized with the regular use of all of the following except:

   A. acetaminophen.

   B. ibuprofen.

   C. naproxen sodium.

   D. estrogen supplements.

27. When can a woman safely conceive after discontinuing CHC or LARC use?

   A. immediately

   B. after 1 to 2 months

   C. after 3 to 4 months

   D. after 5 to 6 months

28. When prescribing the contraceptive patch (Xulane®) or vaginal ring (NuvaRing®), the nurse practitioner (NP) considers that:

   A. these are progestin-only products.

   B. candidates include women who have difficulty remembering to take a daily pill.

   C. there are significant drug interactions with both products.

   D. contraceptive efficacy is less than with COC.

29. When considering the use of etonogestrel subdermal implant (Nexplanon®) for contraception, the NP realizes that:

   A. insertion requires referral to an OB/GYN physician.

   B. this method provides effective contraception for up to 2 years.

   C. the use of this method is discouraged in women who are overweight or obese.

   D. this method is considered acceptable (U.S. MEC category 2) for select women with a history of thrombophilia forms.

30. Which of the following is false regarding the use of Nexplanon®?

   A. consists of a single rod

   B. fertility returns immediately after removal

   C. can be self-administered

   D. is visible on x-ray

31. When considering the use of self-administered DMPA (Depo-subQ®), the NP acknowledges all of the following except:

   A. a self-injection is given every 3 months.

   B. there is no risk of bone loss with long-term use of this DMPA formulation.

   C. it can be started immediately postpartum.

   D. it contains a smaller amount of active ingredient than the IM formulation.

32 to 34. Answer the following questions True or False.

   _____ **32.** The use of COC reduces menstrual volume by approximately 60%, thereby reducing the risk of iron-deficiency anemia.

   _____ **33.** Nausea with COC use can be minimized by taking the pill on an empty stomach.

   _____ **34.** Calcium and vitamin D supplementation is recommended for those taking DMPA (Depo-Provera®) injections to support bone density during its use.

35. Which of the following statements is true concerning vaginal diaphragm use?

A. When the device is in place, the woman is aware that the diaphragm fits snugly against the vaginal walls.

B. This is a suitable form of contraception for women with recurrent UTI.

C. After the device is inserted, the cervix should be smoothly covered.

D. The device should be removed within 2 hours of coitus to minimize the risk of infection.

36. By using a diaphragm with spermicide nonoxynol-9 for contraception, a woman is likely at increased risk for:

A. cervical stenosis.

B. UTI.

C. increased perivaginal lactobacilli colonization.

D. ovarian malignancy.

37. What is the expected rate of failure with the use of a male condom alone for contraception?

A. less than 1%

B. 5%

C. up to 10%

D. up to 20%

38. When used properly, which of the following barrier methods is most effective in preventing transmission and acquisition of STIs?

A. vaginal diaphragm with spermicide

B. contraceptive sponge

C. male condom

D. cervical cap

For answers and rationales, see end of chapter.

Emergency Contraception

Overview

As previously mentioned, nearly half of all pregnancies are unplanned. Emergency contraception (EC), used after coitus to minimize the risk of unintended pregnancy when a contraceptive method fails or is not used, is an effective method of minimizing the number of unintended pregnancies (Table 9-5). An estimated 640,000 annual pregnancy terminations could be avoided if knowledge of and access to EC were more widely available. Numerous methods are available, including the use of oral levonorgestrel (LNG), oral ulipristal acetate, and Cu-IUD.

> **CLINICAL CONCEPT**
> With all EC methods, menstrual bleeding should be expected within 3 to 4 weeks of using EC. If none occurs, a pregnancy test should be done.

HORMONAL EMERGENCY CONTRACEPTION OPTIONS

Oral hormonal agents, such as LNG and ulipristal, are highly effective EC options, reducing the risk of pregnancy by 75% or more, according to the following model: if 100 fertile women have unprotected heterosexual intercourse in the second to third weeks of their cycles, eight typically become pregnant. One or two typically become pregnant when using EC. Efficacy of LNG EC is reduced obesity.

The most likely mechanism of action to reduce pregnancy risk with LNG is by inhibiting or delaying ovulation or impairing ovum or sperm transport; LNG EC is unlikely to prevent pregnancy by impeding the implantation of a fertilized ovum. Progestin-only EC (e.g., Plan B®, Plan B One-Step®, Next Choice®, Next Choice One Dose®, others) includes LNG 1.5 mg total dose, optimally taken within 72 hours of unprotected coitus but can be effective up to 120 hours postintercourse. Single-pill, single-dose options are most popular. These products are available as OTC medication, regardless of the age or gender of the purchaser.

TABLE 9-5 Emergency Hormonal Contraception: Indications and Mechanism of Action

CANDIDATES FOR EMERGENCY CONTRACEPTION

Any time unprotected heterosexual intercourse occurs including potential method failure (e.g., late for or missed pills, late for DMPA, dislodged or misplaced diaphragm, condom break or slippage, expelled intrauterine device)

EMERGENCY CONTRACEPTION MECHANISM OF ACTION WITH LEVONORGESTREL (PLAN B®, PLAN B ONE STEP®, NEXT CHOICE®) OR ULIPRISTAL (ELLA®) USE

Depending on time taken during menstrual cycle

- Inhibit or delay ovulation (most likely effect)
- Inhibit tubal transport of egg or sperm
- Interfere with fertilization
- Possible effect on endometrium:
  - With levonorgestrel use as emergency contraception, minimal to no alteration to endometrium; therefore, unlikely to inhibit implantation of a fertilized egg.
  - With ulipristal use as emergency contraception, changes in the endometrium can potentially alter likelihood of fertilized egg implantation.
- Emergency hormonal contraception use results in minimal to no alteration to endometrium and is unlikely to inhibit implantation of a fertilized egg

EMERGENCY CONTRACEPTION MECHANISM OF ACTION WITH COPPER-CONTAINING INTRAUTERINE DEVICE (PARAGARD®)

- Mechanism of action not completely understood
- Insert within 5 days after unprotected intercourse
- Provides ongoing contraception when left in place
- When used as emergency contraception, unlikely to work as an abortifacient

Source: Trussell J, Bimla Schwarz E. Emergency contraception. In: Hatcher RA, Trussell J, Nelson AL, Cates W, Kowal D, Policar MS, eds. Contraceptive Technology. 21st ed. Atlanta, GA: Managing Contraception; 2018.

An alternative to progestin-only EC is ulipristal acetate (ella®). This product works as a progesterone agonist/antagonist and thus has a direct inhibitory effect on follicular development and ovum release. In contrast with LNG, ulipristal remains effective when administered immediately before ovulation around the time of LH surge. Ulipristal is approved for use up to 5 days (120 hours) after unprotected sexual intercourse. Endometrial alterations associated with ulipristal use could impact embryo implantation. This option is only available through a prescription and is administered as one tablet (though a repeat dose should be taken if vomiting occurs within 3 hours of the dose).

Use of all oral hormonal EC will not interrupt an established pregnancy or increase risk of early pregnancy loss. If pregnancy does occur, use of this therapeutic method does not appear to be teratogenic.

Emergency Contraception with Copper-Containing Intrauterine Device

A Cu-IUD such as the ParaGard® (Copper T 380A) can be inserted within 5 days after intercourse as a form of EC. Because of the risk of upper reproductive tract infections, use of a Cu-IUD is contraindicated in the presence of STI and should be avoided in women with a history of cervicitis. In addition to providing ongoing contraception, Cu-IUD insertion provides a hormone-free EC option.

Discussion Sources

Centers for Disease Control and Prevention. US Medical Eligibility Criteria (USMEC) for contraceptive use, 2016. *MMWR.* 2016;65(3):1–103. http://www.cdc.gov/reproductivehealth/contraception/usmec.htm

Office of Population Research at Princeton University. Emergency Contraception, 2019. http://ec.princeton.edu

Trussell J, Bimla Schwarz E. Emergency contraception. In: Hatcher RA, Trussell J, Nelson AL, Cates W, Kowal D, Policar MS, eds. *Contraceptive Technology.* 21st ed. Atlanta, GA: Managing Contraception; 2018.

QUESTIONS

39. An 18-year-old woman requests EC after having unprotected vaginal intercourse approximately 18 hours ago. Today is day 12 of her normal 27- to 29-day menstrual cycle, and she has no contraindications to the use of any currently available forms of EC. You advise her that:

   A. emergency hormonal contraception use reduces the risk of pregnancy by approximately 33%.

   B. all forms of EC must be used within 12 hours after unprotected intercourse.

   C. the likelihood of conception is minimal.

   D. insertion of a Cu-IUD offers an effective form of emergency and ongoing contraception.

40. Which of the following is likely not among the proposed mechanisms of action of all forms of oral EC?

   A. inhibits ovulation

   B. acts as an abortifacient

   C. slows sperm transport

   D. slows ovum transport

41. A 24-year-old woman who requests EC in oral form wants to know the effects if pregnancy does occur. You respond that:

   A. there is an increased risk of spontaneous abortion.

   B. a distinct pattern of congenital health issues has been noted in the offspring of women who have used all forms of hormonal EC.

   C. placental abruption in the third trimester is noted more often in women who used hormonal EC.

   D. there appears to be no correlation with EC and problematic outcomes if pregnancy occurs.

42. In contrast to progestin-only EC, a possible additional mechanism of action of ulipristal (ella®) is:

   A. inhibiting fertilized egg implantation.

   B. impairing sperm transport.

   C. through inducing abortion.

   D. impairing ovum transport.

43. You see a 34-year-old woman who reports having unprotected sexual intercourse 5 days ago and requests EC. She has a current history of mucopurulent cervicitis. The most acceptable and effective option in this clinical scenario is:

   A. progestin-only EC.

   B. ulipristal.

   C. Cu-IUD.

   D. none as 5 days is beyond the limit of EC effectiveness.

44. Concerning EC, which of the following statements is false?

   A. Progestin-only EC can be taken as one or two doses.

   B. Ulipristal is available by prescription only.

   C. Progestin-only EC is usually available without prescription.

   D. Ulipristal is taken in two doses, 12 hours apart.

45. A woman who has used any form of EC should be advised that if she does not have a normal menstrual period within _____ weeks, a pregnancy test should be obtained.

   A. 1 to 2

   B. 2 to 3

   C. 3 to 4

   D. 4 to 5

For answers and rationales, see end of chapter.

Menopause

Overview

A woman's life is characterized by a series of shifts: first, a woman transitions to the reproductive years, then to the premenopausal period, and then to the menopausal and postmenopausal years. Each transition is normal, expected, and not a disease state. Perimenopause and menopause are often symptom-producing events, however.

> **CLINICAL CONCEPT**
>
> Perimenopause lasts an average of 4 years but can range from a few months to 10 years.

Perimenopause is the time surrounding menopause; its onset is marked by the beginning symptoms of menopause and ends with the cessation of menses. The average age of onset of perimenopause is 40 to 45 years; this occurs earlier in women who are cigarette smokers.

Menopause, when the final menstrual period occurs, marks another transition in a woman's reproductive life. By definition, a woman is in menopause when she has had no naturally occurring menstrual period for 12 months. The average age for a North American woman at menopause is 51.3 years, with many women living one-third of their lives after this time. Approximately 60% of women will consult a health-care provider regarding perimenopausal and menopausal symptoms.

Clinical Presentation

During perimenopause, menstrual irregularity is common, with the interval between periods becoming longer or shorter and flow becoming altered, either heavier or lighter. Ovulation becomes more erratic, but pregnancy is still possible. Hot flashes and sleep problems are usually worse in the week before the menses and are reported by approximately 65% to 75% of women during perimenopause. As mentioned, the woman often notes hot flashes or flushes during the week before the onset of the menses, a time when hormonal shifts are most dramatic. Because most women associate menopause symptoms with irregular or absent menstrual bleeding, these perimenopausal symptoms can be confusing as the woman is menstruating on a regular basis. Although low estrogen levels have often been thought to be the cause of perimenopausal symptoms, usually levels are normal. The shifting levels of multiple biological substances, including elevated FSH, are likely implicated.

As the menopausal period progresses, LH and FSH levels increase dramatically as the anterior lobe of the pituitary sends out an abundance of these substances in an attempt to induce ovulation; the ovaries fail to respond with ovulation, sometimes leading to heavy, anovulatory menstrual bleeding. Levels of estrogen forms (estradiol, estrogen) and androgens (testosterone, progesterone, androsterone, and dehydroepiandrosterone) are reduced. Hot flashes now usually become more frequent and severe, in part induced by the FSH surge. About 80% of women going through menopause have hot flashes, ranging in severity from mildly bothersome to debilitating.

Estrogen receptors are found in high concentrations in the vulva, vagina, urethra, and trigone of the bladder. As a result, symptoms of urogenital atrophy from estrogen shifts are a common perimenopausal and menopausal problem. These receptors are found in lower concentrations in the vascular bed, heart, brain, bone, and eye—areas of the body that also exhibit changes during perimenopause and menopause.

Vasomotor symptoms can be debilitating, causing disturbed sleep, avoidance of social situations in which hot flashes occur, and numerous other problems. Compared with naturally occurring menopause, women with surgical menopause usually have more severe symptoms, likely because the hormonal shifts are more rapid and dramatic.

Diagnostic Testing

An evaluation for menopause should be tailored to the individual woman and include medical, social, and family history as well as a review of symptoms. Hormone measurements are not routinely recommended as changes to the menstrual cycle are the best predictor of menopause stage. Evaluation of FSH and anti-müllerian hormone (AMH) can be considered if menopausal symptoms are atypical or are occurring at an early age. Abnormal bleeding should also be carefully evaluated, such as via transvaginal ultrasound or endometrial biopsy. Saliva testing of reproductive hormones lacks accuracy and is not indicated for the diagnosis of menopause.

Treatment

Women often seek advice from their health-care provider about minimizing vasomotor symptoms. Numerous lifestyle modifications can be quite helpful (Table 9-6). When these measures are inadequate, the addition of pharmacological intervention is often appropriate.

Prescription Medications for Menopausal Symptoms

HT, usually in the form of an estrogen supplement prescription, is likely one of the most commonly used and also one of the most effective therapies that has been extensively studied for hot flash management.

All types and routes of administration of estrogen are effective. Although the benefit appears to be related to the dose, even low doses of estrogen are often effective. Higher doses (equivalent of 1 mg of oral estradiol) usually provide relief in about 4 weeks, whereas lower doses usually take about 8 to 12 weeks to provide a similar hot flash effect. Lower-dose HT is usually better tolerated with less breast tenderness and uterine bleeding. The FDA, the American College of Obstetricians and Gynecologists (ACOG), and the North American Menopause Society (NAMS) recommend using the lowest dose of HT that is effective; the length of therapy should be dictated by clinical response and kept as short as possible (Table 9-7).

As with all medication use, HT comes with the possibility for adverse effects. Endometrial cancer risk with unopposed estrogen use is considerable, with the rate of 4 to 5 per 1,000 users per year, with a 5-year use risk of 2% and a 10-year use risk of 4%. As a result, unless a woman taking HT has undergone a hysterectomy, she should also take a progestin to minimize this risk. An observed increased risk of breast cancer in women who use HT has also been noted, particularly with long-term use. Supplemental systemic estrogen use should be avoided in women who have a history of or are at high risk for cardiovascular disease, breast cancer, uterine cancer, or venous thromboembolic events and in women with active liver disease. Long-term use of HT (greater than 10 years) has also been associated with an increased risk of dementia. Compared with the oral form, transdermal estrogen use is associated with a lower thromboembolic risk in short-term studies. The prescriber and the patient need to be aware of the risks of estrogen

> **CLINICAL CONCEPT**
>
> When given during the first years after menopause, reduction of hot flashes by 80% to 95% is expected with HT therapy.

TABLE 9-6 Lifestyle Modifications to Minimize Hot Flash Triggers

Hot flashes can often be reduced in number and minimized in severity with simple lifestyle changes.

HOT FLASH TRIGGER	INTERVENTION
Spicy foods, chocolate, other foods	Keep food diary to track triggers. Avoid triggers or eat in small amounts.
Alcohol use	Note whether certain amounts of types of alcohol trigger hot flashes. Restrict or avoid use.
Elevated ambient temperature and humidity	Control room temperature and humidity. Using climate control to achieve a cool room with low humidity is particularly helpful in improving sleep quality.
Tight, restrictive clothing	Dress in layers that can be removed and replaced in response to hot flashes.
Cigarette smoking	Tobacco use is associated with a marked increase in hot flashes. Smoking cessation improves overall health and reduces hot flash frequency and severity.
Hot baths or showers	Well-known hot flash trigger. Also tends to worsen dry skin, a common complaint during perimenopause and menopause. Taking a cool shower or bath minimizes hot flash risk.
Relaxation techniques, self-hypnosis	In many smaller studies, shown to be helpful in reducing hot flash severity and frequency.

Source: Nelson AL. Perimenopause, menopause and postmenopause: health promotion strategies. In: Hatcher RA, Trussell J, Nelson AL, Cates W, Kowal D, Policar MS, eds. *Contraceptive Technology*. 21st ed. Atlanta, GA: Managing Contraception; 2018.

TABLE 9-7 Estrogen Forms, Dosage, and Reported Relief

The three most commonly used prescription hormone therapy agents include oral conjugated equine estrogen and oral and transdermal estradiol-17β. The amount of hot flash relief women get from each form and dose differs.

ESTROGEN FORM	DOSE (MG)	REPORTED HOT FLASH RELIEF (%)
Oral conjugated estrogen	0.625	94
	0.4	78
	0.3	78
Oral 17– estradiol	2	96
	1	89
	0.5	79
	0.25	55
Transdermal 17– estradiol	0.1	96
	0.05	96
	0.025	86

supplementation; as with all medications, the use of HT should be approached with caution and is contraindicated in some women (Box 9-1).

Occasionally, a woman with significant vasomotor symptoms does not want to or cannot use HT for relief. Low-dose antidepressant (selective serotonin reuptake inhibitors [SSRIs] and selective serotonin and norepinephrine reuptake inhibitors [SNRIs]) therapy can reduce the frequency and severity of hot flashes by 35%. Examples of options include the SNRI venlafaxine (Effexor®) and the SSRIs sertraline (Zoloft®) and paroxetine (Paxil®). Typically, the doses given to minimize vasomotor symptoms are less than the doses used for the treatment of depression. The usual adverse effects associated with the use of these medications can be anticipated; sexual dysfunction including anorgasmia is common with SSRI and SNRI use. Gabapentin (Neurontin®) has also demonstrated efficacy in reducing vasomotor symptoms. Older antihypertensives, such as methyldopa (Aldomet®) and clonidine (Catapres®), have been used for this purpose but demonstrate limitations of use owing to undesirable adverse effects and low efficacy.

In a woman who continues to menstruate but is having significant perimenopausal symptoms, lower-dose COCs can be helpful for symptom relief and for cycle regulation. COCs contain approximately three to four times the estrogen dose of the usual HT dose.

Estrogen deficiency is a potent risk factor in the development of osteoporosis, which is most common in postmenopausal women. By age 80 years, the average woman has lost greater than 30% of her premenopausal bone density. When taken with calcium supplements, postmenopausal HT can help reduce the risk of postmenopausal fracture by 50% by minimizing further bone loss. However, HT should not be used solely for this purpose because of the greater observed rate of venous thrombotic events with short-term and long-term HT use and invasive breast cancer with longer-term use, as well as the availability of other medications to minimize or treat bone thinning such as the bisphosphonates.

Many women who use oral HT continue to have symptoms of genitourinary syndrome of menopause (GSM), including symptoms of atrophic vaginitis; the addition of topical estrogen, via an estrogen-containing vaginal cream, ring, or tablet, can be helpful. Increasing the dose of oral estrogen is seldom helpful and likely increases HT adverse effects. With low-dose vaginal estrogen therapy, the use of progestogen is not recommended though periodic endometrial surveillance should be considered, particularly in those with increased risk of endometrial cancer or using higher than normal doses of estrogen. Low-dose vaginal estrogen therapy can also be considered to treat GSM in women with a history of breast cancer, as studies show no significant increase in risk of recurrence due to low systemic absorption of the hormone. Some women using HT continue to need topical or local estrogen in the form of a vaginal cream,

BOX 9-1 Contraindications to and Caution With Postmenopausal Estrogen Therapy

Absolute contraindication

- Unexplained vaginal bleeding
- Acute liver disease
- Chronic impaired liver function
- Thrombotic disease
- Neuro-ophthalmological vascular disease
- Endometrial cancer (controversial—short-term use for management of severe menopausal symptoms occasionally acceptable)
- Breast cancer current, past, or suspected (controversial—short-term use for management of severe menopausal symptoms occasionally acceptable)

Use with caution, considering whether benefit outweighs risk

- Seizure disorder (owing to potential drug-drug interaction)
- Dyslipidemia, particularly hypertriglyceridemia (transdermal, intravaginal hormone therapy has limited lipid impact)

Source: Goodman NF, Cobin RH, Ginzburg SB, Katz IA, Woode DE. American Association of Clinical Endocrinologists medical guidelines for clinical practice for the diagnosis and treatment of menopause. Endocr Pract. 2011;17(suppl 6):1–25. https://journals.aace.com/doi/pdf/10.4158/EP.17.S6.1

tablet, or estrogen-impregnated ring (Estring®) to help minimize urogenital atrophy symptoms. Topical or local estrogen use also helps reduce the risk of recurrent UTIs in postmenopausal women, likely through increasing periurethral and perivaginal colonization with lactobacilli and other protective organisms. If a woman in peri- or postmenopause has issues with vaginal dryness with sexual activity as her major issue, the use of OTC vaginal lubricants and moisturizers can also afford great relief.

Vitamin and Botanical Products for Menopausal Symptoms

Due to the potential for serious adverse effects with hormonal options, approximately 50% of women seek nonhormonal alternatives for the treatment of menopausal symptoms. Women approaching and during menopause are among the greatest users of botanical and other natural-based therapies. Although a wide variety of these therapies are available for this indication, relatively few high-quality studies have been done on the safety and efficacy of these products. At the same time, many authorities, including the NAMS, view the use of botanical and other natural-based therapies as an option for assisting a woman through the menopause transition.

Phytoestrogens (aka, isoflavones) are chemical substances similar to estrogen, in particular estradiol, that are found in more than 300 plants, including apples, carrots, coffee, potatoes, yams, soy products, flaxseed, ginseng, bean sprouts, red clover sprouts, sunflower seeds, rye, wheat, sesame seeds, linseed, black cohosh, and bourbon. These are active substances that bind to estrogen receptor sites and have mild estrogenic effects and some antiestrogenic activity in some areas by binding and blocking to sites in the breast, colon, and rectum. OTC topical creams made of wild yam, a phytoprogesterone, are available and commonly used by women seeking relief from hot flashes. Because of poor bioavailability, however, little of the product actually reaches circulation.

Few high-quality studies support the use of nutritional supplements for management of menopausal symptoms. Women often view these supplements as a safe alternative to drug therapy, however. Guidelines from NAMS support the use of isoflavones (derived from soy foods and extracts), as these have demonstrated benefits in alleviating vasomotor symptoms. NAMS does not recommend the use of other herbal and vitamin supplements due to a general lack of supportive evidence.

> **CLINICAL CONCEPT**
>
> In smaller studies, high-dose vitamin E—800 IU/day—modestly reduced the number of hot flashes.

Discussion Sources

American College of Obstetricians and Gynecologists (ACOG). ACOG Practice Bulletin No. 141: management of menopausal symptoms. *Obstet Gynecol.* 2014;123(1):202–216.

Goodman NF, Cobin RH, Ginzburg SB, Katz IA, Woode DE. American Association of Clinical Endocrinologists medical guidelines for clinical practice for the diagnosis and treatment of menopause. *Endocr Pract.* 2011;17(suppl 6):1–25. https://www.aace.com/files/menopause.pdf

Nelson AL. Perimenopause, menopause and postmenopause: health promotion strategies. In: Hatcher RA, Trussell J, Nelson AL, Cates W, Kowal D, Policar MS, eds. *Contraceptive Technology*. 21st ed. Atlanta, GA: Managing Contraception; 2018.

North American Menopause Society. The 2017 Hormone Therapy Position Statement of the North American Menopause Society. *Menopause*. 2017;24(7):728–753.

Santen RJ, Allred DC, Ardoin, SP, et al. Postmenopausal hormone therapy: an Endocrine Society Scientific Statement. *J Clin Endocrinol Metab*. 2010;95(suppl 1):S34.

QUESTIONS

46. The average onset of perimenopause in North American women is between the ages of:

  A. 35 to 40 years.

  B. 40 to 45 years.

  C. 45 to 50 years.

  D. 50 to 55 years.

47. Which of the following statements regarding perimenopause is false?

  A. Menstruation ceases during perimenopause.

  B. Hot flashes and flushes are common during the week before menses.

  C. Though low likelihood, pregnancy is still possible during perimenopause.

  D. Ovulation becomes erratic during perimenopause.

48. In advising a woman about menopause, the NP considers that:

  A. the average age at last menstrual period for a North American woman is 47 to 48 years.

  B. hot flashes and night sweats occur in about 60% to 90% of women.

  C. women with surgical menopause usually have milder symptoms.

  D. FSH and LH levels are suppressed.

49. Findings in estrogen deficiency (atrophic) vaginitis include:

  A. a malodorous vaginal discharge.

  B. an increased number of lactobacilli.

  C. a reduced number of white blood cells (WBCs).

  D. a pH greater than 5.

50. A 53-year-old woman who is taking HT with conjugated estrogen, 0.45 mg/day, with medroxyprogesterone acetate (MPA), 1.5 mg, has bothersome symptoms of GSM. You advise that:

  A. her oral estrogen dose should be increased.

  B. the addition of a topical estrogen can be helpful.

  C. the MPA component should be discontinued.

  D. baking soda douche should be tried.

51. For a woman with bothersome hot flashes who cannot take HT, alternative options with demonstrated efficacy and limited adverse effects include the use of all of the following except:

  A. venlafaxine.

  B. sertraline.

  C. gabapentin.

  D. clonidine.

52. Absolute contraindications to postmenopausal HT include:

  A. unexplained vaginal bleeding.

  B. seizure disorder.

C. dyslipidemia.

D. migraine without aura.

53. A 50-year-old woman with well-controlled hypertension presents with a complaint of recent onset of hot flashes and night sweats. A friend told her about starting HT, but she is concerned about possible health risks. In advising this woman about HT, you consider that it can:

A. reduce the risk of venous thrombotic events.

B. significantly reduce serum triglyceride levels.

C. worsen hypertension in most women.

D. help preserve bone density.

54. A 52-year-old woman with rheumatoid arthritis presents with a chief complaint of hot flashes that have increasingly worsened over the past 2 years. In counseling the woman, the NP advises that the use of HT can result in:

A. a reduction in the rate of cardiovascular disease.

B. an increase in the severity of rheumatoid arthritis symptoms.

C. a reduction in the severity of vasomotor symptoms.

D. a disturbance in sleep patterns.

55. The progestin component of HT is given to:

A. counteract the negative lipid effects of estrogen.

B. minimize endometrial hyperplasia.

C. help with symptoms of GSM.

D. prolong ovarian activity.

56. A 49-year-old woman in perimenopause complains of vaginal dryness and painful intercourse. She has a history of breast cancer that was resolved with a lumpectomy of the right breast. The NP advises that:

A. HT would be an appropriate option to treat symptoms of GSM.

B. vaginal estrogen is contraindicated.

C. a vaginal lubricant can provide relief.

D. this is a transient condition and will resolve over time.

57. Concerning selective estrogen receptor modulator (SERM) therapy such as raloxifene (Evista®), which of the following statements is correct?

A. Concurrent progestin opposition is needed.

B. Hot flashes are reduced in frequency and severity.

C. Use is contraindicated when a woman has a history of breast cancer.

D. Osteoporosis risk is reduced with use.

58. During perimenopause, which of the following is likely to be noted?

A. The length of the menstrual cycle and duration of menstrual flow are often unpredictable.

B. The length of the perimenopausal period is fairly predictable, lasting about 2 years.

C. Symptoms are less severe in women who smoke tobacco.

D. Hot flashes are infrequently reported until menses have ceased for 6 months or more.

59. Expected physiological changes to occur during menopause include all of the following except:

A. increased levels of LH.

B. elevated levels of testosterone.

C. reduced levels of estradiol.

D. increased levels of FSH.

60. Which of the following is most accurate regarding the diagnosis of menopause?

A. Hormone measurements should be routinely used to screen for menopause.

B. Measurement of human chorionic gonadotropin (hCG) is most useful in determining menopause stage.

C. An evaluation of menstrual cycle changes is the best predictor of menopause stage.

D. Saliva hormone testing can provide an accurate determination of menopause stage.

61. Which of the following is likely to be noted with short-term (less than 1 to 2 years) HT use in a post-menopausal woman?

A. reduction in dementia risk

B. significant increase in breast cancer risk

C. minimized hot flashes

D. increase in cardiovascular risk

62. Which body area has the greatest concentration of estrogen receptors?

A. vulva

B. vascular bed

C. heart

D. brain

63. When counseling a 46-year-old woman who is experiencing debilitating hot flashes, you advise all of the following regarding higher- and lower-dose hormone replacement therapy except:

A. current clinical guidelines recommend using the lowest effective dose possible.

B. higher-dose HT will relieve hot flashes faster than lower-dose regimens.

C. lower-dose HT is better tolerated than higher-dose HT.

D. the duration of lower-dose HT is usually shorter than that of higher-dose regimens.

64. You see a 51-year-old woman who is considering HT. She has a family history of endometrial cancer, hyperlipidemia, and VTE in first- and second-degree relatives. You advise her on all of the following except:

A. the use of progestin can minimize the risk of endometrial cancer for a woman on HT and who has not undergone hysterectomy.

B. supplemental oral estrogen should be avoided in women who are at high risk of breast cancer or uterine cancer.

C. high-dose oral estrogen is associated with a higher risk of stroke compared with low-dose or trans-dermal estrogen therapy.

D. short-term studies demonstrate that oral HT is associated with lower thromboembolic risk than transdermal forms of HT.

65. A 49-year-old woman presents with a complaint of recent-onset hot flashes. She expresses a desire to avoid HT and asks about the use of phytoestrogens. The NP advises that all of the following are sources of phytoestrogens except:

A. red clover.

B. ginseng.

C. almond milk.

D. soy products.

66. The typical HT regimen contains _____ or less of the estrogen dose of COC.

   A. one-eighth

   B. one-fourth

   C. one-half

   D. three-fourths

67. For the 48-year-old woman with a history of DVT who is having significant vasomotor symptoms, which of the following oral agents can be used for symptom management?

   A. conjugated estrogen

   B. drospirenone

   C. estrone

   D. paroxetine

68. Long-term calcium supplementation is recommended in postmenopausal women who are taking HT as its use reduces the risk of fracture by approximately:

   A. 25%.

   B. 50%.

   C. 65%.

   D. 80%.

69. In postmenopausal women, a major benefit from the use of topical or local vaginal estrogen is:

   A. reduction in frequency of night sweats.

   B. reduced risk of recurrent UTIs.

   C. reduced risk of type 2 diabetes.

   D. increased levels of androgens.

70. When reviewing the use of nutritional supplements for the management of menopausal symptoms, the NP considers that:

   A. few high-quality studies support the use of these products.

   B. the use of these products is consistently reported to be helpful.

   C. the products can be safely used as long as blood hormone levels are carefully evaluated.

   D. the use of these products is associated with a greater reduction in menopausal symptoms than with prescription HT.

71. Which of the following statements is true?

   A. Many over-the-counter progesterone creams contain sterols that the human body is unable to use.

   B. All progesterone forms are easily absorbed via the skin.

   C. Alfalfa is an example of a phytoprogesterone.

   D. Progesterones, whether synthetic or plant based, should not be used by a woman who has undergone a hysterectomy.

For answers and rationales, see end of chapter.

Benign Prostatic Hyperplasia

Overview

Benign prostatic hyperplasia (BPH) is a common disorder in older men. Based on autopsy studies, the prevalence of BPH increases from approximately 8% in men 31 to 40 years old to approximately 50% in men 51 to 60 years old and to more than 80% in men 80 years old and older. Far fewer men have clinically symptomatic disease. This enlargement of the prostate, not associated with or a precursor to malignancy, can lead to bladder outlet obstruction, likely as a result of an enlargement in prostatic connective tissue and an increase in the number of epithelial and smooth muscle cells. To empty the bladder effectively in the face of increasing outflow tract obstruction, bladder detrusor hypertrophy occurs with occasional notation of subsequent diverticula. Chronic incomplete bladder emptying causes stasis and predisposes to calculus formation and infection with secondary inflammatory changes, including prostatitis and UTI.

Clinical Presentation

Common signs and symptoms in men with BPH usually include increased urinary frequency and urgency, and nocturia (increased frequency of urination at night, interrupting sleep). Difficulty in initiating urinary stream as well as the stream being weaker and starting and stopping during micturition is a common problem. End-void dribbling and sensation of incomplete bladder emptying are also commonly reported. Less commonly, the man with BPH will present with UTI or acute urinary retention.

Digital rectal examination (DRE) is an integral part of the evaluation where prostate size and contour can be assessed, nodules can be evaluated, and areas suggestive of malignancy can be detected. On rectal examination, the hypertrophic prostate usually is enlarged, has a rubbery consistency, and in many cases has lost the median sulcus or furrow. DRE of prostate size is often misleading, however; a prostate that is apparently small on DRE can be found in a man with significant symptoms.

Diagnostic Testing

Diagnosis of BPH is based on numerous components of the evaluation. The use of a validated tool such as the American Urological Association (AUA) Symptom Index for Benign Prostatic Hyperplasia increases the likelihood of an accurate diagnosis. Other tests can be used to rule out infection or other conditions that can cause similar symptoms. These include a urinalysis (to assess for the presence of blood, leukocytes, bacteria, protein, or glucose) and/or urine culture. Additional diagnostic procedures used to confirm that an enlarged prostate is causing the symptoms include urinary flow test, postvoid residual volume test, and transrectal ultrasound. A systematic evaluation for prostate cancer must be done on any man who has an abnormal prostate examination with or without urinary symptoms. Referral to urology is advised, particularly if there is a suspicion of prostate cancer and prostate biopsy is needed.

Prolonged urinary outflow obstruction can lead to hydronephrosis and compromised renal function; this is the etiology of postrenal azotemia, a potentially life-threatening condition. Postrenal azotemia accounts for about 5% of all renal failure. It is characterized by urea nitrogen and creatinine elevation and evidence of urinary retention and outflow tract obstruction; other reasons for renal failure should be ruled out. Intervention in postrenal azotemia is focused on relieving the urinary outflow tract obstruction. When postrenal azotemia is promptly detected, renal function returns to baseline after treatment.

Treatment

Patient education about BPH should include information on measures to avoid making symptoms worse. Drugs with anticholinergic effect, such as tricyclic antidepressants and first-generation antihistamines (e.g., diphenhydramine [Benadryl®], chlorpheniramine [Chlor-Trimeton®]), can cause acute urinary retention in men with BPH; opioid use and inactivity also increase the risk of urinary retention. In addition, urinary frequency occasionally becomes worse with ingestion of certain bladder irritants, such as caffeine, alcohol, and artificial sweeteners. Although men with BPH are often tempted to limit fluid intake to minimize urinary frequency, this can yield more concentrated and perhaps irritating urine, possibly leading to increased symptoms.

The prostate and bladder base contain numerous α_1 receptor sites. When these receptor sites are stimulated, the prostate contracts, increasing outflow tract obstruction. As a result, treatment with α_1 receptor antagonists (alpha blockers) including tamsulosin (Flomax®) can be helpful in improving the symptoms of BPH. The use of finasteride (Proscar®) and dutasteride (Avodart®), 5-α-reductase inhibitors that block the conversion of testosterone to dihydrotestosterone, helps to reduce the size of the prostate and ameliorate symptoms. Tadalafil (Cialis®), a phosphodiesterase-5 (PDE-5) inhibitor most commonly prescribed for erectile dysfunction (ED), is also approved for the treatment of BPH with or without finasteride. PDE-5 inhibitors help mediate smooth muscle relaxation in the lower urinary tract.

Surgical intervention in BPH should be considered when medication and lifestyle modification therapy are ineffective and any of the following are present and clearly secondary to the condition: recurrent UTI, recurrent or persistent gross hematuria, bladder stones, or renal insufficiency. Surgical options can include transurethral resection of the prostate or open prostatectomy. A number of minimally invasive therapies, including thermal and laser interventions, are now available and offer an attractive alternative to more aggressive surgery, although less is known about long-term outcomes.

Herbal and nutritional therapies, including saw palmetto, rye, and pumpkin, are considered emerging therapies by the AUA, pending further study. The observed effect of these plant-based therapies is usually attributed to a mechanism of action similar to approved prescription BPH therapies. As with other herbal and nutritional therapies available OTC, issues of product purity and strength and potential interaction with prescription and other OTC products remain a concern.

Discussion Sources

Deters LA, Leveillee RJ, Patel VR, Costabile RA, Moore CR, Patel VR. Benign prostatic hypertrophy. Medscape. http://emedicine .medscape.com/article/437359-overview

Foer HE, Barry MJ, Dahm P, et al. Surgical management of lower urinary tract symptoms attributed to benign prostatic hyperplasia: AUA guideline. https://www.auanet.org/guidelines/benign-prostatic-hyperplasia-(bph)-guideline

QUESTIONS

72 to 77. A 62-year-old man complains of a weak urine flow and dribbling at the end of urination. In suspecting BPH, indicate (*Yes or No*) which of the following would be expected:

_____ **72.** obliterated median sulcus

_____ **73.** size larger than 2.5 cm × 3 cm

_____ **74.** glucose in urine

_____ **75.** sensation of incomplete emptying

_____ **76.** boggy gland

_____ **77.** pain with palpation of the prostate

78. When assessing a 68-year-old man with suspected BPH, the NP considers that:

A. prostate size does not correlate well with severity of symptoms.

B. BPH affects less than 50% of men of this age.

C. he is at increased risk for prostate cancer.

D. limiting fluids is a helpful method of relieving severe symptoms.

79. Which of the following medications can contribute to the development of acute urinary retention in an older man with BPH?

A. amitriptyline

B. loratadine

C. enalapril

D. lorazepam

80. A 78-year-old man with a history of BPH presents with a 3-day history of new-onset fatigue and difficulty with bladder emptying. Examination reveals a distended bladder but is otherwise unremarkable. Blood urea nitrogen level is 88 mg/dL (31.4 mmol/L); creatinine level is 2.8 mg/dL (247.5 μmol/L). The most likely diagnosis is:

A. prerenal azotemia.

B. acute glomerulonephritis.

C. tubular necrosis.

D. postrenal azotemia.

81. Surgical intervention in BPH should be considered with all of the following except:

    A. recurrent UTI.

    B. bladder stones.

    C. persistent obstruction despite medical therapy.

    D. acute kidney injury.

82. Finasteride (Proscar®, Propecia®) and dutasteride (Avodart®) are helpful in the treatment of BPH because of their effect on:

    A. bladder contractility.

    B. prostate size.

    C. activity at select bladder receptor sites.

    D. bladder pressure.

83. Tamsulosin (Flomax®) is helpful in the treatment of BPH because of its effect on:

    A. bladder contractility.

    B. prostate size.

    C. activity at select bladder receptor sites.

    D. bladder pressure.

84. When considering the use of tadalafil (Cialis®) for the treatment of BPH, the NP advises that this agent:

    A. can be used with or without finasteride.

    B. should be used in combination with an alpha blocker for maximum effectiveness.

    C. should only be considered when surgical intervention is not an option.

    D. is safe to use concomitantly with a nitrate.

85. Concerning BPH, which of the following statements is true?

    A. DRE is accurate in diagnosing the condition.

    B. The use of a validated patient symptom tool is an important part of diagnosing the condition.

    C. Urodynamic testing is of little use in the diagnosis.

    D. Bladder distention is usually present in early disease.

86. Concerning herbal and nutritional therapies for BPH treatment, which of the following statements is false?

    A. The mechanism of action of the most effective and best studied products is similar to prescription medications for this condition.

    B. These therapies are currently considered emerging therapies by the AUA.

    C. Major areas of concern with use of these therapies include issues of product purity and quality control.

    D. These therapies are safest and most effective when used with prescription medications.

For answers and rationales, see end of chapter.

Acute Epididymitis

Overview

Acute epididymitis is a male upper reproductive tract infectious disease caused by various pathogens. In men younger than age 35 years, it is usually caused by *Chlamydia trachomatis* or *Neisseria gonorrhoeae*; the organism is acquired through sexual contact. In men older than age 35 years, acute epididymitis is often seen secondary to prostatitis and is typically caused by a gram-negative organism. In men who have sex with men (MSM; i.e., the insertive partner in anal intercourse), sexually transmitted acute epididymitis is more likely caused by enteric organisms (such as *Escherichia coli* and *Pseudomonas* spp).

Clinical Presentation

Acute epididymitis manifests with a patient history of acute-onset irritative voiding symptoms, fever, and an acutely painful, enlarged epididymis. Pain often radiates up the spermatic cord to the ipsilateral lower abdomen.

Urethritis, scrotal swelling, and mucoid penile discharge are often found. As the disease progresses, the ipsilateral testes are occasionally involved, swelling so that the two testes cannot be distinguished; this is known as epididymo-orchitis.

Diagnostic Testing

Diagnosis of acute epididymitis involves a urinalysis along with urine culture. A complete blood count (CBC) would normally find elevated WBCs with a left shift. For those at risk of gonorrheal or chlamydial infection, a urethral swab culture or nucleic acid amplification test (NAAT) should be performed. If the patient has systemic symptoms, a blood culture should be considered. Color Doppler ultrasonography can help to confirm epididymitis as well as to rule out testicular torsion, which is a medical emergency. In pediatric patients, abdominopelvic ultrasonography is recommended to evaluate for a possible underlying congenital anomaly.

Treatment

Treatment options differ according to age and risk factors. In younger men with low risk for epididymo-orchitis as a complication of UTI, particularly with risk for STI, antimicrobials effective against gonorrhea and chlamydia such as ceftriaxone followed by doxycycline should be used (Table 9-8). In men at risk for epididymo-orchitis as a complication of UTI, the choice of antimicrobial agent should be directed by urine culture results. An oral fluoroquinolone is likely to be effective. In MSM and likely infected with an enteric organism, the recommended treatment is oral levofloxacin or ofloxacin.

> **CLINICAL CONCEPT**
>
> The Prehn sign, a reduction in pain when the scrotum is elevated above the symphysis pubis, is usually noted in acute epididymitis.

TABLE 9-8 Male Genitourinary Infections

CONDITION	TREATMENT OPTIONS
Epididymitis Epididymo-orchitis Age ≤35 years old	Primary: Ceftriaxone 250 mg intramuscularly (IM) as a single dose plus doxycycline 100 mg PO bid × 10 days. Advise scrotal elevation to help with symptom relief.
Epididymitis Epididymo-orchitis Age older than 35 years old or insertive partner in anal intercourse	Primary: Ofloxacin 300 mg PO bid or levofloxacin 500 to 750 mg IV/PO qd × 10 to 14 days. Alternative: IV ampicillin with sulbactam, third-generation cephalosporin, other parenteral agents as indicated by severity of illness.
Acute bacterial prostatitis (younger than 35 years old)	Primary: One-time dose of ceftriaxone 250 mg IM, then doxycycline 100 mg PO bid × 10 days.
Acute bacterial prostatitis (age 35 years old or older, or men who have sex with men)	Levofloxacin 500 to 750 mg IV/PO qd or ofloxacin 300 mg PO bid × 10 to 14 days or TMP-SMX 1 DS tablet (160 mg TMP) PO bid × 10 to 14 days.
Chronic bacterial prostatitis	Ciprofloxacin 500 mg PO bid × 4 to 6 weeks or levofloxacin 750 mg PO qd × 4 weeks. Alternative: TMP-SMX DS 1 tab PO bid × 1 to 3 months. With treatment failure, consider prostatic stones.

Sources: Centers for Disease Control and Prevention. *Sexually transmitted diseases treatment guidelines, 2015.* MMWR. *2015;64(3):1–137;* Gilbert DN, Chambers HF, Eliopoulos GM, Saag MS, Pavia AT. The Sanford Guide to Antimicrobial Therapy. *50th ed. Sperryville, VA: Antimicrobial Therapy, Inc.; 2020:22–27.*

As with all STIs, a critical part of care is discussion of preventive strategies, including using condoms and limiting the number of sexual partners. NPs should offer and encourage testing for other STIs, including human immunodeficiency virus (HIV), hepatitis B, and syphilis. Consideration should also be given to offering testing for hepatitis C and human herpes type 2 (herpes simplex type 2) serology. If not previously immunized, immunization that provides protection against hepatitis A, hepatitis B, and human papilloma-virus (HPV) should be offered and encouraged.

Discussion Source

Gilbert DN, Chambers HF, Eliopoulos GM, Saag MS, Pavia AT. *The Sanford Guide to Antimicrobial Therapy*. 50th ed. Sperryville, VA: Antimicrobial Therapy, Inc.; 2020:27.

QUESTIONS

87. The presentation of acute epididymitis in an otherwise-well 22-year-old man includes:

    A. the presence of a positive Prehn sign.

    B. low back pain.

    C. absent cremasteric reflex.

    D. diffuse abdominal pain.

88. A 26-year-old man presents with acute epididymitis. He states that his female partner was recently diagnosed with "some kind of an infection and was told I should get treated." The most likely causative organisms include (more than one answer may apply):

    A. *E coli.*

    B. *P aeruginosa.*

    C. *C trachomatis.*

    D. *N gonorrhoeae.*

89. A likely causative pathogen in a 37-year-old man who has sex with men with acute epididymitis:

    A. *E coli.*

    B. *Mycoplasma* spp.

    C. *Haemophilus influenzae*

    D. *Acinetobacter baumannii.*

90. A 30-year-old man who has sex with women and has acute epididymitis presents without gastrointesti-nal upset and will be treated as an outpatient. Which of the following is a reasonable treatment option?

    A. PO doxycycline with IM ceftriaxone

    B. PO azithromycin with IM penicillin G benzathine

    C. PO metronidazole with PO linezolid

    D. PO clindamycin with PO cefixime

91. Appropriate treatment of acute epididymitis for a 32-year-old man who is an insertive partner in anal intercourse is:

    A. IM ceftriaxone.

    B. PO azithromycin.

    C. PO levofloxacin.

    D. IV trimethoprim-sulfamethoxazole (TMP-SMX).

92 to 97. Indicate (*Yes or No*) whether each finding would be present in acute epididymitis.

_____ **92.** Irritative voiding symptoms

_____ **93.** Penile discharge

_____ **94.** Ulcerative lesion

_____ **95.** Scrotal swelling

_____ **96.** Boggy prostate

_____ **97.** Bilateral findings possible with later stages or with untreated disease

For answers and rationales, see end of chapter.

Acute and Chronic Bacterial Prostatitis

Overview

The term *prostatitis* is used to describe inflammation of the prostate gland, whether caused by a pathogen or other reason. Acute bacterial prostatitis implies that the inflammation is caused by a bacterial infection. Infection with a gram-negative rod such as *E coli* and *Pseudomonas* species usually causes acute bacterial prostatitis in older men. In men younger than 35 years or men at risk for STIs, gonorrhea or chlamydia or both are most often implicated. Less often, gram-positive organisms such as enterococci are implicated. In men older than 35 years, Enterobacteriaceae (coliforms) are more commonly implicated. Other risk factors include having a past episode of prostatitis, history of bladder or urethral infection, pelvic trauma, dehydration, or use of a urinary catheter.

Chronic bacterial prostatitis is a persistent bacterial infection that lasts more than 3 months. It most commonly affects men 36 to 50 years of age and is caused by *E coli* or other Enterobacteriaceae. Following an episode of acute bacterial prostatitis, about 5% will progress to chronic bacterial prostatitis.

Clinical Presentation

Acute bacterial prostatitis presents acutely, with fever, chills, malaise, and arthralgia. Irritative voiding symptoms, suprapubic pain, and perineal pain are typically reported. Often, obstructive urinary tract symptoms including urinary frequency, urgency, nocturia, difficulty initiating urine stream along with a sensation of incomplete voiding, and weak urinary stream are reported. Objective findings include fever and, on DRE, the notation of a tender, boggy (sponge-like) prostate.

In patients with chronic bacterial prostatitis, irritative voiding symptoms and low back and perineal pain are typically reported along with a history of UTI. Objective findings include a tender, boggy, or indurated prostate. Symptoms persist for at least 3 months.

Diagnostic Testing

In acute bacterial prostatitis, a midstream urine culture should be performed to identify the causative organism. For those suspected of an STI, a urine-based NAAT is preferred to detect gonococcal or chlamydial infection. Urinalysis should yield greater than 10 WBCs per high-power field with neutrophilia. Other diagnostic tests such as CBC, blood culture, and electrolytes can be considered based on severity of illness and presence of systemic symptoms.

> **CLINICAL CONCEPT**
> Prostatic massage should be avoided in acute prostatitis, and imaging studies are typically not needed for diagnosis in uncomplicated cases.

In chronic bacterial prostatitis, a diagnosis can be made in most cases with patient history, physical examination, and urine or prostatic secretion culture. Preprostatic massage urinalysis results are usually normal from a freshly voided specimen. Urinalysis and culture after prostatic massage usually yield leukocytes and the causative organism. A urine dipstick test can also indicate the presence of infection and hematuria. Urodynamic and imaging studies can be considered to assess for obstruction secondary to prostatic enlargement but have limited usefulness for a chronic bacterial prostatitis diagnosis.

Treatment

Treatment for acute bacterial prostatitis is similar to treatment for acute pyelonephritis—an antimicrobial agent with activity against gram-negative organisms and excellent tissue penetration. In men younger than 35 years, when the condition is most likely the result of an STI, a single dose of IM ceftriaxone followed by a course of PO doxycycline is recommended; causative organisms are usually the sexually transmitted organisms *C trachomatis* and *N gonorrhoeae*. Length of doxycycline therapy is usually 10 to 14 days. In men 35 years old and older or MSM, antimicrobial therapy with a higher-dose oral fluoroquinolone, such as ciprofloxacin or levofloxacin, for 10 to 14 days is advised. In chronic bacterial prostatitis, oral antimicrobial therapy for 4 to 12 weeks using a product with excellent tissue penetration and strong gram-negative coverage is usually required (see Table 9-8).

When prostatitis is caused or suspected to be caused by an STI, a critical part of care is discussion of preventive strategies, including using condoms and limiting the number of sexual partners. NPs should offer and encourage testing for other STIs, including HIV, hepatitis B, and syphilis. Consideration should also be given to offering testing for hepatitis C and human herpes type 2 (herpes simplex type 2) serology. If not previously immunized, immunization that provides protection against hepatitis A, hepatitis B, and HPV should be offered and encouraged.

Discussion Sources

Centers for Disease Control and Prevention. Sexually transmitted diseases treatment guidelines, 2015. *MMWR.* 2015;64(3):1–140.

Gilbert DN, Chambers HF, Eliopoulos GM, Saag MS, Pavia AT. *The Sanford Guide to Antimicrobial Therapy.* 50th ed. Sperryville, VA: Antimicrobial Therapy, Inc.; 2020:27.

Turek PJ, Hedayati T, Stehman CR. Prostatitis. Medscape. https://emedicine.medscape.com/article/785418-overview

QUESTIONS

98. Risk factors for acute bacterial prostatitis include all of the following except:

    A. having unprotected intercourse.

    B. use of a urinary catheter.

    C. prior bladder infection.

    D. diminished prostate-specific antigen (PSA) level.

99. The most common causative organisms of acute bacterial prostatitis in men younger than 35 years are:

    A. *E coli* and *Klebsiella pneumoniae.*

    B. *N gonorrhoeae* and *C trachomatis.*

    C. *Pseudomonas* and *Acinetobacter* species.

    D. enterococci.

100. When choosing an antimicrobial agent for the treatment of chronic bacterial prostatitis, the NP considers that:

    A. gram-positive organisms are the most likely cause of infection.

    B. cephalosporins are the first-line choice of therapy.

    C. choosing an antibiotic with gram-negative coverage is critical.

    D. length of antimicrobial therapy is typically 5 days.

101. All of the following are likely to be reported by patients with acute bacterial prostatitis except:

    A. perineal pain.

    B. irritative voiding symptoms.

    C. penile discharge.

    D. fever.

102. During acute bacterial prostatitis, the DRE usually reveals a gland described as:

    A. boggy.

    B. smooth.

    C. irregular.

    D. cystic.

103. A 30-year-old man with acute prostatitis presents with a fever of 102.3°F (39.1°C). What would be the expected CBC findings from this patient?

    A. WBC = 15,000/mm³; neutrophils = 4,000/mm³

    B. WBC = 18,000/mm³; neutrophils = 11,500/mm³

    C. WBC = 7,200/mm³; neutrophils = 3,200/mm³

    D. WBC = 4,000/mm³; neutrophils = 1,200/mm³

104. Appropriate antimicrobial treatment for a 25-year-old man with acute bacterial prostatitis is a course of:

A. oral azithromycin with oral metronidazole.

B. a single dose of IM ceftriaxone followed by oral doxycycline.

C. oral levofloxacin as a solo therapy.

D. oral amoxicillin-clavulanate with oral clarithromycin.

105. Appropriate antimicrobial treatment for a 65-year-old man with acute bacterial prostatitis is a course of oral:

A. doxycycline.

B. cefepime.

C. TMP-SMX.

D. ciprofloxacin.

106. Symptoms in chronic bacterial prostatitis often include:

A. fever.

B. gastrointestinal upset.

C. low back pain.

D. penile discharge.

107. The most common causative organisms in chronic bacterial prostatitis include:

A. gram-negative rods.

B. gram-positive cocci.

C. gram-negative cocci.

D. gram-positive coccobacilli.

108. Which of the following is the best choice of therapy in chronic bacterial prostatitis?

A. oral TMP-SMX for 2 weeks

B. parenteral ampicillin for 4 weeks

C. oral ciprofloxacin for 4 weeks

D. injectable gentamicin for 2 weeks

109. The best diagnostic test to identify the offending organism in acute bacterial prostatitis in a 60-year-old man who has a single long-term female partner is:

A. a urine culture.

B. a urine-based NAAT.

C. serologic antibody testing.

D. a urine Gram stain.

For answers and rationales, see end of chapter.

Vulvovaginitis

Overview

Vulvovaginitis is one of the most common gynecological problems; a variety of causes can result in this condition. When caused by infection, the most common causes of symptomatic vaginitis in women of reproductive age include bacterial vaginosis (approximately 40% to 50%), vaginal candidiasis (20% and more), and trichomoniasis (15% and more); this information is derived from studies of women who seek care for this condition, keeping in mind that a significant number of women will not seek care or will self-treat.

BACTERIAL VAGINOSIS

Overview

Bacterial vaginosis occurs when there is a disruption of the normal vaginal flora, typically lactobacilli, allowing for overgrowth of anaerobes, including *Gardnerella* species and *Mycoplasma hominis.* This is not considered an STI and can be caused by a number of factors including recent antimicrobial use, douching, tub bathing (especially with bubble bath), using OTC intravaginal hygiene products, IUD, frequent sexual intercourse, and the presence of other STIs.

Clinical Presentation

The most common symptom is an amine or fishy odor, particularly after sexual intercourse. Other findings can include increased volume of vaginal discharge that is thin, gray, and homogeneous. Vulvar irritation occurs less commonly, while dysuria and dyspareunia occur rarely.

Diagnostic Testing

Diagnosis of bacterial vaginosis relies on patient history, physical examination, and microscopic examination. Vaginal examination findings include a thin, gray discharge with minimal inflammation.

Other findings include few WBCs, a vaginal pH less than 4.5, and a positive whiff test. Vaginal cultures, as opposed to STI testing, are not needed except for refractory cases.

> **CLINICAL CONCEPT**
>
> On microscopic examination, the presence of clue cells on a saline smear is the most specific finding for bacterial vaginosis.

Treatment

Antimicrobial therapy is the preferred treatment of symptomatic bacterial vaginosis and can include metronidazole (oral tablet or vaginal gel) or clindamycin (oral or vaginal cream or ovules) (Table 9-9). Secnidazole (Solosec™) offers a single-dose oral treatment. Uncomplicated cases can be treated with either oral or topical/localized therapy. During pregnancy, a 7-day regimen of oral metronidazole or clindamycin is recommended. In nursing mothers, intravaginal therapy might be preferred over oral therapy to minimize antimicrobial exposure to the newborn, though there is no definitive evidence suggesting oral therapy poses a risk to the child.

CANDIDA VULVOVAGINITIS

Overview

Vulvovaginal candidiasis can be acute or chronic and can involve a number of *Candida* species, most commonly *C albicans* but also *C glabrata, C krusei,* and *C tropicalis.* Nearly 75% of women will develop at least one episode of vulvovaginal candidiasis during their lifetime, with approximately 50% of college-aged women experiencing an episode. The condition is not considered an STI and occurs most frequently in women of childbearing age. Recent antimicrobial use is a major risk factor as it disrupts the normal bacterial flora in the vulvovaginal region and allows colonization by pathogenic organisms. Other risk factors include pregnancy, high-dose estrogen therapy, immunosuppression (e.g., HIV/AIDS), and diabetes mellitus. Women with recurrent or severe vulvovaginal candidiasis should be screened for diabetes mellitus.

Clinical Presentation

The most common complaints of vulvovaginal candidiasis include itching and burning. A thick white-to-yellow adherent, curd-like discharge is usually present along with vulvovaginal excoriation and erythema and dyspareunia. The rash can extend to the thighs and perineum.

Diagnostic Testing

Diagnosis of vulvovaginal candidiasis includes patient history, physical examination, and microscopic examination. On microscopic examination, hyphae and pseudohyphae are present (observed with wet-mount test or potassium hydroxide preparation). The pH remains relatively normal at less than 5, with few WBCs. Fungal culturing is not routinely needed for diagnosis.

TABLE 9-9 Female Genitourinary Infections

CONDITION	TREATMENT OPTIONS
Bacterial vaginosis	Metronidazole 500 mg PO bid × 7 days or metronidazole vaginal gel once daily × 5 days or 2% clindamycin vaginal cream 5 g intravaginally at bedtime × 7 days
	Alternatives: Clindamycin 300 mg PO bid × 7 days or clindamycin ovules 100 mg intravaginally at bedtime × 3 days or secnidazole 2 g packet (granules mixed with food) one dose over 30 minutes
Candidiasis	Single-day therapy options: fluconazole (Diflucan®) 150 mg PO as single dose); itraconazole 200 mg PO bid; butoconazole 2% SR cream (Gynazole-1®); tioconazole 6.5% (Vagistat-1®); miconazole (Monistat®) 1,200 mg, as single dose vaginally
	Various 3- and 7- to 14-day therapies with azole antifungal vaginal creams, suppositories, tablets (miconazole, butoconazole, clotrimazole, terconazole [Terazol®], tioconazole).
Trichomoniasis	Metronidazole 2 g PO as single dose or 500 mg PO bid × 7 days or tinidazole 2 g PO as single dose
Pelvic inflammatory disease	Recommended therapy for outpatient treatment: ceftriaxone 250 mg IM/IV as a single dose plus doxycycline 100 mg bid for 14 days with or without metronidazole 500 mg PO bid for 14 days, or cefoxitin 2 g IM with probenecid 1 g PO both as single doses plus doxycycline with metronidazole both × 14 days
	Fluoroquinolones not recommended due to increasing resistance.

Sources: Centers for Disease Control and Prevention. Sexually transmitted diseases treatment guidelines, 2015. MMWR. 2015;64(3):1–137; Gilbert DN, Chambers HF, Eliopoulos GM, Saag MS, Pavia AT. The Sanford Guide to Antimicrobial Therapy. 50th ed. Sperryville, VA: Antimicrobial Therapy, Inc.; 2020:26.

Treatment

Azole compounds are preferred for the treatment of vulvovaginal candidiasis and are available in oral form as well as vaginal creams or suppositories (see Table 9-9). Depending on the agent and route, treatment can vary from 1, 3, to 7 days. Treatment selection should be based on patient preference. Topical agents are effective in uncomplicated cases and should be considered when there is a potential for drug interaction. The use of oral azole agents is also associated with potential adverse effects, such as nausea, abdominal pain, and headaches.

TRICHOMONIASIS

Overview

Trichomoniasis is one of the most common STIs in the United States and is caused by the motile protozoan *Trichomonas vaginalis*. Spread is predominantly through sexual intercourse, and infection is associated with adverse pregnancy outcomes, infertility, postoperative infections, and cervical neoplasia. *T vaginalis* infection has also been shown to increase the risk of HIV transmission. Partners of infected women should also be treated and both partners should refrain from sex until pharmacological therapy is completed and symptoms have resolved.

Clinical Presentation

In females, symptoms commonly include dysuria, itching, vulvovaginal irritation, dyspareunia, yellow-green vaginal discharge, and cervical petechial hemorrhages ("strawberry spots") in about 30%.

Diagnostic Testing

Diagnosis relies on microbiological examination. A saline wet mount of vaginal discharge will reveal flagellated, motile organisms along with a large number of polymorphonuclear leukocytes (PMNs). This test is associated with a low sensitivity and is more likely to be positive in women with high organism loads. Wet mount microscopy is not a useful test in the diagnosis for men.

CLINICAL CONCEPT

Males with trichomoniasis are typically without symptoms, with treatment usually triggered by a female partner's diagnosis.

Treatment

The recommended therapy is oral metronidazole (Flagyl®) or tinidazole (Tindamax®) as a one-time dose, or alternatively, metronidazole for 7 days (see Table 9-9). Patients should be advised to avoid consuming alcohol during treatment with oral metronidazole or tinidazole. Abstinence from alcohol use should continue for 24 hours after completion of metronidazole or 72 hours after completion of tinidazole.

Discussion Sources

Girerd PH. Bacterial vaginosis. Medscape. https://emedicine.medscape.com/article/254342-overview
Krapf JM. Vulvovaginitis. Medscape. https://emedicine.medscape.com/article/2188931-overview
Marrazzo JM, Cates W. Reproductive tract infections, including HIV and other sexually transmitted infections. In: Hatcher RA, Trussell J, Nelson AL, Cates W, Kowal D, Policar MS, eds. *Contraceptive Technology*. 20th ed. New York, NY: Ardent Media; 2011:602.

QUESTIONS

110. Which of the following is not a normal finding in a woman during the reproductive years?

    A. vaginal pH of 4.5 or less

    B. *Lactobacillus* as the predominant vaginal organism

    C. thick, white vaginal secretions during the luteal phase

    D. vaginal epithelial cells with adherent bacteria

111. Physical examination of a 19-year-old woman with a 3-day history of vaginal itch reveals moderate perineal excoriation, vaginal erythema, and a white, clumping discharge. Expected microscopic examination findings include:

    A. a pH greater than 6.

    B. an increased number of lactobacilli.

    C. hyphae.

    D. an abundance of WBCs.

112. Women with bacterial vaginosis most often present with:

    A. vulvitis.

    B. pruritus.

    C. dysuria.

    D. malodorous discharge.

113. Treatment of vulvovaginitis caused by *Candida albicans* includes:

    A. metronidazole gel.

    B. tioconazole cream.

    C. oral tinidazole.

    D. clindamycin cream.

114. A 24-year-old woman presents with a 1-week history of thin, green-yellow vaginal discharge with perivaginal irritation. Physical examination findings include vaginal erythema with petechial hemorrhages on the cervix, numerous WBCs, and motile organisms on microscopic examination. These findings most likely represent:

    A. motile sperm with irritative vaginitis.

    B. trichomoniasis.

    C. bacterial vaginosis.

    D. chlamydia cervicitis.

115. The preferred treatment option for trichomoniasis is:

    A. oral metronidazole.

    B. clindamycin vaginal cream.

    C. oral acyclovir.

    D. oral azithromycin.

116 to 119. Treatment options for bacterial vaginosis include (*Yes or No*):

_____ **116.** Oral metronidazole.

_____ **117.** Clindamycin cream.

_____ **118.** Oral clindamycin.

_____ **119.** Oral azithromycin.

120 to 123. Indicate if the following diagnostic findings are expected in bacterial vaginosis, vulvovaginal candidiasis, or trichomoniasis.

_____ **120.** Presence of clue cells

_____ **121.** Abundance of PMNs

_____ **122.** Positive whiff test

_____ **123.** Presence of hyphae on KOH prep

For answers and rationales, see end of chapter.

Common Sexually Transmitted Infections

CHLAMYDIAL INFECTION

Overview

Chlamydial infection is the most commonly reported STI, affecting primarily adolescents and adults younger than 25 years. The causative organism, *C trachomatis* immunotype D–K, is an obligate intracellular parasite closely related to gram-negative bacteria. The organism has an incubation period of approximately 7 to 14 days. Approximately 20% of sexually active women are carriers of this organism.

Clinical Presentation

This infection causes cervicitis in most infected women (Figs. 9-1 and 9-2). About one-half have urethral infection, and one-third have endometrial involvement; despite this, many women are asymptomatic, although mucopurulent vaginal discharge, dysuria, dyspareunia, and postcoital bleeding are

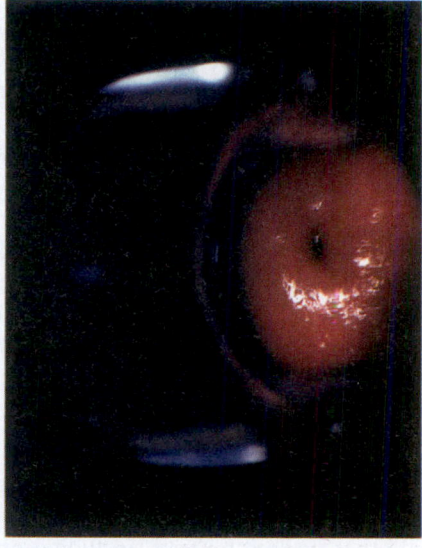

FIGURE 9-1 Normal cervix.
Dillon PM. Nursing Health Assessment: The Foundation of Clinical Practice. 3rd ed. Philadelphia, PA: F.A. Davis; 2016.

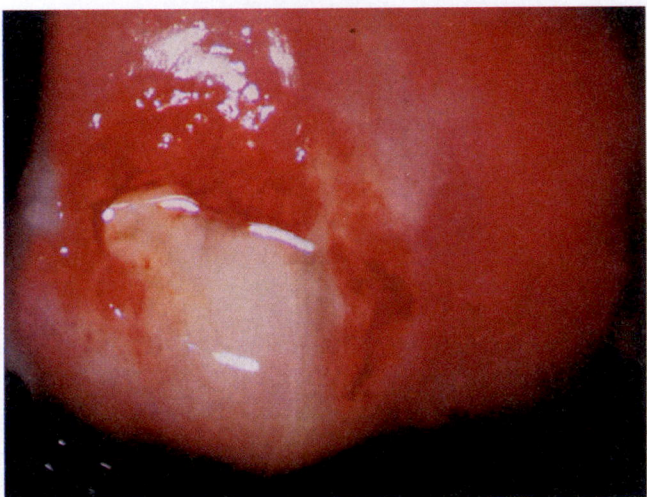

FIGURE 9-2 Chlamydial cervicitis.
Handsfield H. Color Atlas and Synopsis of Sexually Transmitted Diseases. 3rd ed. New York, NY: McGraw-Hill; 2011. (Courtesy of Claire E. Stevens.)

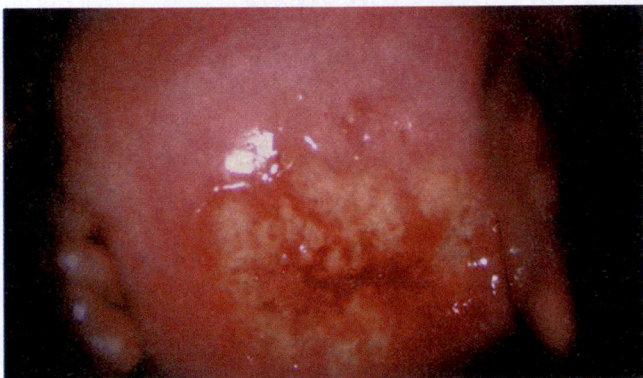

FIGURE 9-3 Friable cervix (erosive cervicitis).
Handsfield H. Color Atlas and Synopsis of Sexually Transmitted Diseases. 3rd ed. New York, NY: McGraw-Hill; 2011. (Courtesy of Claire E. Stevens.)

often reported. Clinical presentation of *C trachomatis* genitourinary (GU) infection in women typically includes the presence of mucopurulent discharge, often adherent to a friable cervix (Fig. 9-3). Cervical motion and adnexal tenderness are usually present when there is an upper reproductive tract infection such as PID.

Chlamydial infection in men is associated with irritative voiding symptoms with occasional mucopurulent penile discharge. However, many men are asymptomatic and act as reservoirs to spread infection. Chlamydial rectal infection can occur in receptive partners of anal intercourse of either gender. This can lead to proctitis, or inflammation of the inner lining of the rectum, resulting in pain and rectal discharge. Other infections caused by *C trachomatis* include salinities, endometritis, urethritis, epididymitis, and conjunctivitis. Signs of chlamydial conjunctivitis include unilateral mucopurulent discharge and redness. GU infections caused by the organisms *Ureaplasma urealyticum* and *M genitalium* present similarly as chlamydial infection and should be considered when making the differential diagnosis.

Diagnostic Testing

Diagnostic testing includes NAAT of endocervical, urethral, rectal, or oropharyngeal samples. A voided urine sample will also capture organisms for NAAT, which is the most sensitive test for detecting *C trachomatis* and has largely replaced other nonculture tests, including direct fluorescent antibody (DFA), enzyme-linked immunosorbent assay (ELISA), or DNA probe kits.

For uncomplicated chlamydial infection, a test-of-cure following completion of the antimicrobial course is not needed unless the patient has persistent symptoms or is pregnant. In pregnancy, testing for cure should be performed 3 weeks after completion of treatment. Because reinfection is common, all women with chlamydial infection should be retested 3 to 4 months after completing antimicrobial treatment. If a woman presents within 12 months of the initial infection and has not been previously screened, she should be reassessed for infection regardless of whether she says the partner was treated or not.

Routine screening—that is, testing that is encouraged and offered to all in a given group even in the absence of signs and symptoms—for C trachomatis infection is recommended annually for all sexually active females aged 25 years and younger as well as older women who are at higher risk of infection. Increased risk includes those who have a new sex partner, more than one sex partner, a sex partner with concurrent partners, or a sex partner with an STI. Evidence is insufficient to recommend routine screening for C trachomatis infection in sexually active men based on feasibility, efficacy, and cost-effectiveness. Screening of sexually active young men should be considered in clinical settings associated with high prevalence of chlamydial infection, including adolescent practices, correctional facilities, and STI clinics. Additionally, all pregnant women under 25 years as well as pregnant women 25 years and older who are at increased risk should be screened. MSM should be screened at least annually, and more frequently, as often as every 3 to 6 months, if remaining at increased risk.

Treatment

Treatment options for uncomplicated C trachomatis infection include oral antimicrobials that act against intracellular organisms, such as doxycycline, erythromycin, and azithromycin. Azithromycin is preferred, given in a highly efficacious, well-tolerated, single-dose oral therapy. In patients diagnosed with chlamydia or gonorrhea, providing prescriptions or medication for the patient to take to his/her partner without a clinical visit, known as expedited partner therapy (EPT), should be considered (though in gonococcal infection, IM ceftriaxone is the preferred treatment option and would require a visit to a health-care provider).

GONORRHEA

Overview

Gonorrhea, caused by the gram-negative diplococcus N gonorrhoeae, is also a common STI. This organism has a short incubation period of 1 to 5 days and is likely to cause infection in approximately 20% of men who have sexual contact with infected women and approximately 80% of women who have sexual contact with men with this infection.

Data from the Centers for Disease Control and Prevention (CDC) demonstrate that the higher percentage of total gonorrhoea cases occurs in MSM (approximately 45%), followed by women (approximately 35%), and men who have sex with women (approximately 30%).

> **CLINICAL CONCEPT**
> Manifestations of gonococcal infection can be found outside the GU system and commonly occur in the pharynx, rectum, and eye.

Clinical Presentation

Most men with gonococcal infection have no symptoms. In symptomatic men, presentation typically includes dysuria with a milky, occasionally blood-tinged penile discharge (Fig. 9-4). In women, presentation typically includes dysuria with a milky to purulent, occasionally blood-tinged, vaginal discharge (Fig. 9-5). Intermenstrual bleeding, dyspareunia, and mild lower abdominal pain can also be present, particularly with development of PID. With anal-insertive sex, rectal infection leading to proctitis is often seen that can present with pruritus, discharge, and tenesmus (cramping rectal pain).

Gonococcal pharyngitis can develop with orogenital contact. Though this is often asymptomatic, signs can include exudative pharyngitis with cervical lymphadenopathy. Gonococcal conjunctivitis is usually unilateral and can present with purulent discharge, eye pain, and photophobia. Without proper treatment, the condition can result in loss of the eye.

Diagnostic Testing

Though bacterial culture has been considered the gold standard for diagnosis, this test is not practical in the clinical setting. The NAAT assay is the test of choice to evaluate urogenital infections in both males and females and provides high specificity and sensitivity. A first-catch urine sample or vaginal swab should be sufficient to detect N gonorrhoeae. A Gram stain is still used in some clinical settings and can provide a high positive predictive value. However, a negative finding on Gram stain is not sufficient to rule out gonococcal infection.

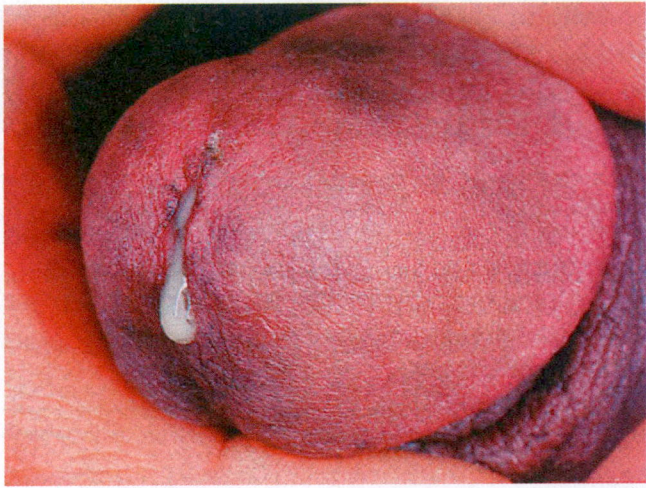

FIGURE 9-4 Gonorrhea (male).
Handsfield H. Color Atlas and Synopsis of Sexually Transmitted Diseases.
3rd ed. New York, NY: McGraw-Hill; 2011.

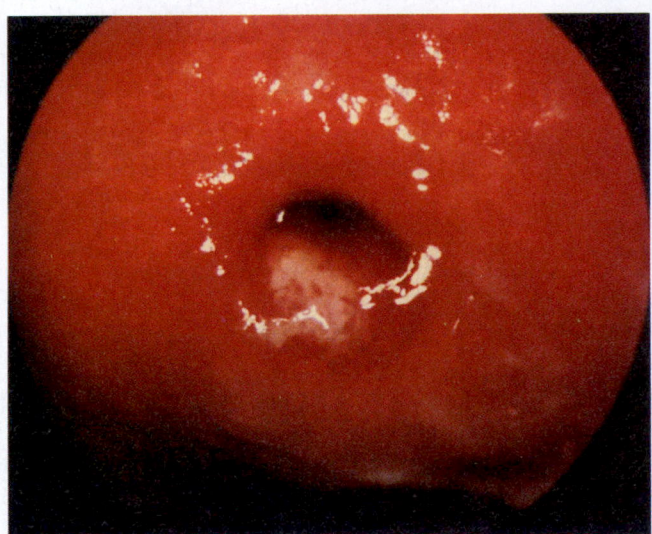

FIGURE 9-5 Gonococcal cervicitis.
Handsfield H. Color Atlas and Synopsis of Sexually Transmitted Diseases.
3rd ed. New York, NY: McGraw-Hill; 2011. (Courtesy of King. K. Holmes, MD, PhD.)

Treatment

Because *N gonorrhoeae* frequently produces beta-lactamase, the choice of a therapeutic agent should include agents with beta-lactamase stability, such as injectable ceftriaxone (as a single IM dose). Because of increasing rates of resistance, the use of the fluoroquinolones to treat this infection is no longer recommended. A single dose of oral cefixime can also be used if ceftriaxone is not available. In cases of severe cephalosporin allergy, gentamicin IM plus oral azithromycin (both as a single dose) can be used, though the effectiveness is less well studied. A test-of-cure is recommended 1 week following completion of therapy.

GENITAL HERPES

Overview

Genital herpes is a result of infection with an HHV (human herpes virus, also known as herpes simplex virus [HSV]). Most often, HSV-2 is the causative organism; HSV-1, the virus form that causes cold sores (herpes labialis), is more commonly acquired in childhood by contact with saliva that contains the virus. HSV-2 can also infect the perioral area.

HSV-2 can be spread through contact with vesicular skin lesions, mucosal surfaces, genital secretions, or oral secretions. The virus can also be shed from skin that looks normal.

Transmission most commonly occurs from an infected partner who does not have a visible sore and may not know that he or she is infected.

> **CLINICAL CONCEPT**
>
> In those with asymptomatic infections, genital shedding of HSV-2 occurs on 10% of days, even in the absence of any signs or symptoms.

Clinical Presentation

The clinical presentation usually includes a painful ulcerated genital lesion, often accompanied by inguinal lymphadenopathy. In women, the most common sites include the external genitalia, labia majora, labia minora, vaginal vestibule, and introitus (Fig. 9-6). If lesions involve the vagina or its introitus, a thin, usually watery, sometimes profuse discharge accompanies the infection. In men, the most common sites of lesions include the glans penis, the shaft of the penis, and sometimes the scrotum, thighs, and buttocks (Fig. 9-7). The initial infection tends to be more severe than subsequent recurrent infections, with higher pain levels associated with lesions and longer duration of

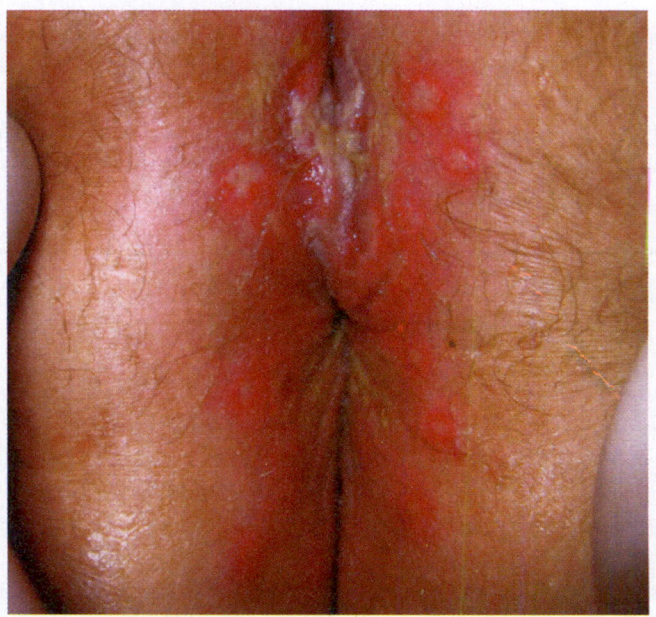

FIGURE 9-6 Genital herpes (female).
Handsfield H. Color Atlas and Synopsis of Sexually Transmitted Diseases. 3rd ed. New York, NY: McGraw-Hill; 2011.

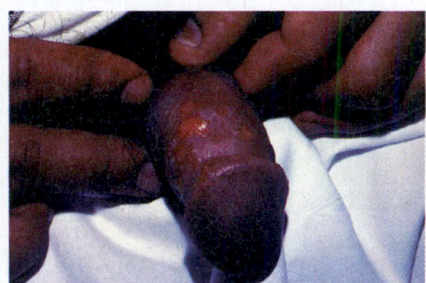

FIGURE 9-7 Genital herpes (male).
Dillon PM. Nursing Health Assessment: A Critical Thinking, Case Studies Approach. 2nd ed. Philadelphia, PA: F.A. Davis; 2007.

symptoms. An initial outbreak can also be associated with flu-like symptoms, including fever, body aches, and lymphadenopathy. Subsequent episodes are milder and shorter.

Diagnostic Testing

Diagnosis can be performed through direct (virological) or indirect (serological) testing. Viral culture is the standard for diagnosing genital herpes, which requires a collection of a sample from a sore. Polymerase chain reaction (PCR) can also be used to test for the presence of viral DNA or RNA from symptomatic patients and may allow for more rapid and accurate results. A Tzank smear can check for morphological changes associated with HSV infection but will not be able to distinguish between HSV-1 and HSV-2. Direct fluorescent antibody testing of cells scraped from a lesion can be used to distinguish HSV-1 and HSV-2. Serological approaches can detect for the presence of antibodies in the blood and can be used in both symptomatic and asymptomatic patients. In symptomatic patients, the use of direct and indirect assays can differentiate between a new infection and a newly recognized older infection. A positive virological test with a negative serological test would suggest a new infection. Positive results for both tests would indicate a recurrent infection. Approximately 15% of the adult population in the United States is seropositive for HHV-2; at the same time, only about 10% to 20% of the seropositive population have clinically evident disease in the form of genital herpes.

Treatment

Though there is no definitive cure for herpes, antiviral therapy for recurrent outbreaks can be given as suppression therapy to reduce the frequency of recurrences, or episodically to shorten the duration of lesions. Treatment with an antiviral such as acyclovir, famciclovir, or valacyclovir for acute infection, recurrence, or suppression is highly effective (Table 9-10). Topical penciclovir can also be a useful option, particularly for cold sores; its use for genital lesions is not recommended. Suppressive therapy reduces the frequency

TABLE 9-10 Sexually Transmitted Infections

CONDITION	TREATMENT OPTIONS
Genital herpes	For primary infection (initial episode): Acyclovir (Zovirax®) 400 mg PO tid × 7 to 10 days or ganciclovir (Famvir®) 250 mg PO tid × 7 to 10 days or valacyclovir (Valtrex®) 1 g PO bid × 7 to 10 days.
	For episodic recurrent infection (all PO; non-HIV patients): Acyclovir 800 mg tid × 2 days or 400 mg tid × 5 days or ganciclovir 1,000 mg bid ×1 day or 125 mg bid × 5 days or valacyclovir 1 g qd × 5 days or 500 mg bid × 3 days.
	For suppression of recurrent infection: Acyclovir 400 mg PO bid or ganciclovir 250 mg PO bid or valacyclovir 1 g PO qd or 500 mg PO qd*
	*Valacyclovir 500 mg qd is likely less effective than other regimens in persons with frequent recurrences (i.e., ≥10 episodes per year).
Nongonococcal urethritis and cervicitis	Primary therapy: azithromycin 1 g PO as a single dose; or doxycycline 100 mg PO bid × 7 days.
	Alternative therapy: erythromycin base 500 mg PO qid × 7 days; or ofloxacin 300 mg bid × 7 days; or levofloxacin 500 mg qd × 7 days.
Gonococcal urethritis and cervicitis	Recommended therapy: Combination therapy for uncomplicated infection.
	Single-dose ceftriaxone 250 mg IM plus single-dose azithromycin 1 g PO.
	Alternative therapy in the presence of severe beta-lactam allergy: gemifloxacin 320 mg PO single dose plus azithromycin 2 g PO as a single dose or combination of gentamicin 240 mg IM single dose plus azithromycin 2 g PO as a single dose.
	Oral cephalosporins no longer recommended.
Genital warts (condyloma acuminata)	Location of lesion can guide choice of treatment. Patient-applied therapy: Podofilox 0.5% solution or gel or imiquimod 5% cream or sinecatechins 15% ointment.
	Provider-applied therapy: Cryotherapy with liquid nitrogen or cryoprobe, trichloroacetic acid, or surgical removal.

Sources: Gilbert DN, Chambers HF, Eliopoulos GM, Saag MS, Pavia AT. The Sanford Guide to Antimicrobial Therapy. 50th ed. Sperryville, VA: Antimicrobial Therapy, Inc.; 2020:22–27; 176–180; Centers for Disease Control and Prevention. Sexually transmitted diseases treatment guidelines, 2015. MMWR. 2015;64(3):1–137.

of genital herpes recurrences by 70% to 80% in those who have frequent recurrences, though treatment is also effective in those who have less frequent recurrences. Suppression therapy also has the advantage of decreasing the risk for viral transmission to susceptible partners.

As with all STIs, a critical part of care is discussion of preventive strategies, including using condoms and limiting the number of sexual partners. NPs should offer and encourage testing for other STIs, including HIV, hepatitis B, and syphilis. Consideration should also be given to offering testing for hepatitis C and HHV type 2 (HSV type 2) serology. Immunization that provides protection against hepatitis A, hepatitis B, and HPV, if not previously immunized, should be offered and encouraged.

Discussion Sources

Centers for Disease Control and Prevention (CDC). *Sexually Transmitted Diseases Surveillance 2017*. Atlanta, GA: CDC; updated October 15, 2018. https://www.cdc.gov/std/stats17/default.htm

Centers for Disease Control and Prevention (CDC). Genital herpes—CDC fact sheet. https://www.cdc.gov/std/herpes/STDFact -Herpes.htm

Centers for Disease Control and Prevention. Sexually transmitted diseases treatment guidelines, 2015. *MMWR*. 2015;64(3):1–137. https://www.cdc.gov/std/tg2015/tg-2015-print.pdf

Marrazzo JM, Cates W. Reproductive tract infections, including HIV and other sexually transmitted infections. In: Hatcher RA, Trussell J, Nelson AL, Cates W, Kowal D, Policar MS, eds. *Contraceptive Technology*. 21st ed. Atlanta, GA: Managing Contraception; 2018.

QUESTIONS

124. Chlamydial infections occur most frequently among women in which age group?

   A. younger than 25 years

   B. 25 to 35 years

   C. 40 to 50 years

   D. over 60 years

125. Common sites of *C trachomatis* infection in women include all of the following except:

   A. ovaries.

   B. cervix.

   C. endometrium.

   D. urethra.

126. The incubation period for *C trachomatis* is approximately:

   A. 24 hours.

   B. 3 days.

   C. 7 to 14 days.

   D. 24 days.

127. Which of the following best describes the characteristics of a friable cervix?

   A. the presence of vesicular lesions

   B. a constant burning sensation felt deeply in the vagina

   C. the presence of multiple cyst-like lesions on cervix

   D. easily irritated and prone to bleeding, especially following intercourse

128 to 133. According to the CDC's recommendations, screening for *C trachomatis* infection is recommended for (*indicate Yes or No*):

_____ **128.** All sexually active women regardless of age.

_____ **129.** Sexually active women 25 years of age and younger.

_____ **130.** Sexually active women with a partner who has an STI.

_____ **131.** All sexually active men 25 years of age and younger.

_____ **132.** MSM regardless of age.

_____ **133.** All pregnant women 25 years and younger.

134. *N gonorrhoeae* are best described as:

    A. gram-positive cocci.

    B. gram-positive rods.

    C. gram-negative diplococci.

    D. gram-negative bacilli.

135. What is the approximate incubation period for *N gonorrhoea*?

    A. 1 to 5 days

    B. 7 to 10 days

    C. 18 days

    D. 28 days

136. The preferred treatment for uncomplicated gonococcal proctitis is:

    A. ceftriaxone 500 mg IM as a single dose.

    B. oral clarithromycin 500 mg bid for 7 days with a single dose of oral cefixime 400 mg.

    C. oral ofloxacin 400 mg bid with metronidazole 500 mg bid for 3 days.

    D. azithromycin 1 g PO as a single dose followed by 1 week of oral cefpodoxime 100 mg.

137. Which of the following is recommended by the CDC as therapy for uncomplicated urethritis caused by *N gonorrhoeae* when an oral product is the most appropriate option?

    A. cefixime PO 800 mg × 1 dose

    B. metronidazole PO 2 g daily × 3 days

    C. fosfomycin PO 3 g × 1 dose

    D. amoxicillin PO 2 g with doxycycline PO 100 mg daily for 3 days

138. You see a 42-year-old man with uncomplicated urogenital gonorrheal infection. His medical records indicate a severe allergic reaction to penicillin and cephalosporins that includes difficulty breathing and diffuse urticaria. You recommend treatment with:

    A. oral cefixime.

    B. oral levofloxacin.

    C. oral azithromycin plus IM gentamicin.

    D. parenteral tigecycline plus oral metronidazole.

139 to 142. Indicate (*Yes or No*) whether each finding normally would be present in symptomatic gonorrheal urethritis in an otherwise well 28-year-old man.

_____ 139. Dysuria

_____ 140. Milky penile discharge

_____ 141. Scrotal swelling

_____ 142. Fever

143. A 30-year-old woman presents without symptoms but states that her male partner has new-onset dysuria without penile discharge. Examination reveals a friable cervix covered with thick, yellow discharge. This description is most consistent with an infection caused by:

    A. *C trachomatis*.

    B. *N gonorrhoeae*.

    C. HSV.

    D. *T vaginalis*.

144. Which of the following agents is active against *N gonorrhoeae*?

    A. IM ceftriaxone

    B. oral metronidazole

    C. oral ketoconazole

    D. oral ciprofloxacin

145. Which of the following is recommended as the first-line therapy against *C trachomatis*?

    A. penicillin

    B. metronidazole

    C. azithromycin

    D. ceftriaxone

146. Which of the following statements is true of gonococcal infection?

    A. The risk of transmission from an infected woman to a male sexual partner is about 80%.

    B. Most men have asymptomatic infection.

    C. The incubation period is about 2 to 3 weeks.

    D. The organism rarely produces beta-lactamase.

147. Complications of gonococcal and chlamydial GU infection in women include all of the following except:

    A. PID.

    B. tubal scarring.

    C. acute pyelonephritis.

    D. acute peritoneal inflammation.

148. GU infections caused by *C trachomatis* present similarly to infections caused by (select all that apply):

    A. *T vaginalis*.

    B. *U urealyticum*.

    C. *M genitalium*.

    D. *C difficile*.

149. Which of the following is most likely found in chlamydial conjunctivitis?

    A. clear, watery discharge

    B. mucopurulent discharge

    C. bilateral cute eye pain

    D. decreased peripheral vision

150. Signs and symptoms of gonococcal or chlamydial proctitis include all of the following except:

    A. rectal discharge.

    B. external hemorrhoid.

    C. tenesmus.

    D. pruritus.

151. All of the following are likely reported in a woman with an initial episode of genital HSV-2 (HHV-2) infection except:

    A. painful ulcerated vulvar lesions.

    B. inguinal lymphadenopathy.

C. thin vaginal discharge.

D. pustular lesions.

152 to 155. A 28-year-old woman presents with a history of HSV-2 infection. She is currently free of typical signs and symptoms associated with this condition. She asks in which ways she could likely spread the virus. You respond that HSV-2 virus can be transmitted through contact with (*indicate Yes or No*):

_____ **152.** genital secretions.

_____ **153.** oral secretions.

_____ **154.** intact skin.

_____ **155.** sharing of bath towels or similar items.

156. When lesions caused by HSV-2 involve the vagina and its introitus, this is usually accompanied by:

A. adnexal tenderness.

B. a friable cervix.

C. rash extending to the upper thighs.

D. a thin profuse discharge.

157. Approximately what percentage of sexually active adults has serological evidence of HHV-2 or HSV type 2?

A. 5%

B. 15%

C. 25%

D. 40%

158. HSV-1, the virus form that causes cold sores (herpes labialis), is more commonly acquired in which of the following situations? Choose all that apply.

A. in childhood

B. in adulthood

C. by sexual contact

D. by contact with oral secretions.

159. During asymptomatic HSV-2 infections, genital shedding of virus occurs during approximately up to _____ of days.

A. 5%

B. 20%

C. 50%

D. 100%

160 to 162. For each patient, indicate the most appropriate diagnostic approach to identify HSV-2 infection (PCR, serological, or both).

_____ **160.** A 32-year-old man with a 2-year history of recurrent, self-resolving, painful penile lesions who currently has one cluster of vesicles on the penile shaft

_____ **161.** A 27-year-old woman with an initial outbreak of vulvar vesicles

_____ **162.** A 41-year-old man who reports having outbreaks in the past but has not had any in the past 3 years

163. The preferred treatment options for a 28-year-old woman who presents with HSV-2 genital infection with vulvar vesicles include:

A. oral ribavirin.

B. oral indinavir.

C. oral famciclovir.

D. topical acyclovir.

164. Suppressive therapy reduces the frequency of genital herpes recurrences by:

A. 5% to 10%.

B. 20% to 25%.

C. 40% to 50%.

D. 70% to 80%.

165. Recommended comprehensive STI testing includes testing for all of the following except:

A. hepatitis B.

B. syphilis.

C. hepatitis A.

D. HIV.

E. hepatitis C.

F. HSV-2

For answers and rationales, see end of chapter.

Pelvic Inflammatory Disease (PID)

Overview

PID is an infectious disease noted only in women, consisting of endometritis, salinities, and oophoritis. The condition is caused by various pathogens, including *C trachomatis*, *N gonorrhoeae*, *H influenzae*, *Streptococcus* species, select anaerobes, *Mycoplasma* species, and *Ureaplasma* species; approximately 60% of infections are acquired through sexual transmission. The majority of STIs cause lower reproductive tract infection, such as urethritis and/or cervicitis, but not the upper reproductive tract infection as noted in PID.

> **CLINICAL CONCEPT**
> Approximately 30% to 40% of PID infections are polymicrobial.

Clinical Presentation

Clinical presentation usually includes a chief complaint of lower abdominal pain that is usually present for a number of days and worsens during this time period. Other signs and symptoms can include abnormal vaginal discharge, dyspareunia, fever, gastrointestinal upset, and/or abnormal vaginal bleeding. An adnexal mass can be palpable when tubo-ovarian abscess is present. PID should be considered when a woman presents with new-onset lower abdominal or pelvic pain coupled with at least one of the following findings on clinical examination: cervical motion tenderness, uterine tenderness, or adnexal tenderness.

Diagnostic Testing

Supporting laboratory findings in PID include elevated erythrocyte sedimentation rate or C-reactive protein level and leukocytosis with neutrophilia. Although diagnosis can usually be made from clinical findings, transvaginal pelvic ultrasound, if obtained, will typically demonstrate tubal thickening with or without free pelvic fluid or tubo-ovarian abscess. Pelvic ultrasound offers an acceptable imaging option and avoids the radiation burden and increased cost associated with pelvic computed tomography (CT) (Box 9-2). Laparoscopy is rarely needed but offers high specificity and sensitivity in diagnosing PID with findings of tubal wall edema and hyperemia of the tubal surface. Testing for *C trachomatis* and *N gonorrhoeae* should be performed with culture, DNA probe, or NAAT assay.

Treatment

Treatment options differ according to patient presentation. When a woman with PID is severely ill, is pregnant, or has tubo-ovarian abscess, hospitalization for hydration and parenteral antibiotic therapy is indicated. In most situations, outpatient therapy with oral and parenteral antibiotics is sufficient. Ceftriaxone, 250 mg IM as a one-time dose, followed by oral doxycycline, 100 mg bid for 2 weeks with or without oral metronidazole 500 mg, is likely the most commonly used treatment regimen and is highly

> ## BOX 9-2 Diagnostic Criteria for Pelvic Inflammatory Disease (PID)
>
> Empiric treatment for PID should be initiated in sexually active young women and other women at risk for sexually transmitted infections if they are experiencing pelvic or lower abdominal pain, if no cause for the illness other than PID can be identified, and if one or more of the following minimum criteria are present on pelvic examination:
>
> ■ Cervical motion tenderness
>
> *or*
>
> ■ Uterine tenderness
>
> *or*
>
> ■ Adnexal tenderness
>
> One or more of the following additional criteria can be used to enhance the specificity of the minimum criteria and support a diagnosis of PID:
>
> ■ Oral temperature greater than 101°F (greater than 38.3°C)
> ■ Abnormal cervical or vaginal mucopurulent discharge
> ■ Presence of abundant numbers of white blood cells on saline microscopy of vaginal fluid
> ■ Elevated erythrocyte sedimentation rate
> ■ Elevated C-reactive protein
> ■ Laboratory documentation of cervical infection with *N gonorrhoeae* or *C trachomatis*

effective. Keeping in mind that 30% to 40% of infections are polymicrobial, the addition of metronidazole is helpful in the treatment of bacterial vaginosis or anaerobic organisms that are often found in the woman with PID. Injectable cefoxitin plus probenecid along with doxycycline and metronidazole offers an alternative oral treatment option. For inpatient treatment, IV cefotetan or IV cefoxitin plus doxycycline (IV/PO) can be used. With severe penicillin or cephalosporin allergy, IV clindamycin plus IV gentamicin followed by oral doxycycline can be used. IV therapy should be continued until there is an adequate response for at least 24 hours before switching to oral treatment. Fluoroquinolones, whether oral or injectable, are no longer recommended for PID due to high resistance rates found in *N gonorrhoeae*.

As with all STIs, a critical part of care is discussion of preventive strategies, including using condoms and limiting the number of sexual partners. NPs should offer and encourage testing for other STIs, including HIV, hepatitis B, and syphilis. Consideration should also be given to offering testing for hepatitis C and HHV type 2 (HSV type 2) serology. Immunization that provides protection against hepatitis A, hepatitis B, and HPV, if not previously immunized, should be offered and encouraged.

Discussion Sources

Centers for Disease Control and Prevention. Sexually transmitted diseases treatment guidelines, 2015. *MMWR*. 2015;64(3):1–137. https://www.cdc.gov/std/tg2015/tg-2015-print.pdf

Marrazzo JM, Cates W. Reproductive tract infections, including HIV and other sexually transmitted infections. In: Hatcher RA, Trussell J, Nelson AL, Cates W, Kowal D, Policar MS, eds. *Contraceptive Technology*. 21st ed. Atlanta, GA: Managing Contraception; 2018.

QUESTIONS

166. Women with PID typically present with all of the following except:

    A. dysuria.

    B. leukopenia.

    C. cervical motion tenderness.

    D. abdominal pain.

167. A 22-year-old woman complains of a 3-day history of progressively worsening pelvic pain. Physical examination reveals cervical motion tenderness and uterine tenderness. Which of the following would further support a diagnosis of PID?

A. 3-day history of loose stools

B. small number of WBCs in vaginal fluid

C. mucopurulent vaginal discharge

D. laboratory documentation of cervical infection with *E coli*

168. The most likely causative pathogen in a 23-year-old woman with PID is:

A. *E coli.*

B. Enterobacteriaceae.

C. *C trachomatis.*

D. *Pseudomonas.*

169. The presence of an adnexal mass in the woman with PID most likely indicates the presence of:

A. uterine fibroids.

B. an ectopic pregnancy.

C. ovarian malignancy.

D. a tubo-ovarian abscess.

170. Up to what percent of PID infections are polymicrobial?

A. less than 1%

B. 15%

C. 40%

D. 75%

171. Expected laboratory findings for the woman with PID include all of the following except:

A. elevated erythrocyte sedimentation rate (ESR).

B. elevated C-reactive protein (CRP).

C. decreased hemoglobin.

D. leukocytosis.

172. A transvaginal ultrasound in the woman with PID will likely show:

A. tubal thickening with or without free pelvic fluid.

B. cervical thickening.

C. endometrial thinning.

D. inflammation of the ovaries.

173. Which of the following is most consistent with a woman with PID?

A. temperature 99.6°F (37.6°C); total WBC 8,000/mm³

B. temperature 101.4°F (38.6°C); WBC total 6,000/mm³

C. temperature 99.0°F (37.2°C); total WBC 14,000/mm³

D. temperature 101.5°F (38.6°C); total WBC 16,000/mm³

174. Which of the following is a treatment option for a 28-year-old woman with PID who has no history of medication allergy and has undergone a bilateral tubal ligation?

A. PO ofloxacin with PO metronidazole

B. IM gentamicin with PO cefpodoxime

C. IM ceftriaxone with PO doxycycline

D. PO clindamycin with PO azithromycin

175. Which of the following is a treatment option for a 30-year-old woman with PID with a tubo-ovarian abscess and a history of severe hive-form reaction with wheezing when taking a penicillin or cephalosporin?

A. PO ofloxacin with PO metronidazole

B. IM cetriaxone with PO doxycycline

C. IV cefotetan with IV vancomycin

D. IV clindamycin plus IV gentamicin then PO doxycycline

For answers and rationales, see end of chapter.

Additional Sexually Transmitted Infections

HUMAN PAPILLOMAVIRUS INFECTION

Overview

HPV is a small DNA virus with more than 120 known types; this virus usually infects the epithelium. A variety of benign and malignant diseases are caused by HPV infection. Infection with multiple HPV types is the rule. Route of transmission is via direct contact with a person who has HPV, whether or not signs and symptoms of the infection are present.

Anal, penile, and cervical carcinomas are largely the consequences of HPV infection. Over 99% of cervical cancer is attributed to HPV infection, as well as about 90% of anal cancers and 60% of penile cancers. HPV has also been implicated in causing up to 70% of oropharyngeal cancers. HPV types with high malignancy risks include types 16, 18, 31, 33, 35, 39, and 45.

Not all HPV types are correlated with malignancy, however. Largely benign, often self-limiting disease is seen with infection with types 6, 11, 40, 42, 43, 44, 54, 61, 70, 72, and 81. Condyloma acuminatum describes the verruciform lesion seen in genital warts. The causative agent is HPV, and infection with multiple HPV types is usually seen with genital infection (Fig. 9-8). More than 90% of genital warts are caused by HPV types 6 and 11.

Clinical Presentation

In genital warts, also known as condyloma acuminata, verruciform lesions are noted. These usually vary in size, shape, and number. The skin-colored lesions can be raised or flat with a smooth or rough feel,

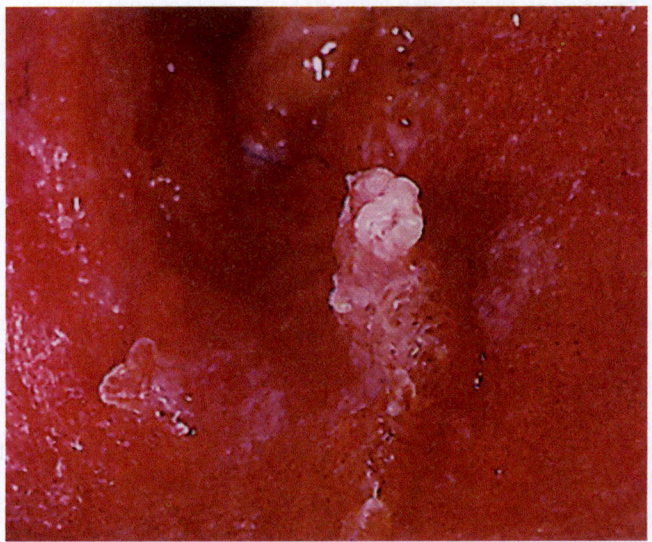

FIGURE 9-8 Condylomata acuminate.
Handsfield H. Color Atlas and Synopsis of Sexually Transmitted Diseases. 3rd ed. New York, NY: McGraw-Hill; 2011.

often presenting with a cauliflower-like appearance. Though lesions can present without other symptoms, some people will report pain, itching, burning, or bleeding. The most common sites in females include the vulva, vagina, cervix, and groin area. In males, lesions can appear on the penis, scrotum, and thigh and groin areas. Lesions can also appear in the mouth and throat of those who have had oral sex with an infected person, as well as around the anus for those who have anal intercourse with a partner who carries the virus.

Clinical presentation and diagnosis of cervical and anogenital cancer are discussed later in this chapter.

Diagnostic Testing

A diagnosis of genital warts can usually be made with patient history and physical examination. A biopsy might be needed for atypical presentation of lesions or patients with recurrent or resistant infection. Routine screening for women for precursors to cervical cancer is done through cytology assays (i.e., Pap test or Pap smear) and HPV testing. (See the Cancer Screening section later for more information.) Anal cancer caused by HPV has similar pathophysiological aspects as cervical cancer, and screening with a Pap test can be considered in high-risk populations. High-risk populations include MSM, men who are immunocompromised (e.g., living with HIV), as well as women with a history of anogenital HPV infection. As there is a lack of evidence demonstrating the value of routine screening with anal Pap tests, there are currently no formal recommendations to screen for abnormal anal cells. However, given the success of Pap smears in detecting and preventing cervical cancer, the use of anal Pap smears can likely provide similar benefits in high-risk populations.

Treatment

About 50% of patients have spontaneous regression of genital warts without intervention. The most common treatment options for genital warts include podofilox, imiquimod, trichloroacetic acid, or cryotherapy. The location of lesions can dictate therapeutic choices; imiquimod use is only indicated for external lesions. Prescribing patient-administered therapies, such as imiquimod (Aldara®) or podofilox, saves the cost and inconvenience of office visits. Surgical intervention and laser ablation are typically reserved for complicated, recalcitrant lesions.

Primary prevention of HPV disease is available through immunization. Gardasil®9 (protects against HPV strains 6, 11, 16, 18, 31, 33, 45, 52, 58) is approved for males and females aged 9 to 45 years. The Advisory Committee on Immunization Practices (ACIP) recommends vaccination for all males and females up to age 26 years, though immunization is preferred at younger ages due to higher immunogenicity and earlier protection from infection. Vaccination in older adults (27 to 45 years) can be considered following shared clinical decision making between the patient and health-care provider. Vaccination involves a series of IM injections and should ideally be started at age 11 to 12 years, prior to onset of sexual activity. Only two doses are needed for those younger than 15 years, while three doses are required when immunization is given after 15 years of age. (See Chapter 2 and Chapter 17 for recommended immunization schedules.)

SYPHILIS

Overview

Caused by the spirochete *Treponema pallidum*, syphilis is a complex, multiorgan disease. Sexual contact is the usual route of transmission. The initial lesion forms about 2 to 4 weeks after contact; contagion is greatest during the secondary stage (Fig. 9-9).

Clinical Presentation

Syphilis is divided into four stages: primary, secondary, latent, and tertiary. Each stage occurs during a time period after acquisition of the causative organism.

Primary syphilis occurs 3 to 90 days after initial exposure and is characterized by the development of a chancre, a firm, round, painless genital and/or anal ulcer(s) with clean base and indurated margins, accompanied by localized lymphadenopathy. The location of the chancre correlates with the site of infection acquisition. As a result, more than 90% of chancres are in the anogenital region, and the remaining are oral lesions. This stage lasts for about 3 weeks.

While the chancre itself resolves, the causative organism for the condition remains in circulation.

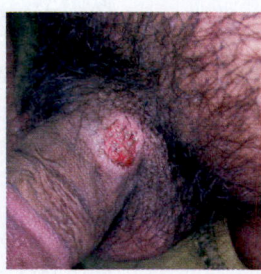

FIGURE 9-9 Typical chancre of primary syphilis.
Venes D. Taber's Cyclopedic Medical Dictionary. 22nd ed. Philadelphia, PA: F.A. Davis; 2013.

Secondary syphilis occurs 4 to 10 weeks after initial infection. This is characterized by a nonpruritic skin rash, often involving the palms and soles, as well as mucous membrane lesions. Fever, lymphadenopathy, sore throat, patchy hair loss, headaches, weight loss, muscle aches, and fatigue commonly are reported. Resolution without treatment is possible.

Latent syphilis is the stage when secondary syphilis resolves though the patient remains seroreactive. A recurrence of skin lesions similar to those observed during secondary syphilis can occur periodically. An early latent syphilis diagnosis can be made if, during the year preceding the diagnosis, the individual had: (1) a documented seroconversion or sustained fourfold or greater increase in nontreponemal test titers; (2) unequivocal symptoms of primary or secondary syphilis; or (3) a sex partner documented to have primary, secondary, or early latent syphilis. In the absence of these conditions, the patient is assumed to have late latent syphilis. Whereas most remain asymptomatic without treatment, about one-third will progress to tertiary syphilis.

Tertiary syphilis occurs 3 to 15 years after initial infection and primarily affects the cardiovascular system and central nervous system. Three categories of tertiary syphilis include gummatous syphilis, cardiovascular syphilis, and neurosyphilis. Gumma (granulomatous lesions involving skin, mucous membranes, and bone) present as a center of necrotic tissue with a rubbery texture that eventually break down to form an ulcer. Cardiovascular syphilis occurs at least 10 years following the primary infection and can cause aortic insufficiency and aortic aneurysm, possibly resulting in aortic valve insufficiency. Neurosyphilis can present in various forms depending on the site of infection. Syphilitic meningitis is an early condition, usually presenting within 6 months of primary infection. Meningovascular syphilis results in damage to blood vessels in the meninges, brain, and spinal cord that causes neurological impairment. Damage to the brain can cause symptoms that mimic dementia, including impairment of memory and speech, personality changes, irritability, and psychotic symptoms. Seizures as well as the Argyll-Robertson pupil (a pupil that does not react to light) can also be present.

Diagnostic Testing

Several laboratory tests are available to screen or diagnose syphilis using blood, body fluid, or tissue samples. Screening tests include the rapid plasma reagin (RPR) test, the rapid immunochromatographic test, or Venereal Disease Research Laboratory (VDRL) test, that each check for antibodies against syphilis. The VDRL is not specific for syphilis. With a positive result from a screening test, a second test should be performed to confirm the diagnosis.

Confirmatory tests that check for antibodies against syphilis include enzyme immunoassay (EIA), the fluorescent treponemal antibody absorption (FTA-ABS) test, and the *Treponema pallidum* particle agglutination assay (TPPA). The FTA-ABS test is only useful after 3 to 4 weeks of exposure. Additionally, darkfield microscopy can identify syphilis in a sample of fluid or tissue from an open sore. Microhemagglutination assay (MHA-TP) can also be used to confirm syphilis when another test had a positive result.

Treatment

Treatment is guided by the stage of disease and clinical manifestations (Table 9-11; Figs. 9-10 and 9-11). Given the significant complications associated with untreated syphilis, adherence to therapy is critical.

HIV Testing, PrEP, and PEP

Overview

HIV and acquired immunodeficiency syndrome (AIDS) remain leading causes of morbidity and mortality in the United States. However, the annual number of new HIV cases has decreased substantially since 1994, partially attributed to limiting the spread of the virus through improved HIV treatment and HIV screening. Approximately 16 to 22 million individuals between the ages of 18 and 64 years are tested annually for HIV, which potentially helps limit the unknowing spread of the virus, particularly since people living with HIV are usually well for many years after initial infection.

The CDC recommends screening for HIV infection should be performed at least once as part of routine health care for all patients aged 13 to 64 years in all health-care settings, including hospital emergency departments, urgent care clinics, correctional health-care facilities, inpatient services, and STI clinics or other venues offering STI services. HIV screening is recommended for all individuals who seek evaluation

TABLE 9-11 Stages of Syphilis and Recommended Treatment

STAGE OF SYPHILIS	TREATMENT OPTIONS	COMMENT
Primary syphilis	Recommended therapy: ■ Benzathine penicillin G 2.4 million U IM as a one-time dose Alternative therapy in penicillin allergy: ■ Doxycycline 100 mg PO bid for 2 weeks or tetracycline 500 mg PO qid × 14 days or ceftriaxone 1 g IM/IV qd × 10 to 14 days (follow-up mandatory)	Azithromycin 2 g PO as a one-time dose has been suggested, although issues of emerging resistance are concerning
Secondary syphilis	Recommended therapy: ■ Benzathine penicillin G 2.4 million U IM as a one-time dose Alternative therapy in penicillin allergy: ■ Doxycycline 100 mg PO bid for 2 weeks or tetracycline 500 mg PO qid × 14 days or ceftriaxone 1 g IM/IV qd × 10 to 14 days (follow-up mandatory)	Also treatment for latent syphilis of less than 1-year duration
Late or tertiary syphilis (more than 1 year's duration or indeterminate duration, cardiovascular effects, gumma)	Recommended therapy: ■ Benzathine penicillin G 7.2 million U IM total, administered as three doses of 2.4 million U IM each at 1-week intervals Alternative therapy in penicillin allergy: ■ Doxycycline 100 mg PO bid for 4 weeks or tetracycline 500 mg PO qid × 28 days Expert consultation advisable, especially in the face of neurosyphilis	With neurosyphilis: penicillin G 18 to 24 million units per day, either as continuous infusion or 3 to 4 million units IV q4h × 10 to 14 days

Sources: Centers for Disease Control and Prevention. Sexually transmitted diseases treatment guidelines, 2015. MMWR. 2015;64(3):1–137; Gilbert DN, Chambers HF, Eliopoulos GM, Saag MS, Pavia AT. The Sanford Guide to Antimicrobial Therapy. 50th ed. Sperryville, VA: Antimicrobial Therapy, Inc.; 2020:24.

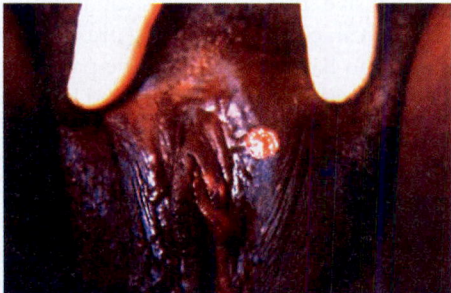

FIGURE 9-10 Syphilitic lesions around the vagina.
Centers for Disease Control and Prevention. https://phil.cdc.gov/Details.aspx?pid=5340

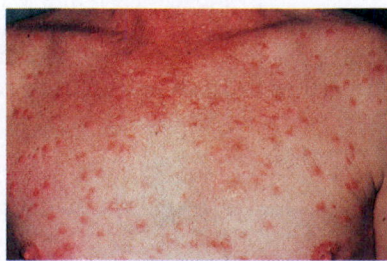 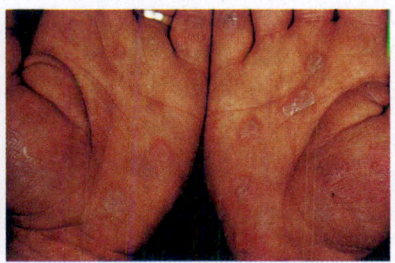

FIGURE 9-11 Rash on chest and palms due to secondary syphilis.
Goldsmith, LA, Lazaraus GS, Tharp MD. Adult and Pediatric Dermatology: A Color Guide to Diagnosis and Treatment. Philadelphia, PA: F.A. Davis; 1997.

or treatment of STIs. HIV testing should be performed after notifying the patient that the test will be performed and giving the patient the opportunity to decline or defer testing. Screening should be voluntary, and individuals should have an opportunity to opt out of testing.

Diagnostic Testing

HIV infection can be detected by serological tests that detect antibodies (Ab) against HIV-1 and HIV-2 or by virological tests that detect HIV antigens (Ag) or RNA. Serological tests are highly sensitive and specific, and rapid antibody tests (e.g., OraQuick HIV Test®) can allow clinicians to make a preliminary diagnosis within 30 minutes. However, it can take 3 to 12 weeks for an HIV-positive person to make enough antibodies to be detected by Ab tests; a negative result during this window period requires repeat testing 3 months following the possible time of HIV exposure. Therefore, the use of Ag/Ab combination tests is encouraged (window period of 2 to 6 weeks), especially if the individual is unlikely to review his or her test results. A preliminary positive test result must be followed by additional testing with an antibody immunoassay (e.g., HIV-1/HIV-2 antibody differentiation test, Western blot, or indirect immunofluorescence assay) to definitively establish the diagnosis.

Repeat screening should be performed at least annually for high-risk individuals who have a negative test result. These include injection-drug users and their sex partners, persons who exchange sex for money or drugs, sex partners of HIV-infected persons, and MSM or heterosexual persons who themselves or whose sex partners have had more than one sex partner since their most recent HIV test.

Ideally, a positive HIV test result should be communicated confidentially through personal contact by a clinician, counselor, or staff member appropriately educated in providing this information. For patients with limited English proficiency, when the health-care provider is not proficient in the patient's primary language, family or friends should not be used as interpreters to disclose HIV-positive test results. Health-care providers should strongly encourage patients to disclose their HIV status to their spouses, current and future sex partners, and previous sex partners and recommend these partners be tested for HIV infection. Health departments can assist patients in notifying these partners without disclosing the patient's identity. For individuals who get a positive result from a home test, they should be instructed to see a health-care provider for follow-up testing.

Treatment

Comprehensive risk transmission instruction is critical. HIV/AIDS treatment should be done in consultation with experts in the comprehensive treatment of this condition.

Individuals at high risk for HIV can consider initiating pre-exposure prophylaxis (PrEP). Those at high risk of HIV include MSM men who have an HIV-positive partner or multiple partners, a partner with multiple partners, or a partner with unknown HIV status and have anal sex without a condom or recently had an STI. Heterosexual individuals are at high risk if they have an HIV-positive partner or have multiple partners, a partner with multiple partners, or a partner with unknown HIV status and do not always use a condom for sex with individuals who inject drugs or with MSM. Those who inject drugs and share needles, syringes, or other equipment to inject drugs are also at high risk.

> **CLINICAL CONCEPT**
>
> PrEP typically uses a combination of standard HIV medications and should be continued as long as the individual remains at high risk for HIV.

Postexposure prophylaxis (PEP) is recommended for individuals who have been potentially exposed to HIV to prevent becoming infected. PEP should be started within 72 hours of an individual's possible exposure, and treatment should continue for 28 days with standard HIV medications; see CDC.gov for more information on PrEP and PEP.

As with all STIs, a critical part of care is discussion of preventive strategies, including using condoms and limiting the number of sexual partners. NPs should offer and encourage testing for other STIs, including chlamydia, gonorrhea, hepatitis B, and syphilis. Consideration should also be given to offering testing for hepatitis C and HHV type 2 (HSV type 2) serology. For those not previously immunized, immunization that provides protection against hepatitis A, hepatitis B, and HPV should be offered and encouraged.

Discussion Sources

Centers for Disease Control and Prevention. Sexually transmitted diseases treatment guidelines, 2015. *MMWR*. 2015;64(3):1–137. https://www.cdc.gov/std/tg2015/tg-2015-print.pdf

Centers for Disease Control and Prevention. Revised recommendations for HIV testing of adults, adolescents, and pregnant women in health-care settings. *MMWR*. 2006;55(RR14):1–17.

Gilbert DN, Chambers HF, Eliopoulos GM, Saag MS, Pavia AT. *The Sanford Guide to Antimicrobial Therapy*. 50th ed. Sperryville, VA: Antimicrobial Therapy, Inc.; 2020:24.

Marrazzo JM, Cates W. Reproductive tract infections, including HIV and other sexually transmitted infections. In: Hatcher RA, Trussell J, Nelson AL, Cates W, Kowal D, Policar MS, eds. *Contraceptive Technology*. 21st ed. Atlanta, GA: Managing Contraception; 2018.

QUESTIONS

176. Which of the following best describes lesions associated with condyloma acuminatum?
    A. verruciform
    B. plaque-like
    C. vesicular form
    D. bullous

177. Sequelae of genital HPV infection in a man can include:
    A. anorectal carcinoma.
    B. low sperm count.
    C. paraphimosis.
    D. Reiter's syndrome.

178. Treatment options for patients with condyloma acuminatum include all of the following except:
    A. topical acyclovir.
    B. cryotherapy.
    C. podofilox.
    D. trichloroacetic acid.

179. Which HPV types are most likely to cause genital condyloma acuminatum in a 24-year-old woman?
    A. 1, 2, and 3
    B. 6 and 11
    C. 16 and 18
    D. 35 and 39

180. Which HPV types are most often associated with cervical and anogenital cancer?
    A. 1, 2, and 3
    B. 6 and 11
    C. 16 and 18
    D. 40 and 42

181. What percentage of anogenital and cervical cancers can be attributed to HPV infection?
    A. less than 30%
    B. at least 50%
    C. at least 70%
    D. 90% or greater

182. Anal Papanicolaou (Pap) tests can be considered for all of the following patient populations except:
    A. men with HIV.
    B. MSM.
    C. women with a history of anogenital HPV infection.
    D. all males under age 25 years.

183. Which of the following terms describes the mechanism of action of imiquimod (Aldara®)?
    A. keratolytic
    B. immune modulator
    C. cryogenic
    D. cytolytic

184. How long after contact do clinical manifestations of syphilis typically occur?
    A. less than 1 week
    B. 1 to 3 weeks
    C. 2 to 4 weeks
    D. 4 to 6 weeks

185 to 192. Indicate if each of the following symptoms is found during the primary, secondary, or tertiary stage of syphilis.
    _____ 185. Painless ulcer
    _____ 186. Diffuse lymphadenopathy
    _____ 187. Gumma
    _____ 188. Spontaneously healing lesion
    _____ 189. Aortic insufficiency
    _____ 190. Arthralgia
    _____ 191. Macular or papular lesions involving the palms and soles
    _____ 192. Flu-like symptoms

193. Syphilis is most contagious during which of the following?
    A. before onset of signs and symptoms
    B. at the primary stage
    C. at the secondary stage
    D. at the tertiary stage

194. First-line treatment options for primary syphilis include:
    A. IM penicillin.
    B. PO ciprofloxacin.
    C. PO doxycycline
    D. IM ceftriaxone.

195. A 26-year-old woman with a history of injection drug use is diagnosed with chlamydial infection and undergoes STI testing. An RPR test is positive for syphilis. The NP recommends:
    A. initiating treatment with IM penicillin.
    B. initiating treatment with PO metronidazole.
    C. performing a second test (e.g., TPPA) to confirm the diagnosis.
    D. referral to an infectious diseases specialist.

196. A 22-year-old male presents with a diffuse maculopapular rash extending to his palms along with flu-like symptoms. He reports having a sore on his penis about a month ago that eventually healed by itself. A TPPA assay is performed and returns positive. The next best course of action is:
    A. repeat testing with the VDRL test.
    B. confirm the diagnosis with darkfield microscopy.

C. initiate treatment with IM penicillin.

D. initiate treatment with PO TMP-SMX.

197 to 200. HIV screening is recommended for which of the following (*indicate Yes or No*):

_____ **197.** A 17-year-old female who states she has no risk factors for HIV and who requests the test

_____ **198.** A 47-year-old male seeking treatment for syphilis

_____ **199.** A 36-year-old pregnant woman

_____ **200.** A 24-year-old male who is an injection-drug user

201. A 32-year-old female reports that she believes she was exposed to HIV via sexual activity 4 weeks ago and requests testing. She is given a rapid antibody test (OraQuick® HIV Test) and the results are negative. The NP recommends:

A. no further testing is necessary.

B. repeat testing in 2 weeks.

C. repeat testing in 2 months.

D. repeat testing in 1 year.

202. When a positive HIV test result is obtained, which of the following statements is most accurate in communicating the results to the patient?

A. Optimally, communication of positive results should be done through in-person contact.

B. An English-speaking first-degree relative can be used as a translator when the patient is not proficient in the English language.

C. Text messaging or e-mail can be used to communicate results if the contact information is provided by the patient and the patient agrees to this at the time of testing.

D. It is appropriate to inform the spouse or partner of a positive test result if the patient is unavailable.

203. A 32-year-old injection-drug user is tested for HIV and has a negative test result. In addition to recommending HIV-prevention counseling and offering PrEP, you advise:

A. repeat testing every month.

B. repeat testing within 1 year.

C. repeat testing in 2 years.

D. that no repeat testing is needed unless new-onset symptoms develop.

For answers and rationales, see end of chapter.

Testicular Torsion

Overview

The male with testicular torsion who reports a sudden onset of scrotal pain is a urological emergency. The condition is caused by a twisting of the testis and spermatic cord around a vertical axis; experimental modeling of the event reveals that a 720° twist is needed to occlude arterial and venous blood flow and cause the resulting testicular swelling and testicular tissue death. The left testicle is most often affected.

This condition is most often found in the adolescent; one hypothesis is that the increasing testicular weight noted during puberty increases the torsion risk. Less commonly, neonates and men in their 40s and 50s develop this condition. Occasionally the condition is associated with recent scrotal trauma, such as an injury during a sporting event, but most will occur spontaneously. Approximately 50% of men presenting with torsion report intermittent unilateral testicular pain in the past, perhaps caused by partial, reversible torsion.

Clinical Presentation

Patients with testicular torsion report a sudden onset of severe unilateral scrotal pain with noticeable swelling of the ipsilateral testicle. On examination, the affected testicle is held high in the scrotum, there is an absent cremasteric reflex, and a lack of pain relief with scrotal elevation.

Diagnostic Testing

Often, with classic testicular torsion presentation, diagnostic testing is not done, and prompt intervention is sought. When diagnostic confirmation is warranted, Doppler ultrasound is the first-line study in testicular torsion and can also help rule out the condition. This study will show reduction of blood flow.

Components of TWIST include testis swelling (2 points), hard testis (2 points), absent cremasteric reflex (1 point), nausea/vomiting (1 point), and high-riding testis (1 point). Using a cut-off value of 2 points provides a 100% negative predictive value, suggesting ultrasound is not needed. A score of 5 to 6 indicates high-risk patients that should proceed directly to surgery, while intermediate-risk patients should undergo ultrasound for further evaluation.

Treatment

Prompt referral to a urological surgeon for detorsion of the organ and restoration of testicular blood flow is indicated. Testicular survival surpasses 85% if detorsion is accomplished within 6 hours. Manual manipulation of the testicle to unwind the torsion is occasionally helpful, largely as a gap measure until surgical intervention is able to be accessed. A bilateral orchiopexy, a procedure in which both testes are brought down and tacked lower in the scrotum, is usually performed to avoid subsequent torsion.

Discussion Source

Rupp TJ. Testicular torsion in emergency medicine. Medscape. http://emedicine.medscape.com/article/778086-overview

QUESTIONS

204. A 24-year-old man presents with sudden onset of left-sided scrotal pain. He reports having intermittent unilateral testicular pain in the past but not as severe as this current episode. Confirmation of testicular torsion would include all of the following findings except:

    A. unilateral loss of the cremasteric reflex.

    B. the affected testicle held higher in the scrotum.

    C. testicular swelling.

    D. relief of pain with scrotal elevation.

205. In assessing a man with testicular torsion, the NP is most likely to note:

    A. elevated PSA level.

    B. WBCs reported in urinalysis.

    C. left testicle most often affected.

    D. increased testicular blood flow by Doppler ultrasound.

206. Anticipated organ survival exceeds 85% with testicular decompression within how many hours of torsion?

    A. 1

    B. 6

    C. 16

    D. 24

207. Optimal management of testicular torsion would consist of which of the following?

    A. systemic corticosteroids

    B. manual detorsion

    C. surgical intervention

    D. watch and wait until swelling diminishes

208. To prevent a recurrence of testicular torsion, which of the following is recommended?

    A. use of a scrotal support

    B. avoidance of testicular trauma

    C. orchiopexy

    D. limiting the number of sexual partners

209. Which of the following is not a component of the TWIST scoring system when determining testicular torsion risk?

    A. scrotal pain

    B. testis swelling

    C. nausea/vomiting

    D. high-riding testis

For answers and rationales, see end of chapter.

Varicocele

Overview

A varicocele is an abnormally dilated spermatic vein within the scrotum. Varicocele usually starts to develop at puberty and is found in approximately 15% of healthy men and up to 35% of men with primary infertility.

Clinical Presentation

Typically described as an asymptomatic "bag of worms" mass and most often found in the left scrotum, a varicocele is usually noted only while the man is standing and disappears in the supine position. The mass is nontender and easily compressed. Rarely, the man with varicocele will report a sensation of scrotal heaviness or ache.

The remainder of the GU examination is within normal limits. A varicocele that cannot be reduced or sudden-onset right-sided varicocele should be more intensely evaluated; spermatic cord compression from increased retroperitoneal pressure, a pathological condition caused by a variety of serious conditions, could be the cause.

> **CLINICAL CONCEPT**
> Approximately one-third of men with varicocele will have bilateral varicocele visible on ultrasound but not detected clinically.

Diagnostic Testing

Varicocele is largely a clinical diagnosis. When the diagnosis is in question, Doppler ultrasound should be obtained. More in-depth evaluation is advised with sudden-onset right-sided or nonreducible varicocele.

Treatment

Treatment of varicocele is likely not necessary unless the lesion causes pain or testicular atrophy. Varicocele repair involves surgery that aims to seal off the affected vein to redirect blood flow into normal veins. Varicocele repair can involve open surgery, laparoscopic surgery, or percutaneous embolization (not as commonly used as surgery). A scrotal support can be helpful for relief of discomfort associated with varicocele.

A decreased sperm count with an increase in abnormal forms is noted in about two-thirds of men with the condition. Although varicocele has historically been considered one of the most common correctable forms of male infertility, many men with the condition have normal fertility. The impact of varicocele repair on infertility usually results in an increase in sperm count and reduction in abnormal forms; in limited study, this has resulted in higher subsequent pregnancy.

Discussion Sources

Mayo Clinic Staff. Varicocele. https://www.mayoclinic.org/diseases-conditions/varicocele/symptoms-causes/syc-20378771
White WM. Varicocele. Medscape. https://emedicine.medscape.com/article/438591-overview

QUESTIONS

210. A 23-year-old man has a nontender "bag of worms" mass within the left scrotum that disappears when he is in the supine position. He reports this has been present since he was an early teenager and has not changed over this time period. When assessing the patient for varicocele, the NP recommends:

    A. no additional diagnostic testing is needed.

    B. Doppler ultrasound.

    C. CT scan.

    D. immediate referral to a urological surgeon.

211. Which of the following is a common finding in a man with varicocele when compared to a man without varicocele?

    A. lower sperm count with increased number of abnormal forms

    B. increased rate of testicular cancer

    C. recurrent scrotal pain

    D. BPH

212. Treatment options for varicocele repair include all of the following except:

    A. an open surgical procedure.

    B. laparoscopic surgery.

    C. treatment with a thrombolytic agent.

    D. percutaneous embolization.

213. For a man with a preoperative altered semen analysis, varicocele repair is correlated with which of the following two answers?

    A. an increase in sperm count and normative sperm forms

    B. no change in fertility

    C. an increase in fertility in limited study

    D. an increased risk of congenital health issues in children conceived after surgical repair

For answers and rationales, see end of chapter.

Erectile Dysfunction

Overview

ED, also known as impotency, is defined as the repeated inability to achieve or maintain a penile erection firm enough for sexual intercourse. The spectrum of ED includes the total inability to achieve erection, an inconsistent ability to do so, and a tendency to sustain only brief erections. Achieving and sustaining a penile erection require a precise sequence of events that depends on healthy nervous system function (brain, spinal column, and penile innervation), appropriate muscle response, and intact blood flow via patent veins and arteries in and near the corpora cavernosa. Any disorder that causes injury to the nerves or impairs blood flow in the penis has the potential to cause ED. Diabetes mellitus, kidney disease, chronic alcohol abuse, vascular disease, tobacco use, neuropathy, and urological surgery such as radical prostatectomy are implicated in at least 70% of cases of ED. Treatment of hypertension, diabetes mellitus, and smoking cessation can contribute to improved erectile function. Certain medications, such as antihypertensives, antidepressants, and cimetidine, can produce ED as an adverse effect. The presence of a mood disorder significantly contributes to the risk of ED.

The incidence of ED increases with age; it is found in about 5% of 40-year-old men and 15% to 25% of 65-year-old men. ED should not be thought to be an inevitable consequence of aging, however. Although most ED in older men has a physical cause, such as disease, injury, or adverse effects of drugs, treatment can often help the patient regain satisfactory sexual function.

> **CLINICAL CONCEPT**
> Hormonal disorders, particularly testosterone deficiency, pose a significant but uncommon ED risk.

Clinical Presentation

The GU examination in most men with ED is unremarkable, save for signs of the underlying cause, if present. The diagnosis is made clinically, largely by health history.

Diagnostic Testing

The diagnosis of ED is largely made by health history and patient report. A standardized questionnaire such as the International Index of Erectile Function can be helpful in assuring that a comprehensive history has been obtained. Diagnostic testing is aimed at evaluating and treating underlying causes, if present.

Treatment

Intervention in ED starts with treating or minimizing the underlying cause, if present. With currently available therapies, effective treatment can be provided for most men with ED. Medications such as the phosphodiesterase-5 (PDE-5) inhibitors, sildenafil, vardenafil, avanafil, and tadalafil, work by enhancing the effects of nitric oxide, a chemical that relaxes smooth muscles in the penis during sexual stimulation and allows increased blood flow. Use of these agents does not trigger an automatic erection, and they should be taken about 1 hour before the anticipated onset of sexual activity. The half-life of sildenafil, avanafil, and vardenafil is approximately 4 to 5 hours, whereas tadalafil has a longer half-life of approximately 17 hours; as a result of its long $T_{1/2}$, tadalafil is the only ED medication recommended for lower-dose daily use. The clinical effect of these medications is delayed by 2 to 3 hours if taken with a high-fat meal.

The concomitant use of an ED medication with a nitrate is contraindicated because of the risk of profound hypotension; the duration of an adverse effect of a PDE-5 inhibitor is likely to persist for a period related to the drug's duration of action and half-life.

Drugs injected directly into the penis, such as alprostadil (Caverject®), cause vasodilation and are highly effective. An alprostadil pellet inserted into the urethra (Muse®) can achieve the same effect. Mechanical vacuum devices cause erection by creating a partial vacuum, which draws blood into the penis, engorging and expanding it. An elastic band is placed around the base of the penis to maintain the erection after the cylinder is removed and during intercourse by preventing blood from flowing back into the body. This mechanical method of ED treatment is particularly helpful when other methods fail to achieve desired results. Surgical options include vessel repair to treat the underlying ED; it should be kept in mind, however, that atherosclerosis, if a contributor to ED, is a widespread disease, and outcomes are unpredictable. Implantation of devices such as prostheses or pumps is another option, albeit with the associated risks and costs of any surgical procedure.

Discussion Sources

Grant P, Jackson G, Baig I, Quin J. Erectile dysfunction in general medicine. *Clin Med.* 2013;13:136–140.
Irwin GM. Erectile dysfunction. *Prim Care.* 2019;46:249–255.
Shamloul R, Ghanem H. Erectile dysfunction. *Lancet.* 2013;381:153–165.

QUESTIONS

214. Which of the following is not a common risk factor for ED?

   A. diabetes mellitus

   B. hypertension

   C. cigarette smoking

   D. testosterone deficiency

215. Patient education about the use of sildenafil (Viagra®) includes the following:

   A. A spontaneous erection occurs about 1 hour after taking the medication.

   B. This medication helps regain erectile function in nearly all men who use it.

   C. With use of the medication, sexual stimulation also is needed to achieve an erection.

   D. Nitrates can be safely used concurrently.

216. When discussing ED with a 70-year-old man, the NP considers that:

   A. it is a normal consequence of aging.

   B. most cases have an underlying contributing cause.

C. although depression is common in older men, it is usually not correlated with increased rates of ED.

D. treatment options for younger men are seldom effective in older men.

217. When considering the use of ED medications, tadalafil (Cialis®) can be used on a daily dosing regimen because of its:

A. unique mechanism of action.

B. superior safety profile.

C. longer half-life.

D. more rapid elimination from the body.

218. For patients with ED who fail therapy with a PDE-5 inhibitor, alternative approaches include all of the following except:

A. alprostadil injection into the penis.

B. mechanical vacuum devices.

C. insertion of a nitroglycerin pellet in the urethra.

D. implantation of a prosthetic device.

For answers and rationales, see end of chapter.

Cervical and Anogenital Cancer Screening

Cervical Cancer

Cervical cancer impacts approximately 12,000 women in the United States each year, most commonly occurring in women over the age of 30 years. The main cause of cervical cancer is HPV, which is a common virus that is transmitted through sexual intercourse. At least half of sexually active women acquire HPV at some point in their lives, though few will develop cervical cancer. In a woman with cervical cancer or precancerous lesions, the cervix often looks normal.

Through routine screening, follow-up, and the availability of the HPV vaccine, death from cervical cancer is highly preventable. There are two types of tests available for screening: cytology (Pap test or Pap smear) and HPV testing. The Pap test is used to detect precancers or cell changes on the cervix that can be identified and treated early before cancer development. The Pap test is recommended for women between 21 and 65 years of age (Table 9-12). Co-testing with a Pap test and HPV testing should be done every 5 years beginning at age 30 years until age 65 years. If only a Pap test is performed, this should be repeated every 3 years. Additionally, most young women clear HPV infection within 1 to 2 years of acquisition, and HPV-related precancerous lesions (i.e., dysplasia) will typically resolve on their own. Please see ASCCP.org for additional advice on the management of an abnormal pap test as well as evaluation of the presence of high-risk HPV types.

> **CLINICAL CONCEPT**
> Cervical cancer screening should be avoided in women under age 21 years as they are at very low risk of cervical cancer and screening can lead to unnecessary and potentially harmful evaluation and treatment.

Anal Cancer

Screening for anal cancer is not routinely recommended for men, although some experts recommend anal cancer screening every 1 to 3 years via anal Pap tests for MSM and men living with HIV. The rate of anal cancer among HIV-negative MSM is 20 times higher than for the general population; among HIV-positive MSM, the rate is 80 times higher. Anal Pap tests can also be considered for women with a history of anogenital HPV infection, anal-receptive intercourse, multiple sexual partners, and a history of STI or anal condyloma. In anal cancer, visual examination is often normal. Occasionally, a nonhealing, painless anal lesion is reported by the patient.

Prostate Cancer

Prostate cancer is the most common noncutaneous cancer in men in the United States. Although clinically detectable prostate cancer is a cause of considerable mortality and morbidity, most cancers are likely occult and limited to the prostate with little risk of metastasis. Prostate cancer has been found on autopsy

TABLE 9-12 Cervical Cancer Screening Recommendations

PATIENT CLASSIFICATION	RECOMMENDATIONS
Ages 20 years or less: Should *not* be screened (*no Pap test should be done*)	Regardless of age onset of sexual activity, sexual orientation, history of sexually transmitted infection (STI), or human papillomavirus (HPV) immunization status. Pelvic examination and appropriate STI screening *should be performed* as indicated by clinical presentation and risk assessment.*
Ages 21 to 29 years: Should be screened every 3 years (*Pap test should be done*)	Screening with *cytology only.* HPV testing should *not* be used, either as a stand-alone test or co-test to include reflex. *Pelvic examination and appropriate STI screening *should be performed* as indicated by clinical presentation and risk assessment.*
Ages 30 to 65 years: Should be screened at a maximum every 5 years (*Pap test should be done*)	Screening with *cytology and HPV* "co-test" (preferred). Screening with *cytology alone is acceptable* every 3 years. *Pelvic examination and appropriate STI screening *should be performed* as indicated by clinical presentation and risk assessment.*
Age older than 65 years: Should *not* be screened (*no Pap test should be done*)	If evidence of negative prior screening (*three consecutive cytology or two consecutive co-test results within 10 years before ceasing screening, with the most recent test occurring within the past 5 years*) and no history of cervical intraepithelial neoplasm (CIN) 2 or greater within the past 20 years. Once screening is discontinued, it should *not* be resumed. *Pelvic examination and appropriate STI screening *should be performed* as indicated by clinical presentation and risk assessment.*
Has undergone a hysterectomy with removal of cervix regardless of age: Should *not* be screened (*no Pap test should be done*) **History of CIN2, CIN3, or adenocarcinoma *in situ*** Should be screened (*Pap test should be done*) **HPV vaccination status (*positive or negative*)** (*see recommendation*)	If no history of CIN 2 or greater, no evidence of adequate negative prior screening is needed. Once screening is discontinued, it should *not* be resumed. *Pelvic examination and appropriate STI screening *should be performed* as indicated by clinical presentation and risk assessment.* Routine screening should continue for at least 20 years, even if this time frame extends past age 65 years. Regardless of immunization status, screening should be done based on the practice recommendations.

Source: Massad LS, Einstein MH, Huh WK, et al. Updated consensus guidelines for the management of abnormal cervical cancer screening tests and cancer precursors. Available at http://www.asccp.org/management-guidelines

in two-thirds of men 80 to 89 years old. The average American man has a 40% lifetime risk of latent prostate cancer, an approximate 10% risk of clinically significant disease, and an approximate 3% risk of dying of prostate cancer; prostate cancer is the second leading cause of male cancer death in the United States, after lung cancer. Risk factors include older age, African American ancestry, a family history of prostate cancer, and obesity.

Most cases of prostate cancer are asymptomatic unless the disease is advanced. Consequently, a high level of vigilance for prostate cancer is important. Although periodic DRE and PSA testing are advised for some men, this screening protocol has limitations in effectiveness. The prostatic DRE can reveal a discrete, painless lesion or area of induration in the posterior lobe of the prostate but is often normal until disease is advanced. PSA is a glycoprotein produced in benign and malignant prostate cells. Nearly two-thirds of men with PSA levels greater than 10 ng/mL (normal PSA less than 4 ng/mL in an older man, less than 2.5 ng/mL in a younger man) have

CLINICAL CONCEPT

PSA level can also be elevated transiently in conditions other than prostate cancer, including prostatitis or immediately after prostatic instrumentation such as cystoscopy.

prostate cancer, whereas about 25% of men with PSA values between 4 and 10 ng/mL have disease, and approximately the same percentage of men in the at-risk age group have evidence of prostate cancer with a normal PSA. Correlating an abnormal prostate examination finding with an abnormal PSA level increases the likelihood of a diagnosis of prostate cancer.

Levels often remain chronically elevated in patients with BPH. Serial increases even in the presence of a normal prostate examination should be evaluated further.

The American Cancer Society recommends that a discussion about screening should take place at age 50 years for men who are at average risk of prostate cancer and expected to live at least 10 more years. For men at higher risk (such as those with African ancestry and men who have a first-degree relative [father, brothers] diagnosed with prostate cancer at less than 65 years of age), the discussion should take place at age 45 years. Men at even higher risk because of multiple first-degree relatives affected at an early age should have the discussion at age 40 years. Following the discussion, those men who want to be screened should be tested with the PSA blood test. The DRE can also be done as part of screening. If no cancer is detected, the frequency of future screenings depends on the result of the PSA test. If the PSA level was less than 2.5 ng/mL, retesting should occur every 2 years. If the PSA was ≥2.5 ng/mL, testing should be conducted annually.

Because of its low sensitivity and specificity, transrectal ultrasound should not be used as a first-line screening test for prostate cancer. This test can be helpful, however, when coupled with PSA and DRE findings and for guiding prostatic biopsy, the usual next step when a diagnosis of prostate cancer is considered. Pathology and disease staging guide prostate cancer treatment options. Watchful waiting is often a reasonable option for older men with local disease.

Discussion Sources

American Cancer Society. American Cancer Society recommendations for prostate cancer early detection. http://www.cancer.org /cancer/prostatecancer/moreinformation/prostatecancerearlydetection/prostate-cancer-early-detection-acs-recommendations

Massad LS, Einstein MH, Huh WK, et al. 2012 updated consensus guidelines for the management of abnormal cervical cancer screening tests and cancer precursors. *J Lower Genital Tract Dis.* 2013;17:S1–S27. http://www.asccp.org/Assets/405b4550 -593f-40a7-ae25-0c783de95b0d/635912114192570000/asccp-updated-guidelines-3-21-13-pdf

Sanda MG, Chen RC, Crispino T, et al. Clinically localized prostate cancer: AUA/ASTRO/SUO Guideline. *J Urol.* 2018;199:683–690. https://www.auanet.org/guidelines/prostate-cancer-clinically-localized-guideline

QUESTIONS

219. You see an 18-year-old woman with a history of *C trachomatis* infection and a total of five male lifetime partners. You recommend:

A. Pap test only.

B. Pap test and HPV testing.

C. Pap test and STI testing.

D. STI testing only.

220. During well-women visits for 21- to 29-year-old sexually active women who report more than one sex partner without condom use within the past 6 months, all of the following are appropriate screening tests except:

A. Pap test if not done within past 3 years.

B. HPV testing.

C. pelvic examination.

D. STI screening.

221. A 45-year-old woman recently had a normal Pap test result and has an absence of high-risk HPV. You recommend her next Pap test in:

A. 1 year.

B. 3 years.

C. 5 years.

D. 7 years.

222. You see a 48-year-old woman who underwent an abdominal hysterectomy with cervical removal for uterine fibroids 6 months ago. She last had a normal Pap test 1½ years ago. You recommend her next Pap test:

A. immediately.

B. in 1½ years.

C. in 3½ years.

D. neither now nor in the future.

223. You see a 24-year-old woman who received a full series HPV vaccine as a teenager. She had a normal Pap test 3 years ago. You recommend:

A. conducting a Pap test.

B. conducting a Pap test and HPV testing.

C. waiting 2 years for the next Pap test.

D. ceasing future Pap tests until she turns 30 years old.

E. referral for select lesion biopsy.

224. You perform a DRE on a 72-year-old man and find a lesion suspicious for prostate cancer. The findings are described as:

A. a rubbery, enlarged prostatic lobe.

B. an area of prostatic induration.

C. a boggy gland.

D. prostatic tenderness.

225. A 54-year-old white man with no obvious risk for prostate cancer opted to undergo PSA screening and DRE testing. The DRE findings are normal, and his PSA is 3.7 ng/mL (normal PSA less than 2.5 ng/mL at this age). You recommend:

A. repeating the PSA test immediately.

B. repeat screening in 1 year.

C. repeat screening in 2 years.

D. repeat screening in 5 years.

226. Risk factors for prostate cancer include all of the following except:

A. African ancestry.

B. history of genital trauma.

C. family history of prostate cancer in first- and second-degree relatives.

D. high-fat diet.

227. The average American man has an approximately _____% lifetime risk of prostate cancer and an approximately _____% likelihood of clinical disease.

A. 15, 5

B. 25, 8

C. 40, 10

D. 60, 15

228. All of the following can cause an elevated PSA level except:

A. current prostate infection.

B. recent cystoscopy.

C. BPH.

D. prostatectomy.

229. According to recent epidemiological studies, prostate cancer is the number _____ cause of cancer death in men residing within the United States.

A. 1

B. 2

C. 3

D. 4

For answers and rationales, see end of chapter.

QUESTION ANSWERS AND RATIONALES

Family Planning

1. **Correct: C. presence of factor V Leiden mutation**
   For those considering the use of a CHC, known thrombotic mutations are listed as U.S. MEC category 4, as these present significant risk for thrombophilia that can lead to the formation of blood clots (C). Thrombotic mutations include factor V Leiden mutation, prothrombin mutations, and protein S, C, or antithrombin deficiency.
   Incorrect:
   Family history of breast cancer is U.S. MEC category 1 (no restriction) (A). Cigarette smoking in individuals younger than 35 years of age is U.S. MEC category 2 (advantages outweigh risks) (D). Though acute hepatitis is U.S. MEC category 4, there are no precautions for the use of CHCs in women with a past history of hepatitis A (B), as this is a condition that resolves without residual liver problems.

2. **Correct: A. take the last pill missed immediately and continue taking the remaining pills at the usual time, even if this means taking two pills today.**
   Missed pills are an expected occurrence for those taking COCs and so it is important for NPs to be knowledgeable of the appropriate actions to continue contraceptive treatment. If two or more consecutive pills have been missed (48 hours or longer), then the patient should take the most recent pill missed as soon as possible and continue taking the remaining pills at the usual time, even if this means taking two pills on the same day (A). Backup contraception should be used or sexual intercourse avoided until hormonal pills have been taken for 7 consecutive days.
   Incorrect:
   In this scenario, the most recent pill missed should be taken immediately followed by normal dosing of the remaining pills, even if this means taking two pills on the same day (D). Thus, only one pill will be discarded (B) while utilizing the remainder of the pack (C).

3. **Correct: D. premenstrual syndrome symptoms are often improved with use of CHCs.**
   The use of CHCs is associated with a number of noncontraceptive benefits. These include reduced menstrual volume and associated iron-deficiency anemia, improvement in acne, reduced risk of several types of cancer, and diminished premenstrual syndrome symptoms (D).
   Incorrect:
   CHCs can be used for a prolonged period of time without a need for a "rest" period (A). Prolonged use is not associated with reduced fertility or other health problems. If a woman desires to become pregnant, discontinuation of CHCs usually returns fertility fairly quickly (B). CHC use is associated with lower rates of benign breast tumors as well as decreased rates of endometrial, ovarian, and colon cancers (C).

4. **Correct: C. cervicitis.**
   The use of CHCs results in thickened endocervical mucus that limits the motility of organisms past the uterus and into the fallopian tubes or ovaries, thus preventing PID. However, changes are not evident at the cervix; thus, CHCs will not prevent cervicitis or other STIs (C).
   Incorrect:
   The thickened endocervical mucus associated with CHC use will limit the motility of microorganisms past the uterus and into the fallopian tubes and ovaries, thus preventing the development of PID (B). CHC use decreases menstrual volume and will reduce the risk of developing iron-deficiency anemia (A). CHCs have been associated with a reduced risk of developing certain types of cancer, including endometrial, ovarian, and colon cancer (D).

5. **Correct: C. a 32-year-old woman with adequately controlled hypertension**
   POPs are well suited for women with certain chronic medical conditions, such as hypertension (C), as CHC use among those with hypertension can be U.S. MEC category 2, 3, or 4, depending on the extent of hypertension.
   Incorrect:
   For POP to be effective, it must be used consistently each day and so would not be recommended for an individual who frequently forgets to take a daily dose (A). For a woman with multiple sexual partners, a barrier method would be preferred for the prevention of STIs, perhaps along with a POP or CHC (B). POPs are not preferred for those with irregular cycles, as this method is frequently associated with bleeding irregularity (D).

6. Correct: B. inconvenience of use.

Discontinuation of COCs most frequently occurs within the first 3 months of use due to BTB and the inconvenience of taking a daily pill (B). For those who desire more convenient contraception, other options can include CHC ring or patch, DMPA, or LARCs.

Incorrect:

Nausea is a common adverse effect of CHCs but is usually transient and can be minimized if dosed with food or at bedtime (A). COCs are relatively inexpensive at a cost under $10 per month in some cases (C). When used appropriately, COCs are highly effective in preventing unwanted pregnancies (D).

7. Correct: D. vaginal diaphragm with spermicide

Due to the woman's age and smoking habit, a CHC would not be recommended as this option would be U.S. MEC category 4. A barrier method such as a vaginal diaphragm with spermicide would present an appropriate choice (D). A POP would also be appropriate as this approach is U.S. MEC category 1.

Incorrect:

For women who are 35 years and older and smoke 15 or more cigarettes per day, the use of a CHC is U.S. MEC category 4. This includes the use of a COC (B), patch (C), or vaginal ring (A).

8. Correct: B. a 31-year-old woman with a history of naturally occurring multiple gestation pregnancy.

Prior naturally occurring multiple gestation pregnancy is not associated with increased VTE risk (U.S. MEC category 1); thus, the use of CHCs would be an appropriate option (B).

Incorrect:

The presence of multiple risk factors for cardiovascular disease (e.g., diabetes mellitus and high LDL) would place the 42-year-old woman in U.S. MEC category 3 or 4 (A). Cigarette smoking is a key risk factor for thrombosis and would place the 33-year-old in U.S. MEC category 2 (C), though she is approaching age 35 years where smoking at this rate and CHC use is a U.S. MEC category 4. A family history of VTE would also place the woman in U.S. MEC category 2 (D). Though the advantages outweigh the risks in U.S. MEC category 2, other effective options, such as progestin-only contraceptives, should be considered for those individuals, particularly when the VTE risk will increase over time (e.g., continued cigarette smoking).

9. Correct: B. current PID

IUDs can provide a highly effective contraceptive option for many women with health issues who would not be able to safely use CHCs. However, initiation of a Cu-IUD in a woman with active PID would be U.S. MEC category 4 and so should be avoided until the episode is resolved (B).

Incorrect:

Cu-IUD can be considered for many women with chronic health issues. This type of contraceptive is generally safe for those with cardiovascular conditions such as uncomplicated valvular heart disease (U.S. MEC category 1; A) and hypertension (U.S. MEC category 1; C) and can be considered for those with severe dysmenorrhea (U.S. MEC category 2; D).

10. Correct: C. "Depo-Provera® (medroxyprogesterone acetate in a depot injection [DMPA]) use will likely not interact with your seizure medication."

For individuals taking antiepileptic medications, such as phenytoin, the use of CHCs is not recommended as the estrogen component will potentially interact and diminish the activity of the AED. However, the progestin-only DMPA is a valuable choice as it provides effective contraception without drug interaction to phenytoin (C).

Incorrect:

The patient is specifically asking about hormonal contraceptive options and so focusing on a barrier method is not optimal, particularly when other hormonal options are available (A). A COC should be avoided due to potential interaction of phenytoin with the estrogen component of this contraceptive (B). There may be precautions with the use of a LNG-IUD in this patient, but it is not contraindicated in individuals taking phenytoin (D).

11. Correct: A. weight gain

DMPA can offer a convenient and effective option for contraception as it is given as an injection every 3 months. However, long-term use of DMPA is associated with bone loss as well as weight gain, with an average of about 11 pounds (5 kg) over 3 years of use (A).

Incorrect:

A significant proportion of women who use DMPA will report amenorrhea, not hypermenorrhea, after the first year of use (B). Once DMPA is discontinued, it can take 6 to 12 months to resume fertility, and so this option should be reserved for those who do not wish to become pregnant for at least 18 months (D). There is no association with DMPA use and the development of acne (C). Typically, acne will improve when using estrogen-containing contraceptives, which is not included in DMPA.

12 to 16. Indicate U.S. MEC category (1, 2, 3, or 4)

12. Correct: 3

U.S. MEC category 3 is given for women 35 years or older who smoke less than 15 cigarettes per day. For those who smoke 15 or more per day, the U.S. MEC category is 4.

13. Correct: 1

The use of COCs might protect against PID due to endocervical mucous thickening but will not protect against HIV or lower genital tract STIs.

14. Correct: 4

Menstrual migraine is considered a subtype of migraine with aura. Migraine without aura is given a U.S. MEC category of 2.

15. Correct: 2

Use of CHCs in breastfeeding women after 42 days' postpartum is given U.S. MEC category 2, primarily due to a lack of studies to determine if there is a risk of serious or subtle long-term effects of exogenous estrogen in infants exposed to CHCs through breastmilk.

16. Correct: 2

Without vascular disease, the presence of type 1 or type 2 diabetes mellitus is U.S. MEC category 2. In the presence of vascular disease, the U.S. MEC category increases to 3/4.

17 to 20. Indicate U.S. MEC category (1, 2, 3, or 4)

17. Correct: 4 (both)

Uterine cavity distortion, defined as any congenital or acquired uterine abnormality distorting the uterine cavity in such a way that is incompatible with IUD insertion, is given U.S. MEC category 4. Uterine fibroids by itself is assigned U.S. MEC category 2.

18. Correct: 1 (both)

Contrary to CHCs, the use of a Cu-IUD or LNG-IUD is considered safe regardless of smoking history.

19. Correct: 1 (both)

The use of a Cu-IUD is considered safe in the presence of adequately controlled hypertension as well as elevated blood pressure. LNG-IUD is safe for adequately controlled hypertension but is given a U.S. MEC category 2 once blood pressure exceeds 160/100 mm Hg.

20. Correct: 1 (both)

The Cu-IUD is safe to use among women with a personal or family history of breast cancer. The LNG-IUD is also safe for those with a family history of breast cancer but is given U.S. MEC category 2 if there is an undiagnosed mass present, U.S. MEC category 4 if breast cancer is present, and U.S. MEC category 3 if a past personal history of breast cancer and no evidence of disease for 5 years.

21. Correct: C. "Avoid using potassium-containing salt substitutes."

Drospirenone is an analogue of an aldosterone antagonist and has potassium-sparing qualities. Therefore, to minimize the risk of hyperkalemia, potassium-containing salt substitutes should be avoided (C).

Incorrect:

There is no specific need to take this contraceptive on a full stomach unless the patient reports nausea with dosing (A). There are no specific warnings on the use of acetaminophen with these products (B). The original belief was that the use of drospirenone-containing products would improve premenstrual syndrome symptoms. However, with greater use of these products, it was determined that the effects were consistent with other COCs (D).

22. Correct: B. the POP is a more effective contraceptive than COC.

POPs can provide a useful alternative to COCs in women with certain health conditions and nursing mothers, as well as provide gap coverage before starting a LARC. However, with failure rates up to 13%, POPs are less effective than COCs (B).

Incorrect:

POPs must be taken every day for full effectiveness (A). Since POPs do not contain an estrogen component, they will not alter the quality or quantity of breast milk and provide a useful contraceptive option for nursing mothers (C). Bleeding irregularity is a major disadvantage of this type of contraceptive (D).

23. Correct: D. reduction in menstrual flow

With the use of LNG-IUD, light or no menstrual flow is often reported after 6 months of use (D). After 2 years of use, about 50% of women are amenorrheic.

Incorrect:

Long-term use of LNG-IUD will typically lead to endometrial thinning rather than endometrial hyperplasia (A) and will more likely lead to amenorrhea rather than hypermenorrhea (B). Due to endocervical mucous thickening, PID rates are often lower with the use of these products (C).

24. Correct: B. acne vulgaris.

The use of COCs has been noted to improve acne vulgaris after about 3 months of use (B). This is likely related to a reduction in free androgens and an increase in levels of SHBG. The benefit persists throughout the duration of taking COCs but is reversible once the COC is discontinued.

Incorrect:

COC use can lead to improvement in cycle control (A), premenstrual syndrome symptoms (e.g., breast tenderness) (C), and even rheumatoid arthritis (D). However, these benefits are not likely due to a reduction in free androgens.

25. Correct: B. no more than 2 years.

Long-term use of DMPA has been associated with bone loss, and so it is recommended that use should be limited to no more than 2 years (B). Calcium and vitamin D supplementation is recommended for women who use this option for contraception. Bone loss is usually reversible once DMPA is discontinued.

Incorrect:

DMPA can be continued up to 2 years as a safe and effective contraceptive option (A) but should be discontinued after 2 years of use due to risk of bone loss (C). The use of this contraceptive approach is not dependent on lipid response (D).

26. Correct: A. acetaminophen.

Irregular bleeding is a common adverse effect during the first few months of DMPA use. This can be minimized with the use of a prostaglandin inhibitor or estrogen supplement. However, acetaminophen will not be helpful for this adverse effect (A).

Incorrect:

Irregular bleeding during the first few months of DMPA use can be minimized with the use of ibuprofen 400 mg tid (B) or naproxen sodium 375 to 540 mg bid (C) for 3 to 5 days. Alternatively, an estrogen supplement can be used for 7 to 10 days (D).

27. Correct: A. immediately

When selecting an optimal contraceptive, it is important to note when a woman might want to start a family. Fertility returns rapidly in women who discontinue use of CHC or LARC (A). For DMPA users, a delay in a return to fertility can last 6 to 12 months, so this would be appropriate for women who do not wish to conceive for at least 18 months.

Incorrect:

In general, there is no delay in the ability to conceive following discontinuation of CHC or LARC use (B, C, D).

28. Correct: B. candidates include women who have difficulty remembering to take a daily pill.

The contraceptive patch and vaginal ring provide convenient options for women who do not wish to take a pill every day or for those who frequently forget to take a pill (B).

Incorrect:

The contraceptive patch and vaginal ring are CHC products and contain both estrogen and progestin (A). These products offer higher contraceptive effectiveness compared to COCs as adherence issues are reduced compared to taking a daily pill (D). As these hormones do not travel through the liver, they are associated with few drug interactions (C).

29. Correct: D. this method is considered acceptable (U.S. MEC category 2) for select women with a history of thrombophilia forms.

Nexplanon® is a progestin-only product that is a single rod insert and does not contain estrogen. Therefore, it is generally safe to use in women with thrombotic risk factors, such as those with a history of thrombophilia (D).

Incorrect:

Subdermal insertion of the Nexplanon® rod is fairly simple and can be performed in the primary care setting by a trained health-care provider without referral to an OB/GYN physician (A). Nexplanon® is effective for up to 3 years, at which point it should be replaced due to a diminished level of hormone released (B). Nexplanon® remains an option in overweight and obese women, though some evidence has shown diminished serum levels of the hormone (C). The reduced hormone level is not clinically significant as failure rates remain low.

30. Correct: C. can be self-administered

Nexplanon® consists of a single rod that is placed subdermally by a trained health-care provider. It cannot be self-administered (C).

Incorrect:

Nexplanon® is a single subdermal rod that can remain in place for up to 3 years (A). The rod is visible on x-ray, which can help with removal (D). As with other LARCs, fertility returns rapidly with removal of the rod (B).

31. Correct: B. there is no risk of bone loss with long-term use of this DMPA formulation.

A self-administered version of DMPA has been approved by the FDA. Similar to the original version, bone loss is a possible adverse effect of this contraceptive and so use should be limited to no longer than 2 years, and calcium and vitamin D supplementation is recommended (B).

Incorrect:

Similar to the original version of DMPA, a self-administered version is dosed every 3 months (A) and can be given immediately postpartum (C). Self-administered DMPA contains about 70% of the amount of the IM formulation, but effectiveness is not impacted (D).

32 to 34. True or False

32. Correct: True

33. Correct: False

34. Correct: True

A noncontraceptive benefit of COC use is reduced menstrual flow, which can reduce the risk of iron-deficiency anemia (32). Nausea is a common adverse effect for women initiating COCs. To minimize nausea, dosing can be done with food or the dose can be taken at bedtime (33). DMPA is associated with bone loss, and duration of use is limited to no longer than 2 years. To prevent bone loss, women should take calcium and vitamin D supplements when taking DMPA (34).

35. Correct: C. After the device is inserted, the cervix should be smoothly covered.

A vaginal diaphragm provides barrier protection against contraception. The diaphragm is fitted by a health-care provider, and once inserted, it should fit snugly in the vagina to smoothly cover the cervix (C). The woman and her partner should not be aware of the diaphragm once in place.

Incorrect:

A properly fitted diaphragm should not be noticed by the woman once it is in place (A). If the woman or the partner can feel the diaphragm, then it is either the wrong size or not properly inserted. A diaphragm is used with spermicide, which can increase the risk of UTI. Therefore, this would not be a suitable choice for women predisposed to UTIs (B). The device should remain in place at least 6 hours after coitus (D).

36. Correct: B. UTI.

The use of spermicide can increase the risk of UTIs (B). This is likely due to the antimicrobial effect of spermicides, which lowers lactobacilli in the lower GU tract of women. Lactobacilli produce lactic acid and hydrogen peroxide that creates an unfavorable environment for uropathogens and helps prevent UTIs.

Incorrect:

The use of spermicides will decrease the perivaginal presence of lactobacilli rather than increase colonization by this organism (C). There is no indication that the use of a diaphragm with spermicide will increase the risk for cervical stenosis (A) or ovarian malignancy (D).

37. **Correct: D. up to 20%**

The success of male condoms in preventing conception and spread of STIs depends on their proper use. Contraception failure rates can approach 20%, though this rate can be improved with the addition of spermicide (D).

Incorrect:

Highly effective forms of contraception will have a failure rate of 1% or less (A). However, the use of male condoms alone can have failure rates up to 20% (B, C).

38. **Correct: C. male condom**

When used properly, a male condom provides protection against the spread of STIs (C).

Incorrect:

Barrier methods such as a vaginal diaphragm (A), contraceptive sponge (B), and cervical cap (D) can be effective in preventing sperm from passing through the cervix for conception. However, these approaches are not effective in preventing the spread of STIs.

Emergency Contraception

39. **Correct: D. insertion of a Cu-IUD offers an effective form of emergency and ongoing contraception.**

EC options can include hormonal treatment with oral LNG or ulipristal as well as insertion of a Cu-IUD for a hormone-free option (D). Insertion of the Cu-IUD can occur within 5 days of unprotected intercourse.

Incorrect:

EC can reduce the risk of pregnancy by at least 75%, likely significantly higher when used appropriately (A). Optimally, oral LNG should be administered within 3 days of unprotected intercourse, while oral ulipristal or Cu-IUD can be used up to 5 days after intercourse (B). For this individual in her second week of the menstrual cycle, she is at a high likelihood of getting pregnant and so EC is a viable option to prevent an unwanted pregnancy (C).

40. **Correct: B. acts as an abortifacient**

None of the oral EC forms available work as an abortifacient (B). Ulipristal can cause endometrial alterations that could impact embryo implantation. However, oral LNG or ulipristal would not interrupt an established pregnancy or increase the risk of early pregnancy loss.

Incorrect:

The key mechanisms of oral EC forms include inhibiting or delaying ovulation (A) or causing changes in the endocervical mucus to slows sperm transport (C) or slow ovum transport (D).

41. **Correct: D. there appears to be no correlation with EC and problematic outcomes if pregnancy occurs.**

The use of oral EC during an established pregnancy does not cause any problematic outcomes, including early termination or teratogenic effects (D).

Incorrect:

Oral EC does not affect an established pregnancy and would not result in early spontaneous abortion (A).

EC use is not associated with any teratogenic effects if a pregnancy occurs (B). There is also no correlation between EC use and placental abruption (C).

42. **Correct: A. inhibiting fertilized egg implantation.**

Oral LNG will likely have minimal impact on the endometrial lining. However, ulipristal can cause alterations in the endometrium that can prevent implantation of a fertilized egg (A).

Incorrect:

Both oral LNG and ulipristal can work by impairing sperm (B) and ovum (D) transport. Neither hormonal EC forms will induce abortion of an established pregnancy (C).

43. **Correct: B. ulipristal.**

In this case the most appropriate option would be oral ulipristal as it is effective up to 5 days following unprotected intercourse (B).

Incorrect:

Oral LNG is recommended to be taken up to 3 days after unprotected intercourse. Though it can be taken up to 5 days after intercourse, this is toward the end of its effectiveness and will have a higher risk of failure (A). The Cu-IUD should be avoided in this patient due to a history of cervicitis (C). Ulipristal is effective even after 5 days of unprotected intercourse (D) and is considered the appropriate option.

44. **Correct: D. Ulipristal is taken in two doses 12 hours apart.**

Ulipristal is taken as a single tablet (D). However, if vomiting occurs within 3 hours of the dose, a repeat dose should be taken.

Incorrect:

There are various dosing options for oral LNG. Some are available as a single-pill option, while others can be taken in two pills, either at the same time or separated by 12 hours (A). Ulipristal is available only by prescription (B), while oral LNG is available OTC (C).

45. **Correct: C. 3 to 4**

A woman should anticipate menses around the time when they would normally occur, typically within 3 to 4 weeks of taking the EC (C). If menses does not occur by that time, a pregnancy test is warranted.

Menopause

46. **Correct: B. 40 to 45 years.**

In North America, the average age of onset of perimenopause is between 40 and 45 years and can last an average of 4 years (B). Menopause, as defined as the time when there is no naturally occurring menstrual period for 12 months, occurs at age 51.3 years on average.

47. **Correct: A. Menstruation ceases during perimenopause.**

Perimenopause is the time surrounding menopause (when the menstrual period ceases). Menstruation still occurs during perimenopause (A), though it can occur irregularly with heavier or lighter flow.

Incorrect:
During perimenopause, vasomotor symptoms including hot flashes are common during the week prior to menses (B). Though ovulation becomes more erratic during this period (D), pregnancy is still possible, and contraceptive use is recommended to prevent pregnancy (C).

48. **Correct: B. hot flashes and night sweats occur in about 60% to 90% of women.**
Vasomotor symptoms, including hot flashes and night sweats, are experienced by a majority of women during menopause, and 60% of women will consult a healthcare provider for treatment options (B).
Incorrect:
In North America, the average age of menopause is approximately 51.3 years (A). For women with surgical menopause, more severe symptoms are reported possibly due to more rapid and dramatic shifts in hormonal levels (C). During menopause, the pituitary gland secretes increased levels of LH and FSH in an attempt to induce ovulation (D).

49. **Correct: D. a pH greater than 5.**
GSM, including atrophic vaginitis, is a common complaint during menopause. Symptoms and findings of atrophic vaginitis can include vaginal dryness, a scant, white discharge without a distinct odor, and a higher pH (D), possibly due to a decreased number of lactobacilli that produce lactic acid.
Incorrect:
Atrophic vaginitis is characterized by a scant, white vaginal discharge without a distinctive odor (A). The number of perivaginal lactobacilli decreases (B), which can diminish the protective effects against colonization and infection by uropathogens. There is usually no impact on the level of WBCs (C).

50. **Correct: B. the addition of a topical estrogen can be helpful.**
For women experiencing bothersome symptoms of GSM, the use of a topical estrogen can be helpful (B). This can include a vaginal cream, ring, or tablet that provides a low dose of estrogen in areas with a high concentration of estrogen receptors.
Incorrect:
For women who experience symptoms of GSM while taking oral HT, increasing the HT dose typically does not help (A). The MPA component should be continued with oral estrogen therapy as this helps decrease the risk of endometrial hyperplasia (C). As GSM is related to changes in hormone levels, a baking soda douche would not be helpful for this situation (D).

51. **Correct: D. clonidine.**
Several nonhormonal options are available to minimize vasomotor symptoms associated with menopause. However, clonidine should be avoided for this purpose due to the potential for undesirable adverse effects and the availability of more effective and safer options (D).

Incorrect:
Nonhormonal options to treat vasomotor symptoms can include a low dose of an SSRI (e.g., sertraline [B]) or SNRI (e.g., venlafaxine [A]). The SSRI/SNRI doses used to treat vasomotor symptoms are typically lower than what is used to treat depression. Gabapentin, an antiepileptic medication, has also been shown to be helpful for this purpose (C).

52. **Correct: A. unexplained vaginal bleeding.**
Unexplained vaginal bleeding is an absolute contraindication for the use of HT (A). It would be necessary to identify the cause of the bleeding prior to considering the use of HT.
Incorrect:
HT can be used with caution in individuals with seizure disorder because of a potential interaction with antiepileptic medications (B). Additionally, caution should be used among those with dyslipidemia due to potential cardiovascular risks with estrogen therapy (C), as well as those who experience migraine with aura. There is less risk for those who experience migraine without aura (D). The impact of transdermal or transvaginal estrogen is much less compared with oral estrogen therapy.

53. **Correct: D. help preserve bone density.**
Estrogen deficiency is a potent risk factor for osteoporosis, as estrogen receptors are found in bone. HT along with calcium supplementation can help reduce bone loss and prevent fractures in postmenopausal women (D). However, since other safer and effective options are available to prevent and manage bone loss, HT should not be selected solely for this purpose.
Incorrect:
HT can increase the risk of thrombotic events largely because of the estrogen component (A). Estrogen can also cause an increase in triglyceride levels and so should be used with caution among individuals with dyslipidemia (B). There is no clinically significant effect of HT on blood pressure, and it may actually reduce blood pressure in some women (C).

54. **Correct: C. a reduction in the severity of vasomotor symptoms.**
Successful use of HT should result in a reduction in the frequency and severity of vasomotor symptoms, including hot flashes, flushing, and night sweats (C).
Incorrect:
HT is associated with an increase in cardiovascular disease risk as well as an increased risk of venous thrombosis (A). HT will sometimes diminish the symptoms of rheumatoid arthritis but not resolve disease (B) and will typically improve sleep patterns and diminish the frequency and severity of night sweats (D).

55. **Correct: B. minimize endometrial hyperplasia.**
For women taking HT, the progestin component is needed to minimize endometrial hyperplasia and reduce the risk of endometrial cancer development associated with estrogen therapy (B). The progestin component is not needed for women who have had a hysterectomy.

Incorrect:
Estrogen can have positive effects on lipid levels, particularly in increasing HDL-cholesterol levels (A). Treatment of GSM symptoms will require localized estrogen therapy, such as via vaginal cream, rather than oral HT (C). The progestin component will not have any impact on prolonging ovarian activity (D).

56. **Correct: C. a vaginal lubricant can provide relief.**
For the patient experiencing symptoms of GSM, a topical estrogen is an appropriate treatment approach. For women with a history of breast cancer, a nonhormonal option can include the use of vaginal lubricants or moisturizers to relieve dryness that can interfere with sexual activity (C).
Incorrect:
Systemic HT should be avoided in women with a history of breast cancer as an increased risk of breast cancer has been noted with long-term use (A). However, vaginal estrogen can be considered as there is little systemic absorption of estrogen, and studies indicate no increase in breast cancer risk with this approach (B). The vaginal dryness is related to decreased levels of estrogen, which will not improve over time in perimenopausal women (D).

57. **Correct: D. Osteoporosis risk is reduced with use.**
SERMs selectively work on estrogen receptors in bone to prevent bone loss and minimize the risk of osteoporosis (D).
Incorrect:
SERMs specifically work on estrogen receptors in bone and thus would not cause endometrial hyperplasia. Thus, the concurrent use of progestin is not needed (A). This class of agents does not have any effect on vasomotor symptoms such as hot flashes (B) and will not stimulate estrogen receptors in the breast, thus not increasing the risk of breast cancer (C).

58. **Correct: A. The length of the menstrual cycle and duration of menstrual flow are often unpredictable.**
Perimenopause can last about 4 years on average and is characterized by menstrual irregularity (A), with the interval between menses becoming longer or shorter, as well as having heavier or lighter flow. Ovulation during this period becomes erratic.
Incorrect:
The duration of perimenopause can range anywhere from a few months to 10 years but lasts an average of 4 years (B). Tobacco use is associated with an increase in hot flashes, while smoking cessation will tend to decrease the frequency and severity of hot flashes (C). Hot flashes are reported by up to 75% of women during perimenopause (D).

59. **Correct: B. elevated levels of testosterone.**
During menopause, the most significant physiological change is a decrease in circulating estradiol, which rapidly declines over a period of 4 years. However, total serum testosterone does not change during this period (B).

Incorrect:
During menopause, there is an increase in levels of FSH and LH in an attempt to induce ovulation (A, D). Circulating estradiol rapidly declines during the menopause transition (C).

60. **Correct: C. An evaluation of menstrual cycle changes is the best predictor of menopause stage.**
When evaluating a woman with menopause, an assessment of menstrual cycle changes offers a practical approach to determine menopause stage (C). Additional laboratory testing, including hormone measurements, is not generally needed for a diagnosis.
Incorrect:
According to the NAMS, routine screening of women for menopause should be individualized and based on physical examination, family history, lifestyle choices, and other factors. Hormone measurements are not routinely needed (A). FSH and anti-müllerian hormone are most helpful in determining menopause stage. The hCG hormone is produced by the placenta during pregnancy and would not be helpful in evaluating menopause (B). Saliva hormone testing is not an accurate approach and not recommended in diagnosis (D).

61. **Correct: C. minimized hot flashes**
HT is indicated for the reduction of vasomotor symptoms such as hot flashes (C). The effect can be observed fairly quickly, with high-dose estrogen therapy providing relief in about 4 weeks, and low-dose treatment providing relief in about 8 to 12 weeks.
Incorrect:
HT is associated with an increased risk of breast cancer and cardiovascular disease. Data from the Women's Health Initiative (WHI) demonstrated an increased risk of breast cancer with 3 to 5 years of estrogen-progestogen therapy but no increase in breast cancer risk after 7 years of estrogen-alone therapy (B). The WHI study also demonstrated an increased risk of stroke and pulmonary embolism with HT use during the 5 years of follow-up (D). An increased risk of dementia has also been observed in large population-based studies of women who take HT for at least 10 years (A).

62. **Correct: A. vulva**
The greatest concentration of estrogen receptors is found in the vulva (A), vagina, urethra, and trigone of the bladder. These areas tend to have the most noticeable symptoms of menopause.
Incorrect:
Lower concentrations of estrogen receptors are found in the vascular bed (B), heart (C), brain (D), bone, and eye. These areas are also impacted by the hormonal changes of menopause, though to a lesser degree compared to areas with higher concentrations of estrogen receptors.

63. **Correct: D. the duration of lower-dose HT is usually shorter than that of higher-dose regimens.**
When considering the use of HT for the treatment of vasomotor symptoms, clinicians should aim to use the

lowest effective dose possible. High-dose treatment will lead to faster resolution of symptoms but is associated with a higher incidence of adverse effects. Whether using a high- or low-dose regimen, the duration of therapy will be the same (D).

Incorrect:

The lowest effective dose possible should be the goal when using HT for menopausal symptoms (A). High-dose HT can provide relief in about 4 weeks, while a low-dose regimen can take up to 8 to 12 weeks for symptom relief (B). Lower doses of HT are better tolerated; thus, high-dose regimens are generally not recommended (C).

64. **Correct: D. short-term studies demonstrate that oral HT is associated with lower thromboembolic risk than transdermal forms of HT.**

Caution should be used when considering the use of oral HT for women at increased risk of cardiovascular disease and certain types of cancer. Oral HT should be avoided in women with risk factors for thrombosis, as this can increase the risk of a thromboembolic event. Transdermal and transvaginal estrogen is considered safe as there is no increase in thromboembolic risk due to little systemic absorption of the hormone (D).

Incorrect:

For women who have not undergone a hysterectomy, HT should include the use of progestin to prevent endometrial hyperplasia and endometrial cancer associated with estrogen therapy (A). Oral estrogen therapy should also be avoided in women with a history of breast cancer or at high risk of breast or uterine cancer (B). Though low-dose and transdermal estrogen has been found to decrease thromboembolic and stroke risk, standard- or high-dose oral estrogen can increase the risk of these conditions (C).

65. **Correct: C. almond milk.**

Phytoestrogens are chemical substances that are similar to estrogen and are found in a variety of plants and plant products. However, almond milk is not a good source of phytoestrogens (C).

Incorrect:

Soy products and extracts are considered excellent sources of phytoestrogens (D). Other good sources of this compound include apples, carrots, red clover sprouts (A), flaxseed, ginseng (B), rye, and wheat, among others.

66. **Correct: B. one-fourth**

When considering using HT to minimize symptoms of menopause, it is important to use products specifically designed for this purpose and not contraceptive products due to the much higher doses of estrogen found in COCs. HT regimens typically contain about one-fourth the dose of estrogen as what is found in COCs (B). A main goal of HT is to utilize the lowest effective dose possible to minimize the risk of adverse effects.

Incorrect:

Menopausal hormone therapy only contains a fraction of the amount of estrogen used in COC regimens. This is typically 25% of the COC dose (A, C, D).

67. **Correct: D. paroxetine**

For a woman with a history of VTE, a nonhormonal treatment option would be most appropriate. Among the answer choices, paroxetine, an SSRI, is an appropriate choice (D). Other options can include other SSRIs or SNRIs (e.g., venlafaxine), as well as gabapentin.

Incorrect:

Estrogen-containing regimens should be avoided in this patient with a history of DVT in order to prevent further thromboembolic events. Oral conjugated estrogen and 17β-estradiol should be avoided in this patient (A, C). Drospirenone, a synthetic progestin, is used as a contraceptive but would not be used as HT for relief of vasomotor symptoms (B).

68. **Correct: B. 50%.**

Estrogen deficiency after menopause can lead to bone loss and is a strong risk factor for the development of osteoporosis. HT along with calcium supplementation can decrease the risk of fracture by 50% by minimizing bone loss (B).

69. **Correct: B. reduced risk of recurrent UTIs.**

GSM is associated with physiological changes, such as atrophic vaginitis as well as decreased perivaginal colonization by lactobacilli. These organisms provide protection against UTIs by creating an unfavorable environment for common uropathogens. The use of topical or local vaginal estrogen can help promote colonization and growth by lactobacilli and reduce the risk of UTIs (B).

Incorrect:

There is very little systemic absorption of local or topical estrogen and so would not provide relief of vasomotor symptoms, such as night sweats (A). Local or topical estrogen is not associated with a reduced risk of type 2 diabetes (C) and will not affect levels of androgens (D).

70. **Correct: A. few high-quality studies support the use of these products.**

The NAMS suggests that certain nonpharmacological approaches can be useful in some women for alleviating vasomotor symptoms, including phytoestrogens derived from soy isoflavones and extracts. However, caution should be used when considering the use of supplements, as there is a lack of strict regulations on the quality of supplements and little clinical evidence supporting the benefits of these products (A).

Incorrect:

There is a lack of clinical evidence that demonstrates the consistent benefits of supplements in relieving vasomotor symptoms (B), and none that shows superiority of these products compared to prescription HT (D). These products are generally safe, though consultation with a health-care provider should be done prior to initiating supplements to ensure minimal drug-drug interactions. Blood hormone levels are not typically needed during supplement use (C).

71. **Correct: D. Progesterones, whether synthetic or plant based, should not be used by a woman who has undergone a hysterectomy.**

Progesterones are used to counteract the effect of estrogen in causing endometrial hyperplasia and increasing the risk of endometrial cancer. However, progesterone treatment is not needed in women who have undergone a hysterectomy (D).

Incorrect:

Topical creams with phytoprogesterone are available, typically derived from wild yam and not alfalfa (C). However, due to poor bioavailability (B, A), little of the product actually reaches systemic circulation.

Benign Prostatic Hyperplasia

72 to 77. Yes or No

72. **Correct: Yes**

73. **Correct: Yes**

74. **Correct: No**

75. **Correct: Yes**

76. **Correct: No**

77. **Correct: No**

Upon DRE, signs of BPH can include loss of the median sulcus or furrow (72), an enlarged prostate (typically larger than 2.5 cm × 3 cm) (73), and a prostate with a rubbery rather than a boggy consistency (76). There should not be pain with palpation as this could indicate another disorder, such as prostatitis (77). End-void dribbling and sensation of incomplete bladder emptying are also commonly reported (75). Glucose in urine is not an indication of BPH but could be a sign of diabetes mellitus (74). It is important to note that the size of the prostate as determined by DRE can be misleading, as apparently small prostates can still cause significant symptoms.

78. **Correct: A. prostate size does not correlate well with severity of symptoms.**

Though prostate size is frequently enlarged when examined by DRE, this can be misleading as small prostates can also cause significant symptoms of BPH (A).

Incorrect:

BPH typically affects about 50% of men from 51 to 60 years of age, and this increases to 80% of men 80 years and older (B). There is no correlation between BPH and prostate cancer risk (C). Limiting fluids is not a recommended approach for BPH as this can lead to higher concentrated urine that can lead to more irritating symptoms (D).

79. **Correct: A. amitriptyline**

Medications with anticholinergic effect, such as tricyclic antidepressants (e.g., amitriptyline), can contribute to the development of acute urinary retention (A).

Incorrect:

Loratadine (B), enalapril (C), and lorazepam (D) are not associated with clinically significant anticholinergic effect and would not likely contribute to acute urinary retention.

80. **Correct: D. postrenal azotemia.**

Prolonged bladder outlet obstruction can lead to postrenal azotemia characterized by elevated blood urea nitrogen and creatinine levels (D). Renal function returns to baseline soon after the obstruction is relieved.

Incorrect:

Bladder outlet obstruction associated with BPH can lead to postrenal azotemia. Prerenal azotemia (A) is typically caused by decreased renal perfusion often associated with volume depletion. Intrinsic renal azotemia is caused by a condition within the kidneys, such as glomerulonephritis (B) or tubular necrosis (C). Prerenal and intrinsic renal azotemia are not likely related to the presence of BPH.

81. **Correct: D. acute kidney injury.**

Acute kidney injury is not likely to be caused by BPH as another medical condition should be investigated (D).

Incorrect:

Surgical intervention can be considered for the alleviation of BPH symptoms, particularly if medication and lifestyle modifications are not effective (C). Additionally, surgery is appropriate when secondary conditions develop because of BPH, including recurrent UTIs (A), recurrent or gross hematuria, bladder stones (B), or renal insufficiency.

82. **Correct: B. prostate size.**

The 5-α-reductase inhibitors finasteride and dutasteride block the conversion of testosterone to dihydrotestosterone. This has been shown to decrease the size of the prostate after about 6 months of use (B).

Incorrect:

Finasteride and dutasteride have been shown to reduce prostate size. These agents do not have activity at bladder receptor sites (C) and are unlikely to affect bladder contractility (A) or bladder pressure (D).

83. **Correct: C. activity at select bladder receptor sites.**

Alpha blockers such as tamsulosin have activity at the α_1 receptor sites that are located on the prostate and bladder base (C). When these receptors are activated, this can cause the prostate to contract and increase outflow tract obstruction. An alpha blocker will prevent this and improve symptoms of BPH.

Incorrect:

Alpha blockers used in the treatment of BPH do not have an effect on prostate size (B), bladder contractility (A), or bladder pressure (D). These agents prevent prostate contraction that can cause bladder outflow obstruction.

84. **Correct: A. can be used with or without finasteride.**

Sildenafil, a PDE-5 inhibitor that is commonly used to treat erectile dysfunction, has been shown to relieve symptoms of BPH. The medication is approved for the treatment of BPH with or without finasteride (A) and can be used in patients with both BPH and erectile dysfunction.

Incorrect:
Due to cardiovascular risk, the concomitant use of tadalafil with an alpha blocker (B) or nitrate (D) should be avoided. Tadalafil can be considered as a first-line agent (especially for those who also have erectile dysfunction) or can be used when response to other medications is inadequate, and it should not be limited to those in whom surgical intervention is not an option (C).

85. **Correct: B. The use of a validated patient symptom tool is an important part of diagnosing the condition.**
An accurate diagnosis of BPH requires a combination of patient history and review of symptoms, physical examination, and laboratory testing. A useful tool in diagnosis is the American Urological Association Symptom Index (AUA-SI), which provides a standardized assessment tool to improve the accuracy of a BPH diagnosis (B).

Incorrect:
A combination of approaches should be used in making a BPH diagnosis. A DRE can identify an enlarged prostate. However, this can be misleading as small prostates can also cause symptoms of BPH (A). Urodynamic testing, including urinary flow test and postvoid residual volume test, can be helpful in assessing urinary flow obstruction (C). Bladder distension is not typically seen in the early stages of BPH but can be a manifestation in late disease (D).

86. **Correct: D. These therapies are safest and most effective when used with prescription medications.**
The use of herbal supplements is considered an emerging therapy by AUA for the treatment of BPH, and a major concern with their use is a potential for drug interactions when used concomitantly with prescription medications (D). A health-care provider should be consulted prior to initiating herbal supplements.

Incorrect:
Some commonly used herbal supplements for the treatment of BPH include saw palmetto, rye, and pumpkin, though these agents are considered emerging therapies by the AUA (B). The mechanism of action of these plant-based supplements is believed to be similar to prescription medications, though there is a general lack of well-controlled clinical studies to assess their effectiveness (A). In addition to the potential for drug interactions when using supplements, another major concern is a lack of standards in ensuring the purity and quality control of these products (C).

Acute Epididymitis

87. **Correct: A. the presence of a positive Prehn sign.**
A positive finding for the Prehn sign is frequently noted in the patient with epididymitis (A). The Prehn sign is characterized by a reduction in pain when the scrotum is elevated above the symphysis pubis.

Incorrect:
The cremasteric reflex is elicited when the inner part of the thigh is stroked, causing the cremaster muscle to contract and pull up the ipsilateral testicle. This reflex remains present during epididymitis (C). Diffuse abdominal pain is usually not noted in early disease but might be observed as a complication of late disease and bilateral epididymo-orchitis (D). Pain with acute epididymitis can radiate up the spermatic cord to the ipsilateral lower abdomen but does not cause low back pain (B).

88. **Correct: C. *C trachomatis*, and D. *N gonorrhoeae***
Men younger than 35 years are more likely to have epididymitis caused by a STI, which is further supported by his partner's reported infection. The most likely causes of STI-related epididymitis are *C trachomatis* (C) and *N gonorrhoeae* (D).

Incorrect:
Epididymitis caused by enteric organisms, such as *E coli* and *P aeruginosa*, is more commonly found in MSM (A, B).

89. **Correct: A. *E coli*.**
MSM (that is, the insertive partner in anal intercourse) are more likely to have acute epididymitis caused by enteric organisms, such as *E coli* (A).

Incorrect:
Infections by *Mycoplasma* (B) and *H influenzae* (C) are more likely to occur in the respiratory tract rather than the GU system. Similarly, *A baumannii* can cause serious lower respiratory tract infections and bacteremia (D).

90. **Correct: A. PO doxycycline with IM ceftriaxone**
This patient is at higher risk of an STI-related epididymitis caused by *C trachomatis* or *N gonorrhoeae*. Effective treatment against these pathogens is IM ceftriaxone followed by oral doxycycline (A).

Incorrect:
Azithromycin and penicillin are not recommended treatment options for acute epididymitis due to any organism (B). Metronidazole is effective against anaerobic infections, while linezolid is an effective choice for serious gram-positive skin and respiratory tract infections and bacteremia (C). Clindamycin and cefixime are not recommended for treatment of *C trachomatis* or *N gonorrhoeae*, the most likely cause of this patient's infection (D).

91. **Correct: C. PO levofloxacin.**
Acute epididymitis in MSM is likely caused by enteric organisms, such as *E coli*. Therefore, the infection should be treated similarly as a UTI, with agents that have excellent activity against these gram-negative bacteria. Among the answer choices, a fluoroquinolone such as levofloxacin would be the most appropriate selection (C).

Incorrect:
Epididymitis caused by enteric organisms should be treated with a fluoroquinolone as the first-line treatment.

Ceftriaxone would be preferred for infections caused by STI organisms (A). Azithromycin is not indicated for the treatment of epididymitis (B). TMP-SMX can be considered for some GU infections, though the use of the IV formulation in this case is not warranted (D).

92 to 97. Yes or No

92. Correct: **Yes**

93. Correct: **Yes**

94. Correct: **No**

95. Correct: **Yes**

96. Correct: **No**

97. Correct: **Yes**

Common symptoms of epididymitis include irritative voiding symptoms (92), fever, penile discharge (93), and acutely painful epididymis. The condition is not associated with an ulcerative lesion (typically seen with syphilis) (94) or a boggy prostate (seen with acute or chronic prostatitis) (96). Scrotal swelling can occur (95), and in later stages, particularly with untreated disease, epididymo-orchitis can develop, where the ipsilateral testes becomes involved and swelling occurs to the extent where the two testes cannot be distinguished (97).

Acute and Chronic Bacterial Prostatitis

98. Correct: **D. diminished prostate-specific antigen (PSA) level.**

Several risk factors have been identified for acute bacterial prostatitis. However, PSA level has not been associated with risk of acute bacterial prostatitis. Those with acute bacterial prostatitis commonly have elevated PSA levels, but this should not be used to screen patients for the condition. Following antimicrobial therapy, PSA levels typically decrease, though this has been observed in men with or without symptoms of prostatitis.

Incorrect:

Common risk factors for acute bacterial prostatitis include having unprotected intercourse (A), prior episodes of prostatitis, history of bladder or urethral infection (C), and the use of a urinary catheter (B). About 5% of those with acute bacterial prostatitis will progress to chronic bacterial prostatitis.

99. Correct: **B. *N gonorrhoeae* and *C trachomatis*.**

For younger men, the cause of acute bacterial prostatitis is more likely due to STI caused by *N gonorrhoeae* and *C trachomatis* (B). Diagnosis and treatment of men younger than 35 years should target these pathogens.

Incorrect:

Infections caused by Enterobacteriaceae (e.g., *E coli*, *K pneumoniae*, *P aeruginosa*) are more likely to occur in older men and those who have sex with other men (A, C). *Acinetobacter* is not a common pathogen for these types of infections. Enterococci and *S aureus* are more commonly found in men undergoing prolonged catheterization, such as in a hospital or long-term care facility setting (D).

100. Correct: **C. choosing an antibiotic with gram-negative coverage is critical.**

Gram-negative pathogens are the most common causative pathogens in chronic bacterial prostatitis and so antimicrobial therapy should exhibit activity against these pathogens (C).

Incorrect:

The gram-negative Enterobacteriaceae (e.g., *E coli*, *K pneumoniae*) are the most common pathogens for chronic bacterial prostatitis (A). First-line therapy is usually a fluoroquinolone (B), such as ciprofloxacin or levofloxacin, with treatment lasting at least 4 weeks (D).

101. Correct: **C. penile discharge.**

Penile discharge is not a common finding for those with acute bacterial prostatitis, including those with STI-related prostatitis (C).

Incorrect:

Frequent clinical findings in the patient with acute bacterial prostatitis include perineal pain (A), irritative voiding symptoms (B), and fever (D). A prostatic massage should not be performed as part of the diagnostic process as this can be painful and harmful to the patient.

102. Correct: **A. boggy.**

A DRE of a patient with acute bacterial prostatitis typically reveals a tender, enlarged, boggy (i.e., soft and sponge-like) prostate (A).

Incorrect:

Acute bacterial prostatitis is typically characterized by a tender, boggy prostate. A normal prostate is usually described as rubbery and smooth (B). Prostates described as irregular (C) and/or with cystic (D) or hard spots should be evaluated further for possible malignancy.

103. Correct: **B. WBC = 18,000/mm³; neutrophils = 11,500/mm³**

This patient presents with systemic symptoms indicating a significant bacterial infection. Typical CBC findings during an acute bacterial infection include leukocytosis (elevated WBC; greater than 10,800 cells/mm³) and neutrophilia (elevated neutrophils; absolute neutrophil count of greater than 8,000 cells/mm³). This is best illustrated with answer choice B.

104. Correct: **B. a single dose of IM ceftriaxone followed by oral doxycycline.**

Acute bacterial prostatitis in a younger man (younger than 35 years) is likely to be caused by an STI, typically *N gonorrhoeae* or *C trachomatis*. First-line therapy in these cases is an initial dose of ceftriaxone followed by doxycycline (B).

Incorrect:

Acute bacterial prostatitis suspected to be caused by enteric (coliform) bacteria would be treated with a fluoroquinolone, such as levofloxacin (C). However, these would not be appropriate choices for acute bacterial prostatitis caused by STI pathogens. Metronidazole (A), an anti-anaerobic agent, amoxicillin-clavulanate (D), or the macrolides are not recommended options for the treatment of acute bacterial prostatitis.

105. Correct: D. ciprofloxacin
Acute bacterial prostatitis in older men (older than 35 years), suspected to be caused by enteric (coliform) bacteria, would be treated similarly as a UTI with first-line therapy with a fluoroquinolone, such as ciprofloxacin (D).
Incorrect:
Doxycycline can be considered in acute bacterial prostatitis suspected to be caused by an STI pathogen when given after IM ceftriaxone (A). Cefepime (B) and TMP-SMX (C) are not recommended treatment options for acute bacterial prostatitis.

106. Correct: C. low back pain.
Patients with chronic bacterial prostatitis are not acutely ill but can present with symptoms of irritative voiding symptoms and low back and perineal pain (C). Unexplained low back pain can be an important finding when making a differential diagnosis of chronic bacterial prostatitis.
Incorrect:
Penile discharge is not a typical finding with acute or chronic bacterial prostatitis, including those caused by STI pathogens (D). Patients with chronic bacterial prostatitis are not acutely ill and will not normally present with fever (A) or gastrointestinal upset (B).

107. Correct: A. gram-negative rods.
Similar to UTIs, the most common pathogens to cause chronic bacterial prostatitis are gram-negative rods, such as *E coli* and *K pneumoniae*. Treatment should focus on targeting these organisms and should include the fluoroquinolones.

108. Correct: C. oral ciprofloxacin for 4 weeks
Treatment of chronic bacterial prostatitis requires a long course of fluoroquinolone therapy, such as ciprofloxacin or levofloxacin for 4 weeks (C). This ensures adequate penetration in the prostatic tissue to eradicate the infection.
Incorrect:
When considering antimicrobial therapy, the least invasive route is preferred; thus, oral medications are preferred over intravenous or injectable dosing when efficacy is unaffected (B, D). Fluoroquinolones are preferred for the treatment of chronic bacterial prostatitis. TMP-SMX can be considered as an alternative but will require 1 to 3 months of treatment to ensure eradication of the infection (A).

109. Correct: A. a urine culture.
For an older patient with acute bacterial prostatitis likely caused by Enterobacteriaceae (coliform), a urine culture is adequate for identification of the organism (A).

Incorrect:
A NAAT would be preferred when an infection is suspected to be caused by an STI pathogen, such as *N gonorrhoeae* or *C trachomatis* (B). Given the patient's older age and having a single partner, his infection is more likely to be caused by coliform bacteria, when a urine culture is sufficient. Serologic antibody testing (C) is not useful in this case, and a urine Gram stain often fails to identify the causative pathogen (D).

Vulvovaginitis

110. Correct: D. vaginal epithelial cells with adherent bacteria
The presence of vaginal epithelial cells with adherent bacteria is a sign of bacterial vaginosis and not a normal finding (D).
Incorrect:
Normal findings in a woman during the reproductive years include an acidic pH (less than 4.5) (A) as well as an abundance of lactobacilli (B). These organisms help maintain an unfavorable environment for colonization by uropathogens and help prevent UTIs. During the luteal phase of the menstrual cycle, a thick, white vaginal secretion is a normal finding (C).

111. Correct: C. hyphae.
The presence of perineal excoriation along with a white, clumping discharge suggests vulvovaginal candidiasis (C). Confirmation of this diagnosis would include a finding of hyphae upon microscopic examination as well as a normal pH.
Incorrect:
A more neutral pH of 6 is more likely to be found with bacterial vaginosis or trichomoniasis (A). All forms of vaginitis typically result in a decrease in lactobacilli that would normally protect against uropathogenic infections (B). An abundance of WBCs is more commonly found with infections caused by *N gonorrhoeae* and *C trachomatis* (D).

112. Correct: D. malodorous discharge.
Bacterial vaginosis is characterized by the presence of an amine or fishy odor that is more evident following heterosexual intercourse (D). Diagnosis includes a positive finding on the whiff test, which is the presence of an amine odor when exposing vaginal discharge to potassium hydroxide (KOH).
Incorrect:
Pruritus (itching) and vulvitis (irritation and inflammation of the vulva) are more commonly associated with vulvovaginal candidiasis (A, B). Dysuria, or painful urination, is a more common finding with *C trachomatis* and *N gonorrhoeae* infections (C).

113. Correct: B. tioconazole cream.
Treatment of vulvovaginal candidiasis is the use of an oral or topical antifungal azole agent. Commonly prescribed azoles include fluconazole, tioconazole (B), and miconazole.

Incorrect:

Metronidazole is effective against anaerobic bacteria and used for the treatment of bacterial vaginosis and trichomoniasis (A). Oral tinidazole is also used to treat bacterial vaginosis and trichomoniasis but is not effective against candidiasis (C). Clindamycin cream is used to treat bacterial vaginosis (D).

114. Correct: B. trichomoniasis.

The presence of petechial hemorrhages ("strawberry spots") and motile organisms on microscopic examination are consistent with the diagnosis of trichomoniasis, an infection caused by the flagellated *T vaginalis*.

Incorrect:

Bacterial vaginosis is characterized by a thin, gray vaginal discharge and few WBCs, along with a fishy odor and clue cells (C). Chlamydial cervicitis would not include findings of "strawberry spots" or motile microorganisms but would include a friable cervix along with high numbers of WBCs (D). In microscopic examination, sperm are much smaller than *T vaginalis* (A).

115. Correct: A. oral metronidazole.

The preferred treatment for trichomoniasis is oral metronidazole or oral tinidazole (A).

Incorrect:

Oral therapy is needed for maximum effectiveness in treating trichomoniasis in both men and women (B). Acyclovir is an antiviral agent used to treat herpes simplex virus (C). Oral azithromycin is used to treat infection caused by *C trachomatis* (D).

116 to 119. Indicate Yes or No

116. Correct: Yes

117. Correct: Yes

118. Correct: Yes

119. Correct: No

Treatment of bacterial vaginosis can include oral or topical treatment with metronidazole or clindamycin (116, 117, 118). A 1-day dose of secnidazole is another option for treatment. Oral azithromycin is used to treat *C trachomatis* (119).

120 to 123. Indicate bacterial vaginosis, vulvovaginal candidiasis, or trichomoniasis

120. Correct: bacterial vaginosis

121. Correct: trichomoniasis

122. Correct: bacterial vaginosis

123. Correct: vulvovaginal candidiasis

Key findings in bacterial vaginosis include a pH less than 4.5, a positive whiff test (122), clue cells (120), and few WBCs. In vulvovaginal candidiasis, hyphae and pseudohyphae are found on the KOH test (123), a pH less than 5, and few WBCs. Trichomoniasis is characterized by the presence of mobile microorganisms and an abundance of PMNs (121).

Common Sexually Transmitted Infections

124. Correct: A. younger than 25 years

Chlamydia is the most commonly reported STI and primarily affects adolescents and young adults 24 years and younger (A). Because of this, the U.S. Preventive Services Task Force (USPSTF) recommends screening of all women 24 years and younger for chlamydia.

Incorrect:

Though women 25 years and younger are at highest risk of chlamydial infection, this can occur in women of all ages (B, C, D), particularly in women who have multiple sexual partners.

125. Correct: A. ovaries.

Chlamydia infection occurs most frequently in the lower GU tract. Salpingitis, or infection of the fallopian tubes, can sometimes occur, though infection of the ovaries is rare (A).

Incorrect:

C trachomatis can cause various types of infection in women, including cervicitis (B), endometritis (C), and urethritis (D). The endometrium is often involved in infection, even without signs of PID. *C trachomatis* can also infect other non-GU areas, including the pharynx and eyes.

126. Correct: C. 7 to 14 days.

C trachomatis has an incubation period of about 1 to 2 weeks (C). This can be useful when trying to determine the origin of the infection in women with symptoms. However, many women will be asymptomatic.

127. Correct: D. easily irritated and prone to bleeding, especially following intercourse

A friable cervix is a common finding in women with chlamydial infection. This is characterized by a cervix that is easily irritated and prone to bleeding (D).

Incorrect:

A friable cervix does not pertain to the presence of vesicular lesions (A) (as seen with herpes infection) or cysts (C). A friable cervix will not necessarily be associated with a deep burning sensation, though it can be overly sensitive (B).

128 to 133. Yes or No

128. Correct: No

129. Correct: Yes

130. Correct: Yes

131. Correct: No

132. Correct: Yes

133. Correct: Yes

The CDC recommends annual chlamydia screening for all sexually active females aged 25 years and younger (129) as well as older women who are at higher risk of infection, but not all sexually active women regardless of age (128). Increased risk includes those who have a new sex partner, more than one sex partner, a sex partner with concurrent partners, or a sex partner with an STI (130). Screening of sexually active young men should be considered in clinical settings associated with high prevalence of chlamydial infection, but routine screening of all men 25 years and younger is not routinely recommended (131). Additionally, all pregnant women under 25 years as well as older pregnant women at increased risk should be screened (133). MSM should be screened at least annually (132).

134. Correct: C. gram-negative diplococci.

Knowing the causative organism of an infection is critical to safe practice. Gonorrhea is caused by the organism, *N gonorrhoeae*, a gram-negative diplococcus (C). The organism frequently produces beta-lactamase and so should be treated with agents with beta-lactamase stability, such as ceftriaxone and macrolides.

Incorrect:

Gram-positive cocci can include staphylococci or streptococci (A). Gram-positive rods can include *Bacillus* spp. and *Clostridioides* spp. (B). Gram-negative bacilli can include *Klebsiella* spp. and *Escherichia coli* (D).

135. Correct: A. 1 to 5 days

N gonorrhoeae is associated with a relatively short incubation time of 1 to 5 days (A). This can be important for individuals who wish to know the origin of their infection and possibly prevent further spread.

Incorrect:

The incubation time for *N gonorrhoeae* is usually no longer than 5 days (B, C, D).

136. Correct: A. ceftriaxone 500 mg IM as a single dose.

Treatment of *N gonorrhoeae* infection requires agents with excellent activity against gram-negative pathogens. The preferred treatment is a single IM injection of ceftriaxone (A).

Incorrect:

N gonorrhoeae frequently produces beta-lactamase that would result in resistance to penicillins, such as amoxicillin. Fluoroquinolones are also not recommended due to increasing resistance to this class of agents (C). Clarithromycin is not a recommended treatment option for this type of infection (B), nor is the use of oral cephalosporins, such as cefpodoxime (D).

137. Correct: A. cefixime PO 800 mg × 1 dose

IM ceftriaxone is the preferred treatment regimen for gonorrhea. In situations when ceftriaxone therapy is not appropriate or IM treatment is refused, an acceptable oral treatment option is a single dose of cefixime (A).

Incorrect:

Amoxicillin is not appropriate due to a high rate of beta-lactamase production by *N gonorrhoeae* (D). Fosfomycin is used for the treatment of UTIs but not

gonorrhea (C). Metronidazole is the typical therapy for trichomoniasis (B).

138. Correct: C. oral azithromycin plus IM gentamicin.

IM ceftriaxone is the preferred treatment regimen for gonorrhea. In situations of severe allergic reaction to cephalosporins, an acceptable treatment option is gentamicin with azithromycin, though this has not been as extensively studied (C).

Incorrect:

Cefixime is a cephalosporin that would be inappropriate to use with severe allergic reaction (A). Oral cephalosporins are also not recommended, along with fluoroquinolone treatment, due to high rates of resistance to this class by *N gonorrhoeae* (B). Metronidazole is typically used for anaerobic infections or trichomoniasis, while tigecycline is not well studied for gonococcal infections (D).

139 to 142. Indicate Yes or No

139. Correct: Yes

140. Correct: Yes

141. Correct: No

142. Correct: No

Most men with gonorrheal infection are typically asymptomatic. However, symptoms can include dysuria (139) along with a milky, occasionally blood-tinged penile discharge (140). Scrotal swelling (141) and fever (142) are not anticipated findings of gonorrheal urethritis.

143. Correct: A. *C trachomatis*.

This offers a classic case of significant physical examination findings without symptoms. A friable cervix is a typical finding in women with chlamydial infection (A).

Incorrect:

Infection caused by *N gonorrhoeae* typically results in purulent vaginal discharge (B). HSV is characterized by the presence of ulcerated genital lesions (C). Trichomoniasis can be detected by the presence of cervical petechial hemorrhages or "strawberry spots" (D).

144. Correct: A. IM ceftriaxone

Agents effective against gram-negative bacteria with beta-lactamase stability are preferred in the treatment of *N gonorrhoeae*. IM ceftriaxone is the preferred agent for these types of infections (A).

Incorrect:

Fluoroquinolones should be avoided in the treatment of gonorrhea due to elevated rates of resistance (D). Metronidazole is effective against anaerobic bacteria (B), while ketoconazole is an antifungal agent (C).

145. Correct: C. azithromycin

First-line therapy for *C trachomatis* includes agents effective against intracellular pathogens and includes either one dose of azithromycin or doxycycline for

7 days (C). Given the convenience and high tolerability of azithromycin, this is usually the preferred choice.
Incorrect:
Penicillin and metronidazole are not recommended treatment options for *C trachomatis* infection (A, B). Ceftriaxone is often given to patients diagnosed with chlamydial infection as there is an assumption of concomitant *N gonorrhoeae* infection (D).

146. **Correct: B. Most men have asymptomatic infection.**
Symptoms associated with gonococcal infection in men can include irritative voiding symptoms and occasional purulent discharge. However, most men with this infection are asymptomatic (B).
Incorrect:
Though male-to-female transmission of gonococcal infection is high (approximately 80%), the transmission of infection from female to male is fairly low at about 20% (A). The incubation period for gonococcal infection is relatively short at about 1 to 5 days (C). This organism frequently produces beta-lactamase, making the organism resistant to certain beta-lactam antimicrobials such as amoxicillin (D).

147. **Correct: C. acute pyelonephritis.**
Gonococcal and chlamydial infections can be associated with various complications of the GU system. However, infection of the upper urinary tract, such as acute pyelonephritis (C), or infection of the kidneys, is not a typical finding with these pathogens.
Incorrect:
Chlamydial and gonococcal infections can impact the upper and lower reproductive tracts in women. Complications can include PID (A), tubal scarring (B) that can lead to infertility or ectopic pregnancy, and acute peritoneal inflammation (D).

148. **Correct: B. *U urealyticum*, and C. *M genitalium*.**
When making a differential diagnosis of GU infections, it is important to consider that chlamydial infections present similarly as infections caused by *U urealyticum* and *M genitalium*. A *C trachomatis* infection can be identified with NAAT that provides high specificity and sensitivity. Recommended treatments of GU infections caused by *U urealyticum* and *M genitalium* are similar to those used in chlamydial infection.
Incorrect:
Identifying the correct pathogen is critical in guiding appropriate treatment of the infection. *T vaginalis*, the causative pathogen of trichomoniasis, can produce a yellow-green vaginal discharge along with cervical petechial hemorrhages (A). *C difficile* is not known to cause GU infections but can cause severe diarrhea and colitis (D).

149. **Correct: B. mucopurulent discharge**
Conjunctivitis caused by *C trachomatis* is typically unilateral and associated with redness and a mucopurulent discharge (B).

Incorrect:
Clear, watery discharge is more likely caused by viral conjunctivitis rather than a bacterial infection (A). The infection is typically unilateral rather than bilateral (C) and is not associated with decreased peripheral vision (D).

150. **Correct: B. external hemorrhoid.**
Gonococcal and chlamydial proctitis are commonly found in the receptive partner of anal intercourse. External hemorrhoids are not associated with this condition (B).
Incorrect:
Proctitis caused by *C trachomatis* or *N gonorrhea* can be characterized by rectal discharge (A) and pain. Signs of gonococcal proctitis can also include pruritus (D) as well as tenesmus (C).

151. **D. pustular lesions.**
Lesions caused by HSV-2 are typically ulcerated vesicles and not pustular lesions (D).
Incorrect:
The clinical presentation of HSV-2 infection includes painful ulcerated lesion (A), lymphadenopathy (B) (especially with the initial outbreak), and a thin vaginal discharge, especially if lesions involve the vagina and introitus (C).

152 to 155. Indicate Yes or No

152. **Correct: Yes**

153. **Correct: Yes**

154. **Correct: Yes**

155. **Correct: No**
Herpes can be spread through contact with lesions, mucosal surfaces, and genital or oral secretions (152, 153). The virus can also be spread through normal, intact skin (154). However, the virus cannot be transmitted from inanimate objects such as towels, toilet seats, bed sheets, or silverware (155).

156. **Correct: D. a thin profuse discharge.**
A thin profuse discharge usually accompanies HSV-2 infection when lesions involve the vagina and introitus (D).
Incorrect:
HSV-2 infection is not typically associated with adnexal tenderness (A) or a friable cervix (B), which is more commonly found with *C trachomatis* infection. Also, HSV-2 infection will not cause a rash extending to the upper thighs, though lesions in men can sometimes extend to the thighs and buttocks regions (C).

157. **Correct: B. 15%**
Approximately 15% of the adult population in the United States is seropositive for HHV-2 (B). However, only about 10% to 20% of the seropositive population will have symptomatic disease in the form of genital herpes.

Incorrect:

The estimated prevalence of HHV-2 seropositivity in sexually active adults is greater than 5% (A) but less than 25% (C, D).

158. Correct: A. in childhood, and D. by contact with oral secretions

Many adults have had acquired HSV-1, the cold sore virus, through saliva contact in childhood. However, a small percentage will manifest with herpes labialis, or cold sores.

Incorrect:

Unlike HSV-2, acquisition of HSV-1 is less likely to occur during adulthood (B) or through sexual contact (C).

159. Correct: B. 20%

During the asymptomatic period, HSV-2 can be spread through viral shedding. This can occur in 5% to 20% of days in individuals with long-term infection, even if there are no signs or symptoms of infection (B).

Incorrect:

Viral shedding of HSV-2 generally occurs in more than 5% of days during asymptomatic periods (A) but less than 50% on average (C, D).

160 to 162. Indicate PCR, serological, or both

160. Correct: both

161. Correct: both

162. Correct: serological

Direct assays can be used in patients with active lesions and can include the use of viral culture or PCR assay to detect viral DNA or RNA. Serological assays that detect the presence of antibodies can be used to determine if an outbreak is an initial infection or recurrent episode. In the 32-year-old, both types of assays can be used to confirm HSV-2 in the current outbreak, while a positive result in the serological test would confirm a recurrent episode (160). For the 27-year-old, PCR will confirm HSV-2 infection, while a negative result on serological assay will indicate that this is an initial episode of HSV-2 infection (161). In the 41-year-old, the absence of lesions will not make the use of a direct assay possible. A serological assay can confirm prior HSV-2 episodes (162).

163. Correct: C. oral famciclovir.

Treatment of herpes can include the use of oral antiviral therapy such as acyclovir, famciclovir (C), or valacyclovir. Systemic treatment is preferred, as this will suppress levels of herpes virus and reduce the rate of recurrent episodes. Topical penciclovir can be used in the treatment of cold sores and provides an option for those who do not wish to or cannot take systemic antiviral medication.

Incorrect:

Systemic antiviral treatment is preferred for the treatment of vulvar vesicles over topical treatment (D).

Ribavirin is an antiviral used in the treatment of hepatitis C infection (A), while indinavir is used to treat HIV (B).

164. Correct: D. 70% to 80%.

Daily use of an oral antiviral agent can be effective in reducing genital herpes recurrences by 70% to 80% in those who have frequent recurrences (D). Treatment will also diminish viral shedding and help prevent the transmission of the virus through direct contact.

165. Correct: C. hepatitis A.

Hepatitis A results in an acute infection that either resolves or leads to death (i.e., there is no chronic hepatitis A infection). Since there is no chronic condition of hepatitis A infection, screening for this infection is not needed (C).

Incorrect:

Comprehensive STI testing should include HBV (A), HCV (E), syphilis (B), HIV (D), and HSV-2 (F). For those who have not been previously vaccinated and are eligible, immunization should be encouraged for HAV, HBV, and HPV.

Pelvic Inflammatory Disease

166. Correct: B. leukopenia.

An expected finding of bacterial infections such as PID is elevated WBC count, or leukocytosis, rather than diminished levels of WBCs or leukopenia (B).

Incorrect:

Other common signs and symptoms of PID include dysuria (A), cervical motion tenderness (C), adnexal tenderness, and abdominal pain that worsens over time (D).

167. Correct: C. mucopurulent vaginal discharge

A common finding of PID is abnormal vaginal discharge that contains high numbers of WBCs, indicating the presence of a bacterial infection (C).

Incorrect:

Loose stools is not an anticipated finding in PID (A). Mucopurulent vaginal discharge is common that contains a high concentration of WBCs due to the bacterial infection (B). Though PID can be caused by a variety of organisms, E coli is an uncommon pathogen for this type of infection (D). Laboratory testing should be performed to identify the presence of STI pathogens, particularly C trachomatis and N gonorrhoeae.

168. Correct: C. C trachomatis.

PID infections are often polymicrobial, necessitating the use of combination antimicrobial therapy to provide adequate coverage of gram-positive, gram-negative, and anaerobic organisms. The most common pathogens include C trachomatis (C), N gonorrhoeae, H influenzae, Streptococcus species, Mycoplasma species, and Ureaplasma species, along with select anaerobic species.

Incorrect:

PID is not typically caused by coliform bacteria such as the Enterobacteriaceae (B) and *E coli* (A). *Pseudomonas* can be a significant pathogen in certain UTIs as well as respiratory tract infections but is not commonly found in PID (D).

169. **Correct: D. tubo-ovarian abscess.**

Transvaginal ultrasound can often detect the presence of an adnexal mass in women with PID. This would indicate the likely presence of a tubo-ovarian abscess (D). This is a serious condition that will require hospitalization and parenteral antimicrobial treatment.

Incorrect:

In a woman with PID, the presence of an adnexal mass identified by transvaginal ultrasound is likely due to a tubo-ovarian abscess. This is less likely to be caused by uterine fibroids (A), an ectopic pregnancy (B), or ovarian malignancy (C).

170. **Correct: C. 40%**

Polymicrobial infections are found in approximately 30% to 40% of women with PID (C). This necessitates the use of multiple antimicrobial agents that provide adequate coverage against gram-negative, gram-positive, and anaerobic organisms.

171. **Correct: C. decreased hemoglobin.**

A finding of decreased hemoglobin is consistent with anemia, which is not an anticipated finding with PID (C).

Incorrect:

Elevated ESR (A) and CRP (B) are expected findings during conditions of inflammation such as PID. Elevated levels of WBCs are also anticipated in the presence of an acute bacterial infection (D).

172. **Correct: A. tubal thickening with or without free pelvic fluid.**

During a transvaginal ultrasound in a woman with PID, an anticipated finding would include the presence of tubal thickening (A). This can occur with or without free pelvic fluid or identification of a tubo-ovarian abscess.

Incorrect:

Cervical thickening (B) and endometrial thinning (C) are not anticipated findings in PID. Oophoritis, or inflammation of the ovaries, as well as ovaries with multiple cysts can occur during PID but are less common than the anticipated finding of tubal thickening (D) that is used in making the diagnosis.

173. **Correct: D. temperature 101.5°F (38.6°C); total WBC 16,000/mm³**

Anticipated findings in PID are fever (temperature greater than 101°F [greater than 38.3°C]) and leukocytosis (WBC greater than 10,800/mm³). Among the answer choices, choice D is most consistent with these findings (D).

Incorrect:

PID is generally associated with the presence of fever (A, C) and elevated levels of WBCs (B).

174. **Correct: C. IM ceftriaxone with PO doxycycline**

First-line treatment of PID in the outpatient setting can include IM ceftriaxone with PO doxycycline (C). This will provide adequate coverage of most gram-negative and gram-positive organisms. The addition of metronidazole can also be considered for coverage against anaerobes.

Incorrect:

Fluoroquinolones are not recommended in the treatment of PID due to rising rates of resistance (A). Gentamicin is typically administered IV rather than IM and is not recommended for outpatient treatment (B). Azithromycin is not recommended in the treatment of PID (D).

175. **Correct: D. IV clindamycin plus IV gentamicin then PO doxycycline**

Because of the presence of a tubo-ovarian abscess, this patient should undergo inpatient management with parenteral antimicrobial therapy. Due to severe allergic reaction to cephalosporins, a combination of IV clindamycin and IV gentamicin is appropriate. Once an adequate clinical response is sustained for at least 24 hours, treatment can be switched to oral doxycycline for 14 days.

Incorrect:

Parenteral antimicrobial treatment is necessary for this patient with tubo-ovarian abscess (A, B). Additionally, fluoroquinolones are not recommended for the treatment of PID due to rising resistance rates. A regimen of IV cefotetan plus IV/PO doxycycline can be an option to treat PID in the inpatient setting. However, this would not be recommended in a patient with severe cephalosporin allergy (C). IV vancomycin is also not recommended for PID treatment.

Additional Sexually Transmitted Infections

176. **Correct: A. verruciform**

Condyloma acuminatum is characterized by the presence of genital warts described as verruciform lesions (A). These can consist of small, flesh-colored lesions with a cauliflower appearance.

Incorrect:

Vesicular lesions are more commonly found with HSV infections (C). Bullous lesions are typically found with certain bacterial skin infections, such as those caused by *S aureus* (D). Plaque-like lesions are consistent with a number of skin conditions, including psoriasis (B).

177. **Correct: A. anorectal carcinoma.**

Certain types of HPV are associated with a higher malignancy risk, particularly HPV types 16 and 18. In men, particularly MSM, HPV infection can increase the risk of anorectal carcinoma (A).

Incorrect:

HPV infection will not impact fertility and sperm count in men (B). Paraphimosis, or when the foreskin becomes trapped beneath the glans penis, can be a medical emergency but is not caused by HPV infection (C). Reiter's syndrome, or reactive arthritis, can cause inflammation of certain joints as well as the eyes and urethra. This is usually caused by a bacterial infection and not associated with HPV (D).

178. Correct: A. topical acyclovir.
Acyclovir is the recommended treatment of genital herpes most commonly caused by HSV-2. Acyclovir would not be used for the treatment of HPV infection (A).
Incorrect:
Treatment of genital warts can include the use of patient-applied treatment such as topical podofilox (C) or imiquimod cream. Treatment by health-care providers can include the application of trichloroacetic acid (D) as well as cryotherapy (B) or surgical removal.

179. Correct: B. 6 and 11
The most common causes of genital warts are HPV types 6 and 11 (B). These types have a low potential for malignancy. The HPV vaccine provides coverage against these types as well as several HPV types associated with malignancy.
Incorrect:
HPV types 16 and 18 are the most common HPV types associated with malignancy (C). HPV types 1, 2, and 3 are likely causes of common warts (A). HPV 35 and 39 also have a high potential for malignancy but are encountered less frequently than HPV types 16 and 18 (D).

180. Correct: C. 16 and 18
HPV types 16 and 18 are the most common HPV types associated with malignancy (C). The HPV vaccine provides coverage against these types along with other HPV types associated with malignancy and genital warts, particularly HPV types 6 and 11.
Incorrect:
HPV 1, 2, and 3 are likely associated with common warts (A). The most common causes of genital warts are HPV types 6 and 11 (B). HPV types 40 and 42 also have a low potential for malignancy and are a less common cause of genital warts compared to HPV types 6 and 11 (D).

181. Correct: D. 90% or greater
In the United States, HPV is the cause of over 99% of all cervical cancers as well as about 90% of anal cancers (D). Additionally, HPV is the leading cause of oropharyngeal cancers (60% to 70%), vaginal cancers (75%), vulvar cancers (69%), and penile cancer (63%). HPV types 16 and 18 are the leading cause of cervical cancer, while other HPV types include 31, 33, 35, 39, 45, 51, 52, and 58.

182. Correct: D. all males under age 25 years.
The use of an anal Pap test to screen for anal cancer precursors can be considered in populations at high risk for anogenital cancers. However, given the generally small numbers of anal cancers that occur each year, routine screening of all men under 25 years would not

be an efficient and cost-effective approach in identifying these cancers (D).
Incorrect:
Screening with anal Pap tests should be considered in populations at high risk of anal cancer. These populations include MSM (B), immunocompromised men, such as those living with HIV (A), as well as women with a history of anogenital HPV infection (C).

183. Correct: B. immune modulator
Various approaches can be used to treat genital warts caused by HPV. Topical imiquimod acts as an immune modulator that stimulates the body's immune system to penetrate and destroy the diseased tissue (B).
Incorrect:
Keratolytic agents can be used to treat genital warts and include trichloroacetic acid (A). Liquid nitrogen can be used in cryogenic treatment to remove lesions (C) by thermal-induced cytolysis (D). Podofilox exhibits cytotoxic and antimitotic effects that can cause tissue necrosis of the lesions.

184. Correct: C. 2 to 4 weeks
Syphilis is caused by the *Treponema pallidum* spirochete and will cause the initial lesion about 2 to 4 weeks after contact (C). Localized lymphadenopathy can also occur during the initial presentation.
Incorrect:
The general amount of time for the appearance of the initial lesion following *T pallidum* exposure is longer than two weeks (A, B) but less than 4 weeks (D).

185 to 192. Indicate primary, secondary, or tertiary syphilis

185. Correct: primary

186. Correct: secondary

187. Correct: tertiary

188. Correct: primary

189. Correct: tertiary

190. Correct: secondary

191. Correct: secondary

192. Correct: secondary
Symptoms of primary syphilis occur about 2 to 4 weeks after infection and consist of a painless genital ulcer (185) that spontaneously heals (188). Localized lymphadenopathy can also occur. Secondary syphilis occurs approximately 4 to 10 weeks after initial infection and can include a diffuse maculopapular rash that can involve the palms and soles (191), diffuse lymphadenopathy (186), arthralgia (190), and generalized flu-like symptoms (192). After a latency period, tertiary syphilis can develop 3 to 15 years after initial infection with the presence of gumma (187) (granulomatous lesions on skin, bone, and mucous membranes) as well as cardiovascular (189) and neurological complications.

193. Correct: C. at the secondary stage
Syphilis is most contagious during the secondary stage of disease (C). This occurs about 4 to 10 weeks

after initial infection and is characterized by a diffuse maculopapular rash, generalized lymphadenopathy, and flu-like symptoms (i.e., low-grade fever, malaise, arthralgias, myalgia, and headache).

194. Correct: A. IM penicillin.

The preferred treatment of primary syphilis is IM penicillin given as a one-time dose (A).

Incorrect:

Alternative treatment options to penicillin can include IM ceftriaxone for 8 to 10 days (D) or oral doxycycline for 2 weeks (C). Fluoroquinolones, such as ciprofloxacin, are not recommended treatment for syphilis (B).

195. Correct: C. performing a second test (e.g., TPPA) to confirm the diagnosis.

For an individual who does not present with obvious symptoms of syphilis but tests positive on a screening assay, a second positive result is needed to confirm a syphilis diagnosis. This can include the use of EIA, the FTA-ABS test, the TPPA, darkfield microscopy, or MHA-TP.

Incorrect:

Treatment for syphilis should not be initiated until the diagnosis is confirmed with a second test (A). When indicated, the preferred treatment is IM penicillin, while metronidazole is not a recommended treatment option for syphilis at any stage (B). A referral is not needed for this patient, as there are no obvious complications from the disease, and treatment is simple (D).

196. Correct: C. initiate treatment with IM penicillin.

This patient presents with characteristic symptoms of secondary syphilis and reports an initial painless genital ulcer about 1 month ago that is likely due to primary syphilis. With the positive finding from the TPPA test, this individual likely has syphilis, and immediate treatment with IM penicillin should be given (C).

Incorrect:

Due to the patient history and presentation consistent with syphilis, along with a positive finding on TPPA, confirmatory testing is not needed (A, B). Preferred treatment of secondary syphilis is IM penicillin. TMP-SMX is used for certain UTIs but is not recommended for syphilis (D).

197 to 200. Yes or No

197. Correct: Yes

198. Correct: Yes

199. Correct: Yes

200. Correct: Yes

HIV testing is recommended at least once for all patients aged 13 to 64 years in all health-care settings. Routine HIV testing should be performed for individuals at higher risk of HIV, including injection drug users (200) and those being treated for other STIs (198). The CDC recommends all pregnant women be tested for HIV in the first trimester as part of routine

prenatal care (199). HIV testing should be performed for anyone who requests testing regardless of risk factors (197).

201. Correct: C. repeat testing in 2 months.

Rapid HIV tests check for the presence of antibodies against HIV. However, it can take up to 12 weeks to make enough antibodies to be detected by these tests. If a rapid test result is negative, then a repeat test should be performed approximately 3 months after the time of possible exposure (C). Alternatively, an early detection HIV test can be performed, which detects genetic material or protein from the virus that is produced within the first few weeks of infection.

Incorrect:

Since antibodies can take up to 3 months following exposure to HIV, a repeat test should be performed at that time to confirm a negative result (A). Testing prior to 3 months can still result in a negative test result despite infection (B). Repeat testing one year later is too long and can result in exposure to others to HIV (D).

202. Correct: A. Optimally, communication of positive results should be done through in-person contact.

The CDC recommends that health-care providers have protocols in place to notify patients about positive HIV results. Optimally, this should be done confidentially and person-to-person (A). In some states, this is required by law.

Incorrect:

Direct person-to-person communication is the preferred method to inform a patient about a positive HIV result. This provides the opportunity to reassure the patient about the benefits of proper medical care and treatment, and the patient should immediately be linked with the next level of structured care. This would not be accomplished with the use of text messaging and e-mails (C). Communication of HIV test results should be done confidentially and not through a spouse or partner (D), though notification and testing of partners should be encouraged as part of the management plan. For patients who are not fluent in English, the use of an interpreter is preferred, while using a friend or relative to translate should be avoided (B).

203. Correct: B. repeat testing within 1 year.

The CDC recommends HIV testing of all individuals between 13 and 64 years at least once, with repeat testing for those at higher risk of infection. These include injection-drug users and their sex partners, persons who exchange sex for money or drugs, sex partners of HIV-infected persons, and MSM or heterosexual persons who themselves or whose sex partners have had more than one sex partner since their most recent HIV test. Though the optimal interval between testing is not fully determined, the CDC recommends repeat testing at least annually (B), though some higher-risk individuals should consider repeat testing every

3 to 6 months. Similar recommendations have been made by the USPSTF.

Testicular Torsion

204. Correct: D. relief of pain with scrotal elevation.

For patients with testicular torsion, relief of pain with scrotal elevation, also known as the Prehn sign, is not evident (D). This is an anticipated finding in patients with acute epididymitis.

Incorrect:

Anticipated findings with testicular torsion include a sudden onset of scrotal pain, testicular swelling (C), and a finding of the affected testicle held higher in the scrotum (B). Additionally, there is a loss of the cremasteric reflex (A), which is observed when the inner thigh is stroked, causing the ipsilateral testicle to be pulled up.

205. Correct: C. left testicle most often affected.

Testicular torsion occurs by the twisting of the testis and spermatic cord around a vertical axis. In most cases, the left testicle is affected (C).

Incorrect:

Elevated PSA level (A) and WBCs in urine (B) are not expected findings related to testicular torsion. If a Doppler ultrasound is performed, it will likely reveal decreased testicular blood flow due to the twisting of the testis (D).

206. Correct: B. 6

Testicular torsion is a urological emergency that requires immediate surgical intervention. There is a high chance of full recovery if surgical intervention is able to restore blood flow within 6 hours of the torsion (B). Delay beyond this time frame can lead to ischemia of the testicle and potential testicular loss.

Incorrect:

Testicular decompression should be performed within 6 hours of torsion to prevent testicular loss (A). Intervention beyond 6 hours places the patient at high risk of testicular loss (C, D).

207. Correct: C. surgical intervention

Testicular torsion is a urological emergency that requires immediate surgical intervention (C). If the condition is not corrected within 6 hours of torsion, this can lead to tissue ischemia and risk of testicular loss.

Incorrect:

Testicular torsion is a urological emergency that requires immediate attention (D). Systemic corticosteroids to reduce inflammation are not warranted in this situation (A). Manual detorsion can be attempted, mainly as a gap measure before surgical intervention, but this will not prevent a recurrent episode (B).

208. Correct: C. orchiopexy

The best measure to prevent a recurrence of testicular torsion is a bilateral orchiopexy, where both testes are brought down and tacked lower in the scrotum (C).

Incorrect:

Testicular trauma is a common cause of testicular torsion, but recurrence can occur in the absence of further trauma (B). Limiting the number of sexual partners is generally recommended to prevent STIs but would not impact testicular torsion recurrence (D). Use of a scrotal support is not as helpful in preventing recurrence compared to bilateral orchiopexy (A).

209. Correct: A. scrotal pain

The TWIST scoring system can be used to determine the risk of testicular torsion and the need for an ultrasound. However, scrotal pain is not a component of this evaluation tool (A).

Incorrect:

Components of TWIST include testis swelling (B) (2 points), hard testis (2 points), absent cremasteric reflex (1 point), nausea/vomiting (C) (1 point), and high-riding testis (D) (1 point). Those at low risk (2 points or less) would not need ultrasound and should be evaluated for another cause of symptoms. Those at high risk (greater than 5 to 6 points) should proceed directly to surgery, while those at intermediate risk should undergo ultrasound for further evaluation.

Varicocele

210. Correct: A. no additional diagnostic testing is needed.

Varicocele is largely a clinical diagnosis that does not require further diagnostic testing (A) in the absence of atypical presentation or risk of complications, such as the presence of a nonreducible varicocele or the development of a sudden-onset right-sided varicocele.

Incorrect:

When evaluating varicocele, Doppler ultrasonography can be considered in certain situations, such as a sudden-onset right-sided or nonreducible varicocele (B). A CT scan is not warranted for diagnosis and should be avoided due to radiation exposure (C). In uncomplicated cases, varicocele is not a medical emergency that requires surgery referral, though surgical intervention can be considered if associated with pain or atrophy, or if fertility is affected (D).

211. Correct: A. lower sperm count with increased number of abnormal forms

Varicocele has been associated with increased infertility in men due to low sperm count and a high number of atypical (e.g., immobile) sperm. An impaired sperm count of less than 20 million/mL may be found, compared to 40 to 300 million/mL in normal males. Surgical correction of varicocele often results in restoration of sperm counts and improved fertility.

Incorrect:

Varicocele typically results in a nontender and easily compressed mass, with rare reports of scrotal heaviness or ache (C). Varicocele is not associated with an increased risk of testicular cancer (B) or BPH (D).

212. **Correct: C. treatment with a thrombolytic agent.**
The use of a thrombolytic agent is not warranted in the treatment of varicocele as the condition is not caused by a thrombus or blood clot in the vein (C).
Incorrect:
When treatment of varicocele is desired due to pain, atrophy, or infertility, interventions can include an open surgical procedure (A), laparoscopic surgery (B), or percutaneous embolization (D). These approaches seal off the affected vein to redirect blood flow to other normal veins.

213. **Correct: A. an increase in sperm count and normative sperm forms, and C. an increase in fertility in limited study**
For men with varicocele and altered semen analysis (e.g., low sperm count and/or abnormal/immotile forms), surgical intervention can help to restore sperm counts to normal levels and reduce the numbers of abnormal forms (A). Limited clinical studies have shown some supporting evidence demonstrating a higher chance of spontaneous pregnancy following surgical intervention (C).
Incorrect:
Surgical intervention of varicocele can improve male fertility and increase the probability of spontaneous pregnancy due to restoration of sperm count and reducing abnormal forms (B). There is no evidence that there is an increase in congenital health issues of children conceived following surgical intervention for varicocele (D).

Erectile Dysfunction

214. **Correct: D. testosterone deficiency**
The most common risk factor for ED is the presence of an underlying condition that causes neurological or cardiovascular damage that impedes the normal physiology needed to achieve and maintain a penile erection. Hormonal disorders, such as testosterone deficiency, can potentially be a cause of ED but is not a common risk factor (D).
Incorrect:
Disorders that impair blood flow or cause nerve damage have the potential to cause ED. The most common disorders include diabetes mellitus (A), kidney disease, chronic alcohol abuse, vascular disease (B), tobacco use (C), and neuropathy. Certain types of medications, such as antihypertensives and antidepressants, can also contribute to ED.

215. **Correct: C. With use of the medication, sexual stimulation also is needed to achieve an erection.**
With the use of sildenafil, an erection can occur after about 1 hour but will require sexual stimulation and will not occur spontaneously (C).

Incorrect:
Sildenafil can provide effective treatment of ED in many men. However, it will have limited effect in men whose ED is caused by underlying atherosclerosis or neuropathy (B). After use of this agent, an erection will typically need sexual stimulation and will not occur spontaneously (A). PDE-5 inhibitors such as sildenafil are contraindicated with the concurrent use of nitrates due to the risk of dangerous hypotension (D).

216. **Correct: B. most cases have an underlying contributing cause.**
Most cases of ED are attributed to underlying disorders that impair blood flow or cause nerve damage (B). The most common disorders include diabetes mellitus, kidney disease, chronic alcohol abuse, vascular disease, tobacco use, and neuropathy. Symptoms of ED are often improved by controlling the underlying disorder.
Incorrect:
Though ED occurs more frequently in older men, this should not be considered a normal age-related condition as the condition commonly manifests from other underlying causes (A). Depression is a treatable cause of ED (C). However, certain antidepressive medications can also contribute to ED, and so consideration should be given to medications with minimal sexual adverse effects. The same medications used in younger men can be used for older men for effective treatment (D). However, older men are more likely to have underlying conditions that would lessen the effectiveness of these medications. Managing the underlying disease can help improve ED symptoms.

217. **Correct: C. longer half-life.**
Tadalafil has a half-life of approximately 17 hours, which is substantially longer than the 4 to 5 hours observed with the other PDE-5 inhibitors. Due to this longer half-life, it can be given as a daily low-dose schedule rather than timing the dose on an as-needed basis (C).
Incorrect:
Tadalafil belongs to the class of PDE-5 inhibitors and does not have a unique mechanism of action (A). All PDE-5 inhibitors are generally well tolerated, though they are contraindicated with the concomitant use of nitrates (B). The longer half-life of tadalafil would suggest less rapid elimination from the body compared to agents with a shorter half-life (D).

218. **Correct: C. insertion of a nitroglycerin pellet in the urethra.**
Alternative approaches can be considered if there is an inadequate response with PDE-5 inhibitors. An alprostadil pellet, rather than nitroglycerin, can be inserted into the urethra, which will cause localized vasodilation (C).
Incorrect:
The use of alternative approaches to treat ED will often require specialty referral. These options include

an alprostadil injection directly into the penis (A), mechanical vacuum devices (B), or the implantation of a prosthetic device or pump (D).

Cervical and Anogenital Cancer Screening

219. Correct: D. STI testing only.

Cervical cancer screening is not recommended for women under the age of 21 years as cervical abnormalities related to HPV infection and dysplasia commonly resolve on their own among adolescents and young women. STI testing is strongly recommended due to her history of past STI and multiple sex partners (D).

Incorrect:

Cervical cancer screening is not recommended among women under the age of 21 years. This includes screening for HPV (B) or performing a Pap test (A, C).

220. Correct: B. HPV testing.

HPV testing is recommended as part of cervical cancer screening in women beginning at age 30 years. In younger women, HPV infection typically clears within 1 to 2 years of acquisition, and dysplasias resolve on their own. HPV testing in these younger women can lead to unnecessary and harmful evaluation and treatment.

Incorrect:

A Pap test is recommended for women every 3 years beginning at age 21 years (A). A pelvic examination should be performed as part of routine health care (C). Women with multiple sex partners and who practice unprotected sex should be tested for STIs as they are at higher risk (D).

221. Correct: C. 5 years.

Current recommendations suggest testing every 5 years when co-testing with a Pap test and HPV test are done (C). If only a Pap test is done, then repeat testing should be performed every 3 years when there are no abnormal results.

Incorrect:

When co-testing is performed, repeat testing is needed every 5 years. With only a Pap test performed, repeat testing should be done every 3 years (B). Annual testing is unnecessary (A) while every 7 years is too long of an interval between testing for any recommended approach (D).

222. Correct: D. neither now nor in the future.

Pap tests should be repeated every 3 years if done alone, and every 5 years when co-testing is performed with HPV testing. However, for a woman who has had her cervix removed for noncancer reasons, a Pap test is no longer needed (D).

Incorrect:

With complete removal of the cervix, further Pap testing is not needed (A, B, C).

223. Correct: A. conducting a Pap test.

For women between the ages of 21 and 29 years old, a Pap test should be performed every 3 years to screen for cervical cancer and so should be tested today (A). HPV testing should not be performed until age 30 years, regardless of whether the patient has been vaccinated against HPV.

Incorrect:

For women between the ages of 21 and 29 years old, a Pap test should be performed every 3 years, and so she should be tested today (C, D). HPV testing should not be done until 30 years of age regardless of immunization status against HPV (B). With an abnormal Pap test, the usual course is a colposcopy. A biopsy is not warranted at this time for this patient (E).

224. Correct: B. an area of prostatic induration.

A prostatic DRE can be used to evaluate for prostate cancer, but the technique has limitations. In patients with prostate cancer, the prostate is often normal until late stages of disease, where a painless lesion or area of induration in the posterior lobe of the prostate can be found.

Incorrect:

A normal prostate is described as having a rubbery texture (A). A boggy prostate, thus having a soft and spongy feel, best describes a prostate with inflammation (i.e., prostatitis) (C). Prostate cancer is typically associated with the presence of a painless lesion rather than prostatic tenderness, which might be associated with acute prostatitis (D).

225. Correct: B. repeat screening in 1 year.

The normal PSA value in younger men is less than 2.5 ng/mL and less than 4 ng/mL in the elderly. For men with a normal DRE and PSA less than 2.5 ng/mL, repeat testing can be performed every 2 years. However, if the PSA is greater than or equal to 2.5 ng/mL in a man of this age, then testing should be repeated annually.

Incorrect:

Due to the elevated PSA level for this patient, a repeat test should be performed in 1 year rather than waiting 2 years (C) or longer (D). Immediately repeating the test is not necessary (A).

226. Correct: B. history of genital trauma.

When evaluating patients for prostate cancer, it is important to recognize patient factors that increase risk that would further support the need for cancer screening. However, a history of genital trauma is not a recognized risk factor for prostate cancer (B).

Incorrect:

Common risk factors for prostate cancer include older age, African ancestry (A), a family history of prostate cancer (C), and high-fat diet (D).

227. Correct: C. 40, 10

Prostate cancer is the most common noncutaneous cancer in men in the United States. However, most prostate cancers are likely occult and have little risk of metastasis. It is estimated that the average American man has a 40% lifetime risk of prostate cancer, with an approximately 10% risk of clinically significant disease, and a 3% risk of dying from prostate cancer (C).

Incorrect:

The lifetime risk of prostate cancer can approach up to 40% (A, B) in average American men. Clinical disease can develop in up to 10% of men but estimates do not exceed this value (D).

228. **Correct: D. prostatectomy.**

The PSA test to detect prostate cancer has significant limitations, particularly that other conditions can cause elevations in PSA. However, a prostatectomy, or removal of the prostate, will actually cause low levels of PSA, not elevated levels (D).

Incorrect:

Conditions or procedures that can lead to an elevated PSA level include prostatitis (A) or immediately following cystoscopy (B). PSA levels can also remain chronically elevated among men with BPH (C).

229. **Correct: B. 2**

Prostate cancer is the second leading cause of male cancer death in the United States, only trailing lung cancer (B). It is the leading cause of gender-related cancer death in men.

Musculoskeletal Disorders

10

Bursitis

Overview

The human body contains more than 150 bursae. These fluid-filled sacs act as a cushion between tendons and bones.

> **CLINICAL CONCEPT**
>
> Bursitis develops when the synovial tissue that lines the sac becomes thickened and produces excessive fluid, leading to swelling and resulting pain.

The bursae are lined by synovial tissue, which produces fluid that lubricates and reduces friction between these structures. The most commonly affected bursae are the subdeltoid, olecranon, ischial, trochanter, and prepatellar. Risk factors for acute bursitis include joint overuse, trauma, infection, or arthritis conditions such as rheumatoid arthritis (RA) or osteoarthritis (OA).

Clinical Presentation

In contrast to most forms of arthritis, where the discomfort is often long term and more gradual in onset, bursitis typically presents with an abrupt onset with focal tenderness and swelling. The joint range of motion (ROM) is usually intact but is often limited by pain. The specific risk factors and presentation of bursitis by its location are outlined in Table 10-1 and Figure 10-1. Other conditions to consider when making the differential diagnosis include cellulitis, gout and pseudogout, RA, soft tissue knee injury, and tendonitis.

Diagnostic Testing

The diagnosis of bursitis is usually made clinically by risk factors, history, and physical examination. Laboratory studies are typically not helpful except in cases of septic bursitis where elevations in erythrocyte sedimentation rate (ESR)

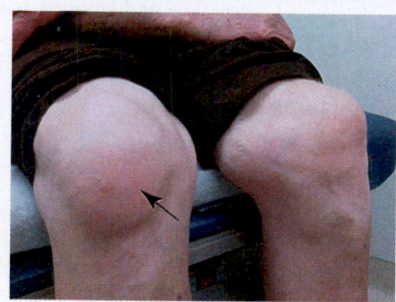

FIGURE 10-1 Prepatellar bursitis.
Venes D. Taber's Cyclopedic Medical Dictionary. 23rd ed. Philadelphia, PA: F.A. Davis; 2017.

and white blood cell (WBC) count can be observed. Imaging is usually not needed for a diagnosis but can be used to rule out other conditions. If diagnosis is unclear, magnetic resonance imaging (MRI) can be used to rule out tumor or other mass, while plain x-ray can detect osteophytes or possible fractures. Ultrasonography can help differentiate solid versus cystic masses and is used to help guide procedures. If septic bursitis is suspected, joint aspiration of fluid should be performed for cell culture. This procedure can also be therapeutic in bursitis.

Treatment

With prepatellar bursitis, bursal aspiration should be considered as a first-line therapy because this procedure affords significant pain relief and allows the bursa to reapproximate. Ultrasonography can be used to help guide injections in bursa. In other sites, first-line therapy includes minimizing or eliminating the offending activity, applying ice to the affected area for 15 minutes at least four times per day, elevating, and taking NSAIDs. If these conservative measures have not worked after approximately 4 to 8 weeks, intrabursal corticosteroid injection should be performed. Before injection, patients should be informed of the risks of this procedure, especially the most common problem, soreness at the injection site. After intrabursal corticosteroid injection, infection, tissue atrophy, and inflammatory reaction are possible, but

TABLE 10-1 Clinical Presentation of Bursitis

LOCATION OF BURSITIS	CLINICAL PRESENTATION	COMMENTS
Prepatellar (knee)	Knee swelling and pain in the front of the knee, normal ROM	Risk factors include frequent kneeling (also known as housemaid's knee). Bursal aspiration offers most effective relief.
Olecranon (elbow)	Pain, swelling behind the elbow, swelling in same area, often described as ball or sac hanging from the elbow	Risk factors include prolonged pressure or trauma to the elbow (also known as draftsman's elbow).
Trochanter (hip)	Gait disturbance, local trochanter tenderness, pain on hip rotation, and resisted hip abduction with normal hip ROM	Risk factors include back disease, leg-length discrepancy, and leg problems that lead to altered gait. OA seldom implicated.
Subscapular (shoulder)	Local tenderness under superomedial angle of the scapula over the adjacent rib, normal shoulder ROM, no nerve root impingement	Risk factors include repeated back-and-forth motion. Common in assembly-line workers.
Pre-Achilles (heel)	Pain and localized swelling behind the heel, minimal pain with dorsiflexion, normal ankle ROM	Usually not disabling and does not contribute to tendon rupture. Often confused with Achilles tendinitis
Retrocalcaneal (heel)	Pain behind ankle worsened by walking. Patient often runs fingers along both sides of Achilles tendon	Risk factors include wearing high-heeled shoes and repetitive ankle motion such as stair-climbing, running, jogging, and walking

OA, osteoarthritis; ROM, range of motion.

Sources: Anderson B. Office Orthopedics for Primary Care: Diagnosis. Philadelphia, PA: Saunders; 2006; Anderson B. Office Orthopedics for Primary Care: Treatment. 3rd ed. Philadelphia, PA: Saunders; 2006.

rarely encountered, complications. For those suspected of septic bursitis, antimicrobial therapy should be initiated while awaiting culture results.

Discussion Sources

Khodaee M. Common superficial bursitis. *Am Fam Physician*. 2017;95:224–231.

Lohr KM, Talbott-Stern JK, Gonsalves A, Root L. Bursitis. Medscape. http://emedicine.medscape.com/article/2145588

QUESTIONS

1. The most common cause of acute bursitis is:

   A. inactivity.

   B. joint overuse.

   C. fibromyalgia.

   D. bacterial infection.

2. A 42-year-old man presents with complaints of sudden-onset swelling and severe pain in both knees. He reports that he went for a run the day before for the first time in "a long while." Suspecting bursitis, a first-line treatment option would include:

   A. corticosteroid bursal injection.

   B. heat to area.

   C. weight-bearing exercises.

   D. oral NSAIDs.

3. Patients with olecranon bursitis typically present with:
   A. swelling and redness over the affected area.
   B. limited elbow ROM.
   C. nerve impingement.
   D. destruction of the joint space.

4. Patients with subscapular bursitis typically present with:
   A. limited shoulder ROM.
   B. heat over affected area.
   C. localized tenderness under the superomedial angle of the scapula.
   D. cervical nerve root irritation.

5. Patients with gluteus medius or deep trochanteric bursitis typically present with:
   A. increased pain from resisted hip abduction.
   B. limited hip ROM.
   C. sciatic nerve pain.
   D. heat over the affected area.

6. When diagnosing bursitis, a plain radiograph is most useful in:
   A. detecting septic bursitis.
   B. identifying the presence of osteophytes.
   C. detecting uric acid crystals in bursal fluid.
   D. guiding the injection site for aspiration.

7. When diagnosing bursitis, MRI is most useful in:
   A. detecting the presence of RA.
   B. guiding the site for corticosteroid injection.
   C. ruling out suspected solid tumors.
   D. detecting possible fracture at the joint.

8. Likely sequelae of intrabursal corticosteroid injection include:
   A. irreversible skin atrophy.
   B. infection.
   C. inflammatory reaction.
   D. soreness at the site of injection.

9. One of the most effective therapies for prepatellar bursitis is:
   A. bursal aspiration.
   B. application of a topical analgesic to the affected area.
   C. acetaminophen use.
   D. knee splinting.

10. When making a diagnosis of bursitis, other similar conditions to consider in the differential diagnosis include all of the following except:
    A. RA.
    B. tendonitis.
    C. osteoporosis.
    D. pseudogout.

For answers and rationales, see end of chapter.

Tendonitis, Tendinopathy, and Tendinosis

Overview

Tendon injury (tendinopathy) is most commonly caused by either inflammation of the tendon (tendinitis) or degradation of the tendon's collagen in response to chronic overuse (tendinosis). There is often confusion when trying to differentiate between tendonitis and tendinosis, and many injuries believed to be due to tendinitis are actually tendinosis. Recognizing the differences between the two types of injuries is important in setting healing timelines and treatment goals.

The most common sites for tendonitis are the rotator cuff, elbow, biceps (shoulder), wrist, and heel. In most cases, a microscopic tear causes tendon inflammation; the resulting swelling and inflammation in the tendon are a result of overuse. The clinical presentation usually includes a report of reduced ROM caused by joint stiffness and discomfort and a dull, aching pain over the affected tendon, especially with joint use. This pain can become sharp and acute when the tendon is squeezed.

Clinical Presentation

Rotator cuff tendonitis is often associated with repetitive overhead activities, such as throwing, raking, or washing cars or windows, or it can be the result of injury. Symptoms include a dull pain radiating from the outer arm to several inches below the top of the shoulder. With rotator cuff involvement, abduction and elevation of the shoulder joint worsen symptoms.

> **CLINICAL CONCEPT**
>
> A clicking in the shoulder can occur when raising the arm above the head in rotator cuff tendinopathy.

In the elbow region, tendonitis can occur as either biceps tendinitis or triceps tendinitis. Biceps tendonitis occurs through repetitive overhead activity, including throwing a baseball, swimming, or playing tennis or golf (see also the section on Epicondylitis, this chapter). Symptoms include pain when the arm is overhead or bent and localized tenderness where the tendon passes over the groove in the upper arm bone.

Wrist tendonitis, or tenosynovitis, typically occurs at points where the tendons cross each other or pass over a bony prominence. The condition is caused by overuse, such as repetitive motions during sports or work-related activities (e.g., writing, typing, and assembly-line work). Wrist tendonitis is associated with pain over the area of inflammation with swelling of the surrounding soft tissue. Reduced ROM and muscle weakness are also common.

Diagnostic Testing

With initial presentation, the diagnosis of tendonitis is usually straightforward, with no special studies required. If these signs and symptoms occur with a history of recent trauma, plain radiographic films of the affected area occasionally reveal calcium deposits on the tendon. Because bursitis and tendonitis often occur concurrently, assessment often reveals both conditions. MRI is generally not recommended for routine diagnosis of tendonitis. However, if there is a question about accompanying soft tissue injury or suspected tendon tear, or for chronic tendonitis sufferers even after rehabilitation, MRI can be helpful in detecting damage to the tendon.

Treatment

Treatment of tendonitis includes limiting or discontinuing the contributing activity. Applying ice to the region is helpful. NSAIDs can be used to reduce pain. When the hand or wrist is affected, splinting can be beneficial. Achilles tendonitis often necessitates treatment with a posterior splint to immobilize the heel, and heel cord stretching and orthotics after the acute phase to prevent recurrence. There is a 10% risk of tendon rupture with recurrent Achilles tendonitis; the risk can exceed 12% with biceps tendonitis. With rotator cuff involvement, the likelihood of concurrent bursitis is high; treatment includes limiting overhead movement and intrabursal corticosteroid injection.

Healing time for tendinitis can range from several days to 6 weeks, whereas healing of tendinosis is generally longer (6 to 10 weeks if caught at an early stage, and up to 9 months if chronic). Use of NSAIDs (e.g., ibuprofen) or corticosteroid injections, though helpful in tendinitis, can actually inhibit collagen repair needed to heal tendinosis. Physical therapy can be helpful in strengthening muscles around the injury or performing muscle-stimulating techniques to improve healing. Extracorporeal shock-wave therapy (ESWT) can also be considered for tendinosis, which uses sound waves to create microtrauma to the tendon that promotes the body's natural healing process.

Discussion Sources

Anderson B. *Office Orthopedics for Primary Care: Diagnosis.* Philadelphia, PA: Saunders Elsevier; 2006.

Anderson B. *Office Orthopedics for Primary Care: Treatment.* 3rd ed. Philadelphia, PA: Saunders Elsevier; 2006.

Bass E. Tendinopathy: why the difference between tendinitis and tendinosis matters. *Int J Ther Massage Bodywork.* 2012;5:14–17. http://www.ncbi.nlm.nih.gov/pmc/articles/PMC3312643/

Turner S. Musculoskeletal system. In: Goolsby M, Grubbs L, eds. *Advanced Assessment: Interpreting Findings and Formulating Differential Diagnoses.* 4th ed. Philadelphia, PA: F.A. Davis; 2018:435–476.

QUESTIONS

11. Which of the following statements about tendonitis is false?

    A. Tendonitis is typically the result of overuse.

    B. Tendonitis is the result of a macroscopic or partial tear of the tendon.

    C. Acute pain results when firm pressure is applied to the tendon.

    D. Signs of tendonitis include reduced ROM caused by stiffness and discomfort.

12. Activities that commonly contribute to the development of rotator cuff tendonitis include all of the following except:

    A. swimming.

    B. throwing a football.

    C. bowling.

    D. pitching a baseball.

13 to 18. Indicate (*Yes or No*) which of the following are common symptoms of wrist tendonitis.

    _____ 13. Muscle cramping

    _____ 14. Reduced ROM

    _____ 15. Swelling of the wrist

    _____ 16. Pain radiating to the shoulder

    _____ 17. Muscle weakness

    _____ 18. Dupuytren's contracture

19. With initial presentation, the diagnosis of tendonitis is usually made from:

    A. clinical presentation.

    B. plain radiographic films.

    C. a computed tomography (CT) scan of the area.

    D. a laboratory diagnosis.

20. Complications of Achilles tendonitis include:

    A. tendon rupture.

    B. neurological sequelae.

    C. stress fracture.

    D. bursitis.

21. Which of the following is often found with rotator cuff tendonitis?

    A. OA

    B. tendon rupture

    C. bursitis

    D. arm numbness

22. First-line therapy for biceps tendonitis usually includes:

    A. applying ice to the area.

    B. local corticosteroid injection.

    C. orthopedic referral.

    D. nerve block.

23. A 36-year-old man has experienced shoulder pain associated with tendonitis for the past 4 weeks despite the use of ice and analgesics (NSAIDs) and undergoing physical therapy. An appropriate next step would include:

    A. systemic corticosteroid use.

    B. x-ray of the shoulder.

    C. MRI of the shoulder.

    D. use of an upper arm sling.

24. Which of the following approaches is aimed at improving the healing process in tendinosis?

    A. corticosteroid injection

    B. oral NSAIDs

    C. adalimumab

    D. ESWT

For answers and rationales, see end of chapter.

Epicondylitis

Overview

Epicondylitis is a term used to describe a painful inflammation of a tendon surrounding an epicondyle, or protuberance above or on the condyle of a long bone, especially at the elbow end of the humerus. One contributing factor to tendinosis development is the relative avascularity of the tendon proximal to its insertion site.

    Epicondylitis that arises as a result of injury to the extensor tendon at the lateral epicondyle is called tennis elbow or lateral epicondylitis. Medial epicondylitis, often called golfer's elbow, is similar to lateral epicondylitis but occurs on the inside of the elbow. Differentiating between the two types of injuries is important in setting timelines and treatment goals.

Clinical Presentation

With either tennis elbow or golfer's elbow, the history includes the triggering activity plus select health history and physical examination findings. With either condition, the elbow of the dominant arm is affected at least 75% of the time.

- *Tennis elbow*: Most commonly found in people in their 30s to 50s, and the majority are not caused by playing tennis but rather another repetitive activity. The patient complains of pain over the lateral epicondyle or outer aspect of the lower humerus. This pain increases with resisted wrist extension, particularly when lifting an object in front of the person, especially with the elbow. Tenderness to palpation over the lateral epicondyle is present and a hallmark of the condition, but the area is usually without increased heat or redness. With the elbow in extension, the patient will complain of pain. Elbow ROM usually is normal.
- *Golfer's elbow*: Most commonly found in people in their 30s to 50s, usually without a history of trauma, and most do not play golf. The condition is associated with racquet sports as well as bowling, archery, and weight lifting. The patient complains of pain over the medial epicondyle or inner aspect of the lower humerus. Presentation includes local epicondylar tenderness, elbow pain, wrist and forearm weakness, pain aggravated by wrist flexion, and pronation activities with decreased grip strength and full ROM. Pain worsens with gripping activities and is localized to the medial aspect of the elbow.

Other conditions to consider when making the differential diagnosis for tennis elbow include radial tunnel syndrome, fractures (associated with trauma), growth plate injuries, or cartilage or bone lesions. Conditions similar to golfer's elbow include cubital tunnel syndrome, medial collateral ligament injury, fractures, growth plate injury, and bone lesions.

Diagnostic Testing

The diagnosis is made clinically, though radiograph of the elbow is done to rule out fracture. Tendon calcification is often noted on plain film. Advanced imaging such as MRI is not warranted unless there is no or limited response to therapy and another diagnosis needs to be considered. MRI can determine if tendon tear is present. Ultrasound can also be used to determine intra-articular pathology if MRI cannot be done.

Treatment

Healing time for a simple tendinitis can range from several days to 6 weeks, whereas healing of tendinosis is generally longer (6 to 10 weeks if caught at an early stage, and up to 9 months if chronic or present for many months). Topical or oral NSAIDs as well as corticosteroids can provide short-term pain relief (up to 4 weeks). Though use of these agents can be helpful in tendinitis, they can actually inhibit collagen repair needed to heal tendinosis. Rest, applying ice (15 to 20 minutes several times per day), and avoidance of the precipitating activity for up to several weeks is the first course of treatment. For sports-related injuries, con-ducting an equipment check and working with an expert on proper form can reduce the risk of aggravating the injury. Physical therapy can be helpful in strengthening muscles in the arm or performing muscle-stimulating techniques to improve healing. Physical therapy can include the use of ultrasound and ionto-phoresis with a steroid cream, which involves applying a topical steroid and then using a mild electric charge to drive the steroids into the tendon. If these first-line approaches offer no improvement after 6 weeks, then steroid injection at the site of maximal tenderness can be considered. This can provide acute improvement in symptoms but does not affect long-term outcomes.

For lateral epicondylitis, a counterforce brace centered over the back of the forearm can help relieve symptoms. In medial epicondylitis, counterforce bracing during activ-ities can be useful, and cock-up wrist splints can be considered for those who awaken with elbow pain. Vasodilators, such as nitroglycerin patches, and platelet-rich plasma have also been studied with mixed results.

Approximately 80% to 95% of patients with epicondylitis can be successfully treated without surgery. Efforts for prevention of both tennis and golfer's elbow recurrence include using palm-up lifting, minimizing precipitating causes, ensuring proper use of tools, using proper body mechanics, and developing flexibility and strength of the involved musculature.

> **CLINICAL CONCEPT**
>
> ESWT can also be considered, which uses sound waves to create microtrauma to the elbow that promotes the body's natural healing process.

Discussion Sources

Bass E. Tendinopathy: why the difference between tendinitis and tendinosis matters. *Int J Ther Massage Bodywork*. 2012;5:14–17. http://www.ncbi.nlm.nih.gov/pmc/articles/PMC3312643/

Walrod BJ. Lateral epicondylitis. Medscape. http://emedicine.medscape.com/article/96969-overview

QUESTIONS

25. Patients with lateral epicondylitis typically present with:
    A. electric-like pain elicited by tapping over the median nerve.
    B. reduced joint ROM.
    C. pain that is worst with elbow flexion.
    D. decreased hand grip strength.

26. Risk factors for lateral epicondylitis include all of the following except:
    A. repetitive lifting.
    B. playing tennis.
    C. hammering.
    D. gout.

27. Up to what percentage of patients with medial or lateral epicondylitis recover without surgery?
    A. 35%
    B. 50%
    C. 70%
    D. 95%

28 to 30. Match each imaging technique with its most appropriate role in the diagnosis of epicondylitis.
    _____ 28. Plain radiograph
    _____ 29. MRI
    _____ 30. Ultrasonography
        A. an option when MRI is not appropriate
        B. to assess for tendon tear
        C. to assess for fracture

31. Initial treatment of lateral epicondylitis includes all of the following except:

  A. rest and activity modifications.

  B. corticosteroid injections.

  C. topical or oral NSAIDs.

  D. counterforce bracing.

32. ESWT can be used in the treatment of epicondylitis as a means to:

  A. improve ROM.

  B. build forearm strength.

  C. promote the natural healing process.

  D. stretch the extensor tendon.

33. Patients with medial epicondylitis typically present with:

  A. forearm numbness.

  B. reduction in ROM.

  C. pain on elbow flexion.

  D. decreased grip strength.

34. Risk factors for medial epicondylitis include participating in all of the following except:

  A. soccer.

  B. golf.

  C. archery.

  D. weight lifting.

For answers and rationales, see end of chapter.

Gouty Arthritis (Gout)

Overview

Gouty arthritis, often simply called gout, manifests as acute monoarticular arthritis, usually triggered by a disorder causing a decrease of uric acid excretion that allows an accumulation of urates in joints, bones, and subcutaneous tissues. Urate precipitates out of biological fluids when levels are elevated, a condition that usually follows the inability of the kidney to eliminate uric acid.

Gout risk factors include obesity, diabetes mellitus, and a family history of the condition. Less often, acute gout is caused by excessive uric acid production, usually coupled with decreased urate excretion. The use of select medications, including thiazide diuretics, niacin, aspirin, and cyclosporine, can precipitate gout by causing hyperuricemia; alcohol use is also a possible precipitant, usually in a person who has other risk factors. Other causes of secondary gout include conditions characterized by increased catabolism and purine turnover, such as psoriasis (possibly due to the inflammatory process), myeloproliferative and lymphoproliferative diseases, and chronic hemolytic anemia, and conditions with decreased renal uric acid clearance, such as chronic kidney disease.

> **CLINICAL CONCEPT**
>
> About 90% of patients presenting with primary gout are men; the condition is rarely seen in women before menopause.

Clinical Presentation

Gout is an acutely painful condition that most often affects the metacarpophalangeal joint of the great toe. Less common locations include the instep of the foot, wrist, finger joints, and knee. The onset is sudden and is accompanied by significant distress. Although the disease manifests acutely, the metabolic disorder behind the problem is typically present for months to years before the clinical presentation.

When the base of the great toe is affected, the patient reports the inability to walk, move the joint, or even tolerate the weight of a bed sheet on the affected joint because of severe pain. The entire great toe is usually reddened and enlarged, with the greatest amount of swelling noted along the medial border of the joint; this usually is also the point of greatest discomfort. Although the clinical presentation of gout can mimic that of an acutely infected joint, gout is 100 times more common than monoarticular septic arthritis (Fig. 10-2).

With repeated episodes, nontender firm nodules known as tophi can develop in soft tissue. Because the gouty crystals that fill tophi precipitate more easily in cooler areas of the body, these lesions often develop in the external ear; less common locations include nasal cartilage, extensor surfaces of the hands and feet, and over the elbows.

Diagnostic Testing

The diagnosis of acute gouty arthritis is usually done clinically, particularly with repeated episodes. With the first episode, an initial uric acid level is obtained in most cases but is usually normal. Uric acid levels are often reduced during the acute phase, or the etiology of the attack is largely poor urate excretion. Analysis of joint aspirate for urate crystals is diagnostic; monosodium urate crystals appear as needle-shaped intracellular and extracellular crystals. Joint fluid should also be analyzed for complete blood count (CBC) with differential, Gram stain, and culture to rule out septic arthritis. The ESR or C-reactive protein (CRP) is usually high, but these findings are neither sensitive nor specific for gout and simply reflect the inflammation associated with the condition. Radiographs of the affected joint should be performed, though this is not diagnostic. Radiographs are usually normal in early disease (first year of onset), while punched out erosions with overhanging edges are observed in later disease.

After the acute flare has subsided, a 24-hour urine collection for uric acid helps assess whether the patient overproduces or undersecretes uric acid. Long-term care to avoid future attacks is directed by the result; undersecretors benefit from probenecid, and overproducers benefit from allopurinol or febuxostat. Other medications not specifically designated for gout treatment, including fenofibrate and losartan, have been studied and found to be helpful with urate excretion and can be used as therapeutic adjuncts as part of a comprehensive uric acid–lowering strategy.

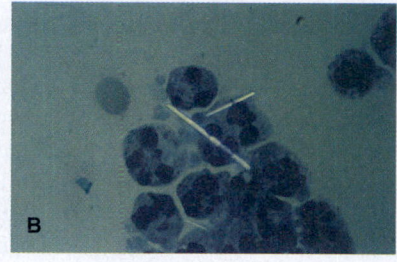

FIGURE 10-2 (A, B) Gout.
Venes D. Taber's Cyclopedic Medical Dictionary. 23rd ed. Philadelphia, PA: F.A. Davis; 2017; Strasinger S, DiLorenzo M. Urinalysis and Body Fluids. 3rd ed. Philadelphia, PA: F.A. Davis; 1994.

Treatment

The treatment of acute gouty arthritis should include minimizing or removing contributing factors, such as alcohol use or use of certain medications. Treatment should be aimed at reducing inflammation first and then treating hyperuricemia. A rapid reduction in serum uric acid can make the gouty episode worse and so should be avoided. A loading dose of an NSAID, such as 750 mg of naproxen followed by lower doses, can be helpful.

Colchicine, once the treatment of choice, is now less commonly used because it is often poorly tolerated, as therapeutic doses often lead to significant gastrointestinal (GI) symptoms. A short course of a systemic corticosteroid, such as oral prednisone (0.5 mg/kg/day for 5 to 10 days, or 0.5 mg/kg/day for 2 to 5 days, then taper for 7 to 10 days), is a helpful alternative to colchicine. Local injection with corticosteroids can provide significant relief and offers a treatment alternative to NSAIDs, particularly in the presence of warfarin use, advanced renal failure, or peptic ulcer disease. Anakinra (Kineret®), an interleukin-1 (IL-1) receptor antagonist, has also been used with favorable results in acute gout when other treatment options are not possible due to comorbidities.

Several medications are available to prevent gout attacks by blocking uric acid production or improving uric acid removal. Prior to using these medications, treatment with an NSAID or colchicine for at least 6 months is needed to prevent precipitating an acute gouty attack due to changes in tissue uric acid level. Xanthine oxidase inhibitors (XOIs), including allopurinol (Aloprim®, Lopurin®, Zyloprim®) or febuxostat (Uloric®), limit the amount of uric acid the body produces. Common adverse effects of allopurinol include rash and low blood counts, whereas febuxostat is associated with rash, nausea, and reduced liver function. Lesinurad (Zurampic®), a selective uric acid reabsorption inhibitor, can be used in combination with an XOI for those who do not achieve target levels of serum uric acid. Probenecid (Probalan®) improves the kidney's ability to remove uric acid from the body. Probenecid use leads to higher concentrations of uric acid in the urine, resulting in a greater risk of kidney stones. Other adverse effects include rash and abdominal pain.

For patients with chronic gout that is refractory to other medications, pegloticase (Krystexxa®) is an option. Pegloticase contains a uric acid–specific enzyme that catalyzes the oxidation of uric acid to allantoin,

CLINICAL CONCEPT
Because aspirin use can precipitate gout, its use in the presence of the condition is contraindicated.

which is an inert water-soluble metabolite that is readily eliminated from the body, thereby reducing serum uric acid. Pegloticase is administered via IV infusion every 2 weeks. There are warnings on its use regarding anaphylaxis and infusion reactions, as well as congestive heart failure (CHF) exacerbation. Gout flare prophylaxis is recommended for at least 6 months, though this can be extended depending on patient findings, such as the presence of tophi. The use of chronic therapy is somewhat controversial. The American College of Rheumatology (ACR) recommends that once all tophi have resolved along with acute and chronic gout symptoms, serum uric acid levels should be maintained below 6 mg/dL indefinitely. Levels should be monitored at 6-month intervals to guide the use or adjustment of pharmacological therapy.

Dietary modification to avoid foods with high purine content is an important and often overlooked intervention to minimize the risk of future gout episodes. Some high-purine foods to be avoided in gout include certain seafood (scallops, mussels), organ and game meats, beans, spinach, asparagus, oatmeal, and baker's and brewer's yeasts when taken as dietary supplements.

Pseudogout, also called calcium pyrophosphate deposition (CPPD) disease, presents similarly to gout but is caused by the presence of calcium pyrophosphate dehydrate crystals in the joint. The knees are most commonly affected, but the wrists and ankles also can be involved, with symptoms of swollen, warm, and severely painful joints. Risk factors include older age, joint trauma, family history of the condition, and mineral imbalances (e.g., hemochromatosis, hypercalcemia, or hypomagnesemia). Pseudogout has also been associated with hypothyroidism or hyperparathyroidism.

Proper diagnosis of pseudogout involves detecting calcium pyrophosphate crystals in the affected joint. Blood tests can detect abnormal thyroid or parathyroid function and abnormal mineral levels linked to pseudogout. The goal of treatment is primarily to relieve pain and improve joint function and includes the use of NSAIDs, colchicine, and oral corticosteroids.

Discussion Sources

Cassagnol M, Saad M. Pharmacologic management of gout. *US Pharmacist.* 2013;38:22–26. https://www.uspharmacist.com/article/pharmacologic-management-of-gout

Khanna D, Fitzgerald JD, Khanna PP, et al. 2012 American College of Rheumatology guidelines for management of gout. Part 1: systematic nonpharmacologic and pharmacologic therapeutic approaches to hyperuricemia. *Arthritis Care Res (Hoboken).* 2012;64:1431–1446.

Qaseem A, Harris RP, Forciea MA, et al. Management of acute and recurrent gout: a clinical practice guideline from the American College of Physicians. *Ann Intern Med.* 2017;166:58–68.

QUESTIONS

35. Risk factors for acute gouty arthritis include:

  A. obesity.

  B. female gender.

  C. RA.

  D. joint trauma.

36. The use of all of the following medications can trigger gout except:

  A. aspirin.

  B. statins.

  C. thiazide diuretics.

  D. cyclosporine.

37. Secondary gout can be caused by all of the following conditions except:

  A. psoriasis.

  B. hemolytic anemia.

  C. bacterial cellulitis.

  D. chronic kidney disease.

38. The clinical presentation of acute gouty arthritis affecting the base of the great toe includes:

  A. slow onset of discomfort over many days.

  B. greatest swelling and pain along the median aspect of the joint.

C. improvement of symptoms with joint rest.

D. fever.

39. The most helpful diagnostic test to perform during acute gouty arthritis is:

A. measurement of ESR.

B. measurement of serum uric acid.

C. analysis of aspirate from the affected joint.

D. joint radiography.

40. First-line therapy for treating patients with acute gouty arthritis usually includes the use of oral:

A. aspirin.

B. naproxen sodium.

C. allopurinol.

D. febuxostat.

41. Tophi are best described as:

A. ulcerations originating on swollen joints.

B. swollen lymph nodes.

C. abscesses with one or more openings draining pus onto the skin.

D. nontender, firm nodules located in soft tissue.

42. Which of the following patients with acute gouty arthritis is the best candidate for local intra-articular corticosteroid injection?

A. a 66-year-old patient with a gastric ulcer

B. a 44-year-old patient taking a thiazide diuretic

C. a 68-year-old patient with type 2 diabetes mellitus

D. a 32-year-old patient who is a binge drinker

43. The most common locations for tophi include all of the following except:

A. the auricles.

B. the elbows.

C. the extensor surfaces of the hands.

D. the shoulders.

44. Which of the following foods is least likely to trigger acute gouty arthritis?

A. mussels

B. beef liver

C. hard cheese

D. spinach

45 to 47. Indicate whether each medication is used for prevention (P) or treatment (T) of gout.

_____ 45. Probenecid

_____ 46. Colchicine

_____ 47. Allopurinol (Aloprim®)

48. Pegloticase (Krystexxa®) reduces serum uric acid levels by:

A. reducing the production of urea.

B. converting uric acid to an inert water-soluble metabolite that is readily eliminated from the body.

C. blocking conversion of urea to uric acid.

D. binding to uric acid and facilitating elimination through the GI system.

49. Which of the following dietary supplements is associated with increased risk for gout?

   A. vitamin A

   B. gingko biloba

   C. brewer's yeast

   D. glucosamine

50. A 62-year-old man is diagnosed with acute gout and initiated on oral NSAID treatment. Gout prophylaxis therapy should begin:

   A. immediately.

   B. in 1 month.

   C. in 6 months.

   D. when signs of a subsequent gouty attack begin.

51. A 57-year-old woman with a history of recurrent gout is being treated with probenecid. She is currently without symptoms, and all tophi have resolved. The nurse practitioner (NP) recommends:

   A. discontinuing probenecid treatment immediately.

   B. switching from probenecid to allopurinol.

   C. testing uric acid levels every 6 months to determine treatment course.

   D. continuing probenecid treatment indefinitely.

52. Pseudogout is caused by the formation of what type of crystals in joints?

   A. uric acid

   B. calcium oxalate

   C. struvite

   D. calcium pyrophosphate dihydrate

53. The most common location for pseudogout is:

   A. neck.

   B. big toe.

   C. knee.

   D. low back.

54. Pseudogout has been linked with abnormal activity of the:

   A. liver.

   B. kidneys.

   C. parathyroid.

   D. adrenal gland.

55. Differentiation between gout and pseudogout can involve all of the following diagnostic approaches except:

   A. analysis of minerals in the blood.

   B. analysis of joint fluid.

   C. x-ray of the affected joint.

   D. measuring thyroid function.

56 to 59. Indicate (*Yes or No*) if the following can be used in the treatment of pseudogout.

_____ 56. NSAIDs

_____ 57. Colchicine

_____ **58.** Allopurinol

_____ **59.** Oral corticosteroids

For answers and rationales, see end of chapter.

Osteoarthritis

Overview

OA is the most common joint disease in North America. It is a condition that usually manifests without systemic manifestations or acute inflammation. In OA, the articular cartilage becomes rough and wears away. Bone spurs often form, and the synovial membrane thickens. Consequently, the joint space narrows. Although the distal interphalangeal joint is the most common OA site, the most problematic joint involvement is in the hip and knee.

Risk factors for OA include a positive family history of the condition and contact sport participation. Obesity is likely the most common personal risk factor, especially with hip and knee OA involvement.

Clinical Presentation

The clinical presentation in patients with OA includes an insidious onset of symptoms, including use-related joint pain that is relieved by rest and joint stiffness that occurs with rest but resolves with less than 15 minutes of activity. A reduced ROM with crepitus is often found. Physical examination usually reveals smooth, cool joints, and symptoms worsen with joint use.

Particularly when the knee is affected, joint effusion is common and can be minimal to severe with up to 20 mL of fluid. Patients cannot achieve full knee flexion in the effused joint; physical examination usually reveals smooth, cool joints, and coarse crepitus. The knee often locks, or a pop is heard, which suggests a degenerative meniscal tear.

OA of the hip is associated with hip pain that develops gradually over time or can have a sudden onset. Pain and stiffness of the joint can develop with rest that resolves with movement. As the disease progresses, pain and stiffness occurs more frequently, even with rest and at night. Locking of the joint and crepitus can interfere with smooth hip motion, and decreased ROM can affect the ability to walk or impact gait.

OA of the hand most often affects the distal interphalangeal (DIP) joints but can also affect the proximal interphalangeal (PIP) joints. Among elderly patients with OA of the hand, palpable osteophytes, called Heberden's nodes, are found in the DIP joints. Similarly, Bouchard's nodes are deformities located in the PIP joints in elderly patients.

Diagnostic Testing

X-rays of the affected joint(s) are usually done to help confirm the diagnosis. Radiological findings in patients with OA include narrowing of the joint space and increased density of subchondral bone. Bone cysts and osteophytes are often present, developed as part of the body's repair process; however, only about 50% of patients with radiological findings have symptoms (Fig. 10-3). In many cases, an x-ray is performed for another reason, such as trauma, only to reveal the presence of OA without manifestation of symptoms. Because OA is typically without systemic inflammation, ESR and CRP levels, both markers of inflammation, are typically normal. In contrast to RA and systemic lupus erythematosus (SLE), antinuclear antibodies (ANAs), rheumatoid factor (RF), and other markers of systemic arthritis syndromes are absent from the serum unless there is concomitant disease.

Treatment

Therapeutic goals for patients with OA include preventing further articular cartilage destruction, minimizing pain, and enhancing mobility. Therapies for symptom control include lifestyle modifications, such as weight loss in overweight and obesity,

> **CLINICAL CONCEPT**
> With OA, discomfort typically increases as the day progresses, and there is minimal morning stiffness; in contrast, with RA, morning stiffness is usually most problematic.

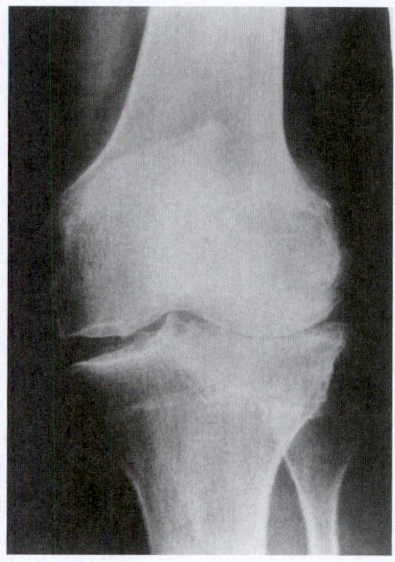

FIGURE 10-3 Osteoarthritis.
Blessing JD. Clinical Problem Solving for Physician Assistants. Philadelphia, PA: F.A. Davis; 2002

TABLE 10-2 Exercise Regimens in Osteoarthritis

JOINT CONDITION	EXERCISE REGIMEN	COMMENTS
Osteoarthritis in the knee	■ Straight-leg raises without weights, advance to using weights as tolerated ■ Quadriceps sets ■ Non-weight-bearing or limited weight-bearing aerobic activity	Avoid squatting and kneeling, high-impact exercise
Osteoarthritis of the hip	■ Straight-leg raises without weights, advance to using weights as tolerated ■ Stretching exercises of adductors, rotator, and gluteus muscles ■ Isometric exercises of iliopsoas and gluteus muscles ■ Non-weight-bearing or limited weight-bearing aerobic activity	Avoid high-impact exercise

exercise with minimal weight-bearing, such as swimming or water-based activities, and physical activity to maintain joint flexibility and enhance strength in the surrounding muscles (Table 10-2). Application of heat to minimize pain and stiffness in the morning before activity can be helpful, and applying ice to the joint after activity can minimize discomfort; the use of heat or ice should be directed by patient response.

Although NSAIDs also have potential anti-inflammatory activity, this mechanism of drug action is seldom needed in OA therapy because inflammation is a minor contributor to symptoms. Because of the gastropathy potential associated with long-term use of NSAIDs, a trial of acetaminophen is warranted for symptom control in less severe cases of OA, recognizing that NSAIDs are usually associated with superior analgesic effect. If long-term use of NSAIDs is anticipated, a gastroprotective agent such as a proton pump inhibitor should be considered. NSAIDs have also been linked to increased risk of cardiovascular disease and so the lowest effective dose or intermittent dosing should be used. NSAIDs can increase mean arterial pressure by about 5 mm Hg with the greatest effect in the elderly and those with diabetes mellitus and chronic kidney disease. NSAIDs can also decrease the blood pressure-lowering effects of many antihypertensive agents, including diuretics, angiotensin-converting enzyme (ACE) inhibitors, angiotensin receptor blockers, and beta blockers. As an alternative, duloxetine (Cymbalta®) has been approved for the treatment of chronic musculoskeletal pain (including chronic pain due to OA).

Topical analgesics can be considered for superficial joints, such as the knee or hands, though these will not work for deeper joints, such as the hip. Capsaicin provides the most effective relief, though the agent must be used for at least 2 weeks before the full effects are realized.

Glucosamine, an amino acid, is usually used as first-line treatment for OA in many European nations and is available as an over-the-counter nutritional supplement in the United States. The results of research studies have differed on the effectiveness of its use, with many reporting no improvement in arthritis symptoms; others reporting a reduction in pain, increased joint flexion, and increased articular function; and some showing no clinical effect. Glucosamine must be used consistently for a minimum of 2 weeks and likely 3 months before any therapeutic effect is seen. Although no drug interactions or hepatotoxicity have been noted with its use, glucosamine should be used with caution because there is a risk of bronchospasm. Chondroitin is often used in conjunction with glucosamine because the two appear to have synergistic activity, although this has been disputed in limited studies. The mechanism of action of these products is not well understood. Although chondroitin is generally well tolerated, it should be used with caution because of a potential anticoagulant effect. As with all nutritional supplements, using a preparation that is supplied by a manufacturer with *United States Pharmacopeia* (USP) or other similar verification is advised.

Intra-articular corticosteroid joint injection is often recommended when conservative therapy has failed. The American Academy of Orthopaedic Surgeons (AAOS), however, does not recommend for or against the use of intra-articular corticosteroid injections because of a lack of compelling evidence comparing the benefits with the risks. AAOS also does not recommend using hyaluronic acid injections for treating symptomatic OA of the knee because of lack of efficacy observed in clinical trials.

Treatment of OA of the hip is similar to treating OA of the knee. Resting the hip, physical therapy to strengthen the muscles surrounding the hip, and decreasing body mass if overweight can be helpful. Oral analgesics with acetaminophen or NSAIDs can be used to control pain. Hip injection of corticosteroids is a technically challenging procedure that can be done with fluoroscopic guidance. In advanced stages of disease, arthroplasty can be considered in certain individuals.

Knee and hip joint replacement should be considered when pain cannot be adequately controlled, when function is severely compromised, or when more than 80% of the articular cartilage is worn away. The ideal candidate for joint replacement in OA is able to tolerate a surgical procedure that lasts for several hours, followed by an aggressive postoperative course of rehabilitation.

Joint replacement in the hand is becoming more common to reduce pain and restore joint motion. Joint replacement can involve the PIP, metacarpophalangeal joint, and wrist joints. Rehabilitation following joint replacement is critical to restore flexibility of the joint and strengthen muscles needed for normal functioning.

> **CLINICAL CONCEPT**
> Many patients with OA who have been debilitated by poor mobility have improved health when ambulation becomes possible after hip or knee replacement.

Discussion Sources

American Academy of Orthopaedic Surgeons. *Treatment of Osteoarthritis of the Knee: Evidence-Based Practice Guidelines, 2013.* 2nd ed. Rosemont, IL: American Academy of Orthopaedic Surgeons; 2013. https://www.aaos.org/globalassets/quality-and-practice-resources/osteoarthritis-of-the-knee/osteoarthritis-of-the-knee-2nd-editiion-clinical-practice-guideline.pdf

American Academy of Orthopaedic Surgeons. *Treatment of Osteoarthritis of the Hip: Evidence-Based Practice Guidelines, 2017.* 2nd ed. Rosemont, IL: American Academy of Orthopaedic Surgeons; 2017. https://aaos.org/globalassets/quality-and-practice-resources/osteoarthritis-of-the-hip/oa-hip-cpg_6-11-19.pdf

Lespasio MJ, Sultan AA, Piuzzi NS, et al. Hip osteoarthritis: a primer. *Perm J.* 2018;22:17-084. https://www.ncbi.nlm.nih.gov/pmc/articles/PMC5760056/pdf/17-084.pdf

National Center for Complementary and Integrative Health. Glucosamine/Chondroitin Arthritis Intervention Trial (GAIT). https://files.nccih.nih.gov/s3fs-public/Glucosamine_and_Chondroitin_11-12-2015.pdf

QUESTIONS

60. Which of the following joints is most likely to be affected by OA?
    A. wrists
    B. elbows
    C. metacarpophalangeal joint
    D. DIP joint

61. Changes to the joint during OA can typically include all of the following except:
    A. widening of the joint space.
    B. wearing away of articular cartilage.
    C. formation of bone spurs.
    D. synovial membrane thickening.

62. Clinical findings of the knee in a patient with OA include which of the following? Choose all that apply.
    A. coarse crepitus
    B. joint effusion
    C. warm joint
    D. knee often locks or a pop is heard
    E. redness and heat over the anterior and posterior knee

63. Radiographic findings of OA of the knee in a 65-year-old man with obesity who has a 10-year history of knee pain would be anticipated to reveal:
    A. microfractures.
    B. decreased density of subchondral bone.
    C. osteophytes.
    D. no apparent changes to the joint structure.

64. Approximately what percentage of patients with radiological findings of OA of the knee will report having symptoms?

     A. 25%

     B. 50%

     C. 70%

     D. 95%

65. Deformity of the PIP joints found in an elderly patient with OA is known as:

     A. Heberden's nodes.

     B. Bouchard's nodes.

     C. hallux valgus.

     D. Dupuytren's contracture.

66. Which of the following best describes the presentation of a patient with OA?

     A. worst symptoms in weight-bearing joints later in the day

     B. symmetrical early morning stiffness

     C. sausage-shaped digits with associated skin lesions

     D. back pain with rest and anterior uveitis

67. As part of the evaluation of patients with OA, the NP anticipates finding:

     A. anemia of chronic disease.

     B. elevated CRP level.

     C. no disease-specific laboratory abnormalities.

     D. elevated ANA titer.

68. First-line pharmacological intervention for milder OA in a 58-year-old woman with hypertension should be a trial of:

     A. acetaminophen.

     B. tramadol.

     C. ibuprofen.

     D. intra-articular corticosteroid injection.

69. In caring for a 55-year-old man with body mass index (BMI) within acceptable range who also has OA of the knee, you advise that:

     A. straight-leg raising should be avoided.

     B. heat should be applied to painful joints after exercise.

     C. quadriceps-strengthening exercises should be performed.

     D. physical activity should be minimized.

70. The mechanism of action of glucosamine and chondroitin is:

     A. via increased production of synovial fluid.

     B. through improved cartilage repair.

     C. via inhibition of the inflammatory response in the joint.

     D. largely unknown.

71. A potential adverse effect associated with the use of glucosamine is:

     A. elevated alanine aminotransferase (ALT) and aspartate aminotransferase (AST).

     B. bronchospasm.

C. increased bleeding risk.

D. QT prolongation.

72. A 72-year-old man presents at an early stage of OA in his left knee. He mentions that he heard about the benefits of using glucosamine and chondroitin for treating joint problems. In consulting the patient, you mention all of the following except:

A. at least 3 months of consistent use may be needed before benefit is observed.

B. glucosamine is not associated with any drug interactions.

C. clinical studies have consistently shown benefit of long-term use of glucosamine and chondroitin for treating OA of the knee.

D. chondroitin should be used with caution because of its anticoagulant effect.

73. The AAOS favors all of the following in the management of symptomatic OA of the knee except:

A. low-impact aerobic exercises.

B. weight loss for those with a BMI ≥25 kg/m².

C. acupuncture.

D. strengthening exercises.

74. The AAOS strongly recommends all of the following therapeutic agents for the management of symptomatic OA of the knee except:

A. oral NSAIDs.

B. topical NSAIDs.

C. tramadol.

D. opioids.

75 to 78. Indicate (*Yes or No*) whether the following surgical and procedural interventions are recommended for the management of symptomatic OA of the knee.

_____ **75.** Intra-articular corticosteroid injection

_____ **76.** Hyaluronic acid injection

_____ **77.** Arthroscopy with lavage and/or débridement

_____ **78.** Platelet-rich plasma

79. You see a 67-year-old woman who has been treated for pain due to OA of the hip for the past 6 months and who asks about hip replacement surgery. She complains of pain even at night when sleeping and avoids walking even moderate distances unless absolutely necessary. In counseling the patient, you mention all of the following except:

A. hip replacement can be considered when pain is not adequately controlled.

B. hip replacement is not indicated if the patient can walk short distances.

C. hip replacement candidates must be able to tolerate a long surgical procedure.

D. rehabilitation following surgery is essential to achieve maximal function of the joint.

80. Recommended exercises for patients with OA of the knee include all of the following except:

A. squatting with light weights.

B. straight-leg raises without weights.

C. quadriceps sets.

D. limited weight-bearing aerobic exercises.

81. Recommended exercises for patients with OA of the hip include all of the following except:

A. stretching exercises of the gluteus muscles.

B. straight-leg raises without weights.

    C. isometric exercises of the iliopsoas and gluteus muscles.

    D. weight-bearing aerobic exercises.

82. Which of the following criteria will favor a knee or hip replacement surgery for a patient with OA? Choose all that apply.

    A. Pain control requires daily use of NSAID therapy.

    B. More than 80% of articular cartilage is worn away.

    C. Physical functioning is severely compromised.

    D. The patient can tolerate the surgical procedure and rehabilitation.

For answers and rationales, see end of chapter.

Autoimmune Diseases

RHEUMATOID ARTHRITIS

Overview

RA is an autoimmune disease that causes chronic systemic inflammation, including the synovial membranes of multiple joints. As with most autoimmune diseases, RA is more common in women than in men (ratio approximately 3:1); RA is often seen in people with other autoimmune diseases.

    A family history of RA and other autoimmune diseases is often noted. Although in the past, RA was believed to be a debilitating condition with little impact on longevity, more recent research shows that RA is now known to potentially shorten the life span while producing considerable disability, particularly without optimal treatment. Approximately 40% of all deaths in individuals with RA are attributed to cardiovascular causes, including ischemic heart disease and stroke.

> **CLINICAL CONCEPT**
> Although new-onset RA can occur at any age, peak age at onset is 20 to 40 years.

Clinical Presentation

Initial RA presentation is often with acute polyarticular inflammation. A clinical picture of slowly progressive malaise, weight loss, and stiffness is more common, however. The stiffness is symmetrical, is typically worst on arising, lasts about 1 hour, involves at least three joint groups, and can recur after a period of inactivity or exercise. RA is more often a small joint disease. The hands (with sparing of the DIP joints), wrists, ankles, and toes are most often involved, as opposed to OA where larger joints such as hips and knees are involved. In RA, soft tissue swelling or fluid is also present, as are subcutaneous nodules (Fig. 10-4). The disease is characterized by periods of exacerbation and remission. A set of classification criteria was developed to help identify newly presenting patients with RA (Table 10-3).

Diagnostic Testing

The diagnosis of RA can be made only when clinical features are supported by laboratory testing. Usually initial diagnostic tests include ANA, ESR, CRP, anticitrullinated protein antibody (ACPA), and RF measurements and radiographs, with additional testing often ordered because of diagnostic uncertainty. When interpreting results, the NP should bear in mind the following:

■ Radiographs typically reveal joint erosion and loss of normal joint space. X-rays can help in detecting RA but often do not show any signs at the early stages of disease. Classic radiographic changes are not present in about 30% at disease onset. Musculoskeletal ultrasound and joint MRI are helpful in revealing RA-associated erosions and determining the severity of disease. Ultrasound can reveal areas of inflammation to support an RA diagnosis and track disease progression. MRI can detect a buildup of fluid in the bone marrow that can be used to predict future bone erosion. Radiographic imaging at the early stages of disease can be helpful in determining disease progression.

■ ESR and CRP are nonspecific tests of inflammation. In general, the higher the values are, the greater will be the degree and intensity of the inflammatory process. Although ESR and CRP are frequently elevated in patients with RA, abnormal results are not diagnostic of this or other conditions. In addition, a single elevated ESR or CRP is seldom helpful; however, following trends during flare and regression of disease often aids in charting the therapeutic course and response.

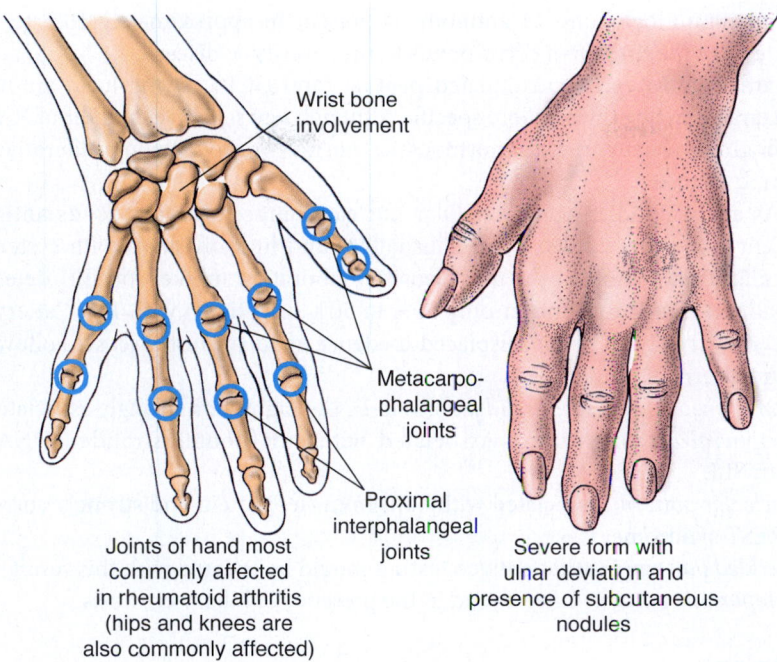

Wrist bone
involvement

Metacarpo-
phalangeal
joints

Proximal
interphalangeal
joints

Joints of hand most
commonly affected
in rheumatoid arthritis
(hips and knees are
also commonly affected)

Severe form with
ulnar deviation and
presence of subcutaneous
nodules

FIGURE 10-4 Rheumatoid arthritis.
Venes D. Taber's Cyclopedic Medical Dictionary. 21st ed. Philadelphia, PA: F.A. Davis; 2009.

TABLE 10-3 American College of Rheumatology/European League Against Rheumatism Classification Criteria for Diagnosis of Rheumatoid Arthritis in Newly Presenting Patients

CRITERION	SCORE
Test patients who:	
1. have at least one joint with definite clinical synovitis	
2. have synovitis not better explained by another disease	
A score of ≥6 out of 10 is needed for classification of a patient as having RA.	
A. Joint involvement:	
1 large joint	0
2 to 10 large joints	1
1 to 3 small joints (with or without involvement of large joints)	2
4 to 10 small joints (with or without involvement of large joints)	3
More than 10 joints (at least 1 small joint)	5
B. Serology (at least one test result is needed for classification)	
Negative RF and negative ACPA	0
Low-positive RF or low-positive ACPA	2
High-positive RF or high-positive ACPA	3
C. Acute-phase reactants (at least one test result is needed for classification)	
Normal CRP and normal ESR	0
Abnormal CRP or abnormal ESR	1
D. Duration of symptoms	
Less than 6 weeks	0
Six weeks or more	1

After adding scores from A to D, a score of greater than or equal to 6/10 indicates RA.
ACPA, anticitrullinated protein antibody; CRP, C-reactive protein; ESR, erythrocyte sedimentation rate; RF, rheumatoid factor.

Source: Adapted from American College of Rheumatology. 2010 rheumatoid arthritis classification criteria. Arthritis Rheum. 2010;62:2569–2581.

- RF, an immunoglobulin M antibody, is present in approximately 50% to 90% of patients with RA. The level of the titer often corresponds to the severity of disease.
- An antibody to cyclic citrullinated peptide (anti-CCP), a ring-form amino acid that is usually not measurable in health, is a more specific, although less sensitive, marker of RA.
- Hemogram usually reveals normocytic, normochromic, hypoproliferative anemia associated with chronic disease.
- ANAs are antibodies against cellular nuclear components that act as antigens. ANA is occasionally present in healthy adults, but it is usually found in individuals with systemic rheumatic or collagen vascular disease. ANA is the most sensitive laboratory marker for SLE, detected in approximately 95% of patients, but it is found in only 30% to 50% of patients with RA. Patterns of immunofluorescence vary and have been given misplaced credence as to type of disease. Following are some examples of ANA patterns:
  - *Homogeneous, diffuse, or solid pattern to DNA*: High titers strongly associated with SLE
  - *Peripheral or rim pattern*: Associated with anti–double-stranded DNA and strongly correlated with SLE
  - *Nucleolar pattern*: Associated with antiribonucleoprotein and strongly correlated with scleroderma or CREST syndrome
  - *Speckled pattern*: Further antigen testing should be ordered with this result
  - *Cytoplasmic pattern*: Often found in the presence of biliary cirrhosis

Treatment

The goal of treatment of patients with RA is to reduce inflammation and pain while preserving function and preventing deformity. NSAIDs have been the backbone of RA drug treatment for years. These medications are helpful in controlling inflammation and pain. Aspirin and ibuprofen are two more commonly used products. With many of the NSAIDs, the half-life of the drug is increased as the dose is increased.

A significant amount of peptic ulcer disease, particularly gastric ulcer and gastritis, is caused by NSAID use. NSAIDs inhibit synthesis of prostaglandins from arachidonic acid, yielding an anti-inflammatory effect. This effect is caused in part by the action of these products against cyclooxygenase (COX). COX-1 is an enzyme found in gastric mucosa, small and large intestine mucosa, kidneys, platelets, and vascular epithelium. This enzyme contributes to the health of these organs through numerous mechanisms, including the maintenance of the protective gastric mucosal layer and proper perfusion of the kidneys. COX-2 is an enzyme that produces prostaglandins important in the inflammatory cascade and pain transmission. The standard NSAIDs and corticosteroids inhibit the synthesis of COX-1 and COX-2, controlling pain and inflammation, but with gastric and renal complications. NSAIDs such as celecoxib (Celebrex®) that spare COX-1 and are more COX-2 selective afford control of the potential for arthritis symptoms. The GI benefit of the COX-2 inhibitors is likely attenuated with long-term use, whereas the cardiovascular risk associated with their use is increased.

> **CLINICAL CONCEPT**
>
> Nonbiological and biological disease-modifying antirheumatic drugs (DMARDs) can help minimize the risk of joint damage and disease progression and should be started as soon as the diagnosis of RA is made (see Table 10-4).

As helpful as NSAIDs are in symptom control, these products do not alter the underlying disease process in RA; joint destruction continues despite control of symptoms and reduction in swelling. As the number and types of nonbiological and biological DMARDs available increase, knowledge of current RA therapy is critical in providing optimal patient care. Expert consultation with rheumatology is indicated to ensure optimal care and to achieve disease remission.

Nonbiological DMARDs are the agents traditionally used to slow disease progression and consist of agents such as methotrexate, leflunomide, sulfasalazine, and hydroxychloroquine, among others. In early RA or with low-to-moderate disease activity, methotrexate monotherapy is the preferred first-line agent unless contraindicated. Sulfasalazine or leflunomide are appropriate options when methotrexate cannot be used. Disease progression should be monitored every 3 to 6 months with adjustment to therapy made.

With moderate-to-high disease activity despite monotherapy, either combination nonbiological DMARD therapy can be considered, or the addition of a biological DMARD can be used, preferably a tumor necrosis factor (TNF) inhibitor. With continued disease activity despite anti-TNF therapy, switching to a non-TNF biological DMARD should be considered. Expert consultation is important when selecting the optimal biological DMARD, as there are substantial differences regarding dosing administration

TABLE 10-4 Treatment of Rheumatoid Arthritis

MEDICATION	EXAMPLES
Anti-inflammatory agents	NSAIDs, COX-2 inhibitors, corticosteroids
Analgesics	Oral–NSAIDs, COX-2 inhibitors, acetaminophen, opioids
	Topical agents–NSAIDs, lidocaine, capsaicin, salicylates, menthol, camphor
DMARDs	Nonbiological DMARDs–methotrexate, leflunomide, sulfasalazine, hydroxychloroquine, minocycline, others
	Biological DMARDs–
	Non-TNF: abatacept, rituximab, anakinra, tocilizumab, sarilumab, others
	Anti-TNF: infliximab, adalimumab, etanercept, certolizumab, golimumab, others
	Oral JAK inhibitors: tofacitinib, baricitinib

COX-2, cyclooxygenase-2; DMARDs, disease-modifying antirheumatic drugs; JAK, Janus kinase; TNF, tumor necrosis factor.

Source: Singh JA, Furst DE, Bharat A, et al. 2012 Update of the 2008 American College of Rheumatology recommendations for the use of disease-modifying antirheumatic drugs and biologic agents in the treatment of rheumatoid arthritis. Arthritis Care Res. 2012;64:625–639.

(e.g., IV infusion, oral), dosing frequency, adverse effects, and cost. As expected, biological DMARDS are generally more expensive than nonbiological DMARDs.

A major adverse effect of biological DMARDs is an increased risk for infection with some dormant infections (such as tuberculosis) activating once treatment begins. Vaccinations should be considered for patients considering initiating DMARD therapy, including immunization against pneumococcal disease, seasonal influenza, hepatitis B, human papillomavirus, and herpes zoster (when indicated). Other vaccines to consider include Tdap and meningococcal vaccine (if considered at higher risk). Ideally, immunizations should be performed prior to the start of DMARD therapy.

If an adequate trial of a DMARD or biological and an NSAID fails to achieve control of pain or symptoms, additional therapy should be added. One option is intra-articular corticosteroid injection. This therapy can be quite helpful but should be limited to not more than two to three injections per joint per year to minimize risk of joint deterioration. Systemic corticosteroids can be most helpful in relieving inflammation, but use should not exceed 2 to 8 weeks, if possible, because of adverse reactions associated with these agents.

Physical therapists can help develop a reasonable activity plan. Maintenance of physical activity through appropriate exercise is of greatest importance. Water exercise in particular is helpful because it includes mild resistance and buoyancy. Splints can provide joint rest while maintaining function and preventing contracture. Behavioral management is important because physiological and psychological stress precipitate RA flares. Allowing for proper rest periods is critical.

SYSTEMIC LUPUS ERYTHEMATOSUS

Overview

SLE is a chronic autoimmune disease that can affect any organ system, including joints, skin, kidneys, blood cells, brain, heart, and lungs. Antibodies are produced against nuclear and cytoplasmic antigens, resulting in systemic inflammation in a relapsing and remitting fashion. The condition predominantly affects women (greater than 90%), with disease onset frequently occurring after puberty. Black women have the highest rate of SLE followed by Asian women and then white women. Complications associated with SLE vary depending on the organ system that is affected. For pregnant women, SLE is a major risk factor for miscarriage; the condition increases the risk of preeclampsia, HELLP (hemolysis, elevated liver enzyme, low platelet count) syndrome, and preterm birth. With better control of SLE, there is generally a better outcome with pregnancy. Though a specific cause of SLE is unknown, there is a strong genetic component.

Clinical Presentation

SLE diagnosis can be difficult because signs and symptoms often mimic other conditions. Symptoms of SLE are highly variable and can include malar rash (covering the cheeks and nasal bridge but sparing the nasolabial folds), fever, unexplained fatigue, headaches, involuntary weight loss, and joint pain, stiffness, and swelling.

In more severe conditions, findings can include acute or chronic renal failure, seizures and psychosis, pulmonary hypertension, pericarditis and myocarditis, and anemia.

Diagnostic Testing

Diagnosis of SLE depends on findings from multiple laboratory and radiographic tests. Common findings include anemia, elevated ESR, proteinuria, and a positive ANA test. A chest x-ray often reveals inflammation in the lungs, whereas an echocardiogram will detect any changes to the heart. A kidney biopsy can be used to detect damage to these organs. The European League Against Rheumatism (EULAR)/ACR criteria items for SLE are presented in Table 10-5. The presence of

TABLE 10-5 European League Against Rheumatism/American College of Rheumatology Diagnostic Criteria for Systemic Lupus Erythematosus

CRITERION	DESCRIPTION
Antinuclear antibodies (ANA)	Titer of ≥1:80 on HEp-2 cells or an equivalent test at least once
Fever	Temperature greater than 38.3°C (100.9°F)
Leukopenia	WBC less than 4,000/mm³
Thrombocytopenia	Platelet count less than 100,000/mm³
Autoimmune hemolysis	Evidence of hemolysis, such as reticulocytosis, low haptoglobin, elevated indirect bilirubin, elevated lactate dehydrogenase, *and* positive Coombs' test
Delirium	Characterized by (1) change in consciousness or level of arousal with reduced ability to focus, (2) symptom development over hours to less than 2 days, (3) symptom fluctuation throughout the day, and (4) either acute/subacute change in cognition or change in behavior, mood, or affect
Psychosis	Delusions and/or hallucinations without insight, or absence of delirium
Seizure	Primary generalized or partial/focal seizure
Nonscarring alopecia	As observed by clinician
Oral ulcers	As observed by clinician
Subacute cutaneous or discoid lupus	Annular or papulosquamous cutaneous eruption, usually photodistributed (subacute cutaneous), *or* Erythematous-violaceous cutaneous lesions with secondary changes of atrophic scarring, dyspigmentation, often follicular hyperkeratosis/plugging, leading to scarring alopecia on the scalp (discoid)
Acute cutaneous lupus	Malar rash or generalized maculopapular rash observed by the clinician
Pleural or pericardial effusion	Imaging evidence of pleural or pericardial effusion, or both
Acute pericarditis	Two or more of (1) pericardial chest pain, (2) pericardial rub, (3) EKG with new widespread ST elevation or PR depression, (4) new or worsened pericardial effusion on imaging

Continued

TABLE 10-5 European League Against Rheumatism/American College of Rheumatology Diagnostic Criteria for Systemic Lupus Erythematosus—cont'd

CRITERION	DESCRIPTION
Joint involvement	Either (1) synovitis involving two or more joints, characterized by swelling or effusion; or (2) tenderness in two or more joints and at least 30 minutes of morning stiffness
Proteinuria	Greater than 0.5 g/24 hours by 24-hour urine or equivalent spot urine protein-to-creatinine ratio
Class II or V lupus nephritis	Based on renal biopsy according to ISN/RPS 2003 classification
Class III or IV lupus nephritis	Based on renal biopsy according to ISN/RPS 2003 classification
Positive antiphospholipid antibodies	Anticardiolipin antibodies at medium or high titer or positive anti-β_2GPI antibodies or positive lupus anticoagulant
Low C3 or low C4	C3 or C4 below lower limit of normal
Low C3 and low C4	Both C3 and C4 below their lower limits of normal
Anti-dsDNA antibodies or anti-Sm antibodies	Immunoassay for anti-dsDNA antibodies with demonstrated 90% or greater specificity for SLE against relevant disease controls, or anti-Sm antibodies

SLE diagnosis requires a positive finding for ANA and then scoring of the remaining criteria based on the American College of Rheumatology classification system found in: Aringer M, Costenbader K, Daikh D, et al. 2019 European League Against Rheumatism/American College of Rheumatology classification criteria for systemic lupus erythematosus. Arthritis Rheum. 2019;71:1400–1412. https://www.rheumatology.org/Portals/0/Files/Classification-Criteria-Systemic-Lupus-Erythematosus.pdf

criteria items can then be entered into the EULAR-ACR classification scoring system to determine a diagnosis of SLE (https://www.rheumatology.org/Portals/0/Files/Classification-Criteria-Systemic-Lupus-Erythematosus.pdf).

Treatment

Similar to RA, treatment of SLE will depend on the manifestation of the disease. If possible, pregnancy should be delayed until SLE is under control for at least 6 months.

Mild disease that waxes and wanes is often controlled with oral NSAIDs. The antimalarial drug hydroxychloroquine has been shown to be effective for the long-term treatment of SLE. Systemic corticosteroids are used to counter the inflammation caused by SLE, although caution is necessary with long-term use of these agents because of their potential adverse effects. For more severe disease or those who do not respond to initial therapy, immune suppressants can be beneficial. These include cyclophosphamide (Cytoxan®), azathioprine (Imuran®), mycophenolate (Cellcept®), leflunomide (Arava®), and methotrexate (Trexall®). These agents are associated with increased risk of infection, liver damage, decreased fertility, and increased risk of cancer. Belimumab (Benlysta®), a parenteral B-lymphocyte stimulator-specific inhibitor, is a biological agent for adults with SLE and may provide added benefits when added to current treatments. Serious adverse effects of this medication include infections, progressive multifocal leukoencephalopathy (PML), and depression and suicidality.

SJÖGREN SYNDROME

Overview

Sjögren's syndrome is an autoimmune disease that usually occurs in conjunction with another chronic inflammatory condition, such as RA or SLE. The condition can affect all organs, but most frequently affects the eyes, mouth, parotid gland, lungs, kidneys, skin, and nervous system. The condition primarily affects women (9:1) with age of onset typically around 50 to 60 years.

Clinical Presentation

Patient presentation includes those of the underlying disease such as SLE or RA with additional complaints related to decreased oral and ocular secretions. These include complaints of dry eyes (xerophthalmia) and dry mouth (xerostomia) along with bilateral parotid swelling. Dry mouth, oral ulcers, and dental caries are common in Sjogren's syndrome, often leading to the "lipstick on the teeth" sign. Angular cheilitis can also be present.

Diagnostic Testing

A salivary gland biopsy for the presence of mononuclear cell infiltration is useful. A positive Schirmer's test that measures tear formation can help support suspicion of Sjögren's syndrome. ESR is elevated in more than 90% of patients. ANAs are typically present in individuals with the condition, while about half will also be positive for RF. Other diagnostic criteria are listed in Table 10-6.

Treatment

Treating the underlying disease is critical. Treatment can include NSAIDs or medications that suppress the immune system (e.g., methotrexate). Hydroxychloroquine has also been found to be helpful. Intervention for patients with Sjögren's syndrome includes management of presenting symptoms with appropriate lubricants. Dry eyes can be alleviated with tear supplementation as well as medications to control inflammation of the lacrimal gland and increase tear production. Dry mouth can be alleviated with liberal sips of water, artificial saliva (e.g., Salivart®, Mouth Kote®), or sugar-free mouth drops to stimulate salivary secretion. Routine dental care and fluoride treatment should be encouraged, while toothpaste without detergent (e.g., Biotene®) can help reduce mouth irritation.

Discussion Sources

American College of Rheumatology. Fast facts on rheumatoid arthritis. http://www.rheumatology.org/I-Am-A/Patient-Caregiver/Diseases-Conditions/Rheumatoid-Arthritis

Aringer M, Costenbader K, Daikh D, et al. 2019 European League Against Rheumatism/American College of Rheumatology classification criteria for systemic lupus erythematosus. *Arthritis Rheum.* 2019;71:1400–1412. https://www.rheumatology.org/Portals/0/Files/Classification-Criteria-Systemic-Lupus-Erythematosus.pdf

Bartels CM. Systemic lupus erythematosus (SLE). Medscape. http://emedicine.medscape.com/article/332244-overview

Ferri, FF. *Ferri's Best Test: A Practical Guide to Laboratory Medicine and Diagnostic Imaging.* 3rd ed. Philadelphia, PA: Elsevier Saunders; 2015.

Ranatunga SK. Sjögren syndrome. Medscape. https://emedicine.medscape.com/article/332125-overview

Singh JA, Saag KG, Bridges Jr SL, et al. 2015 American College of Rheumatology guideline for the treatment of rheumatoid arthritis. *Arthritis Care Res.* 2016:68:1–25.

TABLE 10-6 American College of Rheumatology/European League Against Rheumatism Classification Criteria for Diagnosis of Primary Sjögren's Syndrome

CRITERION	SCORE
Labial salivary gland with focal lymphocytic sialadenitis and focus score of 1 or more	3
Anti-SSA (Ro) +	3
Ocular staining score or 5 or more (or van Bijsterfeld score of 4 or more) on at least one eye	1
Schirmer less than or equal to 5 mm/5 min on at least one eye	1
Unstimulated whole saliva flow rate less than or equal to 0.1 mL/min	1

After adding scores, a score of greater than or equal to 4/9 indicates primary Sjögren's syndrome.

Source: Shiboski CH, Shiboski SC, Seror R, et al. 2016 ACR-EULAR classification criteria for primary Sjögren's syndrome: a consensus and data-driven methodology involving three international patient cohorts. Arthritis Rheum. 2017;69:35–45. https://www.rheumatology.org/Portals/0/Files/ACR-EULAR-2016-Sjogrens-Classification-Criteria.pdf

QUESTIONS

83. Which of the following is not characteristic of RA?

A. It is more common in women than in men at a 3:1 ratio.

B. Family history of autoimmune conditions often is reported.

C. Peak age for disease onset in individuals is age 50 to 70 years.

D. Wrists, ankles, and toes often are involved.

84. The leading cause of death among individuals with RA is:

A. infection.

B. cardiovascular events.

C. cancer.

D. renal failure.

85. Which of the following best describes the presentation of a person with RA?

A. worst symptoms in weight-bearing joints later in the day

B. symmetrical early morning stiffness

C. sausage-shaped digits with characteristic skin lesions

D. back pain with rest and anterior uveitis

86. NSAIDs cause gastric injury primarily by:

A. direct irritative effect.

B. slowing GI motility.

C. thinning of the protective GI mucosa.

D. enhancing prostaglandin synthesis.

87. Of the following individuals, who is at highest risk for NSAID-induced gastropathy?

A. a 28-year-old man with an ankle sprain who has taken ibuprofen for the past week and who drinks four to six beers every weekend over a 2- to 3-day period of time

B. a 40-year-old woman who smokes and takes about six doses of naproxen sodium per month to control dysmenorrhea

C. a 43-year-old man with dilated cardiomyopathy who uses ketoprofen one to two times per week for low back pain (LBP)

D. a 72-year-old man who takes aspirin four times a day for pain control of OA

88. Which of the following is the preferred method of preventing NSAID-induced gastric ulcer?

A. a high-dose histamine-2 receptor antagonist

B. timed antacid use

C. sucralfate (Carafate®)

D. omeprazole (Prilosec®)

89 to 91. Match each autoimmune condition with its most likely clinical presentation.

_____ **89.** RA

_____ **90.** SLE

_____ **91.** Sjögren's syndrome

A. renal involvement

B. subcutaneous nodules

C. oral involvement

92. Which of the following statements is most accurate concerning RA?

    A. Joint erosions are often evident on radiographs or MRI.

    B. RA is seldom associated with other autoimmune diseases.

    C. A butterfly-shaped facial rash is common.

    D. Parvovirus B_{19} infection can contribute to its development.

93. Which of the following hemograms would be expected for a 46-year-old woman with poorly controlled RA?

    A. Hb = 11.1 g/dL (12 to 14 g/dL); MCV = 66 fL (80 to 96 fL); reticulocytes = 0.8% (1% to 2%); RDW = 18.2% (11.5% to 15%)

    B. Hb = 10.1 g/dL (12 to 14 g/dL); MCV = 103 fL (80 to 96 fL); reticulocytes = 1.2% (1% to 2%); RDW = 17.4% (11.5% to 15%)

    C. Hb = 9.7 g/dL (12 to 14 g/dL); MCV = 87 fL (80 to 96 fL); reticulocytes = 0.8% (1% to 2%); RDW = 13.5% (11.5% to 15%)

    D. Hb = 11.4 g/dL (12 to 14 g/dL); MCV = 84 fL (80 to 96 fL); reticulocytes = 2.3% (1% to 2%); RDW = 12.8% (11.5% to 15%)

94. X-rays will fail to show changes in affected joints in approximately what percentage of patients with RA at disease onset?

    A. 30%

    B. 50%

    C. 75%

    D. 95%

95 to 97. Match each imaging technique with the most appropriate use in determining RA disease progression.

_____ 95. X-ray

_____ 96. MRI

_____ 97. Ultrasound

    A. detection of accumulation of fluid in bone marrow

    B. detecting loss of normal joint space

    C. identifying areas of inflammation

98. Mrs. Sanchez is a 42-year-old mother of three who reports pain and stiffness in multiple joints that have lasted for more than 6 months. She is diagnosed with RA. She has no other clinical conditions of significance. You anticipate that which of the following will likely be used as a first-line therapy? Choose all that apply.

    A. a topical analgesic

    B. an oral NSAID

    C. an oral nonbiological DMARD

    D. an injectable biological DMARD

99. A significant adverse effect of biologic DMARDs (e.g., abatacept) for treating RA is:

    A. myopathy.

    B. infection.

    C. renal impairment.

    D. elevated liver enzymes.

100. Prior to initiating a biological DMARD in a 50-year-old woman with RA, vaccination against all of the following is recommended except:

    A. pneumococcal disease.

    B. hepatitis B.

C. *Haemophilus influenzae* type B.

D. influenza.

101. Which of the following tests is most specific to the diagnosis of RA?

A. elevated levels of RF

B. abnormally high ESR

C. leukopenia

D. positive ANA titer

102. A positive ANA test is a sensitive marker for the presence of:

A. hyperparathyroidism.

B. SLE.

C. Kawasaki disease.

D. leukocytosis.

103. Long-term effects of SLE can include all of the following except:

A. increased rate of congenital fetal anomaly when occurring in a woman during pregnancy.

B. chronic kidney disease.

C. avascular necrosis.

D. pericarditis.

104. A 52-year-old woman has RA. She now presents with decreased tearing, "gritty"-feeling eyes, and a dry mouth. You consider a diagnosis of:

A. dry eye syndrome.

B. vasculitis.

C. Sjögren's syndrome.

D. scleroderma.

105 to 108. Indicate if each of the following is a function of cyclooxygenase-1 (COX-1) or COX-2.

_____ 105. Inflammatory response

_____ 106. Pain transmission

_____ 107. Maintenance of gastric protective mucosal layer

_____ 108. Perfusion of the kidneys

109. Management of Sjögren's syndrome can include all of the following except:

A. treat the underlying cause.

B. eye lubrication drops.

C. routine dental care.

D. febuxostat therapy.

110. Which of the following special examinations should be periodically obtained during hydroxychloroquine sulfate use?

A. dilated eye retinal examination

B. bone marrow biopsy

C. pulmonary function tests

D. exercise tolerance test

111. Common physical findings of SLE include all of the following except:

A. weight gain.

B. joint pain and swelling.

    C. fatigue despite adequate opportunity to sleep.

    D. facial rash.

112. Which type of anemia is most often found in a 42-year-old woman with SLE who has undergone endometrial ablation and continues to have significant signs and symptoms despite treatment?

    A. macrocytic, normochromic

    B. microcytic, hypochromic

    C. normocytic, normochromic

    D. hemolysis in origin

113. First-line disease-modifying treatment of SLE in a patient with mild symptoms is:

    A. systemic corticosteroids.

    B. hydroxychloroquine.

    C. anakinra.

    D. methotrexate.

114. Serious adverse effects associated with the use of belimumab (Benlysta®) include all of the following except:

    A. increased suicidal ideation.

    B. thrombocytopenia.

    C. PML.

    D. life-threatening infections.

115. You see a 26-year-old woman who has been recently diagnosed with SLE and has initiated therapy to control moderate symptoms of the disease, including fatigue and joint pain. She mentions that she and her husband are hoping to start a family soon. In counseling her about pregnancy, you consider that which of the following are true? Choose all that apply.

    A. When possible, conception should be delayed until lupus disease control is optimized, preferably for at least 6 months.

    B. Expert consultation should be sought from rheumatology and high-risk obstetrics, optimally prior to attempting pregnancy.

    C. SLE is associated with a high risk of preeclampsia.

    D. Pregnancy is often associated with lupus flares.

For answers and rationales, see end of chapter.

Meniscal Tears

Overview

A meniscal tear results from a disruption of the meniscus, the C-shaped fibrocartilage pad located between the femoral condyles and the tibial plateaus. This injury is often seen in athletes in contact sports because of a twist-type injury to the knee. This condition can also be found in older, sedentary adults; in this case, the injury is usually due to degenerative changes. The condition occurs more often in men than women (ratio ranging from 2.5:1 to 4:1).

Clinical Presentation

Meniscal tears are typically classified as complex or partial; traumatic or degenerative; lateral, posterior, horizontal, or vertical; and radial, parrot-beak, or bucket-handle. Patients with partial, horizontal, and anterior tears often have relatively normal examination findings because the knee's mechanics are relatively unchanged even though these patients continue to have knee locking and pain with certain positions.

    Because the purpose of the fibrocartilage pad is shock absorption and smooth joint mobility, patients with larger tears often report that the knee locks, makes a popping sound, or "gives out." Effusion is also common, especially immediately postinjury,

> **CLINICAL CONCEPT**
>
> Over a third of all meniscal tears involve the anterior cruciate ligament, with peak incidence occurring between 21 and 30 years of age in men and between 11 and 20 years in women.

with the patient reporting a sensation of knee tightness and stiffness. With certain positions, there is often sudden-onset, sharp, localized pain, usually on the medial aspect of the knee. Over time, premature OA is often seen as the normal joint space is compromised.

There are a number of specific clinical examination maneuvers where results help to rule in or out the condition. The McMurray test, a palpable popping on the joint line, is highly specific but poorly sensitive for a meniscal tear (Fig. 10-5); the Apley grinding test gives similar results (Fig. 10-6). The Bragard sign, where an examiner extends and externally rotates the tibia, is positive with tenderness along the anterior medial joint line. Other tests include the bounce home test, Childress test, Merkel sign, and modified Helfat test, among others, that can be used to specify meniscal tear location and ligament involvement. Squatting or kneeling is nearly impossible for patients with a large, complete, or bucket-handle meniscal tear. Joint effusion is typical, with ROM being limited by discomfort. Other conditions that can present similarly include collateral ligament injuries, loose bodies in the knee, and osteochondritis dissecans.

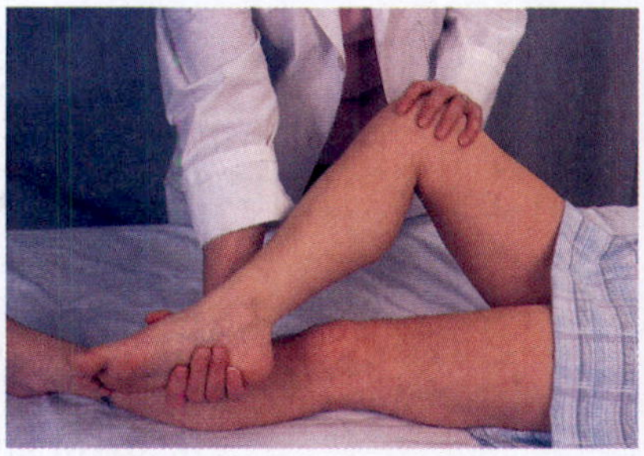

Diagnostic Testing

Knee radiographs, which can reveal osteoarthritic changes, foreign bodies, or other injuries, are reasonable as initial evaluation. Because the meniscus does not contain calcium, the structure is not visible on a plain film. MRI can identify the type and extent of the tear and should be considered if milder symptoms do not resolve within 2 to 4 weeks or if severe symptoms do not resolve earlier.

Treatment

Initial treatment includes rest, ice, compression, elevation (RICE) and analgesia. Because joint effusion is nearly always present but is relatively mild, aspiration should be considered only if there is no improvement after 2 to 4 weeks of conservative therapy. Crutch walking should be encouraged, and a patellar stabilizer is often needed when significant knee instability is present. Straight-leg–raising exercises help strengthen the quadriceps and stabilize the joint. Arthroscopy, which provides the most accurate diagnosis with the possibility of concurrent treatment through débridement and repair, should be considered at 4 to 6 weeks if there is no improvement and earlier if joint locking, giving out, and effusion are particularly problematic.

Though many cases of meniscal tears are not preventable, some steps can be taken to reduce the risk of this condition. These include strengthening exercises of the quadriceps, stretching exercises before and after physical activity, and ensuring proper footwear is used for sports activities.

FIGURE 10-5 The McMurray test assesses the menisci. The medial meniscus is tested with the hip flexed and the knee externally rotated as the examiner moves the knee from full flexion to extension. To test the lateral meniscus, the knee is internally rotated during the procedure. A snap heard or felt during this maneuver suggests a tear of the tested meniscus.
Dillon P. Nursing Health Assessment: The Foundation of Clinical Practice. 3rd ed. Philadelphia, PA: F.A. Davis; 2016.

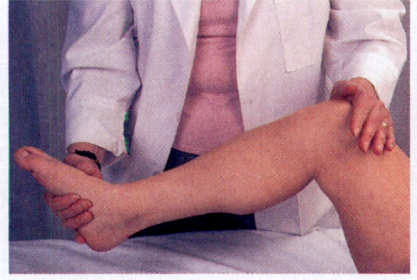

FIGURE 10-6 Apley test.
Dillon PM. Nursing Health Assessment: The Foundation of Clinical Practice. 3rd ed. Philadelphia, PA: F.A. Davis; 2016.

Discussion Sources

Anderson B. *Office Orthopedics for Primary Care: Diagnosis.* Philadelphia, PA: Saunders Elsevier; 2006.

Anderson B. *Office Orthopedics for Primary Care: Treatment.* 3rd ed. Philadelphia, PA: Saunders Elsevier; 2006.

Andrew ST, Porter DO. Common sports injuries. In: Bope ET, Kellerman RD, eds. *Conn's Current Therapy 2018.* Philadelphia, PA: Saunders Elsevier; 2017:864–873.

QUESTIONS

116. The McMurray test is performed by:

    A. compressing the knee while externally or internally rotating the tibia.

    B. moving the knee from full flexion to extension with hip flexed and knee externally rotated.

    C. having the individual attempt to "duck walk."

    D. having the patient stand with knee fully extended and then rotate the trunk.

117. The most common type of injury causing a sport-related meniscal tear involves:

    A. twisting of the knee.

    B. hyperextension of the knee.

C. repetitive striking impact on the knee (e.g., running on hard surface).

D. an unknown origin in most cases.

118. Which of the following best describes the presentation of a patient with complete medial meniscus tear?

A. joint effusion

B. heat over the knee

C. inability to kneel

D. loss of smooth joint movement

119. Which of the following statements about meniscal tears is false?

A. Meniscal tears occur more frequently in males compared to females.

B. Older, sedentary adults are at risk of degenerative meniscal tears.

C. The peak incidence of sports-related meniscal tears in men occurs in their 20s.

D. The peak incidence of sports-related meniscal tears in women occurs in their 30s.

120. When making a diagnosis of meniscal tear, other similar conditions to consider can include all of the following except:

A. osteoporosis.

B. osteochondritis dissecans.

C. collateral ligament injury.

D. loose body in the knee.

121. To help prevent meniscal tear, you advise:

A. limiting participation in sports.

B. quadriceps-strengthening exercises.

C. using a knee brace.

D. applying ice to the knee before exercise.

122. For a patient with a suspected meniscal tear with a knee radiograph that does not reveal acute changes, the preferred next step is:

A. order an MRI of the knee.

B. order an ultrasound of the knee.

C. advise the patient that arthroscopy is the next step in diagnosis.

D. to consider an alternative diagnosis as meniscal tear is unlikely.

123. Initial treatment for meniscal tear includes all of the following except:

A. NSAID use.

B. applying ice to the affected area.

C. elevation of the affected limb.

D. joint aspiration of the affected knee.

124. A 32-year-old male with a diagnosis of meniscal tear shows no improvement after 4 weeks of standard conservative therapy. He also complains of joint locking and effusion. An appropriate next course of action for this patient is:

A. intra-articular corticosteroid injection.

B. application of a topical anti-inflammatory four times a day.

C. referral for arthroscopy and likely surgical intervention.

D. to watch and wait an additional 4 weeks.

For answers and rationales, see end of chapter.

Carpal Tunnel Syndrome

Overview

Carpal tunnel syndrome (CTS) is a painful condition caused by compression of the median nerve between the carpal ligament and other structures within the carpal tunnel. This compression leads to an entrapment neuropathy, causing symptoms in the distribution of the median nerve. The resulting symptoms are likely caused by nerve ischemia rather than nerve damage.

The most common risk factor is repetitive motion; the condition is common with protracted computer keyboard use and in workers such as cake decorators and soldiers, who must consistently grasp a small object. CTS can also be part of the manifestation of a systemic disease, such as RA and sarcoidosis.

Clinical Presentation

Patients with CTS, the most commonly encountered peripheral compression neuropathy, usually report a burning, aching, or tingling pain radiating to the forearm in the distribution of the median nerve and occasionally to the shoulder, neck, and chest. Symptoms are often worse at night. A classic finding is the report of acroparesthesia, awakening at night with numbness and burning pain in the fingers. Physical examination findings occasionally include positive Tinel and Phalen tests, although the carpal compression test, in which symptoms are induced by direct application of pressure over the carpal tunnel, is likely a more sensitive and specific test (Figs. 10-7 and 10-8). In later disease, muscle weakness and thenar atrophy are often noted.

Diagnostic Testing

Diagnostic tests for patients suspected to have CTS include electromyography (EMG) and nerve conduction studies that can confirm the median neuropathy. EMG is used to measure the electrical discharges produced by the muscles. Electrodes are used to measure the electrical activity of the muscles at rest and during contraction and will indicate whether muscle damage is present. In a nerve conduction study, electrodes are taped to the skin, and a small shock is passed through the medial nerve to assess whether electrical impulses are slowed in the carpal tunnel, indicating damage to the nerve. Although plain x-rays are of little diagnostic value, MRI and high-resolution ultrasound results often support the diagnosis and can eliminate other causes of wrist pain, such as space-occupying lesions, arthritis, or a fracture.

Treatment

Treatment of patients with CTS includes limiting the activity that caused the condition and elevating the affected extremity. Nighttime use of a volar splint to keep the wrist in a neutral position helps relieve the increase in intracanal pressure caused by wrist flexion and extension. NSAIDs and acetaminophen provide pain relief. Corticosteroid injection into the carpal tunnel at 6-week intervals can help reduce swelling and symptoms but should be performed only by a skilled practitioner. A short course of oral corticosteroids has been shown to provide some benefit, though further research is needed. Physical therapy is often quite helpful and should be encouraged not only for treatment of acute symptoms but also to prevent CTS recurrence.

Surgery to release the transverse carpal ligament provides symptom relief in most patients whose CTS does not respond to conservative therapy. About 10% who have surgery do not respond, however, because of nerve damage or new pressure within the carpal tunnel that results from recurrent compression caused by scar formation. Diuretics, vitamin B_6, and other nutraceutical therapies have been reported as helpful in minimizing CTS symptoms, although clinical studies have shown these agents to be no more effective than placebo.

Pregnancy-induced CTS usually resolves quickly after the woman gives birth. The use of thyroxine supplements quickly ameliorates CTS caused by hypothyroidism. In the interim, splinting, ice, and analgesia can be helpful.

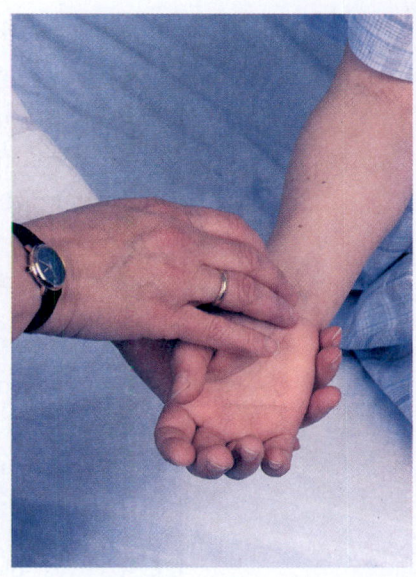

FIGURE 10-7 Tinel test.
Dillon PM. Nursing Health Assessment: The Foundation of Clinical Practice. 3rd ed. Philadelphia, PA: F.A. Davis; 2016.

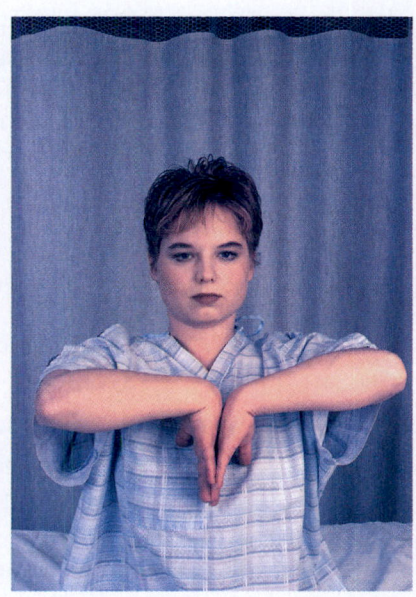

FIGURE 10-8 Phalen test.
Dillon PM. Nursing Health Assessment: The Foundation of Clinical Practice. 3rd ed. Philadelphia, PA: F.A. Davis; 2016.

There is little evidence on strategies to prevent CTS. When the condition is associated with a repetitive activity, individuals should be counseled to limit time spent on these activities when possible, ensuring proper work breaks, and encouraging toning and stretching exercises. BMI and poor fitness level have been linked to the development of CTS, and so individuals should be encouraged to maintain fitness and a healthy body weight.

Discussion Sources

Anderson B. *Office Orthopedics for Primary Care: Diagnosis*. Philadelphia, PA: Saunders Elsevier; 2006.

Anderson B. *Office Orthopedics for Primary Care: Treatment*. 3rd ed. Philadelphia, PA: Saunders Elsevier; 2006.

Turner S. Musculoskeletal system. In: Goolsby M, Grubbs L, eds. *Advanced Assessment: Interpreting Findings and Formulating Differential Diagnoses*. 4th ed. Philadelphia, PA: F.A. Davis; 2019;435–476.

Wipperman J, Goerl K. Carpal tunnel syndrome. *Am Fam Physician*. 2016;94:993–999.

QUESTIONS

125. The Phalen test is described as:

    A. reproduction of symptoms with forced flexion of the wrists.

    B. abnormal tingling when the median nerve is tapped.

    C. pain on internal rotation.

    D. palmar atrophy.

126. The Tinel test is best described as:

    A. reproduction of symptoms with forced flexion of the wrists.

    B. abnormal tingling when the median nerve is tapped.

    C. pain on internal rotation.

    D. palmar atrophy.

127. A 35-year-old woman who is a computer programmer presents with symptoms consistent with carpal tunnel syndrome. The NP explains that an EMG can be helpful in confirming the diagnosis as this procedure does all of the following except:

    A. measures electrical impulses caused by muscles.

    B. compares results of the muscles at rest versus contraction.

    C. can detect muscle damage.

    D. involves sending a small electrical impulse through the muscle tissue.

128. Risk factors for CTS include which of the following? Choose all that apply.

    A. latter half of pregnancy

    B. untreated hypothyroidism

    C. repetitive motion

    D. multiple sclerosis

129. Which of the following is least likely to be reported by patients with CTS?

    A. worst symptoms during the day

    B. burning sensation in the affected hand

    C. tingling pain that radiates to the forearm

    D. nocturnal numbness

130. Acroparesthesia, frequently reported in patients with CTS, is best described as:

    A. constant pain radiating from the elbow.

    B. a transient inability to move the fingers.

    C. waking up at night with numbness and burning pain in the fingers.

    D. muscle spasms that cause fist clenching.

131. Aside from eliminating or minimizing the triggering activity, initial therapy in a 42-year-old man who is a cake decorator and has newly diagnosed CTS includes:

A. referral for intra-articular injection.

B. nighttime use of a volar splint to keep the wrist in a neutral position.

C. a 5-day course of a higher-potency topical corticosteroid to the area twice a day.

D. referral for surgery.

132. A 36-year-old woman who is 32 weeks' pregnant is diagnosed today with CTS after a sudden onset of classic signs and symptoms for the past 2 weeks. You advise that she:

A. is unlikely to benefit from standard CTS therapies while she is pregnant.

B. will likely see significant improvement of CTS signs and symptoms within weeks of giving birth.

C. be referred for surgery to be planned after she gives birth.

D. have vitamin B_6 injections in the carpal tunnel to help with symptom relief.

133. When considering interventions to prevent CTS, all of the following should be encouraged except:

A. maintaining fitness and BMI.

B. daily use of low-dose aspirin.

C. stretching and toning exercises.

D. taking scheduled breaks from repetitive activities.

For answers and rationales, see end of chapter.

Sarcoidosis

Overview

Sarcoidosis is an inflammatory condition that results in the production of noncaseating granulomas in various sites of the body, predominantly in the lungs, lymph nodes, eyes, and skin. Although the exact cause of sarcoidosis is unknown, this disease is likely the result of an exaggerated immune response to an unidentified antigen, possibly inhaled from the air. The condition often occurs in adults between the ages of 20 and 40 years, with a slightly higher incidence in women than men. Individuals of African ancestry are also more likely to have the disease than other ethnic groups and tend to have more severe disease that can cause pulmonary issues. A family history of the disease is also a risk factor.

Clinical Presentation

Symptoms depend on the organs involved and severity of the disease. Sarcoidosis can develop gradually with symptoms that last for years, whereas others can have more rapid progression and resolution of the disease. Dermatological signs include rash, lesions, color change, and nodule formations just under the skin. Ocular symptoms include blurred vision, eye pain, severe redness, and sensitivity to light.

Diagnosis of sarcoidosis can be difficult because there can be few signs and symptoms in early disease and the symptoms can mimic several other disorders. The diagnostic process aims to exclude other disorders while also determining which organ systems are affected by the disease.

Diagnostic Testing

Select serological markers have also been associated with sarcoidosis, including serum amyloid A (SAA), soluble interleukin-2 receptor, ACE, and glycoprotein KL-6. Patients with sarcoidosis are also more likely to present with hypercalcemia and hypercalciuria.

Imaging studies are a key component of diagnosis. Chest x-ray can be used to check for lung damage or enlarged lymph nodes in the chest. High-resolution CT scanning of the chest can detect the presence of alveolitis or fibrosis. Positron emission tomography (PET) or MRI can detect whether the disease is affecting the heart or central nervous system. Pulmonary function tests and carbon monoxide capacity

> **CLINICAL CONCEPT**
>
> Systemic symptoms of sarcoidosis include fever, fatigue, anorexia, and arthralgias, whereas pulmonary complaints include dyspnea on exertion, cough, and chest pain.

tests are used in evaluation and follow-up to gauge pulmonary involvement and progression of the disease. Confirmation of the disease typically requires biopsy to check for the presence of noncaseating granulomas. This can involve a transbronchial biopsy (which gives a high diagnostic yield regardless of disease stage) or can occur from affected skin or the outer membrane of the eye.

Treatment

Sarcoidosis is often self-limiting. Milder disease can be treated with NSAIDs to help relieve symptoms of arthralgias and other rheumatic complaints. Corticosteroids are the mainstay of treatment, especially for systemic disease, and can be taken orally, as a topical agent applied to affected skin, or inhaled for those with endobronchial disease. Optimal dosing for the treatment of sarcoidosis is unclear; some suggest using a low dose or dose that is tapered to every other day over several weeks to months. Other agents used in the treatment of sarcoidosis include the antimalarial drug hydroxychloroquine and immune-suppressing medications used to treat RA (e.g., methotrexate, azathioprine, and TNF inhibitors [e.g., infliximab]). Other agents include chlorambucil, cyclophosphamide, and cyclosporine. Biologic agents, such as infliximab and adalimumab, have been used with some success in refractory disease. For patients with extensive pulmonary damage resulting from the disease, lung transplantation may be a viable option.

Discussion Sources

Kamangar N. Sarcoidosis. Medscape. http://emedicine.medscape.com/article/301914-overview
Soto-Gomez N, Peters JI, Nambiar AM. Diagnosis and management of sarcoidosis. *Am Fam Physician*. 2016;93:840–848.

QUESTIONS

134. A risk factor for sarcoidosis is:

   A. male gender.

   B. African ancestry.

   C. age older than 60 years.

   D. type 2 diabetes mellitus.

135. Common symptoms of a patient with sarcoidosis include all of the following except:

   A. arthralgia.

   B. dyspnea upon exertion.

   C. blurred vision.

   D. cardiac palpitations.

136. A laboratory finding commonly observed in patients with sarcoidosis is:

   A. hyponatremia.

   B. hypercalcemia.

   C. hypokalemia.

   D. hyperkalemia.

137. Which of the following diagnostic approaches is used for confirmation of sarcoidosis?

   A. chest x-ray

   B. high-resolution CT scan

   C. biopsy

   D. ANA fluorescent staining

138. The primary treatment option for systemic sarcoidosis is the use of:

   A. parenteral methotrexate.

   B. oral corticosteroids.

   C. oral acetaminophen.

   D. oral hydroxychloroquine.

139. You see a 42-year-old woman diagnosed with extrapulmonary sarcoidosis that is refractory to first-line and second-line therapy with nonbiological agents. You consider prescribing which of the following biological agents?

A. etanercept

B. tofacitinib

C. infliximab

D. certolizumab

140. Evaluation for disease progression in a patient with sarcoidosis can involve:

A. pulmonary function test and carbon monoxide capacity test.

B. skin biopsy.

C. check for WBCs in the urine.

D. Finkelstein's test.

141. Serological markers for sarcoidosis can include all of the following except:

A. anticyclic citrullinated peptide.

B. SAA.

C. glycoprotein KL-6.

D. soluble interleukin-2 receptor.

For answers and rationales, see end of chapter.

Low Back Pain and Lumbar Radiculopathy

Overview

With a lifetime prevalence of 60% to 90%, LBP is at least an occasional problem for the majority of adults. In about 90% of patients with LBP, symptoms are short-lived and resolve within 1 month without specific therapy. Some individuals have recurrent or chronic LBP, however, and significant disability.

Lumbosacral strain or disk herniation and resulting lumbar radiculopathy and sciatica can cause musculoskeletal LBP. Most often, contributing factors include muscle or ligamentous strain, degenerative joint disease, or a combination of these factors. Lumbosacral strain is the most common reason for a patient to present to the primary care practitioner with acute LBP. In the typical scenario, the patient complains of stiffness, spasm, and reduced ROM. The erector spinae muscle is most often implicated. Sitting usually aggravates the pain, but there may be some relief if the patient lies supine on a firm surface. A precipitating event is reported by only a few patients because lumbosacral strain is usually the culmination of many events, including repeated use of improperly stretched muscles in patients with overall poor conditioning. In addition, poor posture, scoliosis, and spinal stenosis can be predisposing factors.

Lumbosacral disk herniation usually occurs after years of episodes of back pain caused by repeated damage to the annular fibers of the disk and is less common than lumbosacral strain as a cause of LBP. Risk factors for lumbar radiculopathy include smoking, diabetes, spinal infection, overweight or obesity, male gender, and older age. Lumbar disk herniation often leads to sciatica, neurological changes, and significant distress. Because the intravertebral disks contain less water and are more fibrous, the risk of disk rupture decreases after age 50 years. The most common sites of lumbosacral disk herniation are L4 to L5 and L5 to S1, with the posterolateral aspect of the disk protruding.

Neuralgia along the course of the sciatic nerve is known as sciatica. The cause of sciatica is usually pressure on lumbosacral nerve roots from a herniated disk, spinal stenosis, or a compression fracture. Occasionally, sciatica can be caused by external pressure on the sciatic nerve, such as that often found in people who carry a wallet in a rear pants pocket and develop symptoms after prolonged sitting. Patients with sciatica complain of shooting pain that starts over the hip and radiates to the foot, often accompanied by leg numbness and weakness. The degree of pain can vary according to the degree of nerve

> **CLINICAL CONCEPT**
> Risk factors for LBP include older age, overactivity, overweight or obesity, and certain physiological and degenerative disorders (e.g., spinal stenosis, degenerative spondylolisthesis, and scoliosis).

involvement; it ranges from mildly bothersome, and occasionally reported to be more itchy than painful, to incapacitating pain.

Neck pain, a common clinical complaint that often goes along with LBP, can result from abnormalities in the soft tissues, such as muscles, ligaments, and nerves, and in bones and joints of the spine. The most common causes of neck pain are soft tissue abnormalities caused by injury, poor posture, or prolonged wear and tear; cervical vertebral sprain is a frequent injury observed in athletes and victims of motor vehicle accidents, resulting in acute sprains and strains of neck muscles as well as soft tissue contusions. The most common site for a cervical disk lesion, leading to cervical radiculopathy, is at the level of C6 to C7. Rare causes of neck pain include infection and tumor.

Clinical Presentation

In LBP, health history is usually consistent with a history of aching sensation in the lumbar sacral area but without leg weakness or other neurological complaint. The physical examination usually reveals a straightening of the lumbosacral curve, paraspinal muscle tenderness, spasm worst at the level of L3 to L4, and decreased lumbosacral flexion and lateral bending. The neurological examination findings are typically normal in lumbar sacral strain; if there is a neurological abnormality demonstrated on a well-performed clinical examination on a person presenting with LBP, then the diagnosis of lumbar radiculopathy needs to be considered.

Individuals with lumbar radiculopathy will often report a sudden onset of pain that can include LBP. The pain often travels below the knee and can worsen when the patient coughs, sneezes, stands, or sits. Numbness, weakness, or tingling in the back of the legs is common. Radiculopathy that involves L1 to L3 will have pain radiating to the thigh but not below the knee. Loss of the posterior tibial reflex can indicate a lesion at L5, while loss of the Achilles tendon reflex likely indicates a lesion at L5 to S1. The straight-leg–raising maneuver reproduces pain. The straight-leg raise, also called Lasègue's sign or Lazarević's sign, can be done during a physical examination to determine if LBP is associated with an underlying herniated disc. The maneuver evaluates for tension in L5 and S1.

With cauda equina involvement in lumbar radiculopathy, there is compression of the lower portion of the nerve root inferior to the spinal cord, usually secondary to disk herniation. This compression can lead to rectal or perineal pain and disturbance in bowel and bladder function. Cauda equina syndrome constitutes a medical emergency, with prompt expert consultation needed.

An acute cervical sprain can be associated with a jammed-neck sensation with localized pain. After the injury, pain, swelling, and tenderness can become evident as local bleeding occurs in the muscle fibers. Neck motion can become painful, with peak pain occurring several hours later or the next day. However, the patient should have no radiation of pain to the extremities with cervical strain only.

In cervical radiculopathy, the patient presents with neck and arm discomfort that can range from a dull ache to severe burning pain. The pain is commonly referred to the medial border of the scapula, and the chief complaint is shoulder pain. With progression, the pain can radiate to the upper and lower arm and into the hand. For patients presenting with cervical radiculopathy, the Spurling test can be used to identify cervical nerve root compression. The maneuver involves turning the patient's head to the affected side while applying downward pressure on the top of the head. This should elicit pain and numbness to the upper extremities in the presence of cervical radiculopathy.

Diagnostic Testing

Diagnostic tests in lumbosacral or cervical strain vary according to the length and severity of symptoms. Radiographs are helpful only if there is a high degree of suspicion for spondylolisthesis, scoliosis, cancer, or fracture (Table 10-7). In the absence of these conditions, little is likely to be revealed. Radiography is likely to reveal the presence of lumbar arthritis, which has been observed in more than 90% of adults older than 40 years of age, although most do not report LBP.

CT scanning or MRI should be considered if radiculopathy is present and clinical presentation does not improve after a reasonable trial of conservative therapy, because these studies might reveal contributing factors, such as spinal stenosis and disk herniation. MRI is a superior study for revealing soft tissue problems, whereas CT provides superior information on bony structures.

> **CLINICAL CONCEPT**
>
> In evaluating a person with LBP or cervical strain, lumbosacral radiographs should not be routinely obtained.

Treatment

Management of patients with neck pain or LBP differs according to presentation. In most patients with acute neck pain or LBP and intact neurological examination,

TABLE 10-7 Diagnostic Imaging for Low Back Pain

IMMEDIATE ACTION	SUGGESTIONS FOR INITIAL IMAGING
Immediate Imaging	
Radiography plus ESR,* MRI	Major risk factors for cancer
	Risk factors for spinal infection
	Consider MRI if risk factors for or signs of the cauda equina syndrome; severe neurological deficits, particularly if sudden onset
	Radiograph only with high fracture risk
Defer Imaging After a Trial of Standard Therapy	
Radiography ± ESR	Weaker risk factors for cancer; risk factors for or signs of ankylosing spondylitis; risk factors for vertebral compression fracture
MRI	Signs and symptoms of radiculopathy in patients who are candidates for surgery or epidural steroid injection; risk factors for or symptoms of spinal stenosis in patients who are candidates for surgery
No imaging	No criteria for immediate imaging and back pain improved or resolved after at least a 1-month trial of therapy; previous spinal imaging with no change in clinical status

Consider MRI if the initial imaging result is negative but a high degree of clinical suspicion for cancer remains.
ESR, erythrocyte sedimentation rate; MRI, magnetic resonance imaging.
Source: Chou R, Qaseem A, Owens DK, Shekelle P; for Clinical Guidelines Committee of the American College of Physicians. Diagnostic imaging for low back pain: advice for high-value health care from the American College of Physicians. Ann Intern Med. 2011;154(3):181–189. http://annals.org/article.aspx?articleid=746774

treatment is aimed at maintaining function and minimizing symptoms. Longer periods of immobilization can contribute to deconditioning and are potentially harmful. Intervention for acute neck pain is similar.

Application of cold packs for 20 minutes three to four times a day can help with pain control, and heat applications are often helpful to use before gentle stretching exercise. NSAIDs or acetaminophen should be prescribed for pain control. Muscle relaxants have been shown to be helpful in some patients but should generally be used for a short period of time. These medications are usually sedating and need to be used with caution; occasionally, these are used as drugs of abuse. Opioid medications should be avoided if possible for patients with low back or neck pain. Anticonvulsants, such as gabapentin and pregabalin, have been shown to offer pain relief in some types of neuropathic pain, such as diabetic peripheral neuropathy. However, the effect of these agents in reducing neck pain or LBP and cervical or lumbar radiculopathy has not been consistently demonstrated in clinical trials.

Treatment for neck and back pain should also include initiating aerobic and toning exercises and teaching the patient to minimize musculoskeletal stress through appropriate use of body mechanics. Physical therapy referral is quite helpful in patient evaluation as well as teaching. Therapeutic massage can help improve blood flow and reduce muscle stiffness. These nonpharmacological approaches can also be effective in reducing the risk of recurrent back pain.

Prompt referral to specialty care is needed when there is limb, bowel, or bladder dysfunction. Surgery is usually considered only if severe radiculopathy symptoms persist beyond 3 months. In addition, early referral is indicated in certain conditions that are particularly worrisome (Table 10-8).

Discussion Sources

Chou R, Qaseem A, Owens DK, Shekelle P; for Clinical Guidelines Committee of the American College of Physicians. Diagnostic imaging for low back pain: advice for high-value health care from the American College of Physicians. *Ann Intern Med.* 2011;154(3):181–189. http://annals.org/article.aspx?articleid=746774

Qaseem A, Wilt TJ, McLean RM, et al. Noninvasive treatments for acute, subacute, and chronic low back pain: a clinical practice guideline from the American College of Physicians. *Ann Intern Med.* 2017;166:514–530.

TABLE 10-8 Low Back Pain: Red Flags for a Potentially Serious Underlying Cause

POSSIBLE FRACTURE	POSSIBLE TUMOR OR INFECTION	CAUDA EQUINA SYNDROME
History of recent trauma, particularly fall from significant height or motor vehicle accident	Age younger than 20 years or older than 50 years Constitutional symptoms such as unexplained weight loss, fever	Bladder dysfunction, perineal sensory loss, or anal laxity Neurological deficit in lower extremities
In person with or at risk for osteoporosis, minor trauma, or strenuous lifting	Recent bacterial infection, injection drug use, immunosuppression Increased pain with rest History of cancer	Lower extremity motor weakness

Sources: Chou R, Qaseem A, Owens DK, Shekelle P; for Clinical Guidelines Committee of the American College of Physicians. Diagnostic imaging for low back pain: advice for high-value health care from the American College of Physicians. Ann Intern Med. 2011;154(3):181–189. http://annals.org/article.aspx?articleid=746774; Qaseem A, Wilt TJ, McLean RM, et al. Noninvasive treatments for acute, subacute, and chronic low back pain: a clinical practice guideline from the American College of Physicians. Ann Intern Med. 2017;166:514–530.

QUESTIONS

142. Approximately what percentage of patients experiencing LBP will have the symptoms resolve within 1 month without specific therapy?

A. 33%

B. 57%

C. 78%

D. 90%

143. Risk factors for the development of LBP include all of the following except:

A. older age.

B. carpal tunnel syndrome.

C. scoliosis.

D. spinal stenosis.

144. Most episodes of LBP are caused by:

A. an acute precipitating event.

B. disk herniation.

C. muscle or ligamentous strain.

D. nerve impingement.

145. With the straight-leg–raising test, the NP is evaluating tension on which of the following nerve roots?

A. L1 and L2

B. L3 and L4

C. L5 and S1

D. S2 and S3

146. A patient with a lumbosacral strain will typically report:

A. numbness in the extremities.

B. stiffness, spasm, and reduced ROM in the back.

C. "electric" sensation running down one or both legs.

D. pain at its worst when in supine position.

147. You see a 54-year-old man complaining of LBP and who is diagnosed with acute lumbosacral strain. Which of the following is the best advice to give about exercising?

A. You should not exercise until you are free of pain.

B. Back-strengthening exercises can cause mild muscle soreness.

C. Electric-like pain in response to exercise is to be expected.

D. Conditioning exercises should be started immediately regardless of degree of pain.

148. Risk factors for lumbar radiculopathy include all of the following except:

A. male gender.

B. age younger than 50 years.

C. being overweight.

D. cigarette smoking.

149. A patient with sciatica will typically report:

A. loss of bladder control.

B. stiffness, spasm, and reduced ROM.

C. shooting pain that starts at the hip and radiates to the foot.

D. pain at its worst when lying down.

150. Early neurological changes in patients with lumbar radiculopathy include:

A. loss of deep tendon reflexes.

B. poor two-point discrimination.

C. reduced muscle strength.

D. footdrop.

151. Common causes of sciatica include all of the following except:

A. herniated disk.

B. spinal stenosis.

C. compression fracture.

D. soft tissue abnormality.

152. You see a 48-year-old woman who reports LBP. During the evaluation, she mentions new-onset loss of bowel and bladder control. This most likely indicates:

A. cauda equina syndrome.

B. muscular spasm.

C. vertebral fracture.

D. sciatic nerve entrapment.

153. Loss of posterior tibial reflex often indicates a lesion at:

A. L3.

B. L4.

C. L5.

D. S1.

154. Loss of Achilles tendon reflex most likely indicates a lesion at:

A. L1 to L2.

B. L3 to L4.

C. L5 to S1.

D. S2 to S3.

155. Which test is demonstrated when the examiner applies pressure to the top of the head with the neck bending forward, producing pain or numbness in the upper extremities?

    A. Spurling

    B. McMurray

    C. Lachman

    D. Kemp

156. Immediate diagnostic imaging for LBP should be reserved for all of the following except the presence of:

    A. signs of the cauda equina syndrome.

    B. severe neurological deficits.

    C. risk factors for cancer.

    D. moderate pain lasting at least 2 weeks.

157. Which of the following tests yields the greatest amount of clinical information in a patient with acute lumbar radiculopathy?

    A. lumbosacral radiograph series

    B. ESR measurement

    C. MRI

    D. bone scan

158. A lumbosacral x-ray would be most helpful to aid in the diagnosis of new-onset LBP in which of the following individuals?

    A. a 49-year-old man 1 day after performing rigorous yard work

    B. a 62-year-old woman who slipped on an icy sidewalk

    C. a 54-year-old obese man who reports pain radiating to the buttocks

    D. a 61-year-old woman reporting pain after attempting to lift her grandson

159. The most common site for cervical radiculopathy is:

    A. C3 to C4.

    B. C4 to C5.

    C. C5 to C6.

    D. C6 to C7.

160. The most common sites for lumbar disk herniation are:

    A. L1 to L2 and L2 to L3.

    B. L2 to L3 and L4 to L5.

    C. L4 to L5 and L5 to S1.

    D. L5 to S1 and S1 to S2.

161. You see a 37-year-old man complaining of LBP consisting of stiffness and spasms but without any sign of neurological involvement. You recommend all of the following interventions except:

    A. application of cold packs for 20 minutes three to four times a day.

    B. use of NSAIDs or acetaminophen for pain control.

    C. initiation of aerobic and toning exercises.

    D. bedrest for at least 5 days.

162. When considering the use of gabapentin for LBP, which of the following is true?

    A. recommended as first-line therapy in LBP with or without neurological involvement

    B. provides similar pain relief as opioids for nonneurological pain

C. clinical trials fail to demonstrate consistent benefits in LBP

D. should be avoided due to dependence issues similar to opioids

163. Which of the following nonpharmacological methods is least helpful in preventing LBP recurrence?

A. low-impact aerobic exercises

B. toning exercises

C. weekly ice baths

D. massage therapy

164. When considering the use of muscle relaxants for treatment of LBP in a 46-year-old construction worker, the NP advises all of the following except that:

A. these agents have an abuse potential.

B. these agents must be used consistently for at least 2 weeks before seeing peak effect.

C. use at night can improve sleep.

D. caution should be used when operating heavy machinery while taking these medications.

For answers and rationales, see end of chapter.

Reactive Arthritis

Overview

Reactive arthritis (ReA), formally known as Reiter's syndrome, refers to acute nonpurulent arthritis complicating an infection elsewhere in the body. This condition is typically seen many days to weeks after an episode of acute bacterial diarrhea caused by *Shigella* species, *Salmonella* species, *Campylobacter* species, or a sexually transmitted infection, usually with acute urethritis and/or cervicitis, such as *Chlamydia trachomatis* or *Ureaplasma urealyticum*. When seen with infectious diarrhea, the disease is found equally in both genders. When ReA is seen with urethritis, there is a male predominance of 9:1, with most being HLA-B27 positive (a human leukocyte antigen located on the surface of WBCs).

Clinical Presentation

ReA usually develops about 2 to 4 weeks after a GU or GI infection and, less commonly, after a respiratory infection. Quite often, the underlying infection is largely or completely resolved. The presentation is usually with an acute onset of malaise, fatigue, and fever. Lower extremity arthritis is usually unilateral and involves the knee. More diffuse joint stiffness is reported involving knees, ankles, feet, and wrists. LBP will be commonly reported as well as heel pain and plantar fasciitis signs and symptoms.

Diagnostic Testing

Diagnostic testing is aimed at finding the underlying cause, such as appropriate bacterial urethral or urine testing or stool cultures. If there is fluid in a joint, cultures of joint aspirates in ReA typically have negative results. Because this is an inflammatory condition, ESR is elevated, but this is not particularly sensitive or specific for the condition.

Laboratory tests for rheumatic disease, such as ANA and RF analyses, are not affected by the disease; checking these laboratory markers is not necessary unless the diagnosis of RA or SLE is in question.

Treatment

Most cases of ReA are self-limited and will require no treatment other than symptomatic and supportive care. ReA treatment includes the use of anti-inflammatory drugs such as NSAIDs or systemic corticosteroids. A short course of systemic corticosteroids, such as prednisone, should utilize a low dose, while prolonged treatment should be avoided due to potential adverse effects. Corticosteroid injections in the affected joints can be considered to reduce inflammation. The use of DMARDs can be considered for those with chronic symptoms. Nonbiological DMARDs can include sulfasalazine and methotrexate, while biological DMARDs can include the TNF blockers etanercept or infliximab. Expert consultation is advised.

Because ReA usually occurs weeks after infection, especially when associated with infectious diarrhea, antimicrobial therapy is of limited benefit. However, when ReA occurs with urethritis, the use of an antibiotic can shorten the duration of symptoms. Urethritis can be treated with oral doxycycline for 7 days or a single dose of oral azithromycin. Alternative treatments include 7 days of oral erythromycin, ofloxacin, or levofloxacin. No change in symptoms is usually seen with antibiotic use if infectious diarrhea was the precipitating event.

Discussion Sources

Lozada CJ. Reactive arthritis. Medscape. http://emedicine.medscape.com/article/331347-overview

Schmitt SK. Reactive arthritis. *Infect Dis Clin North Am*. 2017;31:265–277.

QUESTIONS

165. A 22-year-old man presents with new-onset pain in his feet and ankles and conjunctivitis, oral lesions, and dysuria. To help confirm a diagnosis of ReA, the most important test to obtain is:

    A. ANA analysis.

    B. ESR measurement.

    C. rubella titer measurement.

    D. urethral swab or urinary test for select infection.

166. Symptoms commonly associated with ReA include all of the following except:

    A. dactylitis.

    B. bursitis.

    C. enthesitis.

    D. cervicitis.

167. Treatment for ReA (also known as Reiter's syndrome) in a 24-year-old man with urethritis usually includes:

    A. antimicrobial therapy.

    B. corticosteroid therapy.

    C. antirheumatic medications.

    D. immunosuppressive drugs.

168. In reference to ReA (also known as Reiter's syndrome), which of the following statements is false?

    A. When the disease is associated with urethritis, the male-to-female ratio is about 9:1.

    B. When the disease is associated with infectious diarrhea, the male and female incidences are approximately equal.

    C. ANA analysis reveals a speckled pattern.

    D. Results of joint aspirate culture are usually unremarkable.

169. In men with ReA and associated urethritis, a common finding is:

    A. ANA positive.

    B. HLA-B27 positive.

    C. RF positive.

    D. ACPA positive.

170. Which of the following antimicrobial agents is most appropriate to treat ReA in a sexually active man with no report of recent acute diarrheal episode?

    A. amoxicillin

    B. doxycycline

C. trimethoprim-sulfamethoxazole (TMP-SMX)

D. antimicrobial therapy not necessary

For answers and rationales, see end of chapter.

Osteoporosis

Overview

Osteoporosis is a disorder of bone thinning in which bone absorption exceeds bone formation to the degree that bone density is insufficient to meet skeletal needs. Osteoporosis is also defined as bone density more than 2.5 standard deviations below the average bone mass for a healthy young adult. For every reduction of bone mass by one standard deviation, the relative risk of fracture rises by 1.5-fold to 3-fold (Fig. 10-9).

Estrogen deficiency is a potent risk factor, and osteoporosis is most common in postmenopausal women; by age 80 years, the average woman has lost more than 30% of her premenopausal bone density. Men appear to be at significantly less risk; this is partly because of inherently greater bone density. Body habitus and ethnicity can influence the risk of osteoporosis; the condition is most common in small-framed women of Asian and European ancestry, who usually have lower bone density in adulthood. At the same time, all ethnic groups are at risk.

Additional risk factors for osteoporosis include select disorders involving the endocrine, GI, and central nervous systems as well as rheumatological, autoimmune, and hematological diseases; inactivity; and prolonged therapy with certain medications, including select anticonvulsants, excessive amounts of thyroid hormones, and systemic corticosteroids (Box 10-1).

> **CLINICAL CONCEPT**
> Obesity appears to minimize osteoporosis risk, in part because of high endogenous estrogen production by fatty tissue and increased bone weight-bearing.

Clinical Presentation

Early disease usually does not have symptoms, but backache is commonly reported. Although hip fracture is often the first clinical manifestation of osteoporosis, it usually indicates advanced disease, as does loss of terminal adult height. Hip, wrist, and spinal fractures most commonly occur, but all bones are at risk.

Diagnostic Testing

Many tests are available to evaluate osteoporosis risk or detect progression of the disease (see Box 10-1). Dual-energy x-ray absorptiometry (DXA) is considered a reliable measure. Qualitative CT is precise but

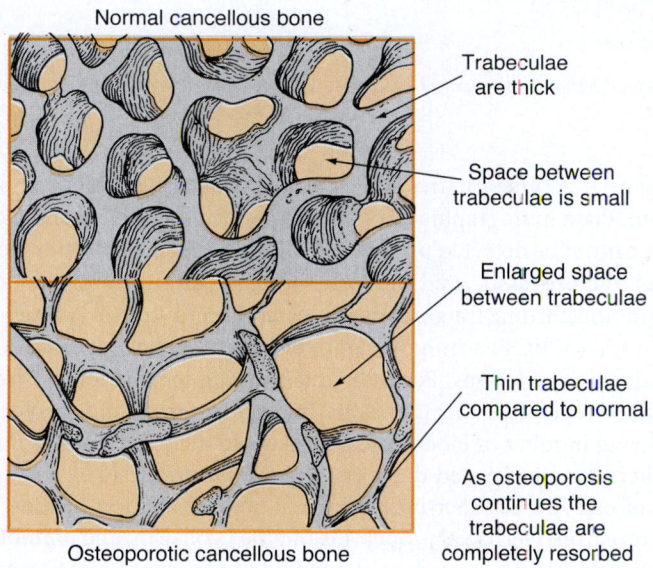

Normal cancellous bone

Trabeculae are thick

Space between trabeculae is small

Enlarged space between trabeculae

Thin trabeculae compared to normal

As osteoporosis continues the trabeculae are completely resorbed

Osteoporotic cancellous bone

FIGURE 10-9 Osteoporosis.
Venes D. Taber's Cyclopedic Medical Dictionary. 21st ed. Philadelphia, PA: F.A. Davis; 2009.

BOX 10-1 Osteoporosis: Risks, Screening Guidelines, and Treatment

Risk Factors for Osteoporosis

- Lifestyle factors (e.g., physical inactivity, low calcium intake, alcohol abuse)
- Genetic factors (e.g., cystic fibrosis, Gaucher disease)
- Hypogonadal states (e.g., androgen insensitivity, hyperprolactinemia)
- Endocrine disorders (e.g., diabetes mellitus, adrenal insufficiency)
- Gastrointestinal disorders (e.g., celiac disease, inflammatory bowel disease)
- Hematological disorders (e.g., multiple myeloma, leukemia)
- Rheumatological and autoimmune disorders (e.g., rheumatoid arthritis, lupus)
- Central nervous system disorders (e.g., epilepsy, multiple sclerosis)
- Miscellaneous other conditions and diseases (e.g., AIDS/HIV, congestive heart failure)
- Use of certain medications (e.g., long-term corticosteroid medications, some anticonvulsants, thyroid hormones)

Recommendations for Osteoporosis Screening

- Women aged 65 and older and men aged 70 and older, regardless of risk factors
- Younger postmenopausal women, women in the menopausal transition, and men aged 50 to 69 with clinical risk factors for fracture
- A woman or man after age 50 years who has broken a bone
- Adults with a condition (e.g., rheumatoid arthritis) or taking a medication (e.g., long-term glucocorticoid) associated with low bone mass or bone loss

Available Screening Tests for Osteoporosis

- Dual-energy x-ray absorptiometry (DXA) of the hip and spine. Using DXA to measure bone density of the hand, wrist, forearm, and heel also seems to detect women who are at increased risk for fracture
- Other tests to measure bone mineral density: Ultrasound, radiographic absorptiometry, single-energy x-ray absorptiometry, peripheral DXA, and peripheral quantitative computed tomography

Osteoporosis Treatment

All to be used with appropriate calcium and vitamin D supplementation

- Bisphosphonates, such as alendronate, ibandronate, risedronate, and zoledronic acid; consider drug holiday after 5 years (low-risk patients) or 10 years (high-risk patients) of treatment
- Other antiresorptive medications including selective estrogen receptor modulators (SERMs), such as raloxifene, calcitonin, estrogen, and RANK ligand inhibitor (denosumab)
- Bone-forming (anabolic) medications such as teriparatide (parathyroid hormone)
- Perform bone mineral density testing 1 to 2 years after initiating treatment for osteoporosis and every 2 years thereafter; more frequent testing may be warranted in certain patients

Source: Cosman F, de Beur SJ, LeBoff MS, et al. Clinician's guide to prevention and treatment of osteoporosis. Osteoporos Int. 2014;25(10):2359. https://cdn.nof.org/wp-content/uploads/2016/01/995.pdf

uses more radiation than DXA. Quantitative ultrasound is relatively inexpensive and can be performed with portable equipment. Plain radiographic films should not be used for screening or evaluation of osteoporosis because disease cannot be detected until 40% to 50% of bone mass is lost. However, plain films can be helpful in diagnosing fractures associated with osteoporosis. MRI is useful in detecting various types of fractures, including acute and chronic fractures of the vertebrae and stress fractures of the proximal femur. Single photon emission CT (SPECT) scanning can offer superior image contrast of the bony structures as well as accurate localization of lesions. For individuals taking medications to treat osteoporosis, bone density scanning should be repeated 1 to 2 years after initiating therapy and then every 2 years thereafter.

There are also a growing number of biochemical markers that can help assess bone formation or bone resorption. These markers can be elevated during high bone turnover states and can help monitor early response to treatment of osteoporosis. Serum markers of bone formation include bone-specific alkaline phosphatase, osteocalcin, carboxyterminal propeptide of type I collagen, and aminoterminal propeptide of type I collagen. Urinary markers of bone resorption include hydroxyproline, free and total pyridinolines, and free and total deoxypyridinolines.

Treatment

Primary prevention of osteoporosis includes ensuring the development of maximal adult bone density. In patients with osteoporosis, the bone loss is from the baseline bone density. A small amount of loss can be of great significance against poor bone density but of little consequence with greater density. Because maximal bone density is achieved in the early adult years, encouraging adequate calcium intake and weight-bearing exercise throughout the teen and adult years is important. According to the recommendations from the National Osteoporosis Foundation (NOF), the calcium intake goal should be the equivalent of 1,000 mg/day for men between 50 and 70 years of age, and the dose should be 1,200 mg/day for women 51 years and older and men older than age 70 years. Vitamin D (minimal dose 800 to 1,000 IU daily) is recommended for all adults older than age 50 years, with higher doses needed for those with vitamin D deficiency. Foods should be one source of this important micronutrient, although few foods are abundant vitamin D sources. Exposing the skin to sunlight is the most important vitamin D source because the body readily synthesizes this nutrient in response to sunlight. Dietary calcium should be the primary source of calcium from dairy and nondairy options (e.g., spinach, sardines, tofu, select nuts, others). Given current lifestyles and dietary habits, supplements are often needed to meet recommended requirements.

When taken with calcium supplements, postmenopausal hormone therapy (estrogen supplementation with or without a progestin) can help reduce the risk of postmenopausal fracture by up to 34% by minimizing further bone loss; the benefit must be balanced against the noted increased risk of breast cancer and other problems with short-term and long-term use. A selective estrogen receptor modulator (SERM) such as raloxifene (Evista®) helps preserve bone density. Because raloxifene does not attach to estrogen receptor sites in the breast or uterus, a SERM is often considered an alternative to hormone therapy. The parathyroid hormone (PTH) teriparatide (Forteo®) is an anabolic agent that can reduce the risk of vertebral fractures by 65% in patients with osteoporosis. This treatment is typically reserved for women with very low bone density or who have had a prior fracture. Treatment with teriparatide should be limited to a 2-year duration because of a potentially increased risk of osteosarcoma.

Bisphosphonates such as alendronate (Fosamax®), ibandronate (Boniva®), risedronate (Actonel®), and zoledronic acid (Reclast®) inhibit the resorptive activity of osteoclasts, can help modestly increase bone mass, and can significantly reduce fracture risk. To minimize the risk of drug-induced esophagitis, patients taking an oral bisphosphonate should be cautioned to take the medication in the morning with a full glass of water. At least 30 minutes must elapse before food, other liquids, or medications are ingested. In addition, patients should remain upright for at least 1 hour. Zoledronic acid is administered as an IV infusion once a year to treat osteoporosis or every 2 years to prevent osteoporosis. In rare cases, low-trauma atypical femoral fractures have been associated with long-term use of bisphosphonates (i.e., more than 5 years). Pain in the thigh or groin area often precedes these fractures. The most robust effects of bisphosphonates occur during the first 5 years of treatment.

The duration of therapy and the drug holiday should be based on fracture risk, with low-risk patients considering stopping treatment after 5 years and remaining off treatment as long as bone mineral density (BMD) is stable. Higher-risk patients can be treated for 10 years and have a drug holiday of no more than 1 to 2 years with consideration of a nonbisphosphonate treatment during that time.

Calcitonin (Miacalcin® or Fortical®) is another antiresorptive medication that is most helpful in building vertebral bone. The U.S. Food and Drug Administration (FDA) advises that the risks associated with calcitonin use outweigh the benefits in treating osteoporosis, largely based on two large studies indicating slightly higher rates of malignancy among patients taking this significant. The FDA supports the continued use of these agents because these medications provide an important option for patients who do not tolerate other treatments.

Denosumab (Prolia®) is a receptor activator of nuclear factor kappa-B ligand (RANKL) inhibitor that reduces the incidence of vertebral fractures by about 68% in patients with osteoporosis. It is given as a subcutaneous injection every 6 months. Romosozumab (Evenity™) is an antibody that inhibits sclerostin, thus increasing bone formation and decreasing bone resorption. It is given as a monthly subcutaneous injection. With all therapies, calcium supplementation should be continued, and vitamin D deficiency should be appropriately treated.

CLINICAL CONCEPT

The bisphosphonates provide a degree of antifracture reduction benefit even when treatment is discontinued; some authorities recommend a drug holiday after 5 to 10 years of therapy.

Discussion Sources

Cosman F, de Beur, SJ, LeBoff MS, et al. Clinician's guide to prevention and treatment of osteoporosis. *Osteoporos Int.* 2014;25(10): 2359. https://cdn.nof.org/wp-content/uploads/2016/01/995.pdf

Watts NB, Diab DL. Long-term use of bisphosphonates in osteoporosis. *J Clin Endocrin Metab.* 2011;95:1555–1565. https://academic .oup.com/jcem/article/95/4/1555/2596477

QUESTIONS

171. All of the following are common sites of fracture in patients with osteoporosis except:

A. the proximal femur.

B. the distal forearm.

C. the vertebrae.

D. the clavicle.

172. Osteoporosis is more common in individuals:

A. with recurrent UTIs.

B. on long-term systemic corticosteroid therapy.

C. who are obese.

D. of African ancestry.

173. Clinical disorders that increase the risk for osteoporosis include all of the following except:

A. RA.

B. celiac disease.

C. hyperlipidemia.

D. hyperprolactinemia.

174. Osteoporosis is defined as having a bone density more than _____ standard deviation(s) below the average bone mass for a healthy young adult.

A. 1

B. 1.5

C. 2.5

D. 4

175. The preferred screening test for osteoporosis is:

A. quantitative ultrasound measurement.

B. DXA.

C. qualitative CT.

D. wrist, spine, and hip radiographs.

176. Osteoporosis prevention measures include all of the following except:

A. calcium supplementation.

B. SERM use.

C. vitamin B_6 supplementation.

D. weight-bearing and muscle-strengthening exercises.

177. All of the following are common signs of osteoporosis except:

A. gradual loss of height with stooped posture.

B. hip or wrist fracture.

C. increase in waist circumference.

D. patient report of back pain.

178. A 52-year-old woman states that she is concerned about osteoporosis and asks about taking calcium supplements. The NP counsels that the recommended daily calcium intake for a woman her age should be:

A. 800 mg.

B. 1,000 mg.

C. 1,200 mg.

D. 1,500 mg.

179 to 183. Indicate (*Yes or No*) whether each of the following nondairy foods is considered a good source of calcium.

_____ **179.** Tofu

_____ **180.** Potato

_____ **181.** Spinach

_____ **182.** Brown rice

_____ **183.** Sardines

184. Long-term bisphosphonate treatment (i.e., more than 5 years) has been associated with:

A. atypical fractures.

B. hyperprolactinemia.

C. OA.

D. bone marrow suppression.

185. Alice, a 68-year-old woman with no history of fracture, is diagnosed with osteoporosis following DXA and is initiated on bisphosphonate treatment. The NP recommends repeated bone density assessment in:

A. 3 months.

B. 6 months.

C. 2 years.

D. 5 years.

186. For Alice in the previous question, a drug holiday from bisphosphonate therapy should be considered after:

A. 1 year.

B. 2 years.

C. 5 years.

D. 10 years.

187. The drug calcitonin should be approached with caution in osteoporosis therapy due to a possible increased risk of which of the following?

A. type 2 diabetes

B. RA

C. malignancy

D. SLE

188. Which of the following patients would be an appropriate candidate for treatment with teriparatide (Forteo®)?

A. a 54-year-old woman with osteopenia

B. a 64-year-old woman with a BMD T-score of –2.9 and prior hip fracture

C. a 67-year-old man with a BMD T-score of –1

D. a 72-year-old woman who has a stable BMD T-score of –1.5 with bisphosphonate treatment for the past 3 years

189. In counseling a postmenopausal woman, you advise her that systemic estrogen therapy users can possibly experience:

A. an increase in breast cancer rates with long-term use.

B. a reduction in high-density lipoprotein cholesterol.

C. a 10% increase in bone mass.

D. no change in the occurrence of osteoporosis.

190. When counseling a patient taking a bisphosphonate such as alendronate (Fosamax®), you advise that the medication should be taken with:

A. a bedtime snack.

B. a meal.

C. other medications.

D. a large glass of water.

For answers and rationales, see end of chapter.

Sprains

Overview

A sprain is a partial or complete injury of a ligament either within the ligament body or at its site of attachment to the bone. Inversion injuries of the ankle cause about 85% of all sprains and are the most common injury sustained while jumping or running. Sprains can also involve the wrist, elbow, and knee. Wearing appropriate footwear, improved conditioning, warm-up exercises, and taping can be helpful in avoiding sprains. Footwear that increases ankle stability includes high-top shoes as well as lace-up or Velcro ankle braces. Supportive shoes will have a firm heel support, a wide toe box, and a rigid or semirigid shank.

> **CLINICAL CONCEPT**
> Sandals, flip flops, and high-heeled shoes offer little ankle stability, while wearing thick-soled shoes can also increase the risk of ankle sprains.

Clinical Presentation

Ankle sprains are often graded according to presentation and proposed underlying degree of ligamentous injury (see Table 10-9). The ankle anterior drawer test is used to assess for excessive laxity of the tibiotarsal joint. Excessive anterior motion is usually seen with a grade III sprain. Immobilization is important in helping appropriate healing and minimizing sequelae. Grades II and III injuries are occasionally associated with persistent joint laxity and a risk of future sprain.

Diagnostic Testing

The decision on the use of plain radiographs to diagnose an ankle sprain should be guided by the Ottawa Ankle Rules criteria. The criteria recommend an ankle radiographic series is necessary only if the patient experiences pain in the malleolar zone along with any one of the following three criteria: bone tenderness at the posterior edge or tip of the lateral malleolus (lower 6 cm of the fibula), bone tenderness at the posterior edge or tip of the medial malleolus, or inability to bear weight immediately after the injury and in the emergency department. An MRI is not indicated for ankle sprains unless there is an unusual feature, such as extensive swelling or ecchymosis.

Treatment

The goal of initial ankle sprain therapy is to decrease pain and swelling by early use of RICE therapy. Patients should avoid activities that increase pain or swelling, while ice should be applied for 15 to 20 minutes three times daily. Patients can use an ACE wrap or elastic ankle sleeve for support, while elevating the ankle above heart level when possible. This will also protect ligaments from further injury. The injured ankle should not bear weight for the first 24 hours after the sprain and even longer depending on the severity of the sprain. Grade II sprains may require an immobilizer or splint, whereas a grade III sprain treatment often requires a short leg cast or a cast-brace for 2 to 3 weeks. Although rarely needed, surgical reconstruction is possible for grade III sprains.

TABLE 10-9 Ligamentous Sprains: Grading, Presentation, and Intervention

GRADE OF INJURY	PATHOLOGY AND PRESENTATION	INTERVENTION
Grade I	Slight stretching or microscopic tear No instability	RICE (rest, ice, compression, elevation) Immobilizer Limit weight-bearing Analgesia Length of disability usually limited to a few days
Grade II	Partial ligamentous tear Moderate joint instability Moderate swelling Mild to moderate ecchymosis	RICE Immobilizer Limit weight-bearing Analgesia Length of disability usually several weeks to a few months Orthopedic referral
Grade III	Complete ligamentous tear Complete ankle instability Significant swelling Moderate to severe ecchymosis	RICE Immobilizer Limit weight-bearing Analgesia Length of disability may be many months

Sources: Anderson B. Office Orthopedics for Primary Care: Diagnosis. *Philadelphia, PA: Saunders; 2006; Anderson B.* Office Orthopedics for Primary Care: Treatment. *3rd ed. Philadelphia, PA: Saunders; 2006; Turner S. Musculoskeletal system. In: Goolsby M, Grubbs L, eds.* Advanced Assessment: Interpreting Findings and Formulating Differential Diagnoses. *2nd ed. Philadelphia, PA: F.A. Davis; 2011:411–449.*

Discussion Sources

Anderson B. *Office Orthopedics for Primary Care: Diagnosis*. Philadelphia, PA: Saunders Elsevier; 2006.
Anderson B. *Office Orthopedics for Primary Care: Treatment*. 3rd ed. Philadelphia, PA: Saunders Elsevier; 2006.
Turner S. Musculoskeletal system. In: Goolsby M, Grubbs L, eds. *Advanced Assessment: Interpreting Findings and Formulating Differential Diagnoses*. 4th ed. Philadelphia, PA: F.A. Davis; 2018:435–476.

QUESTIONS

191. The most common site of sprain is the:
    A. wrist.
    B. shoulder.
    C. ankle.
    D. knee.

192. Risk factors for an ankle sprain include all of the following except:
    A. poor conditioning.
    B. running on paved surfaces.
    C. inappropriate footwear.
    D. lack of a warm-up period prior to exercising.

193. Footwear designed to minimize the risk of ankle sprains will include all of the following characteristics except:
    A. firm heel support.
    B. rigid or semirigid shank.

C. laces above the ankle.

D. narrow toe box.

194. A grade II ankle sprain is best described as:

A. minor swelling and minimal joint instability.

B. moderate joint instability without swelling or ecchymosis.

C. moderate swelling, mild to moderate ecchymosis, and moderate joint instability.

D. complete ankle instability, significant swelling, and moderate to severe ecchymosis.

195. A person with a grade III ankle sprain presents with:

A. minor swelling and minimal joint instability.

B. moderate joint instability without swelling or ecchymosis.

C. moderate swelling, mild to moderate ecchymosis, and moderate joint instability.

D. complete ankle instability, significant swelling, and moderate to severe ecchymosis.

196. Patients with a grade III ankle sprain should be advised that full recovery is likely to take:

A. a few days.

B. 2 to 3 weeks.

C. 4 to 6 weeks.

D. many months.

197. Which of the following is usually not part of treatment of a sprain?

A. immobilization

B. applying ice to the area

C. joint rest

D. local corticosteroid injection

198. For a grade I ankle sprain, weight-bearing should be avoided:

A. for at least 24 hours.

B. for at least 72 hours.

C. for at least 1 week.

D. until full ROM is restored.

199. A short leg cast is often needed for what type of ankle sprain?

A. Grade I

B. Grade II

C. Grade III

D. Grade IV

For answers and rationales, see end of chapter.

Fibromyalgia

Overview

Fibromyalgia is a common, complex disorder composed of a specific set of signs and symptoms that likely affects at least 2% of the general population; the condition is one of the most common central pain-related syndromes. Although its etiology is not fully understood, central nervous system dysfunction and central sensitization are likely the source of the multiple clinical findings associated with this condition. Biochemical changes noted in the central nervous system in a person with fibromyalgia include low serotonin levels, elevated levels of substance P, and other biological markers; these changes likely contribute to the diffuse hypersensitivity to pain signals in the brain.

In other cases, symptoms can gradually develop over time with no apparent triggering event. Genetic factors likely play a role.

Fibromyalgia is four to seven times more common in women than in men; the reason for this finding is not understood. Symptom onset is usually between ages 20 and 55 years. Fibromyalgia is found in all ethnic groups. The presence of RA or lupus increases the risk for fibromyalgia.

CLINICAL CONCEPT
Fibromyalgia symptoms sometimes begin after a physical trauma, surgery, infection, or significant psychological stress.

Clinical Presentation

The diagnosis is made after careful consideration of the patient's health history and physical examination. According to the ACR criteria, the diagnosis of fibromyalgia can be made through a combination of the widespread pain index (WPI) and symptom severity (SS) score. The WPI evaluates 19 body regions in which pain has been experienced during the past week. For the SS score, the patient ranks four symptoms (fatigue, waking unrefreshed, cognitive symptoms, and somatic symptoms) on a scale of 0 to 3. A diagnosis of fibromyalgia is made with a WPI score of at least 7 and an SS score of at least 5, or a WPI score of 3 to 6 and an SS score of at least 9. The tenderness is triggered at the area where pressure, enough to cause the examiner's nailbed to blanch, or about 4 kg pressure, is applied, and there is no referred pain. The pain is often migratory and usually described as burning, aching, soreness, or feeling bruised (without objective evidence of bruising).

Additional patient symptoms often include chronic GI problems, including intermittent diarrhea and constipation, cognitive changes, and/or altered mood. The patient usually presents with a complaint of persistent fatigue combined with nonrefreshing sleep. Many with fibromyalgia also have tension headaches, temporomandibular joint disorder, irritable bowel syndrome, anxiety, and/or depression.

Diagnostic Testing

No particular test is diagnostic for fibromyalgia. Though there are no disease-specific abnormalities noted with laboratory testing, routine laboratory tests can be performed to rule out other conditions with similar manifestations. Routine testing should include CBC with differential, metabolic panel, and urinalysis. ESR, used to measure inflammation, is usually normal in patients with fibromyalgia. Testing for thyroid-stimulating hormone (TSH), 25-hydroxy vitamin D, and vitamin B_{12} can be considered as abnormal levels are associated with fatigue and muscle pain. Iron deficiency is common in fibromyalgia, though anemia of chronic disease is not typically found. Routine imaging is not recommended in fibromyalgia as images would generally show normal findings.

Treatment

Intervention in fibromyalgia is complex and requires a comprehensive, interdisciplinary approach; simply attempting to treat the pain associated with the condition is inadequate. Patient education should include information about the need for physical activity, such as flexibility exercises, progressive stretching, and low-impact activities such as aquatic exercise, which has been shown to reduce pain and increase function. Exercise programs that involve high-intensity and high-impact components such as running or jogging, although not contraindicated, are generally poorly tolerated by the person with fibromyalgia. Stress management techniques can be helpful, and getting sufficient sleep is essential for those with fibromyalgia. Those with fibromyalgia should be encouraged to maintain a healthy lifestyle, including eating healthy foods, limiting caffeine intake, and participating in enjoyable and fulfilling activities each day.

Pharmacotherapy can be used to reduce pain and improve sleep. Trigger point injection has been noted to be helpful in certain patients. Acetaminophen and NSAIDs can be used to alleviate pain, although their effectiveness varies. Medications such as trazodone can be helpful in improving sleep latency and duration. Antidepressants (such as nortriptyline, duloxetine [Cymbalta®], or milnacipran [Savella®]) and antiepileptics (including gabapentin [Neurontin®] and pregabalin [Lyrica®]) have been shown to minimize symptoms in fibromyalgia and numerous other chronic pain conditions; these medications can be helpful in treating the concomitant altered mood that often accompanies, but is not the cause of, fibromyalgia. Some of these medications, particularly the tricyclic antidepressants, help promote sleep. Pregabalin, milnacipran, and duloxetine are approved by the FDA for pain reduction in fibromyalgia. Consistent use of topical treatments such as capsaicin are often helpful treatment adjuncts.

Discussion Sources

Gilliland RP. Rehabilitation and fibromyalgia. Medscape. http://emedicine.medscape.com/article/312778-overview

Mayo Clinic Staff. Fibromyalgia. https://www.mayoclinic.org/diseases-conditions/fibromyalgia/symptoms-causes/syc-20354780

Wolfe F, Clauw DL, Fitzcharles MA, et al. 2016 revisions to the 2010/2011 fibromyalgia diagnostic criteria. *Semin Arthritis Rheum.* 2016;46:319–329.

QUESTIONS

200. Fibromyalgia is caused by:

    A. increased production of serotonin.

    B. an autoimmune reaction following infection.

    C. a genetic autoimmune disorder that targets neuronal axons.

    D. biochemical changes in the central nervous system.

201. Which of the following statements is most consistent with fibromyalgia?

    A. It is predominantly diagnosed in individuals of African ancestry.

    B. It affects less than 1% of the general population.

    C. It is four to seven times more common in women than in men.

    D. It is most often initially diagnosed in adults younger than 20 years old and older than 55 years old.

202. Fibromyalgia is more common in patients with:

    A. type 2 diabetes.

    B. RA and SLE.

    C. migraine headaches.

    D. chronic obstructive pulmonary disorder (COPD).

203. Which of the following is inconsistent with the clinical presentation of fibromyalgia?

    A. widespread body aches

    B. joint swelling

    C. fatigue

    D. cognitive changes

204. The diagnosis of fibromyalgia involves:

    A. a CT scan of the head.

    B. MRI of various joints throughout the body.

    C. calculating a WPI and SS score.

    D. a positive ANA or RF test result.

205. When examining a patient with fibromyalgia, tender points:

    A. are located only above the waist.

    B. can be identified by applying enough pressure to blanch the nailbed of the examiner.

    C. are easily identified through radiography.

    D. can wax and wane throughout the day.

206. The ACR SS score includes assessments of all of the following except:

    A. fatigue.

    B. waking unrefreshed.

    C. a 6-minute walking distance.

    D. cognitive symptoms.

207. When discussing physical activity with a 40-year-old woman with fibromyalgia, you advise that:

    A. limiting exercise is an important component of symptom management.

    B. weight-bearing exercise would be most helpful.

    C. physical activity aimed at increasing flexibility is an important part of treatment.

    D. although possibly helpful in minimizing pain, physical activity usually significantly worsens fatigue.

208. Analgesic approaches used in the management of fibromyalgia include all of the following except:

    A. acetaminophen.

    B. NSAIDs.

    C. a fentanyl patch.

    D. topical capsaicin.

209 to 212. Indicate (*Yes or No*) whether each of the following drug classes can be used to treat symptoms associated with fibromyalgia.

_____ **209.** Tricyclic antidepressants

_____ **210.** Antiepileptics

_____ **211.** SSRIs

_____ **212.** Opioids

213. Patients with fibromyalgia should be encouraged to do all of the following except:

    A. consider adopting a high-intensity aerobic activity such as jogging.

    B. limit caffeine use.

    C. utilize stress management techniques.

    D. participate in a program of exercise focused on maintaining flexibility.

214. Each of the following medications is approved by the FDA for the treatment of fibromyalgia except:

    A. duloxetine (Cymbalta®).

    B. pregabalin (Lyrica®).

    C. phenytoin (Dilantin®).

    D. milnacipran (Savella®).

For answers and rationales, see end of chapter.

Vitamin D Deficiency

Overview

Vitamin D has long been recognized as essential for the efficient utilization of dietary calcium and for bone and muscle health. Recent studies have highlighted this important micronutrient's multiple roles. As an inhibitor of abnormal cellular growth, vitamin D is needed to help with cell differentiation and minimizing abnormal cell proliferation, a key step in cancer development. A stimulator of insulin secretion in response to increased insulin demands, vitamin D plays a role in the maintenance of normoglycemia, possibly minimizing the risk of type 2 diabetes mellitus development. Because vitamin D receptors (VDRs) are expressed by most cells of the immune system, the micronutrient plays an important role as an immunomodulator. When vitamin D is available in physiological amounts, this micronutrient acts as a renin producer, therefore potentially contributing to blood pressure control.

Vitamin D deficiency is a common problem, with studies finding it in 36% of healthy adults aged 18 to 29 in Boston, Massachusetts, by winter's end and in 27% of otherwise healthy Asian ancestry children in the United Kingdom. Additional studies revealed vitamin D deficiency in 57% of patients on a hospital medical ward and in 93% of patients with nonspecific musculoskeletal pain at a Minneapolis pain clinic. Considering this, vitamin D deficiency is a common problem in both the healthy and the sick.

Skin exposure to the sun's rays should supply ≥95% of the daily requirements by triggering the body's natural ability to synthesize this vitamin. The ability of the body's uninduced vitamin D synthesis

CLINICAL CONCEPT

The use of sunscreen, although helpful in minimizing the risk of certain skin cancers and other solar damage, likely increases the risk of vitamin D deficiency.

is determined by a number of factors, including the skin's melanin pigmentation. A person with a darker skin tone will synthesize less vitamin D with sun exposure when compared with a person with a lighter skin tone.

The application of a sunscreen with sun protection factor 8 reduces the capacity of the skin to produce vitamin D by as much as 95%. Obviously, individuals who spend little time outdoors have a significant vitamin D deficiency risk. The time of year and place of residence also influence sun-induced vitamin D synthesis, with winter sun and northern latitudes providing the weakest effect. Even people who are regularly involved in outdoor activities that facilitate exposure to sunshine can have vitamin D deficiency if little skin is exposed to the sun. Exposing the hands, face, arms, or legs daily for about 5 to 15 minutes of sun between the hours of 11 a.m. and 2 p.m. at a strength found in northern latitudes such as Boston will help provide an adequate amount of vitamin D synthesis. This level of sun exposure is unlikely to induce sunburn or increase skin cancer risk. The use of certain medications, including phenytoin (Dilantin®) and phenobarbital, is potentially vitamin D depleting; as a result, patients taking these medications require two to five times the recommended daily amount of vitamin D. Vitamin D deficiency is also common in the presence of hepatic or renal disease after gastric bypass.

In infants and children, severe vitamin D deficiency results in the failure of growing bone to mineralize. The resulting condition is rickets. In contrast, adult bones are no longer growing but are in a state of constant cell renewal and therefore susceptible to problems related to vitamin D deficiency, including persistent, nonspecific musculoskeletal pain. To appreciate this, consider some of the clinical effects of vitamin D deficiency:

◼ Without sufficient amounts of vitamin D, intestinal calcium absorption is inadequate. The resulting calcium deficiency prompts an increase in production and secretion of PTH.

◼ PTH acts at the level of the kidney by facilitating an increase in tubular calcium reabsorption and stimulating renal production of 1,25-dihydroxyvitamin D, the hormonally active form of vitamin D.

◼ With continued deficiency, unusually high levels of PTH allow osteoclast activation so that bone can serve as a calcium source. In addition, the continued presence of high levels of circulating PTH causes phosphate to be wasted via the kidney.

◼ The calcium phosphate product in the circulation decreases and becomes inadequate to mineralize the bone properly, potentially leading to osteopenia and osteoporosis. At the same time, osteoblasts deposit a rubbery collagen matrix layer on the skeleton. This surface cannot provide sufficient structural support. The clinical effect is osteomalacia. This abnormal collagen matrix can absorb fluids and expand. With expansion, pressure builds under the richly innervated periosteal covering.

This process likely, at least in part, explains the origin of the constant dull bone ache often reported in patients with osteomalacia. In these patients, minimal pressure applied with a fingertip on the sternum, anterior tibia, radius, or ulna elicits a painful response. Because vitamin D deficiency symptoms overlap considerably with those of fibromyalgia, one condition is often mistaken for the other.

Clinical Presentation

Vitamin D deficiency has also been long recognized as a cause of muscle weakness and muscle aches and pain in all ages. Aside from osteomalacia and localized bone pain, antigravity muscle weakness, difficulty rising from a chair or walking, and pseudofractures also are noted in the person with vitamin D deficiency. These findings resolve with appropriate treatment. Vitamin D deficiency also contributes to the development of hypocalcemia and hypophosphatemia. In this situation, unless the vitamin D deficiency is addressed, replacing calcium or phosphate alone does not restore the body to homeostasis.

Osteomalacia can occur with severe vitamin D deficiency leading to a softening of the bones. The classic sign is a dull, aching pain originating in the back, pelvis, hips, legs, and ribs. The pain can be worse at night and is aggravated with any pressure to the bone. The condition is also associated with decreased muscle tone and leg weakness that causes individuals to have a slow, waddling gait.

Rickets in children can occur due to inadequate intake of vitamin D. Higher risk can occur in infants fed primarily from breast milk if the mother's vitamin D status is inadequate. Infants with no or low sun exposure as well as those with dark skin can also develop rickets. Characteristic signs include delayed motor milestones, hypotonia, bowing of the long bones, violin case deformity of the chest, and a delay in teeth eruption. Children with rickets also have higher risk of infection due to impaired immune function.

Diagnostic Testing

The preferred test for assessment of vitamin D status is measurement of serum 25-hydroxyvitamin D (25[OH]D). The results of this test are minimally influenced by recent dietary intake or recent sun exposure, and it is considered the most accurate functional indicator of vitamin D stores. Opinions differ on what constitutes vitamin D deficiency. Physiological deficiency is defined as a level of serum 25(OH)D that is sufficiently low to cause an increase in PTH levels. Production and secretion of PTH increases to correct low calcium levels via increased bone turnover and accelerated bone loss, effects that clearly occur later in the disease process. Clinical studies have revealed that increased PTH levels occur with 25(OH)D levels of 20 ng/mL (50 nmol/L). As a result, most laboratories report the normal range to be 20 to 100 ng/mL (50 to 250 nmol/L); however, the preferred minimum level is likely 35 to 40 ng/mL (87.5 to 100 nmol/L). The serum level of the biologically active form of vitamin D, 1,25-dihydroxyvitamin D (1,25[OH]$_2$D), is not an accurate indicator of nutritional vitamin D status because levels of 1,25(OH)$_2$D typically are not altered until vitamin D deficiency is well advanced.

Treatment

The first-line therapy is to avoid vitamin D deficiency. A combination of dietary intake of foods rich in vitamin D in addition to regular periods of skin exposure to the sun should provide the body with an adequate supply of this important micronutrient (Table 10-10). However, with little time spent outdoors and diets replete with highly processed foods, seldom is vitamin D intake and synthesis sufficient to avoid deficiency. Fatty fish and vitamin D–enriched dairy products can supply a small amount of the estimated 3,000 to 5,000 IU/day of vitamin D$_3$ the body needs.

Vitamin D intake recommendations from the Institute of Medicine suggest 400 IU/day for infants (0 to 12 months), 600 IU/day for individuals 1 to 70 years old, and 800 IU/day for those older than 70 years of age. Pregnant and lactating women should intake 600 IU/day.

Vitamin D$_3$ is the preferred form of the micronutrient for the treatment of vitamin D deficiency and for maintenance of vitamin D levels. Because vitamin D$_3$ is stored in fat and has a long half-life, low-dose (400 to 800 IU per day) vitamin D$_3$ supplementation is not sufficient to correct a deficiency. Approximately 100 IU given daily for

> **CLINICAL CONCEPT**
>
> The average U.S. dietary intake is typically less than 5% of the body's daily requirement.

TABLE 10-10 Dietary and Supplemental Sources of Vitamin D

SOURCE	VITAMIN D CONTENT
Sunlight exposure	~3,000 IU of vitamin D$_3$ after 5 to 10 minutes' exposure to arms and legs (dependent on latitude)
Fortified milk	~100 IU/8 oz, usually vitamin D$_3$
Fortified orange juice	~100 IU/8 oz, vitamin D$_3$
Infant formulas	~100 IU/8 oz, vitamin D$_3$
Fortified yogurts	~100 IU/8 oz, usually vitamin D$_3$
Fortified breakfast cereals	~100 IU per serving, usually vitamin D$_3$
Salmon Fresh, wild (3.5 oz) Fresh, farmed (3.5 oz)	~600 to 1,000 IU of vitamin D$_3$ ~100 to 250 IU of vitamin D$_3$ or D$_2$

Continued

TABLE 10-10 Dietary and Supplemental Sources of Vitamin D–cont'd

SOURCE	VITAMIN D CONTENT
Tuna, canned (3.6 oz)	~230 IU of vitamin D_3
Mackerel, canned (3.5 oz)	~250 IU of vitamin D_3
Cod liver oil (1 tsp)	~400 to 1,000 IU of vitamin D_3
Shitake mushrooms Fresh (3.5 oz) Sun-dried (3.5 oz)	 ~100 IU of vitamin D_2 ~1,600 IU of vitamin D_2
Egg yolk	~20 IU of vitamin D_3 or D_2

3 months will increase the 25(OH)D level by just 1 ng/mL (2.5 nmol/L); considered in multiples of 100 IU, 400 IU taken for 3 months will increase the level by 4 ng/mL (10 nmol/L). Vitamin D_2, generally produced by plants and fungi, is not as readily absorbed and utilized by the body as vitamin D_3, and thus will provide diminished effect in the treatment of vitamin D deficiency.

For treatment of vitamin D deficiency in adults, a dose of 50,000 IU of vitamin D_3 by mouth once per week for at least 8 weeks is advised, with extension of this course to 16 weeks if the initial 25(OH)D level was below 30 ng/mL. For long-term prevention, patients should be given 50,000 IU of vitamin D_3 once or twice per month plus 1,000 to 2,000 IU of vitamin D_3 daily. Consuming a diet rich in vitamin D–containing foods and exposing the skin to a sensible and safe level of sunlight can aid in preventing the condition. A confirmation of vitamin D correction should be obtained after the recommended length of high-dose repletion therapy.

Excessive supplementation, but not excessive sun exposure, can cause vitamin D toxicity, leading to a variety of problems, including calcium deposition into solid organs. This is rarely seen and is usually a consequence of chronic use of ≥10,000 IU/day vitamin D_3.

Discussion Sources

Holick MF. The vitamin D deficiency pandemic: approaches for diagnosis, treatment and prevention. *Rev Endocr Metab Disord*. 2017;18:153–165.

Linus Pauling Institute, Micronutrient Information Center. Vitamin D. http://lpi.oregonstate.edu/mic/vitamins/vitamin-D

Moyad MA. Vitamin D: a rapid review. *Medscape Today News*. http://www.medscape.com/viewarticle/589256

Pilz S, Zittermann A, Trummer C, et al. Vitamin D testing and treatment: a narrative review of the current evidence. *Endocr Connect*. 2019;8:R27–R43.

Tangpricha V, Khazai NB. Vitamin D deficiency and related disorders. Medscape. http://emedicine.medscape.com/article/128762-overview

QUESTIONS

215. Which of the following regarding vitamin D is false?

  A. diminishes secretion of insulin

  B. inhibits abnormal cellular growth

  C. encourages the absorption and metabolism of calcium and phosphorus

  D. contributes to blood pressure control

216. Which of the following provides the most abundant source of vitamin D?

  A. fortified dairy products

  B. fatty fish

  C. exposure of the skin to the sun

  D. leafy green vegetables

217. Which of the following statements is false regarding sunlight exposure and vitamin D production?

A. In the continental United States, summertime exposure to sunlight can produce the majority of the body's requirement for vitamin D.

B. One glass of fortified milk has an equivalent amount of vitamin D as that produced after 10 minutes of exposure to summer sunlight in a healthy, young individual.

C. Use of sunscreen can block the majority of solar-induced vitamin D production.

D. A person with a darker skin tone produces less vitamin D with sun exposure compared with a person with a lighter skin tone.

218. The vitamin D needs for a 36-year-old person who is taking phenytoin are best described as:

A. easily met by a well-balanced diet.

B. equivalent to what is required by other adults in this age group.

C. markedly increased by twofold to fivefold from the age norm.

D. reduced from baseline because of the drug's vitamin D–preserving qualities.

219. Clinical manifestations of vitamin D deficiency include all of the following except:

A. pseudofractures.

B. osteomalacia.

C. antigravity muscle weakness.

D. azotemia.

220. Characteristic signs of rickets in a child would include all of the following except:

A. bowing of the legs.

B. delay in teeth eruptions.

C. delayed motor milestones.

D. scoliosis.

221. An indication of osteomalacia in a 47-year-old woman who resides in an extreme northern latitude would include:

A. a diffuse, erythematous rash over the trunk and upper extremities.

B. capillary refill greater than 2 seconds.

C. pain elicited when applying gentle pressure on the sternum.

D. bowing of the legs.

222. Which precursor of vitamin D is the form that is commonly measured in laboratory tests to determine vitamin D status?

A. vitamin D_2

B. 25-hydroxyvitamin D

C. vitamin D_3

D. 1,25-dihydroxyvitamin D

223. Which of the following provides the least amount of vitamin D?

A. fortified milk (8 oz)

B. fortified orange juice (8 oz)

C. one egg yolk

D. infant formula (8 oz)

224. Which of the following servings of fish (3.5 oz) contains the greatest amount of vitamin D?

A. fresh wild salmon

B. fresh farmed salmon

    C. canned tuna

    D. canned mackerel

225. A child must consume _____ oz of fortified milk each day to receive the recommended 400 IU daily of vitamin D_3.

    A. 8

    B. 16

    C. 32

    D. 48

226. For adults 70 years and younger, what is the recommended daily intake of vitamin D_3?

    A. 200 IU

    B. 400 IU

    C. 600 IU

    D. 1,000 IU

227. The daily amount of vitamin D_3 recommended for pregnant or lactating women is:

    A. 300 IU.

    B. 600 IU.

    C. 1,000 IU.

    D. 1,200 IU.

228. You see a 46-year-old woman diagnosed with vitamin D deficiency with a serum 25-hydroxyvitamin D (25[OH]D) level of 18 ng/mL. Treatment should be initiated with which of the following vitamin D_3 dosing regimens?

    A. 400 IU twice a day

    B. 1,000 IU daily

    C. 10,000 IU twice a week

    D. 50,000 IU weekly

For answers and rationales, see end of chapter.

QUESTION ANSWERS AND RATIONALES

Bursitis

1. Correct: B. joint overuse.

Possessing a knowledge of risk factors for a specific condition can be important in guiding patient care and counseling patients on how to prevent the condition in the future. Joint overuse is the most common cause of acute superficial bursitis (B).

Incorrect:

Other common risk factors for bursitis include trauma or arthritic conditions such as RA and OA. Bacterial infection is a cause of septic bursitis, which occurs much less frequently than bursitis caused by joint overuse (D). Inactivity is not a risk factor for bursitis (A) while fibromyalgia does not impact the bursa in joints (C).

2. Correct: D. oral NSAIDs.

First-line treatment of bursitis would commonly utilize conservative approaches, which can include rest, ice to the affected area, and oral NSAIDs (D). Alternative approaches can be considered if conservative treatment does not provide relief within 4 to 8 weeks.

Incorrect:

Conservative approaches should be considered as the initial treatment approach in bursitis. Cold, rather than heat, to the affected area can provide relief from pain and swelling (B). Rest and elevation of the joint should be encouraged, while weight-bearing exercises should be avoided (C). With an inadequate response to conservative therapy, alternative approaches can include corticosteroid injection (A) or aspiration of bursal fluid.

3. Correct: A. swelling and redness over the affected area.

Presentation of bursitis usually includes complaints of pain at the joint as well as redness and swelling (A).

Incorrect:

In bursitis, the ROM of the joint is usually normal, though it can be limited because of pain (B). Bursitis is not typically associated with nerve impingement (C) or destruction of the joint space (D).

4. Correct: C. localized tenderness under the superomedial angle of the scapula.

Knowledge of the most common presentation of disease is critical for safe clinical practice. Common signs of bursitis include pain, redness, and swelling. In subscapular bursitis, this can include tenderness under the superomedial angle of the scapula over the adjacent rib (C).

Incorrect:

Subscapular bursitis will normally present with full ROM of the shoulder (A) without nerve root impingement (D). Heat over the affected area is not a typical finding (B), though this can occur in the presence of infection (septic bursitis).

5. Correct: A. increased pain from resisted hip abduction.

Signs of bursitis in the hip can include gait disturbance, local tenderness, pain on hip rotation, and pain with resisted hip abduction (A).

Incorrect:

Trochanter bursitis is characterized with normal hip ROM (B) without sciatic nerve pain (C). Heat over the affected area is not a typical finding (D), though this can occur in the presence of infection (septic bursitis).

6. Correct: B. identifying the presence of osteophytes.

Imaging studies are not routinely needed for the diagnosis of bursitis but can be important in ruling out other conditions that can be contributing to the signs and symptoms of disease. Plain radiography is most helpful in identifying osteophytes as well as detecting other bony conditions, such as fractures, that can be causing symptoms (B).

Incorrect:

Plain radiography is not helpful in determining the presence of an infection that can cause septic bursitis (A), nor can it detect the presence of uric acid crystals in bursal fluid (C), typically found in acute gouty episodes. Ultrasonography, rather than plain radiograph, is typically used to help guide the injection site for fluid aspiration (D).

7. Correct: C. ruling out suspected solid tumors.

Imaging studies are not routinely needed for the diagnosis of bursitis but can be important in ruling out other conditions that can be contributing to the signs and symptoms of disease. MRI is helpful in visualizing the entire joint including soft tissue and can help rule out the presence of suspected solid tumors and abscesses (C).

Incorrect:

The presence of RA can be detected by the presence of biomarkers in blood tests and plain radiographs of the joint space (A). Ultrasonography is used to guide the site for corticosteroid injection (B), while a plain radiograph can be used to detect a fracture in the joint (D).

8. Correct: D. soreness at the site of injection.

Corticosteroid injection can provide relief of pain from bursitis when conservative approaches have been inadequate. The procedure is generally well tolerated with the most common adverse effect being soreness at the injection site (D).

Incorrect:

Corticosteroid injection is generally well tolerated with the most common adverse effect being soreness at the injection site. Other adverse effects that can occur on a rare occasion include infection (B), tissue atrophy (A), and inflammatory reaction (C).

9. Correct: A. bursal aspiration.

Conservative treatment approaches can be considered for first-line management of prepatellar bursitis, but the effect can take weeks before relief is appreciated. Bursal aspiration, with or without corticosteroid injection, would offer the most effective approach in providing timely relief of the condition (A).

Incorrect:

Conservative approaches for bursitis include application of ice to the affected area, rest, elevation, and oral NSAIDs. A topical analgesic would have limited effectiveness as it would not likely be able to penetrate to the bursa (B). NSAIDs are preferred over acetaminophen due to the anti-inflammatory effect (C). Knee splinting would not provide relief of pain due to bursitis (D).

10. Correct: C. osteoporosis.

Several other conditions can present similarly to bursitis and should be taken into consideration when making the diagnosis. However, osteoporosis, related to a decrease in bone density and an increased risk of fracture, would not normally present similarly to bursitis (C), such as severe joint pain and swelling.

Incorrect:

Other conditions that can present similarly to bursitis include gout and pseudogout (D), RA (A), cellulitis, soft tissue knee injury, or tendonitis (B). Each of these conditions can present with pain and/or swelling of the joint.

Tendonitis, Tendinopathy, and Tendinosis

11. Correct: B. Tendonitis is the result of a macroscopic or partial tear of the tendon.

When evaluating a patient complaining of tendon pain, health-care providers should be adept at differentiating between tendonitis and tendinosis. Tendinitis is caused by inflammation of the tendon usually through overuse. Tendinosis is caused by degradation of the tendon's collagen from chronic overuse (B).

Incorrect:

Tendonitis frequently occurs with overuse (A) and typically presents with joint stiffness, discomfort, and reduced ROM (D). Applying pressure to the affected tendon can elicit acute, sharp pain (C).

12. Correct: C. bowling.

Rotator cuff tendonitis is frequently associated with repetitive overhead activities. As such, bowling, which involves an underhand motion, would not be associated with rotator cuff tendonitis (C).

Incorrect:

Rotator cuff tendonitis is frequently associated with repetitive overhead activities. These can include repeated throwing motion as used in baseball (D) and football (B) as well as some swimming strokes (A).

13 to 18. Yes or No

13. Correct: No

14. Correct: Yes

15. Correct: Yes

16. Correct: No

17. Correct: Yes

18. Correct: No

Wrist tendonitis occurs with overuse of the joint such as in sports or work-related activities. Inflammation of the tendon is associated with pain over the area as well as swelling (15). The condition is also associated with reduced ROM (14) and sometimes muscle weakness (17). The pain associated with wrist tendonitis is typically limited to the area of the tendon and does not radiate to the shoulder (16). Muscle cramping is not a characteristic finding (13), nor is Dupuytren's contracture (18), which is a slowly progressive hand deformity of unknown cause.

19. Correct: A. clinical presentation.

A diagnosis of tendonitis is usually made from clinical presentation without the need for imaging or laboratory studies in the absence of atypical findings or a report of recent trauma to the area (A).

Incorrect:

Plain radiograph of the affected area can be considered if there is a report of recent trauma to the affected area (B). Plain films will sometimes reveal calcium deposits on the tendon. CT scan and MRI are generally not recommended for routine diagnosis (C), though MRI can be used to detect or rule out soft tissue injury or a suspected tendon tear. There are no routine laboratory tests performed to support a diagnosis of tendonitis (D).

20. Correct: A. tendon rupture.

With Achilles tendonitis, there is an approximately 10% risk of tendon rupture with recurrent episodes (A). Therefore, treatment should include the use of a posterior splint to immobilize the heel. Heel cord stretching exercises and the use of orthotics can prevent recurrence after the acute phase of tendonitis.

Incorrect:

Tendon rupture is a major concern with Achilles tendonitis. The condition is not associated with neurological sequalae (B), stress fracture (C), or bursitis (D).

21. Correct: C. bursitis

Bursitis and tendonitis often occur together and are usually both identified when performing imaging studies (C).

Incorrect:

Rotator cuff tendonitis is not associated with OA (A) or tendon rupture (B). Additionally, arm numbness is not a classic sign of the condition (D), though a dull pain can radiate from the outer arm to several inches below the top of the shoulder.

22. Correct: A. applying ice to the area.

First-line management of biceps tendonitis can include conservative interventions such as limiting or discontinuing the contributing activity and applying ice to the region to control pain and swelling (A).

Incorrect:

Biceps tendonitis can initially be managed with conservative approaches. NSAIDs can be used for pain relief and to reduce inflammation, rather than using a nerve block (D). A local corticosteroid injection can be helpful in tendonitis, but only after initial treatments have provided inadequate response (B). Orthopedic referral is rarely indicated in uncomplicated cases (C).

23. Correct: C. MRI of the shoulder.

For individuals who have no response to initial treatment options, further evaluation is needed to confirm the diagnosis. An MRI will provide the best approach in identifying soft tissue injury as well as in detecting a suspected tendon tear (C).

Incorrect:

After 4 weeks of an inadequate response, further evaluation is needed to confirm the diagnosis prior to changing the management strategy, such as corticosteroid use (A). MRI will provide superior visualization of the joint compared with x-ray (B). An upper arm sling can be used if it offers relief of symptoms, though this will not necessarily help with healing and recovery (D).

24. Correct: D. ESWT

There is growing use of ESWT for the treatment of tendinosis. The procedure applies shock waves to the affected area with the belief that this causes microtrauma to the tendon and promotes the body's natural healing process (D).

Incorrect:

Though the anti-inflammatory effects of NSAIDs and corticosteroid injections can be helpful in the treatment of tendonitis, these agents can actually deter the healing process needed for tendinosis (A, B). Adalimumab, a TNF inhibitor, is often used in the treatment of autoimmune disorders such as RA but is not warranted for the treatment of tendinosis (C).

Epicondylitis

25. Correct: D. decreased hand grip strength.

Common signs and symptoms of lateral epicondylitis (i.e., tennis elbow) include pain over lateral epicondyle that increases with resisted wrist extension and a weakened hand grip on the affected side (D).

Incorrect:

An electric-like pain that is elicited by tapping over the median nerve is characteristic of carpal tunnel syndrome rather than lateral epicondylitis (A). Tennis elbow is not associated with reduced ROM unless limited by the patient's reaction to pain (B). The pain is worse with resisted wrist extension rather than elbow flexion (C).

26. Correct: D. gout.

Lateral epicondylitis typically occurs from repetitive activity and playing sports that use a tight grip. Gout is not a risk factor for this condition (D).

Incorrect:

Activities that can result in lateral epicondylitis include repetitive lifting (A), use of certain tools (C) or playing a sport (B) that requires a tight grip.

27. Correct: D. 95%

Up to 95% of patients with epicondylitis can recover without surgery (D). First-line intervention involves rest and avoidance of the precipitating activity for several weeks.

Incorrect:

The vast majority of patients with epicondylitis will recover without surgery, with the rate of recovery exceeding 35% (A), 50% (B), and 70% (C).

28 to 30. Matching Questions

28. Correct: C. to assess for fracture

29. Correct: B. to assess for tendon tear

30. Correct: A. an option when MRI is not appropriate

Imaging studies are typically not needed in the diagnosis of epicondylitis but can be important in ruling out other conditions. A plain radiograph can be used to detect a bone fracture or tendon calcification (28). MRI can be considered if there is limited response to therapy and can evaluate the extent of a tendon tear (29). An ultrasound can also assess intra-articular pathology and provides an option when MRI is not available or not appropriate for the patient (30).

31. Correct: B. corticosteroid injections.

The use of corticosteroid injections should be considered when first-line approaches result in limited effectiveness after several weeks (B). Though corticosteroid injection can provide rapid short-term relief, this treatment does not impact long-term outcomes of epicondylitis.

Incorrect:

First-line treatment of epicondylitis includes rest, physical therapy, and ensuring the proper use of tools and body mechanics (A). Anti-inflammatories can include the use of topical or oral NSAIDs to provide short-term relief of pain (C). Additionally, a counterforce brace centered over the back of the forearm can alleviate symptoms (D).

32. Correct: C. promote the natural healing process.

Though not completely understood, ESWT is believed to stimulate soft-tissue healing and inhibit pain through an unknown mechanism. Some studies show beneficial results with this treatment in reducing pain, though further study is needed.

Incorrect:

The exact mechanism of ESWT is unknown, but studies suggest some benefits in improving pain in those with epicondylitis. ROM is usually normal in patients with epicondylitis, and any improvement might result from decreased pain (A). The technique will not build forearm strength, though this can occur with physical therapy (B). The mechanism of ESWT is not related to stretching the extensor tendon (D).

33. Correct: D. decreased grip strength.

Typical presentation of medial epicondylitis (i.e., golfer's elbow) includes local epicondylar tenderness, elbow pain,

forearm weakness, pain aggravated with wrist flexion, and decreased grip strength (D).

Incorrect:

A sign of forearm numbness is not typically associated with medial epicondylitis but more likely found with carpal tunnel syndrome (A). Full ROM is possible in medial epicondylitis with limited ROM likely related to the patient's reaction to pain and not specific for this condition (B). Pain is aggravated on wrist flexion rather than elbow flexion (C).

34. Correct: A. soccer.

Medial epicondylitis is often associated with a variety of sports that require repetitive motions and a tight grip. However, soccer is not typically associated with this condition (A).

Incorrect:

Some of the more common activities that are associated with medial epicondylitis include golf (B), archery (C), bowling, and weight lifting (D).

Gouty Arthritis (Gout)

35. Correct: A. obesity.

Recognizing patient risk factors can be critical in the timely diagnosis and management of a condition. Common risk factors for gout include obesity (A), diabetes mellitus, and family history of the condition. The use of certain medications can also increase the risk of gout, including thiazide diuretics, niacin, and aspirin.

Incorrect:

Approximately 90% of individuals with gout are male (B). Joint trauma (D) and RA (C) can be part of the differential diagnosis but are not risk factors for gout.

36. Correct: B. statins.

Certain medications can precipitate a gout episode by causing hyperuricemia. However, the use of statins is not associated with increased risk of gout (B).

Incorrect:

Medications that can increase the risk of gout include thiazide and loop diuretics (C), aspirin (A), cyclosporine (D), and niacin. These medications can cause hyperuricemia, precipitating the formation of urate crystals and causing gout. Alcohol use can also precipitate a gout episode.

37. Correct: C. bacterial cellulitis.

Secondary gout can be caused by conditions that affect purine catabolism or turnover. However, bacterial infection is not correlated with the development of gout (C).

Incorrect:

Comorbid conditions that reduce purine catabolism and turnover can contribute to hyperuricemia and the development of gout. These can include inflammatory conditions such as psoriasis (A) as well as conditions that reduce urate excretion, such as in chronic kidney disease (D). Hemolytic anemia can cause hyperuricemia and trigger a gout episode (B).

38. Correct: B. greatest swelling and pain along the median aspect of the joint.

The most common site of gout is the metacarpophalangeal joint of the great toe. The condition has a rapid onset with the great toe reddened and swollen, with the greatest swelling occurring along the median aspect of the joint (B).

Incorrect:

An acute gout episode typically has a rapid onset (A), and symptoms do not improve with rest (C). The joint can be red, warm, and swollen, but systemic fever is not a usual sign of the condition (D). If fever is present, the patient should be evaluated for septic arthritis or other bacterial infection.

39. **Correct: C. analysis of aspirate from the affected joint.**

    A definitive diagnosis of gout involves evaluation of joint aspirate fluid that should reveal needle-like intracellular and extracellular crystals (C).

    Incorrect:

    For a patient with acute gout, ESR and CRP are usually elevated due to inflammation, but this is not a specific or sensitive test for the condition (A). Serum uric acid levels are usually reduced during an acute episode and so would not be helpful (B). Joint radiography can be performed to rule out other causes of the condition, such as joint trauma, but findings are normal during the early stage of disease (within 1 year of onset) (D). At later stages, radiographic abnormalities can be evident, including the presence of tophi.

40. **Correct: B. naproxen sodium.**

    First-line treatment of an acute gout episode can include the use of NSAIDs, such as naproxen sodium (B), as well as colchicine or systemic corticosteroids.

    Incorrect:

    Aspirin can precipitate a gouty attack and is contraindicated in individuals with a current gout episode (A). Allopurinol (C) and febuxostat (D) are used to prevent future gout episodes but not to treat an acute episode. Typically, these agents are started after at least 6 months of treatment with an NSAID or colchicine to prevent a rapid decline in serum uric acid levels that can trigger or worsen an episode.

41. **Correct: D. nontender, firm nodules located in soft tissue.**

    Tophi are best described as nontender, firm nodules that form on soft tissue, usually on cooler parts of the body such as the outer ear or nasal cartilage. Tophi typically form after multiple gouty episodes.

    Incorrect:

    Tophi form on soft tissue and do not originate on joints (A) or lymph nodes (B). Tophi consist of firm nodules rather than pus-filled abscesses (C).

42. **Correct: A. a 66-year-old patient with a gastric ulcer**

    For an individual with a history of gastric ulcer, the use of oral NSAIDs or systemic corticosteroids should be avoided as this can worsen the gastric ulcer and lead to GI bleeding (A). A corticosteroid injection would be preferred in this situation.

    Incorrect:

    Oral NSAIDs can be used without special precautions in individuals taking a thiazide diuretic (B) or with

diabetes mellitus (C). Though NSAIDs would be used with caution in individuals with chronic alcoholism due to risk of GI bleeding, these agents can generally be used in binge drinkers, though counseling should be provided on the risks associated with binge drinking (D).

43. **Correct: D. the shoulders.**

    Tophi typically form in cooler parts of the body that are more likely to allow precipitation of urate crystals. The shoulders would be an unlikely area for the formation of tophi (D).

    Incorrect:

    Cooler parts of the body that would favor the formation of tophi include the auricles or outer part of the ear (A), elbows (B), extensor surfaces of the hands (C), and nasal cartilage.

44. **Correct: C. hard cheese**

    Foods high in purine should be avoided in individuals with a history of gout. Dairy products, including hard cheese, are not high in purines and would not trigger a gouty episode (C).

    Incorrect:

    Foods that are high in purine and should be avoided in individuals with a history of gout include certain seafoods (A), organ and game meats (B), beans, spinach (D), asparagus, oatmeal, and baker's and brewer's yeasts when taken as supplements.

45 to 47. Indicate prevention (P) or treatment (T)

45. **Correct: Prevention**

46. **Correct: Treatment**

47. **Correct: Prevention**

    During an acute gouty episode, treatment should first focus on reducing inflammation and then treating hyperuricemia. NSAIDs are typically used for treatment, while colchicine (46) is used less commonly due to adverse effects. Because a rapid reduction in serum uric acid can make an episode worse, treatment with an NSAID or colchicine should last at least 6 months before prophylactic agents are used. Prophylaxis can include the use of xanthine oxidase inhibitors, such as allopurinol (47) or febuxostat, which block uric acid production, or the use of probenecid (45), which improves the kidney's ability to remove uric acid in the urine.

48. **Correct: B. converting uric acid to an inert water-soluble metabolite that is readily eliminated from the body.**

    Pegloticase can be considered for individuals who fail to achieve target uric acid levels with prior therapy. The agent contains a uric acid–specific enzyme that catalyzes the oxidation of uric acid to allantoin. This is an inert water-soluble metabolite that is readily eliminated from the body, thereby reducing serum uric acid (B).

    Incorrect:

    Uric acid is a by-product of purines found in nucleic acids in food. Urea is a normal by-product of amino acids found in proteins. Medications that affect the production or conversion of urea would not have an impact on uric acid levels, which is a determinant for the development of gout (A, C). Uric acid is excreted via the kidneys and would not be eliminated through the GI system (D).

49. Correct: C. brewer's yeast
Foods and supplements that contain a high concentration of purines would increase the risk of a gouty episode. Supplements containing brewer's or baker's yeast can increase the risk of gout (C).
Incorrect:
Supplements of vitamin A (A), gingko biloba (B), and glucosamine (D) do not have high levels of purines and are not associated with increasing the risk of a gouty episode.

50. Correct: C. in 6 months.
For an individual with acute gout, a rapid reduction in serum uric acid levels can exacerbate the gouty episode. Therefore, treatment with an NSAID or colchicine should continue for at least 6 months before initiating prophylaxis treatment that aims to reduce serum levels of uric acid (C).
Incorrect:
Gout prophylaxis should not be initiated prior to 6 months of NSAID treatment (A, B), nor should prophylaxis be delayed until a subsequent attack begins (D).

51. Correct: C. testing uric acid levels every 6 months to determine treatment course.
The optimal duration of treatment for gout is undetermined, but treatment should be continued until all signs and symptoms of gout are resolved, including the presence of tophi. According to the American College of Rheumatology guidelines, once this is accomplished, serum uric acid levels should be checked every 6 months to ensure a level below 6 mg/dL is achieved, with treatment adjusted accordingly to meet this target.
Incorrect:
Discontinuation of treatment can be considered once serum uric acid levels are maintained below the target value of less than 6 mg/dL (A). Treatment does not necessarily need to be continued indefinitely once target levels are achieved (D), and switching from probenecid to allopurinol might not be appropriate depending on whether the individual is an overproducer or undersecretor of uric acid (B).

52. Correct: D. calcium pyrophosphate dihydrate
Pseudogout can present similarly as gout but is caused by the formation of calcium pyrophosphate dihydrate crystals (D) rather than uric acid crystals.
Incorrect:
Uric acid crystals are present in gout (A). Calcium oxalate (B) and struvite (C) crystals are commonly found in kidney stones.

53. Correct: C. knee.
Unlike gout that most commonly presents in the big toe, pseudogout most commonly occurs in the knees (C). Other locations can involve the joints of the wrist and ankle.
Incorrect:
The neck (A), big toe (B), and low back (D) are not typically involved in pseudogout.

54. Correct: C. parathyroid.
It is important for clinicians to be aware of risk factors for specific conditions to aid in proper diagnosis and management. Pseudogout is associated with mineral imbalances, such as hemochromatosis, hypercalcemia, and hypomagnesemia, and is linked to hypothyroidism and hyperparathyroidism (C).
Incorrect:
Abnormal activity of the liver (A), kidneys (B), and adrenal glands (D) are not typically associated with the development of pseudogout.

55. Correct: C. x-ray of the affected joint.
Differentiating between gout and pseudogout is essential in ensuring appropriate management strategies are utilized. However, an x-ray of the affected joint will not be useful, as x-rays typically appear normal in early disease (C).
Incorrect:
Several diagnostic approaches can be used to differentiate gout and pseudogout. Analysis of joint fluid can detect the presence and type of crystals causing the condition (B). Blood analysis can detect abnormal levels of minerals linked to pseudogout (A). Abnormal thyroid function has also been associated with pseudogout and would be a useful diagnostic approach (D).

56 to 59. Yes or No

56. Correct: Yes

57. Correct: Yes

58. Correct: No

59. Correct: Yes
Treatment of pseudogout is aimed at relieving pain and improving joint function. First-line treatment can include the use of NSAIDs (56), colchicine (57), or oral corticosteroids (59). Allopurinol, an agent that blocks uric acid production, is used in the treatment of gout but would be ineffective for the treatment of pseudogout (58).

Osteoarthritis

60. Correct: D. DIP joint
Knowledge of the epidemiology and pathophysiology of disease is important in its management. OA most frequently affects the DIP joint of the hand (D). However, the most problematic sites of OA involve the knee and hip joints.
Incorrect:
OA can impact a variety of joints in the body. The most common manifestations involve the DIP and PIP joints in the hand as well as the knee and hip. The wrist (A),

elbows (B), and metacarpophalangeal joints (C) in the hand are less frequently affected by this condition.

61. **Correct: A. widening of the joint space.**
A key finding in OA upon radiographic imaging is a narrowing, rather than widening, of the joint space and increased density of subchondral bone (A). This sometimes creates a "bone on bone" rubbing at the joint.
Incorrect:
Key findings in OA include the development of bone spurs and osteophytes as part of the body's repair process in the joint (C). There is a gradual wearing away of the articular cartilage (B) along with a thickening of the synovial membrane (D). This, consequently, leads to joint space narrowing and eventual bone-on-bone contact.

62. **Correct: A. coarse crepitus, B. joint effusion, and D. knee often locks or a pop is heard**
In knee OA, a coarse crepitus is often found on physical examination, observed as a crackling sound with movement at the joint (A). Joint effusion is common and can impact ROM (B). The knee can also lock or make a popping sound, which would suggest a degenerative meniscal tear (D).
Incorrect:
Physical inspection of the affected knee should reveal smooth, cool joints rather than a joint with redness and warmth (C, E).

63. **Correct: C. osteophytes.**
Long-standing disease will typically find the development of bone spurs or osteophytes upon radiographic evaluation (C). This is the body's natural response to repair the joint.
Incorrect:
Long-standing OA will be apparent upon radiographic evaluation (D), primarily with joint space narrowing and the presence of osteophytes. There is often an increased density of subchondral bone, rather than decreased density (B). Microfractures are not a typical finding in OA (A).

64. **Correct: B. 50%**
Only about 50% of individuals who have radiographic evidence of OA of the knee will report symptoms (B). In many cases, an x-ray is performed for another reason, such as trauma, only to reveal the presence of OA without manifestation of symptoms.
Incorrect:
Only about half of those with radiographic evidence of OA of the knee will report symptoms. This rate is lower than 70% (C) and 95% (D), but higher than 25% (A).

65. **Correct: B. Bouchard's nodes.**
Among elderly patients with OA of the hand, deformities can develop at the affected joints. Bouchard's nodes occur on the PIP joints of the hand (B).
Incorrect:
Similar to Bouchard's nodes, Heberden's nodes form on the DIP joints among elderly patients with OA of the

hand (A). Hallux valgus, also known as a bunion, is a foot deformity located on the first metatarsophalangeal joint (C). Dupuytren's contracture is a hand deformity caused by tightening and thickening of tissue on the palm that can eventually pull and bend one or more fingers (D).

66. **Correct: A. worst symptoms in weight-bearing joints later in the day**
The classic presentation of OA in weight-bearing joints is increased pain and discomfort with use of the joints, typically getting worse as the day progresses (A). There is usually minimal morning stiffness.
Incorrect:
A report of symmetrical early morning stiffness more closely resembles RA (B). The presence of sausage-shaped digits with associated skin lesions is characteristic of psoriatic arthritis (C). Back pain with rest and anterior uveitis more closely resembles findings associated with ankylosing spondylitis (D).

67. **Correct: C. no disease-specific laboratory abnormalities.**
OA is a localized, rather than systemic, condition and is not associated with inflammation. As such, laboratory analyses will typically not yield abnormal findings (C). Diagnosis of OA is most accurately performed with radiographic analysis of the affected joint.
Incorrect:
Elevated ANA is a finding typically seen with RA (D). Elevated CRP as well as ESR is found in the presence of an inflammatory reaction, which is not present with OA (B). Anemia of chronic disease would not be present with OA but is more likely with RA, among other conditions (A).

68. **Correct: A. acetaminophen.**
The use of acetaminophen is an acceptable first-line treatment option for mild OA (A). An agent with anti-inflammatory activity is not needed as inflammation is not a typical part of the disease process.
Incorrect:
Due to the presence of hypertension, NSAIDs such as ibuprofen should be avoided as they can diminish the effect of antihypertensive medications as well as increase cardiovascular disease risk (C). Tramadol and opioid medications should be avoided in mild-to-moderate cases of OA as they are potentially habituating and associated with serious adverse effects (B). Intra-articular corticosteroid injection can offer effective pain relief in larger joints but is typically not considered first-line treatment (D).

69. **Correct: C. quadriceps-strengthening exercises should be performed.**
For individuals with OA of the knee, certain exercises should be encouraged to build muscle strength that supports the knees. These include exercises that strengthen the quadriceps (C).
Incorrect:
For those with OA of the knee, high-impact activities should be avoided to prevent progression of the

condition. Physical activity with low-impact exercises should be encouraged to maintain skeletal muscle strength and flexibility (D). Straight-leg raising is a low-impact exercise that can help to strengthen leg and abdominal muscles (A). Following exercise, ice applied to the joints will offer better pain control than applying heat (B).

70. Correct: D. largely unknown.

As with many nutritional supplements, the mechanism of action of glucosamine and chondroitin is largely unknown (D). Clinical study results with these supplements have largely been mixed, and it is recommended that several months of consistent use are needed to observe any effect. AAOS does not recommend the use of these supplements for symptom relief of OA of the knee.

Incorrect:

The mechanism of action of glucosamine (an amino acid) and chondroitin is not well understood. Though these supplements are often used as first-line therapy in some European countries, clinical studies have revealed mixed results on their effectiveness in treating OA of the knee. There are no consistent studies demonstrating that these supplements will increase production of synovial fluid (A), improve cartilage repair (B), or reduce inflammation in the joint (C).

71. Correct: B. bronchospasm.

Though the mechanism of action is unknown for glucosamine, it should be used with caution due to an increased risk of bronchospasm (B).

Incorrect:

Glucosamine is generally well tolerated with no known drug interaction or hepatotoxicity, and will not result in elevated levels of ALT or AST (A). Chondroitin, not glucosamine, is associated with an anticoagulation effect that can increase bleeding risk (C). There is no known link between glucosamine and QT prolongation (D).

72. Correct: C. clinical studies have consistently shown benefit of long-term use of glucosamine and chondroitin for treating OA of the knee.

Though these supplements have been considered first-line treatment in many European countries, there is no consistent clinical trial data supporting its use for the management of OA of the knee (C).

Incorrect:

For individuals who desire to use glucosamine and chondroitin to manage symptoms of OA of the knee, they should be counseled that at least 3 months of consistent use is needed to see any effects (A). Glucosamine is not linked to any drug interactions but can increase the risk of bronchospasm (B). Chondroitin is associated with anticoagulant effect and can increase the risk of bleeding (D).

73. Correct: C. acupuncture.

The AAOS recommends a number of nonpharmacological and nonsurgical options for managing symptoms of

OA of the knee. However, the use of acupuncture is not recommended given a lack of compelling evidence supporting its use for this condition (C).

Incorrect:

Exercise and lifestyle modifications can help to provide relief of symptoms of OA of the knee. These include building strength and flexibility through low-impact aerobic exercises (A) and strengthening exercises that help to support the knee (D). For individuals who are overweight or obese, weight loss is highly recommended to reduce the impact on the weight-bearing joint (B).

74. Correct: D. opioids.

When considering pharmacological therapy for OA of the knee, guidelines from AAOS cannot recommend for or against the use of acetaminophen, opioids (D), or pain patches. This is largely due to a general lack of clinical studies demonstrating the benefits of these treatment modalities when weighed against the risks in managing symptomatic OA of the knee.

Incorrect:

The AAOS guidelines recommend the use of oral or topical NSAIDs (A, B) as well as tramadol (C) for patients with symptomatic OA of the knee. These recommendations were based on a number of well-controlled studies that showed benefits of these agents in relieving symptoms of OA of the knee. Tramadol should be used with caution due to the possibility of abuse, habituation, and adverse effects.

75 to 78. Yes or No

75. Correct: No

76. Correct: No

77. Correct: No

78. Correct: No

Several surgical and procedural interventions commonly used in the management of symptomatic OA of the knee are not supported by the clinical evidence as being able to provide substantial benefits for the patient. As a result, the AAOS could not recommend the use of these procedures, including intra-articular corticosteroid injections (75), hyaluronic acid injection (76), arthroscopy with lavage with or without débridement (77), or the use of platelet-rich plasma (78). In addition, for individuals with a torn meniscus, the AAOS cannot recommend for or against the use of arthroscopic partial meniscectomy. For individuals with advanced disease that significantly impacts daily living, joint replacement should be considered for patients who can tolerate the procedure and rehabilitation course.

79. Correct: B. hip replacement is not indicated if the patient can walk short distances.

Joint replacement can be considered when OA is severe enough to significantly impact daily living, such as limiting mobility that impairs activities of daily living (B).

Incorrect:

Joint replacement surgery is a viable option for those with uncontrolled pain (A) and when function is severely compromised. The ideal candidate will be able to tolerate a long surgical procedure (C) as well as undergo intensive rehabilitation to restore flexibility to the joint and strengthen muscles needed for normal functioning (D).

80. **Correct: A. squatting with light weights.**

For individuals with OA of the knee, physical activity should be encouraged that is low impact and can improve flexibility and strength around the joint. Squatting exercises, however, can put unnecessary strain on the knee joint, causing pain and potentially further damaging the joint (A).

Incorrect:

Limited weight-bearing exercise, such as swimming, can help maintain fitness and weight control without aggravating OA of the knee (D). Quadricep exercises are important to help strengthen the muscle around the knee joint (C), while straight-leg raises are a low-impact exercise (B).

81. **Correct: D. weight-bearing aerobic exercises.**

For individuals with OA of the hip, physical activity should be encouraged that is low impact and can improve flexibility and strength around the joint. However, weight-bearing aerobic exercises can put unnecessary strain on the hip joint, causing pain and potentially furthering damage (D).

Incorrect:

Stretching exercises are important for maintaining flexibility around the joint (A). Straight-leg raises and isometric exercises are important to help strengthen the muscles around the joint with low impact (B, C).

82. **Correct: B. More than 80% of articular cartilage is worn away, C. Physical functioning is severely compromised, and D. The patient can tolerate the surgical procedure and rehabilitation.**

Joint replacement surgery can be considered for patients with advanced OA of the knee or hip. These criteria include when pain is not adequately controlled with pharmacological agents, even at night, when physical functioning is severely compromised (C), or when over 80% of the articular cartilage is worn away (B). Additionally, candidates for surgery must be able to tolerate the long surgical procedure as well as the intensive rehabilitation period needed to restore flexibility and strength to the joint (D).

Incorrect:

Joint replacement can be considered when pain is inadequately controlled with pharmacological agents. The procedure would not normally be considered for the individual who has adequate pain control with daily use of NSAIDs (A). However, as the disease progresses, this might be a viable option.

Autoimmune Diseases

83. **Correct: C. Peak age for disease onset in individuals is age 50 to 70 years.**

RA occurs predominantly in women with a peak age of onset of between 20 and 40 years, not in the range of 50 to 70 years (C).

Incorrect:

RA occurs predominantly in women (A). Though there is no known cause of the condition, there is a strong association with a family history of RA or other autoimmune conditions (B). Unlike OA that primarily affects large joints, RA most frequently affects the smaller joints of the hands, wrists, ankles, and toes (D).

84. **Correct: B. cardiovascular events.**

Though it was once believed that RA had little impact on mortality and life span, more recent evidence suggests that the condition is associated with increased mortality. A leading cause of death in individuals with RA is from cardiovascular events, possibly related to chronic inflammation (B).

Incorrect:

RA is not linked to higher rates of cancer (C), while renal failure is more frequently associated with SLE (D). A greater risk of infection can occur with the use of certain DMARDs for the treatment of RA, but is not due to the disease itself (A).

85. **Correct: B. symmetrical early morning stiffness**

A characteristic sign of RA is stiffness in the joints that is symmetrical and typically worst when first arising (B). The stiffness can last about 1 hour and can recur following a period of inactivity.

Incorrect:

Symptoms that are worst in weight-bearing joints later in the day is more consistent with OA (A). The presence of sausage-shaped digits and skin lesions is more likely due to psoriatic arthritis (C). Ankylosing spondylitis is characterized by back pain with rest and anterior uveitis (inflammation of the middle layer of the eye) (D).

86. **Correct: C. thinning of the protective GI mucosa.**

NSAIDs work by blocking COX-1 and COX-2 enzymes. COX-1 is found in gastric mucosa and contributes to the health of these organs through numerous mechanisms, including the maintenance of the protective gastric mucosal layer (C).

Incorrect:

NSAIDs do not have any effect on GI motility (B) and act by reducing prostaglandin synthesis rather than enhancing synthesis (D). Though there may be a direct irritative effect of NSAIDs on the GI tract, the predominant mechanism of gastric injury is through the thinning of the protective mucosa (A).

87. **Correct: D. a 72-year-old man who takes aspirin four times a day for pain control of OA**

Increased age and frequency of NSAID use are major contributors to gastric injury. Among the answer choices, the elderly man who takes aspirin, an NSAID form, four times per day for an extended period of time would be at highest risk (D).

Incorrect:

For the 28-year-old man, concomitant use of NSAIDs with alcohol can increase the risk of gastric injury, though this is not likely due to his younger age and limited duration of taking NSAIDs (A). The 40-year-old woman takes NSAIDs relatively infrequently to cause gastric injury (B), while the 43-year-old also does not take NSAIDs on a consistent basis (C).

88. **Correct: D. omeprazole (Prilosec®)**

The most effective method to prevent NSAID-induced gastropathy is with the use of a proton pump inhibitor, such as omeprazole (D).

Incorrect:

The use of an antacid (B) or histamine-2 receptor antagonist (A) can help minimize symptoms of GI upset with NSAID use. However, these will not protect the individual from gastric injury as effectively as consistent PPI use. Sucralfate is used for the short-term treatment of an active ulcer but would not be used long term to prevent the formation of an ulcer (C).

89 to 91. Matching Questions

89. **Correct: B. subcutaneous nodules**

90. **Correct: A. renal involvement**

91. **Correct: C. oral involvement**

RA typically presents with soft tissue swelling as well as subcutaneous nodules (89) along with complaints of early morning stiffness. SLE is a chronic autoimmune disease that can affect any organ in the body but frequently presents with acute or chronic renal dysfunction (90). Sjögren's syndrome is frequently characterized by dry eye and dry mouth, which can lead to oral manifestations (91).

92. **Correct: A. Joint erosions are often evident on radiographs or MRI.**

In evaluating a patient with RA, radiographs typically reveal joint erosion and loss of normal joint space. MRI can also be used to reveal joint erosions and determine the severity of disease (A).

Incorrect:

RA is often seen in individuals with other autoimmune diseases, such as SLE and Sjögren's syndrome (B). A butterfly-shaped facial rash is characteristic of SLE rather than RA (C). Parvovirus B_{19} is associated with the development of fifth disease but not RA (D).

93. **Correct: C. Hb = 9.7 g/dL (12 to 14 g/dL); MCV = 87 fL (80 to 96 fL); reticulocytes = 0.8% (1% to 2%); RDW = 13.5% (11.5% to 15%)**

Anemia of chronic disease (ACD) can occur in patients with poorly controlled RA due to prolonged duration of inflammation. ACD is characterized by a normocytic, normochromic, hypoproliferative anemia that is best

illustrated in answer choice C. Usually, ACD can be resolved by controlling the underlying disease.

Incorrect:

ACD often seen in patients with RA is characterized as normocytic, not microcytic (A) or macrocytic (B). ACD is also a hypoproliferative condition rather than hyperproliferative (D).

94. **Correct: A. 30%**

Approximately 30% of patients at the early stage of RA will not present with radiographic evidence of disease (A). Therefore, if RA is suspected, it is important to utilize other diagnostic approaches to confirm the diagnosis. This can include the detection of several biological markers, such as RF or antibodies to anti-CCP or ANA.

95 to 97. Matching Questions

95. **Correct: B. detecting loss of normal joint space**

96. **Correct: A. detection of accumulation of fluid in bone marrow**

97. **Correct: C. identifying areas of inflammation**

Various imaging techniques can be used to support a diagnosis of RA and evaluate disease progression over time. Plain x-rays are most useful in visualizing the loss of normal joint space and can reveal joint erosions (95). MRI can also be used to detect joint erosions and has the ability to detect accumulation of fluid in bone marrow (96). This can be an important tool in predicting future erosion at the joint. Ultrasound is effective in detecting inflammation around a joint, which is important in evaluating progression of disease (97).

98. **Correct: B. an oral NSAID, and C. an oral nonbiological DMARD**

Initial management of RA typically involves the use of an oral NSAID to control pain and inflammation (B) along with a nonbiological DMARD (C), such as methotrexate. The DMARD is important in slowing or stopping disease progression and preventing further damage to the joint.

Incorrect:

An oral NSAID is preferred over topical analgesic due to its anti-inflammatory activity (A). If there is concern for gastric injury due to long-term NSAID use, a COX-2 inhibitor can be used or a gastroprotective agent can be used concomitantly with the NSAID. A biological DMARD is typically reserved for more severe disease and when disease activity is not adequately controlled with a nonbiological DMARD (D).

99. **Correct: B. infection.**

As biological DMARDs work by suppressing the immune system, a major adverse effect associated with these products is an increased risk of infection (B), particularly the activation of some dormant infections, such as tuberculosis. To provide adequate protection for these patients and minimize risk of vaccine-preventable disease, health-care providers should ensure that they are up to date on all vaccinations prior to initiating DMARD treatment.

Incorrect:
Biological DMARDs are not associated with myopathy (A), renal impairment (C), or clinically significant elevations in liver enzymes (D).

100. **Correct: C. *Haemophilus influenzae* type B.**
To provide adequate protection for these patients, health-care providers should ensure that they are up to date on all vaccinations prior to initiating DMARD treatment due to suppression of the immune system. However, the HiB vaccine is not commonly administered outside of childhood (C) due to the low risk of this disease.
Incorrect:
Prior to initiating biological DMARD therapy, individuals should be vaccinated against pneumococcal disease (A) and hepatitis B (B) and be encouraged to receive the annual influenza vaccine (D). They should also be up to date with the Tdap vaccine and be considered for meningococcal vaccination if they are determined to be at high risk for infection.

101. **Correct: A. elevated levels of RF**
The most specific test for RA is the presence of RF, which is present in about 50% to 90% of individuals with RA (A). Generally, the higher the titer, the greater is the severity of disease.
Incorrect:
Elevated ESR is an anticipated finding for various inflammatory conditions and is not specific for RA (B). Similarly, leukopenia occurs in a variety of clinical conditions, including viral infections (C). A positive ANA titer is more specific for SLE, as it is found in approximately 95% of these patients, while it is positive in only 30% to 50% of individuals with RA (D).

102. **Correct: B. SLE.**
A positive ANA titer is a specific test for SLE as it is found in approximately 95% of these patients (B). This test is less specific in RA as only 30% to 50% of these patients will be positive for ANA. Immunofluorescence analysis can further support an SLE diagnosis, with a homogenous, diffuse, or solid pattern strongly correlating with SLE, as well as a peripheral or rim pattern.
Incorrect:
A positive ANA test can be used to support a diagnosis of SLE or RA. It is not used to make a diagnosis of hyperparathyroidism (A), Kawasaki disease (C), or leukocytosis (D).

103. **Correct: A. increased rate of congenital fetal anomaly when occurring in a woman during pregnancy.**
SLE can impact a variety of organ systems including joints, skin, kidneys, and heart. The condition can be particularly problematic in pregnant women as it is a major risk factor for miscarriage and increases the risk of preeclampsia and preterm birth. However, SLE is not associated with an increase in the risk of congenital fetal abnormalities (A).

Incorrect:
Organ systems that are affected by SLE can include cardiovascular (D), renal (B), and musculoskeletal (C) systems.

104. **Correct: C. Sjögren's syndrome.**
Sjögren's syndrome frequently occurs in conjunction with RA and is associated with a decrease in oral and ocular secretions (C). For individuals with other chronic inflammatory conditions who complain of dry eye and dry mouth, Sjögren's syndrome should be suspected with appropriate diagnostic evaluation.
Incorrect:
Dry eye syndrome can be a mimic for Sjögren's syndrome but would not explain the report of dry mouth (A). Vasculitis is also more commonly present with autoimmune diseases but presents with generalized complaints of fever, headache, fatigue, general aches and pains, and weight loss (B). Scleroderma, characterized by a hardening or tightening of the skin and connective tissues, typically presents as hardening or tightening of patches of skin, GI problems, and symptoms of Raynaud's disease (D).

105 to 108. Matching Questions

105. **Correct: COX-2**

106. **Correct: COX-2**

107. **Correct: COX-1**

108. **Correct: COX-1**
COX-1 is found in the gastric mucosa, small and large intestines, platelets, kidneys, and vascular epithelium. An important function of COX-1 is maintenance of the protective mucosal layer of the stomach (107) as well as perfusion of the kidneys (108). COX-2 enzymes are involved in the inflammatory cascade (105) and pain transmission (106). Long-term use of NSAIDs that inhibit both COX-1 and COX-2 can lead to gastric injury; thus, gastroprotective agents are recommended to prevent ulcers and GI bleeding. The use of a COX-2-specific inhibitor, such as celecoxib, can provide pain relief and anti-inflammatory effects with less effect on the GI mucosa.

109. **Correct: D. febuxostat therapy.**
Sjögren's syndrome is an autoimmune disease that often occurs in conjunction with other inflammatory conditions. A key aspect of management is to treat the underlying condition as well as the symptoms of dry eye and dry mouth. Febuxostat, used in the prevention of gout, is not a recommended treatment for Sjögren's syndrome (D).
Incorrect:
Treating the underlying cause of disease is critical and can include NSAIDs or medications that suppress the immune system (e.g., methotrexate) (A). Intervention for patients with Sjögren's syndrome includes management of presenting symptoms with appropriate

lubricants of the eye and mouth (B). Routine dental care is important due to the increased risk of oral ulcers and dental caries with this condition (C).

110. **Correct: A. dilated eye retinal examination**

Hydroxychloroquine is associated with retinal toxicity and retinopathy. This is more likely to occur with long-term use of the agents, typically for over 5 years. Routine examination of the retina should be performed in those taking this medication for extended periods of time (A).

Incorrect:

The use of hydroxychloroquine is not known to affect bone marrow cells (B) nor is there a need to perform pulmonary function tests (C) or exercise tolerance tests (D) when taking this agent.

111. **Correct: A. weight gain.**

SLE is a chronic autoimmune disease that can affect any organ system. A common finding in individuals with the disease is unexplained weight loss rather than weight gain (A).

Incorrect:

Common signs and symptoms of SLE include fever, fatigue (C), headaches, joint pain, and swelling (B). SLE is also characterized by a malar rash that covers the cheeks and nasal bridge (D).

112. **Correct: C. normocytic, normochromic**

Individuals with poorly controlled SLE and RA are at risk of anemia of chronic disease. This is characterized as a normocytic, normochromic, hypoproliferative anemia (C).

Incorrect:

A macrocytic, normochromic anemia is characteristic of vitamin B_{12} or folate deficiency anemia (A). A microcytic, hypochromic anemia can be due to iron-deficiency anemia (IDA), which would not be associated with SLE. Since the patient has undergone endometrial ablation, she likely experiences no to scant menses, placing her at low risk for IDA (B). SLE is not associated with hemolytic anemia (D).

113. **Correct: B. hydroxychloroquine.**

For patients with mild symptoms of SLE, the antimalarial drug hydroxychloroquine has been shown to be effective for long-term treatment (B). The use of oral NSAIDs can also be considered to manage symptoms, especially in individuals where the condition waxes and wanes.

Incorrect:

Systemic corticosteroids can be used to manage inflammation associated with SLE. However, long-term use of these agents is not recommended due to adverse effects (A). Nonbiological DMARDs, such as methotrexate (D), and biological DMARDs, such as anakinra (C), are not typically used as first-line therapy but can be considered in more severe disease or when there is inadequate response to first-line treatments.

114. **Correct: B. thrombocytopenia.**

Belimumab, a B-lymphocyte stimulator-specific inhibitor, is the first biological agent approved for SLE. However, it is associated with significant adverse effects, though thrombocytopenia is not among them (B).

Incorrect:

Similar to other biological immunosuppressants, the use of belimumab is associated with an increased risk of serious infections (D). PML, a rare but often fatal viral infection, can also occur with the use of belimumab as well as other biological DMARDs used in the treatment of SLE and RA (C). Depression and increased suicidal ideation are adverse effects more specific to the use of this agent (A).

115. **Correct: A. When possible, conception should be delayed until lupus disease control is optimized, preferably for at least 6 months; B. Expert consultation should be sought from rheumatology and high-risk obstetrics, optimally prior to attempting pregnancy; and C. SLE is associated with a high risk of preeclampsia.**

SLE is a major concern for women of child-bearing age due to a high risk of miscarriage, preeclampsia (C), HELLP syndrome, and preterm birth. When possible, pregnancy should be delayed for at least 6 months after SLE is well controlled (A). Due to the high rate of pregnancy loss, expert consultation should be sought in these scenarios (B). Usually better control of SLE generally results in a better outcome during pregnancy.

Incorrect:

Though there are increased risks of pregnancy in women with SLE, there is a general decrease in the frequency of SLE flares during pregnancy (D).

Meniscal Tears

116. **Correct: B. moving the knee from full flexion to extension with hip flexed and knee externally rotated.**

The McMurray test assesses the menisci by having the hip flexed and the knee externally rotated. As the knee is moved from full flexion to extension, a snap heard or felt during the maneuver would suggest a medial meniscus tear (B). If a snap is heard or felt while the knee is internally rotated, then the lateral meniscus is likely involved.

Incorrect:

A maneuver that compresses the knee while externally or internally rotating the tibia is part of the Apley grinding test (A). The Childress test has the individual squat with knee fully flexed and then attempt to "duck walk" across the room (C). Pain elicited while the patient is standing with knees extended and rotating the trunk is positive for the Merkel sign (D).

117. Correct: A. twisting of the knee.
Among younger patients, the most common cause of meniscal tears is through contact sports injuries. This typically involves a twist-type injury to the joint, especially with a blow while in the twisting motion (A).
Incorrect:
Meniscal tear is not typically a result of hyperextension of the knee, though this type of injury can cause ligament damage at the joint (B). Repetitive striking can cause bursitis of the knee (C). In most trauma-related cases, the event of injury is clearly noted at the time of injury (D).

118. Correct: C. inability to kneel
For individuals with a complete or bucket-handle meniscal tear, it is nearly impossible to squat or kneel due to the injury (C).
Incorrect:
Joint effusion (A) and the loss of smooth joint movement (D) are common findings with meniscal tears and are not specific to complete meniscal tears. Warmth and heat at the joint are not typical findings with meniscal tears (B).

119. Correct: D. The peak incidence of sports-related meniscal tears in women occurs in their 30s.
Meniscal tears can result from sports-related injury or in older adults through degeneration of the joint. In women, the peak incidence of sports-related meniscal tears occurs between 11 and 20 years of age (D).
Incorrect:
In general, meniscal tears occur more frequently in men than women (A), with a peak incidence in men from between 21 and 30 years of age (C). Meniscal tears can also occur in older, sedentary adults through degenerative disease (B).

120. Correct: A. osteoporosis.
When making a differential diagnosis for meniscal tear, it is important for clinicians to be aware of other conditions that present similarly in order to ensure proper management of the condition. Osteoporosis, associated with reduced bone mass and an increase in fracture risk, does not present with specific symptoms at the knee, particularly joint effusion or loss of smooth motion at the joint (A).
Incorrect:
Other conditions that present similarly to a meniscal tear include osteochondritis dissecans (B), collateral ligament injury (C), and loose or foreign body in the knee (D).

121. Correct: B. quadriceps-strengthening exercises.
Certain steps can be used to reduce the risk of meniscal tears. These include quadriceps-strengthening exercises (B), stretching before and after exercise, and proper footwear.
Incorrect:
Though a large portion of meniscal tears are associated with sports participation, the benefits of sports and exercise outweigh the risk and should not be discouraged (A). A knee brace (C) and ice (D) can be part of the therapy of a meniscal tear. However, they will not necessarily prevent a meniscal tear from happening.

122. Correct: A. order an MRI of the knee.
MRI is better than radiographic analysis at detecting soft tissue damage and is the preferred imaging study when a meniscal tear is suspected (A).
Incorrect:
MRI is preferred over an ultrasound in detecting soft tissue damage (B). Arthroscopy is generally reserved for severe injury resulting in joint locking or the knee giving out, or when there is no improvement after 4 to 6 weeks with conservative therapy (C). A radiograph is not sensitive in detecting a meniscal tear since the meniscus does not contain calcium and is not readily visible on plain film (D).

123. Correct: D. joint aspiration of the affected knee.
Though effusion is a common finding with meniscal tears, aspiration is typically not needed as it will resolve over time (D). Aspiration can be considered with inadequate improvement after 2 to 4 weeks of conservative therapy.
Incorrect:
Management of meniscal tears typically involves conservative approaches with rest, ice (B), and elevation (C). The use of NSAIDs can be considered for pain relief (A).

124. Correct: C. referral for arthroscopy and likely surgical intervention.
For patients who do not improve following 4 to 6 weeks of conservative therapy, further specialty evaluation is needed (C). This can include arthroscopy to confirm the diagnosis as well as débridement and repair performed at the joint.
Incorrect:
Corticosteroid injection (A) and topical anti-inflammatories (B) are not recommended treatment options for meniscal tears. After 4 to 6 weeks of conservative treatment without improvement, further evaluation is needed by a specialist without further delay (D).

Carpal Tunnel Syndrome

125. Correct: A. reproduction of symptoms with forced flexion of the wrists.
The Phalen sign is positive when tingling along the median nerve is induced by full flexion of the wrists for up to 60 seconds (A). This test has about 80% specificity to CTS.
Incorrect:
Abnormal tingling when the median nerve is tapped is a positive finding of the Tinel test (B). This test has low specificity and sensitivity for CTS. Pain on internal rotation (C) and palmar atrophy (D) are not

specific tests used in the diagnosis of CTS. Muscle weakness and thenar atrophy are signs of advanced disease.

126. Correct: B. abnormal tingling when the median nerve is tapped.

Abnormal tingling when the median nerve is tapped is a positive finding of the Tinel test (B). Though this test is still commonly used in the diagnosis of CTS, it is associated with low specificity and sensitivity.

Incorrect:

The Phalen sign is positive when tingling along the median nerve is induced by full flexion of the wrists for up to 60 seconds (A). This test has about 80% specificity to CTS. Pain on internal rotation (C) and palmar atrophy (D) are not specific tests used in the diagnosis of CTS. Muscle weakness and thenar atrophy are signs of advanced disease.

127. Correct: D. involves sending a small electrical impulse through the muscle tissue.

An EMG is able to measure electrical impulses of the muscles and is used in the diagnosis of CTS. However, the procedure does not send electrical impulses through the muscle tissue (D).

Incorrect:

During EMG, electrodes are used to measure electrical activity of the muscles (A) at rest and during contraction (B) and can detect if muscle damage is present (C).

128. Correct: A. latter half of pregnancy; B. untreated hypothyroidism; and C. repetitive motion

Pregnancy-induced CTS is often observed, typically toward the latter half of pregnancy, and quickly resolves after childbirth (A). Untreated hypothyroidism can also increase the risk of CTS, which can be treated with thyroxine supplements (B). More commonly, CTS development is associated with repetitive motion, frequently in workplace settings (C).

Incorrect:

Several risk factors have been associated with the development of CTS. However, multiple sclerosis is not linked with this condition (D).

129. Correct: A. worst symptoms during the day

Individuals with CTS commonly report worst symptoms occurring at night rather than in the day (A).

Incorrect:

Signs and symptoms consistent with CTS include burning, aching, or tingling pain that radiates to the forearm and hand (B) and occasionally to the shoulder, neck, and chest (C). Awakening at night with numbness and burning pain in the hand can also be reported (D).

130. Correct: C. waking up at night with numbness and burning pain in the fingers.

Acroparesthesia is a classic finding among individuals with CTS and refers to awakening at night with numbness and burning pain in the fingers (C).

Incorrect:

Acroparesthesia is not associated with pain radiating from the elbow (A), the inability to move fingers (B), or muscle spasms (D).

131. Correct: B. nighttime use of a volar splint to keep the wrist in a neutral position.

An appropriate first-line treatment option for CTS is the nighttime use of a volar splint that maintains the wrist in the neutral position (B). This helps to relieve any increase in intracanal pressure caused by the flexion and extension of the wrist.

Incorrect:

Intra-articular injection (A) as well as referral for surgery (D) can be considered once more conservative approaches have failed to provide adequate results. Topical corticosteroids are not recommended for the treatment of CTS (C). Some evidence has shown a short course of oral corticosteroid can provide benefits, though additional research is needed.

132. Correct: B. will likely see significant improvement of CTS signs and symptoms within weeks of giving birth.

For those with pregnancy-induced CTS, the symptoms typically resolve soon after childbirth (B). Because of this, only conservative management approaches, such as the use of a volar split, should be considered during pregnancy.

Incorrect:

Therapies, such as splinting, can offer some relief for CTS during pregnancy, though they may not be as effective compared to when used in individuals who are not pregnant (A). Given that the symptoms of CTS will likely resolve soon after childbirth, surgery should not be considered at this point (C). Oral or injections of vitamin B_6 have not been shown to be useful in alleviating symptoms of CTS (D).

133. Correct: B. daily use of low-dose aspirin.

Certain strategies can be used to minimize the risk of CTS development. However, the daily use of low-dose aspirin has no demonstrated benefit in reducing CTS risk.

Incorrect:

Fitness and a healthy BMI have been shown to diminish the risk of CTS development (A). For those who perform repetitive functions, scheduling routine breaks (D) along with stretching and toning exercises (C) can be beneficial.

Sarcoidosis

134. Correct: B. African ancestry.

Individuals of African ancestry have a higher incidence of sarcoidosis compared to other ethnic groups and are also more likely to have more severe disease with pulmonary complications (B).

Incorrect:

There is a higher incidence of sarcoidosis in women compared to men (A), and it is more likely to occur between 20 and 40 years of age rather than in older age (C). A family history of the disease is also a strong risk factor, though type 2 diabetes mellitus is not linked to this condition (D).

135. **Correct: D. cardiac palpitations.**
Sarcoidosis can affect a variety of organ systems resulting in a range of symptoms of disease. Cardiac manifestations can include heart block and sudden death, though palpitations are not anticipated (D).
Incorrect:
Systemic symptoms of sarcoidosis include fever, fatigue, anorexia, and arthralgia (A). Pulmonary complaints can include dyspnea on exertion (B), cough, and chest pain. Ocular symptoms can include blurred vision (C), eye pain, severe redness, and sensitivity to light.

136. **Correct: B. hypercalcemia.**
Laboratory markers can help to support a diagnosis of sarcoidosis. Individuals with the condition are more likely to present with hypercalcemia (B) and hypercalciuria. Serum markers found in patients with sarcoidosis include SAA, soluble interleukin-2 receptor, ACE, and the glycoprotein KL-6.
Incorrect:
Findings of hyponatremia (A), hypokalemia (C), or hyperkalemia (D) are not typically found in individuals with sarcoidosis.

137. **Correct: C. biopsy**
Confirmation of sarcoidosis typically requires a biopsy to check for the presence of noncaseating granulomas (C).
Incorrect:
Though a biopsy is needed to confirm a diagnosis, other tests can be used to support the sarcoidosis diagnosis. Chest x-ray can detect for lung damage with pulmonary manifestation of disease (A). CT scan can detect for the presence of alveolitis or fibrosis in pulmonary disease (B). The ANA test is not helpful in the diagnosis of sarcoidosis but can be used to support a diagnosis of SLE (D).

138. **Correct: B. oral corticosteroids.**
Though many with mild disease can be treated with NSAIDs, the use of corticosteroids remains the mainstay of treatment. Oral corticosteroids can be used for systemic manifestation of disease (B), topical corticosteroids on affected skin, or inhaled corticosteroids for endotracheal disease.
Incorrect:
Corticosteroids are the mainstay of treatment for sarcoidosis. Other agents that can be considered include oral methotrexate (A), oral hydroxychloroquine (D), and certain biological agents, among others. NSAIDs are preferred over acetaminophen for symptom control (C).

139. **Correct: C. infliximab**
Biological agents have been shown to provide benefits for individuals with refractory sarcoidosis. The two most studied agents for this condition are infliximab (C) and adalimumab.
Incorrect:
Infliximab and adalimumab have been shown in clinical trials to offer some benefit in the treatment of refractory sarcoidosis. Biological DMARDs used in the treatment of RA include etanercept (A), tofacitinib (B), and certolizumab (D). However, these agents have not been well studied and/or demonstrated benefit in clinical trials for individuals with sarcoidosis.

140. **Correct: A. pulmonary function test and carbon monoxide capacity test.**
The use of a pulmonary function test and carbon monoxide capacity test can be used to support a diagnosis of sarcoidosis as well as in follow-up visits to assess progression of disease (A).
Incorrect:
A skin biopsy can be used to confirm the diagnosis of sarcoidosis (B). The presence of WBCs in the urine is not a helpful test for sarcoidosis (C). Finkelstein's test is used to help diagnose de Quervain's tenosynovitis of the wrist (D).

141. **Correct: A. anticyclic citrullinated peptide.**
Serological markers can be used to support the diagnosis of sarcoidosis. However, the presence of anticyclic citrullinated peptide is used as a marker for RA and not sarcoidosis (A).
Incorrect:
Markers that can be used in the diagnosis of sarcoidosis include SAA (B), glycoprotein KL-6 (C), and soluble IL-2 receptor (D). The diagnosis requires a biopsy for confirmation, which will detect the presence of noncaseating granulomas.

Low Back Pain and Lumbar Radiculopathy

142. **Correct: D. 90%**
About 9 of every 10 individuals with LBP will have their symptoms resolve within a month without any specific therapy (D). In these cases, no special interventions are needed to treat the condition beyond what can be offered in the primary care setting.
Incorrect:
The vast majority of individuals with low back pain will have the symptoms resolve within one month of onset without specific therapy. This rate exceeds 33% (A), 57% (B), and 78% (C).

143. **Correct: B. carpal tunnel syndrome.**
Several patient factors have been identified that can increase the risk of LBP. However, the presence of carpal tunnel syndrome is not associated with the development of LBP (B).
Incorrect:
Risk factors for LBP can include older age (A), overactivity, and overweight or obesity. Also, certain physiological or degenerative disorders can increase the risk,

including spinal stenosis (D), degenerative spondylolisthesis, and scoliosis (C).

144. Correct: C. muscle or ligamentous strain.

In most cases of LBP, the cause is muscle or ligamentous strain, a degenerative disease, or a combination of both (C). Lumbosacral strain is usually the result of a culmination of many events, including repeated use of improperly stretched muscles in patients with overall poor conditioning.

Incorrect:

For patients with LBP, a specific precipitating event is reported in only a minority of cases (A). LBP is usually the result of a culmination of events leading to lumbosacral strain. Disk herniation occurs less often and typically happens after years of episodes of back pain caused by repeated damage to the annular fibers of the disk (B). In some cases of herniated disk, sciatica can result from pressure on lumbosacral nerve roots, though this is relatively uncommon (D).

145. Correct: C. L5 and S1

The straight-leg raise, also called Lasègue's sign or Lazarević's sign, can be used to determine if LBP is associated with an underlying herniated disk. The maneuver tests for tension on the L5 and S1 nerve roots (C).

Incorrect:

The straight-leg-raising test is not a useful maneuver to evaluate tension in L1/L2 (A), L3/L4 (B), or S2/S3 (D).

146. Correct: B. stiffness, spasm, and reduced ROM in the back.

Lumbosacral strain is the most common reason for LBP, and the patient usually reports stiffness, spasm, and reduced ROM in the back (B). Neurological examination is typically normal for those with lumbosacral strain without radiculopathy.

Incorrect:

With lumbosacral strain, pain can be aggravated while in the sitting position, while moving to a supine position can bring some relief (D). Lumbar radiculopathy is associated with an "electric" sensation running down one or both legs (C). Numbness or weakness in the extremities can be caused by sciatica (A).

147. Correct: B. Back-strengthening exercises can cause mild muscle soreness.

For patients with LBP and intact neurological findings, exercise should be initiated as soon as tolerated. Prolonged immobilization can lead to deconditioning that will be harmful for the individual. When counseling about exercise, the patient should be aware that mild muscle soreness is to be expected with back-strengthening exercises (B).

Incorrect:

Patients should begin exercise as soon as it is tolerable, though the patient may not necessarily be free of pain (A). Electric-like pain should not be expected with a lumbosacral strain but would be anticipated with radiculopathy (C). Though exercise is not contraindicated with LBP, usually the patient is in too much pain to exercise and should wait until exercise can be better tolerated, though not necessarily until pain free (D).

148. Correct: B. age younger than 50 years.

Lumbar radiculopathy occurs more frequently with older age. Thus, age younger than 50 years would not be a risk factor for this condition (B).

Incorrect:

Lumbar radiculopathy typically manifests after years of LBP. Risk factors include smoking (D), diabetes mellitus, spinal infection, overweight or obesity (C), male gender (A), and older age.

149. Correct: C. shooting pain that starts at the hip and radiates to the foot.

Sciatica can result from pressure on the lumbosacral nerve roots from a herniated disk, spinal stenosis, or a compression fracture. A frequent complaint is a shooting pain that originates at the hip and radiates to the foot (C).

Incorrect:

Loss of bladder control can be due to cauda equina syndrome, which would require prompt referral for specialty care (A). LBP associated with stiffness, spasm, and reduced ROM is the classic presentation of lumbosacral sprain (B). Pain with sciatica is typically not worst in the supine position but can be aggravated in the sitting position, particularly in individuals who carry a wallet in the rear pants pocket (D).

150. Correct: A. loss of deep tendon reflexes.

Patients with lumbar radiculopathy, such as from a herniated disk, can experience a range of neurological involvement, from mild symptoms to loss of extremity function. In these patients, deep tendon reflexes are usually absent (A).

Incorrect:

Reduced muscle strength in the affected limb is more likely a later manifestation of the condition (C). Footdrop (D) and poor two-point discrimination (B) are not typically associated with early neurological changes due to lumbar radiculopathy.

151. Correct: D. soft tissue abnormality.

Sciatica is typically caused by pressure on lumbosacral nerve roots. Soft tissue abnormality is not a typical cause of sciatica (D).

Incorrect:

Causes of nerve impingement leading to sciatica can include a herniated disk (A), spinal stenosis (B), or a compression fracture (C). Sciatica can also be caused by external pressure on the sciatic nerve, such as sitting with a wallet in the rear pants pocket.

152. Correct: A. cauda equina syndrome.

Cauda equina syndrome occurs when there is compression of the lower portion of the nerve root inferior to the spinal cord. This can lead to bladder dysfunction, perineal sensory loss, and anal laxity (A). Prompt referral to specialty care is needed for these patients.

Incorrect:

Loss of bladder function is not a usual finding in patients with muscular spasm (B) or vertebral fracture (C). Those with a vertebral fracture will likely report a traumatic event, such as a fall or motor vehicle accident, that precipitates the onset of symptoms. Sciatic nerve entrapment is characterized by a shooting pain that starts at the hip and radiates to the foot (D).

153. **Correct: C. L5.**

Physical evaluation can provide information about the location of possible lesions associated with radiculopathy. Deep tendon reflexes are often absent in the presence of radiculopathy. The loss of posterior tibial reflex often indicates a lesion at L5 (C).

Incorrect:

The absence of posterior tibial reflex most accurately reflects a lesion at L5 and not L3 (A), L4 (B), or S1 (D).

154. **Correct: C. L5 to S1.**

Physical evaluation can provide information about the location of possible lesions associated with radiculopathy. Deep tendon reflexes are often absent in the presence of radiculopathy. The loss of the Achilles tendon reflex likely indicates a lesion at L5 to S1 (C).

Incorrect:

The absence of the Achilles tendon reflex most accurately reflects a lesion in L5 to S1 and not L1/L2 (A), L3/L4 (B), or S2/S3 (D).

155. **Correct: A. Spurling**

The Spurling test can be used to identify patients with cervical radiculopathy (A). The maneuver should elicit pain and numbness to the upper extremities when the condition is present.

Incorrect:

The McMurray test is used to identify meniscal tears (B), while the Lachman test is used to evaluate the integrity of the anterior cruciate ligament in the knee (C). The Kemp test is used to assess facet joint pain and involves having the patient perform extension combined with rotation of the spinal region of interest, which should reproduce the pain (D).

156. **Correct: D. moderate pain lasting at least 2 weeks.**

For patients who present with signs of lumbosacral strain without neurological involvement or suspicion of cancer or fractures, the use of imaging techniques is not recommended as little is likely to be revealed. This includes patients who present with moderate pain lasting at least 2 weeks and do not have any other risk factors for more serious conditions or a report of trauma that can cause a fracture (D). Imaging can be considered after a 1-month trial of therapy does not yield improvement.

Incorrect:

Patients with signs of cauda equina syndrome (A), characterized by loss of bladder function and perineal sensory loss, as well as those with severe neurological deficits (B), require immediate specialty referral for imaging studies. A history of cancer is a red flag warning sign among those complaining of back pain and should be evaluated with imaging studies for possible lesions (C).

157. **Correct: C. MRI**

Among the answer choices, MRI will provide the greatest detail of bone structures as well as soft tissue problems that can be associated with lumbar radiculopathy (C). MRI is preferred if there is a suspicion of cancer. A CT scan can also offer superior information on bone structures.

Incorrect:

Radiography with or without ESR (A, B) can be an option when there is a suspicion of cancer or spinal infection. However, these will not yield the quality of images obtained from MRI. A bone scan is not recommended for the evaluation of LBP (D).

158. **Correct: B. a 62-year-old woman who slipped on an icy sidewalk**

X-ray imaging is most useful when there is a high suspicion of fracture. This is most likely in the older woman with a recent report of trauma (B).

Incorrect:

Plain radiographs are not useful in evaluating patients with likely lumbosacral strain (A, D). In the presence of suspected radiculopathy (C), a CT scan or MRI is preferred, though imaging should be reserved until after a trial of conservative therapy does not yield adequate results.

159. **Correct: D. C6 to C7.**

The most frequent causes of neck pain include injury, poor posture, and prolonged wear and tear. The most common sites of lesions are at C6 to C7.

Incorrect:

Cervical radiculopathy most frequently involves C6/C7, and will involve to a lesser extent C3/C4 (A), C4/C5 (B), or C5/C6 (C).

160. **Correct: C. L4 to L5 and L5 to S1.**

Lumbosacral disk herniation typically occurs after years of repeated episodes of back pain that cause damage to the annular fibers of the disk. The most common sites of herniation are at L4 to L5 and L5 to S1, with the posterolateral aspect of the disk protruding (C).

Incorrect:

Less common sites for lumbar disk herniation will involve L1/L2 and L2/L3 (A), L2/L3 and L4/L5 (B), or L5/S1 and S1/S2 (D).

161. **Correct: D. bedrest for at least 5 days.**

Long periods of immobilization are not recommended for those with back pain, as this can lead to deconditioning, which is a major problem for these patients. Patients should be encouraged to stay active as tolerated and improve fitness.

Incorrect:

Application of cold packs to the affected area can help with pain control, while application of heat can help prior to gentle stretching exercises (A). NSAIDs and acetaminophen can be used for pain control (B), while light aerobic and toning exercises are encouraged as tolerated by the patient (C).

162. **Correct: C. clinical trials fail to demonstrate consistent benefits in LBP**

Gabapentin and pregabalin are frequently used to treat LBP with or without neurological involvement. However, clinical trials fail to demonstrate consistent benefit in reducing symptoms associated with LBP (C).

Incorrect:

Gabapentin is often used to treat LBP; however, NSAIDs and acetaminophen are first-line treatment options for this condition (A). Gabapentin has not shown consistent benefit in relieving LBP with or without neurological involvement (B). The use of gabapentin is not associated with dependence issues in a similar manner as opioids, which are not generally recommended for the treatment of LBP (D).

163. **Correct: C. weekly ice baths**

Several nonpharmacological approaches can be used to prevent LBP recurrence. However, weekly ice baths have not been demonstrated to prevent LBP (C).

Incorrect:

Approaches to minimize LBP recurrence can include maintaining physical fitness through low-impact aerobic (A) and toning exercises (B). Massage therapy can help to increase circulation to the affected areas and reduce muscle stiffness (D). Patients should also be counseled on techniques to minimize back stress through appropriate body mechanics.

164. **Correct: B. these agents must be used consistently for at least 2 weeks before seeing peak effect.**

Muscle relaxants can provide symptom relief for those with LBP. These agents generally have a rapid onset of action and, thus, do not need to be used for 2 weeks before seeing peak effects (B). However, caution should be used with these agents, as they are associated with substantial adverse effects.

Incorrect:

These agents should be used with caution as there is an abuse potential (A). Muscle relaxants have a sedation effect, which can improve sleep when used at night (C). However, they should not be used prior to driving or operating heavy machinery due to an increased risk of accidents (D).

Reactive Arthritis

165. **Correct: D. urethral swab or urinary test for select infection.**

Diagnostic testing of ReA is aimed at identifying the underlying infection. The condition usually occurs as a result of acute bacterial diarrhea or a sexually transmitted infection. In this patient with dysuria, a urethral swab and urinary test will most likely identify the causative pathogen (D).

Incorrect:

During ReA, ESR is typically elevated, but this finding is not specific for this condition (B). ANA, a marker used to support a diagnosis of RA or SLE, is not affected by ReA (A). Measurement of rubella titer is not helpful in confirming a diagnosis of ReA (C).

166. **Correct: B. bursitis.**

Bursitis develops with excessive fluid in the bursa sacs within joints and is usually a consequence of overuse and repeated impact on the joint. ReA is usually not characterized by fluid buildup in the joint (B).

Incorrect:

The signs and symptoms of ReA can encompass a variety of parts of the body. Common findings include dactylitis, or sausage-shaped fingers (A), and enthesitis (C) (inflammation at the site where tendons and ligaments attach to the bone, causing pain and stiffness of the joint). In women with ReA, cervicitis can develop with signs of abnormal bleeding and pain with intercourse (D).

167. **Correct: A. antimicrobial therapy.**

For individuals diagnosed with ReA with urethritis, the use of an antimicrobial agent can help to reduce the duration of symptoms, as there is likely an active sexually transmitted infection (A). Antimicrobial therapy would likely not be helpful in individuals whose ReA was attributed to a recent episode of acute bacterial diarrhea.

Incorrect:

For individuals with ReA and suspected of a sexually transmitted infection, antimicrobial therapy is typically beneficial to shorten the duration of symptoms. NSAIDs can typically be used for pain relief and reducing inflammation. Corticosteroid therapy, either as a short course of systemic therapy or intra-articular injection, can be considered to reduce inflammation (B). In patients with chronic symptoms, the use of nonbiological and biological DMARDs can be considered (C, D).

168. **Correct: C. ANA analysis reveals a speckled pattern.**

The presence of ReA does not have an impact on markers used for RA or SLE, such as ANA and RF (C).

Incorrect:

There is a similar incidence of ReA between males and females when the condition is associated with acute bacterial diarrhea (B). However, when the condition is associated with urethritis and sexually transmitted infection, males predominate (A). Usually there is no excessive fluid present in the joint during ReA. However, when the fluid is examined, the findings are unremarkable, and cultures are typically negative (D).

169. **Correct: B. HLA-B27 positive.**

When ReA is associated with urethritis, the male-to-female ratio is 9:1. Most of these men are found to be positive for HLA-B27, a human leukocyte antigen located on the surface of WBCs (B).

Incorrect:
ANA (A) and RF (C) are markers used in the diagnosis of systemic inflammatory diseases such as RA and SLE but are unaffected by ReA. Similarly, ACPAs, or anti-citrullinated protein antibodies, are also used in the diagnosis of RA (D).

170. Correct: B. doxycycline
For sexually active men with ReA that is likely attributed to sexually transmitted infection, antimicrobial therapy can be beneficial in shortening the duration of symptoms. Treatment can include a 7-day course of oral doxycycline (B) or a single dose of azithromycin.

Incorrect:
Antimicrobial treatment of ReA that is likely attributed to sexually transmitted infection should have activity against *C trachomatis* and *U urealyticum*. Amoxicillin (A) and TMP-SMX (C) are not recommended treatments for these infections. When ReA is attributed to a recent episode of acute bacterial diarrhea, antimicrobial therapy is not needed (D).

Osteoporosis

171. Correct: D. the clavicle.
Though all bones are at risk of fracture among those with osteoporosis, the clavicle is not a common site of osteoporosis-related fracture (D).

Incorrect:
The most frequent sites of fracture among individuals with osteoporosis include the hip, femur (A), wrist and forearm (B), and vertebrae (C). Hip fracture is usually the first manifestation of disease, but this typically indicates advanced disease.

172. Correct: B. on long-term systemic corticosteroid therapy.
Certain patient factors have been identified that increase the risk of osteoporosis, and it is critical for health-care providers to recognize these risks in disease prevention. Certain medications are associated with increased risk including some anticonvulsants, thyroid hormones, and systemic corticosteroids (B).

Incorrect:
Small-framed women of Asian and European ancestry, rather than African ancestry, are at higher risk of osteoporosis (D). Obesity seems to be protective against osteoporosis, possibly due to high endogenous estrogen produced by adipose tissue as well as increased bone weight-bearing (C). Recurrent UTIs are not linked to a higher risk of osteoporosis (A).

173. Correct: C. hyperlipidemia.
Several chronic medical disorders are associated with a higher risk of osteoporosis. However, dyslipidemia does not have a substantial impact on osteoporosis risk (C).

Incorrect:
Medical conditions associated with increased osteoporosis risk include rheumatological disorders such as RA and SLE (A), GI disorders including celiac disease and IBD (B), and hypogonadal states such as hyperprolactinemia (D).

174. Correct: C. 2.5
Osteoporosis is defined as having a bone density that is more than 2.5 standard deviations below the average bone mass for women who are younger than 35 years of age (C). Osteopenia, or low bone density, is defined as having between 1 and 2.5 deviations below the average bone mass for a healthy young adult. Bone density is typically measured by DXA.

175. Correct: B. DXA.
The preferred method to measure bone density is DXA, typically done on the hip and spine (B). Measurements can also be performed on the hand, wrist, forearm, and heel to identify individuals at higher risk of fracture.

Incorrect:
Radiographs are not recommended to assess bone mass as typically 40% to 50% bone loss is needed to be detected by this imaging technique (D). Radiographs are useful in detecting possible fractures, however. Qualitative CT can also assess bone density but exposes the patient to a higher dose of radiation compared to DXA (C). Another option is quantitative ultrasound that uses no radiation and can be performed with portable equipment (A).

176. Correct: C. vitamin B_6 supplementation.
Vitamin D, rather than vitamin B_6, is important for the prevention of osteoporosis with a recommendation of 800 to 1,000 IU daily for those 50 years and older (C). Important sources of vitamin D can be certain foods as well as exposure to sunlight.

Incorrect:
Interventions aimed at strengthening bone are important in preventing osteoporosis. Calcium supplementation can be important for those who do not achieve daily requirements from food sources, which should be 1,000 to 1,200 mg/day for older adults (A). SERMs can be used to help preserve bone density without the potential adverse effects associated with estrogen therapy (B). Proper fitness including weight-bearing exercises and muscle-strengthening exercises can help preserve bone strength (D).

177. Correct: C. increase in waist circumference.
An increase in waist circumference or BMI is not an indication of osteoporosis (C). Overweight and obesity actually has a protective effect against osteoporosis, possibly due to increased bone weight-bearing.

Incorrect:
Signs of osteoporosis can include gradual loss of height with stooped posture (A) and a patient report of back

pain (D). A hip or wrist fracture can also be a sign of osteoporosis and is usually an indication of advanced disease (B).

178. Correct: C. 1,200 mg.

For women older than 50 years of age as well as men older than 70 years, the recommended dose of calcium is 1,200 mg per day (C). For men between the ages of 50 and 70 years, the recommended daily dose is 1,000 mg. Dietary calcium should be the primary source of calcium, though supplements are often needed to meet these requirements.

179 to 183. Yes or No

179. Correct: Yes

180. Correct: No

181. Correct: Yes

182. Correct: No

183. Correct: Yes

Dairy and nondairy foods should be the primary source of calcium to meet daily requirements. Though calcium is found in a variety of foods, brown rice (182) and potatoes (180) are not important sources of this mineral. Important nondairy sources of calcium include tofu (179), spinach (181), select nuts, and sardines (183).

184. Correct: A. atypical fractures.

Though not a common finding, atypical fractures with low trauma events have been attributed to long-term use of bisphosphonates (A). For individuals at lower risk of fracture, a drug holiday is recommended after 5 to 10 years of therapy. For those at higher risk of fracture, a drug holiday should occur after 10 years of bisphosphonate therapy with consideration of using nonbisphosphonate treatment during that time.

Incorrect:

Long-term use of bisphosphonates is not associated with the development of hyperprolactinemia (B), OA (C), or bone marrow suppression (D).

185. Correct: C. 2 years.

For individuals being actively treated for osteoporosis, bone density scanning should be repeated in 1 to 2 years (C), with repeat measurements every 2 years thereafter. More frequent testing can be considered for patients at higher risk of fracture.

186. Correct: C. 5 years.

Long-term use of bisphosphonates has been associated with rare occurrences of atypical fractures. Because of this, a drug holiday is recommended to reduce this risk. Since most of the benefits of bisphosphonate therapy occur in the first 5 years of treatment, the drug holiday can occur after this period in patients at low risk of fracture (C). For higher-risk patients, the drug holiday can occur after 10 years of bisphosphonate treatment, with consideration on the use of nonbisphosphonate therapy during that time.

187. Correct: C. malignancy

Clinical studies with calcitonin demonstrate a slightly higher risk of malignancy with the use of this agent (C). This treatment can still be a useful option for those who cannot tolerate other medications, though other agents should be considered prior to using calcitonin.

Incorrect:

Calcitonin has not been demonstrated to increase the risk of type 2 diabetes (A), RA (B), or SLE (D).

188. Correct: B. a 64-year-old woman with a BMD T-score of −2.9 and prior hip fracture

Teriparatide is a parathyroid hormone that is typically reserved for women with very low bone density and with a prior history of bone fracture. Among the answer choices, the 64-year-old woman is the only one with osteoporosis and history of fracture, and she would be the best candidate for its use (B).

Incorrect:

Teriparatide is recommended for women with very low bone density. This would not be considered for use in men (C) or those with osteopenia rather than osteoporosis (A, D) where other treatments would be more appropriate.

189. Correct: A. an increase in breast cancer rates with long-term use.

Estrogen deficiency in postmenopausal women can lead to bone mass loss. Estrogen supplementation with or without progestin can help reduce the risk of postmenopausal fracture. However, short- and long-term use of estrogen therapy is associated with serious adverse effects, including an increased risk of breast cancer (A). A safer option can be the use of a SERM that works primarily on the bone and does not attach to receptors in the breast.

Incorrect:

Estrogen therapy can impact cholesterol levels, though treatment typically causes an increase in high-density lipoprotein cholesterol (B). Estrogen therapy can diminish bone density loss but will not likely result in an increase in bone mass (C). Therapy can decrease the risk of postmenopausal fracture by up to 34%; however, other options should be considered to prevent and treat osteoporosis due to potential adverse effects (D).

190. Correct: D. a large glass of water.

The use of bisphosphonates can cause drug-induced esophagitis. Because of this, doses should be taken in the morning with a large glass of water (D) and at least 30 minutes before eating or drinking other foods or taking other medications. It is also recommended to remain upright for at least 1 hour after dosing.

Incorrect:

Bisphosphonates should be taken in the morning (A) at least 30 minutes prior to eating or drinking other foods (B) or other medications (C). Patients should remain upright for an hour after dosing and so should not be taken at bedtime.

Sprains

191. Correct: C. ankle.

The ankle is the most common site of a sprain, with inversion injuries of the ankles accounting for about 85% of all sprains (C).

Incorrect:

Other common sites of sprains include the wrist (A), elbow, shoulder (B), and knee (D).

192. Correct: B. running on paved surfaces.

Several factors can increase the risk of an ankle sprain. Running on an uneven or rocky surface can increase the risk of a sprain, while running on a level paved surface will decrease the risk (B).

Incorrect:

The risk of ankle sprains is increased with poor conditioning (A) or starting intensive exercise without a proper warm-up period (D). Ensuring appropriate footwear for the activity is essential in minimizing risk (C), while taping or using an ankle brace can add support to the joint.

193. Correct: D. narrow toe box.

Wearing appropriate footwear is critical in preventing ankle sprains. Shoes with a wide toe box that allows the toes to move can be important in providing stability to the foot and ankle (D).

Incorrect:

Shoes with firm heel support (A), usually with rigid or semirigid shank under the heel and arch (B), will help to lock the heels in place and provide extra support. High-top shoes with lace-ups that extend over the ankle will provide support for athletic activities (C).

194. Correct: C. moderate swelling, mild to moderate ecchymosis, and moderate joint instability.

A grade II sprain is characterized by a partial ligamentous tear with moderate joint instability and swelling as well as mild-to-moderate ecchymosis (C).

Incorrect:

The mildest sprain is grade I that can involve slight stretching or microscopic tear of the ligament but without instability (A). Complete ankle instability with significant swelling and ecchymosis best describes a grade III sprain (D). A sprain with moderate joint instability but without swelling or ecchymosis is possibly a grade I to II sprain (B).

195. Correct: D. complete ankle instability, significant swelling, and moderate to severe ecchymosis.

Complete ankle instability with significant swelling and ecchymosis best describes a grade III sprain (D).

Incorrect:

The mildest sprain is grade I that can involve slight stretching or microscopic tear of the ligament but without instability (A). A grade II sprain is characterized by a partial ligamentous tear with moderate joint instability and swelling as well as mild-to-moderate ecchymosis (C). A sprain with moderate joint instability but without swelling or ecchymosis is possibly a grade I to II sprain (B).

196. Correct: D. many months.

A grade III sprain is the most severe type of sprain and will likely require the use of a short leg cast or a cast-brace for several weeks. Total time needed to fully recover can likely take many months (D).

197. Correct: D. local corticosteroid injection

Conservative treatment of a sprain typically involves RICE (rest, ice, compression, elevation). The use of corticosteroid injection is not recommended for this type of injury (D).

Incorrect:

RICE is the first-line approach for most ankle sprains. Immobilization can be an important part of the healing process and reduces the risk of further damage to the joint (A). Ice should be applied at least three times daily for 15 to 20 minutes to reduce pain and swelling (B). Depending on the severity of the sprain, the ankle should not bear weight for at least 24 hours after the injury (C).

198. Correct: A. for at least 24 hours.

For mild grade I ankle sprains, the injured ankle should not bear weight for at least 24 hours after the injury (A). For more severe sprains, this amount of time can be even longer, while activities should be avoided that increase pain and swelling during the healing process.

199. Correct: C. Grade III

A grade III sprain is the most serious sprain that can involve a complete ligamentous tear and complete ankle instability. For these injuries, a short leg cast or cast-brace might be used for several weeks (C). Depending on severity, surgical reconstruction can be an option for these types of sprains.

Incorrect:

Grades I and II strains can usually be treated with conservative treatment including RICE and an immobilizer. These injuries tend to heal without the use of a short leg cast (A, B). A grade III sprain is the most severe, as there is no grade IV sprain (D).

Fibromyalgia

200. Correct: D. biochemical changes in the central nervous system.

Though the exact cause of fibromyalgia is unknown, it is likely the result of central nervous system dysfunction and central sensitization (D). Several biochemical changes in the central nervous system are noted in the person with fibromyalgia, including low serotonin levels, elevated levels of substance P, and other biological markers.

Incorrect:

Low levels of serotonin are noted in fibromyalgia rather than increased production (A). Though genetics likely plays a role in this condition, the cause is more likely related to biochemical changes rather than an autoimmune reaction that causes diffuse hypersensitivity to pain signals in the brain (B, C).

201. Correct: C. It is four to seven times more common in women than in men.
Fibromyalgia occurs more frequently in women than in men, though the cause for this is unknown. The female-to-male ratio ranges from 4:1 to 7:1 (C).
Incorrect:
Fibromyalgia is found in all ethnic groups without a predominance in those with African ancestry (A). At least 2% of the population is affected by this condition (B), with symptom onset generally beginning between the ages of 20 and 55 years (D).

202. Correct: B. RA and SLE.
Fibromyalgia has been found to occur more frequently among individuals diagnosed with RA or SLE (B).
Incorrect:
There is no apparent link between the development of fibromyalgia and type 2 diabetes mellitus (A), migraine headaches (C), or COPD (D).

203. Correct: B. joint swelling
The presentation of fibromyalgia typically does not include any physical signs of the condition, such as joint swelling (B).
Incorrect:
Common patient complaints with fibromyalgia include chronic, often migratory, pain described as burning, aching, soreness, or bruising (without signs of bruising) (A). Other symptoms include fatigue and unrefreshing sleep (C) as well as cognitive changes (D), anxiety, and depression.

204. Correct: C. calculating a WPI and SS score.
Imaging and laboratory analyses are not helpful in making a diagnosis of fibromyalgia but can help to rule out other conditions with similar manifestations. Diagnostic criteria for fibromyalgia involve calculating a WPI and SS score. The WPI score is assessed by applying pressure to tender points on specific locations on the body.
Incorrect:
Imaging studies such as MRI (B) and CT scan (A) are not helpful in the diagnosis of fibromyalgia, as these will be normal. Imaging can be used to help rule out other conditions with similar manifestations. The use of the ANA and RF test are not recommended for fibromyalgia unless there is suspicion of RA or SLE (D).

205. Correct: B. can be identified by applying enough pressure to blanch the nailbed of the examiner.
Tender points are found at prespecified locations throughout the body and are used to support a diagnosis of fibromyalgia. Tenderness at these points is assessed by applying approximately 4 kg of pressure to the point, which is the amount of pressure needed to cause the examiner's nailbed to blanch (B).

Incorrect:
Tender points are found at prespecified locations in all four quadrants of the body (A). Radiography is not needed to identify tender points, and there will not be any abnormal findings revealed with imaging at these points (C). The tender points are prespecified, though tenderness at these points can vary among individuals with fibromyalgia. A diagnosis of fibromyalgia is supported with tenderness found in at least 11 of the 18 tender points in all four quadrants of the body and in the axial skeleton for 3 or more months (D).

206. Correct: C. a 6-minute walking distance.
The 6-minute walking distance is not a diagnostic criterion of the SS score for fibromyalgia (C). This assessment tool can be used for other disorders, particularly related to cardiovascular and respiratory disease, such as pulmonary arterial hypertension or peripheral arterial disease.
Incorrect:
The SS score is based on having the patient rank four symptoms that include fatigue (A), waking unrefreshed (B), cognitive symptoms (D), and somatic symptoms.

207. Correct: C. physical activity aimed at increasing flexibility is an important part of treatment.
Maintaining fitness has been found to be beneficial in reducing pain and fatigue associated with fibromyalgia. Physical activity that is most helpful in fibromyalgia includes flexibility exercises (C), progressive stretching, and low-impact activities, such as swimming.
Incorrect:
Exercise is an important part of the therapeutic intervention in fibromyalgia as it decreases pain and fatigue associated with the condition (A, D). Low-impact exercises are generally better tolerated compared to weight-bearing or high-impact exercises, such as jogging (B). Additionally, stress management techniques and addressing sleep disorders can be essential aspects in the management of fibromyalgia.

208. Correct: C. a fentanyl patch.
The use of opioid medications, including fentanyl patch, is not recommended for the treatment of fibromyalgia due to significant adverse effects, risk of dependence, and limited effectiveness in relieving neurological pain (C).
Incorrect:
Several pharmacological agents can be used for the management of pain associated with fibromyalgia. Acetaminophen and NSAIDs can be tried as first-line therapy though their effectiveness is generally limited (A, B). Topical agents, such as capsaicin, can provide some relief though they must be used consistently for optimal effect (D).

209 to 212. Yes or No

209. Correct: Yes

210. Correct: Yes

211. Correct: Yes

212. **Correct: No**

Several classes of agents have been shown to provide some relief of symptoms associated with fibromyalgia. These include antidepressants, such as tricyclic antidepressants (209) and SSRIs (211), as well as antiepileptic agents (210), including gabapentin and pregabalin. TCAs can also be used to help promote sleep. The use of opioid medications is not recommended for the treatment of fibromyalgia due to significant adverse effects, risk of dependence, and limited effectiveness in relieving neurological pain (212).

213. **Correct: A. consider adopting a high-intensity aerobic activity such as jogging.**

Patients with fibromyalgia should be counseled on lifestyle modifications that can be important in minimizing symptoms. Physical activity is an important part of disease management, though low-impact exercise is preferred over high-impact activities, such as jogging, as low-impact exercise will be better tolerated (A).

Incorrect:

Lifestyle interventions aimed at minimizing fibromyalgia symptoms include maintaining physical activity with low-impact exercises as well as flexibility training (D). Individuals should be encouraged to eat healthy foods and limit caffeine use (B). Stress management techniques (C) as well as approaches to improve sleep are also helpful.

214. **Correct: C. phenytoin (Dilantin®)**

Phenytoin, an antiseizure medication, is not approved for the treatment of fibromyalgia (C). Other antiepileptic agents, such as gabapentin and pregabalin, would be preferred to alleviate symptoms associated with fibromyalgia.

Incorrect:

Agents that are approved by the FDA to manage symptoms of fibromyalgia include the SSRI duloxetine (A), the SNRI milnacipran (D), and the antiepileptic drug pregabalin (B). Several other agents are frequently used off-label for this condition.

Vitamin D Deficiency

215. **Correct: A. diminishes secretion of insulin**

Vitamin D plays a variety of physiological roles in the body. Vitamin D stimulates insulin secretion in response to increased insulin demands, possibly playing a role in maintaining normoglycemia (A).

Incorrect:

Vitamin D inhibits abnormal cell growth (B) and is essential in normal cell differentiation and minimizing abnormal cell proliferation. Vitamin D is important in the absorption and metabolism of calcium and phosphorus and maintaining bone integrity (C). Vitamin D can also act as a renin producer and contribute to blood pressure control (D).

216. **Correct: C. exposure of the skin to the sun**

Though many foods contain vitamin D, the best source of this vitamin is endogenous production when skin is exposed to sunlight (C). With adequate sun exposure, the body's natural ability to produce vitamin D typically accounts for at least 95% of the daily requirements.

Incorrect:

Fatty fish, such as salmon and tuna, as well as fortified dairy products are good sources of vitamin D (A, B), though they do not typically provide the amount of vitamin D produced by the body with adequate sunlight exposure on skin. Leafy green vegetables are not typically considered excellent sources of vitamin D (D).

217. **Correct: B. One glass of fortified milk has an equivalent amount of vitamin D as that produced after 10 minutes of exposure to summer sunlight in a healthy, young individual.**

Though foods fortified in vitamin D can be an important source of the nutrient, the amount contained in those foods is usually much lower than what is synthesized by the body when skin is exposed to sunlight. In the continental United States, 5 to 10 minutes of sunlight exposure to the arms and legs can result in the production of 3,000 IU of vitamin D, compared with about 100 IU provided in 8 ounces of fortified milk (B).

Incorrect:

Adequate exposure to sunlight can produce at least 95% of the body's daily requirement of vitamin D (A). Certain factors can decrease the production of vitamin D with sunlight exposure, including covering skin with clothing, the use of sunscreen (which can block as much as 95% of vitamin D production) (C), and darker skin tones (D).

218. **Correct: C. markedly increased by twofold to fivefold from the age norm.**

Certain medications have vitamin D–depleting activity that can increase the risk of vitamin D deficiency. Individuals who take medications such as phenytoin or phenobarbital will require two- to fivefold higher amounts of the recommended daily amount of vitamin D (C).

Incorrect:

The vitamin D–depleting activity of phenytoin will require individuals to take higher amounts of the recommended daily requirements of vitamin D rather than the same (B) or lower amounts (D). In general, the majority of vitamin D is provided through exposure of skin to sunlight, with a well-balanced diet only providing a small portion of what is needed on a daily basis (A).

219. **Correct: D. azotemia.**

Vitamin D plays an important role in maintaining the musculoskeletal system. Azotemia, or an elevation in nitrogen waste products in the blood, is a sign of renal dysfunction and possible nephrotoxicity. This is not normally associated with vitamin D deficiency (D).

Incorrect:

Vitamin D deficiency can lead to insufficient absorption of calcium needed for maintaining bone health. Severe cases can lead to the development of osteomalacia (B), where a rubbery collagen matrix is deposited on the skeleton and is associated with a constant dull ache. Other effects of vitamin D deficiency include muscle pain and weakness (C) as well as the presence of pseudofractures (A).

220. Correct: D. scoliosis.
Rickets occurs when there is vitamin D deficiency during bone growth, as seen in children, and growing bone fails to mineralize. This condition is not associated with the development of scoliosis (D), which can be caused by other factors such as multiple sclerosis and cerebral palsy.
Incorrect:
Characteristic signs of vitamin D deficiency in children who develop rickets include bowing of the legs (A), a delay in teeth eruptions (B), as well as a delay in motor milestones (C).

221. Correct: C. pain elicited when applying gentle pressure on the sternum.
Osteomalacia occurs with severe vitamin D deficiency that is characterized by constant dull bone ache. In these patients, applying gentle pressure to the sternum, anterior tibia, or radius will elicit a painful response (C).
Incorrect:
Osteomalacia is not associated with a diffuse skin rash (A) or prolonged capillary refill (B) as seen during dehydration. Bowing of the legs is a sign of rickets, or vitamin D deficiency in children, while bones are still growing (D).

222. Correct: B. 25-hydroxyvitamin D
The preferred test to assess vitamin D status is 25-hydroxyvitamin D as it is minimally influenced by recent dietary intake or recent sun exposure (B).
Incorrect:
1,25-Dihydroxyvitamin D, the biologically active form of vitamin D, is not the preferred test for vitamin D deficiency since levels typically remain unchanged until deficiency is well advanced (D). Vitamin D_3 is the preferred form of the micronutrient for treatment of vitamin D deficiency and maintenance of vitamin D levels (C). Vitamin D_2 is a form produced by plants and fungi and available in some supplements but is not as readily available for use by the body compared to vitamin D_3 (A).

223. Correct: C. one egg yolk
Among the answer choices, one egg yolk will provide the least amount of vitamin D at about 20 IU.
Incorrect:
Eight ounces of fortified milk (A), fortified orange juice (B), or infant formula (D) will provide about the same amount of vitamin D at about 100 IU. This is much lower than exposure of the arms and legs to sunlight for 5 to 10 minutes in the continental United States, which can provide up to 3,000 IU of vitamin D.

224. Correct: A. fresh wild salmon
Fatty fish can be a good source of vitamin D as part of a well-balanced diet. Among the answer choices, fresh, wild salmon will offer the highest amount of vitamin D_3 at about 600 to 1,000 IU (A).
Incorrect:
Fresh farmed salmon will provide about 100 to 250 IU of vitamin D_3 (B), canned tuna will provide about 230 IU of vitamin D_3 (C), and canned mackerel will provide about 250 IU of vitamin D_3 (D).

225. Correct: C. 32
An 8-ounce serving of fortified milk will provide about 100 IU of vitamin D_3. Therefore, to receive the recommended daily amount of 400 IU will require four 8-ounce servings, or 32 ounces total (C).
Incorrect:
An 8-ounce serving of fortified milk will provide about 100 IU of vitamin D_3 (A), 16 ounces will provide 200 IU (B), and 48 ounces will provide 600 IU (D).

226. Correct: C. 600 IU
According to the Institute of Medicine, the recommended daily intake of vitamin D_3 for individuals from 1 to 70 years of age is 600 IU (C). For infants younger than 1 year, the recommended amount is 400 IU daily. Individuals older than 70 years have a recommended daily intake of 800 IU.
Incorrect:
A daily intake of 400 IU of vitamin D_3 is recommended for infants younger than 1 year (B). A daily intake of 200 IU is too low for individuals over 1 year of age (A), while 100 IU exceeds the recommended amount needed for those 70 years and younger (D).

227. Correct: B. 600 IU.
For pregnant or lactating women, the recommended daily intake of vitamin D_3 is 600 IU, similar to young adults.
Incorrect:
A daily intake of 300 IU is too low for young adults (A) while amounts of 1000 IU (C) or 1200 IU (D) exceed recommended amounts.

228. Correct: D. 50,000 IU weekly
Because vitamin D_3 is stored in fat and has a long half-life, a low-dose regimen is not sufficient to correct deficiency, as this will lead to only small increases in vitamin D levels over the long term. Therefore, recommended treatment is a high dose of 50,000 IU weekly taken by mouth for at least 8 weeks, but usually up to 16 weeks if the 25(OH)D level was below 30 ng/mL. Long-term prevention of vitamin D deficiency can include a regimen of 50,000 IU vitamin D_3 once or twice per month along with 1,000 to 2,000 IU of vitamin D_3 daily.
Incorrect:
Low-dose regimens are not sufficient to correct vitamin D deficiency (A, B). The recommended regimen is 50,000 IU weekly for 8 to 16 weeks, rather than 10,000 IU twice per week (C).

Peripheral Vascular Disease

11

Raynaud's Phenomenon

Overview

Raynaud's phenomenon, also known as Raynaud's disease, is most often found in women, idiopathic in origin, and usually appears between the ages of 15 and 45 years. This condition is characterized by paroxysmal digital vasoconstriction.

> **CLINICAL CONCEPT**
>
> Raynaud's phenomenon presents with episodes of intermittent, bilateral symmetrical pallor, tissue blanching, and/or cyanosis followed by rubor (redness of the skin), nearly always involving the hands and rarely involving the feet (Fig. 11-1).

Clinical Presentation

A period of intense itchiness often follows tissue blanching or pallor. Symptoms tend to be progressive, with vasospasm becoming more frequent and prolonged. Vasoconstriction is most often triggered by exposure to cold, with signs and symptoms resolving with rewarming. Emotional upset is also a trigger.

Secondary Raynaud's phenomenon is seen in the presence of an underlying condition, such as atherosclerosis, collagen vascular disease, and select autoimmune diseases such as scleroderma; in scleroderma, this concomitant condition is a nearly universal finding. In addition, the use of vibrating tools, repeated sharp digit movement such as piano playing or typing, frostbite, tobacco, ergotamine, and beta blocker use can be contributing factors. The degree and length of vasospasm are often more severe than its idiopathic form.

Diagnostic Testing

The diagnosis of Raynaud's phenomenon is made clinically by history and physical examination, when recurrent episodes occur for more than 3 years without notation of associated disease or secondary cause. Diagnostic testing is aimed at the underlying cause, such as collagen vascular disease or scleroderma.

Treatment

Whatever the cause, intervention in Raynaud's phenomenon is aimed primarily at preventing vasospasm by avoiding cold and other known triggers. At the onset of an episode, submerging the hands in warm water can be helpful in limiting the length and severity of vasospasm; hot water should not be used because of risk of burn. Because wound healing is often delayed and infection is common, the hands should be protected from even minor injury. Keeping the skin well lubricated can help avoid small fissures. Tobacco use exacerbates vasospasm; cessation of all forms of tobacco products is usually associated with a stabilization of or improvement in symptoms. Biofeedback can be helpful because the patient can be taught to envision warming the digits, reducing symptoms.

The dihydropyridine calcium channel blockers (-*ipine* suffix, such as amlodipine or nifedipine), the angiotensin-converting enzyme inhibitors (ACEIs, -*pril* suffix, such as lisinopril or fosinopril), and the angiotensin-receptor blockers (ARBs, -*sartan* suffix, such as losartan) can be used for their vasodilator effect when lifestyle modification is inadequate. In patients with secondary Raynaud's phenomenon, treatment of the associated condition is important and often helps minimize episodes. A variety of other medications including topical nitroglycerin, prostaglandin analogs such as iloprost, phosphodiesterase-5 enzyme inhibitors such as sildenafil, and botulinum toxin are also used in select situations with specialty consultation. Surgical intervention with distal digital sympathectomy and arterial reconstruction should be considered when more conservative therapy is unsuccessful in managing the condition.

Discussion Source

Hansen-Dispenza H. Raynaud phenomenon. Medscape. https://emedicine.medscape.com/article/331197-overview

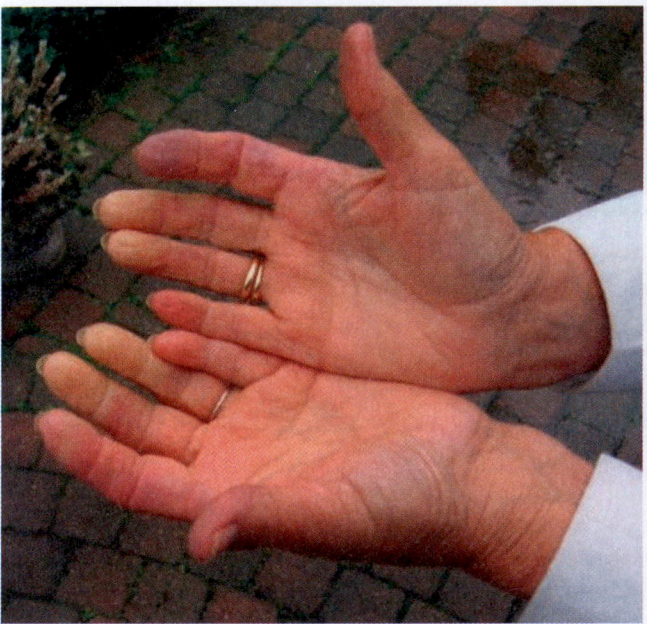

FIGURE 11-1 Raynaud's phenomenon.
(Wikipedia: Courtesy of Jamclaassen.)

QUESTIONS

1. Who is most likely to have new-onset primary Raynaud's phenomenon?
   A. a 68-year-old man with dyslipidemia taking a statin
   B. a 65-year-old woman with type 2 diabetes mellitus taking metformin
   C. a 25-year-old man who is otherwise well taking a vitamin supplement
   D. an 18-year-old woman using combined oral contraceptives

2. All of the following are at risk for the development of secondary Raynaud's phenomenon except:
   A. a 45-year-old woman with well-controlled hypertension.
   B. a 32-year-old woman with scleroderma.
   C. a 45-year-old man who uses vibrating hand tools in his work on a regular basis.
   D. a 28-year-old woman who is taking a beta-adrenergic antagonist for migraine prophylaxis.

3. For a 26-year-old woman with Raynaud's phenomenon, treatment should include advice on which of the following two lifestyle modifications?
   A. Pay attention to hand skin care to avoid dry skin and fissures.
   B. Limit fluid intake.
   C. Place hands in warm water at the onset of symptoms.
   D. Discontinue aspirin use.

4. Medications that are often helpful in relieving symptoms associated with Raynaud's phenomenon include:
   A. NSAIDs.
   B. ACEIs.
   C. beta-adrenergic antagonists.
   D. diuretics.

5. When providing primary care for a 22-year-old woman with Raynaud's phenomenon who lives in the northern U.S. Midwest, which of the following is most likely to be reported?
   A. a history of digital ulceration
   B. worsening of symptoms in summer months

C. a period of intense itchiness after blanching

D. signs and symptoms more intense in the dominant hand

For answers and rationales, see end of chapter.

Varicose Veins

Overview

Varicose veins are seen in 15% of the adult population and are most often found in the lower extremities. Nonmodifiable risk factors for varicose veins include an inherited venous defect (valvular incompetence, weak vessel walls) and female gender (2:1 female-to-male ratio). Modifiable risk factors include leg crossing, wearing of constricting garments, prolonged standing, heavy lifting, and current or prior pregnancy.

Clinical Presentation

Tortuous, dilated, superficial veins are characteristic. The vessel most often affected is the great saphenous vein and its tributaries. With palpation, a varicose vein compresses easily and without pain (Fig. 11-2).

Though often asymptomatic, varicose veins are often associated with aching legs, particularly after prolonged standing, but usually not severe pain. The degree of discomfort is poorly correlated with the number and appearance of the affected veins. Mild edema in the ankle area, particularly at the end of the day and in warmer weather, is common.

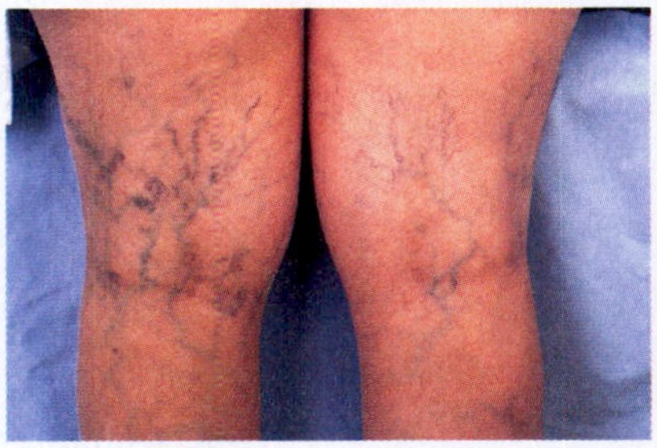

FIGURE 11-2 Spider varicosities.
Dillon P. Nursing Health Assessment: The Foundation of Clinical Practice. 3rd ed. Philadelphia, PA: F.A. Davis; 2016.

Diagnostic Testing

No specific diagnostic tests are needed to establish the diagnosis of varicose veins with typical presentation. Various diagnostic tests are available, however, including duplex ultrasound and magnetic resonance venography; these tests are usually used to rule out deep vein obstruction as a contributor of the severity of varicose veins.

Treatment

With uncomplicated varicose veins, lifestyle modification usually helps minimize the symptoms and disease progression. Attaining and maintaining normal weight help to reduce intravenous pressure and discourage the development and progression of varicose veins. Periodic leg elevation is helpful in minimizing edema and encouraging venous return. The use of medium-weight to heavy-weight elastic support hose such as Jobst™ stockings should be encouraged. Support hose purchased over the counter in a retail outlet do not supply enough compression. Wearing garments that are potentially constricting, such as panty girdles and garters, should be avoided.

Various minimally invasive interventions, including endovenous laser ablation, are also available for varicose vein treatment. Sclerotherapy is a common procedure done for vein obliteration and involves injecting a sclerosing agent into the affected vein followed by a period of compression, which results in vessel obliteration. Surgery is occasionally needed for symptomatic varicose veins that do not respond to more conservative, less invasive therapy. Vessel obliteration with laser or other modalities is helpful in reducing the appearance of spider varicosities and is considered a cosmetic procedure.

> **CLINICAL CONCEPT**
> Spider varicosities are visible surface vessels usually seen with varicose veins. These vessels do not usually cause symptoms and pose no thromboembolic risk.

Discussion Source

Weiss R. Varicose veins and spider veins. Medscape. https://emedicine.medscape.com/article/1085530-overview

QUESTIONS

6. Which of the following does not directly contribute to the development of varicose veins?

   A. leg crossing

   B. pregnancy

   C. heredity

   D. Raynaud's disease

7. The nurse practitioner (NP) sees a 32-year-old woman who works as a hotel housekeeper and who asks about wearing support hose to minimize her varicose vein symptoms. The most appropriate response is to advise the purchase of which of the following types of support hose?

   A. any kind found in the hosiery section of a retail store labeled "support" as long as the top band is not constricting

   B. a lightweight pair and available over the counter

   C. a medium- to heavyweight prescription product

   D. only stockings that are used in the form of pantyhose

8. In patients with varicose veins, which vessel is most often affected?

   A. femoral vein

   B. posterior tibial vein

   C. peroneal vein

   D. saphenous vein

9. When counseling a 26-year-old woman who has developed varicose veins during her second pregnancy, the NP considers:

   A. The degree of venous tortuosity is well-correlated with the amount of leg pain reported.

   B. As the number of affected veins increases, so does the degree of patient discomfort.

   C. Symptoms are sometimes reported with minimally affected vessels.

   D. Lower-extremity edema is usually seen only with severe disease.

10. You see a 38-year-old woman with a history of varicose veins. She has a body mass index (BMI) of 24 kg/m² and works as a registered nurse in the intensive care unit. She reports that she is on her feet for much of her 12-hour shifts and experiences leg aches toward the end of her shifts despite using appropriate support hose. She asks you about any additional measures she can take to reduce her discomfort. You suggest all of the following except:

    A. elevate feet whenever possible.

    B. initiate anticoagulant therapy.

    C. endovenous laser ablation.

    D. sclerotherapy.

11. Spider varicosities are:

    A. usually symptomatic.

    B. a potential site for thrombophlebitis.

    C. responsive to laser obliteration.

    D. caused by sun exposure.

For answers and rationales, see end of chapter.

Deep Vein Thrombosis and Pulmonary Embolism

Overview

Thrombophlebitis, the presence of coagulated blood or thrombus in a vein with resulting inflammation, can occur in superficial (superficial thrombophlebitis) or deep veins (deep vein thrombophlebitis or deep vein thrombosis [DVT]). The lower extremities are most often affected. Virchow's triad of blood stasis, injury to the vascular intima, and abnormal coagulation leading to a clot usually contributes to the development of vessel inflammation and the resulting thrombophlebitis.

Acute DVT usually involves the veins of the lower extremities and pelvis. Long-term sequelae of DVT include chronic venous insufficiency (CVI) and venous ulceration.

CLINICAL CONCEPT

Pulmonary embolism (PE), a potentially fatal condition, is largely a sequela of DVT.

DVT risk factors include local trauma to the leg, prolonged travel or rest, the presence of varicose veins, a history of prior episodes, recent surgery, the use of estrogen-containing hormonal contraceptives or postmenopausal hormone therapy, and the immediate postpartum (within 6 weeks of birth) period. Disorders of coagulation, such as factor V Leiden mutation and proteins C and S and antithrombin III deficiencies, are recognized as a cause of DVT in otherwise healthy adults. The use of estrogen-containing contraceptives (combined [estrogen/progestin] oral contraceptive, topical patch, or vaginal ring) and postmenopausal hormone therapy increases DVT risk, particularly in cigarette smokers, and should be avoided.

Because disordered coagulation tends to occur in multiple locations simultaneously, when superficial thrombophlebitis is present, this condition is often accompanied by DVT in a different location or extremity.

SUPERFICIAL THROMBOPHLEBITIS

Clinical Presentation

In superficial thrombophlebitis, examining the patient after standing for 2 minutes before examination enhances the findings, because less severe cases might be missed on supine examination. Superficial thrombophlebitis is often considered a benign condition; however, this condition is likely a marker of further clotting issues. Extension into a deep vein, the vessels that act as conduits to return blood to the heart, is typically present, however, in 45% of patients with the condition. In particular, superficial, noninfectious thrombophlebitis in hospitalized patients is more likely to be associated with DVT and PE. Until proven otherwise, a patient with superficial thrombophlebitis should be assumed to have deep vein involvement.

Diagnostic Testing

See the DVT section later in the chapter for the proper diagnostic workup for a patient with superficial thrombophlebitis to rule out DVT and PE.

Treatment

After the diagnosis of an initial episode of superficial thrombophlebitis is confirmed, intervention is dictated by DVT risk factors and patient history. In the absence of risk factors and history of similar episodes, warm packs, compression hose, and NSAIDs can be used; anticoagulation is not required in superficial disease. Ambulation should be encouraged because rest promotes stasis and enhances coagulation, although leg elevation when at rest is helpful in managing symptoms and edema. The inflammation associated with superficial thrombophlebitis usually subsides within 2 weeks, with a firm cord remaining for a much longer period. As with DVT, collateral venous flow develops over the next few months. In the presence of prior episodes, more aggressive therapy and evaluation should be considered.

DEEP VEIN THROMBOPHLEBITIS

Clinical Presentation

Because the DVT appearance varies, making the diagnosis from clinical presentation alone is problematic (Table 11-1). Unless the Virchow triad of venous stasis, vessel wall injury, and coagulation abnormalities is present, few patients with suspected DVT have the diagnosis supported by further diagnostics. The Wells Clinical Prediction Guide in Deep Vein Thrombophlebitis (DVT) (Table 11-2) provides a helpful guide for estimating clinical suspicion (Figs. 11-3 and 11-4).

Diagnostic Testing

A compression duplex venous ultrasonography standard imaging test to diagnose DVT should be performed to help rule out concurrent DVT in patients with superficial thrombophlebitis. A compression duplex venous ultrasonography standard imaging test is the most common first-line diagnostic technique in DVT due to its ease of use, absence of irradiation or contrast material, and high sensitivity and specificity. Because disordered coagulation tends to occur in multiple locations simultaneously, the

TABLE 11-1 Clinical Presentation of Deep Vein Thrombophlebitis (DVT)

FINDING	COMMENT
Edema	Usually unilateral (best true-positive finding)
	Bilateral calf measurement with comparative readings helpful in clinical assessment
Leg pain	Usually described as a tugging pain, heaviness, ache
	Present in approximately 50% of patients with DVT with degree of pain not correlating well with extent of thrombus
Homans sign	Pain on dorsiflexion of the foot
	Present only in about one-third of patients with DVT and up to half without DVT
Pulmonary embolus (PE) signs and symptoms	Present in approximately 10% of patients with DVT, but likely PE concurrently present in a higher percentage
Warmth over area of thrombosis	Relatively rare
Venous distention and prominence of subcutaneous veins	Relatively uncommon
Fever	If present, typically mild
Tenderness over and adjacent to the affected area	Found in approximately 75% of patients with DVT
	Also can be found in many conditions other than DVT
	Degree of tenderness does not correlate well with extent of thrombus

Source: Patel K. Deep venous thrombosis. Medscape. https://emedicine.medscape.com/article/1911303-overview

TABLE 11-2 Wells Clinical Prediction Guide in Deep Vein Thrombophlebitis (DVT)

CLINICAL PARAMETER	SCORE
Active cancer (treatment ongoing, within 6 months, or palliative therapy)	1
Paralysis or recent plaster/cast or other similar limb immobilization	1
Recently bedridden for more than 3 days or major surgery less than 4 weeks earlier	1
Localized tenderness along distribution of the deep venous system	1
Entire leg swelling	1
Calf swelling greater than 3 cm compared with asymptomatic leg	1
Pitting edema (greater in the symptomatic leg)	1
Collateral superficial veins (nonvaricose)	1
Alternative diagnosis (as likely as or greater than that of DVT)	−2

TOTAL OF SCORES

High probability: Score greater than or equal to 3

Moderate probability: Score 1 to 2

Low probability: Score 0

Continued

TABLE 11-2 Wells Clinical Prediction Guide in Deep Vein Thrombophlebitis (DVT)—cont'd

Wells clinical prediction guide in pulmonary embolus (PE)

CLINICAL PARAMETER	SCORE
Clinical signs/symptoms of DVT	3
No alternative diagnosis likely or more likely than PE	3
Heart rate greater than 100 bpm	1.5
Immobilization or surgery in the past 4 weeks	1.5
Previous history of DVT or PE	1.5
Hemoptysis	1
Cancer actively treated within past 6 months	1

SCORING

Probability of PE is high if total score greater than 6; moderate, if 2 to 6; and low, if less than 2

Source: Adapted from Anand SS, Wells PS, Hunt D, et al. Does this patient have deep vein thrombosis? JAMA. 1998;279:1094–1099.

study should not be limited to the affected area. Serial studies are often needed if initial examination findings are negative but symptoms persist. Although direct venography is the most sensitive and specific test, its use has been limited because these less invasive tests have become available. Magnetic resonance imaging (MRI) and computed tomography (CT) scan can also provide images of veins and possible blood clots; however, these techniques are not typically used to diagnose DVT. During pregnancy, compression ultrasound remains the initial test of choice, though it is less accurate for detecting pelvic DVT compared to extremity DVT. If the results from compression ultrasound testing are abnormal, then further evaluation with MRI is warranted.

Further evaluation for PE should be undertaken based on clinical findings, such as shortness of breath, tachypnea, and/or pleuritic friction rub. Coagulation studies should be obtained, particularly if there is a history of previous episodes without such evaluation. D-dimer, a degradation product produced by plasmin-mediated proteolysis of cross-linked fibrin, is often elevated in DVT and PE. The test has significant limitations, however, because D-dimer levels can be elevated whenever the coagulation and fibrinolytic systems are activated and are falsely elevated in the presence of high rheumatoid factor levels.

When findings are positive in DVT, the degree of D-dimer elevation depends on the size of the clot. A lower-risk patient with a normal D-dimer level is unlikely to have DVT. An underlying clotting disorder in a person with DVT should be considered, with testing for thrombophilia including protein S, protein C, antithrombin III, fibrinogen, lupus anticoagulant, factor V Leiden, prothrombin 20210A mutation, antiphospholipid antibodies, and other thrombophilia forms.

Treatment

Therapy for patients with DVT should be aimed at minimizing the risk of PE and extension of peripheral thrombus. Anticoagulation therapy should be prescribed. Historically, a heparin form followed by a vitamin K antagonist (VKA; e.g., warfarin) were used. These products are aimed at allowing natural fibrinolysis action and clot resolution to occur and minimizing risk for clot extension; heparin and warfarin

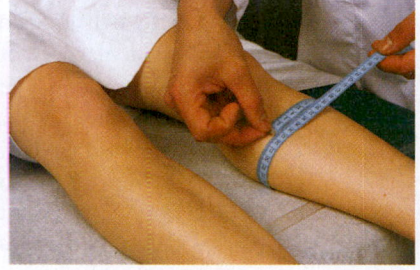

FIGURE 11-3 Measuring calf circumference.
Dillon P. Nursing Health Assessment: A Critical Thinking, Case Studies Approach. 2nd ed. Philadelphia, PA: F.A. Davis; 2007.

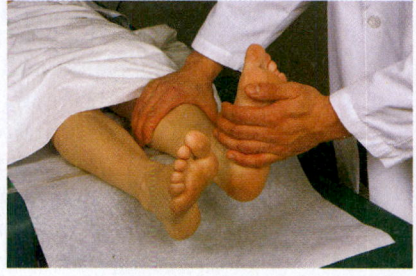

FIGURE 11-4 Assessing for Homans' sign.
Dillon P. Nursing Health Assessment: A Critical Thinking, Case Studies Approach. 2nd ed. Philadelphia, PA: F.A. Davis; 2007.

CLINICAL CONCEPT

An elevated D-dimer level is also found with recent surgery, trauma, myocardial infarction, pregnancy, metastatic cancer, as well as DVT or PE.

do not have intrinsic thrombolytic activity. Current DVT guidelines favor the use of the direct oral anticoagulants (DOACs) as first-line therapy in many individuals. However, DOAC use should be avoided in patients with antiphospholipid antibody syndrome, as well as patients at extremes of weight (less than 50 kg [less than 110 lbs], greater than 120 kg [greater than 265 lbs] or BMI 35 kg/m² or greater) due to changes in the pharmacokinetics of DOACs.

DOACs consist of oral products including direct factor Xa inhibitors (e.g., rivaroxaban [Xarelto®], apixaban [Eliquis®], edoxaban [Savaysa®], and betrixaban [Bevyxxa®]), and the direct thrombin inhibitor dabigatran (Pradaxa®); both are effective for treatment of DVT and PE. The use of these agents, particularly for stroke prevention in rate-controlled atrial fibrillation, has grown because of the ease of use and predictable anticoagulant effect that eliminates the need for ongoing therapeutic monitoring. The ongoing use of these agents can also be considered to reduce the risk of recurrence of DVT and PE. Dose adjustment should be considered in the presence of renal dysfunction. The onset of action with DOACs is much faster than VKAs such as warfarin. The antithrombotic effect is dose dependent, and peak concentration is reached within 0.5 to 4 hours after dosing. Reversal agents are available for some DOACs for when life-threatening or uncontrolled bleeding occurs.

When major bleeding occurs, discontinue use of the DOAC immediately. Given the short half-life of DOACs, DOAC discontinuation is often all that is needed in nonurgent situations. However, for life-threatening major bleeding or nonelective major surgery, aside from DOAC discontinuation, it is imperative to control active bleeding, maintain adequate fluid, oxygen, and hemodynamic support, and follow red blood cell (RBC) transfusion protocols, if necessary.

The use of DOACs has limited but not eliminated the use of heparin in DVT therapy, which continues to be used instead of a DOAC when DOAC therapy is contraindicated. Heparin, a medication given parenterally, inhibits the activity of numerous coagulating factors. Heparin's effect on thrombus formation is immediate. In contrast, warfarin, a VKA, usually requires 3 to 5 days of use before therapeutic levels are reached and clinical effect is seen. Heparin in the unfractionated form, usually given in an IV drip, is available with an average molecular weight of 15,000 daltons, and a low molecular weight heparin (LMWH), with a molecular weight of 4,000 to 6,500 daltons. Enoxaparin (Lovenox®), dalteparin (Fragmin®), and ardeparin (Normiflo®), given via subcutaneous injection, are examples of LMWH. Because of limited bleeding risk, monitoring of partial thromboplastin time (PTT) is not required during LMWH use. When compared to unfractionated heparin, LMWH has additional advantages including superior bioavailability, a longer half-life that allows for once- or twice-daily dosing, ease of calculating dosage, and limited antiplatelet effect. LMWH is often used for DVT prophylaxis for high-risk surgical and medical patients, particularly when DOAC therapy is contraindicated.

Besides the obvious increased risk for bleeding events with its use, another problematic adverse effect of anticoagulation therapy is heparin-induced thrombocytopenia (HIT), a serious condition with potentially life-threatening consequences. Expert consultation on the management of a person who has HIT is required for both immediate management and advice managing future thromboembolic events.

Warfarin acts against coagulation factors II, VII, IX, and X as a result of vitamin K antagonism; hence, it is classified as a VKA (Table 11-3). Warfarin is highly (99%) protein bound, primarily to albumin, and has a narrow therapeutic range; patients must be well informed of the drug-to-drug and drug-to-food interactions (Table 11-4). Because cigarette smoking increases thrombotic risk while reducing efficacy of warfarin, developing a smoking cessation plan is important.

Prothrombin time is used as the measure of the efficacy of warfarin and is reported as an INR (international normalized ratio). INR prolongation is seen in about 48 to 72 hours after the first warfarin dose (Table 11-5). In the presence of a clotting disorder, such as factor V Leiden mutations or antiphospholipid antibodies, anticoagulation should also be lifelong. Given the ease of use, switching from warfarin to a DOAC can be considered for many patients requiring anticoagulation therapy. However, DOACs should be avoided in patients with antiphospholipid antibody syndrome or patients at extremes of weight (see earlier in this chapter).

Approximately 2% to 10% of patients taking warfarin develop a problematic bleeding episode. This complication is rarely seen, however, in patients with an INR of 2 to 3. In the presence of significant bleeding in patients taking warfarin, the drug should be discontinued, and vitamin K should be given promptly. Vitamin K has little effect on hemostasis, however, until 24 hours after its administration. If immediate action is needed, such as in the case of hemorrhage or bleeding into an enclosed space, fresh frozen plasma

TABLE 11-3 Indications and Length of Warfarin Treatment

CONDITION	INR	DURATION OF THERAPY
Acute Venous Thrombosis		
First episode	2 to 3	3 months (extended therapy beyond 3 months in the presence of risk factors)
High risk of recurrence	2 to 3	Indefinitely
With antiphospholipid syndrome or other thrombophilia or coagulopathy	3 to 4	Lifelong
Prevention of Systemic Embolus		
Tissue heart valves	2 to 3	3 months
Valvular heart disease with history of thrombotic event	2 to 3	Indefinitely
Mechanical heart valve (if initially indicated by valve type)	2.5 to 3.5	Indefinitely
Acute myocardial infarction	2 to 3	As deemed by concomitant clinical problems
Atrial Fibrillation		
Chronic or intermittent	2 to 3	Lifelong for chronic or intermittent atrial fibrillation, particularly if not a DOAC candidate
Cardioversion	2 to 3	With cardioversion, for 3 weeks before and 4 weeks after conversion to sinus rhythm

DOAC, direct oral anticoagulant; INR, international normalized ratio.

Source: Moses S. Coumadin protocol. Family Practice Notebook. http://www.fpnotebook.com/HemeOnc/Pharm/CmdnPrtcl.htm

must be given. If anticoagulation therapy is continued after the bleeding crisis, response to warfarin may fluctuate, which necessitates close monitoring.

PULMONARY EMBOLISM

Overview

Pulmonary embolism is the occlusion of one or more pulmonary arteries by thrombi that originate elsewhere, typically in the large veins of the legs or pelvis. With a mortality rate of 20% to 40%, PE is a feared complication of DVT.

Clinical Presentation

The diagnosis of PE is often missed because the presentation is nonspecific. PE presentation usually includes dyspnea, pleuritic chest pain, pleural friction rub, and accentuation of the pulmonic component of S_2 heart sound; tachypnea (respiratory rate greater than or equal to 16/min) and tachycardia are nearly universal findings. DVT signs and symptoms are often noted, but their absence should not eliminate the consideration of PE.

Diagnostic Testing

The use of the Wells predictive scale can be helpful in forming the diagnosis (see Table 11-2). Other clinical scoring systems include the simplified Wells rule, revised

CLINICAL CONCEPT

Hemoptysis, cyanosis, and change in level of consciousness are less commonly encountered but are often considered an expected or classic part of the PE presentation.

TABLE 11-4 Warfarin: Drug and Food Interactions

Note: The concomitant use of warfarin with one of the following medications is not contraindicated. The prescriber and patient need to be aware, however, of the impact of concurrent use on anticoagulation state.

INCREASED ANTICOAGULANT EFFECT	DECREASED ANTICOAGULANT EFFECTS	VARIABLE EFFECT
Alcohol (particularly in the presence of liver disease)	Barbiturates	Phenytoin–increased and decreased effects noted, and increase in phenytoin level
Ingestion of large amounts of dark green leafy vegetables	Carbamazepine	
Amiodarone	Chlordiazepoxide	
Cimetidine	Cholestyramine	
Clofibrate	Griseofulvin	
Cotrimoxazole	Rifampin	
Erythromycin	Sucralfate	
Clarithromycin	Azathioprine	
Fluconazole	Cyclosporine	
Isoniazid	Trazodone	
Metronidazole		
Miconazole		
Proton pump inhibitors		
Piroxicam		
Propranolol		
Acetaminophen (inconsistent)		
Fluoroquinolone antimicrobials		
Disulfiram		
Itraconazole		
Quinidine		
Tamoxifen		
Tetracyclines including doxycycline, minocycline		

Source: Indiana University School of Medicine Division of Clinical Pharmacology. P450 drug interaction table. http://medicine.iupui.edu/clinpharm/ddis/table.asp

TABLE 11-5 Warfarin: Initiation of Therapy and Long-Term Management

■ Warfarin's anticoagulation effect takes at least 3 days of use to achieve. If immediate anticoagulation effect is needed, initiate LMWH therapy while also starting warfarin 5 to 10 mg qd for 2 days, then reduce to 5 mg qd. Check INR daily; when at goal, discontinue heparin.

■ If there is no need for immediate anticoagulation, warfarin should be initiated at 5 mg/day, anticipating therapeutic effect in approximately 4 days. In older adults, initiate warfarin at 4 mg/day, anticipating therapeutic effect in 6 to 7 days.

■ If INR is not within goal during warfarin therapy, check for adherence to recommended therapy before adjusting dose and use of medications or foods that may interfere with warfarin effect.

INR GOAL 2.0 TO 3.0	ACTION
At desired range	Repeat INR at interval determined by duration of therapeutic INR and underlying condition
	■ 4 to 6 weeks if stable condition and typically therapeutic INR
	■ At least weekly when underlying condition can affect coagulation state (e.g., malignancy, clotting disorder, use of medications that can influence warfarin effect)
INR less than 2.0	■ Increase total weekly dose by 5% to 20%
	■ Repeat INR two to three times per week until within desired range

Continued

TABLE 11-5 Warfarin: Initiation of Therapy and Long-Term Management—cont'd

INR 3.0 to 3.5	■ Decrease total weekly dose by 5% to 15% ■ Repeat INR two to three times per week until within desired range
INR 3.6 to 4.0	■ Consider withholding one daily dose, decrease total weekly dose by 10% to 15% ■ Repeat INR two to three times per week until within desired range
INR greater than 4.0 without complications and no indication for rapid reversal of anticoagulation effect	■ Consider withholding one daily dose, decrease total weekly dose by 10% to 20% ■ Repeat INR two to three times per week until within desired range
INR greater than 4.0 and need for rapid reversal of anticoagulant effect	■ Vitamin K 2.5 to 5 mg PO × 1 to 2 doses or 3 mg subcutaneous (SC) or slow intravenous (IV) route
INR GOAL 2.5 TO 3.5 At desired range	**ACTION** ■ Repeat INR at interval determined by duration of therapeutic INR and underlying condition 4 to 6 weeks if stable. ■ 4 to 6 weeks if stable condition and typically therapeutic INR ■ At least weekly when underlying condition can affect coagulation state (e.g., malignancy, clotting disorder, use of medications that can influence warfarin effect)
INR less than 2.0	■ Increase weekly dose by 10% to 20% ■ Repeat INR two to three times per week until within desired range
INR 2.0 to 2.4	■ Increase weekly dose by 5% to 15% ■ Repeat INR two to three times per week until within desired range
INR 3.5 to 4.6	■ Decrease weekly dose by 5% to 15% ■ Repeat INR two to three times per week until within desired range
INR 4.7 to 5.2	■ Consider withholding one dose, decrease weekly dose by 10% to 20% ■ Repeat INR two to three times per week until within desired range
INR greater than 5.2 without complications and no indication for rapid reversal of anticoagulation effect	■ Withhold one to two doses, decrease weekly dose by 10% to 20% ■ Repeat INR two to three times per week until within desired range
INR greater than 5.2 or need for rapid reversal of anticoagulant effect	■ Vitamin K 2.5 mg PO × 1 to 2 doses or 3 mg SC or slow IV route

INR, international normalized ratio; LMWH, low molecular weight heparin.

Source: Moses S. Coumadin protocol. Family Practice Notebook. http://www.fpnotebook.com/HemeOnc/Pharm/CmdnPrtcl.htm

Geneva score, and simplified revised Geneva score, which all show similar ability in excluding acute PE when combined with a normal D-dimer result. The use of D-dimer testing in PE diagnosis has the same limitations as noted in DVT diagnosis. Pulmonary angiography is the historical standard for diagnosing PE; however, with advances in CT scanning, this method is increasingly being preferred for initial testing over angiography as it is noninvasive and less expensive.

Treatment

The American College of Chest Physicians (ACCP) recommends long-term (3 months) anticoagulant therapy for the treatment of DVT or PE. In patients with DVT of the leg or PE and without cancer, a DOAC is preferred over warfarin. Parenteral anticoagulant (i.e., LMWH) use is usually not needed; expert consultation should be obtained. Although 3 months is the recommended duration of treatment for DVT and PE, this is often extended if significant clot risk persists. There is no need to change the choice of anticoagulant after the first 3 months. Patients who experience a recurrent venous thromboembolism (DVT or PE) while on anticoagulant therapy (i.e., warfarin or DOAC) should temporarily switch to treatment with LMWH for at least 1 month. It is unusual for a recurrent episode to occur while on a therapeutic dose of an appropriate anticoagulant therapy. In these cases, the patient should be reevaluated to determine whether there truly was a recurrent venous thromboembolism (VTE), checked for compliance to anticoagulant therapy, and/or considered for an underlying malignancy or previously undiagnosed clotting disorder.

Discussion Sources

Ferri F. Pulmonary embolism. In: Ferri F. *Practical Guide to the Care of the Medical Patient.* 9th ed. Philadelphia, PA: Elsevier Mosby; 2014:358–362.

Kearon C, Akl EA, Ornelas J, et al. Antithrombotic therapy for VTE disease. CHEST Guideline and Expert Panel report. *Chest.* 2016;149:315–352.

Mir MA. Nonplatelet hemostatic disorders. Medscape. https://emedicine.medscape.com/article/210467-overview

Ouellette DR. Pulmonary embolism. Medscape. https://emedicine.medscape.com/article/300901-overview

Patel K. Deep venous thrombosis. Medscape. https://emedicine.medscape.com/article/1911303-overview

QUESTIONS

12. Which of the following is not a contributing factor to the development of venous thrombophlebitis?

A. venous stasis

B. injury to vascular intima

C. malignancy-associated hypercoagulation states

D. history of performing isometric exercise on a regular basis

13. A 28-year-old woman is being evaluated for superficial venous thrombophlebitis. Clinical presentation usually includes:

A. positive Homans sign.

B. diminished dorsalis pedis pulse.

C. a dilated vessel.

D. dependent pallor.

14. The standard treatment of superficial venous thrombophlebitis in a low-risk, stable patient includes use of:

A. compression stockings.

B. DOAC.

C. oral warfarin.

D. parenteral heparin.

15. In providing care for a patient with superficial thrombophlebitis, the NP considers that:

A. it is a benign, self-limiting disease.

B. the linear pattern of induration can help differentiate the process from cellulitis or other inflammatory processes.

C. a chest radiograph should be obtained.

D. limited activity enhances recovery.

16. A 45-year-old woman presents with suspected DVT. Which of the following is most likely to be noted on her physical examination?

A. unilateral leg edema

B. leg pain

C. warmth over the affected area

D. positive obturator sign

17. A positive Homans sign is present in approximately what percentage of patients with DVT?

A. 25%

B. 33%

C. 50%

D. 75%

18. The NP sees a clinically stable 38-year-old woman taking combined oral contraceptives who has a suspected DVT. The initial diagnostic evaluation in this situation is:

A. an impedance plethysmography.

B. an iodine-125 fibrinogen scan.

C. a contrast venography.

D. a duplex ultrasonography.

19. When considering the use of a DOAC for the treatment of VTE, the NP considers all of the following about reversal agents except:

A. reversal agents can be used when life-threatening or uncontrolled bleeding occurs.

B. given the short half-lives of DOACs, reversal agents are not usually needed once DOAC therapy has been discontinued.

C. vitamin K is not a reversal agent for DOACs.

D. protamine sulfate can be used as a reversal agent for multiple DOACs.

20. Which of the following is the preferred medication to reverse or minimize the anticoagulant effects of warfarin?

A. oral or injectable vitamin K

B. injectable protamine sulfate

C. platelet transfusion

D. plasma components

21. The onset of the anticoagulation effect of warfarin usually occurs how soon after the initiation of therapy?

A. immediately

B. 1 to 2 days

C. 3 to 5 days

D. 5 to 7 days

22. Compared with unfractionated heparin, characteristics of LMWH include:

A. more antiplatelet effect.

B. decreased need for monitoring of anticoagulant effect.

C. shorter half-life.

D. need for more frequent dosing.

23. A 36-year-old otherwise well woman who is taking combined oral contraceptives and recently completed a 14-hour plane trip presents with possible diagnosis of PE. Which of the following is least likely to be found in this patient?

A. pleuritic chest pain

B. tachypnea

C. DVT signs and symptoms

D. hemoptysis

24. One of the most commonly used and effective method of preventing venous thromboembolism in higher-risk surgical patients is the routine use of:

A. oral vitamin K.

B. injected LMWH.

C. insertion of a vena cava filter.

D. oral warfarin.

25. When considering other medications in a 56-year-old woman who is starting warfarin therapy, the NP considers that the concomitant use of which of the following will result in a possible increased anticoagulant effect?

A. clarithromycin

B. carbamazepine

C. pravastatin

D. sucralfate

26. When taken concomitantly with warfarin, which of the following oral medications causes a possibly decreased anticoagulant effect?

A. cholestyramine

B. allopurinol

C. cefpodoxime

D. zolpidem

27. What is the INR range recommended during warfarin therapy as part of the management of a patient with DVT?

A. 1.5 to 2

B. 2 to 3

C. 2.5 to 3.5

D. 3 to 4

28. A 57-year-old female experiences a recurrent DVT while taking a DOAC. An appropriate treatment option for this patient is to switch to:

A. oral warfarin.

B. PO edoxaban.

C. PO prasugrel.

D. injected LMWH.

29 to 34. True or False

_____ **29.** During the first 6 weeks of the postpartum period, the childbearing woman is at increased risk for venous thrombus formation.

_____ **30.** In a patient with suspected superficial thrombophlebitis in the calf, the abnormalities in the lower-extremity examination are potentially enhanced by having the patient stand for approximately 2 minutes.

_____ **31.** Idarucizumab should be used for a patient taking rivaroxaban and experiencing uncontrolled bleeding.

_____ **32.** Prescribing a DOAC is an acceptable therapeutic option to reduce the risk of recurrent DVT in many patients who meet certain criteria.

_____ **33.** One of the potential serious adverse effects of unfractionated heparin is thrombocytopenia.

_____ **34.** An abnormally elevated D-dimer test is highly sensitive and specific for the diagnosis of thromboembolic disease.

For answers and rationales, see end of chapter.

Peripheral Vascular Disease

Overview

Peripheral vascular disease (PVD) refers to a group of conditions in which there is a reduction of blood flow to the extremities. With PVD, the venous, arterial, and/or lymphatic system is usually affected.

PERIPHERAL ARTERIAL OCCLUSIVE DISEASE

Overview

Peripheral arterial occlusive disease (PAOD), almost exclusively involving the lower extremities, is usually caused by diffuse and extensive atherosclerosis. Risk factors for PAOD include diabetes mellitus, hypertension, and hyperlipidemia; tobacco use is the most potent risk factor, particularly in progressive disease. In the absence of these risk factors, PAOD is rare except in advanced age; the condition is found in 10% of older adults.

Clinical Presentation

Clinical presentation of PAOD usually includes a patient complaint of claudication, which is a reproducible ischemic calf muscle pain wherein pain is worse with exertion and usually responds promptly to cessation of the trigger activity. Claudication is caused by the inability of the diseased vessel to vasodilate and allow for increased blood flow to handle the metabolic demands associated with physical activity such as walking or climbing stairs.

PAOD caused by atherosclerosis in the distal aorta or iliac, femoral, or popliteal arteries results in the most common clinical form. Presentation varies according to the area of vessel disease and dysfunction (Table 11-6). Atherosclerotic and calcific lesions usually cause occlusive disease of the aorta and its branches. Disease is often asymmetrical because the distribution of obstructive lesions usually occurs in segments rather than continuously.

Diagnostic Testing

The PAOD diagnosis in the lower extremities is made from clinical presentation and select diagnostic studies. An ankle-brachial index (ABI) should be performed to determine PAOD presence. An ABI of less than 0.95 is strongly predictive of lower-extremity perfusion compromise. Doppler ultrasonography is often the first-line imaging study to confirm the diagnosis and monitor disease progression. Magnetic resonance angiography and high-definition CT with contrast are also options. In studies that require the use of contrast, assessment of renal function before the procedure is critical because the risk of contrast-induced renal impairment is greatest in the presence of diffuse arterial disease. Radionuclide-based molecular imaging can offer an alternative noninvasive approach to assess angiogenesis and atherosclerosis in the lower extremities.

Treatment

Because patients with lower-extremity arterial occlusive disease usually have other health problems, prevention and intervention measures (such as aggressive cardiovascular risk factor reduction including cessation of tobacco use and blood pressure, glucose, and lipid control) help improve overall well-being. In addition, the presence of concomitant disease, such as cardiovascular or cerebrovascular disease, often limits the patient's ability to be physically active. Exercise such as walking helps to minimize symptoms and should be encouraged; although exercise was previously thought to enhance collateral blood flow, the benefit is now recognized as being a result of improving oxygen extraction for the skeletal muscles. Meticulous skin care is needed to avoid breakdown, and periodic podiatric care is recommended. In the presence of PAOD, skin and nail disruptions are particularly difficult to heal.

Pharmacotherapy in PAOD often yields variable results. The use of pentoxifylline (Trental®), a medication thought to reduce blood viscosity and improve blood flow by altering the ability of RBCs to pass through diseased vessels, can be helpful in increasing exercise tolerance, especially in milder disease. Cilostazol (Pletal®), a medication that impairs platelet aggregation and increases vasodilation, is often helpful but has limitations. Its use is contraindicated in heart failure and carries a high rate of adverse effects, including headache, dizziness, and diarrhea. The use of these medications does not alter the course of the

TABLE 11-6 Clinical Presentation of Lower-Extremity Peripheral Arterial Occlusive Disease (PAOD)

PATIENT PRESENTATION	CLINICAL SIGNIFICANCE
Burning sensation or ache with walking	Usually indicates femoropopliteal arterial disease
Pain in calf, hip, or buttock with activity, relieved by rest	Classic report in intermittent claudication
Foot pain at rest	Blood flow to extremity less than or equal to 10% of normal; indicates profound disease and gangrene risk
Numbness, coldness, pain in extremity	More common than claudication report in the older adult
Absent posterior tibialis pulse	This pulse is always present in a healthy adult Dorsalis pedis pulse absent in approximately 5% of healthy adults
Nail thickening	Because numbness is often also a problem, meticulous nail hygiene while minimizing injury is needed; onychomycosis common
Absent dorsalis pedis and tibial pulses	Absent peripheral pulses usually indicate 10% or less of normal blood flow to extremity; proximal pulses often remain palpable even in the presence of significant occlusive disease
Blanching of foot with elevation, poor capillary return, dependent rubor	Most common in peripheral with long-standing, poorly controlled diabetes mellitus
Ache in anterior tibial muscles, foot, and metatarsal arch with activity	Can be confused with peripheral neuropathy
Sexual dysfunction	Most common in presence of smoking, hyperlipidemia, diabetes mellitus; PAOD contributes to its development but is likely one of many influencing factors

Source: Dominguez JA. Peripheral arterial occlusive disease clinical presentation. Medscape. https://emedicine.medscape.com/article/460178-clinical#a0217

disease, but rather reduces symptoms. Daily aspirin, with clopidogrel (Plavix®) as a replacement in aspirin allergy, and statin therapy are usually indicated as part of a comprehensive plan to reduce cardiovascular risk; concomitant control of diabetes mellitus, which is often present, is critical. Vorapaxar (Zontivity®), a protease-activated receptor-1 (PAR-1) antagonist, can be used in combination with aspirin and/or clopidogrel to reduce the risk of thrombotic cardiovascular events. Historically, warfarin therapy with a goal INR of 2 to 3 was used for certain patients with high thrombus risk, particularly patients who have undergone a vascular procedure. DOACs (e.g., dabigatran, rivaroxaban, apixaban, edoxaban) are used in place of warfarin owing to more convenient dosing, more predictable anticoagulant effect, and elimination of the need for regular therapeutic monitoring (see the DVT/PE section in this chapter).

Surgical evaluation for possible percutaneous or open procedures should be part of the care of patients with lower-extremity arterial occlusive disease; management of concomitant problems, such as cardiovascular risk factors and diabetes mellitus, needs to be optimized preoperatively, and surgical intervention for other forms of vascular disease also needs to be considered. Angioplasty, grafting procedures, and/or vascular stenting can help improve blood flow and minimize symptoms and complications. Owing to the complexity of care, intervention for peripheral arterial ulcers usually requires specialty consultation.

Although lower-extremity arterial occlusive disease is characterized by a predictable, slower, progressive process, acute occlusion can occur. Acute limb ischemia caused by embolic, thrombotic, or traumatic events usually manifests with the so-called six P's:

■ *pain*
■ *paresthesia*
■ *pallor*

- *pulselessness*
- *poikilothermy (variation in limb temperature)*
- *paralysis*

Pain and paresthesia are the two most common manifestations. When acute limb ischemia is caused by arterial embolism, the origin of the clot is usually the heart, with underlying atrial fibrillation. When caused by arterial thrombosis, chronic arteriosclerotic occlusive disease is usually at the core of the problem. Prompt assessment is needed to support the diagnosis. In the presence of acute arterial occlusion, anticoagulation therapy with heparin is standard along with consideration of procedural intervention to relieve the obstruction.

CHRONIC VENOUS INSUFFICIENCY

Overview

CVI is a common sequela of DVT and leg trauma, although the absence of this history is noted in about 25% of patients. There is decreased venous return because of vessel damage, and lower-extremity edema is usually the earliest sign.

Clinical Presentation

CVI symptoms usually include leg aching, cramping, heaviness, itch, and sensation of leg fatigue. Over time, edema develops and becomes progressively worse; this results in the development of thin, shiny, atrophic skin, often with brown pigmentation. Subcutaneous tissue thickens and becomes fibrous. The stage is set for stasis ulceration. Inflamed pruritic patches usually precede the formation of an irregular ulceration with a clean base. Yellow eschar is occasionally found.

Diagnostic Testing

In the primary care setting, initial CVI diagnosis is made clinically. In particular, duplex ultrasonography, used in a variety of venous abnormalities, is the study of choice for the evaluation of venous insufficiency syndromes and guides the choice of therapies.

Treatment

CVI therapies enhancing venous flow (i.e., limb elevation, exercise, and compression therapy) improve oxygen transport to the skin and subcutaneous tissues, decrease edema, and reduce inflammation and can be utilized for any patient with symptoms and signs of chronic venous disease. Compression therapy has long been considered an important part of venous ulcer therapy; high-compression bandages, exerting 30 to 40 mm Hg at the ankle, are most effective. The use of a flexible compression bandage is preferred over a rigid compression dressing such as an Unna boot. If compression therapy is not successful when used alone, high-dose pentoxifylline therapy can be added to compression therapy. Pentoxifylline used as an adjunct to compression is more effective than medication without compression. When used without compression, it is more effective than placebo or no treatment.

> **CLINICAL CONCEPT**
> If venous ulcers occur, wound débridement, through the use of specialized dressings or via a surgical approach, is an essential component in the management of this condition.

The presence of devitalized tissue increases the potential for local bacterial infection and sepsis. Removal of necrotic tissue and fibrinous debris in venous ulcers aids in the formation of healthy granulation tissue and enhances reepithelialization. Specialized occlusive, moisture-retaining dressings improve pain and have utility in autolytic débridement. Surgical débridement is occasionally needed, especially if an advanced therapy such as a bioengineered skin graft is being considered. Hyperbaric oxygen therapy, due to its ability to saturate the tissue and plasma surrounding the venous stasis ulcer, is an option. The aforementioned therapies are usually done in conjunction with specialty consultation. If wound healing continues to be unsuccessful, a biopsy specimen of the lesion should be obtained to rule out malignancy, as the presentation of squamous or basal cell carcinoma can present as a nonhealing ulcerated skin lesion.

Adequate nutrition is an often-overlooked requirement for wound healing, regardless of wound origin. Inadequate protein-calorie nutrition, even after just a few days of starvation, can impair normal wound-healing mechanisms. For healthy adults, daily nutritional requirements are approximately 1.25 to 1.5 g of protein per kilogram of body weight and 30 to 35 calories/kg; these requirements are increased in the presence of sizable wounds.

Discussion Sources

Alguire PC, Mathes BM. Medical management of lower extremity chronic venous disease. UpToDate. https://www.uptodate.com/contents/medical-management-of-lower-extremity-chronic-venous-disease

Chahin C. Imaging in lower-extremity peripheral artery disease (PAD). Medscape. http://emedicine.medscape.com/article/423649-overview

Daley BJ. Wound care treatment and management. Medscape. http://emedicine.medscape.com/article/194018-treatment#a25

de la Torre JI. Chronic wounds. Medscape. http://emedicine.medscape.com/article/1298452-overview

Latham E. Hyperbaric oxygen therapy. Medscape. http://emedicine.medscape.com/article/1464149-overview

QUESTIONS

35. Which of the following is the most potent risk factor for lower-extremity PAOD?

   A. hypertension

   B. older age

   C. cigarette smoking

   D. leg injury

36. Clinical presentation of PAOD includes all of the following except:

   A. resting pain.

   B. absent posterior tibialis pulse.

   C. blanching of the foot with elevation.

   D. skin hyperpigmentation.

37. Typically, the earliest sign of lower-extremity CVI is:

   A. edema.

   B. altered pigmentation.

   C. skin atrophy.

   D. shiny skin.

38. Comprehensive treatment for a person with PAOD and diabetes mellitus includes all of the following except:

   A. daily aspirin use.

   B. lipid-lowering with an HMG-CoA reductase inhibitor (statin).

   C. application of a topical antimicrobial to the affected area.

   D. maintenance of glycemic control.

39. Treatment options to the affected area of venous stasis ulcers in the lower extremities include:

   A. daily cleansing with hydrogen peroxide.

   B. ensuring a topical antimicrobial is applied twice a day.

   C. prescribing a systemic corticosteroid when lesions are most inflamed.

   D. applying an occlusive, moisture-retaining dressing.

40. Cilostazol (Pletal®) should be used with great caution in the presence of which of the following diagnoses?

   A. diabetes mellitus

   B. heart failure

   C. hypertension

   D. dyslipidemia

41. The clinical presentation of PAOD with acute occlusion most likely includes:

   A. pain and paresthesia.

   B. pallor and pulselessness.

C. poikilothermy.

D. paralysis or loss of limb strength.

42. Which of the following patients is most likely to have acute occlusive lower-extremity atherosclerotic arterial disease?

A. a 68-year-old woman with new-onset atrial fibrillation

B. a 75-year-old man with CVI

C. a 28-year-old woman being treated for DVT

D. a 45-year-old man with a recent ankle sprain

43. In ordering imaging studies in a patient with peripheral vascular disease, the use of radiocontrast medium in a 78-year-old who has hypertension, type 2 diabetes mellitus, and dyslipidemia can potentially result in:

A. hepatic failure.

B. renal failure.

C. bone marrow suppression.

D. thrombocytopenia.

44 to 45. True or False

_____ **44.** In the treatment of a venous stasis ulcer that is not responding to standard therapy, additional therapeutic options include hyperbaric oxygen therapy (HBOT).

_____ **45.** As few as 3 days of malnutrition in the form of inadequate protein-calorie intake can impair normal wound-healing mechanisms.

For answers and rationales, see end of chapter.

QUESTION ANSWERS AND RATIONALES

Raynaud's Phenomenon

1. Correct: D. an 18-year-old woman using combined oral contraceptives

Primary Raynaud's phenomenon typically first appears between the ages of 15 and 45 years and is more commonly found in women. Among the answer choices, the 18-year-old woman best fits within the highest risk category.

Incorrect:

The initial onset of primary Raynaud's phenomenon typically occurs in younger adults, and so would be less common in the older population (A, B). This condition is also more common in women than in men (C). The comorbid conditions and medications included in the answer choices are not contributors to Raynaud's phenomenon.

2. Correct: A. a 45-year-old woman with well-controlled hypertension.

Underlying medical conditions associated with secondary Raynaud's phenomenon include atherosclerosis, collagen vascular disease, and select autoimmune diseases, such as scleroderma. The use of vibrating tools as well as certain medications, such as beta blockers, can increase risk. Hypertension is not a risk factor for Raynaud's phenomenon.

Incorrect:

Scleroderma (B), the use of vibrating tools (C), and beta blocker use (D) are all risk factors for the development of secondary Raynaud's phenomenon. Prevention strategies include avoiding known triggers, such as the consistent use of vibrating tools. Additionally, an alternative medication other than a beta blocker can be considered for migraine prophylaxis.

3. Correct: A. Pay attention to hand skin care to avoid dry skin and fissures, and C. Place hands in warm water at the onset of symptoms.

Lifestyle modifications for patients with Raynaud's phenomenon should include prevention of known triggers of vasospasm, such as cold temperatures. At the onset of an episode, submerging the hands in warm water can reduce the duration and severity of symptoms (C). Also, since wound healing can be delayed in these patients, proper skin care is important in reducing the risk of infection (A).

Incorrect:

Lifestyle modifications can be important in preventing episodes and reducing the duration and severity of symptoms associated with Raynaud's phenomenon. These include avoiding triggers of vasospasm, submerging hands in warm water at the start of an episode, and proper skin care to prevent even minor injuries. Limiting fluid intake (B) and discontinuing the use of aspirin (D) play no role in treating or preventing Raynaud's phenomenon or its complications.

4. Correct: B. ACEIs.

Medications with vasodilator effect can be helpful in treating Raynaud's phenomenon when lifestyle modification is inadequate. These can include the dihydropyridine calcium channel blockers and ACEIs (B).

Incorrect:

NSAIDs (A), beta-adrenergic antagonists (C), and diuretics (D) do not exhibit a vasodilator effect and, thus, would not be effective in treating Raynaud's phenomenon.

5. Correct: C. a period of intense itchiness after blanching

The observation of blanching followed by itching (C) is the classic presentation of Raynaud's phenomenon.

Incorrect:

Digital ulceration (A) is an uncommon finding in Raynaud's phenomenon and is usually only in response to a severe insult to the hands, such as prolonged exposure to the cold. Symptoms are usually better during the warm weather months (B), so it is expected that this patient would have worse symptoms during the winter as she lives in a part of the country where it is cold in winter. Symptoms of Raynaud's phenomenon are usually bilateral and fairly symmetrical (D).

Varicose Veins

6. Correct: D. Raynaud's disease

Raynaud's disease (D) is not associated with varicose veins and is a condition that affects the arterial, rather than venous, system.

Incorrect:

Nonmodifiable risk factors for varicose veins include an inherited venous defect (C) and female gender. Modifiable risk factors include leg crossing (A), wearing constricting garments, prolonged standing, heavy lifting, and pregnancy (B).

7. Correct: C. a medium- to heavyweight prescription product

When considering the use of support hose to minimize varicose vein symptoms, the use of medium- to heavyweight elastic support hose (C) is recommended, as these will provide the adequate amount of compression needed. Stockings purchased in drugstores or department stores do not normally supply sufficient compression.

Incorrect:

Lightweight stockings (B) and hosiery found in the department store (A) will not provide adequate compression. Stockings do not need to be in the form of pantyhose (D). When using compression stockings, it is important to ensure the top band is not constricting as this will increase intravenous pressure and reduce circulation in the lower extremities.

8. Correct: D. saphenous vein

Knowledge of anatomy is critical to safe clinical practice. Varicose veins typically involve the superficial great saphenous vein and its tributaries (D).

Incorrect:

Varicose veins typically involve superficial veins that are close to the skin and drain blood from the skin and underlying tissue. The saphenous vein is commonly involved in varicose veins. The femoral vein (A), posterior tibial vein (B), and peroneal vein (C) are deep veins that are closer to the arteries located deep in the muscle.

9. Correct: C. Symptoms are sometimes reported with minimally affected vessels.

When evaluating varicose veins, it is important to note that the amount of visible vein involvement does not predictably correlate with the degree of discomfort experienced by the patient. Thus, symptoms can be reported by patients with minimally affected vessels (C).

Incorrect:

For varicose veins, there is no predictable correlation between the amount of visible problems and the degree of clinical signs and symptoms. Thus, the degree of venous tortuosity (A) or the number of affected veins (B) are not useful tools in estimating the amount of leg pain and discomfort experienced by the patient. Lower-extremity edema (D) is a common sign of varicose veins, particularly toward the end of the day when the patient has been standing or walking a good deal. Periods of leg elevation are recommended during the day to improve comfort and reduce edema.

10. Correct: B. initiate anticoagulant therapy.

The use of anticoagulants (B) is not indicated for the treatment of superficial varicose veins unless the condition extends into the deep venous system. Unnecessary use of anticoagulants will place the patient at increased bleeding risk.

Incorrect:

In addition to the use of compression stockings, several other measures can be used to reduce the discomfort associated with varicose veins. Periodic leg elevation can minimize edema and encourage venous blood return. More aggressive treatment can include minimally invasive procedures, such as endovenous laser ablation (C) or sclerotherapy (D).

11. Correct: C. responsive to laser obliteration.

Spider varicosities are largely a cosmetic issue and respond well to laser obliteration (C), though multiple rounds of treatment are often needed. The condition is typically benign in nature and does not cause symptoms or pose a thromboembolic risk.

Incorrect:

Spider varicosities are largely a cosmetic issue and pose no serious health threat (e.g., thrombophlebitis [B]), are not ecchymotic, and are not associated with any symptoms (A). These varicosities consist of visible surface vessels that usually occur with varicose veins and are not caused by sun exposure (D).

Deep Vein Thrombosis and Pulmonary Embolism

12. Correct: D. history of performing isometric exercise on a regular basis

Performing any type of exercise, including isometric exercise (D), on a regular basis that helps avoid blood stasis is a preventive measure for developing venous thromboembolism.

Incorrect:

Contributing factors for the development of VTE include the Virchow triad of venous stasis (A), injury to the vascular intima (B), and abnormal coagulation leading to clot formation (C). These contribute to vessel inflammation and resulting thrombophlebitis. Physical activity and exercise are important in reducing the risk for thrombophlebitis.

13. Correct: C. a dilated vessel.

Superficial venous thrombophlebitis is typically characterized by a localized, tender, dilated (C), thrombosed vessel causing a linear area of redness.

Incorrect:

The Homans sign (A) (calf pain at dorsiflexion of the foot) is an indicator for DVT (not superficial thrombophlebitis) but has low specificity and sensitivity. A diminished dorsalis pedis pulse (B), as well as dependent pallor (D), would be more indicative of an arterial condition rather than venous thrombophlebitis.

14. Correct: A. compression stockings.

Superficial thrombophlebitis in a low-risk, stable patient is largely considered a benign condition that would not require the use of anticoagulants after evaluation has ruled out DVT. Compression stockings can be used to help venous blood return.

Incorrect:

The use of anticoagulants, such as DOACs (B), warfarin (C), or heparin (D), is not indicated in a stable, low-risk patient with superficial thrombophlebitis where DVT has been ruled out. In higher-risk patients, superficial thrombophlebitis can be a marker for further clotting issues, particularly in hospitalized patients. Other factors that place these patients at higher risk of DVT include presence of prior episodes, a history of DVT, decreased mobility, hypercoagulability, or extensive saphenous vein involvement. General risk factors for DVT include prolonged rest, recent trauma, recent surgery, pregnancy, and the peripartum period.

15. Correct: B. the linear pattern of induration can help differentiate the process from cellulitis or other inflammatory processes.

Superficial thrombophlebitis is typically characterized by a localized, tender, dilated, thrombosed vessel causing a linear area of redness. The linear pattern can help distinguish superficial thrombophlebitis from other conditions, such as cellulitis (B).

Incorrect:

Though superficial thrombophlebitis is often considered a benign condition, it can be a marker for more serious clotting issues that need to be evaluated, such as DVT (A). While the patient with this condition should be carefully evaluated for DVT or PE, a chest radiograph is not warranted (C). Physical activity should actually be encouraged (D) as this decreases venous stasis and enhances blood flow.

16. Correct: A. unilateral leg edema

Though there are many signs to indicate DVT, unilateral leg edema (A) offers the highest sensitivity and specificity.

Incorrect:

When examining a patient with DVT, there is often little to no leg pain (B), and the affected area is not warm (C). A positive obturator sign (D) is noted in the patient with peritoneal inflammation (such as appendicitis) and not DVT.

17. Correct: B. 33%

About one-third (B) of patients with DVT will have a positive Homans sign. A positive Homans sign is exhibited by calf pain at dorsiflexion of the foot. It is important to note that this is not a sensitive or specific test for DVT, as many patients without DVT will also exhibit a positive Homans sign.

18. Correct: D. a duplex ultrasonography.

Initial imaging of DVT is more commonly being performed with duplex ultrasonography (D) as it offers reasonable sensitivity and specificity, is noninvasive, and is less expensive than contrast venography.

Incorrect:

Contrast venography remains the standard diagnostic test for DVT as it provides the highest specificity and sensitivity. However, its higher cost, invasive nature, and risk of allergy to the contrast medium have limited its use in preference to other noninvasive approaches (e.g., duplex ultrasonography). Iodine-125 fibrinogen scanning (B) and impedance plethysmography (A), though once used for the diagnosis of DVT, have been replaced with newer imaging techniques that offer superior specificity and sensitivity.

19. Correct: D. protamine sulfate can be used as a reversal agent for multiple DOACs.

Protamine sulfate can be used to reverse the effects of heparin but would not be effective as a reversal agent for any DOAC.

Incorrect:

Reversal agents can be important in the event of a life-threatening or uncontrolled bleeding event (A). Current reversal agents include idarucizumab (Praxbind®) to counteract the anticoagulation effects of dabigatran and andexanet alfa (Andexxa®) for reversal of rivaroxaban and apixaban. Since DOACs have short half-lives, the use of reversal agents is not usually needed in nonurgent situations, and the DOAC should be discontinued immediately (B). Vitamin K is used to diminish the effects of warfarin, which is not considered a DOAC (C).

20. **Correct: A. oral or injectable vitamin K**

For patients taking warfarin and who are at significant bleeding risk, they should stop taking warfarin and promptly be given vitamin K (A). However, it is important to note that vitamin K has little effect on hemostasis until 24 hours after administration.

Incorrect:

Protamine sulfate (B) can be used to reverse the effects of heparin but not warfarin. Platelet transfusions (C) or plasma components (D) are occasionally used in extreme situations of bleeding but are not routinely used to reverse the effects of warfarin.

21. **Correct: C. 3 to 5 days**

Recognition of a drug's pharmacokinetics and pharmacodynamics is critical to safe prescribing practices. Warfarin's anticoagulation effect takes 3 to 5 days (C) of use to achieve therapeutic levels. If immediate anticoagulation effect is needed, then heparin should be used concomitantly with warfarin for the first few days, checking INR daily.

Incorrect:

The full anticoagulation effect of warfarin will require at least 3 days after initiating therapy (A, B) and is fully appreciated by 5 days of treatment (D).

22. **Correct: B. decreased need for monitoring of anticoagulant effect.**

LMWH has limited antiplatelet effect and limited bleeding risk; thus, regular monitoring of PTT is not required during its use (B).

Incorrect:

Though LMWH is more costly than unfractionated heparin, it offers a number of advantages. In addition to a decreased need for monitoring anticoagulant effect, LMWH has superior bioavailability, limited antiplatelet effect (A), a longer half-life (C) that allows for less frequent once- or twice-daily dosing (D), and greater ease of calculating doses.

23. **Correct: D. hemoptysis**

Though hemoptysis (D), the coughing up of blood or blood-tinged mucus, is often reported as a finding in pulmonary embolism, it is relatively rare and would be the least likely clinical finding among the given answer choices.

Incorrect:

The diagnosis of PE is often difficult as patient presentation is nonspecific. Universal findings in PE include dyspnea, pleuritic chest pain (A), pleural friction rub, tachypnea (B), and tachycardia. DVT signs and symptoms are also frequently noted, though their absence should not be used to rule out consideration of PE.

24. **Correct: B. injected LMWH.**

Injected LMWH (B) provides rapid-onset anticoagulation that is needed in the immediate prevention and treatment of VTE among surgical patients.

Incorrect:

Oral warfarin usually requires 3 to 5 days of use before attaining therapeutic level and so is not useful in immediate prevention of VTE. Warfarin is more appropriately used for the long-term treatment and recurrence prevention of VTE. Oral vitamin K (A) is used to reverse the anticoagulation effect of warfarin if there is excess bleeding risk. A vena cava filter (C) can be used in the presence of extensive thrombosis but not for preventing VTE.

25. **Correct: A. clarithromycin**

Patients must be well informed of potential drug-drug and drug-food interactions when taking warfarin to prevent coagulation issues. Clarithromycin (A) is a potent CYP450 inhibitor, which will reduce the metabolism of warfarin and, thus, will result in greater warfarin exposure and anticoagulation effect.

Incorrect:

Carbamazepine is a CYP450 enzyme inducer, which will result in faster breakdown of warfarin and, thus, less anticoagulation effect. Sucralfate (D), when taken at the same time as warfarin, will result in binding and inactivation of warfarin in the stomach and will limit warfarin's therapeutic effect. Pravastatin (C) will have minimal effect on warfarin as it has no action on CYP450.

26. **Correct: A. cholestyramine**

Patients must be well informed of potential drug-drug and drug-food interactions when taking warfarin to prevent coagulation issues. Cholestyramine (A), when taken at the same time as warfarin, will result in binding and inactivation of warfarin in the stomach and will limit warfarin's therapeutic effect.

Incorrect:

Zolpidem (D) and allopurinol (B) will have minimal impact on the anticoagulation effect of warfarin as they have little impact on CYP450 enzyme. Cefpodoxime, as an antimicrobial, can disrupt gut flora involved in the synthesis of vitamin K, which will increase the anticoagulation effect of warfarin.

27. **Correct: B. 2 to 3**

It is important for clinicians to know the therapeutic goal of patients taking warfarin therapy. The desired INR range for a patient taking warfarin for the treatment of DVT is 2 to 3 (B). A slightly higher goal of 2.5 to 3.5 can be considered in patients with select thrombophilias.

Incorrect:

For patients taking warfarin, routine INR monitoring and dose adjustment are important in attaining and maintaining therapeutic goal. When the INR goal is between 2 and 3, an INR of less than 2 would indicate an increase in total weekly warfarin dose by 5% to 20%. An INR of 3 to 3.5 should result in a decrease of the total weekly dose of warfarin by 5% to 15%. When INR is 3.6 to 4, consider withholding one daily dose and decreasing the total weekly dose by 10% to 15%.

28. Correct: D. injected LMWH.

For a patient who is taking a DOAC or vitamin K antagonist (warfarin), the appropriate treatment option is to switch to LMWH (D) for at least 1 month.

Incorrect:

For a patient who develops recurrent DVT while on a DOAC, switching to another DOAC, such as edoxaban (B), or to warfarin (A) is not recommended. Prasugrel is an antiplatelet agent and is not indicated for prevention or treatment of VTE. Since a recurrent VTE while on a DOAC is uncommon, these patients should be carefully reevaluated as to whether there truly was a recurrent VTE, evaluation of compliance with anticoagulant therapy, and consideration of a possible underlying malignancy.

29 to 34. True or False

29. Correct: True

Increased blood coagulation is a normative response to childbirth to minimize the mother's risk of postpartum hemorrhage. As a result, the mother is at higher risk of VTE during the postpartum period.

30. Correct: True

When examining a patient with superficial thrombophlebitis, the patient should stand for 2 minutes prior to examination as this will enhance clinical findings. This is particularly true in less severe cases that may present with normal findings when in the supine position.

31. Correct: False

Reversal agents can be an important intervention for patients taking anticoagulation therapy and who experience life-threatening or uncontrolled bleeding. However, the reversal agent for rivaroxaban is andexanet alfa (Andexxa®), while idarucizumab (Praxbind®) is a reversal agent for dabigatran.

32. Correct: True

DOACs, which include direct factor Xa inhibitors and direct thrombin inhibitors, can be an acceptable therapeutic option to prevent DVT recurrence and offer several key advantages compared to warfarin, including more rapid onset of action, ease of dosing, predictable anticoagulant effect, and no need for ongoing therapeutic monitoring. However, DOACs should be avoided in patients with antiphospholipid antibody syndrome, as well as those at extremes of weight (less than 50 kg [less than 110 lb], greater than 120 kg [greater than 265 lb] or BMI 35 kg/m² or greater).

33. Correct: True

HIT is a serious and potentially life-threatening condition associated with the use of unfractionated heparin. The risk of HIT can be decreased with the use of LMWH.

34. Correct: False

D-dimer is a degradation product produced by plasmin-mediated proteolysis of cross-linked fibrin. Though D-dimer is often elevated in DVT and PE, the test has

significant limitations. D-dimer levels can be elevated whenever the coagulation and fibrinolytic systems are activated and are falsely elevated in the presence of high rheumatoid factor levels. As such, the test has high sensitivity but poor specificity.

Peripheral Vascular Disease

35. Correct: C. cigarette smoking

Though several risk factors have been identified for the development of PAOD, tobacco use (C) is the most potent risk factor, particularly in progressive disease.

Incorrect:

In addition to cigarette smoking, other risk factors for PAOD include diabetes mellitus, hypertension (A), and hyperlipidemia. In the absence of these risk factors, POAD is relatively rare except in older age (B), where the condition is found in approximately 10% of older adults. Leg injury (D) can also contribute to the development of PAOD but is not the most potent risk factor.

36. Correct: D. skin hyperpigmentation.

Skin hyperpigmentation is more likely associated with CVI and not PAOD. Acute limb ischemia typically manifests with the so-called six P's: pain, paresthesia, pallor, pulselessness, poikilothermy, and paralysis.

Incorrect:

Lower-extremity PAOD usually manifests as a slowly progressive disease, but acute occlusion can occur with resulting symptoms. Acute limb ischemia associated with PAOD typically manifests with the so-called six P's: pain (A), paresthesia, pallor (C), pulselessness (B), poikilothermy, and paralysis.

37. Correct: A. edema.

CVI is associated with decreased venous return due to blood vessel damage, resulting in lower-extremity edema (A) as the earliest sign.

Incorrect:

In addition to edema, early signs of CVI include leg aching and itchiness. As CVI progresses, edema worsens and leads to the development of thin (C), shiny (D) skin, often with brown pigmentation (B). The subcutaneous tissue eventually thickens and becomes fibrous.

38. Correct: C. application of a topical antimicrobial to the affected area.

For the patient with PAOD, management of cardiovascular risk factors is important in the overall treatment plan. This includes measures to properly control glucose, blood pressure, and lipids, as well as antiplatelet therapy to reduce cardiovascular events. Routine use of a topical antimicrobial (C) is not warranted in these patients in the absence of an active skin infection.

Incorrect:

Since PAOD often occurs in patients with other comorbid conditions, interventions should include aggressive control of risk factors to improve overall well-being. For the PAOD patient with diabetes mellitus, this can include daily aspirin (A) or clopidogrel use, statin use (B) for lipid-lowering therapy, antihypertensive medication, and proper maintenance of blood glucose (D). Smoking cessation should also be a key priority for patients who continue to use tobacco products.

39. Correct: D. applying an occlusive, moisture-retaining dressing.

Stasis ulceration of lower-extremity skin is a common finding among patients with CVI. Wound care to improve ulcer healing can include débridement, multilayer compression dressings, and hyperbaric oxygen. Moisture-retaining dressings can improve pain and promote autolytic débridement. They also supply a favorable microenvironment for growth of new tissue.

Incorrect:

Though skin hygiene is important for patients with CVI, the routine use of a topical antimicrobial (B) is not warranted. Repeated exposure to hydrogen peroxide (A) can actually be damaging to the skin. A systemic corticosteroid (C) is not indicated for the treatment of skin ulcers.

40. Correct: B. heart failure

Cilostazol, a PDE-3 inhibitor, can help reduce symptoms associated with PAOD. However, its use is contraindicated in patients with heart failure (B), as it increases vasodilation and can result in arrhythmias, similar to other PDE-3 inhibitors. This class of drugs is associated with increased mortality in patients with class III through IV heart failure.

Incorrect:

Cilostazol can be safely used in patients with other comorbidities beyond heart failure, including diabetes mellitus (A), hypertension (C), and dyslipidemia (D). However, approximately 20% of patients will develop adverse effects, most commonly headache, dizziness, and diarrhea.

41. Correct: A. pain and paresthesia.

Though it is important to recognize the 6 P's associated with PAOD with acute occlusion, the most common symptoms of this condition are pain and paresthesia (A).

Incorrect:

Acute limb ischemia associated with PAOD typically manifests with the so-called six P's: pain, paresthesia, pallor, pulselessness (B), poikilothermy (C), and paralysis (D). Though any combination of these signs and symptoms can be present during an acute episode, pain and paresthesia are the most commonly found, while the other symptoms occur less frequently.

42. Correct: A. a 68-year-old woman with new-onset atrial fibrillation

It is important for clinicians to be cognizant of risk factors associated with given conditions. Arterial embolism associated with atrial fibrillation (A) is the most common etiology.

Incorrect:

The conditions of CVI (B) and DVT (C) are common risk factors for venous disorders but not acute arterial occlusive disease. The presence of arterial or venous trauma (D) is not typically associated with the development of acute arterial occlusion.

43. Correct: B. renal failure.

High-definition CT with contrast medium can be useful in the diagnosis of PVD. However, renal function should be assessed prior to the procedure as the use of contrast can lead to the development of contrast-induced renal impairment (B). This is particularly important in older patients and those with multiple risk factors for vascular dysfunction.

Incorrect:

The use of contrast medium can lead to renal failure, particularly in patients with renal impairment and risk factors for vascular dysfunction. Contrast medium is not typically associated with hepatic failure (A), bone marrow suppression (C), or thrombocytopenia (D), though an allergic reaction can also be a concern.

44 to 45. True or False

44. Correct: True

For patients with CVI, wounds that fail to heal are typically hypoxic. Therefore, the use of HBOT can be an effective approach to wound healing. HBOT increases oxygen saturation of plasma and raises the partial pressure available to tissues. HBOT should be used in conjunction with a complete wound-healing plan.

45. Correct: True

Adequate nutrition is an important requirement of wound healing. Inadequate protein-calorie nutrition, as well as vitamin and mineral deficiency, can impair the normal wound-healing mechanism after only a few days.

Endocrine Disorders 12

Diabetes Mellitus

Overview

Diabetes mellitus (DM) is a chronic disease where the pancreas is no longer able to produce enough insulin to meet the body's needs and/or where the body is unable to appropriately utilize insulin. The net result is a relative or absolute insulinopenia. Insulin, a pancreatic hormone, plays a variety of roles critical to health, regulating the metabolism of dietary carbohydrates that have been converted into glucose and enabling glucose to enter the body's cells, particularly muscle and liver cells.

The two most common forms of diabetes are type 1 (T1DM) and type 2 (T2DM); approximately 95% of individuals with DM have type 2. T2DM is a component of metabolic syndrome, a cluster of cardiometabolic abnormalities.

TYPE 2 DIABETES MELLITUS

Overview

Insulin resistance (IR) is a genetically predetermined and environmentally modified condition that is central to the pathogenesis of T2DM. In IR, there is a reduced sensitivity in the tissues to insulin's action at a given concentration, which causes a subnormal effect on glucose metabolism. Hyperglycemia results, which stimulates pancreatic insulin production in an effort to reduce the blood glucose level. Euglycemia occurs, albeit in the presence of hyperinsulinemia. Elevated fasting insulin levels are noted to be an independent predictor for ischemic heart disease. When coupled with acquired or lifestyle characteristics that contribute to IR, such as obesity, physical inactivity, and high-carbohydrate (more than 60% of total calories) diet, the body has greater difficulty maintaining a normal blood glucose level.

Numerous conditions are seen in conjunction with IR. Increased IR is inversely related to decreased urinary uric acid clearance; this leads to a dramatic increase in the rate of gout. Acanthosis nigricans, hyperpigmentation of the skin often in the neck and axilla, is also correlated with IR (Fig. 12-1). This finding is most common after puberty and in young adults with IR and DM risk. A personal history of birth weight that was low for gestational age is also correlated with increased risk of IR. Polycystic ovary syndrome (PCOS) is largely an IR consequence, and most women with PCOS have IR. As anovulation is a consequence of PCOS, this condition is the leading cause of endocrine-based female infertility. When IR is reduced, ovulation often resumes with resulting enhanced fertility. In addition, when IR is reduced, acne and hirsutism, usually a consequence of hyperandrogenism associated with PCOS, are usually improved.

IR is recognized as contributing to a prothrombotic and proatherogenic state. Plasminogen activator inhibitor, produced by the liver and endothelial cells, inhibits fibrin degradation by plasmin and enhances clot formation; increased levels are found in atherosclerotic lesions. High levels of triglyceride (TG), very low-density lipoprotein (VLDL), and oxidized low-density lipoprotein (LDL) stimulate the production of plasminogen activator inhibitor. Plasminogen activator inhibitor levels are significantly correlated with increased body mass and high plasma insulin levels, whereas levels are reduced when endogenous insulin levels are reduced by exercise, weight loss, or insulin-sensitizing medications, such as metformin and thiazolidinediones.

Although the correlation of obesity with IR and T2DM is well established, not all body fat types and distribution are equally problematic. Some persons with IR and T2DM are of normal weight, whereas others with IR never develop hyperglycemia. Obesity dramatically increases the risk of diabetes in a person with IR, however. "Apple-shaped" or central abdominal obesity comprises metabolically active fat and is associated with high insulin levels, IR, and a high mobilization rate of free fatty acids; high insulin levels are often associated with increased appetite. This genetic makeup helped increase the likelihood of survival in times of famine. In these times of plentiful food, however, IR helps promote fat storage.

Clinical Presentation

Individuals in the early stages of T2DM are often asymptomatic. The classic findings include polyuria (production of large amounts of dilute urine), polydipsia (great thirst), polyphagia (extreme hunger), and unexplained weight loss. This can also be accompanied by blurred vision, lower-extremity paresthesias, and genital and/or dermal yeast infection. Other physical findings, noted regardless of duration of T2DM, include obesity, hypertension, and acanthosis nigricans. More often found after years of disease, physical examination findings can include diabetic retinopathy and resulting vision changes, neuropathic changes in the lower extremities and hands including diminished deep tendon reflexes and loss of sensation of touch, and evidence of peripheral vascular disease including diminished arterial pulses and foot ulcers.

Diagnostic Testing

Patients with T2DM are most often asymptomatic at onset. As a result, the American Diabetes Association (ADA) recommends periodic fasting plasma glucose (FPG) screening every 3 years in all adults, regardless of appearance or risk; the rationale for this testing interval is that T2DM is unlikely to develop in a 3-year interval if initial glucose is normal. Testing should be considered at a younger age or be done more frequently in individuals with or acquisition of T2DM risk factors (Box 12-1).

When a fasting plasma glucose threshold level of 126 mg/dL or greater (7 mmol/L or greater) after an 8-hour fast is used, this testing is 98% specific and 40% to 88% sensitive for T2DM. Typically, wide-scale screening done according to these guidelines yields a 6% true-positive rate. Additional ADA diagnostic

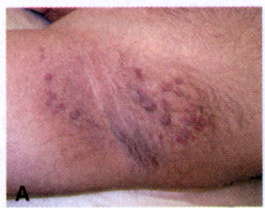 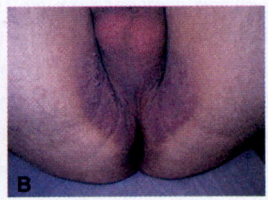

FIGURE 12-1 (A, B) Acanthosis nigricans.
Barankin B, Anatoli F. Derm Notes: Clinical Dermatology Pocket Guide. Philadelphia, PA: F.A. Davis; 2006.

BOX 12-1 Diabetes Mellitus Testing Recommendations

Criteria for Diabetes Testing in Asymptomatic Adults

Testing should be considered in all adults who are overweight (body mass index [BMI] 25 kg/m²* or greater) and have additional risk factors:

■ Physical inactivity
■ First-degree relative with type 2 diabetes mellitus (DM)
■ Members of a high-risk ethnic population (e.g., African American, Latino, Native American, Asian American, Pacific Islander)
■ Women who were diagnosed with gestational DM (GDM) should have lifelong testing at least every 3 years
■ Hypertension (greater than or equal to 140/90 mm Hg or on therapy for hypertension)
■ HDL cholesterol level less than 35 mg/dL (0.90 mmol/L) and/or a triglyceride level greater than 250 mg/dL (2.82 mmol/L)
■ Women with polycystic ovary syndrome
■ Patients with prediabetes (A1c 5.7% or greater [.057 proportion], impaired glucose tolerance [IGT], or impaired fasting glucose [IFG]) should be tested yearly
■ Other clinical conditions associated with insulin resistance (e.g., severe obesity, acanthosis nigricans)
■ History of cardiovascular disease (CVD)

In the absence of these criteria, testing diabetes should begin at age 45 years.
If results are normal, testing should be repeated at least at 3-year intervals, with consideration of more frequent testing depending on initial results and risk status.

*At-risk BMI may be lower in some ethnic groups.

Source: American Diabetes Association. Standards of Medical Care in Diabetes–2019. Diabetes Care. 2019;42(Suppl 1). https://care.diabetesjournals.org /content/42/Supplement_1

criteria for T2DM include a casual (random) plasma glucose level of 200 mg/dL or greater (11.1 mmol/L or greater) with classic diabetic symptoms, or those with an oral glucose tolerance result of 200 mg/dL or greater (11.1 mmol/L or greater) at 2 hours. Glycosylated (or glycated) hemoglobin, also known as hemoglobin A1c (or simply A1c), increases in proportion to the amount of circulating glucose. The most abundant glycohemoglobin subtype of hemoglobin A_1 is A1c, which constitutes about 4% to 6% of the body's total hemoglobin. Glycohemoglobin circulates as part of the red blood cell for about 90 to 120 days, the length of the red blood cell's life span. As a result, measurement of hemoglobin A1c provides a method for evaluating glucose control over time; the measurement best reflects blood glucose trends over the preceding 90 days but best measures glucose control in the past 28 to 42 days. Correlation with average plasma glucose and hemoglobin A1c is an important clinical tool and can be used for reinforcement in patient counseling. The ADA advises that hemoglobin A1c can be used as a tool for diagnosing DM, with a measure equal to or greater than 6.5% consistent with the diagnosis. The test should be repeated in an asymptomatic adult with glucose less than 200 mg/dL (less than 11.1 mmol/L). A repeat test is not needed in the presence of DM symptoms or glucose levels of 200 mg/dL or greater (11.1 mmol/L or greater) (Table 12-1).

With the diagnosis of T2DM, an A1c goal should be set. An A1c goal of less than 7% (0.07) for most is appropriate, but more or less stringent glycemic goals should be considered for individual patients based on such factors as duration of diabetes, age/life expectancy, comorbid conditions (including atherosclerotic cardiovascular disease [ASCVD]), and hypoglycemia unawareness. For example, a goal A1c of 6.5% or less is appropriate for a 35-year-old with T2DM who is highly engaged in her care, has a low risk for hypoglycemic unawareness, and has a high likelihood of being able

CLINICAL CONCEPT

In addition to the appropriate A1c goal, an important marker is the achievement of at least 50% or greater of fasting and postprandial glycemic goals through a combination of therapeutic lifestyle changes and medications.

TABLE 12-1 Diagnosis of Diabetes Mellitus, Categories of Increased Risk for Diabetes

	PLASMA GLUCOSE	ORAL GLUCOSE TOLERANCE TEST (OGTT)	A1C
Diabetes mellitus	Fasting (no caloric intake for 8 hours or more) 126 mg/dL or greater (7 mmol/L or greater) Random 200 mg/dL or greater (11.1 mmol/L or greater) with symptoms including polyphagia, polyuria, polydipsia, and unexplained weight loss or hyperglycemic crisis	2-hour plasma glucose 200 mg/dL or greater (11.1 mmol/L or greater) after a 75 g glucose load	A1c 6.5% or greater No special patient preparation, can be done nonfasting, no protracted time needed to test like OGTT, improved standardization of A1c measurement. A1c repeat recommended in asymptomatic adult with glucose less than 200 mg/dL (less than 11.1 mmol/L) Repeat not needed in presence of DM symptoms and/or glucose levels 200 mg/dL or greater (11.1 mmol/L or greater)
Categories of increased risk for diabetes (impaired fasting glucose [IFG], impaired glucose tolerance [IGT], prediabetes)	IFG = 100 mg/dL (5.6 mmol/L) to 125 mg/dL (6.9 mmol/L)	IGT = 140 to 199 mg/dL (7.8–11 mmol/L) on the 75 g OGTT	A1c = 5.7% to 6.4%

Source: American Diabetes Association. Standards of Medical Care in Diabetes–2019. Diabetes Care. 2019;42(Suppl 1). https://care.diabetesjournals.org/content/42/Supplement_1; International Expert Report on the role of the A1c assay in the diagnosis of diabetes. Diabetes Care. 2009;32(7):1327-1334. http://care.diabetesjournals.org/content/32/7/1327

to actively manage hypoglycemia. A goal A1c of 8% or less is more appropriate for an 83-year-old frail man with ASCVD, osteoarthritis (OA) with limited mobility, high risk for hypoglycemic unawareness, and resulting cognitive dysfunction, falls, and cardiovascular/cerebrovascular events in response to hypoglycemia. Fasting or preprandial blood sugar is recommended at 80 to 130 mg/dL (4.4 to 7.2 mmol/L), while peak postmeal (1 to 2 hours) is recommended at less than 180 mg/dL (10 mmol/L).

DM is a leading cause of chronic renal failure; this is noted in both T1DM and T2DM. After the diagnosis of DM is made, periodic screening of renal function should be done (Table 12-2). Often serum creatinine measurement is used for this purpose. An increase in creatinine is not seen, however, until at least 50% of the nephrons are not functioning. An elevated creatinine level is a latex rather than early indicator of renal damage. A far more sensitive indicator of diabetic nephropathy is the presence of proteinuria, a harbinger of progressive renal failure. Urine protein consists of many forms, including the most abundant, albumin, and immunoglobulin, haptoglobin, and light chains. The standard dipstick test is sensitive to

TABLE 12-2 Guidelines for Adult Diabetes Mellitus Care

		FREQUENCY	DESCRIPTION/COMMENTS
Health History and Physical Examination	Blood pressure (BP), height, and weight	Every 3 to 6 months	Goal BP less than 130 to 140/80 to 90, per American Diabetes Association recommendations; initiate measures to lower at this level with lifestyle modification and medication
	Dilated eye examination	Annual, more often with progressive retinopathy	Refer to eye care specialist
	Foot examination	Initial/annual	Visual examination without shoes and socks every routine diabetes visit
	Comprehensive lower-extremity sensory examination	Initial/annual	Teach protective foot behavior if sensation diminished; refer to podiatrist if indicated
	Dental examination	Every 6 months	Refer to a dentist, reinforce ongoing dental care
	Smoking, tobacco use status	Ongoing	Check every visit; encourage smoking cessation
Laboratory Tests	A1c	Every 3 to 6 months	Goal A1c according to individual benefit/risks
	Fasting/postprandial blood glucose	As indicated	Compare laboratory results with glucose self-monitoring
	Lipid profile	Annual, consider less often with stable levels	As part of comprehensive plan to reduce cardiovascular disease risk
	Urine microalbumin/creatinine	Initial/annual	If abnormal, recheck (2 in a 3-month period, then treat if two out of three collections show elevated levels
	Serum creatinine with estimated glomerular filtration rate (GFR)	Annual	Measure annually for estimation of GFR
	EKG	Initial	If patient 40 years old or older, or has had diabetes mellitus for 10 years or longer
	Thyroid assessment	Initial/as indicated	Thyroid palpitation, thyroid function test(s) if indicated

Continued

TABLE 12-2 Guidelines for Adult Diabetes Mellitus Care—cont'd

		FREQUENCY	DESCRIPTION/COMMENTS
Recommended Immunizations	Influenza vaccine	Annually in anticipation of seasonal influenza	Influenza vaccine form should be guided by standard vaccine practice
	Pneumococcal vaccine	Recommended	Pneumococcal polysaccharide (PCV23, Pneumovax®), pneumococcal conjugate (PCV13, Prevnar®) vaccines as recommended
	Hepatitis B vaccine	If younger than 60 years old at time of diabetes mellitus diagnosis, immunize as soon as possible after diagnosis, if no history of hepatitis B infection or hepatitis B vaccine	If 60 years old or older, at the discretion of the treating clinician based on increased need for assisted blood glucose monitoring in long-term care facilities, likelihood of acquiring hepatitis B infection, its complications, or chronic sequelae, and likelihood of immune response to vaccination
Self-Management Skills and Patient Counseling	Review self-management skills	Initial/ongoing	Reinforce healthy habits, monitoring, sick day care
	Review treatment plan	Initial/ongoing	Check self-monitoring log book, diet, physical activity, and medications
	Review education plan	Initial/ongoing	Refer for diabetes self-management education as indicated
	Review nutrition plan	Initial/ongoing	Refer for medical nutrition therapy as indicated
	Review physical activity plan	Initial/ongoing	Assess/prescribe based on patient's health status
	Tobacco use	Annual/ongoing	Assess readiness, counsel about cessation; refer to smoking cessation program
	Psychosocial adjustment	Initial/ongoing	Suggest diabetes support group; counsel and refer as indicated
	Sexuality/erectile dysfunction	Annual/ongoing	Discuss diagnostic evaluation and therapeutic options
	Preconception/pregnancy	Initial/ongoing	Need for tight glucose control 3 to 6 months preconception; consider early referral to high-risk prenatal care

Source: American Diabetes Association. Standards of Medical Care in Diabetes—2019. Diabetes Care. 2019;42(Suppl 1). https://care.diabetesjournals.org/content/42/Supplement_1

100 to 150 mg/L of urine albumin, an earlier marker of progressive renal failure than serum creatinine, but still a later disease marker. The persistent presence of a small amount of albumin (microalbumin) is considered a predictor of glomerular dysfunction associated with diabetic nephropathy.

Treatment

Lifestyle Modifications

Sadly, patients with increased risk for T2DM are missed due to lack of screening. Patients with impaired glucose tolerance (IGT), impaired fasting glucose (IFG), or an A1c of 5.7% to 6.4% should be identified and treated with lifestyle modifications including a target weight loss of 7% of body weight and an increase in physical activity to at least 150 minutes per week; adding metformin therapy is also a consideration. These treatment options are demonstrated to minimize the risk of progression to T2DM.

Therapeutic lifestyle changes are critically important for a person with DM. Tobacco use in any form should be discouraged owing to its obvious cardiovascular risk. Because approximately 80% of the body's insulin-mediated glucose uptake occurs in muscle and is enhanced by physical activity, a regular program of aerobic exercise such as brisk walking should be prescribed. Exercise reduces IR by approximately 40%, with the effects persisting for up to 48 hours after the activity, and aids in weight maintenance. People with diabetes should be advised to perform at least 150 minutes per week of moderate-intensity aerobic physical activity at 50% to 70% of maximum heart rate. Exercise should be spread over at least 3 days per week with no more than 2 consecutive days without exercise; the insulin-sensitizing effects of physical activity wane after 48 hours. In the absence of contraindications, people with T2DM should be encouraged to perform resistance training at least twice per week. Cardiac stress testing should be considered for the previously sedentary individual at moderate to high risk for cardiovascular disease (CVD) or other patients who are clinically indicated who want to undertake vigorous aerobic exercise that exceeds the demands of everyday living.

For a person with T1DM or T2DM, current ADA recommendations advise a Mediterranean-style diet rich in monounsaturated fats, and foods rich in long-chain omega-3 fatty acids, such as fatty fish. Sodium intake should be limited to less than 2,300 mg/day, whereas alcohol consumption should be limited to one drink per day for women and two drinks per day for men or less.

Weight loss improves insulin sensitivity and reduces blood pressure; improvement is not related to the degree of weight loss. Eating frequent, small, high-fiber meals and foods with a low glycemic index and smaller serving sizes should be encouraged. Dietary fat should be limited, but not eliminated, with emphasis on decreasing saturated fats, while using monounsaturated fat. A pound of fat contains approximately 3,500 stored calories. A deficit of 500 to 1,000 calories per day would lead to a 1 to 2 lb (0.45 to 0.9 kg) weight loss per week (Box 12-2).

Pharmacotherapy

To prescribe these medications appropriately and effectively, the prescriber must know the mechanism of action, indications, anticipated adverse effects, contraindications, and anticipated benefit with the available medications (Table 12-3). Cost and efficacy are considerable factors in choosing the most appropriate drug(s). Metformin along with comprehensive lifestyle modifications is considered first-line treatment of T2DM. If initial A1c is equal to or greater than 2% above goal, at least two drugs will likely be needed.

If A1c persists above target, then a second agent should be added based on patient comorbidities or the compelling need of the patient (e.g., minimize hypoglycemia, weight loss, or minimize costs). Critical to safe practice is the recognition of a given medication's mechanism of action, adverse effect profile, and cost (see Table 12-3 and Fig. 12-2).

Metformin, a biguanide, improves insulin-mediated glucose uptake and metabolic parameters such as fibrinolysis. The anticipated A1c reduction with intensified or maximum safe and tolerated metformin dose is about 1% to 2%; an A1c of 9% prior to metformin initiation can be reduced to 7% or 8% with its use. One of the most commonly reported adverse effects with metformin use is gastrointestinal (GI) upset including diarrhea. This can be minimized by titrating the dose upward over a 2- to 3-week time period, using the extended-release rather than intermediate-release form of the medication and by taking the metformin dose with a meal.

> **CLINICAL CONCEPT**
>
> Metformin use in early metabolic syndrome, as A1c rises above upper limits of normal but is not yet at or greater than 6.5%, helps in delaying the onset of T2DM.

One area of concern with metformin use has been the rare development of lactic acidosis, a potentially fatal illness, during its use. In a patient with normal renal function, lactic acid produced in the body, likely slightly enhanced with metformin use, is excreted via the kidneys without causing harm. In a person with renal impairment, metformin and lactic acid are cleared less effectively. Creatinine should be monitored, and this medication should be used with caution or avoided in those with impaired renal function. Any condition that potentially reduces renal perfusion, including hypovolemia, heart failure, or advanced age, increases the metformin-associated lactic acidosis risk. The time period around the use of radiocontrast and surgery is considered a risk owing to alterations in hydration. With consideration of all of these factors, the risk of lactic acidosis with metformin use is likely overstated; best estimates are a rate of greater than 3 per 100,000 patients treated. At the same time, in order to minimize the risk of lactic acidosis, warnings associated with metformin use include avoiding use in the presence of renal impairment, especially with GFR less than 45 mL/min, heart failure, and age greater than 80 years. In addition, regardless of patient age, metformin use should be discontinued for the day of surgery, radiocontrast use, or other condition potentially impacting hydration status and reintroduced when hydration status and renal function are back to baseline.

BOX 12-2 Type 2 Diabetes Mellitus: Additional Care Considerations

A Aspirin 75 to 162 mg/day (use clopidogrel [Plavix®] 75 mg/day in aspirin allergy) for those with history of atherosclerotic cardiovascular disease (ASCVD); aspirin use can be considered for those at increased cardiovascular risk based on risk-benefit discussion.

Angiotensin-converting enzyme inhibitor, or angiotensin receptor blocker as part of blood pressure control.

Counsel about moderation or abstinence in alcohol and/or recreational drug intake.

B Blood pressure—Treat hypertension to less than 130/80 mm Hg for those with highest ASCVD risk, and, at minimum, less than 140/90 mm Hg.

C Cholesterol—Controlling therapy to reach the following goals:

Moderate-intensity statin therapy to reduce LDL 30% to 50% or high-intensity statin therapy to lower LDL by greater than 50% as determined by patient's estimated 10-year ASCVD risk, with a goal LDL less than 100 mg/dL for most with type 2 diabetes mellitus, or less than 70 mg/dL in highest ASCVD risk.

Check fasting lipid profile annually, consider less often if evidence of stability.

Creatinine (renal function)—Check serum creatinine, calculated glomerular filtration rate (GFR), and urine microalbumin annually.

D Diet—Limit *trans* and saturated fats, healthiest foods in appropriate amounts every meal. Medical nutritional therapy (MNT) with a registered dietician advisable.

Dental care—Reinforce ongoing dental care and treatment of dental disease.

E Exercise/increase physical activity, if not contraindicated, to at least 150 minutes per week of moderate activity such as walking, at least three times per week at 50% to 70% of maximum heart rate with no more than 2 consecutive days without exercise. In addition, resistance training two or more times per week. Vigorous aerobic or resistance activity is potentially contraindicated in the presence of proliferative or severe nonproliferative retinopathy due to the possible risk of vitreous hemorrhage or retinal detachment.

Eye examination (dilated) annually; increase frequency as dictated by developing retinopathy or other eye problems.

F Foot examination (visual) with every visit, teach protective foot behavior, comprehensive lower-extremity sensory examination annually using 10-g monofilament with one or more of the following: vibration using a 128-Hz tuning fork, pinprick sensation, ankle reflexes, or vibration threshold.

G Goals—Periodically review overall goals of care with patient.

Source: American Diabetes Association. Standards of Medical Care in Diabetes–2019. Diabetes Care. 2019;42(Suppl 1). https://care.diabetesjournals.org /content/42/Supplement_1

The sulfonylureas (SUs) are a drug class that includes medication such as glipizide (Glucotrol®), glyburide (DiaBeta®), and glimepiride (Amaryl®). These drugs act as insulin secretagogues, resulting in the release of insulin for pancreatic beta cells. Anticipated A1c reduction with intensified use is approximately 1% to 2%. Because the medication is renally eliminated, the sulfonylurea dose should be adjusted in the presence of renal impairment. The SUs require functioning pancreatic beta cells to be clinically effective. Due to declining beta cell function, these medications are typically less effective after many years post-T2DM diagnosis and in older adults. In addition, the presence of severe hyperglycemia inhibits insulin release. Thus, an SU will appear to be less clinically effective during a hyperglycemic episode, such as during an acute illness, and its original effectiveness will resume once the blood sugar control improves. One of the major SU adverse effects is hypoglycemia, due to the drug classes' mechanism of action, which is to cause insulin release regardless of blood sugar. This risk is particularly profound in the elderly and in individuals who eat on an irregular or unpredictable schedule (see Table 12-3).

The thiazolidinediones (e.g., pioglitazone) work as insulin sensitizers via action on PPAR-γ receptors and can result in an anticipated A1c reduction of 1% to 2%. They are associated with a low risk (less than 0.5%) of hepatic toxicity, and ALT should be monitored periodically. These agents should not be initiated in patients with heart failure, in established ASCVD due to edema risk (especially when combined with insulin or sulfonylurea).

GLP-1 agonists have several mechanisms of action, including stimulating insulin production, inhibiting postprandial glucagon release, and slowing gastric emptying. This class is associated with an anticipated A1c reduction of 1% to 2% with intensified use and can also cause appetite suppression and weight loss.

TABLE 12-3 Medications Used in the Treatment of Type 2 Diabetes Mellitus

MEDICATION	MECHANISM OF ACTION A1C REDUCTION	COMMENT
Sulfonylurea (SU) Examples: Glipizide (Glucotrol®), glyburide (DiaBeta®), glimepiride (Amaryl®)	Insulin secretagogue	Use with caution with sulfonamide allergy, though cross-allergy risk is low. Potentially photosensitizing. Hypoglycemia risk, especially with irregular meal schedule, older adults.
Biguanide Example: Metformin (Glucophage®)	Reduces hepatic glucose production and intestinal glucose absorption, insulin sensitizer via increased peripheral glucose uptake and utilization	Use increases risk of vitamin B_{12} deficiency owing to B_{12} malabsorption; risk appears dependent on dose and length of therapy. Metformin therapy for prevention of type 2 diabetes is encouraged, particularly for those at highest risk, including multiple risk factors, hyperglycemia (i.e., A1c ≥6% [0.06 proportion]) despite lifestyle interventions, those with body mass index greater than 35 kg/m², age older than 60 years, and women with prior gestational diabetes mellitus. Low hypoglycemia risk.
Thiazolidinedione (TZD, glitazones) Examples: Pioglitazone (Actos®), rosiglitazone (Avandia®)	Insulin sensitizer via action at PPAR-γ receptors found in muscle, adipose, and other tissue	In consideration of cardiovascular risk, use with insulin or nitrates not recommended. Low hypoglycemia risk.
Glucagon-like peptide (GLP)-1 agonist (incretin mimetics) Examples: Exenatide (Bydureon®), liraglutide (Victoza®), dulaglutide (Trulicity®), Lixisenatide (Lyxumia®), albiglutide (Tanzeum®) Injection only	Stimulates insulin production in response to increase in plasma glucose; inhibits postprandial glucagon release Slows gastric emptying	Major adverse effect = N/V, usually better with dose adjustment, continued use; contraindicated in gastroparesis. Use with caution in patient with mild-moderate renal impairment (creatinine clearance [CrCl] = 30 to 50 mL/min [0.50–0.835 mL/sec]). Do not use with CrCl less than 30 mL/min (less than 0.50 mL/sec). Low hypoglycemia risk.
Dipeptidyl peptidase-4 (DPP-4) inhibitor Examples: Sitagliptin (Januvia®), saxagliptin (Onglyza®), linagliptin (Tradjenta®), alogliptin (Nesina®), vildagliptin (Galvus®)	Increases levels of incretin, increasing synthesis and release of insulin from pancreatic beta cells and decreasing release of glucagon from pancreatic alpha cells	Dose adjustment required in renal impairment. Monitor patients for the development of pancreatitis after DPP-4 inhibitor initiation or dose increase. Rare adverse effects. Low hypoglycemia risk.
Sodium-glucose cotransporter 2 (SGLT2) inhibitor Examples: canagliflozin (Invokana®), dapagliflozin (Farxiga®), empagliflozin (Jardiance®)	Lowers renal glucose threshold, increased urinary glucose excretion	Use of SGLT2 inhibitors is associated with increased risk of ketoacidosis, hyperkalemia (in patients with impaired renal function), impairment in renal function including acute kidney injury, urosepsis, and pyelonephritis. Low hypoglycemia risk.

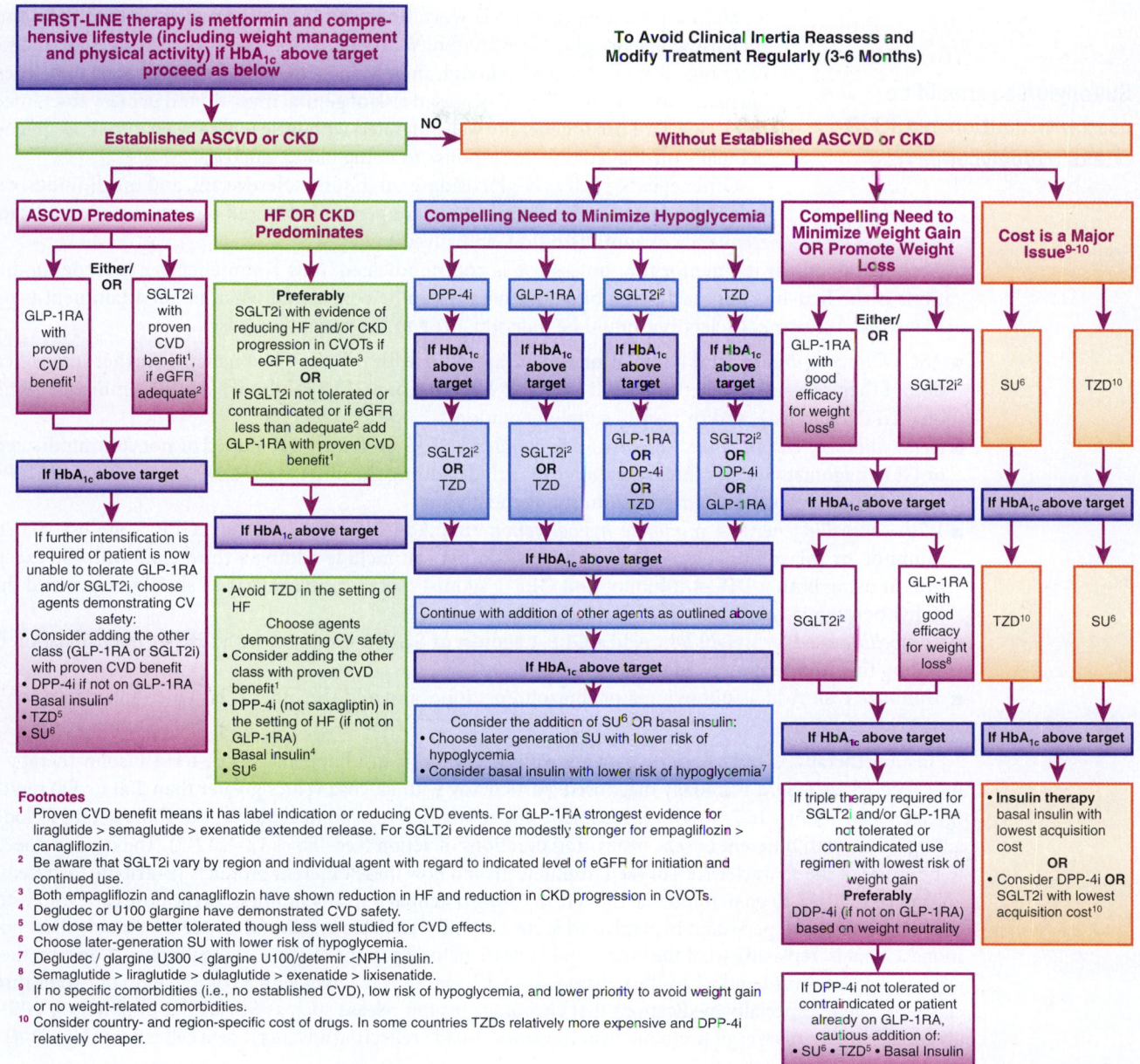

FIGURE 12-2 Algorithm for drug therapy in type 2 diabetes mellitus. *Note:* TZD should not be used with insulin.

American Diabetes Association. Standards of Medical Care in Diabetes–2019. Diabetes Care. 2019;42(Suppl 1):S90–S102. https://care .diabetesjournals.org/content/42/Supplement_1

These agents are associated with nausea and vomiting, which tends to get better with dose adjustment and continued use. However, this drug class is not recommended in patients with a history of gastroparesis, due to the preexisting issue with stomach emptying. Furthermore, the U.S. Food and Drug Administration (FDA) advises clinicians to promptly discontinue GLP-1 agonist use and to advise patients to seek care if acute pancreatitis symptoms (persistent abdominal pain, usually with vomiting) occur with the drug's use. GLP-1 agonists are not recommended with pancreatitis history and should be used with caution in patients with mild-to-moderate renal impairment. The hypoglycemia risk is minimal with GLP-1 agonist use as insulin release increases only in response to rising blood glucose.

DPP-4 inhibitors increase the level of incretin that results in an increase in the synthesis and release of insulin. Anticipated A1c reduction with these agents can range from 0.6% to 1.4%, and these agents are generally weight-neutral. These agents are well-tolerated with little hypoglycemia risk, as the insulin release with DDP-4 inhibitor use occurs only in response to a rise in blood glucose.

CLINICAL CONCEPT

Sulfonylureas should be used with caution in ASCVD due to hypoglycemia risk.

SGLT2 inhibitors (SGLT2-I) work by lowering the renal glucose threshold, thus increasing urinary glucose excretion. With intensified use, anticipated A1c reduction can range from 0.7% to 1%, though there is less effect with renal impairment. These agents are associated with an increased risk of genital mycotic and urinary tract infections. SGLT2-I use is generally well-tolerated with little hypoglycemia risk, as glucose is renally off-loaded only in response to rising blood glucose.

Other agents, such as α-glucosidase inhibitors, colesevelam, and meglitinides, can be tried in specific situations but are not generally favored owing to modest efficacy, frequency of administration, and adverse effects.

As mentioned earlier, metformin, unless use is contraindicated, plus comprehensive lifestyle modifications is the first-line approach. Combination therapy can be considered when target attainment is not achieved, and treatment selection should be individualized to the patient's needs:

- *ASCVD predominates*: Add a GLP-1 or SGLT2 inhibitor with proven CVD benefit. Further intensification of therapy can include the other class (GLP-1 agonist or SGLT2 inhibitor), a DPP-4 inhibitor (if not on a GLP-1 agonist), and/or insulin supplementation.
- *Heart failure or chronic kidney disease predominates*: SGLT2 inhibitor (if tolerated or not contraindicated) or GLP-1 agonist. Further intensification can include adding the other class, a DPP-4 inhibitor (if GLP-1 agonist not being used), and/or insulin supplementation.
- *With compelling need to minimize hypoglycemia risk*: Add a DPP-4 inhibitor, GLP-1 agonist, SGLT2 inhibitor, or thiazolidinedione. Further intensification can include adding a third class with the exception of using both a DPP-4 inhibitor and GLP-1 agonist together. Sulfonylureas should be avoided due to hypoglycemia risk.
- *Compelling need for weight loss*: Add a GLP-1 agonist or SGLT2 inhibitor, with further intensification by adding the other class if needed.
- *Minimize cost*: Add a sulfonylurea or thiazolidinedione, and add the other class when intensification is needed.

Insulin therapy is indicated for patients with T2DM with insulinopenia; short-term insulin therapy is indicated when T2DM is initially diagnosed, particularly with glucose values greater than 250 to 300 mg/dL (greater than 13.9 to 16.7 mmol/L). Insulins come in many forms, from rapid-acting, short-acting to long-acting forms with different onsets, peaks, and durations of action (see Tables 12-4, 12-5). The clinician needs to be aware of the characteristics of each insulin form and how these different products contribute to glycemic control (Fig. 12-3). Keep in mind that the A1c lowering potential is nearly limitless, as the dose can be adjusted easily in response to persistent hyperglycemia. All currently available insulin forms are true bioidentical hormones—that is, replacing what the body would release naturally in the absence of insulinopenia. Insulin therapy can also be considered when the patient fails to achieve an A1c target with a combination of two or three classes of agent, especially medications that encourage insulin release such as SU, DPP-4 inhibitor, or GLP-1 agonists. This is a marker of profound insulinopenia, usually reflecting advanced beta cell failure (Fig. 12-4).

TABLE 12-4 When to Use Insulin in Diabetes Mellitus Treatment

TYPE 1 DIABETES MELLITUS	TYPE 2 DIABETES MELLITUS
■ All patients ■ Basal insulin (50% to 60% of total daily insulin requirements) with adjustments for meals and snacks (40% to 50% of total daily insulin requirements) via multiple injections or pump	■ At time of diagnosis to help achieve initial glycemic control, particularly when glucose values greater than 250 to 300 mg/dL (13.9 to 16.7 mmol/L) ■ When acutely ill ■ In critically ill surgical and nonsurgical patients with type 1 or type 2 diabetes mellitus, blood glucose levels should be kept generally 140 to 180 mg/dL (7.8 to 10 mmol/L). Overtreatment and undertreatment of hyperglycemia represent major safety concerns. ■ When ≥2 insulin secretagogues (SU, GLP-1 agonist, DPP-4 inhibitor) at optimized use are inadequate to maintain glycemic control, indicating progressive pancreatic beta cell's inability to release insulin.

Source: American Diabetes Association. Standards of Medical Care in Diabetes—2019. Diabetes Care. 2019;42(Suppl 1). https://care.diabetesjournals.org/content/42/Supplement_1

TABLE 12-5 Insulin: Type, Onset, Peak, and Duration of Action

INSULIN TYPE	ONSET OF ACTION	PEAK	DURATION OF ACTION
Short-acting, rapid onset of action (lispro insulin solution [Humalog®])	15 to 30 minutes, give within 15 minutes or right after meals	30 minutes to 2.5 hours	3 to 6.5 hours
Short-acting, rapid onset of action (aspart insulin solution [NovoLog®])	10 to 20 minutes, give 5 to 10 minutes before meals	1 to 3 hours	3 to 5 hours
Short-acting, rapid onset of action (insulin glulisine [Apidra®])	10 to 15 minutes, give within 15 minutes or right after meals	1 to 1.5 hours	3 to 5 hours
Rapid-acting inhaled (insulin human [Afrezza®])	15 to 30 minutes, administer at the beginning of a meal	Approximately 53 minutes	2.5 to 3 hours
Short-acting (regular [Humulin R®, Novolin R®])	30 minutes to 1 hour	2 to 3 hours	4 to 6 hours
Intermediate-acting (NPH [Novolin N®, Humulin N®])	1 to 2 hours	6 to 14 hours	16 to 24 hours
Long-acting (insulin glargine solution [Lantus®, Toujeo®])	Clinical effect about 1 hour after injection	None	About 24 hours
Long-acting (insulin detemir solution [Levemir®])	Approximately 1 to 2 hours	6 to 8 hours (minimal peak)	Dose dependent; 12 hours for 0.2 units/kg, 20 hours for 0.4 units/kg; albumin bound
Long-acting (insulin degludec [Tresiba®])	Unknown, not stated in product information	Approximately 12 hours	At least 42 hours (after the last dose of a series of eight once-daily doses)

Source: Comparisons of insulins and injectable diabetes meds. Prescribers Letter. Detail-Document #310302. https://Prescribersletter.therapeuticresearch.com

With insulin use, two conditions that can result in early morning hyperglycemia can occur. The Somogyi effect occurs when an insulin-induced hypoglycemia triggers excess secretion of glucagon and cortisol; this leads to hyperglycemia. Intervention is aimed at lowering the inappropriately high insulin dose, usually the dinnertime dose of intermediate-acting insulin. The dawn phenomenon is a result of reduced insulin sensitivity developing between 5 and 8 a.m., caused by earlier spikes in growth hormone. The net result is cortisol release, which triggers hepatic glucose secretion and early morning hyperglycemia. Intervention for the dawn phenomenon includes splitting the evening intermediate insulin dose between dinner and bedtime. Alternative interventions include switching to a bedtime dose of a basal insulin such as glargine or detemir or an insulin pump.

Daily low-dose aspirin (75 to 162 mg/day) use is recommended for secondary prevention among those with ASCVD. Clopidogrel can be substituted for those with an aspirin allergy (see Box 12-2). Aspirin use can also be considered for primary prevention for those at increased CVD risk, though this should be done after a discussion on the benefits and risks of aspirin therapy (e.g., increased bleeding risk). An angiotensin-converting enzyme inhibitor (ACEI) or angiotensin receptor blocker (ARB) should be part of therapy for hypertension in a person with DM, though hypertension guidelines mention that calcium channel blockers and thiazide diuretics are also acceptable choices, usually in conjunction with an ACEI or ARB.

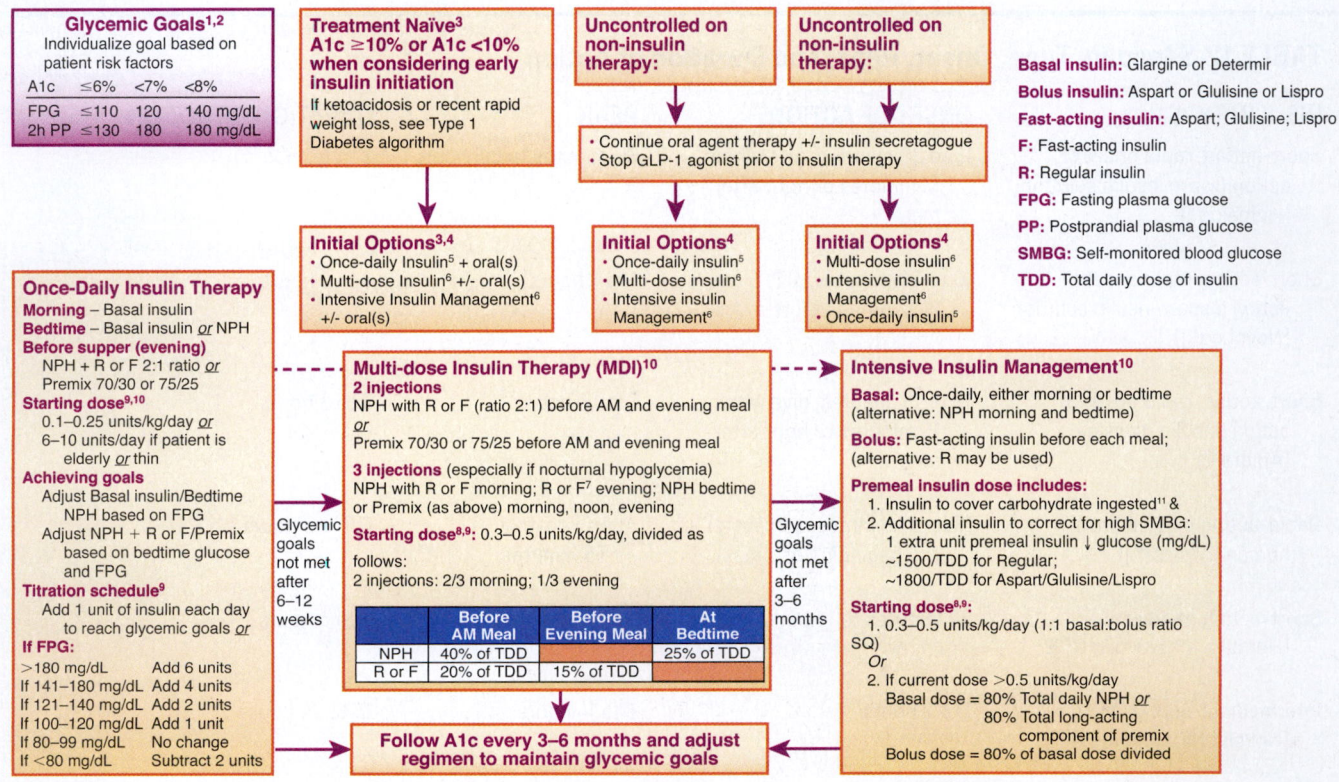

FIGURE 12-3 Insulin algorithm for type 2 diabetes in children and adults.

Texas Diabetes Council. Insulin algorithm for type 2 diabetes mellitus in children and adults. https://www.dshs.texas.gov/txdiabetes/practitioner-resources.shtm

---

TYPE 1 DIABETES MELLITUS

Overview

T1DM is a polygenetic disease that results from autoimmune-induced pancreatic beta cell destruction with resulting profound insulin deficiency. Unlike T2DM, IR is not a significant contributor. T1DM risk factors, though none are as potent as the T2DM risk factors, include the presence of the HLA (human leukocyte antigen) complex, European ancestry, select viral infections, and residence in a northern climate.

Clinical Presentation

T1DM usually occurs in persons younger than 30 years but can occur at any age. In contrast with the usually asymptomatic presentation in T2DM, the person with T1DM usually presents with involuntary weight loss and the classic "polys": polydipsia, polyphagia, and polyuria.

Diagnostic Testing

Diagnosis of T1DM is similar to T2DM with an FPG level greater than 126 mg/dL (7 mmol/L) or a 2-hour plasma glucose level greater than or equal to 200 mg/dL

> **CLINICAL CONCEPT**
>
> When T1DM is associated with ketoacidosis, the presentation can be dramatic, with severe dehydration, abdominal pain, vomiting, and altered level of consciousness.

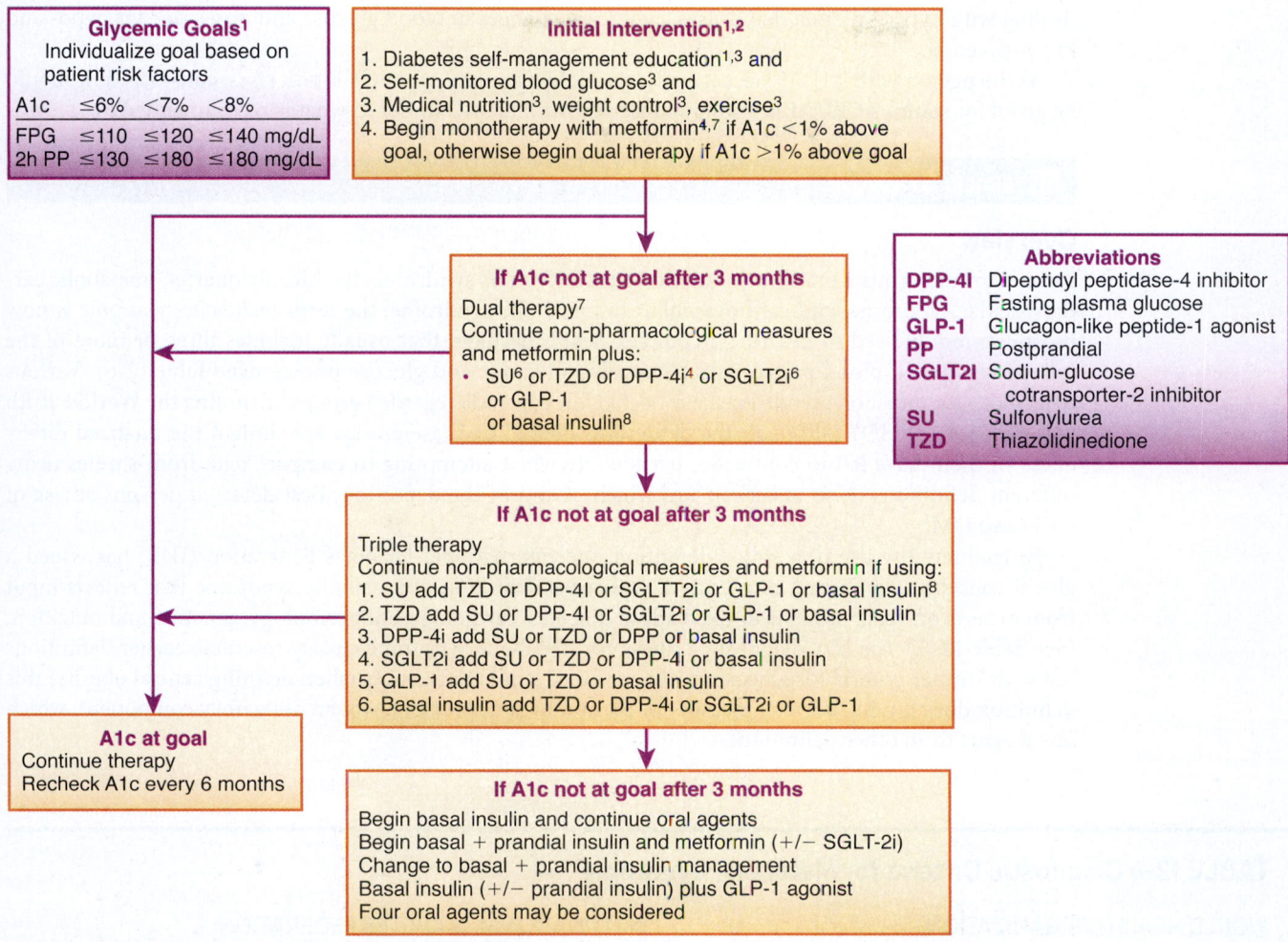

Glycemic Goals[1]
Individualize goal based on patient risk factors

A1c	≤6%	<7%	<8%
FPG	≤110	≤120	≤140 mg/dL
2h PP	≤130	≤180	≤180 mg/dL

Initial Intervention[1,2]
1. Diabetes self-management education[1,3] and
2. Self-monitored blood glucose[3] and
3. Medical nutrition[3], weight control[3], exercise[3]
4. Begin monotherapy with metformin[4,7] if A1c <1% above goal, otherwise begin dual therapy if A1c >1% above goal

If A1c not at goal after 3 months
Dual therapy[7]
Continue non-pharmacological measures and metformin plus:
• SU[6] or TZD or DPP-4i[4] or SGLT2i[6] or GLP-1
  or basal insulin[8]

Abbreviations

DPP-4I	Dipeptidyl peptidase-4 inhibitor
FPG	Fasting plasma glucose
GLP-1	Glucagon-like peptide-1 agonist
PP	Postprandial
SGLT2I	Sodium-glucose cotransporter-2 inhibitor
SU	Sulfonylurea
TZD	Thiazolidinedione

If A1c not at goal after 3 months
Triple therapy
Continue non-pharmacological measures and metformin if using:
1. SU add TZD or DPP-4I or SGLTT2i or GLP-1 or basal insulin[8]
2. TZD add SU or DPP-4I or SGLT2i or GLP-1 or basal insulin
3. DPP-4i add SU or TZD or DPP or basal insulin
4. SGLT2i add SU or TZD or DPP-4i or basal insulin
5. GLP-1 add SU or TZD or basal insulin
6. Basal insulin add TZD or DPP-4i or SGLT2i or GLP-1

A1c at goal
Continue therapy
Recheck A1c every 6 months

If A1c not at goal after 3 months
Begin basal insulin and continue oral agents
Begin basal + prandial insulin and metformin (+/− SGLT-2i)
Change to basal + prandial insulin management
Basal insulin (+/− prandial insulin) plus GLP-1 agonist
Four oral agents may be considered

Footnotes
1 Powers MA et al. Diabetes self management and education support in type 2 DM. Diabetes Care 2015;38:1372-1382.
2 If initial A1c on presentation is ≥10%, consider insulin, with or without oral agents, as the initial intervention (see Insulin Algorithm).
3 These interventions should be maintained life-long (refer to Medical Nutrition, Weight Loss, and Exercise Algorithms).
4 Dose is reduced based on either serum creatinine (metformin, DPP4i's) or calculated/estimated glomerular filtration rates (SGLT2i's).
5 If an SU is selected, glipizide ER or glimepiride are recommended because they have a lower incidence of hypoglycemia than glyburide.
6 SGLT-2 inhibitors are not indicated if the glomerular filtration rate is less than 40%.
7 See package insert for drug contraindica.
8 See Insulin Algorithm.

FIGURE 12-4 Glycemic control algorithm for type 2 diabetes mellitus in adults.
Texas Diabetes Council. Glycemic control algorithm for type 2 diabetes mellitus in adults. https://www.dshs.texas.gov/txdiabetes/practitioner-resources.shtm

(11.1 mmol/L) during a 75-g oral glucose tolerance test, or a random plasma glucose of greater than or equal to 200 mg/dL (11.1 mmol/L) in a patient with classic symptoms of hyperglycemia or in hyperglycemic crisis; the latter describes the most common T1DM presentation. In the absence of T1DM signs and symptoms, routine testing for T1DM is not recommended in low-risk individuals, though annual testing for children under 10 years can be considered for those who have a first-degree relative with T1DM.

Treatment

Prompt intervention with appropriate insulin therapy is indicated, bearing in mind that untreated T1DM is a potentially life-threatening condition. Lifelong insulin therapy is required, most often through the use of basal insulin with boluses of rapid-acting insulin to provide coverage for carbohydrate intake with meals and snacks. This can be done with multiple insulin injections or through the use of an insulin pump (see Table 12-5). The patient should be educated in the role of correction insulin, usually in the form of a rapidly acting insulin (RAI), in response to an unexpected high blood sugar while using a basal and preprandial insulin. The use of sliding-scale insulin, where the blood sugar is allowed to rise post meal or snack and then RAI is given to rapidly lower glucose, is discouraged. Slide scales are a reactive way of dealing with hyperglycemia that causes significant changes in blood glucose and poses risk for hypo- and hyperglycemia.

As the person with T1DM faces the adult/middle-age years, as ASCVD risk rises, consideration should be given for statin, ACEI/ARB, and low-dose aspirin therapy, similar to what is recommended for T2DM.

METABOLIC SYNDROME

Overview

Known by numerous names, such as syndrome X, Reaven's syndrome, the "deadly quartet," metabolic cardiovascular syndrome, and cardiovascular dysmetabolic syndrome, the term *metabolic syndrome* is now most commonly used to describe a complex health problem that usually includes three or more of the following: obesity, blood pressure problems, dyslipidemia, and glucose intolerance (Table 12-6). Various definitions for metabolic syndrome have been offered by well-regarded groups, including the World Health Organization (WHO). Although the definitions offered by these groups are similar, the nuanced differences in them have led to confusion, particularly when attempting to compare data from studies using different definitions. Also uncertain was which, if any, of the definitions best detected persons at risk of CVD and DM.

To facilitate the use of a single definition, the International Diabetes Federation (IDF) has issued a global consensus statement, proposing a consensus definition of metabolic syndrome that reflects input from experts on six continents in the fields of diabetes, cardiology, endocrinology, genetics, and nutrition. (See Table 12-6.) The IDF diagnostic criteria for metabolic syndrome closely resemble earlier definitions but with stricter criteria for glucose intolerance and ethnic differences when defining central obesity; this definition does not include any measure of IR, and hyperglycemia is not an obligatory component, which sets it apart from other definitions.

TABLE 12-6 Diagnostic Criteria for Metabolic Syndrome

WORLD HEALTH ORGANIZATION	INTERNATIONAL DIABETES FEDERATION
Insulin resistance (type 2 diabetes mellitus or impaired fasting glucose) plus two or more of the following	Central obesity, defined as ethnic-specific waist circumference
■ Abdominal/central obesity defined as a waist-to-hip ratio greater than 0.90 (men), greater than 0.85 (women), or BMI 30 kg/m² or greater	European, sub-Saharan African, Eastern Mediterranean, Middle Eastern (Arabic) ancestry
■ Hypertriglyceridemia 150 mg/dL or greater (1.7 mmol/L or greater)	■ Men 94 cm or greater (37 in. or greater)
	■ Women 80 cm or greater (31.5 in. or greater)
■ Low HDL cholesterol less than 35 mg/dL (less than 0.9 mmol/L) for men, or less than 39 mg/dL (less than 1 mmol/L) for women	South Asian, Chinese, ethnic South and Central American ancestry
	■ Men 90 cm or greater (35.5 in. or greater)
■ High BP 140/90 mm Hg or greater or documented use of antihypertensive therapy	■ Women 80 cm or greater (31.5 in. or greater)
	Japanese ancestry
■ Microalbuminuria with urinary albumin-to-creatinine ratio 30 mg/g, or albumin excretion rate 20 mcg/min	■ Men 90 cm or greater (35.5 in. or greater)
	■ Women 80 cm or greater (31.5 in. or greater)
	with two or more of the following
	■ Abnormal triglycerides 150 mg/dL or greater (1.7 mmol/L or greater)
	■ HDL cholesterol less than 40 mg/dL (less than 1.03 mmol/L) in men, less than 50 mg/dL (less than 1.29 mmol/L) in women
	■ BP 130 mm Hg systolic or greater or 85 mm Hg diastolic or greater or treatment of previously diagnosed hypertension
	■ Fasting glucose 100 mg/dL or greater (5.6 mmol/L or greater) or previous diagnosis of type 2 diabetes or impaired glucose tolerance

BMI, body mass index; BP, blood pressure; HDL, high-density lipoprotein.

The majority of individuals with T2DM have metabolic syndrome. Treatment should follow accordingly including encouraging weight loss, proper diet, and increased physical activity as tolerated while controlling dyslipidemia, hypertension, and hyperglycemia.

Discussion Sources

American Association of Clinical Endocrinologists. AACE/ACE comprehensive type 2 diabetes management consensus statement. *Endocr Pract.* 2016;22:84–113.

American Diabetes Association. Standards of Medical Care in Diabetes—2019. *Diabetes Care.* 2019;42(Suppl 1). https://care.diabetesjournals.org/content/42/Supplement_1

International Diabetes Federation. *The IDF Consensus Worldwide Definition of the Metabolic Syndrome.* Brussels: IDF Communications; 2006. https://www.idf.org/e-library/consensus-statements/60-idfconsensus-worldwide-definitionof-the-metabolic-syndrome.html

Redmon B, Caccamo D, Flavin P, et al; Institute for Clinical Systems Improvement. *Diagnosis and Management of Type 2 Diabetes Mellitus in Adults.* https://www.icsi.org/wp-content/uploads/2019/02/Diabetes.pdf

QUESTIONS

1. Which of the following characteristics applies to T1DM?
   A. Significant hyperglycemia and ketoacidosis result from lack of insulin.
   B. This condition is commonly diagnosed on routine examination or workup for other health problems.
   C. Initial response to oral sulfonylureas is usually favorable.
   D. IR is a significant part of the disease.

2. Which of the following characteristics applies to T2DM?
   A. Major risk factors are heredity and obesity.
   B. Pear-shaped body type is commonly found.
   C. Exogenous insulin is needed for control of disease.
   D. Physical activity enhances IR.

3. You consider prescribing insulin glargine (Toujeo®, Lantus®) because of its:
   A. extended duration of action.
   B. rapid onset of action.
   C. ability to prevent diabetic end-organ damage.
   D. ability to preserve pancreatic function.

4. After use, the onset of action of lispro (Humalog®), a rapid-acting insulin, occurs in:
   A. less than 30 minutes.
   B. approximately 1 hour.
   C. 1 to 2 hours.
   D. 3 to 4 hours.

5. The mechanism of action of metformin (Glucophage®) is as:
   A. an insulin-production enhancer.
   B. a product virtually identical in action to sulfonylureas.
   C. a drug that increases insulin action in the peripheral tissues and reduces hepatic glucose production.
   D. a facilitator of renal glucose excretion.

6. Generally, testing for T2DM in asymptomatic, undiagnosed individuals older than 45 years should be conducted every ____.
   A. year
   B. 3 years
   C. 5 years
   D. 10 years

7. You are seeing 17-year-old Amanda. As part of the visit, you consider her risk factors for T2DM would likely include all of the following except:

   A. obesity.

   B. Native American ancestry.

   C. family history of T1DM.

   D. personal history of PCOS.

8. Criteria for the diagnosis of T2DM include:

   A. classic symptoms regardless of fasting plasma glucose measurement.

   B. plasma glucose level of 126 mg/dL (7 mmol/L) as a random measurement.

   C. a 2-hour glucose measurement of 156 mg/dL (8.6 mmol/L) after a 75-g anhydrous glucose load.

   D. a plasma glucose level of 126 mg/dL (7 mmol/L) or greater after an 8-hour or greater fast on more than one occasion.

9. The mechanism of action of pioglitazone is as:

   A. an insulin-production enhancer.

   B. a reducer of pancreatic glucagon output.

   C. an insulin sensitizer.

   D. a facilitator of renal glucose excretion.

10. Which of the following should be the goal measurement in treating a 45-year-old nonsmoking man with DM and hypertension?

    A. blood pressure less than 140 mm Hg systolic and less than 90 mm Hg diastolic

    B. hemoglobin A1c equal to or greater than 7%

    C. TG 200 to 300 mg/dL (11.1 to 16.6 mmol/L)

    D. high-density lipoprotein (HDL) 35 to 40 mg/dL (0.9 to 1.03 mmol/L)

11. In caring for a patient with DM, microalbuminuria measurement should be obtained:

    A. annually if urine protein is present.

    B. periodically in relationship to glycemia control.

    C. yearly.

    D. with each office visit related to DM.

12. The mechanism of action of sulfonylureas is as:

    A. an antagonist of insulin receptor site activity.

    B. a product that enhances insulin release.

    C. a facilitator of renal glucose excretion.

    D. an agent that can reduce hepatic glucose production.

13. When caring for a patient with DM, hypertension, and persistent proteinuria, the nurse practitioner (NP) prioritizes the choice of antihypertension and prescribes:

    A. furosemide.

    B. methyldopa.

    C. fosinopril.

    D. hydrochlorothiazide.

14. Clinical presentation of T1DM usually includes all of the following except:

    A. report of recent unintended weight gain.

    B. ketosis.

C. persistent thirst.

D. polyphagia.

15. Which of the following should be periodically monitored with the use of a biguanide such as metformin?

A. creatine kinase (CK)

B. alkaline phosphatase (ALP)

C. alanine aminotransferase (ALT)

D. creatinine (Cr)

16. Which of the following should be periodically monitored with the use of a thiazolidinedione?

A. CK

B. CrCl

C. ALT

D. Cr

17. All of the following are risks for lactic acidosis in individuals taking metformin except:

A. presence of chronic renal insufficiency.

B. acute dehydration.

C. recent radiographic contrast dye use.

D. history of allergic reaction to sulfonamides.

18. Secondary causes of hyperglycemia potentially include the use of all of the following medications except:

A. high-dose niacin.

B. systemic corticosteroids.

C. high-dose thiazide diuretics.

D. low-dose ARBs.

19. Hemoglobin A1c best provides information on glucose control over the past:

A. 28 to 42 days.

B. 48 to 68 days.

C. 69 to 95 days.

D. 96 to 120 days.

20. Which of the following statements is not true concerning the effects of exercise and IR?

A. Approximately 80% of the body's insulin-mediated glucose uptake occurs in skeletal muscle.

B. With regular aerobic exercise, IR is reduced by approximately 40%.

C. The IR-reducing effects of exercise persist for 48 hours after the activity.

D. Hyperglycemia can occur as a result of aerobic exercise.

21 to 24. With an 8 a.m. dose of the following insulin forms, followed by an inadequate dietary intake and/ or excessive energy use, at approximately what time would hypoglycemia be most likely to occur?

_____ **21.** Lispro_____

_____ **22.** Regular insulin _____

_____ **23.** NPH insulin _____

_____ **24.** Insulin glargine (Toujeo®, Lantus®) _____

25. Risk factors for T1DM include all of the following except:

A. presence of HLA complex.

B. European ancestry.

C. select viral infections.

D. obesity.

26. Which of the following medication classes should not be combined with insulin due to an increased risk of adverse event?

A. GLP-1 agonist

B. thiazolidinediones

C. DPP-4 inhibitor

D. SGLT2 inhibitor

27. Which of the following statements best describes the Somogyi effect?

A. Insulin-induced hypoglycemia triggers excess secretion of glucagon and cortisol, leading to hyperglycemia.

B. Early morning elevated blood glucose levels result in part from growth hormone and cortisol-triggering hepatic glucose release.

C. Late evening hyperglycemia is induced by inadequate insulin dose.

D. Episodes of postprandial hypoglycemia occur as a result of inadequate food intake.

28. Intervention in microalbuminuria for a person with DM includes which of the following? *(More than one can apply.)*

A. improved glycemic control

B. strict dyslipidemia control

C. use of an optimized dose of an ACEI or ARB

D. use of an ACEI with an ARB

29. Hemoglobin A1c should be tested:

A. at least annually for all patients.

B. at least two times a year in patients who are meeting treatment goals and who have stable glycemic control.

C. monthly in patients whose therapy has changed or who are not meeting glycemic goals.

D. only via standardized laboratory testing because of inaccuracies associated with point-of-service testing.

30. The mechanism of action of the DPP-4 inhibitors is as:

A. a drug that increases levels of incretin, increasing synthesis and release of insulin from pancreatic beta cells.

B. a product virtually identical in action to sulfonylureas.

C. a drug that increases insulin action in the peripheral tissues and reduces hepatic glucose production.

D. a facilitator of renal glucose excretion.

31. The mechanism of action of a GLP-1 agonist such as exenatide (Bydureon®) is as:

A. a drug that stimulates insulin production in response to an increase in plasma glucose.

B. a product virtually identical in action to sulfonylureas.

C. a drug that increases insulin action in the peripheral tissues and reduces hepatic glucose production.

D. a facilitator of renal glucose excretion.

32. You see an obese 25-year-old man with acanthosis nigricans and consider ordering:

A. FPG.

B. LFT.

C. RPR.

D. ESR.

33. The use of a thiazolidinedione is not recommended in all of the following clinical scenarios except:

A. a 57-year-old man who is taking a nitrate.

B. a 62-year-old woman with heart failure.

C. a 45-year-old man who is using insulin.

D. a 35-year-old patient with newly diagnosed T2DM.

34. In an older adult with T2DM with gastroparesis, the use of which of the following medications should be avoided?

A. insulin glargine (Toujeo®, Lantus®)

B. insulin aspart (NovoLog®)

C. glimepiride (Amaryl®)

D. liraglutide (Victoza®)

35. Metformin should be discontinued for the day of and up to 48 hours after surgery because of increased risk of:

A. hypoglycemia.

B. hepatic impairment.

C. lactic acidosis.

D. interaction with most anesthetic agents.

36. All of the following medications are recommended as possible first-line medications for treatment of concomitant hypertension when seen with T2DM in a 48-year-old man of European ancestry except:

A. beta blocker.

B. calcium channel blocker.

C. α-adrenergic receptor antagonist.

D. ARB.

37. Which of the following best describes the physical activity recommendations such as brisk walking for a 55-year-old woman with newly diagnosed T2DM? *(More than one can apply.)*

A. The goal should be for a total increased physical activity of 150 minutes per week or more.

B. Increased physical activity is recommended at least three times per week with no more than 48 hours without exercise.

C. Some form of resistance exercise such as lifting dumbbells or using an exercise band should be included at least two times per week.

D. Vigorous aerobic or resistance activity is potentially contraindicated in the presence of proliferative or severe nonproliferative retinopathy because of the possible risk of vitreous hemorrhage or retinal detachment.

38. In teaching a patient with T2DM and taking basal insulin such as degludec (Tresiba®) about using rapid-acting insulin such as aspart (Novolog®) to help with the management of postprandial hyperglycemia, the NP advises first starting an injection of _____ unit(s) prior to the largest meal.

A. 1

B. 4

C. 8

D. 12

39. Which of the following patients has prediabetes?

A. a 70-year-old man with a fasting glucose of 99 mg/dL (6.05 mmol/L)

B. an 84-year-old woman with a 1-hour postprandial glucose of 98 mg/dL (5.44 mmol/L)

C. a 33-year-old man with a hemoglobin A1c of 5.4%

D. a 58-year-old woman with a 2-hour postprandial glucose of 152 mg/dL (8.44 mmol/L)

40. Mr. Samuels is a 58-year-old man with T2DM who is using a single 10-unit daily dose of the long-acting insulin glargine. His fasting blood glucose has been between 141 and 180 mg/dL (7.8 and 10 mmol/L). Which of the following best describes the next step in his therapy?

    A. Continue on the current glargine dose.

    B. Increase his glargine dose by four units per day.

    C. Increase his glargine dose by one unit per day.

    D. Increase his glargine dose by six units per day.

41. Which of the following medications is commonly recommended as part of first-line therapy in the 40-year-old woman with BMI of 26 kg/m^2 with newly diagnosed T2DM (A1c = 7.3%), GFR = 96 mL/min/1.73 m^2, and who has no health insurance?

    A. DPP-4 inhibitor

    B. metformin

    C. GLP-1 agonist

    D. SGLT2 inhibitor

42. Pertaining to the use of sliding-scale insulin in response to elevated blood glucose, which of the following best describes current best practice?

    A. The use of this type of sliding-scale insulin therapy is discouraged as this method treats hyperglycemia after it has already occurred.

    B. Sliding-scale insulin in response to elevated glucose is a safe and helpful method of treating hyperglycemia.

    C. Delivering insulin in this manner is acceptable within the acute care hospital setting only.

    D. The use of the sliding insulin scale is appropriate in the treatment of T1DM only.

43. In a healthy person, what percentage of the body's total daily physiological insulin secretion is released basally?

    A. 10% to 20%

    B. 25% to 35%

    C. 50% to 60%

    D. 75% to 85%

44. Five years or more after T2DM diagnosis, which of the following medications is less likely to be effective in controlling plasma glucose?

    A. metformin

    B. pioglitazone

    C. glipizide

    D. insulin

45. The use of which of the following medications has the potential for causing the greatest reduction in A1c?

    A. a biguanide (metformin)

    B. a thiazolidinedione

    C. a sulfonylurea

    D. an insulin form

46. Which of the following best describes ethnicity and insulin sensitivity?

    A. Little variation exists in insulin sensitivity among different ethnic groups.

    B. African Americans are typically less sensitive to the effects of insulin when compared with people of European ancestry.

C. Mexican Americans are likely the most insulin-sensitive ethnic group residing in North America.

D. The degree of insulin sensitivity has little influence on insulin production.

47. The recommended A1c goal in a 79-year-old woman with a 20-year history of T2DM who has difficulty ambulating, uses a walker, and has a cardiac ejection fraction of 35% and a history of heart failure should be equal to or less than:

A. 7%.

B. 7.5%.

C. 8%.

D. 8.5%.

48. For a 22-year-old man with an 8-year history of T1DM and who has no comorbid conditions, consideration should be given to setting his A1c goal at equal to or less than:

A. 5.5%.

B. 6%.

C. 6.5%.

D. 7%.

49. The use of GLP-1 agonist has been associated with the development of:

A. leukopenia.

B. pancreatitis.

C. lymphoma.

D. vitiligo.

50. The IDF's diagnostic criteria for metabolic syndrome include:

A. an obligatory finding of persistent hyperglycemia.

B. notation of ethnic-specific waist circumference measurements.

C. documentation of microalbuminuria.

D. a family history of T2DM.

51. Metformin has all of the following effects except:

A. improved insulin-mediated glucose uptake.

B. modest weight loss with initial use.

C. diminished fibrinolysis.

D. decreased triglyceride cholesterol production.

52. Cardiovascular effects of hyperinsulinemia include:

A. decreased renal sodium reabsorption.

B. constricted circulating volume.

C. greater responsiveness to angiotensin II.

D. diminished sympathetic activation.

53. Which of the following is an unlikely consequence of untreated metabolic syndrome and IR in a woman of reproductive age?

A. hyperovulation

B. irregular menses

C. acne

D. hirsutism

54. Acanthosis nigricans is commonly noted in all of the following areas except:
    A. groin folds.
    B. axilla.
    C. nape of the neck.
    D. face.

55. A 26-year-old woman was diagnosed with T2DM 2 years ago and is being treated with combination therapy. Her A1c today is 8.4%. She states that she is planning to start a family soon. The NP counsels that:
    A. pregnancy will likely help to control plasma glucose levels.
    B. she is at her target A1c level.
    C. it is important to maintain glucose control prior to and during pregnancy.
    D. her antihyperglycemic medications will likely be discontinued during pregnancy.

56 to 59. For a patient with T2DM who is taking metformin and requires the addition of a second agent, identify the priority medication to add based on the compelling need of the patient. (*Select all that apply.*)
    _____ 56. Patient with heart failure
    _____ 57. Compelling need for weight loss
    _____ 58. Cost is a major issue
    _____ 59. Hypoglycemia is a concern
            A. sulfonylurea
            B. DPP-4 inhibitor
            C. GLP-1 agonist
            D. SGLT2 inhibitor

For answers and rationales, see end of chapter.

Obesity

Overview

Rates of obesity, usually defined as a body mass index (BMI) of 30 kg/m^2 or greater (Table 12-7), are currently at record levels in North America and are projected to double over the next 30 years; this mirrors the overall increase in overweight and obesity rates worldwide. Although no specific endocrine disorder, including thyroid dysfunction, is usually found in obese individuals, the cause of the overweight and obese condition is likely a combination of environmental, genetic, and behavioral influences.

Direct health-care cost increases related to obesity are attributable largely to well-known obesity-related diseases, including gallbladder disease, coronary heart disease, DM, OA, and dyslipidemia. Less commonly known consequences of obesity include an increase in sleep apnea risk, a reduction in female fertility, and nonalcoholic fatty liver including steatohepatitis. Obesity is also associated with increased risks of cancers of the esophagus, postmenopausal breast, endometrium, colon and rectum, kidney, pancreas, thyroid, gallbladder, and possibly other cancer types; the correlation between these cancers and obesity is likely, in part, due to the chronic inflammatory state caused by increased adiposity. Social and workplace discrimination against people with obesity is well-documented.

Often, persons who are overweight or obese assume that only dramatic weight loss can produce healthy results. In reality, a 10% body weight loss yields a nearly immediate improvement of death rates from heart disease and stroke. Clinical improvement in OA and asthma symptoms and a reduction in sleep apnea symptoms are usually noted.

> **CLINICAL CONCEPT**
> Consequences of overweight and obesity include increased risk of all-cause morbidity and mortality, greater health-care cost, lower workforce productivity, and increased workplace absentee rates and employer costs.

Clinical Presentation

The presentation of obesity is usually straightforward with many patients reporting having difficulty maintaining or losing weight despite repeated efforts. Others will present with health conditions or complications related to obesity.

TABLE 12-7 Classification of Overweight and Obesity

BODY MASS INDEX (KG/M²)	INTERNATIONAL CLASSIFICATION	CDC DESCRIPTION
Less than 18.5	Underweight	Underweight
18.5 to 24.9	Normal weight	Healthy weight
25 to 29.9	Overweight	Overweight
30 to 34.9	Class I obesity	Obesity
35 to 39.9	Class II obesity	Obesity
40 or greater	Class III obesity	Extreme or severe obesity

CDC, Centers for Disease Control and Prevention.

Diagnostic Testing

BMI is the most common approach to measure overweight and obesity with the World Health Organization classification commonly used to differentiate the degree of obesity. In this system, grade 1 overweight (or overweight) is given with a BMI of 25 to 29.9 kg/m²; grade 2 overweight (obesity) for BMI between 30 and 39.9 kg/m²; and grade 3 overweight (severe or morbid obesity) for BMI 40 kg/m² or greater. Laboratory studies should include a fasting lipid panel, liver function test, thyroid function test, fasting plasma glucose, and A1c. As a significant portion of obese individuals also have an eating disorder, patients should be screened for these disorders in the patient history.

Treatment

Lifestyle Modifications

The NP is well situated to help a person with obesity. For a person who desires weight loss, a first step is the discussion of achievable, reasonable goals. A first step can be simply to help the person halt weight gain or to lose 5% to 10% of total body weight. Slow, steady weight loss usually leads to long-term health benefits and risk reductions. A pound of fat contains approximately 3,500 stored calories. A deficit of 500 to 1,000 calories per day would lead to a 1 to 2 lb (0.45 to 0.9 kg) weight loss per week. Physical activity is often the most difficult part of a comprehensive weight reduction program. The idea of a protracted walking or other exercise regimen is quite daunting for a person who is obese. Although 30 minutes or more of aerobic activity on 5 days or more per week is typically recommended, an exercise prescription of 3 to 5 minutes of increased physical activity five to six times per day would likely yield the same results and be much better tolerated. A pedometer can also be used to measure objectively the number of steps taken; the goal should be 10,000 steps per day, or the equivalent of walking 4 to 5 miles. A pedometer is one method of quantifying how physically active the patient is in day-to-day behavior and deliberate exercise. In addition, increased physical activity improves overall cardiac health and improves insulin sensitivity.

The use of certain medications can result in weight gain. These medications include atypical or second-generation antipsychotics (risperidone [Risperdal®], olanzapine [Zyprexa®], others), select antiepileptics (valproate [Depakote®], carbamazepine [Tegretol®], others), and systemic corticosteroids (prednisone, methylprednisolone, others). The use of these medications is occasionally necessary in a person with obesity. The patient should be advised about the risk, and weight-controlling efforts would need to be intensified.

A comprehensive approach to obesity treatment that includes behavior modification and pharmacotherapy that results in decreased food intake and increased energy expenditure can lead to long-term success. Asking about readiness for change at every clinical visit can help facilitate success (Table 12-8).

TABLE 12-8 Facilitating Change in the Care of a Person Who Is Overweight or Obese

STAGE	QUESTIONS TO ASK	AS THE PROVIDER, YOU CAN:
Precontemplation (not interested in change)	■ How do you feel about your weight? ■ How does your weight affect you? ■ Are you considering/planning weight loss now? ■ On a scale of 0 to 10, how ready are you to start a weight loss program?	Validate and acknowledge ■ This will take working together, but it can be done. Restate position, leave the door open. ■ It's up to you to make the decision to lose weight. I cannot do this for you, but I am here to help you.
Contemplation (thinking about change)	■ What are the pros and cons of weight loss? ■ Where are you on the scale of 0 to 10 as far as ready? ■ What are barriers/supports you envision? ■ How do you view me as helping?	Praise and validate. ■ I am happy that you want to deal with this issue and feel ready to do so. Try to shift decisional balance. ■ I am here to help you and point you in the direction of other sources of support. Arrange follow-up.
Preparation for change	■ What is your usual food and activity pattern? ■ What is your personal goal for weight loss? ■ Health goal? ■ Cosmetic goal?	Help set small behavioral goals related to diet, physical activity. Assist in compiling food and activity diaries. Begin to negotiate goal weight. Identify support system. Help set a date to start.
Making change	■ How can I help?	Teach nutritional tactics to help control obesity.
Maintaining change	■ What is getting in your way?	Learn energy values of different foods.
Dealing with relapse	■ What is making this work?	Monitor food consumption by keeping a food diary; reduce portion sizes. Read and understand nutrition labels on foods. ■ Learn new habits of food purchasing. ■ Eliminate high-calorie foods from grocery list. Limit fats and oils in cooking, recipes; high-calorie or "calorie-dense" foods. Increase physical activity.

Source: Centers for Disease Control and Prevention. Overweight and obesity. http://www.cdc.gov/obesity/index.html

Pharmacotherapy

Pharmacotherapy is an important tool in weight management. Many antiobesity drugs are available. Orlistat (Xenical®, Alli®) is taken with meals and contributes to weight loss by reducing dietary fat absorption by approximately 30%. The fat passes undigested, and weight loss is facilitated. The medication is taken three times daily with or within 1 hour of a meal that contains fat. The most common adverse effect is GI disturbance, including loose stools and oily anal seepage. Older medications, sympathomimetics such as dexamphetamine and phentermine (Fastin®, others), work with norepinephrine and dopamine, reducing the appetite, with resulting reduction in food intake. Sleep disturbances, nervousness, and elevated heart rate and blood pressure rank among the most frequent adverse effects associated with the use of these medications.

Qsymia® is a fixed-dose combination of phentermine and topiramate that is FDA-approved for weight management in adults with an initial BMI of 30 kg/m² or greater or 27 kg/m² or greater when accompanied by weight-related comorbidities such as hypertension, T2DM, or dyslipidemia. The effect of phentermine is likely mediated by release of catecholamines, including norepinephrine in the hypothalamus, resulting in reduced appetite and decreased food consumption.

Because of the topiramate portion of Qsymia®, women of reproductive potential should have a negative pregnancy test before starting Qsymia® and monthly thereafter during Qsymia® therapy and use a highly effective form of contraception while taking the medication.

Contrave® is a combination of naltrexone (an opioid antagonist) and bupropion (an aminoketone antidepressant). Its mechanism in weight loss is not fully understood but is believed to affect two areas of the brain (hypothalamus and mesolimbic dopamine circuit) involved in the regulation of food intake. FDA-mandated boxed warnings associated with its use include suicidal thoughts and behaviors as well as neuropsychiatric reactions. Patients should be monitored for depression or suicidal thoughts. Contrave® should not be used concomitantly with other bupropion-containing medications, chronic opioid use, or MAOIs. The medication can also cause increases in blood pressure and heart rate and should be used with caution in patients with cardiovascular or cerebrovascular disease.

Liraglutide (Saxenda®) is a GLP-1 receptor agonist. The dose used for chronic weight management is different than what is used to treat T2DM (Victoza®). Similar to other GLP-1 agonists, liraglutide affects areas of the brain involved in appetite regulation and is dosed via daily injections. This agent has a warning associated with increased risk of thyroid C-cell tumors and is contraindicated in patients with a personal or family history of medullary thyroid carcinoma (MTC) or in patients with multiple endocrine neoplasia syndrome type 2 (MEN 2).

As with many other weight loss approaches, weight loss plateaus and then may slowly increase, particularly if lifestyle modification does not include increased activity and decreased caloric intake. With weight loss drugs, the medication should be discontinued if the patient has not achieved a 5% weight loss by week 12 of treatment; in this circumstance, the weight loss medication is unlikely to be helpful in weight reduction.

Surgical

Numerous surgical options are available for obesity intervention. The most common options include gastric bypass, gastric sleeve, and adjustable laparoscopic band. In the United States, the gastric sleeve has become the most common type of bariatric surgery technique, followed by gastric bypass. The ideal candidate for a bariatric surgical procedure is a person with BMI equal to or greater than 40 kg/m² or BMI equal to or greater than 35 kg/m² who also has DM, hypertension, dyslipidemia, obstructive sleep apnea, CVD, gastroesophageal reflux, degenerative joint disease, fatty liver (steatohepatitis), or other obesity-related conditions in whom behavioral and pharmacological therapy has failed. Contraindications to bariatric surgery include untreated or unstable mental health conditions, active substance abuse disorder, poor adherence to advised health regimens, and concomitant health conditions that would pose significant operative risk. Gastric sleeve surgery is a nonmalabsorptive technique that reduces the stomach to about 15% of its original size by surgical removal of the stomach along the greater curvature, leaving a sleeve or tube-like structure. The net result is a marked reduction in calorie intake and less hunger. Unlike in gastric bypass, medications pass through the duodenum with restrictive-only procedures. The Roux-en-Y gastroplasty, or gastric bypass, is one of the more common restrictive/malabsorptive bariatric surgeries. With gastric bypass, not only is the stomach size dramatically reduced, thus limiting intake, but the food that is eaten no longer passes over the duodenum, the part of the GI tract where calories and many medications are normally absorbed. The adjustable laparoscopic band (Lap-Band®) procedure, in which the stomach volume is restricted, is an intervention that does not lead to malabsorption because food and medications still pass through the duodenum, but rather restricts the amount of calories that can be ingested. Given the rate of complications, Lap-Band® procedures are less commonly done.

A noninvasive weight loss option is the gastric balloon, which involves a silicone balloon placed in the stomach endoscopically and filled with saline. At meals, the balloon makes the patient feel full sooner and can lead to significant weight loss. Common adverse effects include nausea, vomiting, and gastric pain, though these usually resolve after 1 to 2 weeks. The balloon is removed after 6 months.

CLINICAL CONCEPT
The precise mechanism of action of topiramate on weight management is not known; the use of this medication has been associated with appetite suppression and satiety.

CLINICAL CONCEPT

With any weight loss surgical procedure, future weight regain can occur if recommended dietary and physical activity guidelines are not followed.

A person considering bariatric surgery must have a realistic idea regarding the anticipated outcome. In a well-selected patient population, the average weight loss with the gastric sleeve can result in approximately 60% excess body weight loss. With gastric bypass, the expected weight loss is approximately 70% to 80% of excess body weight. With either procedure, most of that weight is lost within the first 3 years after surgery, and the most dramatic weight losses are seen in the first months postoperatively.

About 85% of patients lose a great deal of weight without major complications and maintain this loss long term. About 10% have a significant short-term problem after the surgery (e.g., reoperation, long hospital stay, insufficient weight loss, persistent GI upset), but most do well in the long term. Less than 5% have major unresolved problems over time, including, though rarely, death as a direct result of the surgery. With all bariatric surgery, but in particular the malabsorptive procedures, expert consultation on continued micronutrient supplementation should be sought to avoid anemia and other health problems. Postprocedure supplementation usually includes vitamin B_{12}, iron, zinc, calcium, protein, and most fat-soluble vitamins. Given the alteration in the GI tract after gastric bypass, absorption of certain medications is altered. In particular, the use of combined oral contraceptives (COCs; estrogen/progestin-containing) is not recommended after gastric bypass because of the risk of contraceptive failure related to lower drug absorption. However, progestin implants, intrauterine devices, and nonoral combined hormonal contraception such as the patch or vaginal ring are able to be used without difficulty. Study on other medications is ongoing.

Discussion Sources

Centers for Disease Control and Prevention. Overweight and obesity. http://www.cdc.gov/obesity/index.html

Hamdy O, Uwaifo GI. Obesity treatment and management. Medscape. http://emedicine.medscape.com/article/123702-treatment

QUESTIONS

60. Obesity is defined as having a BMI equal to or greater than _____ kg/m².

    A. 25

    B. 30

    C. 35

    D. 40

61. Which of the following is an example of an appropriate question to pose to a person with obesity who is in the precontemplation change stage?

    A. "How do you feel about your weight?"

    B. "What are barriers you see to losing weight?"

    C. "What is your personal goal for weight loss?"

    D. "How do you envision my helping you meet your weight loss goal?"

62. Which of the following is an example of an appropriate question to pose to a person with obesity who is in the contemplation change stage?

    A. "How do you feel about your weight?"

    B. "What are barriers you see to losing weight?"

    C. "What is your personal goal for weight loss?"

    D. "How do you envision my helping you meet your weight loss goal?"

63. When advising a person who will be using orlistat (Xenical®, Alli®) as part of a weight loss program, the NP provides the following information about when to take the medication:

    A. within an hour of each meal that contains fat

    B. before any food with high carbohydrate content

C. only in the morning, to avoid sleep disturbance

D. up to 3 hours after any meal, regardless of types of food eaten

64. Contrave® is believed to effect which part of the brain involved in the regulation of food intake?

A. Cerebellum

B. Hypothalamus

C. Pituitary gland

D. Parietal lobe

65. A pound of fat contains approximately _____ stored calories.

A. 2,500

B. 3,000

C. 3,500

D. 4,000

66. The commonly recommended physical activity level of 10,000 steps per day is roughly the equivalent of walking _____ miles.

A. 1 to 2

B. 2 to 3

C. 3 to 4

D. 4 to 5

67. With the use of weight loss medications, if the patient has not achieved a 5% weight loss by week _____ of treatment, the therapy should be discontinued.

A. 6

B. 12

C. 18

D. 24

68. In a person with obesity, weight loss of _____ % or more yields an immediate reduction in death rates from cardiovascular and cerebrovascular disease.

A. 5

B. 10

C. 15

D. 20

69. When counseling about malabsorptive bariatric surgery such as gastric bypass, the NP provides the following information:

A. Most people achieve ideal BMI postoperatively.

B. The most dramatic weight losses are seen in the first few postoperative months.

C. The death rate directly attributable to surgery is about 10%.

D. Weight loss will continue for years postoperatively in most patients.

70. The use of which of the following medications is often associated with weight gain?

A. risperidone (Risperdal®)

B. topiramate (Topamax®)

C. metformin (Glucophage®)

D. sitagliptin (Januvia®)

71. You are counseling a patient who is considering gastric bypass surgery for weight loss. You advise the following. *(More than one can apply.)*

    A. Calcium absorption will be reduced.

    B. Rapid weight loss after obesity surgery can contribute to the development of gallstones.

    C. Chronic constipation is a common postoperative adverse effect.

    D. Lifelong vitamin B$_{12}$ supplementation is recommended.

72 to 76. Weight loss medications: True or false?

_____ **72.** The same liraglutide dose is used for chronic weight loss management and for management of type 2 diabetes mellitus.

_____ **73.** Phentermine/topiramate (Qsymia®) carries a warning about potential teratogenic effects.

_____ **74.** Phentermine's mechanism of action in weight loss is as a product that reduces GI motility.

_____ **75.** In general, weight lost after gastric bypass is significantly more when compared with the postoperative course of a restrictive procedure such as adjustable gastric band or gastric sleeve.

_____ **76.** Use of naltrexone/bupropion (Contrave®) is associated with an increased risk of suicidal ideation.

77. Which of the following is a possible consequence of obesity? *(More than one can apply.)*

    A. obstructive apnea

    B. steatohepatitis

    C. female infertility

    D. endometrial cancer

For answers and rationales, see end of chapter.

Thyroid Disorders

Overview

Thyroid hormone acts as a cellular energy release catalyst and is essential for normal body function. When assessing a patient with thyroid dysfunction, the NP should look for signs of excessive energy release in hyperthyroidism or decreased energy release in hypothyroidism.

Although thyroid disease likely exists in less than 7% of the population, a high index of suspicion should be maintained for individuals at particular risk. Risk factors and associated conditions include the following:

- Down syndrome: Hypothyroidism
- Elderly: Hypothyroidism or hyperthyroidism with a high propensity for atypical presentation in either situation
- Use of certain medications causing an alteration in thyroid function, including iodide (hypothyroidism), amiodarone, lithium (capable of inducing both hyperthyroidism and hypothyroidism as well as thyroiditis), interferon-α, interleuken-2
- Female gender: Hyperthyroidism or hypothyroidism; because most thyroid dysfunction is autoimmune in nature, these diseases are more common in women than in men, as are most autoimmune diseases
- Postpartum period: A transient hypothyroidism is common, as is a transient thyroiditis
- Personal and/or family history of autoimmune disease, such as pernicious anemia, vitiligo, and T1DM: Hyperthyroidism and hypothyroidism
- History of head and neck irradiation or surgery: Hypothyroidism

Diagnostic Testing in Thyroid Disease

A number of thyroid laboratory tests are available, some with more utility than others. Understanding what information can be obtained from each test helps direct the appropriate diagnosis and intervention in thyroid disease.

The measurement of thyroid-stimulating hormone (TSH; also known as thyrotropin) is the sensitive and specific thyroid test, particularly when diagnosing the condition in the outpatient setting; TSH is the first test that should be obtained with any suspected thyroid disorder. TSH is produced and released by the anterior lobe of the pituitary with secretion stimulated by thyrotropin-releasing hormone through a negative feedback loop in response to the amount of circulating thyroid hormone (T4). Because only a small fraction of T4 circulates free, with 99.7% bound to T4-binding globulin and other plasma proteins, the unbound portion of T4, or free T4, is metabolically active. The measurement of free T4 is the most helpful test to confirm an abnormal TSH level. Approximately 40% of T4 is converted in the periphery to triiodothyronine (T3). Compared with T4, T3 is likely four times more metabolically active; T4 is often referred to as a prodrug for T3.

Serum total T4 is a commonly performed but less than helpful test to assess thyroid function. Numerous factors can cause an increase or decrease in total T4; however, that is not indicative of a change in metabolic status. These factors include a change in thyroxine-binding globulin (TBG) levels, the principal carrier protein of T3 and T4. The use of certain medications, including exogenous estrogen (oral contraceptives, postmenopausal hormone therapy), opioids, and selective estrogen receptor modifiers (tamoxifen, raloxifene) can cause an alteration in TBG levels, resulting in an increase or decrease in total T4 (the total of protein-bound and free T4), but no change in the metabolically active free T4; these results are metabolically insignificant. As a result, the clinical usefulness of total T4 measurement is limited with results that can lead to errors in clinical judgment.

The likelihood of normal free T4 if TSH level is normal is greater than 98%. In the small remainder, pituitary disorder is the likely cause. If the clinician suspects thyroid disorder, and the TSH level is normal, it should be assumed that the hypothalamic-pituitary-thyroid axis is intact, with no further testing required. The TSH level is increased in hypothyroidism; a 50% decrease in T4 concentration can yield a 90-fold increase in TSH. Conversely, the TSH level is decreased in hyperthyroidism. Antimicrosomal thyroid antibodies, also known as thyroid peroxidase (TPO) antibodies, likely reflecting cell-mediated immunity, are found in nearly all patients with hypothyroidism. Given that likely nearly 100% of all patients with hypothyroidism have elevated levels of TPO antibodies, and their presence does not change the treatment plan, routine testing for this marker is not advocated.

Because thyroid disease can produce low-level symptoms attributed to other conditions, especially stress, fatigue, and a variety of self-limiting illnesses, the issue of routine testing for thyroid disorder with TSH has been long debated. U.S. Preventive Services Task Force (USPSTF) guidelines and other authorities advise that there is insufficient evidence to recommend for or against routine screening for all asymptomatic lower-risk adults for thyroid disease.

HYPOTHYROIDISM

Overview

Hypothyroidism is found when the amount of thyroxine (T4) released by the thyroid is inadequate to meet the body's metabolic needs. In North America, hypothyroidism is usually the result of Hashimoto's thyroiditis; this is an autoimmune disease, leading to thyroid failure. Environmental iodine deficiency is the most common cause of hypothyroidism on a worldwide basis but is relatively uncommon in North America due to the use of iodized salt. Other, less common hypothyroidism causes are select medication use, including amiodarone and lithium as well as postradiation exposure; the latter is largely limited to patients who received radioactive iodine to treat Graves' disease or thyroid cancer.

Clinical Presentation

Hypothyroidism signs and symptoms often are present in the history and physical examination (Table 12-9) (Fig. 12-5). Hypothyroidism is most often seen in women 30 to 50 years old; clinical presentation often includes goiter, or chronic, diffuse, nonpainful thyroid enlargement, usually caused by hypertrophic or degenerative changes. Over the years, thyroid enlargement noted in hypothyroidism usually regresses.

CLINICAL CONCEPT

Goiter is also a common finding in many individuals with normal thyroid function or a number of thyroid disease forms.

Diagnostic Testing

In hypothyroidism, given the thyroid is no longer able to secrete sufficient T4 for the body's needs, circulating thyroxine is low. As a result, the pituitary's anterior lobe increases TSH production in an attempt to increase thyroxine production. Due to thyroid failure, the thyroxine level does not increase appreciably. The result is a low serum free T4 and high TSH. Typically, no other diagnostic testing is required in hypothyroidism.

TABLE 12-9 Comparison of Hyperthyroidism to Hypothyroidism

	HYPERTHYROIDISM	HYPOTHYROIDISM
Characteristics	Excessive energy release, rapid cell turnover	Reduced energy release, slow cell turnover
Causes	Graves' disease, thyroiditis, metabolically active thyroid nodule	Post–autoimmune thyroiditis (greater than 95% in North America), primary pituitary failure (rare worldwide) Dietary iodine deficiency most common reason for hypothyroidism worldwide but relatively uncommon in North America
Neurological	Nervousness, irritability, memory problems	Lethargy, uninterest, memory problems
Weight	Weight loss (usually modest, present in approximately 50%, approximately 5 to 10 lb [2.3 to 4.5 kg]), usually quickly regained with euthyroid status	Weight gain (usually 5 to 10 lb [2.3 to 4.5 kg] largely fluid, little fat), quickly lost with initial therapy
Environmental response	Heat intolerance	Chilling easily, cold intolerance
Skin	Smooth, silky skin	Coarse, dry skin
Hair	Fine hair with frequent loss	Thick, coarse hair with tendency to break easily
Nails	Thin nails that break with ease	Thick, dry nails
Gastrointestinal	Frequent, low-volume, loose stools; hyperdefecation	Constipation
Menstrual	Amenorrhea or low-volume menstrual flow	Menorrhagia
Reflexes	Hyperreflexia with a characteristic "quick out–quick back" action	Overall hyporeflexia with characteristic slow relaxation phase, the "hung-up" patellar deep tendon reflex
Muscle strength	Proximal muscle weakness Tachycardia	Usually no change Bradycardia in severe cases

Treatment

In the treatment of hypothyroidism, T4 replacement is needed in the form of levothyroxine (Levothroid®, Levoxyl®, Synthroid®, Unithroid®, generic). The anticipated dosage of thyroid replacement for an adult is 75 to 125 mcg of levothyroxine, or about 1.6 mcg/kg/day; ideal body weight should be used for this calculation as this lean body mass, even in the presence of obesity, best reflects levothyroxine needs; for the person who is underweight, actual body weight should be used. For an elderly person, the anticipated dosage is 75% or less of the adult dosage. Because of its long half-life, the effects of a levothyroxine dosage adjustment would not cause a change in TSH for approximately five to six drug half-lives.

The recommended testing interval after initiation or adjustment of a levothyroxine form is at least 6 to 8 weeks. The levothyroxine dose should be titrated so that TSH is within normal limits. All levothyroxine forms are acceptable, but because of its narrow therapeutic index, the same brand or generic should be taken. If the brand or generic form changes, the TSH should be checked at least 6 to 8 weeks after the adjustment.

Animal-derived desiccated thyroid such as Armour® thyroid contains T4 and T3; drug levels vary substantially throughout the day in those taking desiccated thyroid. The majority of studies on thyroid

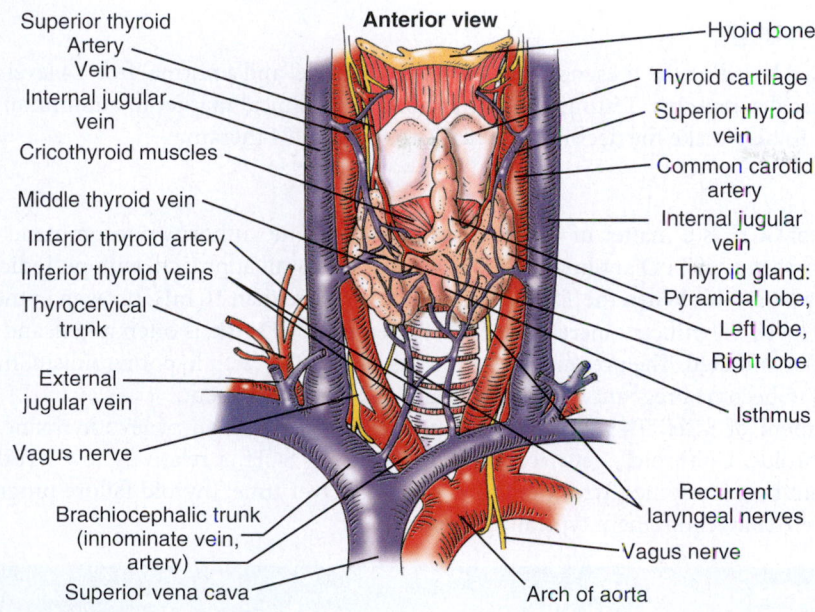

Anterior view

Superior thyroid
Artery
Vein
Internal jugular
vein
Cricothyroid muscles
Middle thyroid vein
Inferior thyroid artery
Inferior thyroid veins
Thyrocervical
trunk
External
jugular vein
Vagus nerve
Brachiocephalic trunk
(innominate vein,
artery)
Superior vena cava

Hyoid bone
Thyroid cartilage
Superior thyroid
vein
Common carotid
artery
Internal jugular
vein
Thyroid gland:
Pyramidal lobe,
Left lobe,
Right lobe
Isthmus
Recurrent
laryngeal nerves
Vagus nerve
Arch of aorta

FIGURE 12-5 Thyroid.
Venes D. Taber's Cyclopedic Medical Dictionary. 21st ed. Philadelphia, PA: F.A. Davis; 2009.

treatment have been done with levothyroxine, a bioidentical hormone. There are no controlled trials supporting the preferred use of desiccated thyroid hormone over levothyroxine in the treatment of hypothyroidism or any other thyroid disease. Desiccated thyroid is animal-sourced, either bovine (cow) or porcine (pig) in nature; the use of the medication would likely pose difficulties for certain ethnic and religious groups as well as individuals following a vegan or vegetarian diet.

In established hypothyroidism, thyroid hormone requirements tend to remain stable over time. Once an adequate replacement dose has been determined, periodic TSH measurements should be done after 6 months and then at 12-month intervals, or more frequently if the clinical situation dictates otherwise. Certain factors can influence thyroid hormone requirements, however. When levothyroxine is taken at the same time as iron, calcium, aluminum-containing antacids, sucralfate, cow or soy milk, and virtually any dairy product, its absorption can be impaired; ingestion of these medications should be separated by several hours. When levothyroxine is taken with rifampin, phenytoin, carbamazepine, and phenobarbital, its metabolism can be increased with resulting reduction of free T4. Levothyroxine should be taken at the same time every day on an empty stomach with water only. If the dose is taken upon arising, no food should be taken for ideally 1 hour after the levothyroxine dose. If this is impractical, taking the medication 4 hours after eating with a 1-hour wait postdose is acceptable.

SUBCLINICAL HYPOTHYROIDISM

Overview

Subclinical hypothyroidism (SCH) is a mild form of early hypothyroidism. The condition is often detected when laboratory testing is done as part of the evaluation of fatigue or mood disorder. With SCH, the thyroid requires more than its typical stimulation with TSH to produce an acceptable amount of thyroid hormone.

After age 60 years, the male-to-female ratio approaches 1:1. As with other thyroid disease, SCH is usually autoimmune in origin. Eventual thyroid failure and resulting hypothyroidism usually follow, particularly if there is evidence of TPO antibodies; there is a 2% to 5% likelihood of development of overt hypothyroidism per year.

> **CLINICAL CONCEPT**
> An estimated 3% to 8% of the population has SCH, with the predominance being women prior to age 60 years.

Clinical Presentation

In SCH, the clinical presentation is often vague and nonspecific, with fatigue, dry skin, and/or constipation complaints often found in individuals with normal thyroid function. Abnormalities on the thyroid examination are rare, as are alterations in deep tendon reflexes.

Diagnostic Testing

SCH is diagnosed based on the presence of an elevated TSH level and a normal free T4 level in the absence of or with minimal symptoms. Testing for TPO antibodies, a clinical marker of autoimmune thyroid disease, is advised to help make the decision of whether to initiate T4 therapy.

Treatment

The treatment of SCH is a matter of differing approaches; some authorities recommend levothyroxine therapy in the presence of TPO antibodies versus a watch-and-wait approach, with periodic TSH and free T4 testing every 6 months. When the TSH level increases to more than 10 mIU/L, even in the presence of a normal free T4 level, a significant increase in LDL, increasing CVD risk, is often noted, and levothyroxine therapy should be initiated. The presence of symptoms compatible with hypothyroidism, infertility, pregnancy, or plans to become pregnant in the near future also favor treatment.

In the treatment of SCH, T4 replacement is prescribed in the form of levothyroxine (Levothroid®, Levoxyl®, Synthroid®, Unithroid®, generic). In the presence of SCH, a relatively low levothyroxine dose is often sufficient because some thyroid function remains. Over time, thyroid failure progresses, and the patient's levothyroxine requirement typically increases.

HYPERTHYROIDISM

Overview

With an 8:1 female-to-male ratio, Graves' disease is the most common form of thyrotoxicosis, or hyperthyroidism. With Graves' disease, thyroid hormone is released in excess. The age at onset is usually 20 to 40 years, and there is a significant correlation with autoimmune diseases such as pernicious anemia, myasthenia gravis, and T1DM.

Clinical Presentation

Hyperthyroidism signs and symptoms often are present in the history and physical examination (see Table 12-9; Fig. 12-5). Clinical presentation of Graves' disease includes diffuse thyroid enlargement, often with a multinodular goiter, exophthalmos, nervousness, tachycardia, and heat intolerance. Thyroid scan reveals a large "hot" (metabolically active) gland with heterogeneous uptake.

Diagnostic Testing

With hyperthyroidism, the TSH is low or undetectable with hyperthyroid state being confirmed with a measurement of free T4. Additional testing, such as thyroid scan or thyroid ultrasound, is occasionally advised, especially in the presence of a toxic adenoma, a benign, T4-releasing thyroid nodule, but not routinely in classic Graves' disease presentation.

Treatment

Graves' disease includes the use of antithyroid preparations such as methimazole or propylthiouracil; the use of both drugs carries a hepatotoxicity warning. Once euthyroid status is achieved, radioactive iodine for thyroid ablation is usually the next step in therapy. Subsequent hypothyroidism is the norm, necessitating the use of levothyroxine. Expert consultation is advised in caring for the person with hyperthyroidism.

THYROID NODULE

Overview

A thyroid nodule is a mass within the gland; the term *nodule* is not specific to any particular thyroid condition. The evaluation of a palpable thyroid nodule presents a challenge. In the absence of hyperthyroidism symptoms, the presentations of benign and malignant thyroid lesions are typically the same; the risk that any thyroid nodule is malignant is about 5%. A history of head or neck irradiation, localized pain, dysphonia, hemoptysis, regional lymphadenopathy, or a hard, fixed mass should raise suspicion for thyroid cancer.

Clinical Presentation

As mentioned, a thyroid nodule, by definition, is a palpable mass, usually larger than 1 cm, held within the gland. The majority of thyroid nodules are nontender and relatively mobile, without heat or redness or adjacent lymphadenopathy.

Diagnostic Testing

Initial testing for a person with a thyroid nodule should include obtaining a TSH measurement. A metabolically active or "hot" thyroid nodule has a low risk of malignancy and can cause a reduction in TSH production from the pituitary. A thyroid scan can identify areas of increased uptake, most commonly noted with a benign toxic adenoma.

Fine-needle aspiration biopsy is advised, regardless of TSH results, and is more helpful and cost-effective in arriving at a definitive diagnosis than ultrasound or thyroid scan. A properly performed fine-needle aspiration biopsy has a false-negative rate of less than 5% and a false-positive rate of about 1%.

Treatment

Intervention in thyroid nodule is dependent on biopsy results. While the majority of thyroid nodules will be nonmalignant, expert consultation is required for biopsy and follow-up.

Discussion Sources

Bahn RS, Burch HB, Cooper DS, et al. Hyperthyroidism and other causes of thyrotoxicosis: management guidelines of the American Thyroid Association and American Association of Clinical Endocrinologists. *Endocrine Practice.* 2011;17:457–520. https://journals.aace.com/doi/pdf/10.4158/EP.17.3.456

Biondi B, Cappola AR, Cooper DS. Subclinical hypothyroidism: a review. *JAMA.* 2019;322:153–160.

Garber JR, Cobin RH, Gharib H; American Association of Clinical Endocrinologists, American Thyroid Association. Clinical practice guidelines for hypothyroidism in adults. *Endocr Prac.* 2012;18(6):989–1028. https://www.aace.com/files/final-file-hypo-guidelines.pdf

Gharib H, Papini E, Garber JR, et al. AACE/ACE/AME guidelines for clinical practice for the diagnosis and management of thyroid nodules—2016 update. *Endocr Prac.* 2016;22(Suppl 1):1–60. https://journals.aace.com/doi/pdf/10.4158/EP161208.GL

QUESTIONS

78. Increased risk of thyroid disorder is found in individuals who are:

A. obese.

B. hypertensive.

C. treated with systemic corticosteroids.

D. elderly.

79. A 48-year-old woman with newly diagnosed hypothyroidism asks about a "natural thyroid" medication she read about online and provides the drug's name: desiccated thyroid. As you counsel her about this medication, you consider all of the following except:

A. this product contains a fixed dose of T3 and T4.

B. the medication is a plant-based product.

C. its pharmacokinetics differ significantly when compared to levothyroxine.

D. the majority of the study on treatment for hypothyroidism has been done using levothyroxine.

80. Hypothyroidism most often develops as a result of:

A. primary pituitary failure.

B. thyroid neoplasia.

C. autoimmune thyroiditis.

D. radioactive iodine exposure.

81. Which of the following is the least helpful test for the assessment of thyroid disease?

A. total T4

B. TSH

C. free T4

D. TPO antibodies

82. Physical examination findings in patients with Graves' disease include:

A. muscle tenderness.

B. coarse, dry skin.

C. eyelid retraction.

D. a delayed relaxation phase of the patellar reflex.

83. The mechanism of action of radioactive iodine in the treatment of Graves' disease is to:

A. destroy the overactive thyroid tissue.

B. reduce the production of TSH.

C. alter the thyroid metabolic rate.

D. relieve distress caused by increased thyroid size.

84. Which of the following medications is a helpful treatment option for relief of tremor and tachycardia seen with untreated hyperthyroidism?

A. propranolol

B. diazepam

C. carbamazepine

D. verapamil

85. In prescribing levothyroxine therapy for an elderly patient, which of the following statements is true?

A. Elderly persons require a rapid initiation of levothyroxine therapy.

B. TSH should be checked about 2 days after dosage adjustment.

C. The levothyroxine dose needed by elderly persons is 75% or less of that needed by younger adults.

D. TSH should be suppressed to a nondetectable level.

86. TSH is released by the:

A. thyroid follicles.

B. adrenal cortex.

C. hypothalamus.

D. anterior lobe of the pituitary.

87. In the report of a thyroid scan done on a 48-year-old woman with a thyroid mass, a "cold spot" is reported. This finding is most consistent with:

A. autonomously functioning adenoma.

B. Graves' disease.

C. Hashimoto's disease.

D. thyroid cyst.

88. You advise a 58-year-old woman with hypothyroidism about the correct use of levothyroxine. She also takes a calcium supplement. All of the following should be shared with the patient except which instruction?

A. "Take the medication on an empty stomach."

B. "To help with adherence, take your calcium supplement at the same time as your thyroid medication."

C. "You should take the medication at approximately the same time every day."

D. "Do not take your medication with soy milk."

89. The findings of a painless thyroid mass and TSH level of less than 0.1 IU/mL in a 35-year-old woman who presents with fine tremor is most consistent with:

A. autonomously functioning adenoma.

B. Graves' disease.

C. Hashimoto's disease.

D. thyroid malignancy.

90. A fixed, painless thyroid mass accompanied by hoarseness and dysphagia should raise the suspicion of:

A. adenomatous lesion.

B. Graves' disease.

C. Hashimoto's disease.

D. thyroid malignancy.

91. Which of the following is the most effective method of distinguishing a malignant from a benign thyroid nodule?

A. ultrasound

B. magnetic resonance imaging (MRI)

C. fine-needle aspiration biopsy

D. radioactive iodine scan

92. Possible consequences of excessive levothyroxine use include:

A. bone thinning.

B. fatigue.

C. renal impairment.

D. constipation.

93. At minimum, at what interval should TSH be reassessed after a levothyroxine dosage is adjusted?

A. 1 to 2 weeks

B. 2 to 4 weeks

C. 4 to 6 weeks

D. 6 to 8 weeks

94. As part of an evaluation of a 3-cm, round, mobile thyroid mass, you obtain a thyroid ultrasound scan revealing a fluid-filled structure. The most likely diagnosis is:

A. adenoma.

B. thyroid cyst.

C. multinodular goiter.

D. internal hemangioma.

95. Periodic routine screening for hypothyroidism is indicated in the presence of which of the following clinical conditions?

A. digoxin use

B. male gender

C. Down syndrome

D. alcoholism

96 to 112. Identify each of the following findings as associated with hyperthyroidism, hypothyroidism, or both.

_____ 96. heat intolerance

_____ 97. smooth, silky skin

_____ 98. goiter

_____ 99. frequent, low-volume, loose stools

_____ 100. secondary hypertriglyceridemia

_____ 101. amenorrhea or oligomenorrhea

_____ 102. coarse, dry skin

_____ **103.** menorrhagia

_____ **104.** hyperreflexia with a characteristic "quick out–quick back" action at the patellar reflex

_____ **105.** proximal muscle weakness

_____ **106.** tachycardia with hypertension

_____ **107.** hyporeflexia with a characteristic slow relaxation phase, the "hung-up" reflex

_____ **108.** coarse hair with tendency to break easily

_____ **109.** thick, dry nails

_____ **110.** constipation

_____ **111.** atypical presentation in an elderly person

_____ **112.** change in mental status

113. The use of which of the following medications can induce thyroid dysfunction?

    A. sertraline

    B. venlafaxine

    C. bupropion

    D. lithium

114 to 116. Match the condition with the laboratory results: hypothyroidism, hyperthyroidism, or SCH.

_____ **114.** TSH = 8.9 mIU/L (0.4 to 4 mIU/L); free T4 = 15 pmol/L (10 to 27 pmol/L)

_____ **115.** TSH less than 0.15 mIU/L (0.4 to 4 mIU/L); free T4 = 79 pmol/L (10 to 27 pmol/L)

_____ **116.** TSH = 24 mIU/L (0.4 to 4 mIU/L); free T4 = 3 pmol/L (10 to 27 pmol/L)

For answers and rationales, see end of chapter.

Dyslipidemia

Overview

Dyslipidemia refers to abnormal levels of circulating total cholesterol (TC), including low-density lipoprotein cholesterol (LDL-C) and TGs, most often with low levels of high-density lipoprotein cholesterol (HDL-C.). In many cases, dyslipidemia is also associated with decreased levels of HDL-C, or beneficial cholesterol. Dyslipidemia can be caused by overproduction or diminished clearance of lipoprotein particles, and can often have a genetic component (e.g., familial hypercholesterolemia). Other risk factors for LDL-C elevation can include a diet rich in saturated fat, sedentary lifestyle, and the use of certain medications (e.g., high-dose thiazide diuretics, progestins, or anabolic steroids). Comorbid conditions with poor control such as DM, hypothyroidism, and excessive alcohol intake contribute to an increase in TGs.

Clinical Presentation

Dyslipidemia in the early stages is not associated with any signs or symptoms but is identified through routine lipid profile screening.

CLINICAL CONCEPT

Prolonged dyslipidemia is associated with an increased risk of ASCVD including coronary artery disease, cerebrovascular disease, as well as peripheral vascular disease.

Diagnostic Testing

The American College of Cardiology (ACC)/American Heart Association (AHA) recommend lipid screening for individuals 20 to 78 years without ASCVD to be performed every 4 to 6 years with a standard lipid profile (TC, HDL-C, LDL-C, TG), either fasting or not, including TC and LDL. If nonfasting TGs are 400 mg/dL or greater (4.5 mmol/L), then a repeat profile in the fasting state should be performed. During treatment for dyslipidemia, the lipid profile should be rechecked approximately 6 weeks after start or adjustment of drug therapy to measure response. If dyslipidemia therapy is focused on lifestyle management without drug therapy, usually a 3- to 6-month time period is recommended prior to rechecking the lipid profile. Follow-up testing is typically done every 1 to 2 years unless clinically indicated to be done more frequently. More complex lipid testing, including apolipoprotein B, is occasionally indicated to detect individuals who might be at higher ASCVD risk.

Treatment

Treatment of dyslipidemia is an important part of cardiovascular and cerebrovascular risk reduction. Intensive therapeutic lifestyle changes should be the first line of therapy. Dietary advice includes reducing saturated fat and cholesterol intake and adding dietary options to enhance LDL lowering, such as adding plant stanols and sterols and increasing intake of viscous or soluble fiber. Most adults achieve only a 5% to 10% reduction in LDL cholesterol with dietary advice as a single intervention. Weight management and a program of regular aerobic exercise should be prescribed for overall health. Dietary lipid improvement is often enhanced if coupled with exercise; because physical activity reduces IR, the anticipated improvement in the lipid profile includes an increase in HDL and reduction of TGs.

Pharmacological intervention in dyslipidemia is likely to be needed in patients with considerable cardiovascular and cerebrovascular risk, including patients with DM, hypertension, and existing vascular disease. The choice of a lipid-lowering agent should be guided by the effect of the agent on the lipid profile.

Recommendations from the ACC and AHA advise statin treatment for four major groups for the prevention of ASCVD risk reduction (Fig. 12-6). These groups include those (1) with LDL-C 190 mg/dL (4.9 mmol/L) or higher; (2) with diabetes who are aged 40 to 75 years; (3) older than 75 years; or (4) aged 40 to 75 years who have LDL-C between 70 and 189 mg/dL. For individuals in the last group, the CVD Risk Estimator Calculator is used to determine the calculated 10-year risk of ASCVD that will help to determine the course of therapy. Prior to initiating statin therapy, baseline hepatic enzyme levels should be measured due to a low risk of severe liver injury. Routine monitoring of liver enzymes is not needed as serious liver injury is usually idiosyncratic and not preventable with routine monitoring.

Specific statin regimens are recommended for high- and moderate-intensity therapy; currently, there is no clinical indication for low-intensity statin therapy.

High-intensity statin therapy will lower LDL-C by 50% or more (e.g., atorvastatin 40 to 80 mg, rosuvastatin 20 to 40 mg), whereas moderate-intensity statin therapy will lower LDL-C by 30% to less than 50% (e.g., simvastatin 20 to 40 mg; atorvastatin 10 to 20 mg; pravastatin 40 to 80 mg; or rosuvastatin 5 to 10 mg). Low-intensity therapy will lower LDL-C by less than 30% and is generally not recommended unless higher statin doses are not tolerated. The ACC/AHA guidelines recommend the following statin intensity for each risk group for primary prevention:

> **CLINICAL CONCEPT**
>
> As a drug class, statin clinical effect is primarily in LDL-C reduction.

- Pretreatment LDL-C of 190 mg/dL or more: high-intensity statin (or moderate-intensity statin if not a candidate for high-intensity statin)
- Diabetes (type 1 or 2) and age 40 to 75 years: moderate-intensity statin
- Age 40 to 75 years, also considering therapy age older than 75 years, and pretreatment LDL-C 70 to 189 mg/dL (1.8 to 4.9 mmol/L): statin treatment based on calculated 10-year ASCVD risk along with risk discussion.
  - With less than 5% risk (low risk), emphasize lifestyle modifications to reduce risk.
  - With 5% to less than 7.5% risk (borderline risk), identify risk enhancers and have a discussion about initiating moderate-intensity statin therapy.
  - With 7.5% to less than 20% risk, initiate moderate-intensity statin therapy.
  - With 20% or higher risk, initiate high-intensity statin therapy.

Once statin treatment is initiated, a repeat lipid profile should be performed in 4 to 12 weeks to determine if dose adjustment is needed, and then repeated every 12 months as needed, more frequently if needed in the presence of increased or new ASCVD risk factors.

ACC/AHA guidelines note that the benefit of statin therapy in the prevention of cardiovascular events is less clear in other patient groups. Causes of secondary dyslipidemia should be considered and eliminated or minimized, usually through lifestyle intervention or treatment of the underlying cause, medication adjustment, or a combination of these efforts.

Combination therapy with statins is an option when optimized dosing does not attain the LDL-C target or the patient cannot tolerate statins at higher doses, such as those needed for high-intensity therapy. Ezetimibe (Zetia®) is a selective cholesterol absorption inhibitor that can result in an additional LDL-C reduction of 15% to 20% when added to statin therapy. The agent has limited systemic absorption and, thus, is associated with few adverse effects. The PCSK9 inhibitors (evolocumab [Repatha®],

> **CLINICAL CONCEPT**
>
> A diet high in saturated fat, obesity, as well as high-dose, but not lower-dose, thiazide diuretics are common contributors to LDL elevation.

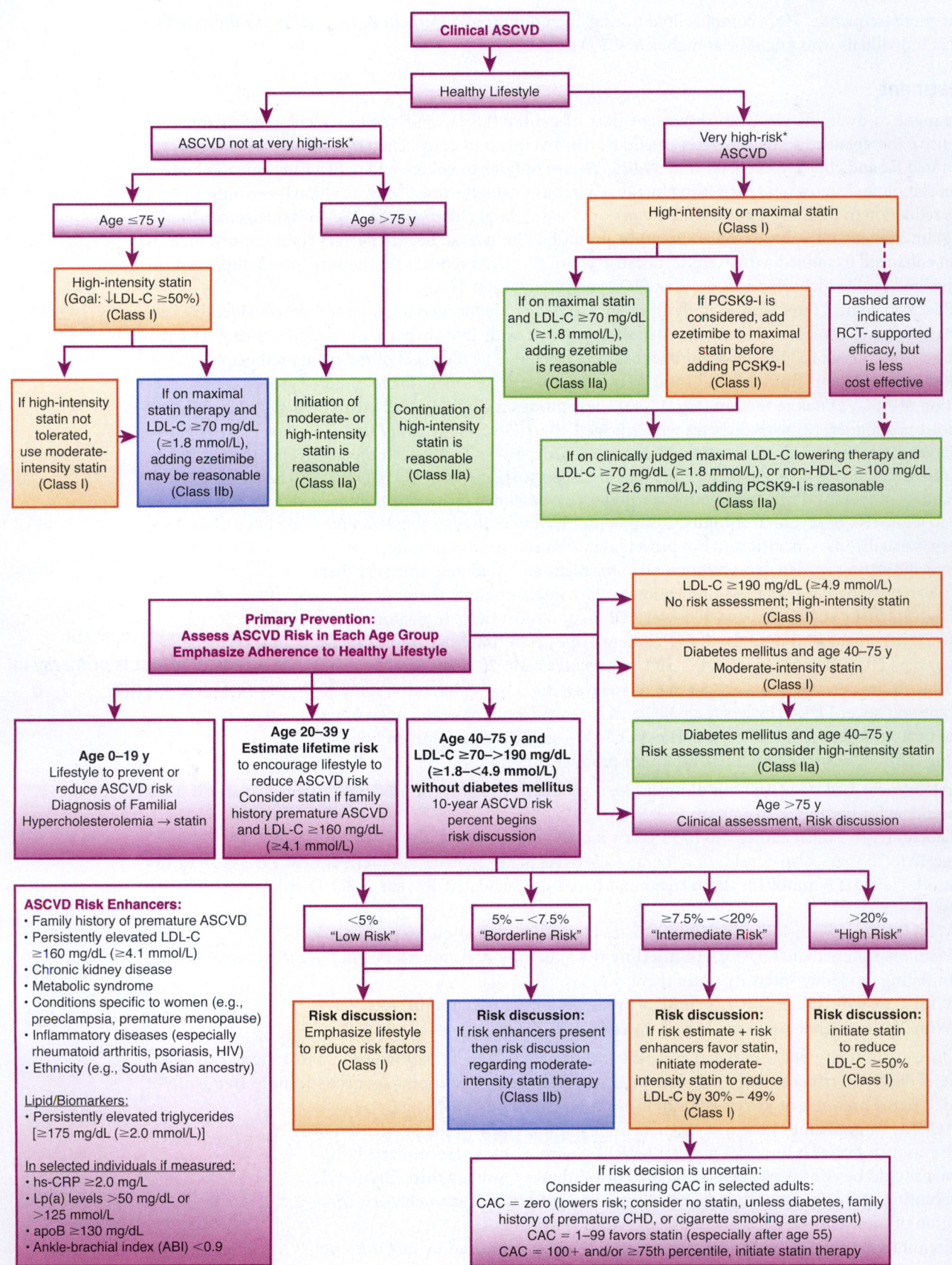

FIGURE 12-6 ACC/AHA 2018 Guideline on the Management of Blood Cholesterol.

Grundy SM, Stone NJ, Bailey AL, et al. 2018 AHA/ACC/AACVPR/AAPA/ABC/ACPM/ADA/AGS/APhA/ASPC/NLA/PCNA Guideline on the management of blood cholesterol. J Am Coll Cardiol. 2018;73:e285–350. http://www.onlinejacc.org/content/73/24/e285?_ga=2.80809173.374917006.1569775649 -2145646910.1569775649

alirocumab [Praluent®]) are a class of agents that consist of a human monoclonal antibody to proprotein convertase subtilisin/kexin type 9. These agents are available as injections only, given biweekly or monthly, and can result in an additional 60% in LDL-C reduction in individuals who are already on optimized statin therapy. These agents are most useful for individuals with a history of CVD and who cannot meet the LDL-C target with optimized statin therapy, though cost could be a limiting factor. Adverse effects include injection site reaction as well as cold and flu-like symptoms. Other treatments historically used to lower LDL-C, including bile acid sequestrants, fibrate, and niacin, are no longer routinely recommended due to a lack of clinical evidence demonstrating improved cardiovascular outcomes with these agents.

In addition to LDL-C, elevated TGs (hypertriglyceridemia) should also be actively treated for the reduction of cardiovascular events. Guidelines from the American Association of Clinical Endocrinologists (AACE)/American College of Endocrinology (ACE) define mild hypertriglyceridemia as a level between 150 and 199 mg/dL (1.7 to 2.3 mmol/L), moderate hypertriglyceridemia as a level between 200 and 999 mg/dL (2.3 to 11.3 mmol/L), severe hypertriglyceridemia as a level between 1,000 and 1,999 mg/dL (11.3 to 22.6 mmol/L), and very severe as above 2,000 mg/dL (22.6 mmol/L). Treatment options include the use of fibrates and prescription-strength omega-3 oil. Fenofibrate can be considered with low- to moderate-intensity statin therapy when TGs are greater than 500 mg/dL or when the benefits of ASCVD reduction are judged to outweigh the potential risks of adverse effects. Prescription-strength omega-3 fatty acids should be considered for treatment in hypertriglyceridemia in the presence of risks for statin-fibrate adverse effects, particularly in renal impairment and advancing age. The use of prescription-strength omega-3 fatty acids is associated with a modest antiplatelet effect; they should be used with caution when taken concomitantly with other antiplatelet medications, such as aspirin or clopidogrel. Dietary supplements of omega-3 oil are not recommended for the treatment of hypertriglyceridemia, given the variability of product quality and dose. As mentioned, evaluation of and intervention in causes for secondary hypertriglyceridemia should be pursued.

Discussion Sources

American Heart Association. Fish oil and omega-3 fatty acids. http://www.heart.org/HEARTORG/HealthyLiving/HealthyEating/HealthyDietGoals/Fish-and-Omega-3-Fatty-Acids_UCM_303248_Article.jsp#.V2lwlrgrJPY

Grundy SM, Stone NJ, Bailey AL, et al. 2018 AHA/ACC/AACVPR/AAPA/ABC/ACPM/ADA/AGS/APhA/ASPC/NLA/PCNA Guideline on the management of blood cholesterol. *J Am Coll Cardiol.* 2018;73:e285–350. http://www.onlinejacc.org/content/73/24/e285?_ga=2.80809173.374917006.1569775649-2145646910.1569775649

Jellinger PS, Handelsman Y, Rosenblitt PD, et al. American Association of Clinical Endocrinologists and American College of Endocrinology guidelines for management of dyslipidemia and prevention of cardiovascular disease. *Endocrine Practice.* 2017;23(Suppl 2):1–87. https://journals.aace.com/doi/pdf/10.4158/EP171764.APPGL

QUESTIONS

117. A 72-year-old woman has hypertension, a 100 pack-year history of cigarette smoking, and reduced renal function (GFR = 47 mL/min/1.73 m²). The TG level is 280 mg/dL (3.164 mmol/L); HDL level is 48 mg/dL (1 mmol/L); and LDL level is 135 mg/dL (3.5 mmol/L). Her calculated 10-year ASCVD risk is 15%. Which of the following represents the most appropriate pharmacological intervention for this patient's lipid disorders?

    A. Owing to her age and comorbidity, no further intervention is required.

    B. Moderate-intensity statin therapy is the preferred treatment option.

    C. Niacin should be prescribed.

    D. The use of ezetimibe (Zetia®) will likely be sufficient to achieve dyslipidemia control.

118. You examine a 46-year-old male who is a one-half pack per day cigarette smoker with hypertension. He has no evidence of clinical ASCVD, and his estimated 10-year ASCVD risk is 10%. His lipid profile is as follows: HDL level is 48 mg/dL (1.24 mmol/L); LDL level is 192 mg/dL (4.9 mmol/L); and TG level is 110 mg/dL (1.3 mmol/L). He had been on a low-cholesterol diet for 6 months when these tests were taken. Which of the following represents the best next step?

    A. No further intervention is required.

    B. A fibrate should be prescribed.

    C. A low-intensity 3-hydroxy-3-methylglutaryl–coenzyme A (HMG-CoA) reductase inhibitor should be prescribed.

    D. A high-intensity HMG-CoA reductase inhibitor (statin) regimen should be initiated.

119. You examine a 64-year-old man with hypertension and T2DM. Lipid profile results are as follows: HDL level is 38 mg/dL (1 mmol/), LDL level is 135 mg/dL (3.5 mmol/L), and TG level is 180 mg/dL (1.9 mmol/L). His estimated 10-year ASCVD risk is 5%. His current medications include a sulfonylurea, a biguanide (metformin), an ACEI, and a thiazide diuretic, and he has acceptable glycemic and blood pressure control. He states, "I really watch the fats and sugars in my diet." Which of the following is the most appropriate advice?

    A. No further intervention is needed.

    B. His lipid profile should be repeated in 6 months.

    C. Lipid-lowering drug therapy with a moderate-intensity statin should be initiated.

    D. The patient's dietary intervention appears adequate.

120. When providing care for a patient taking an HMG-CoA reductase inhibitor (statin), initial evaluation when starting medication includes checking which of the following serological parameters?

    A. potassium

    B. alanine aminotransferase

    C. bilirubin

    D. ALP

121. When prescribing a fibrate, the NP expects to see which of the following changes in lipid profile?

    A. marked increase in LDL level

    B. decrease in HDL level

    C. decrease in TG level

    D. increase in VLDL level

122. When prescribing a PCSK9 inhibitor in combination with statin therapy, the NP expects to see which of the following changes in lipid profile?

    A. marked decrease in LDL level

    B. marked decrease in HDL level

    C. increase in TG level

    D. minimal change to lipid profile

123. The latest guidelines for the management of dyslipidemia do not recommend the use of bile acid sequestrants or niacin for LDL reduction due to:

    A. a high incidence of serious adverse effects.

    B. high cost.

    C. a lack of evidence demonstrating improvement in cardiovascular outcomes with these agents.

    D. no effect in reducing LDL level.

124. With the use of ezetimibe (Zetia®), the NP expects to see:

    A. a marked increase in HDL cholesterol.

    B. a reduction in LDL cholesterol.

    C. a significant reduction in TG levels.

    D. increased rhabdomyolysis when the drug is used in conjunction with HMG-CoA reductase inhibitor.

125. With ezetimibe (Zetia®), which of the following should be periodically monitored?

    A. ALP

    B. lactate dehydrogenase (LDH)

    C. creatinine phosphokinase (CPK)

    D. No special laboratory monitoring is recommended.

126. You see a 63-year-old man with peripheral artery disease and a 42 pack-year smoking history. He is currently taking high-intensity statin therapy plus ezetimibe but has not attained LDL goal. The next best course of action is to:

A. add niacin.

B. switch to a different statin.

C. add a PCSK9 inhibitor.

D. substitute ezetimibe for fibrate.

127. All of the following are risk factors for statin-induced myositis except:

A. advanced age.

B. concomitant use of ezetimibe.

C. low body weight.

D. high-intensity statin therapy.

128. What is the average LDL reduction achieved with a change in diet as a single lifestyle modification?

A. less than 5%

B. 5% to 10%

C. 11% to 15%

D. 16% to 20% or more

129. Which of the following adverse effects is associated with the use of prescription-strength omega-3 fatty acid?

A. antiplatelet effect

B. drug-induced cough

C. immune suppression

D. hyperglycemia

130. Which of the following medications is representative of high-intensity statin therapy?

A. pravastatin 40 mg

B. rosuvastatin 20 mg

C. simvastatin 40 mg

D. lovastatin 20 mg

131. Which of the following daily doses has the lowest lipid-lowering effect?

A. simvastatin 10 mg

B. rosuvastatin 5 mg

C. atorvastatin 10 mg

D. pravastatin 40 mg

132. Untreated hypothyroidism can result in which of the following changes in the lipid profile?

A. increased HDL and decreased TGs

B. increased LDL and TC

C. increased LDL, TC, and TGs

D. decreased LDL and HDL

133. A program of regular aerobic physical activity can yield which of the following changes in the lipid profile?

A. increases HDL, lowers VLDL and TGs

B. lowers VLDL and LDL

C. increases HDL, lowers LDL

D. lowers HDL, VLDL, and TGs

134. The anticipated effect on the lipid profile with high-dose omega-3 fatty acid use includes:

A. increase in HDL.

B. decrease in LDL.

C. decrease in TC.

D. decrease in TGs.

135. The anticipated effect on the lipid profile with plant stanol and sterol use includes:

A. increase in HDL.

B. decrease in LDL.

C. decrease in select lipoprotein subfractions.

D. decrease in TGs.

136. For patients with documented coronary heart disease, the AHA advises intake of approximately _____ of eicosapentaenoic acid (EPA) and docosahexaenoic acid (DHA) per day, preferably from oily fish.

A. 500 mg

B. 1 g

C. 2 g

D. 4 g

137. Which of the following is an example of moderate-intensity statin therapy?

A. fluvastatin 20 mg

B. atorvastatin 10 mg

C. simvastatin 10 mg

D. pravastatin 20 mg

For answers and rationales, see end of chapter.

Select Adrenal Disorders

Overview

The adrenal glands, located on top of each kidney, are responsible for producing a variety of hormones. Glucocorticoid hormones, such as cortisol, play a role in maintaining glucose control, suppressing the immune response, and helping the body respond to stress. Mineralocorticoid hormones, such as aldosterone, regulate sodium and potassium balance. Sex hormones in males (androgens) and females (estrogens) are involved in sexual development and sex drive. While adrenal disorders are not commonly encountered, recognizing these potentially life-threatening and certainly life-altering conditions is critical to safe practice.

ADDISON'S DISEASE

Overview

Addison's disease is a disorder that occurs when there is an inadequate amount of hormones produced by the adrenal glands. The condition occurs in all age groups and has a similar prevalence in male and female genders. Patients with Addison's disease (also called adrenal insufficiency or hypocortisolism) do not produce enough cortisol and, in some cases, aldosterone.

In primary adrenal insufficiency, the adrenal gland is damaged and hinders production of hormones, resulting from an autoimmune response that attacks the glands, infections (such as tuberculosis, HIV, or fungal infections), hemorrhage or blood loss, tumors, or the use of anticoagulants. A key risk factor for the autoimmune type of Addison's disease is the presence of other autoimmune conditions. These include chronic thyroiditis, dermatitis herpetiformis, Graves' disease, hypoparathyroidism, hypopituitarism, myasthenia gravis, T1DM, and vitiligo. Genetic alterations are likely responsible for causing this condition.

Secondary adrenal insufficiency can occur if the pituitary gland is diseased. The pituitary gland produces adrenocorticotropic hormone (ACTH), which stimulates the adrenal cortex to produce its hormones. Inadequate production of ACTH can lead to insufficient production of hormones from the adrenal gland. Secondary adrenal insufficiency can also occur in those who have been taking systemic corticosteroids for a chronic condition (such as asthma or arthritis) for a protracted time period (usually longer than 2 weeks and typically at higher dose) and then abruptly stop taking the corticosteroids.

Clinical Presentation

Symptoms of Addison's disease can be wide and varied and usually develop slowly, often over several months to perhaps years. GI impacts can include chronic diarrhea, nausea and vomiting, or loss of appetite resulting in weight loss. Dermatological changes include paleness or darkening of the skin in some places that causes the skin to have a patchy appearance. Other signs include muscle weakness, fatigue, slow or sluggish movement, hypoglycemia, low blood pressure, fainting, and salt craving.

During an addisonian crisis, or acute adrenal failure, the signs and symptoms appear suddenly. These can include pain in the lower back, abdomen, or legs; severe vomiting and diarrhea leading to dehydration; low blood pressure; loss of consciousness; and hyperkalemia.

Diagnostic Testing

Laboratory evaluation for Addison's disease includes checking blood levels of potassium, sodium, cortisol, and ACTH. An ACTH stimulation test can be used to confirm the diagnosis. This test involves injecting synthetic ACTH and comparing the level of cortisol before and after injection. Damage to the adrenal gland will show limited or no response to synthetic ACTH. An abdominal computed tomography (CT) scan can be used to evaluate the size of the adrenal glands and identify any abnormalities. Additionally, an MRI scan of the pituitary gland can be used to identify secondary adrenal insufficiency.

When considering differential diagnosis, other conditions that present similarly to Addison's disease can include adrenal hemorrhage, eosinophilia, hyperkalemia, and sarcoidosis.

Treatment

Symptoms of the disease are usually controlled with corticosteroid replacement therapy, which can include a combination of glucocorticoids (cortisone, prednisone, or hydrocortisone) and mineralocorticoids (fludrocortisone). Oral treatments are preferred, though injections may be needed if the patient is vomiting and cannot retain oral medications. An ample amount of sodium is also recommended, especially during heavy exercise, in hot climates, and during GI upset, such as diarrhea. During an addisonian crisis, immediate use of parenteral hydrocortisone is needed along with supportive treatment for low blood pressure and a firm plan for seeking health care promptly. With proper hormone replacement therapy, most people with Addison's disease can lead normal lives. Expert consultation is required to provide appropriate care for the person with Addison's disease.

CUSHING'S SYNDROME AND CUSHING'S DISEASE

Overview

Cortisol plays various roles in the body, including regulation of blood pressure, helping the body cope with stress, and regulating the metabolism of proteins, carbohydrates, and fats. Cushing's syndrome occurs when the body is exposed to elevated levels of cortisol for an extended period of time.

An exogenous cause of Cushing's syndrome is the long-term use of high doses of systemic corticosteroids, such as prednisone, for the treatment of inflammatory conditions (e.g., rheumatoid arthritis, systemic lupus, and asthma). Corticosteroid exposure can result from the use of oral or parenteral medications, and, less commonly, inhalers, nasal sprays, and skin creams, or from joint injections.

These drugs have the same effect as cortisol and are often prescribed at doses that attain supraphysiological levels in the body.

> **CLINICAL CONCEPT**
>
> The most common reason for Cushing's syndrome is protracted (greater than 2 weeks) use of higher-dose systemic corticosteroids.

Endogenous causes of Cushing's syndrome can also occur. Overproduction of cortisol can occur from one or both adrenal glands or can result from overproduction of ACTH, which is produced by the pituitary gland and regulates cortisol production. Overproduction of ACTH can occur because of a pituitary gland tumor (pituitary adenoma) or an ectopic ACTH-secreting tumor (such as in the lung). Cushing's disease is a specific form of Cushing's syndrome caused by a benign tumor on the pituitary gland that overproduces ACTH. Overproduction of cortisol can also occur from a benign tumor of the adrenal cortex (adrenal adenoma) or, more rarely, an adrenocortical carcinoma.

Clinical Presentation

The hallmark signs of Cushing's syndrome include progressive weight gain and altered fatty tissue deposits, particularly around the midsection and upper back, in the face (moon face), and between the shoulders (buffalo hump). Other signs include pink or purple stretch marks (striae) on the abdomen, thighs, breasts, and arms; thinning, fragile skin that bruises easily; slow healing of cuts, insect bites, and infections; and acne. Those with Cushing's syndrome often experience fatigue; muscle weakness or myopathy; depression, anxiety, and irritability; new or worsened high blood pressure; glucose intolerance that can lead to diabetes; headache; and bone loss. Women with this condition report thicker and more visible body and facial hair (hirsutism), as well as irregular or absent menstrual periods.

Diagnosis

Diagnosis of Cushing's syndrome can be difficult, particularly when endogenous in origin. For patients with long-term use of high-dose corticosteroids, Cushing's syndrome is usually suspected as a result of this exposure. For patients without a history of long-term corticosteroid use, urine, blood, and saliva tests can evaluate cortisol levels. MRI or CT scans can be used to detect abnormalities of the pituitary or adrenal glands. These tests can also help rule out other medical conditions with similar signs and symptoms, such as PCOS, depression, eating disorders, and alcoholism. Expert consultation is advised.

Treatment

Without intervention, Cushing's syndrome is associated with increased rates of cardiovascular events (heart failure or myocardial infarction) and infection. In addition, this condition can lead to osteoporosis, hypertension, T2DM, frequent and unusual infections, and loss of muscle mass. Treatment is designed to reduce the level of cortisol in the body. For patients taking long-term treatment of systemic corticosteroids, tapering the dose as soon as possible is recommended. Abrupt discontinuation of long-term systemic corticosteroid therapy can lead to adrenal crisis; therefore, reducing its use to a low or maintenance dose is the safest initial intervention.

For endogenous Cushing's syndrome, surgical resection is the primary treatment of choice to remove a tumor of the adrenal gland overproducing cortisol, or to remove a tumor of the pituitary gland or other sites that are overproducing ACTH. For those with Cushing's disease, first-line treatment is transsphenoidal surgery, which results in an approximately 80% cure rate. Often surgery is curative, though radiation therapy may be needed in conjunction. Radiation therapy is also an option for those who are not suitable candidates for surgery. Cortisol replacement therapy is often used following surgery to provide a normal physiological level of cortisol. In most cases, this treatment can be tapered over time as the body returns to normal adrenal hormone production.

Certain medications can be used to control cortisol production. These include mitotane (Lysodren®) and metyrapone (Metopirone®). Mifepristone (Korlym®) has been approved for use in patients with endogenous Cushing's syndrome and T2DM or glucose intolerance and have failed surgery or cannot have surgery. This agent does not impact the production of cortisol but blocks the effects of cortisol on tissues.

Discussion Sources

Barthel A, Benker G, Berens K, et al. An update on Addison's disease. *Exp Clin Endocrinol Diabetes.* 2019;127:165–175. https://www.thieme-connect.com/products/ejournals/html/10.1055/a-0804-2715

Castinetti F, Morange I, Conte-Devolx B, Brue T. Cushing's disease. *Orphanet J Rare Dis.* 2012;7:41. https://www.ncbi.nlm.nih.gov /pmc/articles/PMC3458990/pdf/1750-1172-7-41.pdf

Griffing GT. Addison disease. Medscape. https://emedicine.medscape.com/article/116467-overview

Nieman LK. Diagnosis of Cushing's syndrome in the modern era. *Endocrinol Metab Clin North Am.* 2018;47:259–273.

QUESTIONS

138. A 34-year-old woman presents with a chief complaint of a many month history of progressive weakness, fatigue, poor appetite, and unintended weight loss. She has also noticed the development of hyperpigmentation, mainly on the knuckles, elbows, and knees. All of the following blood tests can be used to help confirm a diagnosis of Addison's disease except:

    A. sodium.

    B. potassium.

    C. cortisol.

    D. folate.

139. The hormone cortisol plays a role in all of the following processes except:

    A. maintaining glucose control.

    B. maintaining thyroid function.

    C. suppressing the immune response.

    D. helping the body respond to stress.

140. Which of the following is a mineralocorticoid?

    A. cortisol

    B. aldosterone

    C. insulin

    D. hydrocortisone

141. Secondary adrenal insufficiency can occur with the presence of a diseased or malfunctioning:

    A. pituitary gland.

    B. thyroid.

    C. pancreatic beta cells.

    D. hypothalamus.

142. A 43-year-old man is experiencing an acute adrenal/addisonian crisis and presents with prominent nausea, vomiting, and low blood pressure. He appears cyanotic and confused. The most appropriate treatment is an injection of:

    A. epinephrine.

    B. insulin.

    C. adrenaline.

    D. hydrocortisone.

143. A 24-year-old woman who is a long-distance runner is diagnosed with Addison's disease. In counseling her about exercise, you recommend:

    A. tapering her running to only 10 minutes per day for 2 to 3 days per week.

    B. ceasing any prolonged strenuous exercise.

    C. ensuring an ample amount of sodium is ingested.

    D. an injection of hydrocortisone prior to exercise.

144. A 46-year-old woman complains of fatigue, weakness, lethargy, decreased concentration and memory, and increased facial hair over the past 12 months. She also reports gaining over 30 pounds (13.6 kg) in the past 2 months. She has a history of asthma with repeated flares during the past 6 months requiring multiple courses of prednisone therapy. A likely diagnosis for this patient is:

    A. T2DM.

    B. Cushing's syndrome.

> **C.** Cushing's disease.
>
> **D.** central obesity.

145. Cushing's syndrome results from an excess of:

> **A.** luteinizing hormone.
>
> **B.** follicle-stimulating hormone.
>
> **C.** cortisol.
>
> **D.** aldosterone.

146. A first-line approach to treating Cushing's syndrome in a 56-year-old woman who has been taking oral corticosteroids to treat rheumatoid arthritis for the past 2 years is:

> **A.** gradually tapering corticosteroid use.
>
> **B.** referral for surgery.
>
> **C.** consideration of radiation therapy.
>
> **D.** prescribing mifepristone.

147. Untreated Cushing's syndrome can lead to all of the following except:

> **A.** rheumatoid arthritis.
>
> **B.** hypertension.
>
> **C.** T2DM.
>
> **D.** osteoporosis.

148. Cushing's disease is the specific type of Cushing's syndrome that is caused by:

> **A.** long-term exposure to corticosteroids.
>
> **B.** a benign tumor of the adrenal gland.
>
> **C.** a benign pituitary tumor.
>
> **D.** an ectopic tumor that produces ACTH.

149. The most commonly recommended treatment for Cushing's disease is:

> **A.** tapering or ceasing systemic corticosteroid use.
>
> **B.** eliminating trigger medications.
>
> **C.** antineoplastic therapy.
>
> **D.** surgical intervention.

For answers and rationales, see end of chapter.

Abnormal Uterine Bleeding

Overview

Abnormal uterine bleeding (AUB, formerly known as dysfunctional uterine bleeding [DUB]) is generally defined as irregular uterine bleeding in the absence of an obvious medical condition or pregnancy. AUB can be acute or chronic and characterized by abnormal bleeding irregularity, volume, frequency, or duration. The cause of AUB can be varied, and the PALM-COEIN system was developed to use standardized terminology to help determine the most likely etiology and guide effective management (Table 12-10). Up to a third of women with heavy menstrual bleeding will have some form of von Willebrand disease or an underlying coagulation disorder.

Clinical Presentation

A woman who is not pregnant with AUB will typically present with unpredictable or episodic heavy or light bleeding despite a normal pelvic examination. In more severe cases, the patient can present with signs of hemodynamic instability and/or

> **CLINICAL CONCEPT**
>
> Causes of AUB are divided into structural (PALM) and nonstructural (COEIN) etiologies.

TABLE 12-10 PALM-COEIN Classification System for Abnormal Uterine Bleeding

Abnormal Uterine Bleeding (AUB) Characterized by Heavy Menstrual Bleeding or Intermenstrual Bleeding

PALM (STRUCTURAL CAUSES)	COEIN (NONSTRUCTURAL CAUSES)
■ Polyp (AUB-P)	■ Coagulopathy (AUB-C)
■ Adenomyosis (AUB-A)	■ Ovulatory dysfunction (AUB-O)
■ Leiomyoma (AUB-L)	■ Endometrial (AUB-E)
• Submucosal leiomyoma (AUB-LSM)	■ Iatrogenic (AUB-I)
• Other leiomyoma (AUB-LO)	■ Not yet classified (AUB-N)
■ Malignancy and hyperplasia (AUB-M)	

Source: Munro MG, Critchley HO, Broder MS, Fraser IS. FIGO classification system (PALM-COEIN) for causes of abnormal uterine bleeding in nongravid women of reproductive age. FIGO working group on menstrual disorders. Int J Gynaecol Obstet. 2011;113:3–13. https://www.figo.org/sites/default/files/uploads/IJGO/papers/AUB%20Classification.pdf

hypovolemia, requiring immediate intervention to stabilize the patient with a blood transfusion and clotting factor replacement.

Diagnostic Testing

AUB is primarily a diagnosis of exclusion, and so patient history, physical examination, and laboratory testing are needed to rule out other causes of anovulatory bleeding. A thorough patient history should be performed with a focus on the PALM-COEIN system to guide evaluation of the current bleeding episode. Laboratory studies should include the following:

- *CBC*: To evaluate for anemia and platelet count
- *Pap test*: If due, largely to be up to date on health maintenance, rarely revealing information that contributes to the AUB underlying cause.
- *Pregnancy test*: To rule in or rule out pregnancy
- *Endometrial sampling via endometrial biopsy*: To evaluate for endometrial hyperplasia or endometrial cancer
- *Thyroid function*: Assessment for hypothyroidism, an occasional cause of menorrhagia
- *Prolactin*: To evaluate pituitary function
- *Liver function tests*: To detect hepatic dysfunction that can impact estrogen metabolism or the availability of coagulation components
- *Coagulation studies*: Including von Willebrand factor antigen test and prothrombin/international normalized ratio to evaluate for contribution of a clotting disorder
- *Pelvic ultrasound*: To detect for pelvic abnormalities

Based on findings, additional evaluation can be considered to detect for PCOS or possible ovarian or adrenal tumors.

Treatment

Interventions for AUB are aimed to control bleeding in the current episode and to reduce menstrual flow in subsequent cycles. Hormonal therapy is the first-line approach in women without known or suspected coagulation disorders. Choice of initial therapy is usually dictated by severity of current vaginal bleeding. The primary treatment for significant acute bleeding is estrogen, given parenterally or orally. For long-term AUB management, progestin-containing options are the mainstay. In women up to age 39 years, COCs or a levonorgestrel intrauterine device (IUD) are options; these are particularly helpful options when contraception is also desired. In pre- and perimenopausal women 40 years and older, cyclic progestin therapy, low-dose COC, levonorgestrel IUD, or cyclic hormone therapy can be considered. In addition, particularly when the primary problem is regular but heavy menses and hormonal therapy is to be avoided or is not desired by the patient, taking an NSAID by-the-clock, such as naproxen bid, for 2 days prior to and for the first 2 days of menses can be helpful. The resulting reduction in menstrual flow with NSAID use is usually in excess of 25%. Antifibrinolytic drugs, such as tranexamic acid, can be helpful in reducing bleeding in women with acute or chronic AUB.

The use of hormone therapy and antifibrinolytic drugs can also be considered in women with a known or suspected bleeding disorder. For women with AUB who have von Willebrand disease, desmopressin can help control acute bleeding. Recombinant factor VIII, von Willebrand factor, or other factor-specific replacement can also help to control severe hemorrhage. Expert consultation with hematology should be obtained, especially when bleeding is difficult to control. NSAIDs should be avoided in these patients with bleeding disorder due to their antiplatelet effect and their impact on liver function needed for the production of coagulation components.

Surgical measures should be reserved for patients who do not adequately respond to medical therapy, when pharmacological therapy is contraindicated, or when the severity of bleeding requires surgery. Surgical treatment can include dilation and curettage (D&C) with hysteroscopy, endometrial ablation, uterine artery embolization, and hysterectomy. The choice of technique will depend on clinical findings, patient preference, and desire for fertility. D&C with hysteroscopy can be effective in the treatment of endometrial polyps. Hysterectomy might be needed for women who failed medical management and when bleeding causes anemia and diminished quality of life. Endometrial ablation provides an option for women who do not wish to undergo hysterectomy. Hysterectomy and endometrial ablation should only be considered for women who do not have plans for future childbearing.

Discussion Sources

ACOG. Committee Opinion No. 557. Management of acute abnormal uterine bleeding in nonpregnant reproductive-aged women. April 2013 (Reaffirmed 2019). https://www.acog.org/clinical/clinical-guidance/committee-opinion/articles/2013/04/management-of-acute-abnormal-uterine-bleeding-in-nonpregnant-reproductive-aged-women

Behara MA. Abnormal (dysfunctional) uterine bleeding. Medscape. https://emedicine.medscape.com/article/257007-overview

QUESTIONS

150. Based on the PALM-COEIN classification system, which of the following is not included as a structural cause of AUB?

    A. malignancy

    B. adenomyosis

    C. PCOS

    D. leiomyoma

151. Based on the PALM-COEIN classification system, which of the following is not included as a nonstructural cause of AUB?

    A. ovulatory dysfunction

    B. neoplasia

    C. coagulopathy

    D. endometrial

152. Laboratory testing for a 34-year-old woman with acute AUB should include all of the following except:

    A. hepatic function test.

    B. Pap test.

    C. creatine kinase.

    D. hemoglobin and hematocrit.

153. Which of the following would not be considered for initial treatment of AUB in a 28-year-old woman without a coagulation disorder?

    A. low-dose COC

    B. levonorgestrel IUD

    C. oral progestin

    D. copper-containing IUD

For answers and rationales, see end of chapter.

QUESTION ANSWERS AND RATIONALES

Diabetes Mellitus

1. **Correct: A. Significant hyperglycemia and ketoacidosis result from lack of insulin.**
T1DM results from destruction of the pancreatic beta cells that reduces or eliminates the production of insulin. The resulting state causes significant hyperglycemia and ketoacidosis (A) that can lead to an urgent medical condition, including severe dehydration, abdominal pain, vomiting, and decreased level of consciousness.
Incorrect:
Individuals with T1DM often present with dramatic symptoms due to insulin deficiency including vomiting, severe dehydration, and abdominal pain (B). Because the condition is caused by a lack of insulin production, lifelong insulin treatment is needed rather than an insulin secretagogue or sensitizer such as a sulfonylurea (C). Unlike T2DM, IR is not a part of the mechanism of disease, but rather T1DM is caused by insulin deficiency (D).

2. **Correct: A. Major risk factors are heredity and obesity.**
IR is a major part of the disease mechanism for T2DM. and heredity and obesity are key risk factors (A).
Incorrect:
Though obesity is a major risk factor for T2DM, not all body fat types are equally problematic. "Apple-shaped" rather than "pear-shaped" individuals are associated with a greater risk of IR (B). Though exogenous insulin can be used to manage hyperglycemia, typically other treatments are used prior to insulin, including various oral medications (C). IR can be decreased with increased physical activity as well as weight loss and the use of insulin-sensitizing medications (D).

3. **Correct: A. extended duration of action.**
Insulin glargine is a long-acting insulin that has a duration of action of at least 24 hours and does not have a substantial peak concentration when used (A).
Incorrect:
Insulin glargine has a relatively slow onset of action of approximately 1 hour after injection, compared to approximately 15 to 30 minutes of onset for other rapid-acting insulins (B). All insulins work in the same manner (though with varying pharmacokinetics) to control hyperglycemia and prevent potential end-organ damage in advanced disease (C). The use of insulin glargine does not have any unique ability among insulins to preserve pancreatic function (D).

4. **Correct: A. less than 30 minutes.**
Lispro is a short-acting insulin with a rapid onset of action. The effects are typically observed within 15 to 30 minutes of injection (A) and should be administered within 15 minutes of meals or immediately following a meal. Its duration of action is approximately 3 to 6.5 hours.
Incorrect:
Insulin that is short-acting but non-rapid onset of action (e.g., Regular insulin) can have an onset of action between 30 minutes and 1 hour (B). Intermediate-acting and long-acting insulin have an onset of action typically between 1 and 2 hours (C). Insulin formulations will have some clinical effect before 3 to 4 hours (D).

5. **Correct: C. a drug that increases insulin action in the peripheral tissues and reduces hepatic glucose production.**
Metformin works by a variety of mechanisms. It reduces hepatic glucose production as well as intestinal glucose absorption. It also acts as an insulin sensitizer by way of increased peripheral glucose uptake and utilization (C).
Incorrect:
GLP-1 agonists and DPP-4 inhibitors work by enhancing insulin production (A). A sulfonylurea works as an insulin secretagogue, which increases the release of insulin from beta cells (B). Facilitation of renal glucose excretion is the mechanism of action of SGLT2 inhibitors (D).

6. **Correct: B. 3 years.**
Testing for DM should be considered for all adults who are overweight and have additional risk factors for disease. For those who are asymptomatic and without risk factors, testing should begin at age 45 years and be repeated at least in 3-year intervals, with adjustment to more frequent testing depending on test results and change in risk status (B).

7. **Correct: C. family history of T1DM.**
A family history of T1DM is not a risk factor for T2DM. T1DM is caused by an autoimmune condition that results in the destruction of pancreatic beta cells. This is a different mechanism of disease compared to T2DM, which is predominantly caused by IR.
Incorrect:
There are several risk factors for T2DM including certain ethnicities (B), obesity (A), and family history of T2DM. Women with PCOS are also at high risk of T2DM (D).

8. **Correct: D. a plasma glucose level of 126 mg/dL (7 mmol/L) or greater after an 8-hour or greater fast on more than one occasion.**
Several criteria can be used to make a diagnosis of T2DM. These include a fasting plasma glucose greater than or equal to 126 mg/dL (7 mmol/L) (D), or a random plasma glucose greater than or equal to 200 mg/dL (11.1 mmol/L) along with classic symptoms of disease. Alternatively, a 2-hour plasma glucose greater than or equal to 200 mg/dL (11.1 mmol/L) after a 75-g glucose load can be used, as well as an A1c 6.5% or greater. The A1c should be repeated in asymptomatic adults with a serum glucose level less than 200 mg/dL (11.1 mmol/L).
Incorrect:
Classic symptoms should be accompanied with a random plasma glucose of greater than 200 mg/dL (11.1 mmol/L) (A, B). A 2-hour plasma glucose after a 75-g glucose load should be greater than 200 mg/dL (11.1 mmol/L) for a T2DM diagnosis (C).

9. **Correct: C. an insulin sensitizer.**
Pioglitazone belongs to the class of thiazolidinediones that work as insulin sensitizers via action at the PPAR-γ receptors found in muscle, adipose, and other tissue (C).
Incorrect:
GLP-1 agonists and DPP-4 inhibitors work by enhancing insulin production (A). DPP-4 inhibitors also decrease the release of glucagon from pancreatic alpha cells (B). Facilitation of renal glucose excretion is the mechanism of action of SGLT2 inhibitors (D).

10. **Correct: A. blood pressure less than 140 mm Hg systolic and less than 90 mm Hg diastolic.**
Individuals with T2DM are at higher risk of CVD and so should be monitored closely for hypertension and dyslipidemia. For those with hypertension, a blood pressure goal of less than 140/90 mm Hg is acceptable, though some may also consider a goal of less than 130/80 mm Hg (A).
Incorrect:
The general recommendation for A1c goal for most nonpregnant adults is a target of less than 7% and not 7% or greater (B). Though this patient was not indicated to have dyslipidemia, the general recommendation for those with T2DM is to maintain a TG level less than 150 mg/dL (1.7 mmol/L) (C), and an HDL level of greater than or equal to 40 mg/dL (1 mmol/L) for men and greater than or equal to 50 mg/dL (1.3 mmol/L) for women (D).

11. **Correct: C. yearly.**
For individuals with T2DM, renal function should be evaluated at least annually (C). This will include serum creatinine, calculated GFR, and urine microalbumin.
Incorrect:
Renal function should be checked at least annually regardless of glycemic control (B). With protein present in the urine, more frequent testing may be needed (A). It is not necessary to routinely check renal function at each office visit unless there is a particular concern (D).

12. **Correct: B. a product that enhances insulin release.**
Sulfonylureas work as an insulin secretagogue, which increases the release of insulin from beta cells (B). These agents are typically less effective with long-term use (5 years or longer) as well as in older adults and those with severe hyperglycemia.
Incorrect:
Facilitation of renal glucose excretion is the mechanism of action of SGLT2 inhibitors (C). One of the actions of metformin is to decrease hepatic glucose production (D). Thiazolidinediones act as an insulin sensitizer via action at the PPAR-γ receptors found in various tissues (A).

13. **Correct: C. fosinopril.**
Concomitant hypertension and T2DM need to be treated aggressively to minimize the risk of CVD. The ADA recommends the use of ACEIs, such as fosinopril (C), as well as ARBs, beta blockers, alpha-beta blockers, and calcium channel blockers.

Incorrect:
Loop diuretics (e.g., furosemide) (A), alpha blockers (e.g., methyldopa) (B), and thiazide diuretics (e.g., hydrochlorothiazide) (D) are not typically chosen as first-line antihypertensive therapy in patients with T2DM. Thiazide diuretics, particularly in higher doses, can contribute to hyperglycemia in patients with T2DM.

14. **Correct: A. report of recent unintended weight gain.**
A classic sign of DM, whether type 1 or type 2, is recent unexplained weight loss rather than weight gain (A).
Incorrect:
In addition to unexplained weight loss, the other classic signs include polyphagia (D), polyuria, and polydipsia (extreme thirst) (C). A state of insulin deficiency can also lead to ketosis in T1DM (B).

15. **Correct: D. creatinine (Cr)**
The use of metformin is not recommended in patients with impaired renal function due to a rare risk of lactic acidosis. The condition is most often seen in the presence of renal dysfunction, hypovolemia, low perfusion state, and older age. As such, creatinine should be periodically monitored to assess any change in renal function (D).
Incorrect:
Metformin is not associated with hepatotoxicity, and so routine monitoring ALP (B) or ALT (C) is not warranted. Creatine kinase is used to detect the presence of a myocardial infarction or muscle damage, and routine monitoring would not be needed with metformin use in the absence of any symptoms (A).

16. **Correct: C. ALT**
The thiazolidinediones are associated with a low risk of hepatic toxicity and so routine monitoring of liver enzymes, such as ALT should be performed (C).
Incorrect:
Creatine kinase is used to detect the presence of a myocardial infarction or muscle damage, and monitoring would not be needed with metformin use (A). The thiazolidinediones are not associated with renal toxicity. Thus, periodic monitoring of renal function via creatinine clearance (CrCl) or creatinine (Cr) is not warranted (B, D). However, renal function should be evaluated at least annually for individuals with T2DM regardless of treatment.

17. **Correct: D. history of allergic reaction to sulfonamides.**
Metformin is associated with a relatively rare risk of lactic acidosis. Certain conditions can increase this risk and should be avoided when using metformin. However, an allergic reaction to sulfonamides is not a risk factor for lactic acidosis (D). The use of sulfonylurea should be avoided in those with an allergic reaction to sulfonamides.
Incorrect:
Risk factors for lactic acidosis when taking metformin include impaired renal function (A), hypovolemia, acute

dehydration (B), advanced age, and low perfusion state. Metformin use should be temporarily stopped with radiocontrast use, surgery, or other condition that can affect the hydration status of the patient (C).

18. Correct: D. low-dose ARBs.

Certain medications can contribute to hyperglycemia and should be used with caution in those with T2DM. However, the ARBs (D) can be safely used among patients with T2DM and concomitant hypertension and is a first-line therapy choice.

Incorrect:

Medications that can contribute to hyperglycemia include high-dose niacin (A), systemic corticosteroids (B), and high-dose thiazide diuretics (C).

19. Correct: A. 28 to 42 days.

The A1c provides an assessment of average glucose control over time. Glycohemoglobin circulates in red blood cells which have an average life span of 90 to 120 days. A1c values provide a good reflection of blood glucose trends over the preceding 90 days but provide a best measure of glucose control over the preceding 28 to 42 days (C). A1c can be an important tool in patient education and reinforcement on the importance of glucose control.

20. Correct: D. Hyperglycemia can occur as a result of aerobic exercise.

Increased physical activity and regular aerobic exercise are important lifestyle modifications that can help manage T2DM and reduce IR. Hyperglycemia will not be a result of aerobic exercise (D).

Incorrect:

A regular regimen of exercise should be prescribed for those with T2DM as approximately 80% of the body's insulin-mediated glucose uptake occurs in skeletal muscles (A). With regular aerobic exercise, IR is reduced by approximately 40% (B). These IR-reducing effects can persist for up to 48 hours after exercise (C). Thus, it is recommended that the interval between exercise should not exceed 48 hours.

21 to 24. Indicate at approximately what time hypoglycemia is most likely to occur.

21. Correct: 8:30 to 10:30 a.m.

22. Correct: 10:00 to 11:00 a.m.

23. Correct: 2:00 to 10:00 p.m.

24. Correct: Hypoglycemia highly unlikely.

Hypoglycemia with insulin use is most likely to occur during the peak of action. For insulin lispro, a short-acting insulin with rapid onset of action, its peak occurs approximately 30 minutes to 2.5 hours after administration, and so hypoglycemia would most likely occur between 8:30 and 10:30 a.m. if administered at 8:00 a.m. (21). For regular insulin, peak occurs 2 to 3 hours after administration, and so hypoglycemia is most likely to occur between 10:00 and 11:00 a.m. (22). NPH insulin has a peak around 6 to 14 hours after administration,

and so hypoglycemia can occur between 2:00 and 10:00 p.m. (23). Insulin glargine is a long-acting insulin with a minimal peak, and so there is little risk of hypoglycemia with this type of insulin (24).

25. Correct: D. obesity.

T1DM is caused by an autoimmune-induced destruction of pancreatic beta cells. Certain patient factors have been identified that are associated with T1DM, though these are not as strongly correlated as some risk factors for T2DM. Obesity is strongly correlated with the development of T2DM but is not linked to T1DM (D).

Incorrect:

Though the exact cause of type 1 diabetes is not known, it is believed to result from an interplay between genetics and exposure to an environmental trigger. Patient risk factors for T1DM include the presence of HLA complex (A), European ancestry (B), select viral infections (C), and residence in a northern climate. Family history (first-degree relative) of T1DM is also linked to the development of this condition. There is currently no known approach to prevent T1DM.

26. Correct: B. thiazolidinediones

Intensification of antihyperglycemic medications is typically needed in the management of T2DM as the disease progresses over time. Intensification can include optimized dosing of current medications or the addition of a new class of medication. Selection of a new class should be based on the compelling need of the patient as well as patient preference. The addition of insulin is usually reserved for patients who cannot maintain glycemic control with a combination of other medication classes. When initiating insulin, it is important to consider that insulin should not be used in combination with a thiazolidinedione due to increased risk of edema and cardiac and vascular events (B).

Incorrect:

Insulin can be used safely in combination with most antihyperglycemic agents, including biguanides, DPP-4 inhibitors (C), GLP-1 agonists (A), and SGLT2 inhibitors (D).

27. Correct: A. Insulin-induced hypoglycemia triggers excess secretion of glucagon and cortisol, leading to hyperglycemia.

Many patients with T2DM and taking insulin therapy will experience early morning hyperglycemia. This can result from insulin-induced hypoglycemia that triggers excess secretion of glucagon and cortisol. This is called the Somogyi effect and can be avoided by lowering an inappropriately high insulin dose, typically around dinnertime (A).

Incorrect:

The Somogyi effect refers to early morning hyperglycemia. The dawn phenomenon can also result in early morning hyperglycemia due to reduced insulin sensitivity during the early morning hours. This can release cortisol that triggers hepatic glucose secretion and hyperglycemia (B). There is no specific term for late evening hyperglycemia caused by inadequate insulin dosing, though this can be easily corrected by adjusting the insulin regimen (C). Similarly, postprandial hypoglycemia can also be corrected with insulin dose adjustment, though there is not a specific term for this condition (D).

28. **Correct: A. improved glycemic control; B. strict dyslipidemia control; and C. use of an optimized dose of an ACEI or ARB**
Microalbuminuria is a risk marker for CVD and can predict the progression of renal dysfunction. The condition should be managed accordingly with a comprehensive treatment plan that aims to improve glycemic control (A), manage dyslipidemia (B), and control hypertension with either an ACEI or ARB (C).
Incorrect:
When managing hypertension, the concomitant use of an ACEI with an ARB should be avoided, as this can increase the incidence of adverse effects, and the combination of agents will decrease the efficacy of each agent compared to when they are used alone (D).

29. **Correct: B. at least two times a year in patients who are meeting treatment goals and who have stable glycemic control.**
The current recommendation is to perform A1c testing at least every 6 months for those who are meeting treatment goals and who have stable glycemic control (B). Testing should be performed more frequently for those who are not meeting treatment goals and/or have had adjustments made to their treatment regimen.
Incorrect:
Patients with stable glycemic control should undergo A1c testing at least every 6 months and not annually (A). As A1c measures average glycemic levels for the past 3 months, there is little value in performing the test on a monthly basis (C). Other tests can be used to measure changes in glycemic control due to medication adjustment, such as FPG or oral glucose tolerance test (OGTT). Standardization of A1c measurements is not an issue, and the test can be performed with point-of-service testing due to eye damage risk (D).

30. **Correct: A. a drug that increases levels of incretin, increasing synthesis and release of insulin from pancreatic beta cells.**
DPP-4 inhibitors block the degradation of incretin, thus allowing for increased levels of incretin. This in turn causes an increase in the synthesis and release of insulin from pancreatic beta cells while also decreasing the release of glucagon from pancreatic alpha cells (A).
Incorrect:
Sulfonylureas work as an insulin secretagogue in a different manner than DPP-4 inhibitors (B). Metformin works as an insulin sensitizer in the peripheral tissues as well as reduces hepatic glucose production (C). SGLT2 inhibitors work by facilitating renal excretion of glucose (D).

31. **Correct: A. a drug that stimulates insulin production in response to an increase in plasma glucose.**
Similar to DPP-4 inhibitors, GLP-1 agonists work via the incretin system to improve glucose control. These agents are able to stimulate insulin production in response to an increase in plasma glucose while also inhibiting postprandial glucagon release (A).
Incorrect:
Sulfonylureas work as an insulin secretagogue in a different manner than GLP-1 agonists (B). Metformin works as an insulin sensitizer in the peripheral tissues as well as reduces hepatic glucose production (C). SGLT2 inhibitors work by facilitating renal excretion of glucose (D).

32. **Correct: A. FPG.**
Overweight/obesity are risk factors for T2DM, while the presence of acanthosis nigricans can be an early sign of the condition. Various plasma glucose tests can be used to check for T2DM, including an FPG (A), random plasma glucose, or OGTT.
Incorrect:
This patient shows signs most indicative of T2DM, and the priority should be on performing plasma glucose testing. There is no indication from the patient description regarding hepatic dysfunction requiring a liver function test (LFT) (B), nor is there any indication of an inflammation disorder requiring an ESR (D). A rapid plasma reagin (RPR) test is used to screen for syphilis and is not indicated for this patient (C).

33. **Correct: D. a 35-year-old patient with newly diagnosed T2DM.**
Thiazolidinediones are an acceptable choice for the treatment of newly diagnosed T2DM, particularly when there is no additional CVD risk or heart failure (D). This class provides a low-cost approach to managing T2DM.
Incorrect:
Thiazolidinediones are not recommended to be used in combination with insulin or sulfonylureas due to increased risk of edema (C). These should also be avoided in patients using insulin and nitrates, as this can increase cardiovascular risk (A). This class can also exacerbate heart failure and should not be initiated in patients in the presence of heart failure (B).

34. **Correct: D. liraglutide (Victoza®)**
One of the mechanisms of GLP-1 agonists, such as liraglutide, is to delay gastric emptying, which can cause appetite suppression and weight loss. However, this class of agents is not recommended in patients with a history of gastroparesis (D).
Incorrect:
Gastroparesis is a condition where the stomach is not able to empty its contents in a normal fashion. GLP-1 agonists are not recommended in patients with severe GI disorders such as gastroparesis. Insulin formulations (A, B) and sulfonylureas (C) are safe to use in patients with gastroparesis.

35. Correct: C. lactic acidosis.

The use of metformin is associated with a risk (though rare) of lactic acidosis (C). Certain conditions can increase this risk, including acute dehydration and hypovolemia. Therefore, individuals undergoing radio-contrast use, surgery, or other conditions that can affect hydration status should stop taking metformin for 24 hours prior to the procedure and at least 48 hours after the procedure, until baseline renal function has been reestablished.

Incorrect:

Metformin is not associated with hepatic toxicity (B) and has a very small risk of hypoglycemia (A). The concern with metformin use during surgery is lactic acidosis and not an interaction with anesthetic agents (D).

36. Correct: C. α-adrenergic receptor antagonist.

Several classes of antihypertensive medications are recommended as first line by the ADA when there is concomitant T2DM and hypertension. An ACEI or ARB should be one of the hypertension medications. However, α-adrenergic receptor antagonists (or alpha blockers) are not among first-line choices (C).

Incorrect:

First-line antihypertensive agents to use in patients with T2DM can include ACEIs, ARBs (D), beta blockers (A), and calcium channel blockers (B).

37. Correct: A. The goal should be for a total increased physical activity of 150 minutes per week or more; B. Increased physical activity is recommended at least three times per week with no more than 48 hours without exercise; C. Some form of resistance exercise such as lifting dumbbells or using an exercise band should be included at least two times per week; and D. Vigorous aerobic or resistance activity is potentially contraindicated in the presence of proliferative or severe nonproliferative retinopathy because of the possible risk of vitreous hemorrhage or retinal detachment.

For patients with T2DM, regular vigorous aerobic exercise should be prescribed as approximately 80% of the body's insulin-mediated glucose uptake occurs in muscle, and exercise can reduce IR by up to 40%. At least 150 minutes of exercise per week is recommended (A), with exercise at least three times per week (B). Resistance exercise should also be included in the regimen at least twice each week (C). However, note that vigorous aerobic or resistance activity should be avoided in patients with proliferative or nonproliferative retinopathy due to eye damage risk (D).

38. Correct: B. 4

For individuals with T2DM and who are taking basal insulin, a rapid-acting insulin may be needed to manage postprandial hyperglycemia. The ADA recommends initiating prandial insulin once per day with the largest meal and starting with a dose of 4 IU per day or about 10% of the basal dose (B). This initial dose can then be titrated by 1 to 2 IU twice weekly until glycemic control is achieved.

39. Correct: D. a 58-year-old woman with a 2-hour postprandial glucose of 152 mg/dL (8.44 mmol/L)

Criteria for prediabetes include an A1c of 5.7% to 6.4%, a fasting plasma glucose of 100 to 125 mg/dL (5.6 to 6.9 mmol/L), or a 2-hour OGTT of 140 to 199 mg/dL (7.8 to 11 mmol/L). Among the patients listed, the 58-year-old woman fulfills the criteria for prediabetes (D).

Incorrect:

The 70-year-old man (A) and 33-year-old man (C) are below the criteria for prediabetes, though they are at the higher end of the normal range and should continue with recommended routine monitoring. The 84-year-old woman does not fit the criteria for prediabetes, though a 2-hour OGTT would provide a better assessment based on the guidelines (B).

40. Correct: B. Increase his glargine dose by four units per day.

The fasting glucose goal in T2DM is between 80 and 100 mg/dL (4.44 and 5.55 mmol/L). For a patient with FPG between 141 and 180 mg/dL, the recommendation is to increase the dose by four units (B).

Incorrect:

No change in his current regimen would be appropriate if he was at FPG goal (A). An increase of one unit would be needed if FPG fell in the range of 100 to 120 mg/dL (5.55 to 6.66 mmol/L) (C). An increase of six units would be recommended for individuals who have an FPG of 180 mg/dL (9.99 mmol/L) or higher (D).

41. Correct: B. metformin

For a patient with newly diagnosed T2DM, initial management will include counseling about lifestyle modifications and pharmacotherapy. The ADA typically recommends the use of metformin as first-line pharmacological therapy (B). This would also be an appropriate choice for a patient without health insurance as it is a low-cost option compared to newer medication classes.

Incorrect:

Metformin is typically considered for first-line therapy in newly diagnosed T2DM. If intensification of therapy is needed for a patient with no health insurance, low-cost options could include the addition of a sulfonylurea or thiazolidinedione. Newer classes of antihyperglycemic agents, such as the DPP-4 inhibitors (A), GLP-1 agonists (C), and SGLT2 inhibitors (D), would generally not be preferred due to their higher cost.

42. Correct: A. The use of this type of sliding-scale insulin therapy is discouraged as this method treats hyperglycemia after it has already occurred.

Sliding-scale insulin therapy is a progressive approach that corrects hyperglycemia through frequent administration of short-acting insulin dosed based on the patient's blood glucose level. Sliding-scale insulin therapy used in many health-care settings is not recommended as it treats hyperglycemia after it has already occurred (A). This reactive approach to insulin therapy can lead to rapid and substantial changes to plasma glucose levels that can increase the risk for hyper- or hypoglycemia.

Incorrect:

The sliding-scale insulin approach is not recommended to manage hyperglycemia as it treats hyperglycemia after it occurs (B). Though this approach has been used in acute care settings, it is also an approach commonly used in other settings, such as skilled nursing facilities and long-term care settings (C). This approach would not be recommended for T1DM as it does not necessarily use basal insulin, which is required in the management of T1DM (D).

43. Correct: C. 50% to 60%

In a healthy person, basal insulin comprises 50% to 60% of the total daily physiological insulin released (C). The remainder of insulin secretion results from meals and snacks.

Incorrect:

Approximately half of the body's total insulin secretion is basal insulin (A, B, D).

44. Correct: C. glipizide

A major disadvantage of the sulfonylureas, such as glipizide, is that they tend to lose effectiveness with long-term use (greater than 5 years) (C). Sulfonylureas require functioning beta cells to be clinically effective. As beta cell function declines over time in T2DM, the effectiveness of these medications also declines. Sulfonylureas also have decreased effectiveness in older patients and in the presence of severe hyperglycemia.

Incorrect:

Metformin (A), the thiazolidinediones (B), and insulin (D) can retain their effectiveness over time in the treatment of T2DM as they do not rely on beta cell function.

45. Correct: D. an insulin form

The A1c reduction potential of insulin is essentially limitless, as the dose can be easily adjusted based on hyperglycemia status (D).

Incorrect:

The anticipated A1c reduction of metformin (A), thiazolidinediones (B), and sulfonylureas (C) with intensified use are all in the range of 1% to 2%.

46. Correct: B. African Americans are typically less sensitive to the effects of insulin when compared with people of European ancestry.

Ethnicity has a large influence on insulin sensitivity and can be a predominant risk factor for T2DM. Certain ethnic groups are less sensitive to the effects of insulin compared to people of European ancestry, and these include African Americans, Latinos, and Native Americans (B).

Incorrect:

There is a substantial variation in insulin sensitivity among ethnic groups (A). Ethnicities that are typically less sensitive to insulin compared to people of European ancestry include African Americans, Native Americans, and Latinos, including Mexican Americans (C). Insulin

sensitivity can have an impact on insulin production, with those who are less sensitive to the effects of insulin requiring greater insulin production to maintain glycemic control (D).

47. Correct: C. 8%.

For most nonpregnant adults, the ADA recommends an A1c goal of less than 7%, though a goal of less than 6.5% can be reasonable for selected individuals if this can be achieved without a significant risk for hypoglycemia or other adverse effects. Less stringent goals are also acceptable for certain individuals, such as those with a history of hypoglycemia, limited life expectancy, advanced microvascular or macrovascular complications, long-standing diabetes, or extensive comorbid conditions. In these cases, an A1c goal less than 8% is acceptable (C).

Incorrect:

For a frail older adult as described in this example, an A1C goal of <8% is acceptable rather than the more stringent goals of <7% (A) or <7.5% (B). An A1C of <8% is achievable in most cases and should be the target with use of antihyperglycemic medications and/or insulin. A1C goals higher than 8% can increase the risk of microvascular and macrovascular complications (D).

48. Correct: C. 6.5%.

Similar to T2DM, the ADA recommends an A1c goal less than 7% for most nonpregnant adults. However, more stringent glycemic control (such as A1c less than 6.5%) can be considered for certain patients as this has been shown to offer additional benefits in preventing microvascular and macrovascular complications (C). In particular, this can be considered for younger patients with no comorbid conditions and no history or little risk of hypoglycemic episodes.

Incorrect:

For younger patients with diabetes mellitus and no comorbidities, a more stringent A1C goal should be considered rather than the general goal of <7% (D). An A1C goal of <6.5% is generally acceptable. More stringent A1C goals of 6% or less, though safely achievable for many patients, can increase the risk of hypoglycemic episodes (A, B).

49. Correct: B. pancreatitis.

The use of GLP-1 agonists has been associated with the development of pancreatitis, and its use is not recommended for patients with a history of pancreatitis (B). Prescribers are advised to discontinue GLP-1 agonist therapy at the first signs of pancreatitis, including persistent abdominal pain usually accompanied by vomiting. These agents are also not recommended in patients with gastroparesis, which is related to the drug's ability to slow gastric emptying.

Incorrect:

GLP-1 agonists have not been linked to the development of leukopenia (A), lymphoma (C), or vitiligo (D).

50. **Correct: B. notation of ethnic-specific waist circumference measurements.**

The diagnostic criteria for metabolic syndrome can vary considerably depending on the particular health promotion group. Criteria developed by the IDF include central obesity defined by ethnic-specific waist circumference measurements that range from greater than or equal to 90 to 94 cm (35.5 to 37 inches) in men and greater than or equal to 80 cm (31.5 inches) in women (B).

Incorrect:

In addition to central obesity, two or more of the following are required for a diagnosis of metabolic syndrome according to IDF criteria: elevated TGs, low HDL-C level, hypertension, and/or elevated FPG or prior diagnosis of T2DM or impaired glucose tolerance. Persistent hyperglycemia is not an obligatory finding for a diagnosis of metabolic syndrome (A). There is no requirement for a family history of T2DM (D) or microalbuminuria (C).

51. **Correct: C. diminished fibrinolysis.**

Metformin is commonly considered first-line pharmacotherapy for T2DM as it provides a variety of beneficial effects. The use of this agent can lead to improved metabolic parameters such as enhanced fibrinolysis that can decrease the risk of vascular disease, particularly in those with coronary artery disease and peripheral vascular disease. The use of metformin does not diminish fibrinolysis (C).

Incorrect:

A mechanism of action of metformin is as an insulin sensitizer that increases peripheral glucose uptake and utilization (A). Use of metformin is associated with some weight loss during the initial period of use (B), and it can decrease the production of TG cholesterol (D).

52. **Correct: C. greater responsiveness to angiotensin II.**

Hyperinsulinemia, often seen in response to IR, is associated with various effects on the cardiovascular system. However, the condition results in diminished responsiveness to angiotensin II, which can contribute to the development of hypertension (C).

Incorrect:

Effects of hyperinsulinemia can include decreased renal sodium reabsorption (A), which can contribute to polyuria, diminished sympathetic activation (D), and constricted circulating volume (B).

53. **Correct: A. hyperovulation.**

Women of reproductive age with IR and metabolic syndrome are at risk of developing PCOS. A consequence of PCOS is anovulation, rather than hyperovulation, and is a leading cause of endocrine-based female infertility (A).

Incorrect:

IR in women of reproductive age can lead to the development of PCOS that will often present with irregular menses (B). Other signs of IR can include acne (C), acanthosis nigricans, and hirsutism (D).

54. **Correct: D. face.**

Acanthosis nigricans is hyperpigmentation of the skin that is correlated with IR. However, the condition does not normally present on the face (D).

Incorrect:

The most common areas for acanthosis nigricans include groin folds (A), axilla (B), and the nape of the neck (C).

55. **Correct: C. it is important to maintain glucose control prior to and during pregnancy.**

For women with T2DM and who are considering pregnancy, it is essential to attain glycemic control prior to and during pregnancy (C). Poorly controlled diabetes (as well as untreated gestational diabetes) during pregnancy can have serious adverse effects, including preterm birth and macrosomia (excessively large fetus).

Incorrect:

The onset of pregnancy does not help to control hyperglycemia (A). Given the younger age and absence of any other comorbidities, the A1c goal for this patient should be less than or equal to 7% (B). Medications used to treat hyperglycemia are not discontinued during pregnancy but may be adjusted to ensure adequate glucose control (D).

56 to 59. Select the appropriate medication.

56. **Correct: C. GLP-1 agonist; and D. SGLT2 inhibitor**

57. **Correct: C. GLP-1 agonist; and D. SGLT2 inhibitor**

58. **Correct: A. sulfonylurea**

59. **Correct: B. DPP-4 inhibitor; C. GLP-1 agonist; and D. SGLT2 inhibitor**

Recommendations from the ADA encourage individualizing treatment selection based on patient needs and preferences. For a patient with heart failure or chronic kidney disease, the use of a SGLT2 inhibitor or GLP-1 agonist with proven cardiovascular benefits should be preferred in combination with metformin (56). When there is a compelling need for weight loss, the use of SGLT2 inhibitor or GLP-1 agonist is preferred as the use of these agents is associated with weight loss (57). For patients with cost concerns, a sulfonylurea or thiazolidinedione can be selected as the least expensive treatment approaches (58). Agents that minimize the risk of hypoglycemia include DPP-4 inhibitors, GLP-1 agonists, SGLT2 inhibitors, and thiazolidinediones (59).

Obesity

60. **Correct: B. 30**

Current definitions of overweight and obesity categorize obesity as having a BMI of 30 kg/m² or greater, with a BMI of 40 kg/m² being severe or morbidly obese (B). Overweight is considered in individuals with a BMI between 25 and 29.9 kg/m².

61. **Correct: A. "How do you feel about your weight?"**

Individuals in the precontemplation stage have not started to think about making a life change or may see no reason to make a change. Asking patients about how they feel about their weight is a neutral approach to better

understand their beliefs on weight status and whether they feel a change is needed or would be attempted (A).
Incorrect:
Asking about barriers to weight change is more appropriate for a patient in the contemplation stage who is considering making a change but needs help to make that change (B). Identifying personal goals is appropriate during the preparation stage where the patient exhibits some change behavior but does not have the tools to proceed (C). Asking the individual about how the provider can help to achieve the weight loss goal is also an important part during the preparation stage (D).

62. **Correct: B. "What are barriers you see to losing weight?"**
Asking about barriers to weight change is more appropriate for a patient in the contemplation stage who is considering making a change but needs help to make that change (B).
Incorrect:
Individuals in the precontemplation stage have not started to think about making a life change or may see no reason to make a change. Asking patients about how they feel about their weight is a neutral approach to better understand their beliefs on weight status and whether they feel a change is needed or would be attempted (A). Identifying personal goals is appropriate during the preparation stage where the patient exhibits some change behavior but does not have the tools to proceed (C). Asking the individual about how the provider can help to achieve the weight loss goal is also an important part during the preparation stage (D).

63. **Correct: A. within an hour of each meal that contains fat**
Orlistat primarily works by reducing dietary fat absorption from the GI tract, which passes through undigested, causing weight loss. Optimal use of this agent is to take the drug with or within 1 hour of a meal that contains fat (A).
Incorrect:
Orlistat diminishes the absorption of fat, not carbohydrates, and so should be taken with meals that contain fat (B). It should be taken three times per day with each meal that contains fat, ideally with the meal or within 1 hour of the meal (D). It is not associated with sleep disturbance, though GI adverse effects are common (C).

64. **Correct: B. Hypothalamus**
Contrave® is a combination of naltrexone and buproprion. Though the exact mechanism of action is not fully understood, it is believed to affect the hypothalamus (B) and mesolimbic dopamine circuit that are involved in regulation of food intake.
Incorrect:
Contrave® is believed to affect the hypothalamus and mesolimbic dopamine circuit, and not the cerebellum (A), pituitary gland (C), or parietal lobe (D).

65. **Correct: C. 3,500**
One pound of fat contains approximately 3,500 calories (C). Restricting calorie intake by 500 calories per day can lead to a loss of approximately 1 pound per week.

Incorrect:
Each pound of fat contains 3500 calories (A, B, D).

66. **Correct: D. 4 to 5**
A pedometer can be a useful tool to measure the number of steps taken in a day and assess the level of physical activity by a patient. The recommendation of 10,000 steps per day is equivalent to walking about 4 to 5 miles (D).
Incorrect:
10,000 steps is equivalent to 4 to 5 miles. One to 2 miles is about 2,500 steps (A), 2–3 miles is about 5,000 steps (B), and 3 to 4 miles is about 7,500 steps (C).

67. **Correct: B. 12**
Weight loss medications can provide an important and useful tool in weight management. However, the medication should be discontinued if the patient has not achieved a 5% weight loss by 12 weeks of treatment (B). In these cases, the weight loss medication is unlikely to be helpful in weight reduction, and an alternative approach should be considered.
Incorrect:
With weight loss medications, a clinical effect should be observed by 12 weeks of use. Six weeks can be too soon to determine adequate effect (A), while the effect should be observed before 18 or 24 weeks (C, D).

68. **Correct: B. 10**
Though there is a common belief by individuals with obesity that a dramatic weight loss is needed to see any health benefits, this is not necessarily true. A loss of approximately 10% body weight (B) can result in immediate improvements in reducing death rates from heart disease and stroke. Other improvements can include symptoms associated with OA, asthma, and sleep apnea.
Incorrect:
Benefits from weight loss can be observed with only a 10% decrease in body weight among individuals with obesity. Though this is higher than 5% loss (A), a 15% or 20% loss is not needed to begin seeing the benefits (C, D).

69. **Correct: B. The most dramatic weight losses are seen in the first few postoperative months.**
Bariatric surgery can be an effective approach to weight loss for certain patients. The procedure can result in up to an 80% loss of excessive body weight. Most of the body weight is lost within the first 3 years following surgery, with the most dramatic weight loss occurring in the first few postoperative months (B).
Incorrect:
Bariatric surgery can result in a loss of 40% to 80% of excessive body weight, though patients may not achieve an ideal BMI (A). About 10% of patients will experience a significant short-term problem after surgery, though death attributed to surgery is rare (C). Most of the weight loss occurs in the first 3 years after surgery. Weight re-gain can occur if diet and physical activity recommendations are not followed (D).

70. Correct: A. risperidone (Risperdal®)
When counseling patients about weight loss, it is important to identify medications that can contribute to weight gain and discontinue or substitute those medications when possible. Some medications that are implicated in weight gain include second-generation antipsychotics (e.g., risperidone) (A), select antiepileptics, and corticosteroids.
Incorrect:
DPP-4 inhibitors such as sitagliptin are generally weight neutral (D), while metformin can be associated with weight loss with initial use (C). Topiramate is used in combination with phentermine as a weight management medication (B).

71. Correct: A. Calcium absorption will be reduced; B. Rapid weight loss after obesity surgery can contribute to the development of gallstones; and D. Lifelong vitamin B$_{12}$ supplementation is recommended.
Gastric bypass surgery is a restrictive/malabsorption-type surgery where food bypasses the duodenum, where calories are normally absorbed. Due to malabsorption, supplementation is needed for nutrients that are normally absorbed in the duodenum, including vitamin B$_{12}$ (D), iron, zinc, calcium (A), and other fat-soluble vitamins. The most dramatic weight loss is usually observed in the first few months following surgery, which can increase the risk of gallstones (B).
Incorrect:
Persistent GI upset is occasionally noted as an adverse effect following bariatric surgery, though chronic constipation is not a typical finding among these patients (C).

72 to 76. True or False

72. Correct: False
The liraglutide dose used for chronic weight loss management (3 mg subcutaneous injection daily) is much higher when compared to the dose used to manage type 2 diabetes mellitus (0.75 mg to 1.5 mg subcutaneously once weekly).

73. Correct: True
Topiramate is Pregnancy Risk Category D and should be avoided in pregnant women. Before initiating Qsymia®, women of reproductive age should test negative on a pregnancy test and be counseled on the use of a highly effective contraceptive while taking the medication.

74. Correct: False
The mechanism of action of phentermine is likely through the release of catecholamines that act to suppress the appetite and decrease food consumption.

75. Correct: True
Gastric bypass surgery can result in approximately 70% to 80% loss of excess body weight, compared to 40% to 60% with the gastric band and approximately 60% with the gastric sleeve.

76. Correct: True
The FDA has mandated a boxed warning related to an increased risk of suicidal thoughts and behaviors with the use of Contrave®, as well as other neuropsychiatric reactions. Patients should be regularly monitored for depression or suicidal thoughts.

77. Correct: A. obstructive apnea; B. steatohepatitis; C. female infertility; and D. endometrial cancer
Obesity increases the risk of a variety of medical conditions beyond the most commonly recognized conditions of CVD, DM, and dyslipidemia. Female infertility can occur via increased risk of PCOS (C). Obesity is linked to several cancers, including postmenopausal breast, endometrial (D), colon and rectum, kidney, and pancreas, among others. Obesity is also associated with obstructive sleep apnea (A) and nonalcoholic fatty liver disease such as steatohepatitis (B).

Thyroid Disorders

78. Correct: D. elderly.
Recognizing patient risk factors for thyroid disorders is important in early detection and management of these conditions. Risk factors include elderly age (D), female gender, postpartum period, or a personal or family history of autoimmune disease.
Incorrect:
Hypertension (B) and obesity (A) are not recognized risk factors for thyroid disorders. Certain medications can increase the risk of thyroid disorders, including iodide, amiodarone, lithium, interferon-α, and interleukin-2. Systemic corticosteroids have not been linked to thyroid disorders (C).

79. Correct: B. the medication is a plant-based product.
Desiccated thyroid is animal derived, usually from bovine or porcine (B). Its use can be limited due to ethnic or religious restrictions as well as for vegetarians or vegans.
Incorrect:
The majority of studies for the treatment of hypothyroidism have used levothyroxine, and so the efficacy of desiccated thyroid is less known (D). Though these products provide a fixed dose of T3 and T4 (A), the pharmacokinetics can vary substantially compared to levothyroxine (C), and drug levels can vary significantly throughout the day.

80. Correct: C. autoimmune thyroiditis.
In parts of the world where iodine deficiency is rare, such as in the United States, autoimmune thyroiditis is the leading cause of hypothyroidism (C). The condition is often linked to other autoimmune disorders.
Incorrect:
Secondary hypothyroidism can be caused by failure of the pituitary to release TSH, but this occurs less frequently than autoimmune thyroiditis, such as Hashimoto's thyroiditis (A). Metabolically active thyroid nodules are a common cause of hyperthyroidism rather than hypothyroidism (B). Radioactive thyroid exposure is a treatment for hyperthyroidism that subsequently leads to hypothyroidism. However, this occurs less frequently than autoimmune thyroiditis (C).

81. **Correct: A. total T4**

Total T4 is a common test performed in the evaluation of thyroid disorders, However, many factors can impact the level of total T4 and so this is not useful in measuring a change in metabolic status (A).

Incorrect:

TSH is a highly sensitive and specific test to diagnose thyroid disorders (B). Only a small portion of T4 is in the metabolically active free T4 form, and this measurement is the most helpful test to confirm an abnormal TSH level (C). The presence of TPO antibodies can result from cell-mediated immunity; they are found in nearly all patients with Hashimoto's thyroiditis (D).

82. **Correct: C. eyelid retraction.**

Graves' disease is a form of hyperthyroidism that is associated with excessive energy release. A common physical finding would include eyelid retraction or exophthalmos, causing the appearance of bulging eyes.

Incorrect:

Hyperthyroidism is associated with muscle weakness but not typically muscle tenderness (A). Hyperthyroidism also presents with smooth, silky skin and hyperreflexia compared with coarse, dry skin (B) and hyporeflexia (D) seen in hypothyroidism.

83. **Correct: A. destroy the overactive thyroid tissue.**

Radioactive iodine is routinely used as part of treatment for hyperthyroidism. The treatment results in ablation of thyroid tissue (A), which subsequently results in hypothyroidism.

Incorrect:

Hyperthyroidism is caused by a metabolically active thyroid gland that causes a reduction in TSH production from the pituitary, so further TSH reduction is not a treatment approach (B). The treatment attempts to eliminate, not alter, the metabolically active thyroid gland (C). An enlarged thyroid gland, such as seen in a goiter, can cause hyperthyroidism (D). Though radioactive iodine can lead to some degree of diminished size of the goiter, surgery or other approaches may be needed. It is also important to note that not all goiters are associated with hyperthyroidism.

84. **Correct: A. propranolol**

For patients with hyperthyroidism, the use of a beta blocker, such as propranolol or nadolol, can be considered to minimize symptoms of tachycardia or tremor (A).

Incorrect:

The beta blockers are the preferred treatment to counteract tachycardia and tremor during hyperthyroidism. Benzodiazepines (e.g., diazepam) (B), anticonvulsants (e.g., carbamazepine) (C), or calcium channel blockers (e.g., verapamil) (D) are not the preferred treatment choice in these cases.

85. **Correct: C. The levothyroxine dose needed by elderly persons is 75% or less of that needed by younger adults.**

Special considerations are needed when prescribing levothyroxine therapy in the elderly. The dose should be calculated based on ideal body weight, but the anticipated dose in the elderly should be 75% or less compared to a younger adult dose (C).

Incorrect:

Other than the dosage amount needed in the elderly, initiation and titration of levothyroxine are similar compared to other adults (A). After drug initiation or dose adjustment, the TSH level should be checked in 6 to 8 weeks rather than 2 days (B). The goal of treatment is to attain a normal TSH level of between 0.4 and 4 mIU/L (D).

86. **Correct: D. anterior lobe of the pituitary.**

The anterior lobe of the pituitary is responsible for the release of TSH (D). Secretion is stimulated by thyrotropin-releasing hormone through a negative feedback loop in response to the amount of T4 produced in the thyroid.

Incorrect:

The thyroid produces T3 and T4 (A). Thyrotropin-releasing hormone is produced in the hypothalamus along with several other hormones (C). The adrenal cortex is responsible for the production of several hormones, including aldosterone, cortisol, and male sex hormones (B).

87. **Correct: D. thyroid cyst.**

A "cold spot" is associated with a metabolically inactive area of the thyroid that would be most consistent with a thyroid cyst (D). Fine-needle aspiration biopsy would be needed to determine if the cyst is benign or malignant to guide further management decisions.

Incorrect:

Contrary to a "cold spot," a "hot spot" would indicate a metabolically active area that could be responsible for hyperthyroidism and Graves' disease (B). A "cold spot" would not be specific for Hashimoto's disease that can present with a diffusely enlarged thyroid with fine nodules (C). A functioning adenoma would present as a "hot spot" in the thyroid scan (A).

88. **Correct: B. "To help with adherence, take your calcium supplement at the same time as your thyroid medication."**

Levothyroxine is commonly used in the treatment of hypothyroidism. However, its absorption can be affected by several factors, including when taken with food, supplements, and medications, particularly those containing calcium, iron, and aluminum. When taking levothyroxine, the administration of a calcium supplement should be separated by several hours (B).

Incorrect:

For optimal absorption of levothyroxine, it should be taken on an empty stomach with a glass of water (A), preferably at the same time each day (C). Soy milk or other foods containing calcium (e.g., dairy products) should be separated by several hours from when levothyroxine is taken (D).

89. **Correct: A. autonomously functioning adenoma.**

A painless thyroid mass and low TSH level suggest a metabolically active nodule that is releasing excess T3 and/or T4 that results in hyperthyroidism. This would most likely be due to an autonomously functioning adenoma (A). A thyroid scan would reveal this as a "hot spot," and a fine-needle aspiration biopsy can be used to confirm the diagnosis and determine if the nodule is benign or malignant.

Incorrect:
Graves' disease is also a form of hyperthyroidism but is not necessarily caused by a metabolically active nodule (B). Hashimoto's disease is hypothyroidism caused by an autoimmune response (C). A metabolically active nodule is not necessarily malignant and would require fine-needle aspiration biopsy to determine whether it is benign or malignant (D).

90. **Correct: D. thyroid malignancy.**
A thyroid mass that is accompanied by hoarseness and dysphagia (difficulty swallowing) is an indication of thyroid malignancy and should be evaluated immediately via biopsy (D). Other signs or patient factors to raise suspicion of thyroid malignancy include history of head or neck irradiation, localized pain, dysphonia (change in voice), hemoptysis (coughing blood or blood-tinged mucus), and/or regional lymphadenopathy.

Incorrect:
Hoarseness and dysphagia are not typical signs of Graves' disease (B) or Hashimoto's disease (C). Though some adenomatous lesions can be malignant, it is rare for a metabolically active nodule to be malignant (A).

91. **Correct: C. fine-needle aspiration biopsy**
A fine-needle aspiration biopsy is the preferred method to differentiate whether a thyroid mass is benign or malignant (C).

Incorrect:
Ultrasound (A) and MRI (B) are able to detect the presence of nodules but are not as effective as a fine-needle aspiration biopsy in determining whether the nodule is malignant. Ultrasound is most useful in differentiating a fluid-filled cyst versus a solid thyroid nodule. A radioactive iodine scan would be able to determine if the nodule is metabolically active but would not be effective in determining if the nodule is malignant or benign (D).

92. **Correct: A. bone thinning.**
When using levothyroxine to treat hypothyroidism, the dose should be titrated to achieve normal TSH levels. Excessive use of levothyroxine will lead to diminished TSH level and signs and symptoms of hyperthyroidism, which can lead to bone thinning (A).

Incorrect:
Excessive levothyroxine can lead to symptoms of hyperthyroidism including nervousness and irritability rather than fatigue (B), and hyperdefecation rather than constipation (D). Renal impairment is not associated with excessive use of levothyroxine (C).

93. **Correct: D. 6 to 8 weeks**
TSH levels should be assessed at least 6 to 8 weeks after initiating or adjusting the dose of levothyroxine (D).

Due to levothyroxine's long half-life, this is the amount of time needed to see any change in TSH levels.

Incorrect:
Due to levothyroxine's long half-life, reassessing TSH before 6 to 8 weeks after dose adjustment will not accurately evaluate the full therapeutic potential of the adjustment (A, B, C).

94. **Correct: B. thyroid cyst.**
A fluid-filled mass is most consistent with the diagnosis of a cyst (B). Surgical removal can be considered, especially if the cyst is associated with pain or difficulty swallowing.

Incorrect:
Goiter is associated with an enlarged thyroid usually as a result of excessive TSH produced by the pituitary. A multinodular goiter would not be characterized by a single large thyroid mass (C). An adenoma is characterized as a solid nodule and not fluid filled (A). Hemangiomas are most commonly found on the skin, such as strawberry spots observed in newborns. An internal hemangioma is a benign tumor of a blood vessel that is solid and not fluid filled (D).

95. **Correct: C. Down syndrome**
Those with Down syndrome are at higher risk of hypothyroidism and should be routinely monitored (C).

Incorrect:
Thyroid disorders are more likely in the female gender rather than the male gender (B). Certain medications can increase the risk of hyper- and hypothyroidism (e.g., iodide, amiodarone, and lithium), though digoxin is not linked to these disorders (A). There is no significant association between alcoholism and thyroid disorders that would require periodic screening (D).

96 to 112. Indicate hyperthyroidism, hypothyroidism, or both.

96. **Correct: Hyperthyroidism**
97. **Correct: Hyperthyroidism**
98. **Correct: Both**
99. **Correct: Hyperthyroidism**
100. **Correct: Hypothyroidism**
101. **Correct: Hyperthyroidism**
102. **Correct: Hypothyroidism**
103. **Correct: Hypothyroidism**
104. **Correct: Hyperthyroidism**
105. **Correct: Hyperthyroidism**
106. **Correct: Hyperthyroidism**
107. **Correct: Hypothyroidism**
108. **Correct: Hypothyroidism**
109. **Correct: Hypothyroidism**
110. **Correct: Hypothyroidism**
111. **Correct: Both**

112. Correct: Both

Timely detection and diagnosis of thyroid disorders requires a thorough understanding of the characteristic signs and symptoms of these conditions. Hyperthyroidism, resulting in excessive energy release, is characterized by heat intolerance (96), smooth, silky skin (97), frequent, low-volume loose stools (99), amenorrhea and oligomenorrhea (101), hyperreflexia (104), proximal muscle weakness (105), and tachycardia with hypertension (106). Hypothyroidism is associated with reduced energy release and characterized by secondary hypertriglyceridemia (100), coarse, dry skin (102), menorrhagia (103), hyporeflexia (107), coarse hair (108), thick, dry nails (109), and constipation (110). Both conditions can include a presentation of goiter (98) as well as altered mental status (112) and have an atypical presentation in the elderly (111).

113. Correct: D. lithium

Certain medications can increase the risk of thyroid disorders, including iodide, amiodarone, lithium (D), interferon-α, and interleukin-2.

Incorrect:

The use of sertraline (A), venlafaxine (B), or bupropion (C) has not been associated with the development of thyroid disorders.

114 to 116. Matching Questions

114. Correct: SCH

115. Correct: Hyperthyroidism

116. Correct: Hyperthyroidism

TSH and free T4 are the most helpful tests to diagnose thyroid disorders. Hyperthyroidism is characterized by elevated TSH and diminished free T4 levels (116). Consequently, hypothyroidism is found in the individual with diminished TSH and elevated free T4 (115). SCH is diagnosed based on the finding of elevated TSH but normal level of free T4 (114). Individuals with SCH typically have minimal or no symptoms.

Dyslipidemia

117. Correct: B. Moderate-intensity statin therapy is the preferred treatment option.

According to the ACC/AHA guidelines, an individual between the ages of 40 and 75 years, with LDL-C between 70 and 190 mg/dL, and with a 10-year ASCVD risk of 7.5% to less than 20% should receive moderate-intensity therapy statin therapy (B). High-intensity statin therapy would be considered with ASCVD risk of 20% or greater.

Incorrect:

Individuals over the age of 75 years and without ASCVD should have a clinical assessment and risk discussion to determine whether statin therapy is appropriate based on a risk-benefit analysis (A). Statin is the preferred initial therapy for LDL-C lowering. Ezetimibe can be considered with statin therapy if there is

an inadequate response with statin alone (D). Niacin is not recommended for LDL-C reduction due to a lack of evidence demonstrating improved cardiovascular outcomes with its use (C).

118. Correct: D. A high-intensity HMG-CoA reductase inhibitor (statin) regimen should be initiated.

According to the ACC/AHA guidelines, any individual without ASCVD and LDL-C of 190 mg/dL or higher should be initiated on high-intensity statin therapy (D).

Incorrect:

High-intensity statin therapy is recommended for this patient (A, C). Fibrate is not recommended for LDL-C lowering due to a lack of evidence demonstrating improved cardiovascular outcomes with its use (B).

119. Correct: C. Lipid-lowering drug therapy with a moderate-intensity statin should be initiated.

According to the ACC/AHA guidelines, individuals between the ages of 40 and 75 years of age with DM and with ASCVD should be initiated on moderate-intensity statin therapy (C). Risk assessment should be performed periodically to determine whether high-intensity statin therapy should be considered.

Incorrect:

Due to a higher risk of CVD among those with DM, statin therapy is recommended for all those with diabetes between the ages of 40 and 75 years (A). Even with his dietary intervention, the patient's LDL-C level is elevated (D). After initiating therapy, a repeat lipid profile should be performed in 4 to 12 weeks (B).

120. Correct: B. alanine aminotransferase

Statin use has rarely been shown to cause mild and reversible hepatic injury demonstrated by elevations in ALT. Prior to starting statin therapy, ALT should be measured to obtain a baseline value (B). Routine monitoring of ALT during statin use is not warranted unless the patient shows signs of hepatotoxicity.

Incorrect:

ALT is the preferred diagnostic measure over bilirubin (C) or ALP (D) to evaluate possible hepatotoxicity with statin use. Statins are not known to impact potassium levels (A). After statin initiation, no further hepatic enzyme monitoring is warranted unless there are signs or symptoms of hepatic dysfunction.

121. Correct: C. decrease in TG level

Fibrates are not preferred over statins for lowering LDL-C but are recommended for the treatment of hypertriglyceridemia, as these agents can result in a 20% to 50% reduction (C).

Incorrect:

The use of fibrates will result in only a mild or modest decrease in LDL or VLDL levels and are not preferred for this purpose (A, D). In addition to decreasing TG levels, the use of fibrates can result in an increase in HDL levels (B).

122. Correct: A. marked decrease in LDL level

PCSK9 inhibitors are the newest class of agents approved to reduce LDL levels in patients with an inadequate response to statin treatment (A). The use of these agents in combination with a statin can result in an additional 60% reduction in LDL compared to statin alone.

Incorrect:

PCSK9 inhibitors are used with the goal of reducing LDL level. These agents when used with a statin will not cause a marked reduction in HDL level (B) or an increase in TGs (C). The addition of a PCSK9 inhibitor to a statin regimen will result in a marked reduction in LDL (D).

123. Correct: C. a lack of evidence demonstrating improvement in cardiovascular outcomes with these agents.

Statins are the recommended first-line treatment option for reduction of LDL cholesterol. Though bile acid sequestrants and niacin have been recommended in the past for the treatment of dyslipidemia, these agents are no longer favored, as there is a lack of clinical evidence demonstrating a beneficial effect of these agents on cardiovascular outcomes (C).

Incorrect:

Bile acid sequestrants are not systemically absorbed and are not typically associated with systemic adverse effects. These agents are most frequently associated with GI adverse effects, such as GI distress, constipation, and flatulence. Niacin is associated with a high incidence of flushing, but this can be minimized with the use of aspirin prior to dosing (A). Bile acid sequestrants and niacin are fairly inexpensive (B) and can result in substantial reduction in LDL (up to 25% to 30%) (D), though there is a lack of clinical evidence demonstrating beneficial cardiovascular outcomes.

124. Correct: B. a reduction in LDL cholesterol.

Ezetimibe is a selective cholesterol absorption inhibitor that is often used in combination with statin therapy to further reduce LDL levels, typically by an additional 15% to 20% (B).

Incorrect:

The addition of ezetimibe to statin therapy might cause a small increase in HDL (3% to 5%), but not a marked increase (A). As a selective cholesterol absorption inhibitor, ezetimibe does not have a significant impact on TG levels (C). The use of ezetimibe will not increase the risk of rhabdomyolysis, which is a rare occurrence with the use of high doses of statins in certain patient populations, such as the elderly (D).

125. Correct: D. No special laboratory monitoring is recommended.

There is very little systemic absorption of ezetimibe; thus, it has a low incidence of adverse effects. Therefore, there is no special laboratory monitoring needed with its use (D).

Incorrect:

Ezetimibe is not associated with any significant systemic adverse effects and, thus, would not require monitoring for ALP (A), LDH (B), or CPK (C).

126. Correct: C. add a PCSK9 inhibitor.

For a patient with a history of ASCVD and who cannot attain LDL goal with statin therapy, the next best option is to add a PCSK9 inhibitor (C). These agents have been demonstrated to reduce the LDL level by up to 60% in patients already receiving dose-optimized statin therapy.

Incorrect:

For a patient already receiving high-intensity statin therapy, switching to another statin will likely not result in any significant improvement in LDL level (B). The addition of niacin will likely result in a small decrease in LDL and is no longer recommended for LDL reduction but can be considered to reduce TGs (A). Fibrates are generally not recommended with high-dose statin therapy due to a risk of myalgia and rhabdomyolysis (D).

127. Correct: B. concomitant use of ezetimibe.

The use of statins is associated with myositis that can result in muscle aches and weakness. In rare circumstances, rhabdomyolysis can occur. The condition is more common with high statin doses, particularly when used in combination with a fibrate. However, the addition of ezetimibe to statin therapy does not increase the risk of myositis (B).

Incorrect:

Risk factors for statin-induced myositis include advanced age (A), high-intensity statin therapy (D), renal impairment, low body weight (C), and concomitant use of a fibrate.

128. Correct: B. 5% to 10%

Lifestyle modifications can be an important aspect of managing dyslipidemia and are an important first-line management approach for individuals with borderline or slightly elevated LDL level. However, modification in diet will usually only have a modest effect in reducing LDL level, typically by as much as 5% to 10% (B). For individuals requiring greater reduction in LDL, pharmacotherapy will be needed, typically with a statin.

Incorrect:

Anticipated LDL reduction from lifestyle modifications is normally in the range of 5% to 10% (A). Pharmacotherapy, such as statin therapy, will be required if a greater LDL reduction is needed (C, D).

129. Correct: A. antiplatelet effect

Prescription-strength omega-3 fatty acid is recommended for lowering TG levels. However, the use of this agent is associated with a modest antiplatelet effect and should be used with caution when taken concomitantly with other antiplatelet medications, such as aspirin or clopidogrel (A). Dietary

supplements of omega-3 fatty acid are not recommended for lowering TG levels.
Incorrect:
Omega-3 fatty acid is not associated with a drug-induced cough (B), immune suppression (C), or hyperglycemia (D).

130. **Correct: B. rosuvastatin 20 mg**
A high-intensity statin therapy can include rosuvastatin 20 mg (B) or atorvastatin 40 to 80 mg.
Incorrect:
Moderate-intensity statin treatments can include pravastatin 40 mg (A) or simvastatin 40 mg (C). Lovastatin 20 mg is a low-intensity statin therapy (D).

131. **Correct: A. simvastatin 10 mg**
Simvastatin 10 mg is a low-intensity statin therapy that will result in about 28% reduction of LDL on average (A).
Incorrect:
Rosuvastatin 5 mg (B), atorvastatin 10 mg (C), and pravastatin 40 mg (D) are all moderate-intensity statin treatments that will result in an approximate 30% to 50% reduction in LDL levels on average.

132. **Correct: C. increased LDL, TC, and TGs**
Hyperlipidemia can be caused by several factors, including lifestyle factors (e.g., high-fat diet and limited physical activity), genetics, certain medications, and comorbid conditions, such as untreated hypothyroidism and DM. Untreated hypothyroidism is associated with elevated levels of LDL, TC, and TGs (C). Proper management of hyperlipidemia in these patients will require appropriate treatment of hypothyroidism along with lipid management.

133. **Correct: A. increases HDL, lowers VLDL and TGs**
Regular aerobic exercise can be an important lifestyle modification to help manage dyslipidemia. Recommendations include aerobic exercise for at least 5 days per week for 30 minutes (150 minutes or more each week) with no more than 48 hours without exercise. Anticipated effects of regular aerobic exercise will include an increase in HDL level and decreases in VLDL and TGs (A).

134. **Correct: D. decrease in TGs.**
Prescription omega-3 oil is recommended for the treatment of hypertriglyceridemia (greater than 500 mg/dL [5.6 mmol/L]) at a dose of 2 to 4 g per day. Dietary supplements of fish oil are not generally recommended and not FDA-approved for the treatment of hypertriglyceridemia.
Incorrect:
Omega-3 oil can result in a negligible increase in HDL, but only by 1% to 5% on average (A). Omega-3 oil will not substantially decrease LDL (B) or TC levels (C) and should not be used for this purpose.

135. **Correct: B. decrease in LDL.**
Plant stanols or sterols, also called phytosterols, are plant-derived products that are sometimes used to decrease LDL. These products have a similar structure as cholesterol and compete with cholesterol for absorption in the digestive system. Consuming phytosterols at recommended doses can reduce LDL levels by up to 14% (B). For those with dyslipidemia, the recommended daily dose is 2 grams per day, which can be consumed with dietary supplements, with food supplements with plant sterol or stanol (e.g., Benecol® spread, Minute Maid® Heart Wise orange juice, Promise Activ™ spread, etc.), or by eating foods high in phytosterols, including vegetable oil, nuts, legumes, whole grains, fruits, and vegetables.
Incorrect:
The greatest effect of plant stanols and sterols is in reducing LDL. These products will have less if any effect in increasing HDL (A) or decreasing select lipoprotein subfractions (C) or TGs (D).

136. **Correct: B. 1 g**
EPA is an omega-3 fatty acid found in fatty fish and has been shown to be effective in reducing TG levels. The AHA recommends that those with coronary heart disease consume 1 g of EPA daily, preferably from oily fish (B). For the treatment of hypertriglyceridemia, AACE recommends prescription omega-3 oil at a dose of 2 to 4 g daily.

137. **Correct: B. atorvastatin 10 mg**
Moderate-intensity statin therapy will result in approximately 30% to 50% reduction in LDL level on average. Atorvastatin 10 mg daily will reduce LDL levels by approximately 38% (B).
Incorrect:
Low-intensity statin therapy will result in less than a 30% reduction in LDL level on average and can include simvastatin 10 mg (C), fluvastatin 20 mg (A), or pravastatin 20 mg (D).

Select Adrenal Disorders

138. **Correct: D. folate.**
Evaluation for Addison's disease can involve laboratory testing along with an ACTH stimulation test for confirmation. However, folate is not a test warranted in the evaluation for this condition (D).
Incorrect:
Addison's disease is characterized by a decrease in the production of mineralocorticoid hormones and cortisol. Mineralocorticoid hormones produced by the adrenal glands, such as aldosterone, are involved in the regulation of sodium and potassium. Laboratory evaluation for Addison's disease can involve checking the levels of sodium (A), potassium (B), and cortisol (C).

139. **Correct: B. maintaining thyroid function.**
Cortisol is a glucocorticoid produced by the adrenal glands that serves a variety of functions in the body. However, it does not have a role in maintaining thyroid function (B), which is typically controlled by TSH produced in the pituitary gland.

Incorrect:
Some functions of cortisol include maintaining glucose control (A), suppressing the immune response (C), and helping the body respond to stress (D).

140. **Correct: B. aldosterone**
Mineralocorticoids are involved in the regulation of salt balance in the body. Aldosterone is a mineralocorticoid hormone produced by the adrenal gland and is involved in sodium and potassium balance (B).
Incorrect:
Cortisol is a glucocorticoid hormone (A). Hydrocortisone is the name of cortisol when it is supplied as a medication (D). Insulin is an anabolic hormone produced by beta cells in the pancreas and is involved in the maintenance of blood glucose levels (C).

141. **Correct: A. pituitary gland.**
Primary adrenal insufficiency occurs when the adrenal gland is damaged, resulting in decreased levels of adrenal hormones. Secondary adrenal insufficiency occurs when the pituitary gland is damaged or diseased, thereby lowering its production of ACTH, a hormone needed to stimulate hormone production by the adrenal cortex (A).
Incorrect:
The thyroid (B), pancreatic beta cells (C), or hypothalamus (D) are not involved in the development of secondary adrenal insufficiency.

142. **Correct: D. hydrocortisone.**
During an acute adrenal or addisonian crisis, severe signs and symptoms can appear rapidly and lead to loss of consciousness. An immediate injection of hydrocortisone is the recommended treatment (D) to boost cortisol levels in the body. Supportive treatment for hypoglycemia and hypotension should also be provided.
Incorrect:
Treatment to increase cortisol levels is the recommended immediate treatment during an addisonian crisis. Epinephrine (A), insulin (B), and adrenaline (C) are not warranted in the treatment of this condition.

143. **Correct: C. ensuring an ample amount of sodium is ingested.**
Management of Addison's disease involves corticosteroid replacement therapy with a combination of oral glucocorticoids and mineralocorticoids. For those who exercise, the individual should ensure an adequate amount of sodium is ingested (C).
Incorrect:
Individuals with Addison's disease do not need to limit exercise when managed appropriately (A, B). For Addison's disease, oral treatment is preferred over injection except in cases where the individual is vomiting or cannot retain oral medications (D).

144. **Correct: B. Cushing's syndrome.**
This patient presents with the classic signs of Cushing's syndrome (B), including progressive weight gain, fatigue, muscle weakness, hirsutism, and difficulty concentrating. Her repeated use of prednisone also supports this diagnosis.
Incorrect:
Cushing's syndrome can increase the risk of T2DM. However, T2DM by itself will not cause many of the signs and symptoms presented by this patient (A). Though the patient may present with central obesity (though this is not specifically described), this does not offer a diagnosis for the cause of progressive weight gain (D). The cause of her condition is likely related to the prolonged and repeated use of corticosteroids rather than to a benign tumor of the pituitary gland, which is required for a diagnosis of Cushing's disease (C).

145. **Correct: C. cortisol.**
Cushing's syndrome is the result of an excessive production of cortisol from the adrenal gland (C). This most likely results from long-term use of high-dose corticosteroids. The classic signs include progressive weight gain, particularly around the midsection and upper back, in the face, and between the shoulders.
Incorrect:
Cushing's syndrome is the result of excessive cortisol production. Excessive production of luteinizing hormone (A) and follicle-stimulating hormone (B) can be the result of an imbalance related to the reproductive system that is often genetic in nature. Excessive aldosterone production by the adrenal gland can result in imbalances of sodium and potassium (D).

146. **Correct: A. gradually tapering corticosteroid use.**
For a patient with Cushing's syndrome related to long-term corticosteroid therapy, first-line treatment is designed to decrease the level of cortisol in the body. The best approach would be to gradually taper the dose of corticosteroids (A). Abrupt discontinuation should be avoided as this can lead to adrenal crisis.
Incorrect:
Surgery is an option for Cushing's disease where the source of excessive cortisol production is a benign tumor of the pituitary gland (B). Radiation therapy can also be considered with surgery for Cushing's disease, but not for Cushing's syndrome caused by an exogenous source (i.e., corticosteroid use) (C). For those with Cushing's disease who failed surgery or when surgery is not an option, mifepristone can be used to block the effects of cortisol on tissue (D).

147. **Correct: A. rheumatoid arthritis.**
Rheumatoid arthritis is an autoimmune disease that is not related to the presence of Cushing's syndrome (A).
Incorrect:
Untreated Cushing's syndrome can increase the risk of several conditions, including cardiovascular events, infection, hypertension (B), osteoporosis (D), T2DM (C), and loss of muscle mass.

148. Correct: C. a benign pituitary tumor.

Cushing's disease is specific to the development of Cushing's syndrome caused by a benign tumor of the pituitary gland that overproduces ACTH (C).

Incorrect:

Excessive cortisol production can be caused by a benign tumor of the adrenal gland that overproduces cortisol (B), or an ectopic tumor that produces ACTH, which signals excessive production of cortisol in the adrenal gland (D). However, these are not specific to Cushing's disease, which is caused by a benign tumor of the pituitary gland. Long-term exposure of corticosteroids can result in Cushing's syndrome but not Cushing's disease (A).

149. Correct: D. surgical intervention.

Cushing's disease is caused by a benign tumor of the pituitary gland. In these cases, surgery is the main intervention for treatment, with or without radiation therapy (D).

Incorrect:

Cushing's disease is caused by a benign tumor and not corticosteroid therapy (A) or other trigger medications (B). The tumor causing Cushing's disease is benign, and thus, antineoplastic therapy is not warranted (C).

Abnormal Uterine Bleeding

150. Correct: C. PCOS

The PALM-COEIN classification system for AUB was developed to use standardized terminology for the various etiologies of AUB. The classification system divides the etiologies into those related to uterine structural abnormalities and those not related to uterine structural abnormalities. The PALM components are related to structural causes of AUB but do not contain PCOS (C). Those with PCOS can present with similar characteristics of AUB, including irregular menses.

Incorrect:

Structural causes of AUB include polyp, adenomyosis (B), leiomyoma (D), and malignancy (A) and hyperplasia.

151. Correct: B. neoplasia

Nonstructural causes identified in the PALM-COEIN classification system for AUB do not include neoplasia (B). Malignancy and hyperplasia are included in the structural causes of AUB.

Incorrect:

Nonstructural causes of AUB that comprise the COEIN component of the classification system include coagulopathy (C), ovulatory dysfunction (A), endometrial (D), iatrogenic, and not yet classified causes.

152. Correct: C. creatine kinase.

An evaluation of creatine kinase measures muscle damage as the enzyme is released from damaged tissue. AUB is not associated with muscle damage; thus, creatine kinase would not be a useful test to perform in these patients (C).

Incorrect:

Liver function tests are useful in detecting hepatic dysfunction that can impact estrogen metabolism or the availability of coagulation components (A). A Pap test is useful in detecting possible uterine malignancy or hyperplasia (B). Hemoglobin and hematocrit will be needed to determine the presence of anemia that can result from acute and chronic blood loss (D).

153. Correct: D. copper-containing IUD

Hormone therapy is typically the first-line approach for the treatment of AUB. A copper-containing IUD is a nonhormonal contraceptive that would not be effective for the treatment of AUB (D).

Incorrect:

Medical intervention is preferred over surgery for the treatment of AUB with hormonal therapy recommended as first-line treatment. Hormonal therapy options can include IV conjugated equine estrogen, low-dose COC (A), oral progestin (C), or levonorgestrel IUD (B).

Renal and Urinary Tract Disorders

13

Acute Kidney Injury and Chronic Kidney Disease

Overview

Kidney disease is the ninth leading cause of death in the United States, and renal failure can be either acute or chronic. In either case, deterioration of renal function can cause an accumulation of toxic wastes and disrupt the body's homeostasis. Diminished renal function is a normal age-related process; thus, chronic kidney disease (CKD) is more prevalent among the elderly. However, other factors can also lead to acute or more progressive kidney dysfunction. A healthy kidney contains about 1 million nephrons where each contributes to the glomerular filtration rate (GFR); other functions include tubular reabsorption and secretion. Damage to a portion of nephrons can be made up by the healthy nephrons; thus, signs and symptoms are not evident during early stages of disease. A measurable increase in urea and creatinine will be observed once the GFR decreases by about 50%.

ACUTE KIDNEY INJURY

Overview

Acute kidney injury (AKI), formerly called acute renal failure, is characterized by an abrupt change and rapid decline in renal function.

The most common reason for AKI is prerenal in nature, where the kidneys are hypoperfused. Reasons for this hypoperfusion include decreased circulating volume, as seen in patients with dehydration (e.g., due to vomiting or diarrhea), overdiuresis, and acute blood loss. Other common reasons include decreased cardiac output, as seen in patients with heart failure, or excessive sequestering of fluid, as seen in patients with burns. When AKI is triggered by a prerenal problem, the underlying renal function is often normal, and renal function returns to baseline when the underlying cause is addressed. At the same time, AKI can also be seen in patients with underlying CKD, wherein baseline renal function is compromised but suddenly worsens when the AKI risk factor is superimposed.

Prerenal AKI can often lead to intrinsic AKI if the underlying condition is not corrected in a timely manner. In intrinsic AKI, there is disease within the kidney at the levels of the renal tubules, glomeruli, interstitium, or vessels. Etiologies include glomerulonephritis and acute interstitial nephritis. Vascular causes of intrinsic AKI include renal artery or vein obstruction, microangiopathy, malignant hypertension, and atheroembolic disease. Certain medications can also cause damage to the renal tubules and interstitium, including aminoglycosides, lithium, amphotericin B, penicillins, cephalosporins, NSAIDs, proton pump inhibitors, mesalamine, and sulfonamides.

When AKI is postrenal in origin, azotemia and resulting deterioration of renal function are caused by obstruction to urine flow; this is an uncommon cause of AKI. Causes of postrenal AKI can include prostatic hypertrophy; obstructing kidney stone; obstructing prostate; cervical, bladder, or colorectal cancer; or another cause resulting in retention of urine into the renal pelvis.

Clinical Presentation

Signs of AKI can be similar to those of CKD, though they occur over a shorter time period (within days versus over a period of months) and can include fatigue, weight loss, anorexia, nocturia, sleep disturbance, and pruritus. Presentation will also depend on the type of AKI (i.e., prerenal, intrinsic, or postrenal failure). Those with prerenal failure often can present with thirst, diminished urine output, dizziness, and orthostatic hypotension. Additional findings are usually consistent with the underlying cause. Intrinsic renal failure can be accompanied with hematuria, edema, and hypertension. Postrenal failure, such as caused by obstruction, can include signs of urgency, frequency, and hesitancy, while flank pain and hematuria are noted when AKI is caused by obstructing renal stones.

Diagnostic Testing

The most commonly obtained tests of renal function include serum creatinine (SCr) along with calculated estimated glomerular filtration rate (eGFR) and blood urea nitrogen (BUN). Creatinine is the end product of creatine metabolism, which arises from skeletal muscle. Because creatinine excretion by a healthy kidney is efficient, measurement of creatinine is used as a surrogate marker of kidney function; creatinine production equals creatinine excretion. With decreased renal function, whatever the cause, SCr increases. When the SCr level doubles, the GFR is considered to have been halved; when SCr increases threefold, the GFR is decreased by 75%. In cases of AKI, the eGFR equation is not as accurate since kidney function is not at a steady state.

With AKI, renal ultrasound or a computed tomography (CT) scan (without contrast) of the abdomen and pelvis can be used to rule in or out outflow tract blockade, particularly if the condition is considered postrenal in origin. The quality of ultrasound images can be limited for individuals who are obese as well as those with abdominal distension or retroperitoneal fluid collection. In particular, a bladder scan is helpful when AKI is noted in an otherwise well older man with known benign prostatic hyperplasia (BPH) who reports new-onset difficulty in bladder emptying.

Treatment

In AKI, treatment is aimed at the correction of underlying, precipitating cause(s). In the outpatient/primary care setting, AKI treatment, no matter its origin, often involves referral for inpatient treatment. Expert consultation in the management of the contributing causes is warranted.

Given the majority (approximately 70%) of AKI is prerenal in origin, circulating volume management is key to treatment. When AKI is postrenal in origin, prompt relief of the urinary tract obstruction is indicated. The most common examples include urinary catherization if obstructive BPH is the trigger, or prompt referral to urology for treatment of the obstructing kidney stone.

CHRONIC KIDNEY DISEASE

Overview

CKD is characterized by a gradual loss of renal function over time, usually months to years. Common causes of CKD, also known as chronic renal failure (CRF), include type 1 (T1DM) or type 2 diabetes mellitus (T2DM), hypertension, cardiovascular disease, increasing age (older than 60 years), history of AKI, obesity, family history of CKD, and member of higher-risk ethnic groups including Native American, African American, and Latino. In African Americans, hypertension and T2DM are the most potent CKD risk factors. CKD is more common in individuals whose contributing conditions have been inadequately controlled for a sustained period of time.

Clinical Presentation

In CKD, clinical presentation differs with its stage. With stages 1 through 3 CKD, when eGFR is greater than 30 mL/min/1.73 m², the patient is usually without specific signs or symptoms. In stages 4 and 5, due to anemia and worsening renal failure, and commonly found comorbidities including heart failure and other cardiovascular conditions, nonspecific signs and symptoms usually include fatigue, lower extremity or diffuse edema, and/or shortness of breath. Urine output is often decreased, and urine becomes foamy with altered color.

Diagnostic Testing

Similar to AKI, measurements of SCr, eGFR, and BUN are important to evaluate renal function. For CKD, the eGFR provides a more accurate assessment of kidney function than SCr alone. The eGFR also decreases with aging due to normal age-related changes in the kidney. This decreased kidney function among older adults also contributes to the higher incidence of CKD among the elderly in the presence of other chronic medical conditions, such as T2DM, hypertension, and dyslipidemia.

BUN is derived from the breakdown of protein from dietary or other sources. The BUN level typically increases (uremia) more rapidly than the creatinine level in response to decreased renal perfusion and can increase from prerenal, renal, and postrenal causes of kidney failure. Upper gastrointestinal (GI) bleeding usually causes a marked increase in BUN level without a corresponding increase in creatinine as the gut digests and absorbs proteins found in the blood.

In addition to eGFR, quantification of albuminuria can also provide an accurate assessment of CKD. A spot albumin-to-creatinine ratio (ACR) provides a more sensitive and specific indicator for CKD than protein-to-creatinine ratio, as ACR is able to detect lower levels of proteinuria. Though small amounts of albumin in the urine were once thought to be a clinically insignificant finding, this is now recognized as an important renal function prognostic factor. An ACR of 30 to 299 mg/g is considered moderately elevated, while values greater than 300 mg/g are considered severely elevated, typically requiring referral to a nephrologist (Table 13-1).

CKD is classified into five stages based on eGFR (see Table 13-1):

■ *CKD stages 1 through 3*: Electrolytes are usually normal and water balance is not disturbed.
■ *CKD stages 4 and 5*: Likely to develop serious complications of CKD, including hypertension, cardiovascular disease, and anemia of chronic disease (resulting from reduced erythropoietin production seen in chronically impaired renal function).

TABLE 13-1 Staging and Management of Chronic Kidney Disease (CKD)

■ All patients with CKD are at increased risk of cardiovascular disease.
  • Nearly all are candidates for lipid-lowering therapy.
  • Add aspirin therapy (for secondary prevention unless bleeding risk outweighs benefits).
■ Ensure vaccinations are up to date, especially influenza and pneumococcal immunizations.

CKD STAGING

CKD Stage by eGFR (mL/min/1.73 m^2)
■ eGFR 90 or greater = stage 1 (normal or high)
■ eGFR 60 to 89 = stage 2
■ eGFR 45 to 59 = stage 3a
■ eGFR 30 to 44 = stage 3b
■ eGFR 15 to 29 = stage 4
■ eGFR less than 15 = stage 5 (kidney failure)

CKD Stage by albumin-to-creatinine (ACR) ratio (mg/g)
■ ACR less than 30 = normal or mildly elevated
■ ACR 30 to 299 = moderately elevated
■ ACR greater than 300 = severely elevated

PATIENT SAFETY CONSIDERATIONS

eGFR less than 60–Patient safety risk
■ Consider eGFR for drug dosing
■ Reduce risk of AKI volume depletion
■ Use measures to prevent contrast-induced AKI

eGFR 45 to less than 60
■ Avoid prolonged NSAID use
■ Continue metformin use

GFR 30 to less than 45
■ Avoid prolonged NSAID use.
■ With metformin use, monitor closely for worsening renal function, prescribe at approximately 50% of recommended dose if no other contraindications to its use. 50% dose

eGFR less than 30
■ Avoid the use of NSAIDs, bisphosphonates, metformin, others

CKD PROGRESSION AND COMPLICATIONS

Hypertension
■ Blood pressure goal less than 130 to 140/80 to 90 mm Hg
  • Consider BP goal of less than 130/80 if ACR greater than 300 mg/g

Diabetes mellitus
■ Target HbA1C 7% or less unless otherwise contraindicated

CKD complications testing
■ Evaluate for anemia
  • Hb less than 13 g/dL for men and less than 12 g/dL for women

Nephrology referral (if not already done)
■ eGFR less than 30 or ACR greater than 300 mg/g
■ 25% decrease in eGFR
■ Persistent hyperkalemia/metabolic acidosis
■ Others

ACR, albumin-to-creatinine ratio; AKI, acute kidney injury; CKD, chronic kidney disease; eGFR, estimated glomerular filtration rate.

Adapted from Vassalotti JA, Centor R, Turner BJ, et al. Practical approach to detection and management of chronic kidney disease for the primary care clinician. Am J Med. 2016;129(2):153-162.e7.

Evaluation of patients at stage 4 or above should include measurements of serum calcium, phosphorus, parathyroid hormone, alkaline phosphatase, and 25-hydroxyvitamin D levels. For those at stage 5 (eGFR less than 15 mL/min) or end-stage renal disease, the kidneys have lost nearly all of their ability to perform, and the person will likely die within a relatively short period of time as a result of the renal impairment or require dialysis or transplantation for survival.

Anemia is often seen in patients with CRF. Erythropoietin, a glycoprotein growth factor produced primarily by the kidneys, is normally released in the bloodstream and binds with receptors in the bone marrow to stimulate the production of erythrocytes (red blood cells [RBCs]). With end-stage renal disease, erythropoietin response is reduced because of limited supply; that is, as the kidney fails, erythropoietin production declines. In addition, as is common in chronic illness, the RBC life span is shortened. These factors result in a normocytic, normochromic anemia with reticulocytopenia, representing a form of anemia of chronic disease.

Since the kidneys play an important role in maintaining homeostasis, CKD and AKI can lead to imbalances of fluid, electrolytes, and acid-base balance. Electrolyte disorders commonly associated with AKI and advanced CKD (particularly stages 4 and 5) include hyperkalemia, hypercalcemia, and hypernatremia. Laboratory assessment should include measurements of serum electrolytes as well as fasting lipids, A1c, and ACR.

Treatment

In CKD, treatment is aimed at minimizing the contributing factors to its development. For example, when CKD is associated with T2DM, hypertension, and dyslipidemia, a critical part of therapy is to enhance control of these conditions to recommended treatment goals to help preserve remaining renal function. By stage 3 CKD, input should be sought as part of managing risk factors, and electrolyte and hematological derangements. Dialysis, also known as renal replacement therapy, and possibly kidney transplantation should be considered for those approaching stage 4 (eGFR = 15 to 29 mL/min) who have advanced kidney damage and are candidates for these interventions; this decision is based on a number of factors and requires expert consultation with a nephrologist.

Discussion Sources

Gaitonde DY, Cook DL, Rivera IM. Chronic kidney disease: detection and evaluation. *Am Fam Physician.* 2017;96:776–783.

Kliger AS, Foley RN, Goldfarb DS, et al. KDOQI US commentary on the 2012 KDIGO clinical practice guideline for anemia in CKD. *Am J Kidney Dis.* 2013;62:849–859. http://www.sciencedirect.com/science/article/pii/S0272638613009785

National Kidney Foundation Kidney Disease Outcomes Quality Initiative (NKF KDOQI). https://www.kidney.org/professionals/guidelines

Vassolott JA, Centor R, Turner BJ, et al. Practical approach to detection and management of chronic kidney disease for the primary care clinician. *Am J Med.* 2016;129:153–162.

QUESTIONS

1. All of the following electrolyte disorders are commonly found in a person with CKD except:

   A. hypernatremia.

   B. hypercalcemia.

   C. hyperkalemia.

   D. hypophosphatemia.

2. All of the following are common precipitating factors in AKI except:

   A. acute hypotension.

   B. sepsis.

   C. hypovolemia.

   D. T1DM.

3. Common causes of CKD include all of the following except:

   A. T2DM.

   B. prior history of AKI.

   C. hypotension.

   D. cardiovascular disease.

4. The use of which of the following medications can precipitate AKI in a patient with bilateral renal artery stenosis?

   A. corticosteroids

   B. angiotensin II receptor antagonists

   C. β-adrenergic antagonists

   D. aminoglycosides

5. A 78-year-old man of Asian ancestry presents with a 2-week history of increasing fatigue and difficulty with bladder emptying. Examination reveals a distended bladder but is otherwise unremarkable. The BUN is 88 mg/dL (31.4 mmol/L); SCr is 2.8 mg/dL (247.5 μmol/L); eGFR is 21 mL/min/1.73 m². Two months ago, his SCr was 1.4 mg/dL and eGFR was 48 mL/min/1.73 m². This clinical assessment is most consistent with:

   A. prerenal azotemia.

   B. acute glomerulonephritis.

   C. acute tubular necrosis.

   D. postrenal AKI.

6. You see a 68-year-old woman with a history of hypertension, T2DM, and dyslipidemia for 20 years. She has a history of an acute coronary syndrome event occurring 2 years ago resulting in heart failure with reduced left ventricular ejection fraction. Her eGFR has held steady at around 42 mL/min/1.73 m². Today she presents with no symptoms, an eGFR of 44 mL/min/1.73 m², SCr of 1.3 mg/dL, and BUN of 24 mg/dL. How would you best categorize her kidney disease?

   A. prerenal AKI

   B. intrinsic AKI

   C. postrenal AKI

   D. CKD

7. The patient in the previous question experiences an exacerbation of heart failure. Today, her blood pressure is 90/68 mm Hg, BUN is 58 mg/dL (20.7 mmol/L), and SCr is 2.4 mg/dL (212.1 μmol/L), and eGFR is 20 mL/min/1.73 m². These changes are most likely caused by:

   A. prerenal AKI.

   B. intrinsic AKI.

   C. postrenal AKI.

   D. CKD.

8. Which of the following is found early in the development of CKD?

   A. persistent proteinuria

   B. anemia

   C. acute uremia

   D. hyperkalemia

9. You see a 63-year-old man with a documented acute upper GI bleed with a resulting 9% drop in hematocrit. He has no renal health issues, and a baseline GFR is within acceptable range for age. Expected laboratory findings would include:

   A. elevated BUN; elevated SCr.

   B. normal BUN; elevated SCr.

   C. elevated BUN; normal SCr.

   D. lowered BUN; elevated SCr.

10. Angiotensin-converting enzyme inhibitors (ACEIs) or angiotensin receptor blockers (ARBs) can limit the progression of some forms of renal disease by:

    A. increasing intraglomerular pressure.

    B. reducing efferent arteriolar resistance.

    C. enhancing afferent arteriolar tone.

    D. increasing urinary protein excretion.

11. Objective findings in patients with glomerulonephritis include all of the following except:

    A. edema.

    B. urinary RBC casts.

    C. proteinuria.

    D. hypotension.

12. A doubling of SCr is typically seen with a GFR reduction of _____.

    A. 25%

    B. 50%

    C. 75%

    D. 100%

13. Creatinine clearance usually:

    A. approximates GFR.

    B. does not change as part of normative aging.

    C. is greater in women compared with men.

    D. increases with hypotension.

14. Creatinine is best described as:

    A. a substance produced by the kidney.

    B. a product related to skeletal muscle metabolism.

    C. produced by the liver and filtered by the kidney.

    D. a by-product of protein metabolism.

15. A referral to a nephrologist should be considered with an ACR of:

    A. less than 1 mg/g.

    B. less than 10 mg/g.

    C. greater than 50 mg/g.

    D. greater than 300 mg/g.

16. Guidelines recommend considering initiating treatment with an erythropoiesis-stimulating agent (ESA) for patients with CRF and a hemoglobin (Hb) level:

    A. less than 8.5 mg/dL.

    B. less than 9 mg/dL.

    C. less than 10 mg/dL.

    D. less than 11.5 mg/dL.

17. Which of the following hemograms would be expected for a 75-year-old woman with stage 4 CKD and related anemia?

    A. Hb = 9.7 g/dL (12 to 14 g/dL); MCV = 69 fL (80 to 96 fL); reticulocytes = 0.8% (1% to 2%).

    B. Hb = 10.2 g/dL (12 to 14 g/dL); MCV = 104 fL (80 to 96 fL); reticulocytes = 1.2% (1% to 2%).

    C. Hb = 9.4 g/dL (12 to 14 g/dL); MCV = 83 fL (80 to 96 fL); reticulocytes = 0.7% (1% to 2%).

    D. Hb = 10.4 g/dL (12 to 14 g/dL); MCV = 94 fL (80 to 96 fL); reticulocytes = 2.6% (1% to 2%).

18. Which of the following is the most likely candidate to initiate dialysis resulting from CKD?

    A. a 46-year-old man with hypertension and eGFR = 42 mL/min/1.73 m^2

    B. a 64-year-old woman with T2DM and eGFR = 28 mL/min/1.73 m^2

    C. a 76-year-old man with anemia and eGFR = 55 mL/min/1.73 m^2

    D. a 58-year-old woman with heart disease and eGFR = 46 mL/min/1.73 m^2

For answers and rationales, see end of chapter.

Glomerulonephritis

Overview

Glomerulonephritis is a condition caused by inflammation of the renal glomeruli. Glomeruli are responsible for removing waste and excess electrolytes and fluid from the bloodstream. Glomerulonephritis can be acute or chronic and is caused by a number of underlying conditions. The acute condition can develop as a result of infection, immune diseases (e.g., lupus, Goodpasture's syndrome, or IgA nephropathy), or vasculitis (e.g., polyarteritis or Wegener's granulomatosis). Poststreptococcal glomerulonephritis can develop 1 to 2 weeks following pharyngitis caused by group A beta-hemolytic streptococcal infection ("strep throat") when an overproduction of antibodies produced from the infection settle in the glomeruli and cause inflammation. Whereas historically, poststreptococcal infection was one of the most common causes of glomerulonephritis, its rate has fallen in developed countries during the past decades. At the same time, poststaphylococcal glomerulonephritis rates have risen. Those with bacterial endocarditis are also at high risk of developing glomerulonephritis, whereas some viral infections have also been implicated (e.g., HIV, hepatitis B or C). If left untreated, glomerulonephritis can lead to kidney failure, high blood pressure, blood electrolyte disorders, and nephrotic syndrome.

Nearly all forms of acute glomerulonephritis have the potential to progress to chronic glomerulonephritis. The condition is the third leading cause of CKD and accounts for about 10% of all patients on dialysis. In many cases, the cause of chronic glomerulonephritis is unclear, though genetics and changes to the immune system can play a role. The chronic condition is often found in young men who are also experiencing hearing and vision loss.

Clinical Presentation

When infection is the trigger, for glomerulonephritis there is usually a lag of a number of weeks between the acute illness, with the infection resolved, and the onset of glomerulonephritis. When an autoimmune condition such as lupus erythematosus is the causal event, the presentation of glomerulonephritis often includes widespread arthralgias and characteristic skin lesions. Other autoimmune conditions include Goodpasture's syndrome and Wegener's granulomatosis. Goodpasture's syndrome is caused by the production of antiglomerular basement membrane antibodies that result in tissue damage to the kidney and lungs. Wegener's granulomatosis (also known as granulomatosis with polyangiitis) is a rare type of vasculitis that limits blood flow to the organs, particularly the kidney.

Regardless of the trigger, the clinical presentation of glomerulonephritis usually includes new-onset edema of the face, hands, feet, and abdomen as well as newly elevated blood pressure or worsening previously present hypertension. With acute glomerulonephritis, regardless of the cause, headache is common, and occasionally shortness of breath is reported, particularly if edema is severe. Urine is reported as being pink or cola-colored due to hematuria; foamy urine is present due to proteinuria.

Diagnostic Testing

Diagnosis involves a urinalysis and blood analysis including SCr and BUN. Urine will typically contain RBCs and RBC casts, as well as white blood cells (WBCs) and elevated levels of protein. Elevated SCr and BUN are typically found and indicate impaired renal function.

Glomerulonephritis can lead to a decline in GFR, though the exact impact can vary considerably among patients, from a rapid, marked decline to a slow progressive decline over years (as seen with chronic glomerulonephritis). Imaging studies, such as a CT scan or kidney ultrasound, can be used to evaluate the status of renal damage. A kidney biopsy is usually needed to confirm the diagnosis.

Treatment

Acute glomerulonephritis is often self-limiting and requires supportive therapy only, though expert consultation is of great importance.

Nephrotic syndrome, where excessive amounts of protein are excreted in the urine, is a serious complication and can lead to infection, thrombus formation, AKI, and death. Renal function, blood pressure, edema, serum albumin, and proteinuria should be closely monitored. Antihypertensive medications can be used to lower blood pressure. Antimicrobials are used if an infection is confirmed or suspected. Systemic corticosteroids can be considered to reduce inflammation (e.g., vasculitis), though the benefits of these agents are unclear. For worsening cases due to an immune disorder, plasmapheresis and immunosuppressive medications can be considered to remove and block production of antibodies as well as remove other toxic proteins from the blood that might be triggering inflammation in the kidney. In cases with associated acute kidney failure, dialysis/renal replacement therapy is sometimes required to remove excess fluid and control high blood pressure. If renal function does not return, dialysis should be continued indefinitely, or renal transplantation can be considered.

Discussion Sources

Couser WG. Pathogenesis and treatment of glomerulonephritis—an update. *J Bras Nefrol*. 2016;38:107–122.

Parmar MS. Acute glomerulonephritis. Medscape. http://emedicine.medscape.com/article/239278-overview

Radhakrishnan J, Cattran DC. The KDIGO practice guideline on glomerulonephritis: reading between the (guide)lines—application to the individual patient. *Kidney Int*. 2012;82:840–856.

QUESTIONS

19. Risk factors for acute glomerulonephritis include all of the following except:

    A. bacterial endocarditis.

    B. Goodpasture's syndrome.

    C. Crohn's disease.

    D. polyarteritis.

20. Poststreptococcal glomerulonephritis typically occurs how long following a bacterial pharyngitis infection?

    A. 4 to 6 days

    B. 1 to 2 weeks

    C. 3 to 4 weeks

    D. 2 months

21. Diagnostic confirmation of glomerulonephritis typically requires:

    A. urinalysis plus a complete blood count (CBC) with WBC differential.

    B. abdominal CT scan.

    C. kidney ultrasound.

    D. kidney biopsy.

22. A 35-year-old man presents with a 4-day history of edema of the face, hands, and ankles along with hypertension (175/115 mm Hg). He reports that he was seen by a health-care provider about 2 months ago and his blood pressure was, "Normal, like it always is." He also describes recent changes in urine, "Looks like dark tea and foams like beer." You suspect acute glomerulonephritis and would expect urinalysis results to include all of the following findings except:

    A. elevated level of protein.

    B. presence of RBCs.

    C. presence of renal casts.

    D. abnormally high glucose levels.

23 to 25. Match each potential cause of glomerulonephritis with the most appropriate treatment option. *(Questions may have more than one answer.)*

_____ **23.** Infective endocarditis

_____ **24.** Vasculitis

_____ **25.** Goodpasture syndrome

    A. systemic corticosteroids

    B. systemic antimicrobials

    C. immunomodulators

    D. plasmapheresis

26. A possible complication of glomerulonephritis is:

    A. T2DM.

    B. nephrotic syndrome.

    C. pyelonephritis.

    D. bladder cancer.

For answers and rationales, see end of chapter.

Urinary Tract Infection

Overview

The urinary tract, adjacent to the bacteria-rich lower GI tract, produces and stores urine. The periurethral area is typically colonized with gut and other flora, some capable of causing urinary tract infection (UTI). Although the process of urination usually flushes bacteria from the urethral orifice, periurethral pathogens occasionally enter the urethra and ascend, reaching the bladder and resulting in UTI. Most UTIs occur via this ascending route. Rarely, hematogenous UTI occurs when a pathogen is delivered to the urinary tract via the bloodstream from a distant source of infection, such as the lungs in a patient with pneumonia and bacteremia. UTIs can involve mucosal tissue and the lower urinary tract (cystitis, most common) or soft tissue and the upper urinary tract (pyelonephritis, relatively uncommon).

Certain factors protect against or increase the risk for UTI. Male gender is recognized as a potent UTI protective factor, in part because of the longer urethral length in men than in women; women with a shorter urethra-to-anus length appear to be at increased UTI risk. In contrast to the periurethral area in women, the male periurethral area does not support bacterial growth. Zinc-rich prostatic secretions are antibacterial, further discouraging pathogens. Factors that alter efficient bladder emptying, such as cystocele, rectocele, and BPH, increase UTI risk.

Multiple factors put a person, particularly a woman, at increased risk for UTI. In either sex, efficient emptying helps prevent urine stagnation and minimizes UTI risk. Exposure to the spermicide nonoxynol-9, either through vaginal use or with a male partner who uses condoms with this spermicide, increases UTI risk, through the spermicide's antibacterial effect, causing a reduction in lactobacilli, a normal component of the periurethral flora. Lactobacilli produce hydrogen peroxide and lactic acid, providing the periurethral area and vagina with a pH that inhibits bacterial growth, blocks potential sites of attachment, and is toxic to uropathogens. In postmenopausal women, estrogen deficiency leads to a marked reduction in lactobacilli colonization in the vaginal-perineal areas; topical estrogen use results in reestablishment of the normal protective flora and a reduction of UTI risk. Recent antimicrobial use potentially increases UTI risk by the same mechanism. UTI risk increases in women with more frequent vaginal intercourse. Women who are nonsecretors of ABO blood group antigens show enhanced adherence of pathogenic *Escherichia coli* to urothelial cells compared with women who are secretors of these antigens.

Factors that predispose older patients to UTIs include the use of urinary catheters and external urine collection devices, as well as age-related conditions that impair bladder emptying. These changes include loss of elasticity of the bladder wall, weakening of the bladder muscles, and blockage of the urethra due to prolapse (women) and enlarged prostate (men). In children and elderly adults, constipation has been noted to contribute to bladder instability and helps encourage UTI development.

Complicated UTI can occur in either the upper or the lower urinary tract but is accompanied by an underlying condition that increases the risk for failing therapy, such as obstruction, urological dysfunction, or multidrug-resistant pathogens. Most episodes of UTI and pyelonephritis are uncomplicated and not accompanied by risk of treatment failure, such as obstruction, urological dysfunction, or a multidrug-resistant uropathogen.

Clinical Presentation

UTI is typically diagnosed by clinical presentation, including history, limited physical examination findings, and urinalysis results. In an otherwise healthy woman with an uncomplicated lower UTI, history of present illness (HPI) usually reveals a complaint of dysuria, often reported as internal discomfort, with urinary frequency and urgency, but without fever or constitutional symptoms.

Back pain, fever, nausea, and vomiting are more often associated with pyelonephritis and, in rare cases, with cystitis. Many patients with pyelonephritis also report lower UTI symptoms. Although vaginal infection and irritation can cause dysuria, most women who have dysuria without vaginal discharge have a UTI, not vaginitis. Other conditions to consider in the presence of dysuria include sexually transmitted infections (STIs; e.g., gonococcal, chlamydial), urethritis, and vaginitis. Examination of discharge from STIs will typically detect a large number of WBCs, while urine will also contain WBCs, but nitrites will be absent. Screening for STIs should be considered when STI risk factors are present, and measures should be implemented to prevent the spread of infection to sexual partners.

UTIs are one of the most common types of infection in the elderly, occurring in both the community and long-term care settings. Symptomatic UTIs in the older adult can include the classic symptoms of dysuria but can also include new-onset urinary incontinence (UI), change in mental status, and/or muscle weakness.

Hemorrhagic cystitis is characterized by large quantities of visible blood in the urine. Its etiology can be bacterial infection or infection with adenovirus types 7, 11, 21, and 35 and influenza A, or it can be a result of radiation, cancer chemotherapy, or certain immunosuppressive medications. The clinical presentation usually depends on its origin; with all causes, irritative voiding symptoms are typically reported. When the disease is infectious in origin, signs and symptoms of infection can also be encountered. Adenovirus is a common cause and is self-limiting in nature. Hemorrhagic cystitis is often confused with glomerulonephritis, but hypertension and abnormal renal function are typically absent in the former.

Acute pyelonephritis is an infection of the renal parenchyma and renal pelvis, caused by ascending cystitis. The condition is most commonly found in women 18 to 40 years old. Irritative voiding symptoms similar to symptoms of cystitis, fever, flank pain, an acutely ill appearance, costovertebral (CVA) tenderness, and pyuria are usually reported; GI upset including vomiting is often noted.

Diagnostic Testing

Urine dipstick testing is commonly done in the inpatient or outpatient setting when UTI is suspected because it is simple and convenient and yields immediate results. Leukocyte esterase, nitrites, protein, and blood are the important features in evaluating for UTI. The presence of leukocyte esterase on a urine dipstick is equivalent to 4 WBCs or more per high-power field (HPF).

Some uropathogens are capable of reducing dietary nitrates in the urine to nitrites; this is an indirect test for bacteriuria. When this finding is coupled with a leukocyte esterase response, the likely offending organism is a gram-negative pathogen (*E coli*, *Proteus* species, *Klebsiella pneumoniae*). The nitrite test result is occasionally falsely negative in UTI with a low colony count or with recently voided or dilute urine. In addition, this test does not detect organisms unable to reduce nitrate to nitrite, such as enterococci, staphylococci, or adenovirus. Small amounts of protein and RBCs can also be positive on dipstick testing in cases of UTI (Table 13-2).

Urine culture is important, especially when diagnosis is unclear or UTI is recurrent. The presence of more than one organism often indicates a contaminated urine specimen, and collection and testing should be repeated. The presence of 10^5 or more colony-forming units (CFUs) per milliliter is the traditional diagnostic indicator for UTI. In the presence of dysuria and other symptoms for UTI, more than 10^2 CFU/mL confirms the diagnosis.

UTIs in younger, otherwise healthy males are fairly uncommon. In these cases, additional diagnostic testing should be considered to identify a potential urinary tract abnormality, such as obstruction, that increases the risk of UTI.

Treatment

Most episodes of community-acquired cystitis in women, the most commonly encountered UTI, are caused by enteric gram-negative rods from the Enterobacteriaceae group, such as *E coli*, *P mirabilis*, and *K pneumoniae*. *Staphylococcus saprophyticus*, a gram-positive organism, and *E coli* account for the majority of cases of cystitis in reproductive-age women.

TABLE 13-2 Common Urinalysis Dipstick Findings in Urinary Tract Infection

FINDING	SIGNIFICANCE	CLINICAL CONSIDERATIONS
Color	Typically pale yellow to colorless	Change in urine color is not synonymous with UTI or disease
Clarity	Typically clear	Pyuria causes urinary turbidity
Odor	Mild characteristic odor	Rancid or ammonia odor in urea-splitting organism (e.g., *Proteus mirabilis*)
SG	Dilute urine: SG ≤1.008 Concentrated urine: SG greater than 1.020	Dilute or concentrated urine can influence results of urine chemical test strip testing
Leukocyte esterase	Test for enzyme present in WBCs	Positive results indicate presence of neutrophils greater than 5 WBCs/HPF, an indicator of UTI, reported sensitivity of 75% to 90%; results not valid in neutropenic patients; decreased sensitivity with increased urinary glucose concentration, high urinary SG, and presence of antimicrobial in urine
Nitrites	Surrogate marker for bacteriuria; presence indicates bacterial reduction of dietary nitrates to nitrites by select gram-negative uropathogens including *E coli, Proteus* spp. Normally absent in sterile urine and infection caused by enterococci, staphylococci	Best done on well-concentrated urine such as first morning void; for nitrites to be present, urine should be held in bladder for 1 hour or more for nitrate-to-nitrite conversion to occur; dietary nitrate intake must be adequate; false-negative result possible with low colony count UTI
Protein	Dipstick testing most sensitive for albumin	Common in febrile response or represents presence of protein-containing substance such as WBCs, bacteria, mucus; in UTI, usually trace to 30 mg/dL (1⁺), seldom ≥100 mg/dL
pH	Average pH 5 to 6 Acid pH 4.5 to 5.5 Alkaline pH 6.5 to 8	If alkaline urine is found in presence of UTI symptoms and positive leukocyte esterase, likely that a urea-splitting organism such as *Proteus* is allowing urea to be split into CO_2 and ammonia, causing increase in urine's normally acid pH
RBCs	Low number of RBCs noted Gross hematuria rare in uncomplicated UTI, but may be present in infection complicated by nephrolithiasis	Microscopic hematuria common with UTI, but not in urethritis or vaginitis

HPF, high-powered field; RBC, red blood cell; SG, specific gravity; UTI, urinary tract infection; WBCs, white blood cells.

Common UTI antimicrobial agents include trimethoprim-sulfamethoxazole (TMP-SMX), nitrofurantoin, fluoroquinolones, and fosfomycin (Table 13-3). In the absence of culture and susceptibility testing, the choice of antimicrobial should be based on the local antibiogram, which provides a profile of local susceptibility testing results of specific bacteria to a range of antimicrobials. Phenazopyridine (Pyridium®) can also be added to antimicrobial therapy to hasten the resolution of dysuria, as this medication exerts an analgesic effect on the mucosa of the urinary tract. However, due to its properties as a dye, its use can interfere with urinalyses that are based on spectrometry or color reactions, including urinary glucose, ketone, nitrates, and leukocytes.

Treatment for pyelonephritis is also focused on coverage of gram-negative pathogens, usually for 5 to 7 days with a fluoroquinolone or 2 weeks with certain other antimicrobials (see Table 13-3). Intact GI function, characterized by lack of vomiting and baseline adequate hydration, is noted in the majority of

TABLE 13-3 Urinary Tract Infection Therapies

TYPE OF INFECTION	USUAL PATHOGENS	REGIMENS
Acute, uncomplicated UTI (cystitis, urethritis) in nonpregnant women	Gram negative: *E coli* (most common), *P mirabilis*, *Klebsiella* spp. Gram positive: *S saprophyticus*	**PRIMARY** If local *E coli* resistance to TMP-SMX less than 20% and no allergy, then TMP-SMX DS 1 tab bid × 3 days; if sulfa allergy, nitrofurantoin 100 mg bid × 5 days or fosfomycin 3 g × one dose. All plus phenazopyridine (Pyridium®). If local *E coli* resistance to TMP-SMX greater than 20% or sulfa allergy, ciprofloxacin (250 mg bid), ciprofloxacin ER (500 mg qd) × 3 days, nitrofurantoin × 5 days or fosfomycin × 1 dose. All plus phenazopyridine (Pyridium®).
Recurrent UTI (3 or more infections in 1 year)	Same as uncomplicated UTI	**PRIMARY** Eradicate organisms, then continuous TMP-SMX 1 SS tablet, or TMP 100 mg, or cephalexin 250 mg, or ciprofloxacin 125 mg (all PO once daily). **ALTERNATIVE** Postcoital: TMP-SMX 1 SS tablet or cephalexin 250 mg or ciprofloxacin 125 mg (all 1 tab PO). For recurrent UTI in postmenopausal women, consider use of estrogen cream; also consider urological factor, such as cystocele, residual urine volume, incontinence.
Acute uncomplicated pyelonephritis suitable for outpatient therapy (Note: Obtain urine and blood cultures before initiating antimicrobial therapy.)	*E coli,* enterococci	**PRIMARY** Ceftriaxone 1 g IV, then (ciprofloxacin 500 mg PO bid, ciprofloxacin ER 1000 mg PO qd, levofloxacin 750 mg PO qd) all for 7 days (levofloxacin 750 mg approved for 5 days). Complicated pyelonephritis requires inpatient management with IV antimicrobial therapy

TMP-SMX, trimethoprim-sulfamethoxazole; UTI, urinary tract infection.

Source: Gilbert DN, Chambers HF, Eliopoulos GM, Saag MS, Pavia AT. The Sanford Guide to Antimicrobial Therapy. 50th ed. Sperryville, VA: Antimicrobial Therapy, Inc.; 2020:34.

patients presenting with uncomplicated pyelonephritis, therefore allowing for outpatient treatment with an oral antibiotic. In this scenario, the use of a parenteral antimicrobial provides no additional benefit.

Although *E coli* is the most common uropathogen in the community and among older adults living in long-term care facilities, *P mirabilis* and *K pneumoniae* account for approximately one-quarter of all infections in this age group. Length of antimicrobial treatment in older adults with uncomplicated UTI should be 7 to 10 days for women and 10 to 14 days for men; short-course therapy is not recommended. First-line therapy includes TMP-SMX or fluoroquinolones; nitrofurantoin should not be used in elderly patients because safe and effective use of the product requires a minimal creatinine clearance of 30 mL/min. In an older adult with impaired renal function, the fluoroquinolone dosage potentially needs adjustment but is considered to be a safe, effective, first-line intervention. TMP-SMX should be used with caution in a person, especially with impaired renal function, who is taking an ACEI or ARB due to the hyperkalemia risk.

Recurrent Urinary Tract Infection and Urinary Tract Infection Prophylaxis

UTI prophylaxis should be considered for women of reproductive age who experience two or more symptomatic UTIs within 6 months or three or more UTIs over 12 months, and for women with fewer infections but with severe discomfort. Continuous prophylaxis with daily TMP-SMX single-strength tablets has been shown to be effective in the management of recurrent uncomplicated cystitis, though other options can be considered (see Table 13-3). Alternatively, prophylaxis with TMP-SMX, cephalexin, or ciprofloxacin can be used postcoitally. Before UTI prophylaxis is initiated, resolution of the previous UTI should be confirmed by a negative urine culture 1 to 2 weeks after treatment. The method prescribed depends on the frequency and pattern of recurrences and on patient preference.

Choice of an antimicrobial agent for recurrent UTI should be based on susceptibility patterns of the strains causing the patient's previous UTIs and on patient history of drug allergies or intolerance. Long-term TMP-SMX or nitrofurantoin therapy has been used successfully for many years. Compared with TMP-SMX, nitrofurantoin has the advantage of lower rates of resistance by the more common UTI pathogens. At the same time, long-term prophylaxis with nitrofurantoin should be used with caution owing to a risk of pulmonary fibrosis. It is important to note that antimicrobial prophylaxis does not appear to change the natural history of recurrences, as most women reestablish their pattern and frequency of UTIs within 6 months of discontinuing prophylaxis.

> **CLINICAL CONCEPT**
>
> UTI prophylaxis in a postmenopausal woman should also include a topical or vaginal estrogen to encourage lactobacilli recolonization in the periurethral area.

Postmenopausal women with recurrent infections should be evaluated for potentially correctable urological factors, including cystocele, incontinence, and an elevated residual urine volume. Though most cases of recurrent UTIs can be managed in the primary care setting, referral to specialists in urology or, less commonly, infectious disease can be considered with complicated UTIs.

Cranberry and blueberry juice or solids intake have been touted as a helpful measure to reduce the rate of recurrent infections. These juices were initially believed to cause high levels of benzoic acid that resulted in urinary acidification and bacteriostatic action. However, additional clinical studies demonstrated that cranberry or blueberry juice is not as effective as initially thought and showed no significant benefit in reducing the occurrence of symptomatic UTIs when compared with placebo, water, or no treatment.

Voiding at regular intervals with efficient bladder emptying, wiping patterns, and postcoital voiding have not been shown to provide UTI protection. Use of hot tubs, wearing pantyhose, douching, and obesity have not been shown to increase UTI risk.

Discussion Sources

Gilbert DN, Chambers HF, Eliopoulos GM, Saag MS, Pavia AT. *The Sanford Guide to Antimicrobial Therapy*. 50th ed. Sperryville, VA: Antimicrobial Therapy, Inc.; 2020:35–36.

Gupta K, Hooton TM, Naber KG, et al. International clinical practice guidelines for the treatment of acute uncomplicated cystitis and pyelonephritis in women: a 2010 update by the Infectious Diseases Society of America and the European Society for Microbiology and Infectious Diseases. *Clin Infect Dis*. 2011;52:e103–e120.

QUESTIONS

27. Which of the following is most likely to be part of the clinical presentation of an otherwise healthy 27-year-old woman with uncomplicated lower UTI?

    A. urinary frequency

    B. fever

    C. suprapubic tenderness

    D. lower GI upset

28. Compared with UTI in younger women, uncomplicated UTI in an elderly woman is more likely to be associated with each of the following signs and symptoms except:

    A. new-onset UI.

    B. delirium.

    C. weakness.

    D. hematuria.

29. A 36-year-old afebrile woman with no health problems presents with dysuria and frequency of urination. Her urinalysis findings include results positive for nitrites and leukocyte esterase. You evaluate these results and consider that she likely has:

    A. purulent vulvovaginitis.

    B. a UTI caused by a gram-negative organism.

    C. cystitis caused by *S saprophyticus*.

    D. urethral syndrome.

30. The most likely causative organism in community-acquired UTI in women during the reproductive years is:

    A. *Klebsiella* species.

    B. *P mirabilis.*

    C. *E coli.*

    D. *S saprophyticus.*

31. You see a 24-year-old man who complains of painful urination, urgency to urinate, and occasional purulent penile discharge. He is without fever or abdominal tenderness. His health history is unremarkable, and he reports a new sexual partner. The most likely diagnosis is:

    A. UTI caused by a gram-positive organism.

    B. pyelonephritis.

    C. gonococcal urethritis.

    D. varicocele.

32. You see a 34-year-old woman with an uncomplicated UTI. She is otherwise healthy but reports having a sulfa allergy, describing the reaction as "breaking out in hives all over and having difficulty breathing." Appropriate first-line therapy includes:

    A. TMP-SMX.

    B. amoxicillin.

    C. azithromycin.

    D. nitrofurantoin.

33. The notation of alkaline urine in a patient with a UTI often points to infection caused by:

    A. *Klebsiella* species.

    B. *P mirabilis.*

    C. *E coli.*

    D. *S saprophyticus.*

34. Which of the following is the most accurate information in caring for a 40-year-old man with cystitis (lower UTI) who is otherwise without chronic health problems?

    A. This is a common condition in men of this age.

    B. A gram-positive organism is the likely causative pathogen.

    C. A urological evaluation should be considered.

    D. Pyuria is rarely found.

35. Evidence-based factors that prevent or minimize the risk of UTIs include all of the following except:

    A. male gender.

    B. longer urethra-to-anus length in women.

    C. timed voiding schedule.

    D. zinc-rich prostatic secretions.

36. In assessing a 24-year-old otherwise well woman who presents with hemorrhagic cystitis, you anticipate encountering which of the following?

    A. patient report of irritative voiding symptoms

    B. persistent microscopic hematuria

C. the presence of new-onset hypertension

D. new onset of elevated creatinine and BUN levels

37. A 44-year-old woman presents with a 3-day history of persistent fever, CVA tenderness, and other findings consistent with pyelonephritis. The report of her urinalysis is least likely to include:

A. WBC casts.

B. positive nitrites.

C. 3+ protein.

D. rare RBCs.

38. An example of a first-line therapeutic agent for the treatment of pyelonephritis in a 35-year-old woman who presents with a 2-day history of back pain with fever and who will be treated as an outpatient is:

A. IM ceftriaxone for 3 days.

B. oral TMP-SMX for 14 days.

C. IM ceftriaxone for one dose plus oral ciprofloxacin for 7 days.

D. IM ceftriaxone for one dose plus oral nitrofurantoin for 5 days.

39. All of the following are normal age-related changes that can increase the risk of UTI in the elderly except:

A. weakened bladder wall muscles.

B. increased elasticity of the bladder.

C. vaginal prolapse in women.

D. enlarged prostate in men.

40. Risk factors for UTI in women include:

A. postvoid wiping back to front.

B. low perivaginal lactobacilli colonization.

C. hot tub use.

D. wearing snug-fitting pantyhose.

41. All of the following can negatively impact perivaginal lactobacilli colonization except:

A. recent antimicrobial use.

B. exposure to the spermicide nonoxynol-9.

C. estrogen deficiency.

D. postcoital voiding.

42. In children and the elderly, which of the following conditions can contribute to bladder instability and increase the risk of a UTI?

A. constipation

B. upper respiratory tract infection

C. chronic diarrhea

D. efficient bladder emptying

43. Which of the following is not a gram-negative organism?

A. *E coli*

B. *K pneumoniae*

C. *P mirabilis*

D. *S saprophyticus*

44. You see a 70-year-old woman in a walk-in clinic with a chief complaint of increased urinary frequency and dysuria. Urinalysis reveals pyuria and positive nitrites. She mentions she has a "bit of kidney trouble, not too bad." Recent evaluation of renal status is unavailable. In considering antimicrobial therapy for this patient, you consider prescribing:

A. nitrofurantoin.

B. fosfomycin.

C. ciprofloxacin.

D. doxycycline.

For answers and rationales, see end of chapter.

Bladder Cancer

Overview

Bladder cancer is the sixth most common type of cancer in the United States and the second most common urological malignancy after prostate cancer. This is usually a disease that occurs later in life—the mean age at diagnosis is 65 years—and it is more common in men. Established risk factors for bladder cancer include cigarette smoking, which accounts for most cases; male gender; family history of bladder cancer; arsenic exposure (mainly occurring outside the United States); and exposure to industrial chemicals, including certain paints, dyes, and solvents. Certain medications, such as the anticancer treatment cyclophosphamide, can also increase the risk for bladder cancer. Primary prevention of bladder cancer through risk reduction is critical.

> **CLINICAL CONCEPT**
> Research is also demonstrating an association of infection by certain human papillomavirus (HPV) types that are associated with other malignancies, such as cervical, anal, and oropharyngeal cancer, with bladder cancer.

Clinical Presentation

Gross painless hematuria, where the patient reports bright to dark red urine without discomfort on voiding, is the most common presenting sign of bladder cancer; persistent microscopic hematuria is the only finding in about 20% of individuals presenting with the disease. Irritative voiding symptoms and urinary frequency without fever are reported occasionally. Abdominal changes, such as a mass that is palpable on examination, are only present with advanced disease.

Diagnostic Testing

The initial test in suspected bladder cancer is a urinalysis, confirming the presence of RBCs in the urine (hematuria). Coupling the patient report of painless gross hematuria with RBCs noted on the urinalysis, particularly in the presence of known bladder cancer risk factors, should prompt referral to urology for further evaluation, including cystoscopy. The diagnosis is usually confirmed by biopsy sample taken via transurethral resection during the cystoscopy for analysis. Cytology can also be used to detect the presence of cancer cells in the urine. With normal urological studies, another diagnosis should be pursued. Other diagnoses to consider in the differential can include UTI, nephrolithiasis, renal cell carcinoma, and ureteral trauma.

Treatment

Most patients with newly diagnosed bladder cancer have superficial disease (non-muscle-invasive bladder cancer). Transurethral resection is used to remove bladder cancers that are confined to the inner lining of the bladder, or a partial cystectomy is occasionally needed to remove the tumor and a small portion of the bladder. Treatment also includes a single immediate instillation of intravesical chemotherapy (e.g., mitomycin C). Subsequent therapy is based on patient risk factors.

Meticulous follow-up in bladder cancer is critical because recurrence is often seen, necessitating repeat procedures. Follow-up can involve urinary cystoscopy and urinary cytology with or without biopsy every 3 to 6 months for 2 years, then at increasing intervals as appropriate. Long-term survival is the norm with the noninvasive form of the disease. With invasive disease, treatment is dictated by type of tumor, degree of invasion, and presence of metastatic disease; long-term survival is based on numerous factors.

Discussion Sources

American Urological Association. Diagnosis, evaluation and follow-up of asymptomatic microhematuria (AMH) in adults: AUA guideline. https://www.auanet.org/education/guidelines/asymptomatic-microhematuria.cfm

Kiragu D, Cifu AS. Evaluation of patients with asymptomatic microhematuria. *JAMA.* 2015;314:1865–1866.

Rodriguez Faba O, Gaya JM, Lopez JM, et al. Current management of non-muscle-invasive bladder cancer. *Minerva Med.* 2013:104:273–286.

Steinberg GD. Bladder cancer. Medscape. https://emedicine.medscape.com/article/438262-overview

QUESTIONS

45. A 72-year-old man with a 35 pack-year smoking history presents with a report of red-tinged urine, stating, "The toilet looks like it is filled with fruit punch after I urinate." Which of the following would be the best approach to confirm a diagnosis of bladder cancer?

   A. urinalysis

   B. cystoscopy with biopsy

   C. abdominal ultrasound

   D. CT scan

46. Which of the following is not a risk factor for bladder cancer?

   A. prolonged occupational exposure to textile dyes

   B. cigarette smoking

   C. occupational exposure to heavy metals

   D. long-term aspirin use

47. A 68-year-old man presents with suspected bladder cancer. You consider that its most common presenting sign or symptom is:

   A. painful urination.

   B. fever and flank pain.

   C. painless gross hematuria.

   D. palpable abdominal mass.

48. In a 70-year-old man diagnosed with superficial bladder cancer without evidence of metastases, you realize that:

   A. the prognosis for 2-year survival is poor.

   B. a cystectomy is indicated.

   C. despite successful initial therapy, local recurrence is common.

   D. systemic chemotherapy is the treatment of choice.

49. Persistent microscopic hematuria would be the primary finding in about ____ % of individuals with bladder cancer.

   A. 10

   B. 20

   C. 30

   D. 40

50. Preferred therapy for non-muscle-invasive bladder cancer without evidence of metastases is:

   A. partial or complete cystectomy.

   B. intravesical chemotherapy as the first-line, solo agent.

   C. transurethral resection with intravesical chemotherapy.

   D. systemic chemotherapy.

For answers and rationales, see end of chapter.

Urinary Incontinence

Overview

UI is the involuntary loss of urine in sufficient amounts to be a problem. This condition is often thought by many women to be a normal part of aging. In reality, numerous treatment options are available after the cause of UI is established (Table 13-4). Certain medications can also exacerbate UI symptoms (Table 13-5).

The most common forms of UI are urge, stress, functional, and transient incontinence. When both urge incontinence and stress incontinence are present, the term mixed UI is used.

> **CLINICAL CONCEPT**
>
> Urge incontinence, also called overactive bladder (OAB), is the most common form of UI in older adults.

Clinical Presentation

A thorough UI history should be taken, documenting duration of the problem, severity, quantity and severity of urine loss episodes, and typical UI pattern. Additional information should be gathered on triggering factors such as coughing, sneezing, lifting, bending, or the sound of running water, among others. Gathering this information will help inform diagnosis and direct treatment.

There are no specific physical examination findings with UI. Occasionally, signs of UI including genital irritation from exposure to urine, urine odor, and evidence of dried drops of urine on footwear are present.

Diagnostic Testing

In all cases, urinalysis and urine culture and susceptibility should be obtained. Further diagnostic testing should be directed by patient presentation. If UTI is present, treatment with the appropriate antimicrobial is indicated. Additional testing, particularly when the etiology of UI is unclear, standard therapy is ineffective, or additional intervention is required, can include cough stress test, measurement of post void residual (PVR) urine volume, cystoscopy, and urodynamic studies. These tests usually require referral to urology.

Treatment

Effective management of UI requires individualizing treatment based on the type of UI that is present. In urge UI/OAB, behavioral therapy, including a voiding schedule and gentle bladder stretching, is helpful. Pharmacological intervention is indicated in conjunction with behavioral therapy (see Table 13-4). Certain medications, including selective muscarinic receptor antagonists that block bladder receptors and limit bladder contraction, are helpful in reducing OAB symptoms, increase voiding volume, and improving bladder control. Examples of these medications include tolterodine (Detrol®), solifenacin succinate (VESIcare®), darifenacin (Enablex®) and fesoterodine fumarate (Toviaz®). Oxybutynin (Ditropan®) is a nonselective muscarinic receptor antagonist that blocks receptors in the bladder and oral cavity. An oxybutynin transdermal patch (Oxytrol® for Women) is available over-the-counter for treatment of OAB in women. While clinically effective, oxybutynin use carries greater risk for systemic anticholinergic effects including dry mouth, constipation, sedation, and change in mental status when compared to the selective muscarinic antagonists. Mirabegron (Myrbetriq®), a beta-3 adrenoceptor agonist, is also an option, particularly when the other OAB medications are not tolerated. Botulinum toxin injections in the bladder have also been approved and can be effective for those who fail or are intolerant of pharmacological treatment.

In stress incontinence, pelvic floor physiotherapy and anti-continence devices are the usual approaches. Topical and systemic estrogen therapy were formerly recommended for this condition, but are now recognized as not helpful and can perhaps contribute to stress incontinence symptoms. Other forms of incontinence can be treated with behavioral therapy (e.g., mixed incontinence), treating the underlying cause of incontinence (e.g., transient incontinence), and/or surgery (e.g., urethral obstruction or stress incontinence) (see Table 13-4). Functional incontinence in individuals with mobility issues or altered cognition is best handled by having an assistant who is aware of voiding cues and helping with toileting activities.

Discussion Sources

Vasavada SP. Urinary incontinence. Medscape Web site. http://emedicine.medscape.com/article/452289.

Gormley EA, Lightner DJ, Burgio KL, et al. Diagnosis and treatment of overactive bladder (non-neurogenic) in adults: AUA/SUFU guideline. Approved May 2014 by the AUA Board of Directors. www.auanet.org/common/pdf/education/clinical-guidance /Overactive-Bladder.pdf.

Potts JM, Payne CK. Urinary urgency in the elderly. *Gerontology*. 2018;64:541–550.

TABLE 13-4 Types of Urinary Incontinence

TYPE OF URINARY INCONTINENCE	ETIOLOGY	CLINICAL PRESENTATION	TREATMENT OPTIONS
Urge incontinence	Detrusor overactivity causing uninhibited bladder contractions. Most common form of incontinence in elderly.	Strong sensation of needing to empty bladder that cannot be suppressed, often coupled with involuntary loss of urine	Behavioral therapy ■ Avoiding stimulants such as caffeine, alcohol ■ Gentle bladder stretching by increasing voiding interval by 15 to 30 minutes after establishing a half-hour voiding schedule ■ Cautious fluid ingestion (sips of fluid rather than large amounts ingested rapidly) Medication to reduce bladder contractility and symptoms ■ Oral selective muscarinic receptor antagonists (see narrative) ■ Alternatives to selective muscarinic receptor antagonists include mirabegron (Myrbetriq®), botulinum toxin injection
Stress incontinence	Weakness of pelvic floor, urethral muscles. Most common form of incontinence in women; rare in men, occasionally noted after prostate/bladder surgery.	Loss of urine with activity that causes increase in intra-abdominal pressure such as coughing, sneezing, exercise	Support to the area through use of a vaginal tampon, urethral stents, periurethral bulking agent injections, pessary use Pelvic floor rehabilitation with biofeedback, electrical stimulation, and bladder training Kegel and other similar exercises most helpful in younger patients Surgical intervention in well-chosen patients
Urethral obstruction	Obstruction of bladder outflow through urethral obstruction (prostatic, stricture, tumor) resulting in urinary retention with overflow, detrusor instability. Most commonly found in older men.	Dribbling postvoid coupled with urge incontinence on presentation	Treatment of urethral obstruction, requiring urological referral
Functional incontinence	Associated with inability to get to the toilet or lack of awareness of need to void.	Usually in person with mobility issues or altered cognition	Ameliorated by having assistant who is available to help with toileting activities; with altered mental status, assistant should also be aware of voiding cues
Transient incontinence	Associated with acute event such as delirium, UTI, medication use, restricted activity.	Presentation consistent with underlying process	Treatment of underlying process, discontinuation of offending medication
Iatrogenic incontinence	Associated with medical or surgical treatment.	Usually in individual starting a new medication or following a medical procedure	Discontinue or switch medication if possible; surgical correction

Source: Khandelwal C, Kistler C. Diagnosis of urinary incontinence. Am Fam Physician. 2013;87:543–550.

TABLE 13-5 Select Medications and Their Effect on Urinary Continence

TYPE OF MEDICATION	EFFECT ON URINARY CONTINENCE
Diuretics	Increase in volume and frequency of voiding. Use in older adult with limited mobility can result in functional urinary incontinence.
Drugs with systemic anticholinergic/ antimuscarinic activity ■ First-generation antihistamines ■ Tricyclic antidepressants ■ Antipsychotics	Urinary retention, overflow incontinence, dry mouth, constipation with increased risk for fecal impaction. Sedation risk, with resulting risk in functional urinary incontinence.
Opioids/opiates	Can contribute to functional incontinence due to alteration in sensorium, sedation, mobility. Additional impact on urinary continence due to constipation with increased risk for fecal impaction.
Alcohol	Increase in volume, frequency, and urgency of voiding, alteration in sensorium.
Sedatives, hypnotics, benzodiazepines	Can lead to functional incontinence due to alteration in sensorium, sedation, reduced mobility.
α-Adrenergic antagonists such as tamsulosin	Relaxing internal urethral sphincter. Desired effect in man with BPH.

BPH, benign prostatic hyperplasia.

Panesar K. Drug-induced urinary incontinence. US Pharm. 2014;39:24–29.

QUESTIONS

51. You see a 71-year-old woman who complains of a strong sensation of needing to void. She reports often having anxiety that she would not make it to a bathroom in time. This best describes:

    A. stress incontinence.

    B. urge incontinence.

    C. functional incontinence.

    D. transient incontinence.

52. A 64-year-old man with a history of BPH complains of urine loss as dribbling after voiding the bladder. This is most likely a result of:

    A. urge incontinence.

    B. stress incontinence.

    C. urethral obstruction.

    D. UTI.

53. A 34-year-old woman who gave birth to three full-term infants and has a body mass index of 40 kg/m² reports loss of small amounts of urine with coughing or sneezing. This would most likely indicate:

    A. urge incontinence.

    B. stress incontinence.

    C. functional incontinence.

    D. transient incontinence.

54 to 58. Match each of the following types of UI with the appropriate risk factors.

_____ **54.** Urge incontinence

_____ **55.** Stress incontinence

_____ **56.** Urethral obstruction

_____ **57.** Transient incontinence

_____ **58.** Functional incontinence

    A. detrusor overactivity

    B. chronic prostatitis

    C. pelvic floor weakness

    D. Alzheimer's dementia

    E. UTI

59. Pharmacological intervention for patients with urge incontinence includes:

    A. tamsulosin (Flomax®).

    B. tolterodine (Detrol®).

    C. finasteride (Proscar®).

    D. pseudoephedrine.

60 to 62. Match the most appropriate behavioral intervention with each form of UI.

_____ **60.** Urge incontinence

_____ **61.** Stress incontinence

_____ **62.** Functional continence

    A. having an assistant who is aware of voiding cues and helps with toileting activities

    B. establishing a voiding schedule and gentle bladder stretching

    C. Kegel exercises and pelvic floor rehabilitation with biofeedback

63. Which form of UI is most common in elderly adults?

    A. stress

    B. urge

    C. iatrogenic

    D. overflow

64. Common adverse effects of oral selective muscarinic receptor antagonists used in OAB treatment include:

    A. dry mouth and constipation.

    B. nausea.

    C. headaches.

    D. syncope.

65. You see an 82-year-old woman with early stage dementia and urge incontinence. Which of the following medications is least likely to contribute to worsening mental status?

    A. oxybutynin (Ditropan®)

    B. tolterodine (Detrol®)

    C. darifenacin (Enablex®)

    D. solifenacin succinate (VESIcare®)

66. A 64-year-old woman presents with urge incontinence and has not been able to tolerate treatment with anticholinergic agents. You recommend the use of which of the following? *(More than one can apply.)*

    A. botulinum toxin injections

    B. fesoterodine fumarate (Toviaz®)

C. mirabegron (Myrbetriq®)

D. finasteride (Proscar®)

67 to 69. Match each diagnostic technique with its contribution in the diagnosis of UI.

_____ **67.** Urinalysis and culture

_____ **68.** Cystoscopy

_____ **69.** Cough stress test

    A. urethral obstruction

    B. UTI

    C. pelvic floor weakness

For answers and rationales, see end of chapter.

Renal Stones

Overview

Renal stones (also known as kidney stones, renal lithiasis, or nephrolithiasis) are one of the most common urinary tract disorders, accounting for more than 1 million annual visits to health-care providers and more than 300,000 visits to emergency departments in the United States.

> **CLINICAL CONCEPT**
>
> Kidney stones form when the urine becomes highly concentrated with mineral and acid salts, such as calcium, oxalate, and phosphorus, which eventually crystallize.

Men are more likely to have renal stones than women. Other risk factors include family history of kidney stones, chronically poor fluid intake, dehydration, certain diets (i.e., high in protein, sodium, and sugar), and being overweight or obese. Health conditions associated with a higher risk of renal stones include hypercalciuria, cystic kidney disease, hyperparathyroidism, renal tubular acidosis, cystinuria, and gout. Certain medications can also increase the risk of renal stones, including calcium-based antacids, select sulfa drugs, indinavir (for HIV infection), and topiramate.

Calcium stones are the most common and can occur in two forms: calcium oxalate (caused by high levels of calcium and oxalate excretion) or calcium phosphate (caused by high levels of urine calcium and alkaline urine). Oxalate is a substance that occurs naturally in some fruits and vegetables as well as nuts and chocolate. Uric acid stones form when urine is persistently acidic. These stones form in people who do not drink sufficient fluids or who lose too much fluid, including overdiuresis, eat a high-protein diet, or have gout. Purines derived from animal protein, including certain shellfish and organ meats, in the diet can cause elevated levels of uric acid in the urine. Other types of stones include struvite stones (resulting from kidney infections) and cystine stones (caused by a genetic disorder that causes cystine to pass through the kidneys and into the urine).

Clinical Presentation

The presentation of the person presenting with nephrolithiasis is dictated by the size of the stone, degree of obstruction caused by the stone, and stone location.

■ *Stone in the ureter*: The classic scenario of sudden onset of severe flank pain that radiates anteriorly and inferiorly, often toward the groin, testicles, or vulva on the side of the stone, and often accompanied by nausea and vomiting. Pain is constant with waves of increased pain; these episodes of increased pain are referred to as renal colic. People who have small stones that pass easily through the urinary tract often have no symptoms. Others can experience pain while urinating; have pink, red, or brown urine; or feel a sharp pain in the back or lower abdomen. Pain is caused by the dilation, stretching, and spasm caused by the obstruction, and the pain is relieved once the stone passes out of the ureter. About 50% of those experiencing renal colic will report nausea and vomiting associated with the pain, which can last a short or long time. Some patients will have a persistent urge to urinate and/or urinate more often than usual.

■ *Stone in the ureteropelvic junction*: This can lead to mild to deep flank pain without radiation to the groin region. Patient complaints can include irritative voiding symptoms, urinary frequency and urgency, dysuria, and bowel symptoms.

■ *Stones in the bladder*: Typically asymptomatic but can sometimes lead to urinary retention.

Diagnostic Testing

Diagnostic testing in kidney stones starts with urinalysis to confirm the presence of hematuria, observed in about 85% of patients with renal colic; this diagnosis is unlikely if urine does not contain RBCs. Infection of an obstructed renal system can result in a life-threatening situation, and thus laboratory testing should include CBC with differential, blood culture, and urine culture and susceptibility testing. In addition, the urine can be tested to check for the presence of substances that form stones and rule out other conditions that can cause similar symptoms, such as infection. SCr should be checked, as obstructing stones can result in loss of renal function and postrenal azotemia.

Imaging with either ultrasound or CT scan (without contrast) can confirm the diagnosis and show stone locations. Ultrasound by itself is often sufficient to detect a kidney stone in slender adults, though this technique can miss smaller stones (less than 5 mm), and visualization of stones can be difficult in obese patients. Ultrasound can also detect hydronephrosis, which is the enlargement of the kidney due to urine obstruction. CT scan has replaced intravenous pyelography (IVP) as the standard in diagnosis, particularly in acute renal colic, as it offers superior sensitivity and specificity in detecting smaller stones (3 mm or larger) and results can be available within minutes. CT scan can also help identify other underlying pathologies if symptoms are not caused by a renal stone. Plain x-rays, such as a KUB (kidney, ureters, bladder), can help assess total stone burden. However, x-rays can miss small renal stones as well as uric acid, indinavir-induced, or cystine calculi, which are radiolucent and not visible on x-ray. Calcium-containing stones are radiopaque and easily visible on x-ray. Ultrasound or CT scan in combination with x-ray can help to determine the presence, location, and composition of the stone.

Stones that pass through the urine can be analyzed to reveal the makeup of the stone. This information can be used to determine a plan for preventing further kidney stones. The stone is harvested via straining the urine or by retrieval via endoscope.

Treatment

In kidney stones, urological consultation is nearly always required. Acute nephrolithiasis treatment depends on the size and location of the stone as well as whether the stones are causing pain and/or blocking the urinary tract.

IV hydration is needed if the patient experiences nausea and vomiting and is unable to maintain hydration with oral intake. Infection should be treated with appropriate antimicrobial therapy.

- *Stones in the ureter*: Small stones (less than 4 mm) typically pass through the urinary tract without treatment, though analgesics (e.g., acetaminophen) can be prescribed to alleviate the pain. An alpha blocker can be used to relax the muscles in the ureter in order to pass the stone more quickly and with less pain. Several options are available if more urgent measures are needed and for stones greater than 8 mm, which will typically not pass without intervention. Extracorporeal shock wave lithotripsy (ESWL) generates shock waves that travel through the body to break up the stones into smaller pieces that more readily pass through the urinary tract. Ureteroscopy via a small endoscope can be used to retrieve the stone or break a stone into smaller pieces with a laser.
- *Stones located in the uteropelvic junction*: Internal ureteral stents can be used to drain the kidney in cases of obstruction and help with the passage of stones more efficiently. When a stent is not appropriate, percutaneous nephrostomy (a catheter is inserted through the skin to drain the kidney) can be used. For larger stones located in the kidney, ESWL can be used to break up the stone followed by the use of a nephrostomy tube to drain urine and stone fragments directly from the kidneys.

A 24-hour urine sample should be collected for stone analysis and to guide the prevention strategy.

Nephrolithiasis Prevention

Proper hydration is the optimal method to prevent renal stones, with a recommendation of drinking, at minimum, 2 to 3 liters (67 to 100 oz) of fluid per day. An increased intake of fruits and vegetables is recommended for patients with calcium stones and low urinary citrate levels. For those with calcium oxalate or calcium phosphate stones, prevention can also include reducing sodium and animal protein while getting enough calcium from food sources. If calcium supplements are used, these should be taken with meals. Calcium oxalate stones can be prevented by reducing intake of oxalate-rich foods, such as rhubarb, beets, okra, spinach, Swiss chard, sweet potatoes, nuts, tea, chocolate, and soy products. For those with uric acid stones, limiting animal protein will help prevent further stone formation.

> **CLINICAL CONCEPT**
> Nephrolithiasis prevention can include a combination of dietary adjustments, nutritional supplements, and medications.

Medications can also help prevent stone formation. Patients with high urine calcium and recurrent calcium stones should consider taking a thiazide diuretic. Potassium citrate can be offered for those with recurrent calcium stones but low urinary calcium. Allopurinol can also be considered for patients with a history of uric acid stones or cystine calculi, as the drug reduces uric acid secretion.

Discussion Sources

Dave CN. Nephrolithiasis. Medscape. http://emedicine.medscape.com/article/437096

Guirguis-Blake J. Preventing recurrent nephrolithiasis in adults. *Am Fam Physician*. 2014;89:461–463.

National Institute of Diabetes and Digestive and Kidney Diseases. Kidney stones in adults. http://www.niddk.nih.gov/health-information/health-topics/urologic-disease/kidney-stones-in-adults/Pages/facts.aspx

QUESTIONS

70. Risk factors for renal stones include all of the following except:

- **A.** male gender.
- **B.** vegetarian diet.
- **C.** family history of renal stones.
- **D.** obesity.

71. Medications known to increase the risk of renal stones include all of the following except:

- **A.** sulfasalazine.
- **B.** moxifloxacin.
- **C.** topiramate.
- **D.** indinavir.

72. The most common renal stones are composed of:

- **A.** calcium.
- **B.** uric acid.
- **C.** sodium.
- **D.** iron.

73 to 75. Match the following locations of a renal stone with its most appropriate clinical presentation.

_____ **73.** Ureter

_____ **74.** Ureteropelvic junction

_____ **75.** Bladder

- **A.** asymptomatic
- **B.** renal colic
- **C.** mild to deep flank pain without radiation to the groin region

76. Common signs and symptoms of renal stones include all of the following except:

- **A.** pink, red, or brown urine.
- **B.** sharp pain in the back or lower abdomen.
- **C.** marked febrile response.
- **D.** pain while urinating.

77 to 79. Match each imaging technique with its role in the diagnosis of nephrolithiasis.

_____ **77.** Ultrasound

_____ **78.** CT scan

_____ **79.** X-ray

- **A.** identify stones during renal colic
- **B.** determine radiopaque total stone burden
- **C.** detect the presence of hydronephrosis

80. You see a 58-year-old man diagnosed with a kidney stone who reports pain primarily during urination. You consider the use of all of the following interventions except:

A. improved hydration.

B. alpha blocker use.

C. ESWL.

D. analgesia.

81 to 83. Match each intervention in the treatment of renal stones with the appropriate location of the stone. *(Answer choice may be used more than once.)*

_____ **81.** Alpha blocker and hydration

_____ **82.** Internal ureteral stent

_____ **83.** Percutaneous nephrostomy

    A. ureter

    B. ureteropelvic junction

    C. bladder

84. The most effective strategy for preventing renal stones is:

A. daily exercise.

B. adequate hydration.

C. limiting coffee consumption.

D. smoking cessation.

85. You see a 58-year-old woman who is being treated for nephrolithiasis. Analysis of a stone passed in the urine reveals that it is composed of calcium oxalate. In counseling the patient about preventing future stones, you consider all of the following except:

A. reducing sodium in her diet.

B. limiting consumption of beets, rhubarb, nuts, and chocolate.

C. encouraging her to get her daily calcium requirements from food.

D. if calcium supplements are needed, this medication should be taken on an empty stomach.

For answers and rationales, see end of chapter.

QUESTION ANSWERS AND RATIONALES

Acute Kidney Injury and Chronic Kidney Disease

1. Correct: D. hypophosphatemia.
The kidneys play an important role in maintaining homeostasis. Thus, CKD can lead to imbalances of fluid, electrolytes, and acid-base balance. A common finding is hyperphosphatemia rather than hypophosphatemia (D).
Incorrect:
Electrolyte disorders commonly associated with AKI and advanced CKD (particularly stages 4 and 5) include hyperkalemia (C), hypercalcemia (B), hyperphosphatemia, and hypernatremia (A). Other conditions can include bicarbonate deficiency (i.e., metabolic acidosis).

2. Correct: D. T1DM.
AKI is characterized by an abrupt change and rapid decline in renal function, often precipitated by a single event that is easily identifiable and potentially correctable. T1DM is a chronic genetic-based condition with

an autoimmune component leading to beta-cell destruction and insulinopenia that will not likely precipitate rapid changes in kidney function, though many years of T1DM, particularly with poorly glycemic control, can lead to CKD.
Incorrect:
AKI can occur when there is decreased blood flow to the kidneys, damage to the kidneys, or urine blockage in the kidneys. Precipitating events that can cause rapid decline in kidney function include acute hypotension (A), sepsis (B) or other infection, and hypovolemia (C) caused by acute blood loss or dehydration.

3. Correct: C. hypotension.
CKD is a gradual loss of renal function over time. One of the most potent risk factors for this condition is hypertension, particularly with poor control, rather than hypotension (C). Hypotension is a risk factor for AKI.

Incorrect:

A number of risk factors have been identified for the development of CKD. These include T1DM and T2DM (A), cardiovascular disease (D), older age, obesity, prior history of AKI (B), as well as belonging to certain high-risk ethnic groups.

4. **Correct: B. angiotensin II receptor antagonists**

Bilateral renal artery stenosis is the narrowing of both renal arteries most commonly caused by atherosclerosis. This can typically lead to secondary hypertension that is often resistant to therapy. ACEIs and ARBs are contra-indicated in patients with bilateral renal artery stenosis because of increased risk of azotemia and resulting AKI.

Incorrect:

Corticosteroids (A) and β-adrenergic antagonists (C) are generally safe to use in patients with bilateral renal artery stenosis. Aminoglycosides (D) are not contraindicated in these patients, though this medication class should be used with caution as they exhibit nephrotoxicity that can lead to AKI in some patients.

5. **Correct: D. postrenal AKI.**

The presence of bladder distention suggests an obstruction to urine flow. This together with findings of an elevated BUN and a rising level of SCr (and decreasing eGFR) suggest postrenal azotemia (D). The eGFR value indicates this patient has existing CKD (stage 3a) that is now superimposed with AKI.

Incorrect:

This patient presents with signs of urine blockage, thus indicating a postrenal cause of AKI and not prerenal azotemia (A). Acute glomerulonephritis (B) and acute tubular necrosis (C) are both intrinsic renal causes of AKI.

6. **Correct: D. CKD**

For this patient with heart failure, her eGFR has held steady for the past 2 years and is stable at this visit, suggesting the absence of acute renal injury (AKI). CKD is present due to heart failure along with her long history of multiple comorbidities, including hypertension, T2DM, and dyslipidemia. She is currently at stage 3b based on her eGFR value.

Incorrect:

There is no report of a rapid change in her renal function and so AKI should not be suspected for this patient. Her reduced renal function is likely a result of heart failure causing CKD due to, in part, chronic renal hypoperfusion that is caused by lower cardiac output.

7. **Correct: A. prerenal AKI.**

In this patient following an exacerbation of heart failure, there is likely hypoperfusion of the kidneys due to a further acute decrease in cardiac output. Thus, this is a prerenal cause of AKI, superimposed on her CKD, leading to azotemia, elevated SCr, and further decreased eGFR.

Incorrect:

The rapid changes in laboratory values and eGFR suggest AKI on top of her CKD (D). The most likely cause resulting from the heart failure exacerbation is hypoperfusion

of the kidneys leading to decreased renal function. This is a predominantly prerenal cause of AKI, thus not related to direct damage to the kidneys (intrinsic AKI [B]) or due to blockage of urine in the kidneys (postrenal AKI [C]).

8. **Correct: A. persistent proteinuria**

Protein in the urine is an early indicator of CKD, and recommendations to screen for CKD include urinalysis, urine albumin/creatinine ratio (ACR), and SCr.

Incorrect:

Uremia (C), or elevated BUN, is a condition of high levels of urea in the blood, and acute uremia will more likely occur during AKI or more advanced CKD. Electrolyte disorders, such as hyperkalemia (D), and anemia (B) are associated with later stages of renal failure and not early development of CKD.

9. **Correct: C. elevated BUN; normal SCr.**

For an individual with normal renal function who experiences an acute GI bleed, there would be no increase in SCr, particularly if the patient remains well hydrated. However, BUN levels can increase markedly as the gut digests and absorbs proteins from the blood (C).

Incorrect:

In this scenario, the BUN can be elevated due to digestion and absorption of excess proteins from the blood (B, D), while SCr will not change since there is no indication of renal dysfunction in this patient (A).

10. **Correct: B. reducing efferent arteriolar resistance.**

Treatment with an ACEI or ARB is recommended for individuals with CKD with or without diabetes mellitus. These agents work by reducing efferent arteriolar resistance (B), thus improving perfusion of the kidneys and reducing albuminuria. Combinations of these agents should not be used as there is greater risk of complications, such as AKI, without added benefit. These agents should also be avoided in patients with bilateral renal artery stenosis.

11. **Correct: D. hypotension.**

Glomerulonephritis is an intrinsic cause of renal disease and can be due to poststreptococcal infection or an autoimmune reaction. As with other forms of AKI, this condition can lead to the development of edema as well as proteinuria and the presence of renal casts in the urine. Hypotension is not a typical finding associated with glomerulonephritis (D), though hypertension is.

Incorrect:

Similar to other forms of AKI, glomerulonephritis can be associated with edema (A) and proteinuria (C). RBC casts can also be present in the urine with this condition (B).

12. **Correct: B. 50%**

Measurement of creatinine is used as a surrogate marker of kidney function; in healthy individuals, creatinine production equals creatinine excretion. With decreased renal function, the SCr value increases. When the SCr level doubles, the eGFR is considered to have been halved; when SCr increases threefold, the eGFR is decreased by 75%.

Incorrect:

An increase in SCr generally indicated a decrease in eGFR. When SCr increases threefold, eGFR will decrease by 75% (C). An increase in SCr of 50% will cause a decrease in eGFR of 25% (A). A decrease of 100% in eGFR will indicate no renal function (D).

13. **Correct: A. approximates GFR.**

Measurement of creatinine is used as a surrogate marker of kidney function, and creatinine clearance approximates GFR (A). With decreased renal function, the SCr value increases while the GFR decreases. When the SCr level doubles, the GFR is considered to have been halved; when SCr increases threefold, the GFR is decreased by 75%.

Incorrect:

Renal function decline is a normal age-related change and, thus, would impact creatinine clearance (B). SCr is proportional to muscle mass, and so males would have higher levels of SCr and higher creatinine clearance when compared to women (C). Hypotension can result is decreased perfusion of the kidneys and diminished renal function, thus lowering creatinine clearance (and GFR) (D).

14. **Correct: B. a product related to skeletal muscle metabolism.**

Creatinine is the end-product of creatine metabolism, which arises from skeletal muscle. Because creatinine excretion by a healthy kidney is efficient, measurement of creatinine is used as a surrogate marker of kidney function.

Incorrect:

Creatinine is not produced by the kidney, but it is excreted by the kidney (A). Creatinine is produced by skeletal muscles, not the liver (C), and is a by-product of creatine metabolism, which is not a protein (D).

15. **Correct: D. greater than 300 mg/g.**

ACR can provide a more sensitive and specific indicator for CKD than protein/creatinine ratio, as ACR is able to detect lower levels of protein in the urine. Even small amounts of albumin in the urine are considered an important prognostic factor. An ACR of 30 to 299 mg/g is moderately elevated, while values greater than 300 mg/g are severely elevated, typically requiring referral to a nephrologist (D).

16. **Correct: C. less than 10 mg/dL.**

Anemia of chronic disease is a common finding among patients with CKD. ESAs such as epoetin-α should be considered when hemoglobin levels fall below 10 mg/dL (C). Treatment should target a hemoglobin level not exceeding 11.5 mg/dL.

17. **Correct: C. Hb = 9.4 g/dL (12 to 14 g/dL); MCV = 83 fL (80 to 96 fL); reticulocytes = 0.7% (1% to 2%).**

Anemia of chronic disease can occur in the presence of CRF. Renal erythropoietin synthesis is reduced, and this results in a hypoproliferative, normochromic, normocytic anemia with a decreased percentage of reticulocytes (C).

Incorrect:

A microcytic anemia is most likely the result of iron-deficiency anemia (A). Macrocytic anemia can be caused by folic acid deficiency or vitamin B_{12} deficiency (B). A normocytic anemia with increased reticulocytosis (D) can occur once the cause of anemia of chronic disease is addressed or following administration of erythropoietic-stimulating therapy.

18. **Correct: B. a 64-year-old woman with T2DM and eGFR = 28 mL/min/1.73 m²**

Dialysis and kidney transplantation can be considered for patients approaching stage 4 CKD (eGFR 15 to 29 mL/min/1.73 m²) and/or who have advanced kidney damage. These patients are more likely to develop severe complications from CKD.

Incorrect:

Dialysis is not warranted for patients at stage 3 or below CKD (A, C, D), though these patients should be monitored closely for any changes in renal function. Patients with advanced renal disease and a limited life expectancy without intervention would also not be considered for renal replacement therapy. Conversely, in the presence of multiple life-shortening or a terminal illness other than CKD, the patient with stages 4 to 5 CKD could make the decision to forgo dialysis.

Glomerulonephritis

19. **Correct: C. Crohn's disease**

Glomerulonephritis can be caused by systemic immunological conditions, vasculitis, and infection. Crohn's disease has not been implicated as a risk factor for glomerulonephritis as it is predominantly localized to the GI tract.

Incorrect:

Infections that can trigger glomerulonephritis include bacterial endocarditis (A), some viral infections, as well as the period following streptococcal pharyngitis. Autoimmune conditions, such as Goodpasture's syndrome (B), as well as vasculitis (e.g., polyarteritis [D] or Wegener's granulomatosis), can lead to glomerulonephritis.

20. **Correct: B. 1 to 2 weeks**

Poststreptococcal glomerulonephritis can develop approximately 1 to 2 weeks following pharyngitis caused by group A beta-hemolytic streptococcal infection. In response to the infection, there is an overproduction of antibodies produced that eventually settle in the glomeruli and cause inflammation.

Incorrect:

There is often a delay of at least 1 week between bacterial pharyngitis infection and poststreptococcal glomerulonephritis (A). The delay does not normally extend beyond two weeks, however (C, D).

21. **Correct: D. kidney biopsy.**

Though glomerulonephritis can be diagnosed clinically in many cases, confirmation of the diagnosis requires a biopsy of the kidney (D). A biopsy can be helpful in determining the prognosis and treatment approach for the patient.

Incorrect:
Confirmation of glomerulonephritis requires a renal biopsy. A urinalysis with CBC and WBC differential can be helpful in detecting the presence of infection as well as evaluating protein in the urine to assess renal damage (A). Imaging studies with an ultrasound (C) or CT scan (B) can be helpful in assessing damage to the kidney but cannot be used to confirm the diagnosis.

22. **Correct: D. abnormally high glucose levels.**
The changes in urine found during glomerulonephritis are typically caused by the presence of RBCs, casts, and protein. Acute glomerulonephritis is not normally associated with glucosuria (D).

Incorrect:
Expected findings during a urinalysis of a patient with glomerulonephritis include the presence of RBCs (B), RBC casts (C), WBCs, and elevated levels of protein (A). Other laboratory findings associated with decreased renal function include elevated SCr and BUN.

23 to 25. Matching Questions

23. **Correct: B. systemic antimicrobials**

24. **Correct: A. systemic corticosteroids**

25. **Correct: C. immunomodulators, and D. plasmapheresis**
Treatment of glomerulonephritis should aim to manage the underlying cause of the condition and prevent further damage to the kidneys. In the presence of a bacterial infection, systemic antimicrobials should be used until the infection is eradicated. Systemic corticosteroids can be used to reduce inflammation present during vasculitis. For autoimmune conditions, such as Goodpasture's syndrome, immunomodulators together with plasmapheresis are important to reduce levels of circulating antibodies and remove toxins from the body.

26. **Correct: B. nephrotic syndrome.**
Nephrotic syndrome (B) is a serious complication of glomerulonephritis that is characterized by excessive amounts of protein excreted in the urine. This can lead to infection, formation of blood clots, and AKI. Proper treatment of glomerulonephritis can reduce the risk of nephrotic syndrome.

Incorrect:
Untreated glomerulonephritis can lead to serious complications related to kidney function. However, these complications do not include T2DM (A), pyelonephritis (C), or bladder cancer (D).

Urinary Tract Infection

27. **Correct: A. urinary frequency**
In otherwise healthy women with UTI, the typical presentation includes a complaint of dysuria, often reported as internal discomfort with increased urinary frequency and urgency (A). Fever or constitutional symptoms are often absent.

Incorrect:
Dysuria with urinary frequency and urgency are the most common complaints of UTI in an otherwise healthy woman. Fever (B) and GI upset (D) are more likely with an upper UTI, such as pyelonephritis. Suprapubic tenderness (C) can be present but is only reported in a minority of women with UTI.

28. **Correct: D. hematuria.**
UTI in the elderly can have an atypical presentation when compared to younger adults. However, older age does not impact the presence of blood in the urine (hematuria) (D), as microscopic hematuria is a common finding with UTIs regardless of age.

Incorrect:
UTIs can trigger mental status changes in the elderly and is a common cause of delirium (B) in the older population. UTIs in the elderly can also lead to new-onset UI (A) as well as overall weakness (C) and increased fall risk. The presence of these findings in the elderly should raise suspicion of a UTI.

29. **Correct: B. a UTI caused by a gram-negative organism.**
Important features of a urinalysis during a UTI include a positive leukocyte esterase test and the presence of nitrites. Gram-negative organisms are able to reduce nitrate to nitrite. Thus, positive leukocyte esterase with the presence of nitrites would indicate a UTI caused by a gram-negative pathogen.

Incorrect:
Gram-positive organisms, such as *S saprophyticus*, are unable to reduce nitrate to nitrite (C). Purulent vulvovaginitis would likely be accompanied by a report of vaginal discharge (A) and vaginal, rather than urinary tract, infection. Urethral syndrome, caused by an inflamed or irritated urethra, is not associated with a bacterial infection and so would not have positive findings of leukocytes and nitrites in the urine (D).

30. **Correct: C. *E coli*.**
Recognizing the various potential pathogens that can cause a UTI is critical in guiding evidence-based practice. For women of reproductive age, the most common pathogen for UTIs is the gram-negative organism, *E coli* (C).

Incorrect:
E coli is the leading cause of UTIs among women of reproductive age. Other common causes of UTIs include the gram-negative organisms *P mirabilis* (B) and *Klebsiella* species (A), as well as the gram-positive organism *S saprophyticus* (D).

31. **Correct: C. gonococcal urethritis.**
UTIs are generally not common among younger, otherwise healthy males. The presence of purulent discharge along with a report of a new sexual partner would indicate a potential STI, such as gonococcal urethritis (C).

Incorrect:
UTIs are not typically associated with purulent urethral or vaginal discharge, which would more likely indicate a

possible STI (A). Pyelonephritis can be associated with fever and abdominal tenderness but not with purulent discharge (B). A varicocele (D), typically described as a "bag of worms" lesion most often found in the left scrotum, would not cause urinary tract symptoms of dysuria and urgency to urinate.

32. **Correct: D. nitrofurantoin.**

For a patient with a history of sulfa allergy, nitrofurantoin would be an appropriate first-line treatment option (D). Ciprofloxacin can also be considered, though there is increasing concern of resistance to the fluoroquinolones by common uropathogens, such as *E coli*; therefore, this should not be used routinely as a first-line UTI medication.

Incorrect:

TMP-SMX (A) should be avoided in this patient due to a history of allergic reaction. Though there is no risk of cross-reactivity with the beta-lactams such as amoxicillin (B), this agent is not recommended because of high levels of resistance by uropathogens. The macrolides such as azithromycin (C) are not recommended for uncomplicated UTIs.

33. **Correct: B. *P mirabilis*.**

The presence of alkaline urine would suggest infection with an organism that is capable of splitting urea into CO_2 and ammonia, which causes an increase in urine pH. *P mirabilis* (B) is an organism that is able to split urea.

Incorrect:

Among the organisms listed, *P mirabilis* is the only one capable of splitting urea and causing alkaline urine. *Klebsiella* spp. (A), *E coli* (C), and *S saprophyticus* (D) do not have this ability.

34. **Correct: C. A urological evaluation should be considered.**

UTIs in otherwise healthy younger men are fairly uncommon; thus, additional urological evaluation should be considered to identify the cause of the UTI (C). This can include diagnostic imaging studies to identify a urinary tract abnormality.

Incorrect:

A UTI is not a common condition in healthy, younger men (A). *E coli*, a gram-negative organism, is the most common cause of UTIs in the community for both men and women (B). UTIs in men, similar to women, would include the presence of WBCs in the urine (pyuria) (D).

35. **Correct: C. timed voiding schedule.**

Certain beliefs that were once thought to prevent UTIs have not been supported by clinical evidence. These include timed voiding schedules (C), wiping patterns, and postcoitus voiding for women.

Incorrect:

Certain factors can protect against the risk for UTI. Male gender is recognized as a potent protective factor (A), in part because of the longer urethral length in men than in women. Women with a shorter urethra-to-anus length appear to be at increased UTI risk (B). Additionally, the

zinc-rich prostatic secretions in men are antibacterial, further discouraging pathogen growth (D).

36. **Correct: A. patient report of irritative voiding symptoms**

Hemorrhagic cystitis is the presence of large quantities of blood in the urine. Common symptoms are bladder pain and irritative voiding symptoms (A).

Incorrect:

Hemorrhagic cystitis can include substantial amounts of blood in the urine, beyond microscopic hematuria (B). The condition can sometimes be confused with glomerulonephritis; however, the latter condition is typically associated with new-onset hypertension (C) and decreased renal function (D), which are not typically observed with hemorrhagic cystitis.

37. **Correct: C. 3+ protein.**

Protein in the urine is a common finding in UTIs due to the presence of WBCs, bacteria, and mucus. However, protein levels typically range from a trace to 30 mg/dL (1+). A protein level of 3+ would not normally be expected.

Incorrect:

Typical findings of pyelonephritis would include the presence of WBC casts (A) in the urine as well as nitrites (B) if the infection is caused by a gram-negative organism. Microscopic hematuria is also a normal finding during a UTI (and rare RBCs are sometimes noted even in normal urine as well) (D).

38. **Correct: C. IM ceftriaxone for one dose plus oral ciprofloxacin for 7 days.**

Treatment of pyelonephritis requires an antimicrobial with potent gram-negative activity and excellent penetration into the renal tissue. Ciprofloxacin provides an appropriate choice for pyelonephritis, and due to its high bioavailability, the oral formulation has similar efficacy as the IV formulation and can be used in patients who tolerate fluids. Ciprofloxacin can be used following one dose of IM ceftriaxone. Traditional duration of therapy with ciprofloxacin was 2 weeks, but more recent research has shown a 7-day duration is just as effective and likely decreases the risk of resistance development. In the presence of a potentially life-threatening infection such as pyelonephritis, the benefit of fluoroquinolone use outweighs its risks, including fear of antimicrobial resistance.

Incorrect:

Nitrofurantoin (D), moxifloxacin, and fosfomycin should not be considered for pyelonephritis due to poor penetration in renal tissue. IM ceftriaxone (A) should be given initially as one dose followed by a 5- to 7-day course of oral ciprofloxacin or levofloxacin. TMP-SMX (B) can be considered, but only if susceptibility results demonstrate this agent will be effective against the causative pathogen.

39. **Correct: B. increased elasticity of the bladder.**

Normal age-related changes can increase the risk of UTIs in the elderly. The bladder actually loses elasticity with aging (B), thus decreasing the amount of urine it can hold that can contribute to UI and infection.

Incorrect:
Other normal age-related changes include weakened bladder wall muscles (A) that can contribute to incomplete voiding of the bladder during urination. Blockage of the urethra can also occur in the presence of an enlarged prostate (D) in men or vaginal prolapse (C) in women.

40. **Correct: B. low perivaginal lactobacilli colonization.**
Lactobacilli are a normal component of the periurethral flora and produce hydrogen peroxide and lactic acid that inhibit bacterial growth in women during the reproductive years. In postmenopausal women, estrogen deficiency reduces lactobacilli colonization, thus increasing the risk of UTIs. Use of topical estrogen can help to reestablish lactobacilli and restore the protective benefits against UTIs.

Incorrect:
Several traditional or long-standing beliefs of the cause of UTI have not been supported by clinical evidence and thus are not considered risk factors. These include wiping habits (A), the use of hot tubs (C), and pantyhose use (D).

41. **Correct: D. postcoital voiding.**
Postcoital voiding will not impact lactobacilli colonization. Once thought to help prevent UTIs, the benefits of this practice have not been supported in clinical studies.

Incorrect:
Lactobacilli is a normal component of the periurethral flora and produces hydrogen peroxide and lactic acid that inhibit bacterial growth. In postmenopausal women, estrogen deficiency reduces lactobacilli colonization (C), thus increasing the risk of UTIs. Spermicides, such as nonoxynol-9, can decrease lactobacilli through their antibacterial effects (B), as will the use of systemic antimicrobials (A).

42. **Correct: A. constipation**
Among risk factors in children and the elderly, constipation (A) has been found to contribute to bladder instability and helps to encourage UTI development.

Incorrect:
Chronic diarrhea (C), upper respiratory tract infections (B), and efficient bladder emptying (D) have not been associated with increased risk for a UTI in these populations.

43. **Correct: D. *S saprophyticus***
S saprophyticus (D) is a gram-positive organism that is a common cause of UTIs.

Incorrect:
Gram-negative organisms that commonly cause UTIs include *E coli* (A), *K pneumoniae* (B), and *P mirabilis* (C). Infections caused by these organisms will result in a positive nitrite urine test.

44. **Correct: C. ciprofloxacin.**
For elderly patients with the potential for reduced renal function, the fluoroquinolones can be a safe and effective first-line choice, though dose adjustment should be considered.

Incorrect:
Nitrofurantoin (A) is not recommended for routine use in the report of reduced renal function, as this drug should not be used in the presence of severe renal impairment. Fosfomycin (B) is not recommended as a first-line agent for the treatment of uncomplicated UTIs. Doxycycline is not recommended for UTIs as the drug is primarily excreted in the feces rather than the urine (D).

Bladder Cancer

45. **Correct: B. cystoscopy with biopsy**
When bladder cancer is suspected, the patient should be referred to a specialist to undergo cystoscopy (B). Usually, a biopsy sample is taken during the procedure to confirm the diagnosis.

Incorrect:
Confirmation of bladder cancer is achieved with a cystoscopy with biopsy. Urinalysis (A) can be helpful in determining the presence of a UTI that can be contributing to the symptoms. While urinalysis will help document the presence of RBCs in the urine, this finding does not confirm the bladder cancer diagnosis. Imaging can be important in assessing the scope of possible lesions, though imaging cannot confirm the diagnosis (C, D). Cytology can also be helpful in the diagnosis to detect for the presence of cancer cells in the urine.

46. **Correct: D. long-term aspirin use**
Several risk factors have been identified for bladder cancer. However, the long-term use of aspirin (D) is not implicated in this disease.

Incorrect:
Cigarette smoking contributes to the development in most cases of bladder cancer (B). Other risk factors include occupational exposure to paints, dyes, and solvents (A, C). Certain medications as well as HPV infection have also been associated with bladder cancer.

47. **Correct: C. painless gross hematuria.**
The most common presenting sign of bladder cancer is painless gross hematuria (C).

Incorrect:
Painful urination is a presenting symptom in only a minority of patients with bladder cancer (A). A palpable abdominal mass will only be present in advanced disease (D). Fever and flank pain are not typical findings for this condition (B).

48. **Correct: C. despite successful initial therapy, local recurrence is common.**
For patients with bladder cancer, recurrence is a major concern even with successful initial therapy. Therefore, meticulous follow-up is necessary to identify new lesions and repeat treatment when necessary.

Incorrect:
With superficial (non-muscle-invasive) bladder cancer, long-term survival is expected with appropriate treatment and follow-up (A). In these cases, surgical treatment can include transurethral resection or partial

cystectomy, though a total cystectomy will likely not be required (B). In addition to surgical management, an immediate postsurgical instillation of intravesical treatment should be administered, as opposed to systemic chemotherapy (D).

49. **Correct: B. 20**

Painless gross hematuria is the most common presenting sign in bladder cancer. Persistent microscopic hematuria is the primary finding in only 20% of individuals with bladder cancer. For patients with risk factors for bladder cancer, the presence of persistent microscopic hematuria should be further evaluated to rule in or out bladder cancer.

Incorrect:

Only a minority of individuals with bladder cancer will present with persistent microscopic hematuria. This finding is typically present in about one-fifth of these patients (A, C, D).

50. **Correct: C. transurethral resection with intravesical chemotherapy.**

For individuals with non-muscle-invasive bladder cancer, surgical treatment can include transurethral resection or partial cystectomy. In addition to surgical management, an immediate postsurgical instillation of intravesical treatment should be administered (C).

Incorrect:

For this type of bladder cancer, a total cystectomy is not required as the lesions can be excised through transurethral resection or, in more severe cases, a partial resection (A). An instillation of intravesical chemotherapy is preferred over systemic therapy to focus the treatment at the site of the lesions (D). Chemotherapy should be performed in conjunction with surgical management (B).

Urinary Incontinence

51. **Correct: B. urge incontinence.**

Urge incontinence is best characterized as having a strong sensation of needing to empty the bladder that cannot be suppressed, often accompanied with involuntary loss of urine (B). This is the most common form of UI in the elderly.

Incorrect:

Stress incontinence is characterized by a loss of urine with activity, such as exercise, coughing, or sneezing (A). This is the most common form of incontinence in women. Functional incontinence occurs in individuals with mobility issues or cognitive dysfunction (C). Transient incontinence occurs in individuals with an acute event, such as delirium, infection, or medication use (D).

52. **Correct: C. urethral obstruction.**

Dribbling following urination is a characteristic sign of urethral obstruction. Men with BPH are at higher risk of urethral obstruction due to the enlarged prostate, and treatment should aim to decrease the size of the prostate, which should help to alleviate the symptoms of incontinence.

Incorrect:

Urge incontinence is best characterized as having a strong sensation of needing to empty the bladder that cannot be suppressed, often accompanied with involuntary loss of urine (A). Stress incontinence is characterized by a loss of urine with activity, such as exercise, coughing, or sneezing (B). UTIs are not typically associated with UI (D).

53. **Correct: B. stress incontinence.**

Stress incontinence is characterized by a loss of urine with activity, such as exercise, coughing, or sneezing (A). This is the most common form of incontinence in women and is caused by a weakness in the pelvic floor and urethral muscles.

Incorrect:

Urge incontinence is best characterized as having a strong sensation of needing to empty the bladder that cannot be suppressed, often accompanied with involuntary loss of urine (A). Functional incontinence occurs in individuals with mobility issues or cognitive dysfunction (C). Transient incontinence occurs in individuals with an acute event, such as delirium, infection, or medication use (D).

54 to 58. Matching Questions

54. **Correct: A. detrusor overactivity**

55. **Correct: C. pelvic floor weakness**

56. **Correct: B. chronic prostatitis**

57. **Correct: E. UTI**

58. **Correct: D. Alzheimer's dementia**

Urge incontinence is the most common form of incontinence in the elderly and is caused by detrusor overactivity that results in uninhibited bladder contractions. Stress incontinence is caused by pelvic floor and urethral muscle weakness and is the most common form of incontinence in women. During urethral obstruction, obstruction of the bladder outflow, such as an enlarged prostate, prolapse, or presence of a tumor, can result in urinary retention with overflow and detrusor instability. Transient incontinence occurs in individuals with an acute event, such as delirium, infection, or medication use. Functional incontinence occurs in individuals with mobility issues or cognitive dysfunction, such as Alzheimer's dementia.

59. **Correct: B. tolterodine (Detrol®).**

Treatment of urge incontinence is aimed at reducing bladder contractions with the use of systemic anticholinergic agents. Tolterodine is one of many different anticholinergic agents that are currently used to treat urge incontinence (B). An alternative to systemic anticholinergics is mirabegron, a β_3-adrenoceptor agonist, which can be effective for individuals who cannot tolerate the systemic anticholinergics.

Incorrect:

Tamsulosin is an alpha blocker used specifically to relieve BPH symptoms, which can cause UI via partial urethral obstruction (A). Similarly, finasteride is used to reduce the size of an enlarged prostate but will not be effective in treating urge incontinence (C). Pseudoephedrine is used to relieve nasal congestion and not to treat urge incontinence (D) but historically has been used, albeit with minimal effect, to treat stress incontinence.

60 to 62. Matching Questions

60. Correct: **B. establishing a voiding schedule and gentle bladder stretching**

61. Correct: **C. Kegel exercises and pelvic floor rehabilitation with biofeedback**

62. Correct: **A. having an assistant who is aware of voiding cues and helps with toileting activities**
Urge incontinence is caused by detrusor overactivity that results in uninhibited bladder contractions. Treatment can include using a voiding schedule along with bladder stretching, as well as pharmacotherapy when necessary. Stress incontinence is caused by pelvic floor and urethral muscle weakness, and the condition can be alleviated with physiotherapy aimed at pelvic floor rehabilitation. Functional incontinence occurs in individuals with mobility issues or altered cognition. This condition can be ameliorated with an assistant who is able to help with toileting activities.

63. Correct: **B. urge**
Urge incontinence (B) is the most common form of incontinence in the elderly and is caused by detrusor overactivity that results in uninhibited bladder contractions.
Incorrect:
Stress incontinence (A) is caused by pelvic floor and urethral muscle weakness and is the most common form of incontinence in women. Iatrogenic incontinence (C) is associated with the use of a medication or following a medical treatment. Urine overflow (D) is associated with urethral obstruction and is most commonly found in older men.

64. Correct: **A. dry mouth and constipation.**
Oral selective muscarinic receptor antagonists work by exerting systemic anticholinergic effect to relieve symptoms of urge incontinence. However, these medications are associated with systemic anticholinergic-related adverse effects, with the most commonly reported being dry mouth and constipation (A).
Incorrect:
Antimuscarinic agents used to treat urge incontinence exert systemic anticholinergic effects and their associated adverse effects. These adverse effects do not typically include nausea (B), headaches (C), or syncope (D).

65. Correct: **C. darifenacin (Enablex®)**
The elderly and those with cognitive dysfunction are more vulnerable to mental status changes with the use of systemic anticholinergic agents. Darifenacin (C) is a newer anticholinergic agent that has been shown to

have fewer adverse effects, such as confusion, and is likely more helpful in older patients with underlying dementia.
Incorrect:
Oxybutynin, tolterodine, and solifenacin succinate (A, B, and D) provide nonspecific systemic antimuscarinic action and will potentially contribute to confusion and functional decline in the elderly and those with underlying dementia.

66. Correct: **A. botulinum toxin injections, or C. mirabegron (Myrbetriq®)**
Botulinum injections in the bladder have been shown to improve symptoms of urge incontinence and offer an alternative to the use of pharmacotherapeutics to treat the condition (A). Mirabegron is a β_3-receptor agonist that can provide an effective alternative for patients who cannot tolerate anticholinergic agents (C).
Incorrect:
Fesoterodine fumarate belongs in the class of systemic anticholinergics and would likely not be tolerated by this patient (B). Finasteride is used to decrease the size of an enlarged prostate that can be causing urethral obstruction and, thus, would not be helpful for this patient (D).

67 to 69. Matching Questions

67. Correct: **B. UTI**

68. Correct: **A. urethral obstruction**

69. Correct: **C. pelvic floor weakness**
When evaluating an individual with signs and symptoms of UI, the first diagnostic approach is typically urinalysis with culture and susceptibility testing to check for the presence of a UTI. When the etiology of UI is unclear or standard therapy is ineffective, further diagnostic evaluation would be needed. A cough stress test, where the bladder is filled with water and the individual is asked to cough or strain to reproduce the incontinence, can help assess the presence of pelvic floor weakness associated with stress incontinence. Cystoscopy can be used to visualize the bladder and identify tumors or obstruction that can contribute to urine outflow issues.

Renal Stones

70. Correct: **B. vegetarian diet.**
Several risk factors have been identified for the development of renal stones. Among these, a diet high in animal protein can increase the risk of uric acid stones. A vegetarian diet would not normally increase the risk of renal stones (B), though a diet high in certain fruits and vegetables rich in oxalate can increase the risk of calcium oxalate stones.
Incorrect:
Known risk factors for renal stones include male gender (A), prior history or family history of kidney stones (C), chronically poor fluid intake, dehydration, and overweight or obesity (D).

71. Correct: B. moxifloxacin.

Certain medications can increase the risk of renal stones. However, the fluoroquinolones, such as moxifloxacin, have not been shown to induce the formation of renal stones.

Incorrect:

Indinavir (D), used to treat HIV, as well as sulfa medications, such as sulfasalazine (A), are poorly soluble drugs that can favor crystallization when they reach sufficient concentrations in the urine. Other drugs, such as topiramate (C), can promote the formation of urinary calculi by altering urinary pH and/or excretion of calcium, phosphate, oxalate, citrate, uric acid, or other purines.

72. Correct: A. calcium.

Calcium stones are the most common form and account for about 75% of renal calculi. These stones are radiopaque and, thus, visible on x-ray.

Incorrect:

Other types of stones include uric acid stones (B), as well as struvite stones and cystine stones. Stones are typically not composed of sodium (C) or iron (D).

73 to 75. Matching Questions

73. Correct: B. renal colic

74. Correct: C. mild to deep flank pain without radiation to the groin region

75. Correct: A. asymptomatic

The clinical presentation of renal stones can depend on the size and location of the stone as well as the degree of obstruction it causes. Stones present in the bladder are typically asymptomatic but can cause some urinary retention. Stones in the ureter cause the typical symptoms of renal stones, including sudden-onset, severe flank pain that can radiate to the groin region. This is referred to as renal colic. When stones are present in the ureteropelvic region, this is associated with mild to deep flank pain that does not radiate to the groin region.

76. Correct: C. marked febrile response.

The most common signs and symptoms of renal stones include acute pain, dysuria, and change in urine color (due to hematuria). Fever is not typically a common finding in these patients, though it could be an indication of an underlying infection that would need immediate further evaluation.

Incorrect:

Signs and symptoms of renal stones will depend on the size and location of the stone. The most frequently reported symptoms include acute back pain, often radiating to the groin region (B), as well as dysuria (D). Nausea and vomiting are common findings among those with renal colic. Hematuria is also frequently present that can cause a change in urine color (A).

77 to 79. Matching Questions

77. Correct: C. detect the presence of hydronephrosis

78. Correct: A. identify stones during renal colic

79. Correct: B. determine radiopaque total stone burden

Imaging techniques used in the diagnosis of renal stones have certain advantages and disadvantages. Plain x-rays can assess the total stone burden of radiopaque stones, which are typically calcium-containing stones. However, this technique can miss small stones or other types of stones that are radiolucent. Ultrasound can detect hydronephrosis but can miss stones less than 5 mm in size. CT scan offers high sensitivity and specificity in the diagnosis of acute renal colic and can detect stones as small as 3 mm in size.

80. Correct: C. ESWL.

Most patients with a kidney stone will pass the stone without any type of treatment. ESWL can be considered for patients with larger stones and more severe symptoms (C). For this patient, supportive therapy with analgesia and improved hydration could be sufficient to resolve the condition without further intervention.

Incorrect:

For patients with mild symptoms of renal stones, conservative management will be sufficient in the majority of cases, as small stones will eventually pass without intervention. The patient should be advised to increase hydration (A) and use an analgesic (e.g., acetaminophen) (D) when needed. An alpha blocker (B) can help to relax the muscles in the ureter to help pass the stone more quickly.

81 to 83. Matching Questions

81. Correct: A. ureter

82. Correct: B. ureteropelvic junction

83. Correct: B. ureteropelvic junction

Intervention in resolving a renal stone will depend on the stone size and placement. Small stones (less than 4 mm) typically pass through the urinary tract without treatment, though analgesics (e.g., acetaminophen) can be prescribed to alleviate the pain, and an alpha blocker can be used to relax the muscles in the ureter. For stones present in the ureteropelvic junction, internal ureteral stents can be used to drain the kidney and help with the passage of stones. When a stent is not appropriate, percutaneous nephrostomy (a catheter is inserted through the skin to drain the kidney) can be used. Percutaneous nephrostomy can be done in conjunction with ESWL when large stones are present.

84. Correct: B. adequate hydration.

Adequate hydration is the optimal method to prevent renal stones (B), with the recommendation to drink 2 to 3 liters of water per day.

Incorrect:

Prevention can include a combination of dietary adjustments, nutritional supplements, and medications. In addition to proper hydration, other strategies can include an increase in fruit and vegetable intake, and reduced sodium and animal protein intake. Medications can include the use of thiazide diuretic, potassium citrate, and allopurinol, depending on the type of renal stone. Though daily exercise (A), limiting excessive coffee consumption (C), and smoking cessation (D) are important in maintaining a healthy lifestyle, they are not necessarily effective strategies to prevent renal stones.

85. **Correct: D. if calcium supplements are needed, this medication should be taken on an empty stomach.** Calcium oxalate stones can be formed with high concentrations of calcium and oxalate in the urine. Oxalate is a substance found in certain fruits and vegetables as well as nuts and chocolate. Individuals with a history of calcium oxalate stones should continue to receive their daily calcium requirements either through diet or calcium supplements. If supplements are needed, these should be taken with meals to prevent a high concentration of excreted calcium (D).

Incorrect:
Strategies to prevent renal stones can include adequate hydration and limiting the amount of sodium and animal protein (A). For calcium oxalate stones, individuals should limit consumption of foods high in oxalate, including nuts and chocolate (B). Individuals should still aim to receive their recommended daily amount of calcium each day, preferably from food (C). If calcium supplements are needed, they should be taken with meals rather than on an empty stomach.

Hematological and Select Immunological Disorders

14

Anemia

Overview

Anemia is defined as a decrease in the oxygen-carrying capability of the blood. This condition is not a disease, but rather a sign of an underlying process. Anemia occurs only in the presence of a clinical insult severe enough to disturb the normal hematological homeostatic mechanisms and exceed the body's ample hematological reserves.

Clinical Presentation

The clinical presentation of anemia is highly variable, and compensation is common because most anemias are usually gradual in onset. In addition, the oxyhemoglobin-dissociation curve is moved to the right as the hemoglobin (Hgb) level decreases, with the oxygen molecule given up more freely by the red blood cell (RBC). As a result, symptoms of anemia seldom occur, unless the Hgb level decreases to less than 10 g/dL.

The health history usually reveals clues about the cause of the anemia (e.g., excessive menstrual flow, acute blood loss). Patients frequently report deep, sighing respiration with activity, often associated with a sensation of rapid, forceful heart rate; this is likely a reflection of the decreased oxygen-carrying capability of the blood and a corresponding compensatory mechanism. Fatigue, headache, and decreased exercise tolerance are often present. Poor school performance and learning difficulties have been reported in children with anemia. In patients at risk for or who have coronary artery disease, anginal symptoms are commonly reported.

The physical examination usually contributes little to the diagnosis, unless the anemia is severe. Pallor of the skin and mucous membranes is an unreliable indicator and is usually seen only when the Hgb is significantly decreased (less than 8 g/dL). In elderly persons and in individuals with coronary artery disease, signs of heart failure (e.g., distended neck veins, rales, tachycardia, right upper quadrant abdominal tenderness, hepatomegaly) are often seen with severe anemia. An early systolic murmur, also known as a hemic murmur, is often heard, owing in part to the increase in blood flow over the heart valves. Neurological findings, such as paresthesia, stocking-glove neuropathy, difficulty with balance, and in extreme cases, confusion, can be found in patients with vitamin B_{12} deficiency. Less commonly, mental status changes are noted in folate-deficiency anemia.

Diagnostic Testing

The first-line test in suspected anemia is the complete blood count (CBC), also known as the hemogram, with RBC indices. In evaluating the CBC of patients with anemia, the following questions should be answered to ascertain the origin of the anemia (Table 14-1):

- *What are Hgb, hematocrit (Hct), and RBC values?* These values should be proportionately decreased. Normally, the Hgb-to-Hct ratio is 1:3, so that in health, 1 g/dL of Hgb is equivalent to 3 percentage points of Hct. Hgb is an iron-containing protein responsible for the transportation of oxygen and other gases. The Hct value reflects the percentage of RBCs in a given volume of blood; the value is influenced by the body's hydration status. The 1:3 Hgb-to-Hct ratio is usually violated only in severe dehydration, where the Hct is artificially elevated (e.g., Hgb 12 g/dL, Hct 42%), or overhydration, where the Hct is artificially decreased (e.g., Hgb 12 g/dL, Hct 32%).

- *What is the RBC size?* This is reflected by the mean corpuscular volume (MCV); the method of categorizing anemia is known as Wintrobe's classification. The RBC maintains its size and color throughout its 90- to 120-day life span.

  - *Is the RBC abnormally small (microcytic or low MCV)?* Ninety percent of the RBC volume is composed of Hgb. As a result, Hgb is the major contributor to cell size; microcytosis is seen in patients with anemia in whom Hgb synthesis is impaired, such as in the presence of iron-deficiency anemia (IDA) and the thalassemias.

  - A microcytic cell will also have a low mean corpuscular hemoglobin (MCH) concentration and mean cell hemoglobin concentration (MCHC).

  - *Is the RBC abnormally large (macrocytic)?* Impaired RNA and DNA synthesis in young erythrocytes most commonly causes macrocytosis. Folic acid and vitamin B_{12} contribute significantly to RNA and DNA synthesis in the developing RBC. A lack of either or both of these micronutrients can result in macrocytic anemia. Because Hgb synthesis is not the issue, macrocytic cells are usually of normal color (normochromic or MCH and MCHC within normal limits).

TABLE 14-1 Hemogram Evaluation in Anemia*

LABORATORY PARAMETER	CLINICAL CONSIDERATIONS
What are Hgb and Hct, RBC count values?	Values should be proportionately decreased. Normally, Hgb:Hct ratio is 1:3. ■ 10 g/dL = 30% ■ 12 g/dL = 36% ■ 15 g/dL = 45%
What is the RBC size?	Wintrobe's classification of anemia by evaluation of MCV ■ Microcytic: Small cell with MCV less than 80 fL ■ Normocytic: Normal-sized cell with MCV 80 to 96 fL ■ Macrocytic: Abnormally large cell with MCV greater than 96 fL
What is the RBC's hemoglobin content?	Reflected by MCH and MCHC ■ Hemoglobin is the source of the cell's color (*chromic*) ■ Normochromic: Normal color–MCHC 31 to 37 g/dL ■ Hypochromic: Pale–MCHC less than 31 g/dL
What is the RDW?	Index of variation in RBC size (normal 11.5% to 15%) Abnormal value: Greater than 15%, indicating that new cells differ in size (smaller or larger) compared with older cells. This is one of the earliest laboratory indicators of an evolving microcytic or macrocytic anemia.
What is the reticulocyte percentage or count?	The body's normal response to anemia is to attempt correction via increasing the number of new cells (reticulocytes). Normal response to anemia is reticulocytosis. Because the reticulocyte MCV is greater than 96 fL, marked reticulocytosis can cause RDW to increase transiently.

*Note: Minor variations in laboratory norms may occur. Hct, hematocrit; Hgb, hemoglobin; MCH, mean cell hemoglobin; MCHC, mean cell hemoglobin concentration; MCV, mean corpuscular volume; RBC, red blood cell; RDW, red blood cell distribution width.

CLINICAL CONCEPT

In addition, because Hgb gives RBCs their characteristic red color, small (microcytic) and pale (hypochromic) go together.

• *Is the RBC of normal size (normocytic)?* In these anemias, the cells are made under ordinary conditions with sufficient Hgb; there is no problem with RNA, DNA, or Hgb synthesis and that the cell was made with sufficient iron, protein, folic acid, and vitamin B_{12}. Acute blood loss and anemia of chronic disease (ACD) result in a normocytic, normochromic anemia.

■ *What is the Hgb content (color) of the cell?* The Hgb content of the cell is reflected in the MCH or MCHC. Because Hgb gives RBCs their characteristic red color, the suffix *-chromic* is used to describe the MCH. When a cell has a normal MCH or MCHC, it is of normal color, or normochromic. When there is an impairment of Hgb synthesis, such as in IDA or thalassemia, the cells are pale or hypochromic, and the MCH or MCHC is low. RBCs seldom are hyperchromic or contain excessive amounts of Hgb.

■ *What is the RDW (RBC distribution width)?* RDW reflects the degree of variation in RBC size; this is often reported as anisocytosis on RBC morphological study. RDW measurement is elevated when RBCs are of varying sizes, which implies that cells were synthesized under varying conditions. For example, in IDA, normal-sized cells produced before iron depletion continue to circulate until their 90- to 120-day life span ends. Meanwhile, new, microcytic, iron-deficient cells containing less Hgb are produced. There is wide variation in cell size (newer cells are smaller, and older cells are larger) and an increase in RDW. The opposite occurs during an evolving macrocytic anemia. Because minor variation in cell size is normal, RDW is considered increased only when it is greater than 15%. An elevated RDW is often the first abnormal finding in the hemogram of a person with an evolving microcytic or macrocytic anemia.

Poikilocytosis refers to a variation in RBC shape and is not specific to any anemia type but usually occurs with more severe anemia.

■ *What is the percentage of reticulocytes?* The body's normal response to anemia is to attempt correction via increasing the number of new cells (reticulocytes). The body's normal response to anemia is reticulocytosis, or an increase in the percentage of circulating reticulocytes to greater than the 1% to 2% noted in health. The notation of reticulocytopenia, or an abnormally low reticulocyte percentage, is evidence of inadequate hemopoiesis.

Treatment

Anemia treatment is focused on treating the underlying cause. As a result, anemia treatment varies according to its etiology. See specific conditions later in this chapter.

IRON-DEFICIENCY ANEMIA

Overview

Men and postmenopausal women require 1 mg of iron each day. During reproductive years, women require 1.5 to 3 mg/day of iron, in part because of the monthly loss of RBCs with menses. In these circumstances, iron requirements are achievable with a well-balanced diet.

Worldwide, iron deficiency is the most common reason for anemia (Table 14-2). Because an estimated 8 years of poor iron intake is needed in adults before IDA occurs, diet is rarely the etiology in many countries, including the United States and Canada. Rather, chronic blood loss causing a wasting of the RBCs' recyclable iron, the body's most important iron source, is the most common cause.

Occult gastrointestinal (GI) blood loss, such as from an oozing gastritis or GI malignancy, is a common cause of IDA in males, especially in those older than 50 years old, and in postmenopausal women. In women during the reproductive years, heavy menstrual flow is the most common IDA etiology.

> **CLINICAL CONCEPT**
> Because 1 mL of packed RBCs contains 1 mg of iron, losses of 2 to 3 mL of blood per day through chronic, low-volume blood loss can lead to iron deficiency.

Diagnostic Testing

The laboratory diagnosis of IDA is supported by the following findings:

■ *Early in the disease process*: Low to normal Hgb, HCT, and RBC count; normocytic, possibly hypochromic; RDW greater than 15% as new, microcytic, iron-deficient cells are produced.
■ *Low serum iron level*: Reflecting iron concentration in circulation. Serum iron is reflective of iron intake during the past 24 to 48 hours and can be falsely elevated because of recent high levels of dietary iron ingestion or self-prescribed oral iron supplementation.
■ *Elevated total iron-binding capacity (TIBC)*: A measure of transferrin, a plasma protein that easily combines with iron. When more transferrin is available for binding, the TIBC level increases, reflecting iron deficiency.
■ *Iron saturation less than 15%*: Calculated by dividing the serum iron level by the TIBC.
■ *Low serum ferritin level*: This is the body's major iron storage protein. Ferritin depletion is one of the first laboratory markers of iron deficiency, as stores are depleted prior to abnormal cells being formed.
■ *Later disease*: Microcytic, hypochromic anemia with low RBC count and elevated RDW greater than 15%. A decrease in Hgb or RBC indices is a late, rather than an early, marker of disease.

Treatment

Therapy for patients with IDA involves not only iron replacement but also treatment of the underlying cause. Iron use without a distinct clinical indication, including the use of iron-fortified multiple vitamins, is not recommended because this can lead to an iatrogenic iron overload. Iron overload has been hypothesized to be a cardiovascular risk factor.

A number of oral iron (Fe) forms are available, including ferrous gluconate and ferrous sulfate. Either is acceptable as a supplement. Enteric-coated iron should be avoided. Although this iron form is often reported as causing less GI upset, iron is best absorbed in the duodenum. The use of enteric-coated iron results in relatively little of the dose being properly absorbed. In addition, the duodenum is relatively refractory to iron absorption for about 6 hours postexposure to a high iron dose. As a result, oral iron should be dosed no sooner than every 6 hours; twice-daily supplementation is usually adequate to correct

TABLE 14-2 Identifying Common Anemias

ANEMIA TYPE	DESCRIPTION	EXAMPLE
Normocytic (MCV 80 to 96 fL), normochromic anemia with normal RDW Most common etiology: Acute blood loss or ACD	Cells made under ordinary conditions with sufficient hemoglobin. This yields cells that are of normal size (normocytic), normal color (normochromic), and about the same size (normal RDW)	72-year-old man with an acute gastrointestinal bleed (acute blood loss) 32-year-old woman with newly diagnosed lupus erythematosus (ACD) Hgb 10.1 g/dL (12 to 14 g/dL) Hct 32% (36% to 43%) RBC 3.2 million mm³ (4.2 to 5.4 million mm³) MCV 82 fL (81 to 96 fL) MCHC 34.8 g/dL (31 to 37 g/dL) RDW 12.1% (11.5% to 15%)
Microcytic (MCV less than 80 fL) hypochromic anemia with elevated RDW Most common etiology: Iron-deficiency anemia	Small cell (microcytic) owing to insufficient hemoglobin (hypochromic) with new cells smaller than old cells (elevated RDW)	68-year-old man with erosive gastritis Hgb 10.1 g/dL (12 to 14 g/dL) Hct 32% (36% to 43%) RBC 3.2 million mm³ (4.2 to 5.4 million mm³) MCV 72 fL (81 to 96 fL) MCHC 26.8 g/dL (31 to 37 g/dL) RDW 18.1% (11.5% to 15%)
Microcytic (MCV less than 80 fL) hypochromic anemia with normal RDW Most common etiology: α- or β-thalassemia minor At-risk ethnic groups for α-thalassemia minor: Asian, African ancestry At-risk ethnic groups for β-thalassemia minor: African, Middle Eastern, Mediterranean ancestry	Through genetic variation, small (microcytic), pale (hypochromic) cells that are all about the same size (normal RDW)	27-year-old man of African ancestry Hgb 11.6 g/dL (14 to 16 g/dL) Hct 36.7% (42% to 48%) RBC 6.38 million mm³ (4.7 to 6.10 million mm³) MCV 69.5 fL (81 to 99 fL) MCH 22 pg (27 to 33 pg) RDW 13.8% (11.5% to 15%)
Macrocytic (MCV greater than 96 fL) normochromic anemia with elevated RDW Most common etiology: Vitamin B_{12} deficiency, pernicious anemia, folate-deficiency anemia	Abnormally large (macrocytic) cell owing to altered RNA: DNA ratio, hemoglobin content normal (normochromic), new cells larger than old cells (elevated RDW)	52-year-old woman with untreated pernicious anemia Hgb 10.2 g/dL (12 to 14 g/dL) Hct 32% (36% to 43%) RBC 3.2 million mm³ (4.2 to 5.4 million mm³) MCV 125.5 fL (81 to 99 fL) MCH 31 pg (27 to 33 pg) RDW 18.8% (11.5% to 15%)

ACD, anemia of chronic disease; Hct, hematocrit; Hgb, hemoglobin; MCHC, mean cell hemoglobin concentration; MCV, mean corpuscular volume; RBC, red blood cell; RDW, red blood cell distribution width.

iron deficiency. Oral iron overdose is the most common cause of fatal childhood overdose. The source of this iron is usually an adult's prescription, most often that of the child's mother. The use of carbonyl iron has been advocated owing to its slow rate of GI absorption, yielding less toxicity in overdose. A typical adult iron dose for anemia correction is 50 to 60 mg of elemental iron taken orally twice a day for 3 to 6 months.

Ascorbic acid (vitamin C) is an enhancer of iron absorption and can reverse the inhibiting effects of substances such as tea and calcium. Ascorbic acid taken at the same time as ferrous sulfate can help with iron absorption. To minimize adverse GI effects, iron supplements are often taken with food; this can result in as much as a two-thirds reduction in iron absorption. Taking iron on an empty stomach allows for maximum absorption. Because of safety concerns and high cost, parenteral iron use should be limited to individuals who are unable to ingest, tolerate, or properly absorb oral iron.

Oral iron has the potential to interact with numerous other medications (Table 14-3). This is a localized interaction, largely limited to when an iron dose is in the stomach around the same time as the target drug.

Laboratory Evaluation During IDA Resolution

During IDA recovery, reticulocytosis begins quickly after initiation of iron therapy, with the reticulocyte percentage peaking 7 to 10 days into therapy. Hgb increases at a rate of 2 g/dL every 3 weeks in response to iron therapy and is likely to take 2 months to correct if the underlying cause of the anemia has been successfully treated. As a result, the following laboratory tests can be used to evaluate the resolution of IDA:

■ Reticulocytes at 1 to 2 weeks to ensure marrow response to iron therapy
■ Hgb at 6 weeks to 2 months to ensure anemia recovery
■ Ferritin at 2 months after measure of normal Hgb (or 4 months after initiation of iron therapy) to ensure documentation of replenished iron stores

TABLE 14-3 Drug Interactions With Oral Iron Therapy

DRUG	EFFECT	THERAPEUTIC CONSIDERATIONS
Antacids	Decreased iron absorption	Separate use by 2 hours or more
Caffeine	Decreased iron absorption	Separate use by 2 hours or more
Fluoroquinolones (ciprofloxacin, moxifloxacin, levofloxacin, others)	Decreased fluoroquinolone effect	Avoid concurrent use or separate doses by 6 hours or more
Levodopa	Decreased levodopa and iron effect	Separate medications by as much time as possible; increase levodopa dose as needed
Select antihypertensives (angiotensin-converting enzyme [ACE] inhibitors, methyldopa)	Decreased antihypertensive effect	Separate medications by 2 hours or more, monitor blood pressure Additional effect with IV iron: When ACE inhibitors are given concurrently, increased risk of systemic reaction to iron (fever, arthralgia, hypotension); concurrent use should be avoided
Tetracyclines including doxycycline	Decreased tetracycline and iron effect	Do not use concurrently, or separate by 3 to 4 hours or more
Levothyroxine (Synthroid®, Unithroid®, Levoxyl®, generic)	Decreased levothyroxine effect	Take levothyroxine 2 or more hours before or 4 hours after iron dose
Histamine-2 receptor antagonists	Decreased dietary iron absorption	Less significant when compared to proton pump inhibitor use
Proton pump inhibitor	Decrease dietary iron absorption	Potentially significant contributor to iron and other micronutrient deficiencies, particularly with protracted use

Source: Iron sulfate (ferrous sulfate) drug interactions. Drugs.com. https://www.drugs.com/drug-interactions/ferrous-sulfate,iron-sulfate.html

THE THALASSEMIAS

Overview

The thalassemias are genetically based blood conditions wherein the body makes an abnormal Hgb form. Hgb is made of two proteins: α-globin and β-globin. In α-thalassemia, the alteration is in the genes or genes related to α-globin, and in beta form, it is an alteration on the β-globin. The α-thalassemias occur most commonly in persons from Southeast Asia, the Middle East, China, and Africa. The β-thalassemias occur in persons of Mediterranean origin and, to a lesser extent, those of Asian and African origins.

The thalassemia majors are life-threatening conditions that are identified in early life; two altered genes are inherited, one from each parent. In North America, the thalassemia majors are relatively rare. The thalassemia minors (thal minor or thal trait), in which one altered gene has been inherited, result in a mild microcytic hypochromic anemia. Because there is no micronutrient deficiency, the RDW and platelets are within normal limits. Given the risk of passing the altered genes to offspring if both members of a couple are affected with thal minor, prior genetic counseling is recommended. Otherwise, people with a thal minor have no particular health risks.

THE MACROCYTIC ANEMIAS

> **CLINICAL CONCEPT**
>
> When macrocytosis with anemia is detected, the usual next step is to obtain a serum vitamin B_{12} and folate.

Overview

In synergy with folic acid (folate), vitamin B_{12} plays an essential role in RBC DNA synthesis. When deficiencies of either of these micronutrients exist, DNA synthesis in the RBC is impaired, which leads to the distinct changes in the RBC, macrocytosis, and bone marrow.

When the diagnosis of macrocytic anemia is uncertain, additional testing is recommended; elevated serum methylmalonic acid (MMA) and homocysteine levels are found with pernicious anemia, whereas elevated homocysteine levels with normal MMA levels are found in folic acid deficiency (FAD).

FOLIC ACID DEFICIENCY ANEMIA

Overview

During times of accelerated tissue growth and repair, such as in childhood, pregnancy, recovery from serious illness, and recovery from hemolytic anemia, folic acid requirements increase from the baseline by twofold to fourfold.

The most common causes of FAD anemia are inadequate dietary intake, seen in the elderly, alcohol abusers, and individuals with poor access to nutritious food. In addition, people with decreased ability to absorb folic acid, occurring with malabsorption syndromes such as sprue and celiac disease, are at increased FAD risk. Repeated pregnancies, particularly those with less than 2 years between births, cause depletion of maternal folate stores. Maternal FAD is a teratogenic state, particularly during neural tube formation, leading to increased risk for fetal spina bifida and anencephaly. Supplementation should continue through lactation because approximately 0.5 mg/day of folic acid is transferred to breast milk. Accumulation of the vitamin in human milk takes precedence over maintaining maternal folate levels. A growing body of knowledge points to genetic factors in metabolizing and using folic acid, rather than dietary FAD, as a possible contributor to the risk of neural tube defect and a factor in treatment-resistant depression.

Diagnostic Testing

Hemogram in FAD, regardless of cause, reveals a macrocytic, normochromic anemia with an elevated RDW. The degree of anemia in FAD is usually modest, as is the degree of macrocytosis.

Confirmatory testing should include initial testing for serum levels of both folic acid and cobalamin (vitamin B_{12}), as a deficiency in either of these B vitamins will result in a macrocytic, normochromic anemia as well as similar neurological symptoms. Laboratories often bundle these tests, though folate deficiency is much less common. If the macrocytic anemia diagnosis is still uncertain, additional follow-up tests can be performed for confirmation, including serum homocysteine (elevated in folate and vitamin B_{12} deficiency) and serum MMA (elevated in vitamin B_{12} deficiency only).

Treatment

FAD can be avoided with a healthy diet featuring folate-rich fruits and vegetables. In addition, many foods, including most flours, are supplemented with folic acid, further reducing risk.

As with all anemias, the first-line therapy is to treat the underlying causes. Recommendations for oral acid replacement for adults range from 0.5 to 1 to 5 mg/day, the usual dose being 1 mg/day. The underlying cause of the folate deficiency must also be treated. To reduce the rate of fetal neural tube defects, a woman planning a pregnancy should be advised to take additional amounts of folic acid, 0.4 mg/day, for 3 months before conception. This recommendation should be extended to all women capable of conception. Over-the-counter multivitamin or diet supplementation with vitamin-fortified foods can easily supply the recommended folate dose. Folate deficiency during pregnancy can be largely avoided through the consistent use of prenatal vitamins, each tablet usually containing 0.8 to 1 mg of folic acid. If a woman has a history of having a pregnancy associated with a neural tube defect, the folic acid dose should be increased to 4 mg/day for 3 months before conception and continued at least through the first 12 weeks of pregnancy. If the pregnancy is unplanned or preconception counseling was not sought, initiating folic acid supplementation during the first 7 weeks of pregnancy seems to offer some neural tube protection.

Folic Acid Deficiency Anemia: Evaluation of Therapy

Reticulocytosis occurs rapidly, with a peak at 7 to 10 days into folic acid therapy. The Hct level increases by 4% to 5% per week and generally returns to normal within 1 month. Leukopenia and thrombocytopenia resolve within 2 to 3 days of therapy. A repeat hemogram in 1 to 2 months assists in monitoring the therapeutic effect. Resolution of the related signs and symptoms generally follows the time frame needed for the resolution of the anemia.

VITAMIN B_{12} ANEMIA

Overview

Vitamin B_{12}, a member of the cobalamin family, is found in abundance in foods of animal origin and is essential to the development of the RBC. When vitamin B_{12} is ingested orally, it binds with intrinsic factor (IF), a glycoprotein produced by the gastric parietal cells critical to B_{12} intestinal absorption; IF production impairment occurs with autoimmune gastric parietal cell destruction. The term *pernicious anemia* is usually given to vitamin B_{12} deficiency secondary to lack of IF. Vitamin B_{12} deficiency from diet alone is uncommon with an omnivore diet but is possible with a plant-based or vegan diet. As a result, B_{12} supplementation is recommended in a vegan diet.

> **CLINICAL CONCEPT**
>
> Proton pump inhibitor (PPI) and metformin use limit dietary B_{12} absorption; protracted use can result in vitamin B_{12} deficiency and a resulting anemia.

Clinical Presentation

The onset of pernicious anemia usually is slowly progressive with vague signs and symptoms including weakness, sore tongue with absent papillae, anorexia with unintended weight loss, and GI disturbance. This anemia develops slowly, allowing for compensation. However, when Hct is less than 20%, cardiac output increases and heart rate accelerates, occasionally with resulting heart failure and angina with preexisting heart disease.

Neurological symptoms of vitamin B_{12} deficiency, including paresthesia, weakness, clumsiness, and unsteady gait, are common as is neuropathy affecting the hands and feet (stocking-glove neuropathy). New-onset mental status changes including forgetfulness are often noted. Physical examination reflects the alterations as noted in the physical examination and includes hypoactive deep tendon reflexes (DTRs), loss of vibratory sense, and tachycardia.

Diagnostic Testing

Hemogram in vitamin B_{12} deficiency, regardless of cause, reveals a macrocytic, normochromic anemia with an elevated RDW. In pernicious anemia, the presenting Hct is usually quite low, less than 28%, and MCV quite high, greater than 115 fL. With B_{12} deficiency from other sources, the Hct is typically not as low and MCV not as high, and neurological findings are usually absent. Confirmatory testing includes documenting B_{12} deficiency with low serum cobalamin (B_{12}). Concomitant folic acid (folate) deficiency is common, and hence, cobalamin testing and folate testing are usually done together.

Treatment

Vitamin B_{12} therapy should be initiated when the diagnosis is made. Vitamin B_{12} is available generically and in oral and injectable forms. The parenteral form of vitamin B_{12} is historically preferred because of its perceived excellent absorption, ability to document treatment adherence, and fear of permanent neurological damage associated with chronic vitamin B_{12} deficiency. However, in oral form, even in pernicious anemia, vitamin B_{12} continues to be absorbed via the GI system.

With the use of oral B_{12}, drug interactions should be noted (Table 14-4). When given parenterally, the usual initial vitamin B_{12} dosage is 1,000 mcg/day intramuscularly (IM) for the first week, then weekly for the first month, and then 1,000 mcg every 1 to 3 months for the rest of the patient's life. In reality, likely as little as 100 mcg per injectable dose is sufficient, as higher amounts exceed the binding capacity of transcobalamin II; the excess is excreted via the kidney and wasted. When vitamin B_{12} deficiency is to be treated orally, a higher dose, 1,000 mcg/day, is needed. Vitamin B_{12} is also available in a nasal gel, usually used weekly at a dose of 500 mcg. Concomitant administration of folic acid, iron, vitamin C, and other micronutrients is often needed to help with hematological recovery.

When the cause of macrocytic anemia has not yet been established, a prudent course of action is to give parenteral vitamin B_{12} initially while giving folic acid, 1 to 2 mg/day. With this plan, no intervention time is lost. After the appropriate diagnosis is established, the correct vitamin supplement is continued; note drug interactions (see Table 14-4).

The hematological response is generally rapid after therapy is begun. Reticulocytosis is brisk and peaks at 5 to 7 days. Hypokalemia, caused by serum-to-intracellular potassium shifts, is common if the anemia was particularly severe and is most likely seen with the peak of reticulocytosis. Monitoring serum potassium frequently during the first week of therapy is important, especially in patients receiving diuretic therapy, at other risk of hypokalemia, or taking digoxin. If hypokalemia occurs, oral potassium replacement at 40 mEq/day is usually sufficient. Concomitant oral iron therapy is indicated if there is an iron deficiency or low iron stores. Full hematological recovery usually takes about 2 months.

Reversal of the signs and symptoms of vitamin B_{12} deficiency is generally rapid. A sense of improved well-being is usually reported within 24 hours of the onset of treatment. Neurological changes, if present for less than 6 months, reverse quickly. Neurological reversal is likely impossible, however, if these changes have been present for a protracted period.

ANEMIA OF CHRONIC DISEASE

Overview

Anemia is often noted in persons with select chronic health problems, such as acute and chronic inflammatory conditions (e.g., infection, or poorly control systemic inflammatory disease such as rheumatoid arthritis and systemic lupus), renal insufficiency, and hypothyroidism. In part, this condition, known as ACD, is caused by reduced erythropoietin response in the marrow, resulting in RBC hypoproliferation.

In ACD, micronutrient deficiency is not an issue, in that the RBCs are made with sufficient iron, vitamin B_{12}, folic acid, and other vitamins and minerals; this yields a normocytic, normochromic anemia.

> **CLINICAL CONCEPT**
>
> Seldom does ACD result in a severe anemia; usually Hct is 24% or greater.

TABLE 14-4 Oral Vitamin B_{12}–Drug Interactions

DRUG	EFFECT
Colchicine	With concomitant use, decreased vitamin B_{12} absorption
Potassium supplements	With concomitant use, decreased vitamin B_{12} absorption
Ascorbic acid	Potential to destroy vitamin B_{12} if taken within 1 hour of oral vitamin B_{12} ingestion
Proton pump inhibitor	With concomitant use, decreased vitamin B_{12} absorption, particularly with protracted use

Source: Vitamin B_{12} (cyanocobalamin) drug interactions. Drugs.com. http://www.drugs.com/drug-interactions/cyanocobalamin,vitamin-b12.html

Worldwide, ACD is second only to iron deficiency in occurrence. Bone marrow can be suppressed as a result of the use of certain drugs, including cancer chemotherapy agents. Because normal RBC death occurs without the production of new RBC forms, anemia can occur. When the glomerular filtration rate (GFR) declines to less than 30 to 40 mL/min, renal erythropoietin synthesis is reduced; a hypoproliferative normochromic, normocytic anemia develops, usually with an Hgb level of 8 g/dL or greater. That is, as the kidney fails, erythropoietin production declines, and ACD develops.

Diagnostic Testing

ACD is largely a diagnosis of exclusion, where other causes of normocytic, normochromic anemia have been eliminated by history, clinical presentation, and diagnostics. If ACD is suspected, serum iron, transferrin, reticulocyte count, and serum ferritin should be measured to check if IDA is also present. At the same time, ferritin can be elevated in the presence of inflammation; the results should be carefully evaluated and correlated with the clinical presentation.

Treatment

As with all other anemia forms, treatment is aimed at the condition's underlying cause. Given there is no micronutrient deficiency, nutritional supplements such as vitamin B_{12}, folic acid, and iron have no impact on ACD resolution. Rather, treatment of the underlying inflammatory disease will help with anemia resolution.

In chronic renal disease, especially when the GFR is less than 45 mL/min per 1.73 m^2 (normal = 90 to 120 mL/min per 1.73 m^2), erythropoetin production is significantly reduced, resulting in ACD. Recombinant human erythropoietin (epoetin alfa) is used to boost RBC production. The drug can only be administered parenterally (subcutaneously or intravenously) three times per week with an expected increase in Hct of approximately 4% over 2 weeks. Iron therapy, as well as supplements with other micronutrients, is also needed, unless iron overload is present. Patient symptoms, such as altered exercise capacity and sexual function, which are often attributed to renal disease, are often attenuated if Hgb level is appropriately corrected to 11 to 12 g/dL with the use of recombinant human erythropoietin (epoetin alfa); correction beyond this Hgb level has been associated with increased thrombotic risk without additional health benefit.

Discussion Sources

Coffey-Vega K. Folic acid deficiency. Medscape. http://emedicine.medscape.com/article/200184-overview

Desai S. *Clinician's Guide to Laboratory Medicine: Pocket.* Houston, TX: MD2B; 2009.

Harper J. Iron deficiency anemia. Medscape. http://emedicine.medscape.com/article/202333

Nagalla S. Pernicious anemia. Medscape. http://emedicine.medscape.com/article/204930

Society for the Advancement of Blood Management. A physician's guide to oral iron supplements. https://www.sabm.org/wp-content/uploads/2018/08/Physician-Guide-to-Oral-Iron-Nov-2013.compressed.pdf

QUESTIONS

1. Worldwide, which of the following is the most common type of anemia?

   A. pernicious anemia

   B. folate-deficiency anemia

   C. ACD

   D. IDA

2. Most of the body's iron is obtained from:

   A. animal-based food sources.

   B. recycled iron content from aged RBCs.

   C. endoplasmic reticulum production.

   D. vegetable-based food sources.

3. Which of the following is most consistent with IDA?

   A. low MCV, normal MCH

   B. low MCV, low MCH

   C. low MCV, elevated MCH

   D. normal MCV, normal MCH

4. One of the earliest laboratory markers in evolving macrocytic or microcytic anemia is:

   A. an increase in RDW.

   B. a reduction in measurable Hgb.

   C. a low MCH level.

   D. an increased platelet count.

5. A 48-year-old woman developed IDA after excessive perimenopausal vaginal bleeding, successfully treated by endometrial ablation. Her Hct level is 25%, and she is taking iron therapy. At 5 days into therapy, one possible observed change in laboratory parameters would include:

   A. a correction of mean cell volume.

   B. an 8% increase in Hct level.

   C. reticulocytosis.

   D. a correction in ferritin level.

6. A healthy 34-year-old man asks whether he should take an iron supplement. You respond that:

   A. this is a prudent measure to ensure health.

   B. IDA is a common problem in men of his age.

   C. use of an iron supplement in the absence of a documented deficiency can lead to iatrogenic iron overload.

   D. excess iron is easily excreted.

7. Which of the following is the best advice on taking ferrous sulfate to enhance iron absorption?

   A. "Take with other medications."

   B. "Take on a full stomach."

   C. "Take on an empty stomach."

   D. "Do not take with vitamin C."

8. A 40-year-old woman with pyelonephritis is taking two medications: ciprofloxacin and ferrous sulfate (for IDA). She asks about taking both medications. You advise that:

   A. she should take the medications with a large glass of water.

   B. an inactive drug compound is potentially formed if the two medications are taken together.

   C. she can take the medications together to enhance adherence to therapy.

   D. the ferrous sulfate potentially slows GI motility and results in enhanced ciprofloxacin absorption.

9. Two months into therapy for pernicious anemia, you wish to check the efficacy of the intervention. The best laboratory test to order at this point is a(n):

   A. Schilling test.

   B. Hgb measurement.

   C. reticulocyte count.

   D. serum cobalamin.

10. A woman who is planning a pregnancy should increase her intake of which of the following to minimize the risk of neural tube defect in the fetus?

    A. iron

    B. niacin

    C. folic acid

    D. vitamin C

11. Risk factors for folate-deficiency anemia include:

    A. menorrhagia.

    B. chronic ingestion of overcooked foods.

    C. use of NSAIDs.

    D. gastric atrophy.

12. Folate-deficiency anemia causes which of the following changes in the RBC indices?

    A. microcytic, normochromic

    B. normocytic, normochromic

    C. microcytic, hypochromic

    D. macrocytic, normochromic

13. Pernicious anemia is usually caused by:

    A. dietary deficiency of vitamin B_{12}.

    B. lack of production of intrinsic factor by the gastric mucosa.

    C. RBC enzyme deficiency.

    D. a combination of micronutrient deficiencies caused by malabsorption.

14. Pernicious anemia causes which of the following changes in the RBC indices?

    A. microcytic, normochromic

    B. normocytic, normochromic

    C. microcytic, hypochromic

    D. macrocytic, normochromic

15. Common physical examination findings in patients with pernicious anemia include:

    A. hypoactive bowel sounds.

    B. stocking-glove neuropathy.

    C. thin, spoon-shaped nails.

    D. retinal hemorrhages.

16. You examine a 47-year-old man who presents with difficulty initiating and maintaining sleep and chronic pharyngeal erythema with the following results on hemogram:

    Hgb = 15 g/dL (normal 14 to 16 g/dL)
    Hct = 45% (normal 42% to 48%)
    RBC = 4.8 million mm³ (normal 4.7 to 6.1 million mm³)
    MCV = 108 fL (normal 81 to 96 fL)
    MCHC = 33.2 g/dL (normal 31 to 37 g/dL)

    These values are most consistent with:

    A. pernicious anemia.

    B. alcohol abuse.

    C. thalassemia minor.

    D. Fanconi anemia.

17. You examine a 22-year-old woman of Asian ancestry. She has no presenting complaint. Hemogram results are as follows:

    Hgb = 9.1 g/dL (normal 12 to 14 g/dL)
    Hct = 28% (normal 36% to 43%)
    RBC = 5.6 million mm³ (normal 4.2 to 5.4 million mm³)

MCV = 68 fL (normal 81 to 96 fL)
MCHC = 28.2 g/dL (normal 31 to 37 g/dL)
RDW = 13% (normal ≤15%)
Reticulocytes = 1.5% (normal 1% to 2%)

This is most consistent with the laboratory assessment of:

A. IDA.

B. Cooley anemia.

C. α-thalassemia minor.

D. Hgb Barts.

18. A 68-year-old man who is usually healthy presents with new onset of "huffing and puffing" with exercise for the past 3 weeks. Physical examination reveals conjunctiva pallor and a hemic murmur. Hemogram results are as follows:

Hgb = 7.6 g/dL
Hct = 20.5%
RBC = 2.1 million mm³
MCV = 76 fL
MCHC = 28 g/dL
RDW = 18.4%
Reticulocytes = 1.8%

The most likely cause of these findings is:

A. poor nutrition.

B. occult blood loss.

C. malabsorption.

D. chronic inflammation.

19. You examine a 57-year-old woman with rheumatoid arthritis who is on a biological disease-modifying antirheumatic drug (DMARD) but continues to have poor disease control, and you find the following results on hemogram:

Hgb = 10.5 g/dL
Hct = 33%
RBC = 3.1 million mm³
MCV = 88 fL
MCHC = 32.8 g/dL
RDW = 12.2%
Reticulocytes = 0.8%

The laboratory findings are most consistent with:

A. pernicious anemia.

B. ACD.

C. β-thalassemia minor.

D. folate-deficiency anemia.

20. You examine a 27-year-old woman with menorrhagia who is otherwise well and note the following results on hemogram:

Hgb = 10.1 g/dL
Hct = 32%
RBC = 2.9 million mm³
MCV = 72 fL
MCHC = 28.2 g/dL
RDW = 18.9%

Physical examination is likely to include:

A. conjunctiva pallor.

B. hemic murmur.

C. tachycardia.

D. no specific anemia-related findings.

21. When prescribing erythropoietin supplementation, the nurse practitioner (NP) considers that:

A. the adrenal glands are its endogenous source.

B. the addition of micronutrient supplementation needed for erythropoiesis is advisable.

C. its use is as an adjunct in treating thrombocytopenia.

D. with its use, the RBC life span is prolonged.

22. In the first weeks of anemia therapy with parenteral vitamin B_{12} in a 68-year-old woman with hypertension who is taking a thiazide diuretic, the patient should be carefully monitored for:

A. hypernatremia.

B. dehydration.

C. hypokalemia.

D. acidemia.

23. Which of the following conditions is unlikely to result in ACD?

A. rheumatoid arthritis

B. peripheral vascular disease

C. chronic renal insufficiency

D. osteomyelitis

24. In health, the ratio of Hgb to Hct is usually:

A. 1:1.

B. 1:2.

C. 1:3.

D. 1:4.

25 to 28. Match each definition with the correct term.

_____ 25. RBCs of unequal size

_____ 26. Variation in RBC shape

_____ 27. Increase in the production of immature RBCs

_____ 28. Abnormal decrease in the production of immature RBCs

A. poikilocytosis

B. anisocytosis

C. reticulocytosis

D. reticulocytopenia

29. Which of the following is not consistent with ACD?

A. Normal limit (NL) RDW

B. NL MCHC

C. Hct less than 24%

D. NL to slightly elevated serum ferritin

30. When counseling a patient about the neurological alterations often associated with vitamin B_{12} deficiency, the NP advises that:

    A. these usually resolve within days with appropriate therapy.

    B. if present for longer than 6 months, these changes are occasionally permanent.

    C. the use of parenteral vitamin B_{12} therapy is needed to ensure symptom resolution.

    D. cognitive changes associated with vitamin B_{12} deficiency are seldom reversible even with appropriate therapy.

31. When the cause of a macrocytic anemia is uncertain, the most commonly recommended additional testing includes which of the following?

    A. haptoglobin and reticulocyte count

    B. Schilling test and gastric biopsy

    C. MMA and homocysteine

    D. transferrin and prealbumin

32. A 66-year-old man is recently diagnosed with advanced colon cancer. A hemogram reveals the following:

    Hgb = 9.7 g/dL
    Hct = 30%
    RBC = 2.7 million mm³
    MCV = 69 fL
    MCHC = 27.2 g/dL
    RDW = 18.4%

    Next-step testing for this patient should be serum:

    A. ferritin.

    B. folate.

    C. cobalamin.

    D. homocysteine.

33. A 46-year-old woman complains of a 2-month history of tiredness as well as a progressive worsening of short-term memory and coordination. Her hemogram is as follows:

    Hgb = 10 g/dL
    Hct = 30%
    RBC = 3.7 million mm³
    MCV = 118 fL
    MCH = 32 pg
    RDW = 19.4%

    Next-step testing for this patient should include:

    A. cobalamin.

    B. ferritin.

    C. thyrotropin (TSH).

    D. head computed tomography (CT).

34. You see a 36-year-old man with a history of depression. He states that he drinks about a six-pack of beer every night and primarily eats from fast-food restaurants. His diet consists of very little consumption of fruits and vegetables. His hemogram is as follows:

    Hgb = 10.4 g/dL
    Hct = 31%
    RBC = 3.8 million mm³
    MCV = 116 fL
    MCHC = 33.1 g/dL
    RDW = 17.6%

Next-step testing for this patient should include:

A. ferritin.

B. folate.

C. Hgb electrophoresis.

D. No further testing is needed.

35. Prolonged use of PPIs can lead to which micronutrient deficiency that can contribute to anemia?

A. vitamin D

B. folate

C. vitamin B_{12}

D. potassium

36 to 40. Anemia: True or False

_____ **36.** Anemia in children is potentially associated with poorer school performance.

_____ **37.** During pregnancy, folic acid requirements increase two- to fourfold.

_____ **38.** The RBC content is approximately 90% Hgb.

_____ **39.** Approximately 90% of the body's erythropoietin is produced by the kidney.

_____ **40.** The body's normative response to anemia is reticulocytopenia.

For answers and rationales, see end of chapter.

Anaphylaxis

Overview

Anaphylaxis is an acute, life-threatening systemic reaction with varied mechanisms, clinical presentations, and severity; this is a manifestation of a type I hypersensitivity. Anaphylaxis usually results from an immunoglobulin E (IgE)-immune-mediated reaction; however, nonimmunological events often cause sudden release of mediators from mast cells and basophils. Vasodilation, increased capillary permeability, and smooth muscle contraction occur; new inflammatory cells are attracted to the area, which then perpetuates the systemic reaction. The more rapidly anaphylaxis develops, the more likely the reaction is to be severe and potentially life-threatening.

> **CLINICAL CONCEPT**
> Increased risks for fatal anaphylactic reactions include being a teen or young adult, having asthma, and failing to administer epinephrine promptly and/or properly.

Clinical Presentation

Clinical presentations are unpredictable, and initial mild symptoms can rapidly progress to a life-threatening situation. Urticaria and angioedema are the most commonly reported findings in anaphylaxis (Table 14-5); however, respiratory compromise and cardiovascular collapse are of greatest concern because these are the most frequent cause of death from anaphylaxis.

Anaphylaxis includes one of three clinical scenarios:

1. The acute onset of a reaction (minutes to hours) with involvement of the skin, mucosal tissue, or both, *and at least one of the following*: (1) respiratory compromise, (2) reduced blood pressure, or (3) symptoms of end-organ dysfunction, *or*
2. Two or more of the following that occur rapidly after exposure to a *likely* allergen for that patient: involvement of the skin/mucosal tissue, respiratory compromise, reduced blood pressure or associated symptoms, and/or persistent GI symptoms, *or*
3. Reduced blood pressure after exposure to a *known* allergen

Diagnostic Testing

Anaphylaxis is a clinical diagnosis. At the same time, testing to determine its cause usually is conducted once the patient is stabilized. Foods are the most common cause of IgE-mediated anaphylaxis. Eight foods account for 90% of all food-allergic reactions in the United States: peanuts, tree nuts, fish, shellfish, milk, eggs, wheat, and soy.

TABLE 14-5 Frequency of Occurrence of Signs and Symptoms of Anaphylaxis

SIGNS AND SYMPTOMS	FREQUENCY OF OCCURRENCE BY PERCENTAGE
Cutaneous	
Urticaria and angioedema	85 to 90
Flushing	45 to 55
Pruritus without rash	2 to 5
Respiratory	
Dyspnea, wheeze	45 to 50
Upper airway angioedema	50 to 60
Rhinitis	15 to 20
Dizziness, syncope, hypotension	30 to 35
Abdomen	
Nausea, vomiting, diarrhea, cramping pain	25 to 30
Miscellaneous	
Headache	5 to 8
Substernal pain	4 to 6
Seizure	1 to 2

Source: Lieberman P, Nicklas RA, Randolph C, et al. Anaphylaxis–a practice parameter update 2015. Ann Allergy Asthma Immunol. 2015;115:341–384. https://www.aaaai.org/Aaaai/media/MediaLibrary /PDF%20Documents/Practice%20and%20Parameters/2015-Anaphylaxis-PP-Update.pdf

Food allergy is more common in children than adults. Food allergy in adults can reflect persistence of childhood allergies or can be a new sensitization. Milk, egg, wheat, and soy allergies often resolve in children; peanut, tree nut, fish, and shellfish allergies can resolve but more likely persist. Fatal food allergic reactions are usually caused by peanuts, tree nuts, fish, and shellfish but have also occurred from milk, egg, seeds, and other foods.

Medications are another potential source for IgE– and non-IgE–mediated anaphylaxis. Antibiotics (particularly penicillin), aspirin, and NSAIDs are the more common medications identified. Insect venoms and latex are other causes for anaphylaxis. Health-care workers, children with spina bifida and genitourinary abnormalities, and workers with occupational exposure to latex via latex gloves are at increased risk for natural rubber latex–induced anaphylaxis. As a result, the majority of gloves used in health care are now latex-free. Cross-sensitivity can occur between natural rubber latex protein and certain fruit proteins, potentially causing a reaction if the patient eats bananas, avocados, kiwi, melons, or chestnuts.

Treatment

Quick recognition of the signs and symptoms of anaphylaxis and immediate implementation of a prioritized action plan are essential.

The initial drug of choice for the management of anaphylaxis is parenteral epinephrine (Table 14-6). This medication reverses the effects of anaphylaxis and inhibits further mediator release and should be administered as soon as the diagnosis is suspected. The time to highest blood concentration (C_{max}) when studied in asymptomatic subjects is shorter when given IM in the vastus lateralis muscle (lateral thigh) than when administered either subcutaneously or IM in the deltoid muscle. Unusually severe or refractory anaphylaxis

TABLE 14-6 Anaphylaxis Treatment Protocol

IMMEDIATE MEASURES

Allergen	Remove the inciting allergen, if possible
Airway	Assess airway, breathing, circulation, and orientation; if needed, support the airway using the least invasive but effective method
Cardiopulmonary resuscitation	Start chest compressions if cardiovascular arrest occurs at any time
Epinephrine intramuscularly (IM)	Inject epinephrine 0.3 to 0.5 mg (0.01 mg/kg for children) IM in the vastus lateralis (lateral thigh)
Get help	Summon appropriate assistance
Position	Place adults and adolescents in recumbent position; place young children in position of comfort; place pregnant patient on left side
Oxygen	Give 8 to 10 L/min through face mask or up to 100% oxygen as needed; monitor by pulse oximetry if available
Epinephrine IM	Repeat IM epinephrine every 5 to 15 minutes for up to three injections if the patient is not responding
Emergency medical system (EMS)	Activate EMS (call 911 or local rescue squad) for transportation to emergency department or other higher level of care, particularly if no immediate response to first dose of IM epinephrine or if anaphylaxis is moderate-to-severe grade
IV fluids	Establish IV line for venous access and fluid replacement; keep open with 0.9 NL saline, push fluids for hypotension or failure to respond to epinephrine using 5 to 10 mg/kg as quickly as possible and up to 30 mL/kg in first hour for children and 1 to 2 L for adults

ADDITIONAL MEASURES

Albuterol	Consider administration of 2.5 to 5 mg of nebulized albuterol in 3 mL of saline for lower airway obstruction; repeat as necessary every 15 minutes
Glucagon	Patients on beta blockers who are not responding to epinephrine should be given 1 to 5 mg of glucagon IV slowly over 5 minutes because rapid administration of glucagon can induce vomiting
Epinephrine infusion	For patients with inadequate response to IM epinephrine and IV saline, give epinephrine by continuous infusion by micro-drip in office setting (infusion pump in hospital setting); add 1 mg (1 mL of 1:1,000) of epinephrine to 1 L of 0.9 NL saline; start infusion at 2 mcg/min (2 mL/min = 120 mL/hr) and increase up to 10 mcg/min; titrate dose continuously according to blood pressure, cardiac rate and function, and oxygenation
Intraosseous access	If IV access is not readily available in patients experiencing refractory anaphylaxis, obtain intraosseous access for administration of IV fluids and epinephrine infusion

REFRACTORY ANAPHYLAXIS

Advanced airway management	Use supraglottic airway, endotracheal intubation, or cricothyroidotomy for marked stridor, severe laryngeal edema, or when ventilation using a bag-valve mask is inadequate and EMS has not arrived

Continued

TABLE 14-6 Anaphylaxis Treatment Protocol—cont'd

REFRACTORY ANAPHYLAXIS—cont'd

Vasopressors	Consider administration of dopamine (in addition to epinephrine infusion) if patient is unresponsive to treatment; this will likely be in the hospital setting where cardiac monitoring is available

OPTIONAL TREATMENTS

H1 antihistamine	Consider giving 25 to 50 mg of IV diphenhydramine for adults and 1 mg/kg (maximum 50 mg) for children; use 10 mg of cetirizine if an oral antihistamine is administered
Systemic corticosteroids	Administer 1 to 2 mg/kg up to 125 mg per dose, IV or orally, of methylprednisolone or an equivalent formulation; no evidence that this medication needs to be continued

OBSERVATION AND MONITORING

Observation in emergency department/hospital	Transport to emergency department (ED) by EMS for further treatment and observation for 8 hours or more

DISCHARGE MANAGEMENT

Education	Educate patient and family on how to recognize and how to treat anaphylaxis
Auto-injectable epinephrine	Prescribe two doses of auto-injectable epinephrine for patients who have experienced an anaphylactic reaction and for those at risk for severe anaphylaxis; train patient, patient provider, and family on how to use the auto-injector
Anaphylaxis action plan	Provide patients with an action plan instructing them on how and when to administer epinephrine

Source: Lieberman P, Nicklas RA, Randolph C, et al. Anaphylaxis—a practice parameter update 2015. Ann Allergy Asthma Immunol. 2015;115:341–384. https://www.aaaai.org/Aaaai/media/MediaLibrary/PDF%20Documents/Practice%20and%20Parameters/2015-Anaphylaxis-PP-Update.pdf

CLINICAL CONCEPT

Recurrence later in the day of similar anaphylactic signs and symptoms (a biphasic reaction) occurs in 1% to 23% of episodes and can occur hours (most within 10 hours) after anaphylactic resolution.

in patients taking β-adrenergic blockers has been reported. This might be due to a blunted response to epinephrine, an increased propensity for bronchospasm, and reduced cardiac contractility with perpetuation of hypotension. H1 antihistamines are second-line agents and do not replace epinephrine. Parenteral or oral diphenhydramine is a common option for an H1 antihistamine. However, other oral first- or second-generation H1 antihistamines can also be used. H2 antagonists, such as ranitidine, added to H1 antihistamines can be helpful and often are used. An inhaled β-adrenergic agent (i.e., albuterol) is indicated for bronchospasms and/or upper airway obstruction. Systemic corticosteroids have not been shown to be effective in altering the course of acute anaphylaxis but can prevent recurrent or protracted anaphylaxis. Length of time for observation is individualized; often it is several hours.

The discharge plan should include the diagnosis, including the suspected cause for the anaphylaxis, avoidance measures, recognition of signs and symptoms, and a treatment plan. A prescription for an epinephrine auto-injector twin package with instructions should be provided, and the patient should be well informed on its use. A bracelet or similar identification, indicating anaphylaxis history, should be worn. After an anaphylactic episode, referral to allergy/immunology to confirm cause and to reduce risk factors for future reactions should be considered.

Discussion Sources

American Academy of Allergy Asthma and Immunology. What primary care givers need to know about the new guidelines for the diagnosis and management of food allergy in the US. January 2012. http://www.aaaai.org/Aaaai/media/MediaLibrary/PDF%20Documents/Practice%20Resources/Food-Allergy-Guidelines-Summary.pdf

Boyce JA, Assa'ad A, Burks AW, et al. Guidelines for the diagnosis and management of food allergy in the United States. *J Allergy Clin Immunol*. 2010;126:S1–58. https://www.ncbi.nlm.nih.gov/pmc/articles/PMC4241964/pdf/nihms247178.pdf

Lieberman P, Nicklas RA, Randolph C, et al. Anaphylaxis—a practice parameter update 2015. *Ann Allergy Asthma Immunol*. 2015; 115:341–384. https://www.aaaai.org/Aaaai/media/MediaLibrary/PDF%20Documents/Practice%20and%20Parameters/2015 -Anaphylaxis-PP-Update.pdf

Simons FER, Ebisawa M, Sanchez-Borges M, et al. 2015 update of the evidence base: World Allergy Organization anaphylaxis guidelines. *World Allergy Organization J*. 2015;8:80. https://waojournal.biomedcentral.com/articles/10.1186/s40413-015 -0080-1

The Food Allergy and Anaphylaxis Network. https://www.foodallergy.org

QUESTIONS

41. Tom is a 19-year-old man who presents with sudden onset of edema of the lips and face and a sensation of "throat tightness and shortness of breath" after a bee sting. Physical examination reveals inspiratory and expiratory wheezing as well as pruritic wheals on his face and arms. Blood pressure is 78/44 mm Hg, heart rate is 102 bpm, and respiratory rate is 24/min. His clinical presentation is most consistent with the diagnosis of:

A. vasculitis.

B. angioedema.

C. anaphylaxis.

D. reactive airway disease.

42. Your priority in caring for Tom, the aforementioned patient, is to:

A. administer a rapidly acting oral antihistamine.

B. administer parenteral epinephrine.

C. initiate vasopressor therapy.

D. administer a parenteral systemic corticosteroid.

43. Which of the following food-based allergies is likely to be found in adults and children?

A. milk

B. egg

C. soy

D. peanut

44. A person with latex allergy also often has a cross-allergy to all of the following except:

A. banana.

B. avocado.

C. kiwi.

D. romaine lettuce.

45. The most common clinical manifestation of systemic anaphylaxis typically is:

A. dizziness.

B. airway obstruction.

C. urticaria.

D. GI upset.

46. Second-line drug intervention in the presence of anaphylaxis should be:

A. oral diphenhydramine.

B. nebulized pentamidine.

C. nebulized epinephrine.

D. oral prednisone.

47. Which of the following is the best answer regarding anaphylaxis?

   A. Adults usually do not develop new anaphylaxis triggers such as food allergies.

   B. Peanuts are the only primary food that can cause a severe allergic reaction.

   C. Future anaphylactic reactions will become increasingly more severe.

   D. Trace amounts of an allergen in a food can cause a severe anaphylactic reaction.

48. Increased risks for fatal reactions from anaphylaxis include all of the following except:

   A. personal history of asthma.

   B. delay in administering epinephrine.

   C. age in the teen years.

   D. delay in administering antihistamines.

49. Which of the following plays an essential role in type 1 hypersensitivity?

   A. immunoglobulin E

   B. immunoglobulin A

   C. immunoglobulin G

   D. immunoglobulin F

50. Of the following medications, which is least likely to be implicated as a trigger for anaphylaxis?

   A. ibuprofen

   B. amoxicillin

   C. acetaminophen

   D. aspirin

51. The time to C_{max} of epinephrine is shorter when the medication is given:

   A. IM in the vastus lateralis.

   B. subcutaneously in the abdominal wall.

   C. IM in the deltoid.

   D. IM into the gluteus.

52. The use of a systemic corticosteroid in the treatment of anaphylaxis is primarily helpful for:

   A. treatment of the most acute symptoms.

   B. minimization of a protracted allergic response.

   C. prevention of future episodes.

   D. reducing the risk of fatality associated with the event.

For answers and rationales, see end of chapter.

QUESTION ANSWERS AND RATIONALES

Anemia

1. Correct: D. IDA

IDA (D) is the leading cause of anemia worldwide, most commonly caused by chronic, low-volume blood loss. Losses of only 2 to 3 mL per day can cause IDA, frequently by GI bleeding, repeated phlebotomy, or persistent excessive menstrual flow.

Incorrect:

ACD (C) is the second leading cause of anemia worldwide and can be attributed to acute and chronic inflammation (infection, arthritis), renal insufficiency, malignancy, and hypothyroidism. Pernicious anemia (A) and folate-deficiency anemia (B) are the most common causes of macrocytic anemia and are most frequently caused by inadequate dietary intake or a malabsorption syndrome.

2. Correct: B. recycled iron content from aged RBCs.

The body's most important source of iron is the recycled iron content from aged RBCs. Because of this, chronic, low-volume blood loss is the leading cause of

IDA as the body is unable to adequately replace this lost iron.

Incorrect:
A well-balanced diet can be an important source of iron. However, in developed countries, diet (A, D) is rarely an etiology for IDA as recycled iron from aged RBCs is the major source of the body's iron. An estimated 8 years of poor iron intake are needed in adults before IDA occurs. Iron is not produced in the endoplasmic reticulum (C).

3. Correct: B. low MCV, low MCH
Iron deficiency will inhibit the normal production of Hgb. As 90% of RBCs consist of Hgb ("heme" = iron; "globin" = protein), diminished production of Hgb will result in smaller RBCs (microcytic) with low MCH (B).

Incorrect:
Wintrobe's classification is used to categorize anemia as microcytic (low MCV), normocytic (MCV within normal limits), or macrocytic (abnormally high MCV). IDA is characterized as a microcytic anemia with low MCH resulting from decreased production of Hgb.

4. Correct: A. an increase in RDW.
RDW reflects the degree of variation in RBC size and is often the first abnormal finding in the hemogram of a person with an evolving microcytic or macrocytic anemia. During an evolving anemia, the new cells can be smaller (microcytic anemia) or larger (macrocytic anemia) than older cells, thus elevating the RDW (A). For example, IDA is characterized by microcytosis as new cells are smaller in size due to iron deficiency and reduced Hgb production.

Incorrect:
An evolving microcytic anemia can be characterized by a reduction in measurable Hgb (B) and/or a low MCH level (C), as is seen in IDA, but this would not be necessarily true for an evolving macrocytic anemia (e.g., pernicious anemia or vitamin B_{12} deficiency anemia). Platelet count (D) is not used as a marker for anemia.

5. Correct: C. reticulocytosis.
For a patient being treated for IDA with iron therapy, an early sign of recovery is reticulocytosis (C), or the production of new immature RBCs (reticulocytes). Reticulocytosis begins quickly after iron therapy and peaks 7 to 10 days into therapy.

Incorrect:
Reticulocytosis is the earliest sign of response to iron therapy in IDA. Hgb can increase at a rate of 2 g/dL every 3 weeks in response to iron therapy, which would correlate with an estimated 6% increase of Hct level (B). A normal ferritin level should be achieved after 4 months of therapy (D). Given the 90- to 120-day life span of RBCs, the correction of MCV should be observed after 2 to 4 months of therapy and the elimination of microcytic cells (A).

6. Correct: C. use of an iron supplement in the absence of a documented deficiency can lead to iatrogenic iron overload.

For healthy men without documentation of iron deficiency, the use of an iron supplement is not recommended due to the risk of iatrogenic iron overload (also called secondary hemochromatosis) (C). This results in the extra iron being deposited within the organs of the body that can have toxic effects, including cirrhosis, diabetes, joint pains, and hypothyroidism.

Incorrect:
Iron supplementation in healthy men is not recommended or needed without documentation of iron deficiency (A). IDA is not a common condition in healthy younger males and so iron supplementation as prophylaxis is not recommended (B). Excess iron can be deposited and stored in the solid organs, rather than be excreted, which can have toxic effects on the body (D).

7. Correct: C. "Take on an empty stomach."
A variety of foods and medications can inhibit the absorption of oral iron. Therefore, iron supplements should be taken on an empty stomach to maximize absorption (C).

Incorrect:
Iron supplements can cause GI upset that can be minimized by taking iron with food. However, this can reduce iron absorption by up to two-thirds (B). Milk, calcium, and antacids can also decrease iron absorption and should not be taken with iron supplements. The bioavailability of a large number of medications can be impacted when taken at the same time as iron (A), including certain antibiotics, bisphosphonates, and levodopa. Iron supplements should be taken at least 2 hours before or after administration of other medications, though concomitant use of certain medications should be avoided (e.g., angiotensin-converting enzyme [ACE] inhibitors, fluoroquinolones). Vitamin C taken with iron supplements can improve absorption (D).

8. Correct: B. an inactive drug compound is potentially formed if the two medications are taken together.
Iron is a strong chelating agent that binds to a number of other medications, including ciprofloxacin, that reduces bioavailability and effectiveness. Therefore, iron supplements and fluoroquinolones should be taken at least 6 hours apart to minimize any drug-drug interaction.

Incorrect:
Due to drug-drug interaction potential, the two medications should not be taken together (A, C), as this will decrease the bioavailability of ciprofloxacin (D). To improve absorption of iron, it should be taken on an empty stomach, though vitamin C can also improve iron absorption. To minimize drug-drug interactions, iron supplements should be taken at least 2 hours before or after other medications, though some medications may require greater spacing or avoidance.

9. Correct: B. Hgb measurement.
Full hematological recovery for pernicious anemia usually takes about 2 months after initiation of therapy with vitamin B_{12}. At the 2-month follow-up, an Hgb

measurement would be the most appropriate test to check for efficacy of treatment (B).

Incorrect:
In pernicious anemia, the hematological response to treatment is generally rapid. Reticulocytosis is brisk and peaks at 5 to 7 days after treatment initiation (C), which would be a more appropriate time to obtain a reticulocyte count as a measure of efficacy early in treatment. Similarly, serum cobalamin should return to normal levels early with vitamin B_{12} treatment (D). The Schilling test is used to determine if the body is absorbing vitamin B_{12} properly and should be performed at the time of diagnosis of pernicious anemia (A).

10. Correct: C. folic acid
Maternal folic acid deficiency is a teratogenic state that can increase the risk of neural tube defects (C). A woman planning a pregnancy should be advised to take an additional 0.4 mg or more per day of folic acid for 3 months prior to conception.

Incorrect:
Maternal folic acid deficiency can lead to fetal neural tube defects, and so supplementation of folic acid is recommended for women planning on pregnancy for at least 3 months prior to conception. For unplanned pregnancies or where prepregnancy counseling was not sought, folic acid supplementation during the first 7 weeks of pregnancy seems to offer some benefit in neural tube protection. Supplementation with iron (A), niacin (B), or vitamin C (D) will not impact the risk of neural tube defect during pregnancy.

11. Correct: B. chronic ingestion of overcooked foods.
Folic acid is a water-soluble B complex vitamin that is found in abundance in peanuts, fruits, and vegetables, as well as folic acid-supplemented foods, such as most flours. However, overheating and overcooking foods rich in folic acid will destroy the vitamin and contribute to folate-deficiency anemia (B).

Incorrect:
The most common causes of folate-deficiency anemia include inadequate dietary intake of folate and a decreased ability to absorb folate, such as with malabsorption syndromes (e.g., sprue, celiac disease). Menorrhagia (A) would be a risk factor for IDA through chronic low-volume blood loss. Gastric atrophy (D) or the use of NSAIDs (C) are not associated with folate-deficiency anemia.

12. Correct: D. macrocytic, normochromic
Folate-deficiency anemia is characterized as a macrocytic, normochromic anemia according to Wintrobe's classification. In this anemia, Hgb production is unaffected as iron levels are normal. However, folate deficiency impairs DNA synthesis within RBCs and causes distinct changes, including macrocytosis.

Incorrect:
Microcytic and/or hypochromic anemias (A, B, C) typically result from decreased Hgb production, often related to iron deficiency. This is not the case with folate-deficiency anemia, where Hgb production is normal. Macrocytosis occurs in folate-deficiency anemia as the micronutrient deficiency impairs DNA synthesis in RBCs within the bone marrow.

13. Correct: B. lack of production of intrinsic factor by the gastric mucosa.
Pernicious anemia is not a result of dietary deficiencies but is related to the inability to absorb vitamin B_{12} that is found abundantly in foods. When vitamin B_{12} is ingested, it must bind with intrinsic factor for intestinal absorption. Failure to produce intrinsic factor by the gastric parietal cells can lead to vitamin B_{12} deficiency and pernicious anemia.

Incorrect:
Dietary deficiency is an uncommon cause of pernicious anemia, as vitamin B_{12} is abundantly found in a variety of foods (A). Pernicious anemia specifically relates to deficiency in vitamin B_{12} due to malabsorption caused by a lack of intrinsic factor production, thus not a combination of micronutrient deficiencies (D). Intrinsic factor is produced by gastric parietal cells and does not involve an enzyme from RBCs (C).

14. Correct: D. macrocytic, normochromic
Similar to folate-deficiency anemia, pernicious anemia is characterized as a macrocytic, normochromic anemia (D) according to Wintrobe's classification. In this anemia, Hgb production is unaffected as iron levels are normal. However, vitamin B_{12} deficiency impairs DNA synthesis within RBCs and causes distinct changes within the bone marrow, including macrocytosis.

Incorrect:
Microcytic and/or hypochromic anemias (A, B, C) typically result from decreased Hgb production, often related to iron deficiency. This is not the case with pernicious anemia, where Hgb production is normal. Macrocytosis occurs with vitamin B_{12} deficiency as the micronutrient deficiency impairs DNA synthesis in RBCs within the bone marrow.

15. Correct: B. stocking-glove neuropathy.
Vitamin B_{12} is an important micronutrient needed for proper neurological function in the body. Pernicious anemia, often caused by malabsorption of vitamin B_{12}, is associated with neurological symptoms that can include stocking-glove neuropathy (B), confusion, short-term memory loss, poor balance, irritability, and in severe cases, hallucinations and delusions.

Incorrect:
Pernicious anemia is associated with neurological signs and symptoms. Hypoactive bowel sounds (A), thin, spoon-shaped nails (C; often seen in IDA), and retinal hemorrhages (D; often observed in poorly controlled hypertension) are not specific to pernicious anemia.

16. Correct: B. alcohol abuse.
Alcohol abuse can result in mild macrocytosis without anemia, as found in this patient. Usually the individual

will have other findings consistent with heavy alcohol use, such as pharyngeal redness and sleep disturbance.
Incorrect:
This patient has a normal Hgb level and so does not present with pernicious anemia (A). Thalassemias are associated with a microcytic anemia according to Wintrobe's classification, while this patient demonstrates mild macrocytosis (C). Fanconi anemia is a rare, genetically linked disease that affects the bone marrow and results in reduced production of all types of blood cells, and so can be ruled out for this patient who has normal RBC production (D).

17. Correct: C. α-thalassemia minor.
Asian and African ethnicities are at risk for α-thalassemia minor, which is characterized by microcytic RBCs, normal RDW, and an elevated number of RBCs. Among the answer choices, the diagnostic findings were most consistent with α-thalassemia minor (C).
Incorrect:
IDA (A) is characterized by microcytic cells and elevated RDW. Cooley's anemia (B), also known as β-thalassemia major, is a severe, life-threatening condition where two defective genes are inherited, leading to a complete lack of beta protein in Hgb. Hgb Barts is found in fetal cord blood and in newborns in association with α-thalassemia (D) but would not be present in a 22-year-old woman.

18. Correct: B. occult blood loss.
A microcytic, hypochromic anemia with elevated RDW is most consistent with IDA. A common cause of IDA is chronic, low-volume blood loss (B).
Incorrect:
Poor nutrition (A) and malabsorption (C) are more consistent with the macrocytic anemias of folate-deficiency anemia and pernicious anemia, respectively. Chronic inflammation can cause ACD, which is characterized as a normocytic, normochromic anemia (D).

19. Correct: B. ACD.
When making a differential diagnosis, it is important to consider all patient factors. The presence of a normocytic (as per Wintrobe's classification), normochromic anemia would suggest ACD. This is consistent with the presence of a chronic inflammatory condition that is not well controlled with medication. Reticulocytopenia also suggests a poor hematological response related to a chronic condition.
Incorrect:
As per Wintrobe's classification, pernicious anemia (A) and folate-deficiency anemia (D) are macrocytic anemias with elevated RDWs that would not be consistent with this patient. β-Thalassemia minor (C) results in a microcytic, normochromic anemia with an elevated number of RBCs.

20. Correct: D. no specific anemia-related findings.
Anemia in a patient with menorrhagia is likely due to IDA from chronic low-volume blood loss. However,

in mild anemia, symptoms may not be evident, and physical examination usually contributes little to the diagnosis.
Incorrect:
Mild cases of anemia will not typically present with obvious signs and symptoms. During more severe cases, such as when Hgb is below 8 g/dL, individuals may present with obvious signs and symptoms, such as pale conjunctiva (A) or a hemic murmur (B). In elderly patients and those with coronary artery disease, symptoms of anemia can include signs of heart failure, such as distended neck veins, rales, tachycardia (C), and hepatomegaly.

21. Correct: B. the addition of micronutrient supplementation needed for erythropoiesis is advisable.
Erythropoietin is a hormone primarily produced in the kidneys that stimulates the production of RBCs in bone marrow. Recombinant human erythropoietin is often used to treat anemia associated with certain diseases, such as end-stage renal disease, HIV infection, and cancer chemotherapy. In anticipation of reticulocytosis, micronutrient supplementation is recommended, such as iron supplementation.
Incorrect:
Endogenous erythropoietin is predominantly produced in the kidneys, not the adrenal glands (A). It is used to stimulate production of RBCs, not platelets that are lacking in thrombocytopenia (C). Erythropoietin will not have any impact on the life span of RBCs, which is typically 90 to 120 days.

22. Correct: C. hypokalemia.
Hypokalemia is common during peak times of reticulocytosis, such as during the first week of vitamin B_{12} therapy in severe anemia. Patients should be monitored daily for hypokalemia, particularly in those with additional risk factors for hypokalemia, such as those taking a diuretic or digoxin.
Incorrect:
Hypokalemia is a common finding during intense reticulocytosis, particularly in those being treated for severe anemia and who have additional risk factors for hypokalemia. Hypernatremia (A) and acidemia (D) are not associated with vitamin B_{12} therapy and reticulocytosis or the use of a diuretic. Though it is important to ensure the patient is adequately hydrated, careful monitoring for dehydration is not needed for a patient who can tolerate fluids (B).

23. Correct: B. peripheral vascular disease
ACD is associated with a number of chronic health conditions, including renal disease, inflammation, and infection. Peripheral vascular disease (B) is not typically associated with ACD.
Incorrect:
ACD is caused by reduced erythropoietin response in the marrow. Select chronic conditions include chronic inflammation (rheumatoid arthritis [A]) and infection

(HIV, osteomyelitis [D]). Chronic renal insufficiency (C) is also a major contributor to ACD as this can lead to decreased production of endogenous erythropoietin that stimulates reticulocytosis.

24. **Correct: C. 1:3.**
The normal Hgb-to-Hct ratio is 1:3. Thus, an Hgb level of 12 g/dL should correspond with an Hct of 36%.
Incorrect:
The normal Hgb-to-Hct ratio is 1:3. The ratio can differ during periods of severe dehydration, where the Hct is elevated (e.g., Hgb of 12 g/dL and Hct of 39%), or during periods of overhydration, where Hct is decreased (Hgb of 12 g/dL and Hct of 32%).

25 to 28. Matching Questions

25. **Correct: B. anisocytosis**
Anisocytosis, where blood cells are of unequal size, is commonly found in certain anemias, particularly IDA.

26. **Correct: A. poikilocytosis**
Poikilocytosis is characterized by RBCs of varying shapes. These can include oval, teardrop, sickle shaped, or irregularly contracted. Genetic causes can include sickle cell anemia and thalassemia, while acquired causes can include IDA, megaloblastic anemia, and auto-immune hemolytic anemias.

27. **Correct: C. reticulocytosis**
Reticulocytosis is the increased production of new RBCs (reticulocytes). This is typically the body's normal response to correct anemia. The normal percentage of circulating reticulocytes is 1% to 2%, while this percent-age will be higher in reticulocytosis.

28. **Correct: D. reticulocytopenia**
Reticulocytopenia is an abnormally low percentage of circulating reticulocytes and is a possible sign of inade-quate hemopoiesis.

29. **Correct: C. Hct less than 24%**
ACD is characterized by a normocytic, normochromic anemia. This is due to a reduced erythropoietic response in the bone marrow resulting in RBC hypoproliferation. However, anemia seldom reaches severe status, with Hct at or above 24% (C).
Incorrect:
ACD is characterized by a normocytic, normochromic anemia. As this is not an evolving anemia, RDW is within normal limits. Micronutrient deficiency is not an issue in ACD, thus ferritin levels (D) and Hgb produc-tion (MCHC [B]) are within normal levels.

30. **Correct: B. if present for longer than 6 months, these changes are occasionally permanent.**
Pernicious anemia is treated with oral or parenteral vitamin B_{12}. Improvement in neurological symp-toms can occur quickly with treatment. However, if neurological abnormalities have been present for 6 months or longer, the changes are occasionally permanent even with appropriate vitamin B_{12} repletion therapy (B).

Incorrect:
The hematological response to vitamin B_{12} therapy for pernicious anemia is rapid, with reticulocytosis peaking in 5 to 7 days. Reversal of neurological symptoms occurs more slowly (A), though some improvement is seen quickly. Neurological symptoms, including cognitive changes, are usually reversible if they were present for less than 6 months (D). Vitamin B_{12} can be administered orally or parenterally (C). However, parenteral therapy is recommended, as the oral form can be absorbed errati-cally and lead to treatment failure.

31. **Correct: C. MMA and homocysteine**
The most common causes of a macrocytic anemia are due to folate-deficiency anemia and pernicious anemia caused by malabsorption of vitamin B_{12} (a member of the cobala-min family). If the diagnosis of a macrocytic anemia is still uncertain following serum folate and cobalamin testing, additional follow-up tests include serum homocysteine (elevated in folate and vitamin B_{12} deficiency) and serum MMA (elevated in vitamin B_{12} deficiency only) (C).
Incorrect:
Tests for serum MMA and homocysteine can be used to differentiate between folate-deficiency anemia and perni-cious anemia when a macrocytic anemia is encountered. The other tests listed are not specific or particularly useful in trying to diagnose a macrocytic anemia.

32. **Correct: A. ferritin.**
A patient diagnosed with advanced colon cancer and anemia is most likely experiencing chronic low-volume blood loss from the GI tract. This will likely cause IDA, which is consistent with the hemogram findings of a microcytic anemia and elevated RDW. A serum ferritin test (A) will help to confirm the diagnosis of IDA.
Incorrect:
Folate-deficiency anemia and pernicious anemia are macrocytic anemias. Initial testing for a macrocytic anemia can include serum folate (B) or cobalamin (C; member of vitamin B_{12} family). If initial testing is incon-clusive, further testing for serum homocysteine (D) and MMA can be used to differentiate between these two types of anemia.

33. **Correct: A. cobalamin.**
The most common macrocytic anemias are folate-deficiency anemia and pernicious anemia. The presence of neurological symptoms would suggest a vitamin B_{12} deficiency. Testing for cobalamin levels (a member of the vitamin B_{12} family) would be most appropriate (A), though folate, homocysteine, and MMA may also be included to make the differential diagnosis.
Incorrect:
Serum ferritin (B) would be appropriate in the presence of a microcytic anemia due to iron deficiency. The pres-ence of anemia would also suggest that the symptoms are related to a hematological disorder and not a thyroid disorder requiring TSH testing (C). A head CT scan is not indicated for this patient (D).

34. Correct: B. folate.

Excessive alcohol consumption can be associated with mild macrocytosis without anemia. The presence of a macrocytic anemia with elevated RDW suggests an evolving disease process beyond excessive alcohol use. Given his poor diet lacking in fruits and vegetables, he is most likely deficient in folic acid. Testing for serum folate would be most appropriate (B). Additional testing to make the differential diagnosis of a macrocytic anemia can include cobalamin, homocysteine, and MMA.

Incorrect:

Serum ferritin (A) would be used to test for IDA that is characterized as a microcytic anemia. Hgb electrophoresis (C) would be used to detect for defective Hgb present in the thalassemias. As this anemia cannot be attributed solely to excessive alcohol consumption, additional testing is needed to make the differential diagnosis (D).

35. Correct: C. vitamin B_{12}

Consistent, prolonged use of PPIs, such as omeprazole and lansoprazole, can result in decreased absorption of vitamin B_{12} (C). PPIs not only block the release of gastric acid but also inhibit the release of intrinsic factor that is required for vitamin B_{12} absorption. PPI use can also decrease absorption of dietary iron.

Incorrect:

PPI use has been associated with an increased risk of vitamin and mineral deficiencies, including vitamin B_{12}, vitamin C, calcium, iron, and magnesium. Though folate deficiency (B) can lead to anemia, absorption of this micronutrient is less likely to be affected by PPI use when compared to vitamin B_{12}. Absorption of potassium (D) and vitamin D (A) is not substantially impacted with PPI use, and deficiencies in these micronutrients are not associated with anemia.

36 to 40. True or False

36. Correct: True

As the signs of anemia can include fatigue, headache, and poor exercise tolerance, these can negatively impact school performance in children.

37. Correct: True

During pregnancy, folic acid is essential in the normal neural tube development by the fetus. Therefore, women planning a pregnancy should take additional amounts of folic acid for 3 months prior to conception, and supplementation should continue through lactation.

38. Correct: True

Approximately 90% of a RBC is composed of Hgb, and the normal MCHC is 31 to 37 g/dL. An MCHC of less than 31 g/dL will lead to pale (hypochromic) RBCs, often seen in IDA as well as thalassemias.

39. Correct: True

The majority of erythropoietin produced in the body is made in the kidneys. During renal impairment (e.g., GFR less than 30 to 40 mL/min), renal erythropoietin production diminishes and can result in a hypoproliferative, normochromic, normocytic anemia.

40. Correct: False

The normative response to anemia is increased production of new RBCs (i.e., reticulocytosis). Reticulocytopenia is a decreased production of RBCs and is indicative of inadequate hemopoiesis.

Anaphylaxis

41. Correct: C. anaphylaxis.

Though the presentation of anaphylaxis can be highly variable, the most common symptoms include urticaria, angioedema, upper airway angioedema, hypotension, and wheeze that develops over a relatively short period of time. The overall physical findings of this patient are most consistent with anaphylaxis.

Incorrect:

Vasculitis (A), or inflammation in blood vessels, can develop over a prolonged period of time (days to months) and can include fever, weight loss, headache, and fatigue. Though this patient is experiencing angioedema (B), or swelling of the lips and face, this is one sign of a larger disease process the patient is experiencing. Though wheezing is a sign of reactive airway disease (D), this diagnosis would not explain the constellation of physical findings of this patient, including angioedema and hypotension.

42. Correct: B. administer parenteral epinephrine.

When anaphylaxis is suspected, first-line treatment is parenteral epinephrine, preferably given IM in the lateral thigh. There is no contraindication to epinephrine in anaphylaxis, and a failure or delay in administration is associated with greater risk of fatality.

Incorrect:

Parenteral or oral antihistamine (A) is considered a second-line treatment for anaphylaxis but should not replace epinephrine. Similarly, vasopressors (C) and IV fluid can be used to maintain circulation following epinephrine administration. Systemic corticosteroids (D) have not been shown to improve the course of acute anaphylaxis but may help in preventing recurrent or protracted anaphylaxis.

43. Correct: D. peanut

Food allergies are more common in children than adults, though persistence of some food allergies can extend into adulthood. Of the most common food allergies, peanut (D), tree nut, fish, and shellfish are most likely to persist in adults.

Incorrect:

Eight foods account for nearly 90% of food allergies and include peanuts, tree nuts, fish, shellfish, eggs, milk, wheat, and soy. Allergies caused by milk (A), egg (B), soy (C), and wheat are more likely to resolve in children.

44. Correct: D. romaine lettuce.

Individuals with an allergic reaction to natural rubber latex protein can experience cross-reactivity to certain fruit proteins. However, romaine lettuce does not contain these proteins for cross-reactivity (D).

Incorrect:
Fruits that contain proteins that can lead to cross-reactivity with a natural rubber latex allergy include bananas (A), avocado (B), kiwi (C), melons, and chestnuts. Individuals with a known allergy to natural rubber latex should be educated on avoidance of these foods to prevent severe allergic episodes.

45. **Correct: C. urticaria.**
The clinical presentation of anaphylaxis can be unpredictable, and an initial mild reaction can rapidly progress to a life-threatening condition. The most common findings in anaphylaxis are urticaria (i.e., hives) and angioedema, found in approximately 85% to 90% of cases.

Incorrect:
Urticaria and angioedema are the most common findings in anaphylaxis; however, respiratory compromise and cardiovascular collapse are of greatest concern as they are the most frequent causes of death. Dizziness (A), syncope, and hypotension occur in 30% to 35% of cases, upper airway angioedema (B) occurs in 50% to 60% of cases, and GI upset (D) is experienced by 25% to 30% of those during an anaphylaxis episode.

46. **Correct: A. oral diphenhydramine.**
When anaphylaxis is suspected, first-line treatment is parenteral epinephrine. Parenteral or oral antihistamine, such as diphenhydramine (A), is considered a second-line treatment for anaphylaxis but should not replace epinephrine.

Incorrect:
Epinephrine (C) is first-line treatment for anaphylaxis, though this should be administered preferably via IM injection in the lateral thigh. Systemic corticosteroids, such as oral prednisone (D), have not been shown to improve the course of acute anaphylaxis but may help in preventing recurrent or protracted anaphylaxis. Pentamidine (B), an antimicrobial, is not recommended for treatment of anaphylaxis.

47. **Correct: D. Trace amounts of an allergen in a food can cause a severe anaphylactic reaction.**
For individuals with food allergies, small amounts of the allergen present in food can elicit a severe IgE-mediated immune reaction that causes anaphylaxis. Following anaphylaxis, individuals should be referred to an allergist or immunologist to confirm the cause of the allergic reaction and reduce risk factors for future episodes.

Incorrect:
Though food allergies are more common in children, adults can have food allergies that reflect either persistence of childhood allergies or the origination of an allergy from a new sensitization (A). Peanuts are one of the most common food sources to cause severe and fatal allergic reactions, which also include tree nuts, fish, and shellfish (B). Many food allergies in children resolve over

time, particularly allergies caused by milk, egg, wheat, and soy (C).

48. **Correct: D. delay in administering antihistamines.**
Severe anaphylaxis can be a life-threatening event and should be treated with parenteral epinephrine to reduce mortality risk. Antihistamines are considered second-line treatment but should not replace the use of epinephrine. A delay in the use of antihistamines is not associated with improved mortality (D).

Incorrect:
Risk factors for fatal anaphylaxis include being a teen or young adult (C), having asthma (A), and failure to administer epinephrine in a timely manner (B).

49. **Correct: A. immunoglobulin E**
Anaphylaxis is a manifestation of a type I hypersensitivity reaction resulting from an IgE-mediated immune reaction. Type I immediate hypersensitivity reactions can involve the rapid release of histamine and other mediators from mast cells and basophils.

Incorrect:
Immunoglobulin A and immunoglobulin G play an important role in the immune system and are involved in fighting bacteria, viruses, and toxins. However, IgA (B) and IgG (C) are not involved in type I hypersensitivity reactions. There is no immunoglobulin F (D).

50. **Correct: C. acetaminophen**
Certain medications have been associated with IgE– and non-IgE–mediated anaphylaxis. However, acetaminophen use is not typically associated with anaphylaxis.

Incorrect:
Medications that have been implicated in anaphylaxis include certain antimicrobials (i.e., members of the penicillin class such as amoxicillin [B]), aspirin (D), and NSAIDs (e.g., ibuprofen [A]).

51. **Correct: A. IM in the vastus lateralis.**
Pharmacokinetic studies in healthy volunteers demonstrate that C_{max} of epinephrine is achieved in the shortest amount of time when it is administered via IM injection to the vastus lateralis (lateral thigh).

Incorrect:
Parenteral epinephrine is the initial drug of choice for the management of anaphylaxis, and a delay in administration can increase the risk of death. Epinephrine is typically given subcutaneously or via IM injection in the lateral thigh or deltoid muscle. However, the fastest C_{max} is achieved when given IM in the lateral thigh.

52. **Correct: B. minimization of a protracted allergic response.**
Systemic corticosteroids in anaphylaxis have been shown to prevent recurrent or protracted episodes.

Incorrect:
Evidence is lacking on the benefits of systemic corticosteroids in altering the course (A) or preventing death (D) during acute anaphylaxis. These agents will also not prevent future anaphylaxis if the individual is exposed to the allergen (C).

Psychosocial Disorders

15

Substance Use Disorder

Overview

The misuse and overuse of various mood-altering products such as alcohol, opioids, simulants, benzodiazepines (BZDs), and other similar products is often referred to as substance abuse or substance use disorder (SUD). SUD is a common problem, with over 10% of individuals 12 years and older reporting any illegal drug or prescription drug for a reason other than its indication use over the past month. When providing health care, the nurse practitioner (NP) should remember that substance abuse and dependence commonly mean misuse of multiple agents, including alcohol, prescription drugs, and illegal agents.

Sedatives, hypnotics, anxiolytics, including the BZDs, and stimulants are the most commonly misused and abused prescription drugs. Young adults (18- to 25-year-olds) are most likely to misuse prescription medications, with 14.4% using prescription drugs for nonmedical purposes in the past year, compared with 4.9% of 12- to 17-year-olds.

Many individuals with SUD have an underlying mental health problem, such as a mood disorder. The TWO 6-PACK mnemonic can be helpful when evaluating a patient for SUD. See Box 15-1.

In providing care, the NP must maintain an attitude that, as with any substance abuse, the patient is capable of changing and achieving sobriety. Change occurs dynamically and often unpredictably. A commonly used change framework is based on the work of James Prochaska, who notes five stages of preparation for change:

- *Precontemplation*: The patient is not interested in change and might be unaware that the problem exists or minimizes the problem's impact.
- *Contemplation*: The patient is considering change and looking at its positive and negative aspects. The person often reports feeling "stuck" with the problem.
- *Preparation*: The patient exhibits some change behaviors or thoughts and often reports feeling that he or she does not have the tools to proceed.
- *Action*: The patient is ready to go forth with change, often takes concrete steps to change, but is inconsistent with carrying through.
- *Maintenance/relapse*: The patient learns to continue the change and has adopted and embraced the healthy habit. Relapse can occur, however, and the person learns to deal with backsliding.

As health counselor, the NP provides a valuable role in continually "tapping," repeating to the patient a message of concern about health and safety, and possibly moving the person in the precontemplation stage to the contemplation stage. When the patient is at this stage, presenting treatment options and support for change is a critical part of the NP's role.

ALCOHOL USE DISORDER

Overview

In the United States, about 18 million people have an alcohol use disorder (AUD), classified as either alcohol dependence or alcohol abuse. Additionally, a growing number of young adults (12 to 20 years of age) participate in underage drinking and are more likely to participate in binge drinking (five drinks or more for men or four drinks or more for women on a single occasion). By the age of 18 years, 80% have consumed alcohol, and 60% have been intoxicated.

Clinical Presentation

Providing care for patients misusing alcohol presents many challenges; this is a complex disorder affecting an individual's family and social function, health, and employment. Often a person who is abusing alcohol minimizes its effect by pointing out that employment has not been affected. In reality, alcoholism is a progressive disease that usually affects family and personal relationships first, then health and, much later, employment. The use of an effective screening tool for alcohol abuse such as the CAGE questionnaire is critical for disease detection. An alcoholic drink is defined as 12 oz (360 mL) beer, 5 oz (120 mL) nonfortified wine, or 0.5 oz (30 to 45 mL) liquor (80 proof).

Diagnostic Testing

For those who test positive with the CAGE questionnaire, a patient interview can be performed to determine if the criteria from the *Diagnostic and Statistical Manual of Mental*

BOX 15-1 TWO 6 PACK Mnemonic for Substance Use Disorder

■ **T**olerance: Reduced response to increasing amounts of substance taken
■ **W**ithdrawal: Characteristic set of signs and symptoms when substance not used
■ **O**ccupational: Social or recreational activities given up or reduced
■ 6
■ **P**ersistent: Desires or unsuccessful efforts to cut down or control substance use
■ **A**mount: Amount of substance use is excessive
■ **C**ontinues: Substance use despite having persistent or recurrent physical or psychological problems
■ **K**eeps: Spends excessive amount of time in search, use, or recovery from the substance

Source: Kumari Mall, S. Deep Mall, G. DRiNK TWO 6 PACK clarifies Substance Use. Current Psychiatry. 2009;8(5):66. https://www.mdedge.com /psychiatry/article/63575/drink-two-6-pack-clarifies-substance-use. For full diagnostic criteria, please see American Psychiatric Association. Diagnostic and statistical manual of mental disorders: DSM-5. 5th ed. Arlington, VA: American Psychiatric Association Publishing; 2013.

CLINICAL CONCEPT

Substance abuse is often a method of self-treatment in patients with an undetected or untreated psychiatric illness.

Disorders, Fifth Edition (DSM-5) are met for substance abuse disorder. Although it is tempting to rely on laboratory markers in assessing a person with alcohol abuse, typically few laboratory markers are abnormal (e.g., alanine aminotransferase [ALT], aspartate aminotransferase [AST], alkaline phosphatase [ALP], γ-glutamyl transferase [GGT]). Evaluation of hepatic function is often ordered by providers, who then have the dilemma of presenting an alcohol-abusing patient with a set of relatively normal test results. This situation can help further reinforce the patient's denial or minimization of the effect excessive alcohol use has on health; as previously mentioned, physical health is negatively affected by alcohol abuse later in the course of the abuse. All currently available hepatic tests indirectly measure liver function or capacity. The most commonly performed tests are measurement of hepatic enzymes (e.g., AST, ALT). Elevated AST can suggest long-standing alcohol abuse, especially when coupled with normal or minimally elevated ALT and mild macrocytosis (mean corpuscular volume [MCV] greater than 100 fL). This finding is noted in about 30% to 60% of men who drink five or more drinks per day and in women who drink three or more drinks per day. The hepatic enzymes generally return to baseline after 2 to 3 months of sobriety. This is an important patient teaching point, because a patient who has abused alcohol for many years often believes that little health benefit is gained from sobriety. The mild macrocytosis seen in alcohol abuse also resolves after about 2 to 3 months of alcohol abstinence.

Treatment

Counseling the patient and family about alcoholism as a lifelong but treatable disease is a helpful clinical approach. In addition, asking about current drinking habits and associated consequences to health with each visit is important. Consistently offering assistance in accessing treatment conveys the seriousness of this life-threatening condition. As with other health problems with a behavioral component, using statements beginning with "I" is important—"I continue to be quite concerned about your health and safety when I hear that you are drinking every day."

In a person who drinks more than 1 pint (16 oz or 475 mL) of hard liquor or six beers (12 oz each) per day or its equivalent, alcohol withdrawal symptoms typically begin about 12 hours after the last drink. Peak symptoms are seen at 24 to 48 hours with abatement over the next few days. Withdrawal symptoms can be divided into three stages:

■ Stage 1 (mild) symptoms develop approximately 8 to 12 hours after the last drink and can include anxiety or nervousness, depression, fatigue, nausea, abdominal pain, vomiting, irritability, jumpiness or shakiness, mood swings, and nightmares.
■ Stage 2 (moderate) symptoms begin to develop after 24 hours and can include hypertension, hyperthermia, rapid and/or irregular heartbeat, elevated respiratory rate, sweating, mental confusion, and heightened mood disturbances.
■ In severe cases, this can be followed by stage 3 symptoms that can lead to potentially life-threatening problems with autonomic hyperactivity (i.e., agitation, hallucinations, disorientation) and seizures. This is the most serious presentation of alcohol withdrawal and is sometimes known as delirium tremens, which has significant mortality in untreated patients.

Treatment of concurrent problems, such as dehydration, malnutrition, and infection, is also warranted. Inpatient treatment is recommended for those with severe symptoms, abnormal laboratory results, absence of a support network, acute illness, at high risk of delirium tremens, history of withdrawal seizures, other serious chronic medical or psychiatric condition, or abuse of other substances.

A highly motivated person with adequate social support systems and a relatively low level of alcohol addiction is likely a suitable candidate for outpatient detoxification. In this type of detoxification, the patient and support person contract with the health-care provider about a safe plan of detoxification. This plan includes daily office visits or contact, ongoing involvement in Alcoholics Anonymous (AA), Employee Assistance Program (EAP) or similar program, counseling services, and use of a limited supply of medications for managing withdrawal symptoms.

Pharmacotherapy is usually required to manage withdrawal symptoms. BZDs have long been used to treat alcohol withdrawal symptoms. Chlordiazepoxide (Librium®) and diazepam (Valium®), therapeutic agents with a long half-life ($t_{1/2}$), are reasonable treatment options for a patient with adequate hepatic function, but agents with shorter half-lives (e.g., lorazepam) or agents that have an absence of active metabolites (e.g., oxazepam) should be used in patients with hepatic dysfunction to prevent prolonged effects. Providing a higher-dose, long-acting BZD, such as diazepam 20 mg on day one, followed by a dosing schedule reduced by 5 mg daily (increased if symptoms are particularly severe), is often effective and is currently favored over a fixed-dosed dosing schedule. If BZD allergy or intolerance is an issue, carbamazepine offers a therapeutic alternative; atypical or standard antipsychotics play no role in managing alcohol withdrawal symptoms.

Adjunctive therapy with an anticonvulsant (e.g., carbamazepine, oxcarbazepine, or divalproex) can help reduce alcohol craving but will have a limited effect in preventing delirium tremens or seizures. The use of these medications does not prevent the progression of alcohol withdrawal, and these should not be used as monotherapy but only with appropriate use of a BZD. Neuroleptic agents such as phenothiazines and haloperidol can help reduce the severity of withdrawal symptoms and uncontrolled agitation but are not as effective as BZDs in preventing delirium and seizures.

> **CLINICAL CONCEPT**
> Alpha-adrenergic agonists (e.g., clonidine) or β-adrenergic antagonists (i.e., propranolol) are helpful in managing the distressing physical manifestations of alcohol withdrawal such as tachycardia and tremor.

Attention must be focused on treating alcohol-induced nutritional deficiencies, in particular with high-dose vitamin B supplementation, including thiamine, pyridoxine, and folic acid, and vitamin C. Magnesium deficiency is a common correctable problem in alcohol abuse. The recommended dietary allowance (RDA) for magnesium in men is 400 to 420 mg/day, whereas for women who are not pregnant or lactating, the RDA is 310 to 320 mg/day. Supportive care, including sufficient fluid intake and frequent clinical reassessment, including vital signs, is important.

In addition to psychosocial support and counseling, many medications are available to assist in preventing relapse in an alcohol-dependent person. These products can be divided into categories by anticipated clinical effect and include medications that modify the intoxicating effects of alcohol, such as naltrexone (Revia®, Vivitrol®); medications that help to reduce alcohol craving, such as acamprosate (Campral®); and medications that induce unpleasant adverse effects if alcohol is ingested, such as disulfiram (Antabuse®). Topiramate (Topamax®) has also shown some potential in preventing relapse by mitigating the euphoric effect of alcohol. Although these medications can be helpful, the therapeutic effect is generally seen only when these products are used in a motivated patient who has adequate psychosocial support and is involved in counseling. Because of its significant adverse effect profile, disulfiram use has largely fallen out of favor. Other agents are being studied to assist alcohol-dependent persons, such as baclofen, metadoxine, nalmefene, and ondansetron. Treatment of underlying mental health problems such as depression and/or anxiety with a selective serotonin reuptake inhibitor (SSRI) can also be helpful in maintaining sobriety.

BENZODIAZEPINE ABUSE

Overview

Compared with men, women have higher rates of misuse of prescription medications including BZDs, which is most likely related to their more frequent use of the health-care system. In addition, women are more likely to have mood disorders, including anxiety and depression, and, consequently, are more likely to have potential drugs of abuse such as BZDs prescribed by a health-care provider (Table 15-1). The NP should keep in mind that first-line treatment for depression and anxiety is SSRIs, not BZDs. (See Anxiety Disorders section later in this chapter.)

Psychological dependence on BZDs is usually associated with a rapid-onset agent, one that possibly gives a sensation of intoxication. In addition, prescribing at dosing intervals beyond duration of action of

TABLE 15-1 Psychotropic Medications Occasionally Prescribed to Treat Anxiety, as Adjunctive Therapy in Depression With Anxiety

MEDICATIONS	PHARMACOKINETICS	INDICATIONS	ONSET OF ACTION	COMMENTS
Buspirone (BuSpar®)	Slow onset of action (greater than 7 days), lipophilic, $t_{1/2}$ of metabolite 16 hours	Generalized anxiety syndrome, social phobia. Can be used as adjunct in OCD, PTSD. Less effective in panic disorder, acute anxiety. Not helpful in alcohol withdrawal.	2 to 4 weeks for some relief of anxiety 4 to 5 weeks for full therapeutic effect	5-HT1A receptor site agonist, not a BZD, not effective as a prn or sleep aid drug. Minimal to no effect on performance, nonsedating. No tolerance, withdrawal syndrome. No potentiation with alcohol. Little abuse potential.
Lorazepam (Ativan®)	Plasma peak in 1 to 6 hours, about half as lipophilic as diazepam (Valium®) No active metabolites $t_{1/2}$ 10 to 20 hours	Generalized anxiety syndrome, social phobia, adjunct in OCD, PTSD, panic disorder. Helpful in acute anxiety, alcohol withdrawal.	Slow onset of action, sustained effect	As with all BZDs, abuse and habituation potential.
Oxazepam (Serax®)	About half as lipophilic as diazepam, slower onset of action Plasma peak in 1 to 4 hours No active metabolites $t_{1/2}$ 3 to 21 hours	Generalized anxiety syndrome, social phobia, adjunct in OCD, PTSD, panic disorder. Helpful in acute anxiety, alcohol withdrawal.	Slow onset of action, relatively sustained effect	Abuse and habituation potential. Preferred choice for elderly patients. With all BZDs, caution with use in older adults due to increased risk of fall and potential for altering mental status.
Alprazolam (Xanax®)	Plasma peak in 1 to 2 hours About half as lipophilic as diazepam Parent compound $t_{1/2}$ 12 to 15 hours	Generalized anxiety syndrome, social phobia, adjunct in OCD, PTSD, panic disorder. Helpful in acute anxiety, alcohol withdrawal.	Slow onset of action, relatively sustained effect	Abuse and habituation potential. When prescribed, sufficient daily doses should be allotted.
Clonazepam (Klonopin®)	Plasma peak in 1 to 2 hours About one-quarter as lipophilic as diazepam No active metabolites $t_{1/2}$ 18 to 50 hours	Generalized anxiety syndrome, social phobia, adjunct in OCD, PTSD, panic disorder. Helpful in acute anxiety, alcohol withdrawal, absence, and petit mal seizures. Anxiety and panic.	Slow onset of action, highly sustained effect	Abuse and habituation potential. Caution when used in elderly due to protracted $t_{1/2}$; helpful in younger adults for consistent anxiety relief.
Diazepam (Valium®)	Plasma peak in 0.5 to 2 hours Highly lipophilic Three active metabolites with various $t_{1/2}$ Desmethyldiazepam $t_{1/2}$ 30 to 200 hours Oxazepam $t_{1/2}$ 3 to 21 hours 3-hydroxydiazepam $t_{1/2}$ 5 to 20 hours	Generalized anxiety syndrome, social phobia, adjunct in OCD, PTSD, panic disorder. Helpful in acute anxiety, alcohol withdrawal. Anxiety Seizures Musculoskeletal pain	Rapid onset of action, relatively sustained effect	Abuse and habituation potential. Protracted $t_{1/2}$ can pose a problem when used in elderly patients.

BZD, benzodiazepine; OCD, obsessive-compulsive disorder; PTSD, post-traumatic stress disorder; $t_{1/2}$, half-life.

Source: Goldberg R, Posner D. Anxiety disorders: diagnosis and management. In: Goldberg R, ed. Practical Guide to the Care of the Psychiatric Patient. 3rd ed. Philadelphia, PA: Mosby; 2007:158–177.

the drug gives alternating periods of drug effect and withdrawal. The perception of difference is significant and possibly perceived as a buildup of unpleasant anxiety followed by a period of relief or rescue provided by the patient, with the cycle repeated with each drug dose. On the occasion that BZD use is considered appropriate, psychological dependence can likely be avoided by using a slow-onset product with a long $t_{1/2}$, such as clonazepam. If using short-acting products, an adequate number of doses per day should be given. If a BZD is being used on an as-needed basis, the practitioner should advise a maximum number of available or prescribed doses per week, such as three to four times per week, rather than once or twice a day. This approach can help avoid BZD tolerance, a situation in which the patient requires increasingly higher doses to reach therapeutic effect. Tolerance usually precedes physical dependence. Expert consultation on appropriate BZD use is critical to safe practice.

> **CLINICAL CONCEPT**
>
> Using a BZD as an "as-needed" product increases the likelihood of abuse, because this heightens the patient's awareness of drug versus no-drug state.

Clinical Presentation

Individuals who abuse prescription medications such as BZDs typically fall into two categories: those who have prescriptions and medical indications for the use of the drugs for treatment of a given disorder, and those who use these drugs for nonmedical purposes. In either case, they will experience, in most cases, similar sedative-hypnotic effects as well as tolerance and withdrawal symptoms.

Diagnostic Testing

The *DSM-5* criteria are used for the diagnosis of sedative, anxiolytic, or hypnotic misuse under SUD and require significant impairment or distress over a 12-month period. At least 2 of the 11 criteria must be fulfilled to make a diagnosis, which include tolerance and withdrawal.

For BZDs, withdrawal symptoms can be detected within hours or days of cessation (depending on the $t_{1/2}$ of the agent used). The characteristic withdrawal symptoms usually include tachycardia, sweating, tremors, insomnia, nausea and vomiting, transient hallucinations or illusions, psychomotor agitation, anxiety, and grand mal seizures.

Treatment

Physical dependence on BZDs is a significant problem. When working with a patient to discontinue BZD use, the practitioner should consider reducing the dose by 25% per week. Rapid withdrawal can lead to tremors, hallucinations, seizures, and a delirium tremens–like state. The onset of withdrawal symptoms occurs a few days after the last dose in a BZD with a shorter $t_{1/2}$ (e.g., lorazepam) and up to 3 weeks in one with a longer $t_{1/2}$ (e.g., clonazepam). The major therapeutic goal of BZD abuse is treatment of the underlying mood disorder. There is no specific treatment for BZD abuse with the exception of the previously mentioned tapering of the medication's dose. Concomitant cognitive behavioral therapy (CBT) is an important part of treatment of BZD abuse.

BZDs rarely cause hepatic or renal impairment. When taken alone in overdose, BZDs have a favorable toxicity profile. Sedation risk is enhanced, however, when BZDs are combined with alcohol and barbiturates, leading to a potentially life-threatening condition. Accidental and intentional fatalities with BZD ingestion with alcohol often occur.

Flunitrazepam (Rohypnol®) is a BZD, also known as "roofies" or the "date-rape drug." Flunitrazepam is particularly potent with a rapid onset of action and is not available for prescription use in North America. This product is a commonly prescribed sleep aid in other countries, however. Flunitrazepam has been misused as a drug to reduce sexual inhibition, often given without the knowledge of the recipient. Because its use can result in amnesia, sexual assault can occur, possibly without the victim recalling the event.

OPIOID USE DISORDER

Overview

Opioid use disorder has become a national epidemic with nearly one in five Americans reported to take an opioid. Each month, nearly 4 million individuals are reported to take prescription pain relievers for nonmedical uses. In drug overdose deaths, on average, more than two-thirds involved an opioid. On average, 130 Americans die each day from an opioid overdose. The desired effects of opioid use include euphoria and central nervous system (CNS) depression followed by sedation. Gabapentin and pregabalin misuse, obtained via prescription or illegally, is increasingly common with opioid use due to these drugs having the potential to enhance opioid effects.

Clinical Presentation

The short-term effects of opioid use include pain relief, drowsiness, nausea, and constipation. Opioid intoxication can involve constricted pupils, respiratory depression, and extreme drowsiness. An overdose is typically characterized by respiratory arrest, unresponsiveness, coma, hypothermia, hypotension, and bradycardia. When used in combination with alcohol, there is an increased risk for respiratory arrest, bradycardia, and death. For suspected opioid overdose, the opioid antagonist naloxone (Narcan®) should be administered immediately.

Diagnostic Testing

Diagnosis of opioid use disorder is based on *DSM-5* criteria with individuals meeting at least 2 of the 11 criteria for SUD. Tolerance and withdrawal would not be considered for those taking opioids for a medical indication.

Treatment

Opioid withdrawal shares many common characteristics with alcohol withdrawal. Hypertension, tachycardia, diarrhea, nausea, temperature dysregulation, fever, papillary dilation, restlessness, myalgia, lacrimation, and rhinorrhea are often reported in addition to intense cravings for opioids. Although quite distressing, the condition is usually not life-threatening, particularly in younger adults, and typically resolves within a few days. However, older adults and individuals with significant comorbidities can develop fluid and electrolyte imbalances with protracted diarrhea and vomiting. Expert management is required.

> **CLINICAL CONCEPT**
>
> Compared with methadone in the treatment of opioid use disorder, the drug combination of buprenorphine with naloxone (Suboxone) has clinically desirable qualities, such as lower abuse potential, less withdrawal discomfort, and greater safety against overdose.

Clonidine, an α-adrenergic agonist, has traditionally been used off-label to help minimize opioid withdrawal symptoms. Lofexidine (Lucemyra™), a central $α_2$-adrenergic agonist, has been approved by the U.S. Food and Drug Administration (FDA) for the treatment of opioid withdrawal syndrome and can help transition those who desire to abstain from opioid use. As with any chemical dependence, long-term rehabilitation therapy is usually needed, necessitating a high level of patient desire for sobriety. Methadone, a long-acting opioid, can help curb the inappropriate use of opioids when used in conjunction with a comprehensive counseling and monitoring program. Buprenorphine with naloxone (Suboxone®) is a fixed-dose combination of an opioid agonist (buprenorphine) and antagonist (naloxone) that offers an alternative to methadone.

When used to treat addiction, methadone can be dispensed only through a qualified opioid treatment program, whereas buprenorphine with naloxone (Suboxone®) can be prescribed in a variety of clinical practices by qualified clinicians. Buprenorphine with naloxone and methadone are helpful options in opioid addiction. These medications are most helpful when used by a motivated patient who is actively involved in a comprehensive treatment program.

MARIJUANA USE DISORDER

Overview

Marijuana has historically been considered a drug that has potential for psychological dependence but with little potential for physical addiction. For adolescents in many communities, daily use of marijuana is more common than daily alcohol use. With greater legalization of marijuana use, adolescents, in particular, are using this drug with greater frequency. When surveying high school students about marijuana use in the past month, a tenfold increase was reported from 1991 (0.6%) to 2017 (6.3%). The number of teens who reported using both marijuana and alcohol at least once per month also increased from 3.6% in 1991 to 7.6% in 2017. Marijuana currently being used in all forms is extremely potent because of its high tetrahydrocannabinol (THC) content. Common methods of consuming marijuana include vaporizing, as edibles (infused into foods), topical preparations, and tinctures (concentrated form of medical cannabis in an alcohol solution and placed under the tongue or mixed with water).

A significant number of states have legalized recreational use of marijuana, and a growing number of states have approved its use for medical purposes. Cannabis can help relieve symptoms of several conditions, including cancer, HIV/AIDS, mood disorders, and chronic pain. Edible and food-based cannabis medicines can be an option for patients who wish to use this plant-based therapy but do not want to ingest smoke. The clinical effect of cannabis edibles typically takes longer than smoking but usually lasts longer. Consuming edibles on an empty stomach will hasten its effect. When considering the use of edibles, patients should be aware of what constitutes one serving (e.g., one cookie can constitute four servings). Patients should also ensure that cannabis edibles are safely stored and out of reach of children, pets, and any other individuals who are likely not to be aware of the content. Topical forms have been reported to be effective for joint diseases (e.g., rheumatoid and osteoarthritis), migraines, psoriasis, and restless leg syndrome. The NP should check the current state legal status of medical marijuana prior to prescribing to patients, to ensure the NP is properly licensed to prescribe cannabis products and is well informed on this growing therapeutic option.

Clinical Presentation

The effects of marijuana include euphoria, relaxation, antinausea, heightened sensitivity to stimuli, and a sensation of slowed time. Short-term effects can include slowed reaction time, balance and coordination issues, increased heart rate and appetite, and problems with learning and memory. Long-term effects can include mental health problems, impairment of higher cognitive functions, chronic cough, and frequent respiratory infections. There is growing evidence demonstrating that smoking both marijuana and tobacco results in a greater risk for chronic obstructive pulmonary disease (COPD) compared to smoking tobacco only. Individuals with marijuana intoxication, when performing activities requiring concentration or physical skills, such as operating a motor vehicle, show significant impairment. When combined with alcohol, marijuana use can result in tachycardia and hypertension.

After a period of abstinence, physical withdrawal symptoms are often reported among daily marijuana users, though the specific characteristics of withdrawal have not been well defined. Chronic inhaled marijuana use can lead to airway obstruction similar to that found in heavy tobacco users.

Diagnostic Testing

A diagnosis of marijuana use disorder is similar to other SUDs and is based on *DSM-5* criteria, with the presence of at least 2 of the 11 criteria within a 12-month period, and can include symptoms of tolerance and withdrawal. However, making a diagnosis of a withdrawal state and physiological dependence with marijuana remain controversial, as these conditions are not as clearly defined when compared with other illicit substances.

Treatment

Withdrawal symptoms typically include irritability, trouble sleeping, decreased appetite, and anxiety. There are no FDA-approved medications to treat marijuana addiction or habituation, though behavioral therapies can be effective. These include CBT, motivational enhancement therapy (MET), as well as contingency management or motivational incentives. It is unclear whether the long-term effects of marijuana use are reversible with abstinence.

STIMULANT USE DISORDER

Overview

One of the most commonly abused stimulants is cocaine. The drug is a potent sympathomimetic and has been used by approximately 15% of individuals 12 years and older.

Amphetamine, able to be prescribed legally for the treatment of attention-deficit hyperactivity disorder and select other disorders, and methamphetamine, an illegal drug, are among the most commonly abused drugs in the United States. These stimulants are rapidly absorbed and have a rapid onset of action (less than 1 hour), causing the desired effects of CNS stimulation, euphoria, mood elevation, and appetite suppression.

MDMA (3,4-methylenedioxy-methamphetamine), also known as ecstasy or Molly (a purportedly pure drug form but often tainted with contaminants or other intoxicating substances), is a psychoactive drug that has similarities to amphetamine and the hallucinogen mescaline. Initially popular with white adolescents and young adults, MDMA use has expanded to broader demographics. The drug increases the activity of the neurotransmitters serotonin, dopamine, and norepinephrine, and the effects can last approximately 3 to 6 hours. In high doses, MDMA can interfere with regulation of body temperature which can lead to hyperthermia, rapid heart rate, excessive sweating, shivering, and involuntary twitching. In rare cases, the effect can lead to a serotonin syndrome-like condition causing extreme hyperthermia with resulting liver, kidney, and cardiovascular system failure and eventual death.

Clinical Presentation

After cocaine ingestion, the user has an increase in heart rate and myocardial contractility and generalized vasoconstriction, causing an increase in blood pressure. The use of cocaine preferentially constricts the coronary and cerebral vessels, creating significant risk for cerebral ischemia and stroke and myocardial ischemia and infarction. Inquiring about chest pain is prudent in caring for a patient with cocaine abuse. Crack cocaine is the freebase form of cocaine that comes in crystal form that can be smoked. It is considered to be a more addictive form of cocaine. Short-term effects of stimulant abuse include enlarged pupils, increased body temperature, increased heart rate and blood pressure, headache, abdominal pain and nausea, increased energy and alertness, insomnia, and restlessness. Psychological signs can include anxiety, erratic and violent behavior, panic attacks, paranoia, and psychosis. Long-term use of methamphetamines can lead to hallucinations and delusions as well as severe dental problems ("meth mouth").

> **CLINICAL CONCEPT**
>
> Behavioral therapies, including CBT, contingency management, and community-based recovery groups, can offer effective options to overcome addiction.

Diagnostic Testing

There is no specific diagnostic testing other than standard drug screening.

Treatment

There are no FDA-approved medications to treat addiction of cocaine, amphetamines, or methamphetamines. Withdrawal can cause depressed mood, fatigue, vivid and disturbing dreams, sleep disturbance, increased appetite, and psychomotor agitation or retardation. For those seeking to overcome addiction, expert consultation should be sought.

Discussion Sources

American Psychiatric Association. *Practice Guideline for the Treatment of Patients With Substance Use Disorders.* 2nd ed. Arlington, VA: American Psychiatric Association Publishing; 2010. https://psychiatryonline.org/pb/assets/raw/sitewide/practice_guidelines/guidelines/substanceuse.pdf

Centers for Disease Control and Prevention. About drugs and addiction. http://www.cdc.gov/pwid/addiction.html

Ferri F. *Ferri's Best Test: A Practical Guide to Clinical Laboratory Medicine and Diagnostic Imaging.* 4th ed. Philadelphia, PA: Elsevier Saunders; 2017.

Ferri F. Management of alcohol withdrawal. In: Ferri F. *Practical Guide to the Care of the Medical Patient.* 9th ed. Philadelphia, PA: Elsevier Mosby; 2014.

Hoffman RS, Weinhouse GL. Management of moderate and severe alcohol withdrawal syndromes, 2019. UpToDate. https://www.uptodate.com/contents/management-of-moderate-and-severe-alcohol-withdrawal-syndromes

Mayo-Smith MF, Beecher LH, Fischer TL, et al. Management of alcohol withdrawal delirium: an evidence-based practice guideline. *Arch Intern Med.* 2004;164:1405–1412.

McHugh RK. Treatment of co-occurring anxiety disorders and substance use disorders. *Harv Rev Psychiatry.* 2015;23:99–111.

Prochaska JO, Redding CA, Evers KE. The transtheoretical model and stages of change. In: Glanz K, Lewis FM, Rimer BK, eds. *Health Behavior and Health Education: Theory, Research, and Practice.* 2nd ed. San Francisco, CA: Jossey-Bass; 1997.

Schreiner AD, Rockey DC. Evaluation of abnormal liver tests in the adult asymptomatic patient. *Curr Opin Gastroenterol.* 2018;34:272–279.

QUESTIONS

1. A 44-year-old man who admits to drinking "a few beers now and then" presents for examination. After obtaining a health history and performing a physical examination, you suspect he is a heavy alcohol user. Your next best action is to:

   A. obtain an evaluation of liver enzymes.

   B. administer the CAGE questionnaire.

   C. confront the patient with your observations.

   D. advise him about the hazards of excessive alcohol use.

2. Which of the following is not a component of the CAGE questionnaire?

   A. Have you ever felt you should cut down on your drinking?

   B. Have you been annoyed by people criticizing your drinking?

    C. Have you ever felt guilty about your drinking?

    D. Have you ever engaged in a violent act while drinking?

3 to 5.   Rank each alcoholic drink from the highest (1) to the lowest (3) amount of alcohol.

_____   **3.** 12 oz (360 mL) beer (9 proof)

_____   **4.** 6 oz (120 mL) wine (22 proof)

_____   **5.** A mixed drink containing 3.5 oz (105 mL) of 80-proof liquor

6. During an office visit, a 38-year-old woman states, "I drink way too much but do not know what to do to stop." According to Prochaska's change framework, her statement is most consistent with a person at the stage of:

    A. precontemplation.

    B. contemplation.

    C. preparation.

    D. action.

7. Lorazepam or oxazepam is the preferred BZD for treating alcohol withdrawal symptoms when there is a concomitant history of:

    A. seizure disorder.

    B. folate-deficiency anemia.

    C. multiple substance abuse.

    D. hepatic dysfunction.

8. Peak symptoms of alcohol withdrawal are usually observed how long after alcohol intake is discontinued?

    A. less than 12 hours

    B. 12 to 24 hours

    C. 24 to 36 hours

    D. more than 48 hours

9 to 11.   Rank the following alcohol withdrawal symptoms from earliest (1) to latest (3) to develop.

_____   **9.** Increased body temperature

_____   **10.** Nausea and vomiting

_____   **11.** Seizure

12. Which of the following is the most helpful first-line approach in the care of a patient with alcohol abuse?

    A. Advise the patient in a straightforward manner to stop drinking.

    B. Counsel the patient that alcohol abuse is a treatable disease.

    C. Inform the patient of the long-term health consequences of alcohol abuse.

    D. Refer the patient to AA.

13. A 42-year-old man who has a long-standing history of alcohol abuse presents for primary care. He admits to drinking 12 to 16 beers daily for 10 years. He states, "I really do not feel like the booze is a problem. I get to work every day." Your most appropriate response is:

    A. "You must be fortunate to still have a job."

    B. "Your family has suffered by your drinking."

    C. "I am concerned about your health and safety."

    D. "Participating in a support group can help you understand why you drink."

14. Which of the following agents offers an intervention for the control of tremor and tachycardia associated with alcohol withdrawal?

    A. phenobarbital

    B. clonidine

    C. verapamil

    D. naltrexone

15. Which of the following is most likely to be noted in a 45-year-old woman with laboratory evidence of chronic excessive alcohol ingestion?

    A. ALT 202 U/L (0 to 31 U/L), MCV 70 fL (80 to 96 fL)

    B. AST 149 U/L (0 to 31 U/L), MCV 81 fL (80 to 96 fL)

    C. ALT 88 U/L (0 to 31 U/L), MCV 140 fL (80 to 96 fL)

    D. AST 80 U/L (0 to 31 U/L), MCV 103 fL (80 to 96 fL)

16. Which of the following is the anticipated clinical effect of acamprosate (Campral®) in the treatment of alcohol dependence?

    A. modifies intoxicating effects of alcohol

    B. causes unpleasant adverse effects of alcohol

    C. helps to reduce the urge to drink

    D. minimizes alcohol withdrawal symptoms

17. When providing primary care for a middle-aged woman with a history of prescription BZD dependence, you consider that:

    A. she is unlikely to have a problem with misuse of other drugs or alcohol.

    B. rapid detoxification is the preferred method of treatment for this problem.

    C. she likely has an underlying untreated or undertreated mood disorder.

    D. she is at significant risk for drug-induced hepatitis.

18. Demographic data indicate which of the following persons is most likely to misuse prescription medications?

    A. a 14-year-old male

    B. a 24-year-old female

    C. a 33-year-old male

    D. a 38-year-old female

19. First-line treatment of anxiety and panic disorders are:

    A. BZDs.

    B. SSRIs.

    C. tricyclic antidepressants (TCAs).

    D. barbiturates.

20. When discontinuing BZD treatment after prolonged use, you recommend:

    A. terminating treatment immediately.

    B. decreasing the dose 20% per day.

    C. decreasing the dose 25% per week.

    D. decreasing the dose 50% per week.

21. When counseling a patient who is about to initiate BZD therapy, the NP cautions that the patient should avoid which of the following?

   A. alcohol

   B. NSAIDs

   C. beta blockers

   D. statins

22. While counseling an adolescent about the risks of marijuana use, the NP considers that:

   A. symptoms of physical and psychological dependency are rarely reported by regular users.

   B. the development of chronic obstructive airway disease is often associated with regular smoking, particularly when combined with inhaled tobacco use.

   C. use among teens is more common than that of alcohol.

   D. driving ability is minimally impaired with its use.

23. A 64-year-old man undergoing chemotherapy for lung cancer asks about the use of medical marijuana to help relieve symptoms of pain and nausea. The NP considers that:

   A. there is no evidence supporting the use of medical marijuana in cancer care for symptom treatment.

   B. smoking would be preferred to edible forms to maximize effect for this patient.

   C. state laws should be consulted to check the legal status of medical marijuana prior to prescribing.

   D. the patient should be evaluated for substance abuse.

24. Which of the following statements about edible medical cannabis is most accurate?

   A. Cooking cannabis will destroy its effect.

   B. The effect of edibles will be faster on an empty stomach.

   C. The effect of edibles generally occurs faster than smoking marijuana.

   D. The effect of edibles is usually shorter than smoking marijuana.

25. When assessing a person with acute opioid withdrawal, you expect to find:

   A. constipation.

   B. hypertension.

   C. hypothermia.

   D. somnolence.

26. An alternative to methadone that can be used to help with maintenance therapy in the treatment of opioid use disorder is:

   A. gabapentin.

   B. buprenorphine plus naloxone.

   C. methylnaltrexone.

   D. topiramate.

27. When providing care for a middle-aged man with acute cocaine intoxication, you inquire about:

   A. feelings of anxiety.

   B. difficulty maintaining sleep.

   C. chest pain.

   D. abdominal pain.

28. Hyperthermia and a racing heart rate are part of a potentially life-threatening presentation for a person using:

 A. cannabis.

 B. MDMA, or "Molly."

 C. LSD.

 D. barbiturates.

29. The use and abuse of flunitrazepam (Rohypnol®) has been associated with:

 A. agitation.

 B. amnesia.

 C. increased appetite.

 D. insomnia.

For answers and rationales, see end of chapter.

Eating Disorders

Overview

Eating disorders are serious and potentially life-threatening conditions that can affect individuals of all genders, ages, ethnicities, and body shapes and weights. It is estimated that approximately 20 million women and 10 million men in the United States will have an eating disorder at some point in their lifetimes. Risk factors can include a broad range of biological, psychological, and sociocultural aspects, including a family history of eating disorders, a history of dieting, perfectionism and body image dissatisfaction, weight stigma, teasing or bullying, and limited social networks. Many individuals with an eating disorder have other psychological disorders that can challenge effective treatment.

> **CLINICAL CONCEPT**
>
> The three most common eating disorders are anorexia nervosa (AN), bulimia nervosa (BN), and binge eating disorder (BED).

Early identification and treatment of eating disorders can help improve outcomes. Some warning signs of an eating disorder include a preoccupation with weight, food, and dieting; food rituals; skipping meals; extreme concern with body size and shape; and extreme mood swings. All adolescents should be screened annually for eating disorders by determining body mass index (BMI) and asking about body image and dieting patterns.

Physical signs of an eating disorder can include fluctuations in weight, nonspecified gastrointestinal (GI) complaints, menstrual irregularities, certain abnormal laboratory findings, dizziness, fainting, dental problems, and muscle weakness, among others. Screening tools are available to detect disordered eating; tools are usually specific to a given condition (Table 15-2).

While each eating disorder has specific characteristics and interventions, there are commonalities. Once diagnosed, treatment involves a combination of psychological and nutritional counseling along with medical and psychiatric monitoring. Referral to specialists in eating disorders is prudent in treatment. Recovery from eating disorders can take months to years, and the process can be divided into three stages:

- *Physical recovery*: Reverse partly or completely the physical effects of the eating disorder, including normalizing weight, electrolytes, and hormone levels, and resuming menstruation
- *Behavioral recovery*: Overcome the tendency to limit food intake, overexercise, purge, or binge-eat
- *Psychological recovery*: Address the cognitive and emotional aspects of the eating disorder, including perfectionism, body image anxiety, and extreme weight monitoring

Unfortunately, relapse is a common occurrence with eating disorders and usually coincides with periods of stress (e.g., going to college, starting a new job, death of a loved one). Anticipating relapses and having a good support system (e.g., nutritionist, psychiatrist) can help individuals continue toward recovery.

ANOREXIA NERVOSA

Overview

AN is a potentially life-threatening disease characterized by weight loss, difficulty maintaining an appropriate body weight, and distorted body image. A denial of the seriousness of the low body weight is often

TABLE 15-2 Screening Tools for Psychosocial Disorders

EATING DISORDERS

SCOFF	Five questions Two or more positive responses: 100% sensitive for detecting AN or BN
Eating Disorder Examination (EDE)	Semistructured interview conducted by a trained clinician
Yale-Brown-Cornell Eating Disorder Scale (YBC-EDS)	Eight-item scale assessing severity of eating-related preoccupations and rituals
Bulimia Test-Revised (BULIT-R)	36-item self-report questionnaire Score range: 29 to 140; score greater than 104 indicative of BN

DEPRESSION

Patient Health Questionnaire (PHQ-9)	Nine-item questionnaire; Score range: 1 to 27 Minimal depression (score 1 to 4) to severe depression (20 to 27)
Beck Depression Inventory (BDI)	21 items Score range: 0 to 63 points; minimal depression (0 to 13 points) to severe depression (29 to 63 points)
Zung Self-Rating Depression Scale	20 items; Score range: 20 to 80 Normal range (20 to 49) to severely depressed (70 or greater)
Geriatric Depression Scale (GDS)	30-item questionnaire (long form) or 15-item questionnaire (short form)
Hamilton Depression Rating Scale	17 to 21 questions performed by expert clinician

ANXIETY

Generalized Anxiety Disorder-7 (GAD-7)	Seven-item self-report questionnaire Score range: 0 to 21; minimal anxiety (0 to 4) to severe anxiety (15 to 21)
Hamilton Anxiety Rating Scale (HAM-A)	14-item questionnaire administered by trained clinician
Zung Self-Rating Anxiety Scale	20 items; Score range: 20 to 80 Normal range (20 to 44) to extreme anxiety (75 or greater)
Primary Care PTSD (PC-PTSD)	Five-item screen designed for use in primary care Positive response to three or more is sensitive for probable PTSD

INTERPERSONAL VIOLENCE

Partner Violence Screen	Three-item questionnaire; conducted by clinician alone with patient
SAFE	Series of questions asked by clinicians to assess patient safety, history of abuse, social support, and emergency/escape plan

AN, anorexia nervosa; BN, bulimia nervosa; PTSD, post-traumatic stress disorder.

found in patients with AN. Often despite extreme thinness, a patient with AN looks in the mirror and comments on the need to lose "just a few more pounds." The usual onset of AN in women is during the teens to early 20s, with ages 14 to 18 years being the most common; men with the condition typically present a few years later. AN is an overwhelmingly female disease (90%), with either gender often involved in an activity that has an emphasis on weight and shape, including wrestling, modeling, dancing, gymnastics, and swimming. Some of the activities are occasionally called appearance as well as performance sports.

Patients with AN usually exhibit one of two types of behavior. With the restricting type, a patient with AN severely limits food intake but does not binge-eat or purge. In the binge-purge type, a patient with AN has cycles of these behaviors.

Clinical Presentation

In contrast to BN, which is a secretive disease with relatively few easily noted clinical findings, AN is usually easy to identify clinically.

Cheilosis (aka, angular cheilitis) can occur in both AN and BN and presents as inflammatory lesions at the corners of the mouth, which can result in deep cracks or splits. This is likely a consequence of malnutrition and the result of repeated episodes of vomiting. Amenorrhea, which is common in women with AN, contributes to establishing the diagnosis.

Diagnostic Testing

Several screening tools are available for detection of eating disorders at an early stage. Examples include SCOFF, the Eating Disorder Examination (EDE), and the Yale-Brown-Cornell Eating Disorder Scale (YBC-EDS) (see Table 15-2). The SCOFF test consists of five simple questions, and two or more positive responses provide a 100% sensitivity for anorexia or bulimia. For those suspected of AN, an interview and physical examination should be conducted to assess patient history, symptoms, behaviors, BMI, vital signs, cardiac function, and blood chemistries.

The *DSM-5* criteria are used for the diagnosis of eating disorders such as AN. The CIDA mnemonic can be helpful in recognizing the signs and symptoms of this disorder:

■ **C**hoosing not to eat, leading to a potentially dangerous weight loss
■ **I**ntense fear of being obese, even when underweight
■ **D**isturbance of weight perception, feeling "fat" when actually being quite thin or underweight
■ **A**menorrhea for three or more cycles when not using a contraceptive method that results in menstrual cessation[1]

Atypical anorexia can occur in individuals who meet the criteria for diagnosis but are not underweight despite significant weight loss.

Treatment

AN is a potentially life-threatening disease with a mortality rate of 5% to 20%. Hospitalization to correct fluid and electrolyte disorders and to initiate refeeding is often needed. When physiological stability is reached, AN treatment usually includes cognitive-behavioral, pharmacological, and ongoing nutritional therapy. In CBT, the focus is the disturbed eating and the patterns of thinking that help perpetuate the binge-purge cycle. To be effective, accessing care with a clinician or treatment team expert in eating disorders is critical.

Acute pharmacological therapy is rarely needed for AN unless there is a coexisting psychological condition. When indicated, pharmacological therapy usually involves the use of antidepressants, which are thought to have an effect because of the high rate of comorbid depression. SSRIs (e.g., sertraline [Zoloft®], fluoxetine [Prozac®]) are preferred with depression or anxiety in patients with AN. The choice of a specific agent should be guided by the principles used in choosing therapy for depression. Anxiolytics are also sometimes used to reduce anxiety associated with eating. Cyproheptadine (Periactin®) can be used before meals to enhance appetite and reduce anxiety. Bupropion should be avoided owing to increased risk of seizure. In addition, second-generation antipsychotics should be avoided if possible; the weight gain that accompanies the use of this drug class can be counterproductive to recovery. As with other complex psychosocial health issues, expert consultation should be sought.

---

1. Adapted from Zebrudaya (2006, November 23). *The Diagnostic Criteria for Anorexia Nervosa* [online forum post]. http://www.rxpgonline.com /medicalmnemonic911033.html

BULIMIA NERVOSA

Overview

BN is more common in women and typically is present for many years before the patient presents for treatment or before the disorder is noted by a health-care provider, usually when seeing the patient for another issue.

Clinical Presentation

Because BN tends to be a secretive disease, few with the disease present directly requesting intervention. A patient with BN is often identified in the clinical setting by problems with erosion of the lingual surface of the upper teeth because of excessive exposure to gastric contents during induced vomiting. Hypokalemia, caused by laxative and diuretic use, is also common. Body weight provides few clues because a patient is typically of average to slightly above average weight.

Diagnostic Testing

Screening for BN can include the use of tools such as SCOFF, Bulimia Test-Revised (BULIT-R), EDE, and YBC-EDS (see Table 15-2). The CECE mnemonic can be a helpful tool in recognizing the signs and symptoms of BN:

- Control—Lack of control in amount and type of food consumed
- Eating binges—Characterized by excessive quantity in a defined period of time (typically within 2 hours)
- Compensatory behavior—Self-induced vomiting, excessive exercise, laxative or diuretic use, or fasting to prevent weight gain
- Excessive influence—Body weight and shape on self-worth

Treatment

Treatment of a patient with BN usually includes cognitive-behavioral and pharmacological therapy. In CBT, the focus is the disturbed eating and the thinking patterns that help perpetuate the binge-purge cycle. To be effective, accessing care with a clinician or treatment team expert in eating disorders is critical.

Pharmacological therapy usually involves the use of antidepressants such as SSRIs. SSRIs are usually highly successful in reducing the frequency and number of binges, partly because of their activity at the 5-HT1A-receptor site. All antidepressants can be used except for bupropion (Wellbutrin®), which can induce further bingeing or seizures in patients with BN. The choice of a specific agent should be guided by the principles used in choosing therapy for depression. As with other complex psychosocial health issues, expert consultation should be sought.

BINGE EATING DISORDER

Overview

BED is characterized as a lack of control over the amount and type of food eaten, occurring two or more times per week for at least 6 months. The bingeing is accompanied by marked distress, self-anger, shame, and frustration as a result of the bingeing.

Clinical Presentation

Typically, there are no specific presentations in BED. Purging activity is not present; as a result, a person with BED is usually overweight or obese.

Diagnostic Testing

BED is defined as eating an abnormally large amount of food in a discrete period of time (e.g., within a 2-hour period) and feeling a lack of control during the episode. Episodes occur at least once per week for 3 months. The CAR FAD mnemonic can be helpful in recognizing the signs of BED:

- Control—Lack of control when eating
- Amount—Abnormally large amounts of food consumed, eating while not hungry
- Rapid—Eating faster than normal

■ **Full**—Eating until uncomfortably full
■ **Alone**—Eating alone due to embarrassment
■ **Depressed**—Experiencing feelings of guilt and disgust afterward

Treatment

As with all eating disorders, treatment requires an interdisciplinary approach with contributions from health-care providers with expertise in this area. CBT is the treatment of choice, while family therapy can also be considered when family dynamics are associated with bingeing events or when children or adolescents are involved.

Lisdexamfetamine (Vyvanse®) is an FDA-approved medication to treat moderate-to-severe BED. Other agents can be used to decrease obsessive and compulsive behavior, such as antiepileptics (e.g., topiramate, zonisamide, and lamotrigine) and medications to decrease compulsive eating (e.g., exenatide, liraglutide). Anti-obesity medications can also be considered to control weight. As with other complex psychosocial health issues, expert consultation should be sought.

CLINICAL CONCEPT

In addition to behavioral therapy, pharmacotherapy can be considered. SSRIs and SNRIs are typically used for the treatment of depression and obsessive-compulsive disorder commonly seen in those with BED.

Discussion Sources

Academy for Eating Disorders. *Eating Disorders: A Guide to Medical Care.* 3rd ed. https://www.aedweb.org/resources/publications/medical-care-standards

Bernstein BE. Anorexia nervosa. Medscape. http://emedicine.medscape.com/article/912187-overview

Bernstein BE. Binge eating disorder (BED). Medscape. https://emedicine.medscape.com/article/2221362-overview

Hilty DM. Bulimia nervosa. Medscape. http://emedicine.medscape.com/article/286485-overview

QUESTIONS

30. Screening tools for eating disorders include all of the following except:

A. SCOFF.

B. PHQ-9.

C. EDE.

D. YBC-EDS.

31. Screening for eating disorders should be considered for:

A. all with a BMI less than 22 kg/m².

B. all with a BMI greater than 30 kg/m².

C. all individuals who express dissatisfaction with body weight.

D. all adolescents.

32. Which of the following statements is true concerning AN?

A. The disease affects men and women equally.

B. Onset is usually in the mid-20s for men and women.

C. Depression is often found concomitantly.

D. Effective treatment rarely needs specialty referral.

33. Initial treatment for a 19-year-old woman with appropriate hydration who has been diagnosed with AN usually includes:

A. referral for parenteral nutrition evaluation.

B. antidepressant therapy.

C. use of psychostimulants.

D. psychoanalysis.

34. Physical examination findings in a 21-year-old woman diagnosed with BN will likely include:

A. BMI less than 75% of anticipated.

B. dental surface erosion.

C. tachycardia.

D. hair that is easily plucked.

35. Cheilosis in a 20-year-old man with BN is best described as:

A. ruptured capillaries in the cornea.

B. deep cracks or splits in the corners of the mouth.

C. inflammatory lesions in the pharynx.

D. hair that is easily plucked.

36. Use of laxatives and diuretics by persons with BN will most commonly result in:

A. hypokalemia.

B. hypercalcemia.

C. proteinuria.

D. hypernatremia.

37. Which of the following is most consistent with the diagnosis of BN?

A. Patients with BN usually present asking for treatment.

B. Periods of anorexia often occur.

C. Hyperkalemia often results from laxative abuse.

D. Most patients with BN are significantly obese.

38. All of the following pharmacological interventions are used in the treatment of patients with BN except:

A. fluoxetine (Prozac®).

B. desipramine (Norpramin®).

C. bupropion (Wellbutrin®).

D. paroxetine (Paxil®).

39. Characteristics of BED include all of the following except:

A. lack of control over the amount and type of food eaten.

B. behavior present for at least 3 months.

C. marked distress, self-anger, shame, and frustration as a result of bingeing.

D. purging activity after an eating binge.

40 to 42. Each of the following patients has been diagnosed as having an eating disorder. Match each patient example with the most likely eating disorder diagnosis listed.

_____ **40.** A 27-year-old male with a BMI of 38 kg/m² who states that he usually eats by himself

_____ **41.** A 16-year-old female with a BMI of 18 kg/m² and deep cracks in the corners of her mouth

_____ **42.** A 21-year-old female with a BMI of 26 kg/m² who complains about not losing weight despite doing 3-hour intense workouts

A. AN

B. BN

C. BED

43 to 47. Identify whether the following characteristics are noted in AN, BN, or both disorders.

_____ **43.** parotid gland enlargement

_____ **44.** electrolyte disorder

_____ **45.** lanugo

_____ **46.** esophageal tears

_____ **47.** dysrhythmias

For answers and rationales, see end of chapter.

Mood Disorders

Overview

Mood disorders (also called affective disorders) are estimated to impact approximately 20% of the general population at any given time. These disorders affect a person's mood to such a degree that they impact normal everyday activities and can include depressive, anxiety, manic, and bipolar disorders. The concept that a person has either depression or anxiety has been largely replaced with the recognition that mood disorders occur on a continuum, with most individuals with mood disorders showing features of depression and anxiety.

Anxiety often occurs in patients with depression, making the differentiation between these two common disorders problematic. A patient with depression that has an anxious component usually reports nervous feelings after the onset of depressed mood. The depressed patient may also have feelings of worthlessness and the feeling that situations are hopeless; patients with anxiety often report feeling "worried sick" and helpless. Physical and mental health evaluations are needed to make a mood disorder diagnosis. Once underlying medical conditions have been ruled out, a mental health assessment determines mood stability.

DEPRESSION

Overview

Depression is a common health problem with at least a 15% lifetime occurrence rate. The *DSM-5* criteria are used for the diagnosis of depression and other mood disorders. The C GASP DIE mnemonic can be a helpful tool in identifying symptoms of depression.

- **C**oncentration difficulties or indecisiveness
- **G**uilt or feeling worthless
- **A**ppetite abnormality or weight change
- **S**leep disturbance
- **P**sychomotor retardation or agitation
- **D**eath or suicide (thoughts or acts of)
- **I**nterest (diminished)
- **E**nergy (loss)[2]

Individuals with depression will normally present with multiple symptoms, with depressed mood and/or loss of interest being key findings. The symptoms cause clinically important distress or impair work, social, or personal functioning and cannot be attributed to another health condition. Other symptoms of depression are often reported.

> **CLINICAL CONCEPT**
>
> Hypochondriasis is found in at least 30% of patients with depression; such patients are unable to process objective information that they have no particular health problems.

Alternatively, a person with hypochondriasis perceives that an existing health problem is far more serious than it is in reality. Suicidal ideation is occasionally present, with the patient voicing thoughts (most common) or a plan (less common) of self-harm. Most patients with depression have a passive idea of death without a plan. The patient often agrees with the statement, "If I could just die in my sleep, that would be all right," but steadfastly denies a plan of self-harm. As with any person with suicidal ideation or plan, a thorough safety evaluation should be completed and appropriate referral facilitated; this can include involuntary hospitalization for a patient who is at risk of self-harm. Inquiring about thoughts or plans of harm to others is also an important part of the patient's safety plan. All patients with a mood disorder should be made aware of local resources for emergency mental health care.

In an older adult, depression is sometimes mistaken for new-onset or worsening dementia. A patient with dementia typically has cognitive changes that are slowly progressive over months to years, however. The cognitive changes reported by older adults with depression usually have evolved over a much shorter period with the patient often accurately reporting what changes have occurred. See further discussion in Chapter 16.

Persistent depressive disorder (formerly known as dysthymia) is found in approximately 3% of the general population and is characterized by low-level daily depression with at least two of the previously identified depressive symptoms for at least 2 years in adults and 1 year in children and adolescents. *DSM-5* consolidates

---

2. Reprinted with permission from the *American Journal of Psychiatry* (Copyright ©2006). American Psychiatric Association. All Rights Reserved. From Abraham PF, Shirley ER (2006). New mnemonic for depressive symptoms [editorial]. *Am J Psychiatry* 2006;163(2):329–330.

dysthymia with chronic major depression to form the "persistent depressive disorder" category. As with people who are depressed, patients with persistent depressive disorder respond well to a combination of interpersonal and pharmacological intervention. A patient who reports a life-changing feeling with antidepressant use, often described as "feeling good to be alive for the first time," is likely suffering from persistent depressive disorder. The person's underlying personality emerges after being suppressed or altered by the debilitating effects of the low-level depression that characterizes persistent depressive disorder.

When a patient who is depressed takes antidepressants while undergoing an ongoing significant life stressor, such as family or marital discord or abuse, depressive symptoms usually subside as the medication takes effect. If the stressor continues, however, the antidepressant can appear to lose its initial effectiveness. Ongoing interpersonal therapy can be highly effective in augmenting pharmacological treatment in such situations.

Depressed mood often follows a significant life stressor, such as death of a loved one or loss of a job; normal sadness or grief is often inappropriately labeled as depression. An important difference is that the person who is sad, as might be reported in an individual who was recently laid off from work, or the person who is grieving, such as an individual whose loved one recently died, can identify the reason for the altered mood. With the passage of time and support, most people with normative sadness or grief find that the altered mood improves. An important role for the health-care provider is to help the bereaved person to identify the difference between the normative sadness of loss and depression. Commonly, the acutely bereaved person will mistake grief for depression. At the same time, if diagnostic criteria for depression are met beyond 1 to 3 months after the precipitating event, particularly if the bereaved is having difficulty with daily basic function, the diagnosis of complicated grief with major depression should be considered. Treatment for adjustment disorder with depressed mood lasting beyond 1 to 3 months is the same as treatment for major depression, recognizing that interpersonal therapy can be highly effective in assisting patients in dealing with loss. Although treating a reactive depression is helpful in lifting mood and restoring function, such treatment would not relieve the normal sadness associated with loss.

Anxiety is often reported by a depressed person and is a common comorbid condition. In individuals with depression, the mood disturbance occurs first, followed in several weeks by the addition of anxiety-related symptoms. Depression should be considered as the diagnosis rather than anxiety if the patient reports feeling worse while taking BZDs. If a patient with depression also has episodes of mania, bipolar I disorder is present.

Psychomotor agitation with fidgeting and irritability is often found in patients with depression, especially in children and adolescents. In these age-groups, this presentation is more likely than psychomotor retardation. This type of increased activity is also found in type A adults with depression.

Clinical Presentation

There is no typical clinical presentation of depression. In milder depression, the patient appears at his or her baseline. With more severe symptoms, speech and reactivity are often slower. Affect is flat, with little emotional expression. Hygiene is often neglected. The person with depression often has a weight change, either increased or decreased.

Diagnostic Testing

Depression is a clinical diagnosis that does not require laboratory tests or neuroimaging. According to the U.S. Preventive Services Task Force, screening for depression should be considered for all adults, particularly older adults as well as pregnant and postpartum women. The most common screening tool is the self-reported Patient Health Questionnaire-9 (PHQ-9), which is a nine-item depression scale. Other self-reported screening tools include Beck Depression Inventory (BDI; a 21-question scale), BDI for primary care (7-item questionnaire), the Zung Self-Rating Depression Scale (a 21-item questionnaire), and the Geriatric Depression Scale (GDS; a 30-item questionnaire) (see Table 15-2). A Hamilton Depression Rating Scale is performed by a specialist rather than self-reported. It is important to recognize that any screening tool has advantages and disadvantages, and further evaluation by a specialist is prudent to make a definitive diagnosis of depression and start treatment.

ANXIETY DISORDERS

Overview

Anxiety is a normal human emotion that is an important part of the fear response and helps a person focus on the issue at hand, such as anxiety associated with taking an important examination or making a presentation. Anxiety can be protective, heightening senses when an individual encounters a dangerous situation. This is a rational, expected emotion when present for an appropriate reason and should dissipate with the cessation of the stressor. Anxiety becomes problematic, however, when it is exaggerated, is prolonged, or interferes with daily function.

Generalized anxiety disorder (GAD) is present in approximately 2% to 4% of the population. The typical age of onset is usually in the teen to young adult years; 15% have a first-degree relative with GAD. Many individuals with GAD experience physical symptoms related to anxiety that lead to health-care visits. Yet, many with GAD remain undiagnosed and untreated.

Panic disorder affects 2% to 4% of the general population. Average age of onset is 27 years; new onset is rare after age 45 years. There is a strong comorbidity with depression. The female-to-male ratio for panic disorder is approximately 1:1 if seen without agoraphobia. Panic disorder with agoraphobia is more common in women, however, with a ratio of 2:1. A strong family history of agoraphobia is often also reported.

Post-traumatic stress disorder (PTSD) is a condition that occurs after a significant single event, such as a natural disaster, being the victim of a crime, or exposure to combat conditions. It can also be precipitated by recurrent trauma, such as serving in combat, living in a war-torn area, or domestic abuse. Trauma can involve direct personal experience of an event that involves actual or threatened death or serious injury or witnessing an event that involves death, injury, or a threat to the physical integrity of another person. Horror and helplessness are expected emotions in response to a traumatic life event for at least 1 month afterward. These emotions last significantly longer in patients with PTSD, however, and are coupled with intrusive recall of the event, numbing of emotions, detachment, hyperarousal, and impaired social and occupational function. When considering military personnel with PTSD, it should be noted that they do not always respond in the same manner as civilians, and criteria for "fear, helplessness, and horror" do not always apply.

Clinical Presentation

The WATCHERS mnemonic can be helpful in identifying symptoms of GAD, with at least three of the following symptoms occurring on most days for 6 or more months:

■ **W**orry—Disproportionate to daily concerns, worry continues after the end of the trigger event
■ **A**nxiety—"On edge" emotionally
■ **T**ension—In muscles, physical manifestation of anxiety
■ **C**oncentration—Difficulty concentrating, "mind going blank"
■ **H**yperarousal—Irritability
■ **E**nergy—Loss
■ **R**estlessness—Feeling of being keyed up
■ **S**leep disturbance—Often difficulty falling asleep[3]

The cardinal presenting signs of anxiety disorder are related to the hypersympathetic state. Physical manifestations include tachycardia, hyperventilation, palpitations, tremors, and sweating.

> **CLINICAL CONCEPT**
>
> Panic attacks can occur with or without agoraphobia and should not be due to a substance or medical condition or accounted for by another mental disorder.

Diagnostic Testing

When establishing the diagnosis of GAD, it is important to rule out many clinical conditions that can mimic the disorder, including thyrotoxicosis, sleep disorders, Addison's disease, alcohol withdrawal, or abuse of sympathomimetic drugs such as caffeine, amphetamines, and cocaine.

Screening for GAD can include the use of the GAD-7 (a seven-question survey), the Hamilton Anxiety Rating Scale (HAM-A), or the Zung Self-Rating Anxiety Scale (see Table 15-2). The PC-PTSD is a four-item questionnaire that can be used in primary care to identify those with possible PTSD.

Diagnostic criteria for panic disorder include recurrent and unexpected panic attacks and one or more of the panic attacks is followed by at least one of the following: worry about an additional attack, pondering implications of attacks, or significant change of behavior related to attacks.

---

3. Adapted from Berber MJ. WATCHERS: recognizing generalized anxiety disorder [editorial]. *J Clin Psychiatry* 2000;61(6):447. https://www.psychiatrist.com/JCP/article/Pages/2000/v61n06/v61n0610.aspx

Panic attack is central to panic disorder. This is a period of intense fear or discomfort developing abruptly and peaking within 10 minutes with at least four characteristic symptoms present. The mnemonic STUDENTS FEAR the 3Cs can be helpful in identifying these symptoms:

- **S**weating
- **T**rembling or shaking
- **U**nsteady, dizziness, light-headed, or faint
- **D**erealization (feelings of unreality) or depersonalization (being detached from one's self)
- **E**xcessive/accelerated heart rate, palpitations, or pounding heart
- **N**ausea or abdominal distress
- **T**ingling, numbness, paresthesia
- **S**hortness of breath
- **F**ear of losing control or "going crazy"
- **E**ar of dying
- **A**r Choking feelings
- **R** Chest pain or discomfort
- Chills or heat sensations[4]

BIPOLAR DISORDER

Overview

When a patient with depression also has episodes of mania, bipolar I disorder is likely present. When episodes of mania are relatively mild and short-lived, then bipolar II disorder is likely. Bipolar disorders occur in approximately 1% of the general population.

In bipolar I disorder, the patient usually presents with cycles of elevated or irritated mood lasting longer than 1 week. Bipolar I disorder is most common in women, with an onset around puberty. If a patient with depression has episodes of mania lasting fewer than 4 days with little social incapacitation, the diagnosis of bipolar II disorder is made. In patients with bipolar II disorder, the episodes of mania are relatively mild (hypomania) and are often quite productive in contrast to the low point of depression.

Further descriptors of bipolar disease include rapid cycling and cyclothymic disorder. In rapid-cycle bipolar disorder, there are four or more hypomanic, manic, mixed, or major depressive episodes in a 1-year period. In cyclothymic disorder, the mood disorder has been present for at least 2 years with episodes of mania lasting fewer than 4 days, too brief to fit standard criteria of mania or hypomania.

The most widely used screening tool for bipolar disorder is the Mood Disorder Questionnaire, which is a brief self-report instrument. A positive screen should be followed up by a comprehensive mental health evaluation by an expert.

Clinical Presentation

The DIG FAST mnemonic can be used to identify characteristics of mania. For at least 1 week, or less if hospitalized, the person's mood is persistently high, irritable, or expansive, coupled with other symptoms:

- **D**istractibility—Easily frustrated, difficulty keeping on task
- **I**rresponsibility—Erratic, uninhibited behavior
- **G**randiosity—Described as "larger than life" feelings of superiority, invulnerability, and often leading to risky behavior
- **F**light of ideas—Verbalizes incomplete thoughts, unable to continue through on common tasks
- **A**ctivity increased—Often with weight loss related to physical activity; increased libido commonly reported
- **S**leep—Decreased, often with reports of going days without sleep but not with a report of excessive fatigue
- **T**alkativeness—Often with overfamiliarity, crossing usual social boundaries[5]

---

4. Adapted from Berber MJ. Panic mnemonic. *Am J Psychiatry* 1997:154(3);438.
5. Adapted from Carlat, M.D., The psychiatric review of symptoms: a screening tool for family physicians. *Am Fam Physician*. 1998 Nov 1;58(7): 1617–1624. https://www.aafp.org/afp/1998/1101/p1617.html

MOOD DISORDER TREATMENT

Overview

Intervention for patients with mood disorders includes a combination of support, counseling, and medication. Interpersonal therapy alone, including counseling and support, has a 40% to 60% efficacy with a high relapse rate. As a single therapeutic modality, interpersonal therapy is most effective for individuals with reactive depression, or depression associated with significant life event. Combined therapy of pharmacological intervention and interpersonal therapy allows the patient to have effective therapy for what is now recognized as a biochemical disorder, while acquiring the cognitive skills that are helpful in dealing with what is often a chronic, relapsing condition. These principles apply to the treatment of nearly all patients with mood disorders.

> **CLINICAL CONCEPT**
>
> Primary care providers write at least 80% of all psychotropic prescriptions, making the acquisition of skill in prescribing these helpful medications crucial to practice.

All prescription antidepressant/psychotropic medications are about equally effective if taken in therapeutic doses for sufficient lengths of time. Primary care providers tend to underdose antidepressants, however, and prescribe them for an insufficient length of therapy. Current treatment guidelines offer recommendations for length of therapy (Box 15-2). Long-term psychotropic medication therapy should be considered when there is a high risk of relapse (Box 15-3).

Choice of Psychotropic Agent

When prescribing a psychotropic agent, the provider should encourage psychotherapy or counseling to work on building skills needed to help manage this usually long-term health problem. In particular, the provider should convey the message to the patient that the use of psychotropics can help facilitate therapy.

When choosing a psychotropic medication, the prescriber should ask the following questions:

■ What has worked in the past? Unless now contraindicated, this medication should be the agent of choice.
■ What has worked for relatives? Certain medications seem to have greater activity at given serotonin receptor sites. Besides having heard positive comments about the medication from family members, relatives often have similar serotonin receptor site activity and response to a given medication.

BOX 15-2 Length of Pharmacological Intervention in Depression

Acute plus continuation phases

■ In acute phase treatment, 4 to 8 weeks of treatment generally are needed before concluding that a patient is partially responsive or unresponsive to a specific treatment.
■ Patients successfully treated during acute phase should continue the same course of treatment for 4 to 9 months, preferably for a minimum of 6 months, typically a minimum of 9 months total treatment.
  ■ Relapse is highest in first 2 months after discontinuation of therapy.
■ With more than two major depressive disorder episodes, 80% relapse in 1 year without treatment.
  ■ Consider maintenance therapy as with any chronic illness.

Source: American Psychiatric Association. Practice Guidelines for the Treatment of Patients With Major Depressive Disorder. 3rd ed. Arlington, VA: American Psychiatric Association Publishing; 2010. https://psychiatryonline.org/pb/assets/raw/sitewide/practice_guidelines/guidelines/mdd.pdf

---

BOX 15-3 Risks in Depression Relapse

Persistent depressive disorder preceding episode
Poor recovery between episodes
Current episode more than 2 years
Onset of depression when younger than 20 years old or older than 50 years old
Family history of depression
Severe symptoms such as suicide and psychosis

■ What are the most bothersome signs and symptoms of the mood disorder? An antidepressant with activity against these or at least one that will not make these worse should be chosen. If insomnia and anxiety bother a person with depression, using a highly energizing medication is a poor choice (Tables 15-3 and 15-4).

■ What are the potential drug-drug interactions? As with all medication use, a careful inventory should be taken so that potential drug-drug interactions can be avoided (Table 15-5).

TABLE 15-3 Selective Serotonin Reuptake Inhibitors (SSRIs)

SSRI	HALF-LIFE (T$_{1/2}$)	LABELED INDICATIONS	ADVERSE EFFECT PROFILE	COMMENTS
Paroxetine (Paxil®)	t$_{1/2}$ 21 hours, no active metabolites	Major depressive disorder, panic disorder with or without agoraphobia, OCD, social anxiety disorder, GAD, PTSD, premenstrual dysphoric disorder	Sedating (HS dosing likely best) Likely most anticholinergic effect of the SSRIs. More constipation (13%) than diarrhea (11%) Can lead to increased appetite	Helpful in depression with anxiety Elimination via renal and hepatic routes Fewer problems with limited renal/hepatic function Low mania induction in bipolar; helpful in treatment of elderly patients (short half-life, lack of active metabolites) Because of short t$_{1/2}$, slow tapering dose when discontinuing medication is recommended to avoid significant withdrawal syndrome
Sertraline (Zoloft®)	t$_{1/2}$ 26 hours Metabolite t$_{1/2}$ 62 to 104 hours	Major depression, OCD, panic disorder, PTSD, premenstrual dysphoric disorder, social anxiety disorder	Equal numbers reporting somnolence and insomnia. Favorable gastrointestinal profile Low rates of agitation and anorexia	Take with food to enhance absorption
Citalopram (Celexa®) Escitalopram (Lexapro®)	Citalopram: Racemic compound t$_{1/2}$ approximately 35 hours for parent compound, metabolite t$_{1/2}$ 2 days for one, 4 days for another Escitalopram: Single isomer of citalopram with shorter t$_{1/2}$ 27 to 32 hours	Major depression, GADs	Energizing, anorexia common Because of risk of QT prolongation with citalopram, for patients older than 60 years of age, the maximum recommended dose is 20 mg/day, maximum 40 mg/day in all others	Escitalopram 10 mg is therapeutically equivalent to citalopram 20 to 40 mg with a possibly superior adverse effect profile
Fluoxetine (Prozac®)	t$_{1/2}$ 24 to 72 hours Metabolite t$_{1/2}$ 4 to 16 days	Major depressive disorder, BN, OCD, premenstrual dysphoric disorder, panic disorder with or without agoraphobia		Morning dosing recommended. Protracted t$_{1/2}$ can present problem in elderly patients; however, less of a problem with missed doses Weight loss of approximately 3 to 5 lb (1.4 to 2.3 kg) common in early months of use, but usually not sustained long term

GAD, generalized anxiety disorder; OCD, obsessive-compulsive disorder; PTSD, post-traumatic stress disorder; SSRI selective serotonin reuptake inhibitor.

Source: Posternak M, Zimmerman M. Antidepressants. In: Goldberg R, ed. Practical Guide to the Care of the Psychiatric Patient. 3rd ed. Philadelphia, PA: Mosby; 2007:108–136.

TABLE 15-4 Selective Serotonin Norepinephrine Reuptake Inhibitors, Tricyclic, Tetracyclic, and Other Antidepressants

AGENT	HALF-LIFE	ADVERSE EFFECTS	COMMENTS
Venlafaxine (Effexor® and Effexor XR®) Desvenlafaxine (Pristiq®) [SSNRI]	5 hours for venlafaxine and 11 hours for its active metabolite (15 hours for venlafaxine extended-release capsules) 11 hours for desvenlafaxine (the major active metabolite of venlafaxine)	Activating in larger amounts Patients often need trazodone or other agent to help with sleep Significant nausea with rapid onset of high dose Dose-dependent increases in diastolic blood pressure (average 5 mm Hg response)	SSRI-like effect only in low doses, with norepinephrine uptake blockade at medium to high doses, similar to TCA effect, but with fewer adverse effects. Withdrawal syndrome similar to SSRIs
Duloxetine (Cymbalta®) [SSNRI]	8 to 17 hours	Rare liver toxicity risk, most often noted in presence of other hepatic risk factors. Few anticholinergic adverse effects	Indicated for treatment of mood disorders and neuropathic pain
Levomilnacipran (Fetzima®) [SSNRI]	12 hours	Nausea, constipation, hyperhidrosis, tachycardia, erectile dysfunction; can increase risk of activation of mania/hypomania (screen for bipolar disorder)	Indicated for treatment of MDD
Bupropion (Wellbutrin®) [SDRI]	9.8 hours (3.9 to 24 hours) Extended-release 29 hours (20 to 38 hours)	Few anticholinergic effects Energizing Possible increased libido, agitation (25%) Avoid with significant manifestation of anxiety, agitation, insomnia	Blocks reuptake of dopamine at presynaptic neuron, especially in high doses, some increase in norepinephrine transmission. Dopamine receptor sites likely stimulated in substance abuse, making bupropion a helpful antidepressant for a person with a history of substance abuse. Nonaddicting and nonintoxicating. Avoid use in presence of eating disorder or if anorexia is a major component of depression. Weight loss often seen (28% greater than 5 lb [2.3 kg]) after initiation of therapy Do not give if history of or risk for seizure, closed head injury history, history of quiescent epilepsy Seizure risk worsens if dose increased rapidly
Mirtazapine (Remeron®) [tetracyclic antidepressant]	20 to 40 hours	Potent H1 inhibitor Weight gain common Major side effect is sedation that is worse in lower doses. Little sexual dysfunction or gastrointestinal side effect	Effect likely due to increase in central noradrenergic and serotoninergic activity Selectively stimulates 5-HT1A while blocking 5-HT2 and 5-HT3 Higher doses more receptor site-selective and associated with fewer adverse effects

Continued

TABLE 15-4 Selective Serotonin Norepinephrine Reuptake Inhibitors, Tricyclic, Tetracyclic, and Other Antidepressants—cont'd

AGENT	HALF-LIFE	ADVERSE EFFECTS	COMMENTS
Tricyclic antidepressants; includes nortriptyline ([Pamelor®, active metabolite of amitriptyline], desipramine [Norpramin®], active metabolic of imipramine)	24 to 32 hours	Weight gain Anticholinergic activity (blurred vision, dry mouth, memory loss, sweating, anxiety, postural hypotension, dizziness, and tachycardia) Constipation a problem, but infrequent nausea. Little sexual dysfunction	Inexpensive, more effective than SSRI in more severe depression, likely owing to its norepinephrine and serotonin activity More bothersome adverse effect profile leads to high dropout rate Primary care providers seldom prescribe sufficient doses to relieve depression Taper off over 2 to 4 weeks to avoid TCA withdrawal symptoms; sleep disturbance, nightmares, gastrointestinal upset, malaise, irritability
Trazodone (Desyrel®, Oleptro®) [triazolopyridine]	5 hours (3 to 9 hours)	Highly sedating, dizziness, favorable gastrointestinal adverse effect profile. Priapism risk found in 1 in 6,000 men using drug. Patient should be informed to go to emergency department promptly for painful erection lasting longer than 30 minutes	Anxiolytic and antidepressant activity 5-HT2 antagonist Clinical use limited by marked sedation Effective hypnotic with little morning drowsiness at doses 25 to 100 mg taken 1 hour before sleep Can use in low, frequent doses as BZD alternative for generalized anxiety
Vilazodone (Viibryd®) [novel class]	25 hours	Diarrhea, nausea, vomiting, and insomnia most common; no apparent effect on weight or cardiac function (e.g., QT prolongation)	Works through enhancement of serotonergic activity in the CNS through selective inhibition of serotonin uptake as well as a partial agonist of serotonergic 5-HT1A receptors
Esketamine (Spravato™)	7 to 12 hours	Nausea, sedation, dizziness, nasopharyngeal irritation	For use in resistant depression as rescue therapy, intranasal delivery, used in conjunction with standard oral antidepressant, only by expert prescribers

BZD, benzodiazepine; CNS, central nervous system; MDD, major depressive disorder; SDRI, selective dopamine reuptake inhibitor; SSNRI, selective serotonin and norepinephrine reuptake inhibitor; SSRI, selective serotonin reuptake inhibitor; TCA, tricyclic antidepressant.

Source: Posternak M, Zimmerman M. Antidepressants. In: Goldberg R, ed. Practical Guide to the Care of the Psychiatric Patient. 3rd ed. Philadelphia, PA: Mosby; 2007:108–136.

Spravato prescribing information available at https://www.janssenlabels.com/package-insert/product-monograph/prescribing-information/SPRAVATO-pi.pdf

When choosing a psychotropic agent, the adverse effect profile is critical. Often a given agent has a desirable adverse effect, such as sedation in a patient having difficulty with sleep or anxiety. In addition, the drug's $t_{1/2}$ influences the therapeutic choice, with products with a shorter $t_{1/2}$ being desirable in elderly patients and patients with hepatic disease. A younger adult could benefit from the use of a drug with a longer $t_{1/2}$ if he or she skips a dose from time to time.

Another consideration in choosing a psychotropic agent is its toxicity when taken in overdose. A patient with suicidal ideation and plan clearly needs hospitalization to ensure safety and appropriate treatment. As with many conditions, however, depression is a disease with episodes of improvement and deterioration. The prescriber should consider the risk of an intentional overdose. A 2-week supply of a TCA in full therapeutic dose would likely be lethal, with significantly smaller amounts capable of causing seizures and dysrhythmias. SSRIs, selective dopamine reuptake inhibitors (SDRIs), and serotonin and norepinephrine reuptake inhibitors (SNRIs) have a significantly better safety profile when taken in overdose; usually more than a 2-month

TABLE 15-5 Cytochrome P450 Isoenzyme Inhibition by Selective Serotonin Reuptake Inhibitors

CYP ISOENZYMES					
	1A2	2C9	2C19	2D6	3A4
Escitalopram	0	0	0	0	0
Citalopram	+	0	0	+	0
Fluoxetine	+	++	+ to ++	+++	++
Paroxetine	+	+	+	+++	+
Sertraline	+	+	+ to ++	+	+

0 = minimal or weak inhibition; +, ++, +++ = mild, moderate, or strong inhibition.

supply of a full therapeutic dose is needed to cause life-threatening effects. BZDs taken as a solo product in overdose are seldom fatal. However, when taken in conjunction with other sedating substances such as opioids, alcohol, and barbiturates, the risk of a fatal outcome with BZD overdose is significant.

Regular monitoring of symptoms is essential in determining the effectiveness of pharmacotherapy and whether medication adjustment is needed. Depression and anxiety rating scales (e.g., PHQ-9, GAD-7) can be used to assess for changes in symptoms and severity. When initiating therapy, follow-up visits should occur every 1 to 2 weeks for at least the first 6 weeks, until a stable, effective dose is achieved. Patients should then be monitored monthly for clinical status as well as any potential drug-drug or drug–disease state interactions.

Antidepressants generally work by causing an increase in availability of certain neurotransmitters, such as serotonin, norepinephrine, and dopamine. This increased availability allows for greater activity at the neurotransmitter's respective receptor sites. There is evidence that interpersonal therapy also increases serotonin availability.

> **CLINICAL CONCEPT**
>
> Adverse effects of the SNRIs and SSRIs are similar, with the most common consisting of nausea, dry mouth, dizziness, and excessive sweating.

SSRIs are generally the first-line agent for the treatment of mood disorders, including depression and anxiety, due to ease of dosing and low toxicity in overdose. When using an SSRI, the phrase "start low, go slow, but get to goal" should guide therapy. The use of SNRIs for the treatment of depression has been increasing (see Table 15-4). These can be considered for patients who fail to respond to SSRIs and are also used to treat other conditions, such as anxiety and chronic pain. These drugs increase the availability of serotonin and norepinephrine in the brain, which changes the balance of these chemicals, thereby boosting mood.

Tiredness, difficulty urinating, anxiety, constipation, insomnia, sexual dysfunction, headache, and loss of appetite have also been reported.

The use of SSRI/SNRIs and other psychotropics is often associated with sexual function problems. Decreased libido and anorgasmia in either gender are often reported; erectile dysfunction in men is also common. If this is a problem, switching the patient to an SDRI, such as bupropion (Wellbutrin®), an SNRI (such as venlafaxine [Effexor®], duloxetine [Cymbalta®], or desvenlafaxine [Pristiq®]), or a TCA can be considered because the use of these products is associated less often with sexual dysfunction. Venlafaxine is associated with a dose-dependent increase in diastolic blood pressure, though the effect is modest at most. Vilazodone (Viibryd®) is a dual-acting serotonergic agent that combines the antidepressant effects of an SSRI with partial serotonin-receptor agonist activity and provides an additional option. Additional options for SSRI/SNRI sexual dysfunction include adding bupropion to the therapeutic regimen; support for this common practice is largely based on anecdotal reports. Taking a 1-day "drug holiday" from SSRI/SNRI use, with sexual activity planned for the end of the drug-free period, offers a reasonable option for a person with relatively infrequent sexual activity.

This practice can lead to SSRI/SNRI withdrawal symptoms toward the end of the drug-free period, however, with all products except fluoxetine. Given its long $t_{1/2}$, this practice is unlikely to be helpful for a person taking fluoxetine.

In early SSRI/SNRI therapy, the patient often complains of drug-related adverse effects, including headache, nausea, and diarrhea; these resolve within 2 to 6 weeks of medication use. Advising the patient that these adverse effects are expected, easily treatable, and transient helps avoid the problem of the patient discontinuing this important therapeutic agent. The headache is usually frontal in location and resolves with acetaminophen. Using an NSAID will likely contribute further to the GI upset often found in the first weeks of SSRI/SNRI use. Taking these medications with food can minimize nausea and diarrhea. Because of the potential chelation effect and impact of altered stomach pH on drug absorptions, taking many medications with an antacid can potentially limit the drug's effectiveness.

Treatment recommendations for pharmacological intervention in anxiety disorders are similar to the guidelines for depression therapy (see Table 15-1). The practitioner should encourage psychotherapy to work on building skills needed to help manage a long-term health problem. In particular, the practitioner should convey the message to the patient that the use of psychotropic agents can help facilitate therapy. This acute care phase, usually lasting 4 to 8 weeks, should be followed with a 6- to 12-month maintenance period, yielding a minimum treatment period of 9 months. With all psychotropics, a receptor site–induced effect is immediate when therapy is initiated. The length of onset of therapeutic action is usually several weeks, however. This length of onset is likely associated with time needed for change in receptor site activity. Longer-term treatment should be considered, especially if symptoms recur with depression. Choice of a therapeutic agent is guided by numerous factors, including asking about what has worked in the past and what has worked in the treatment of relatives with similar conditions.

Trazodone is used to treat depression or anxiety but has the potential to cause priapism (i.e., prolonged, often painful, erection). Its use for mood disorder therapy is limited because it is highly sedating. When used in patients with disordered sleep such as is often noted in mood disorder, trazodone should be administered about 1 hour prior to sleep for maximum effect.

TCAs (e.g., clomipramine, desipramine, nortriptyline) are sometimes used for the treatment of mood disorders, particularly with comorbid chronic pain. In small doses, these agents can also be used as a sleep aid for those with disordered sleep. However, TCAs are not typically used at full therapeutic doses for the treatment of depression or anxiety disorders as they are generally less tolerated compared to SSRIs, and overdose attempts can be fatal.

In antidepressant discontinuation syndrome, there is a sudden change in the amount of serotonin available and an alteration in receptor site action.

Onset of withdrawal is related to the $t_{1/2}$ of the drug, with three to five drug-free half-lives needed before the medication clears fully. Symptoms occur more rapidly after SSRI/SNRI discontinuation with a drug with a short $t_{1/2}$ and may not occur at all in a drug with a protracted $t_{1/2}$ (e.g., fluoxetine). Symptoms of SSRI/SNRI-withdrawal syndrome include dizziness, paresthesia, anxiety, nausea, sleep disturbance, and insomnia. Although disturbing and uncomfortable, this syndrome, in contrast to BZD withdrawal, is not dangerous or life-threatening and generally resolves within days to a few weeks.

> **CLINICAL CONCEPT**
>
> A withdrawal syndrome is often seen with SSRI/SNRI use longer than 5 weeks when the product is rapidly discontinued.

Bupropion is used to treat depression as well as seasonal affective disorder (SAD) and as an aid in smoking cessation. Bupropion blocks the reuptake of dopamine, which makes this agent especially useful for those with a history of substance abuse because dopamine receptor sites are likely stimulated in substance abuse. The drug is nonaddicting and nonintoxicating and is associated with few anticholinergic effects. The most common adverse effects include headache, dry mouth, nausea, weight loss, and insomnia. This medication can be energizing.

Treatment Options in Bipolar Disorder

Ongoing evaluation and treatment of a person with bipolar disorder require significant expertise; expert advice should be sought. If a TCA is given to a person with bipolar disorder, approximately 15% develop mania. This also happens when an energizing SSRI/SNRI such as fluoxetine is given. Treatment will depend on the stage of the bipolar disorder the patient is experiencing and usually includes the use of mood-stabilizing medications. Those experiencing severe mania can be treated with lithium carbonate, valproic acid, carbamazepine, or second-generation antipsychotics such as risperidone. Those with bipolar depression should initiate therapy with olanzapine-fluoxetine combination, quetiapine, or lamotrigine. Patients should be monitored closely for at least the first 6 weeks, with dose adjustments made based on serum concentrations (e.g., lithium carbonate, valproate, carbamazepine) and clinical effect. Combination therapy can be considered for those with only a partial response to monotherapy.

Treatment Options in Panic Disorder

Because of the low abuse potential and favorable adverse effect profile, SSRIs have become the initial treatment of choice for persons with panic disorder. SSRI use helps decrease the number and severity of panic attacks and, to a lesser degree, phobia and anxiety related to the attacks. Individuals with panic disorder usually do not tolerate a rapid induction or change in any therapy because of their heightened sympathetic state. An agent with an early adverse effect profile that the patient is likely to tolerate should be chosen, such as a product that is less rather than more energizing with a lower rate of insomnia, nervousness, and akathisia; such agents include paroxetine (Paxil®), citalopram (Celexa®), or escitalopram (Lexapro®), but a more energizing SSRI such as fluoxetine (Prozac®) is unlikely to be well tolerated. Also, SSRI use can precipitate panic attacks with early use but prevent these episodes after the full therapeutic effect is realized. Due to the chronic nature of panic disorder, BZD use is generally discouraged owing to risk of habituation and abuse. In cases where BZD treatment was initiated due to refractory panic disorder, patients should receive a psychiatric referral to review pharmacological and nonpharmacological options.

Monoamine oxidase inhibitors (MAOIs) are the most potent drugs available for treating patients with panic disorder. Because of adverse effects and the need for dietary restriction while patients take the medications, their use is generally limited to individuals with treatment-resistant panic disorder. Consultation and care by a psychopharmacology team with experience in prescribing these medications are recommended.

> **CLINICAL CONCEPT**
>
> A nighttime dose of prazosin (Minipress®) can be helpful in decreasing nightmares and sleep disturbances in PTSD.

Treatment Options in Post-Traumatic Stress Disorder

Treatment of patients with PTSD requires an interdisciplinary approach of expert providers. First-line pharmacological intervention can include the use of an SSRI or SNRI to treat arousal symptoms and associated depression. Beta blockers, such as propranolol (Inderal®), as well as the α_2-adrenergic agonist clonidine (Catapres®) can also be considered for minimizing the effects of hyperarousal.

Treatment can also include mirtazapine (for insomnia) as well as a second-generation antipsychotic or mood stabilizers. BZDs should be used with caution because substance use disorder is a common comorbid condition in patients with PTSD. Carbamazepine (Tegretol®) and valproic acid (Depakote®) have been used with some success in treating irritability, aggression, and impulsiveness. Trazodone (Desyrel®) offers a nonaddicting option to enhance sleep.

Nutritional Supplements

Patients often choose to treat mood disorder with nutritional supplements, which are available over the counter in unlimited supply. Although encouraging and facilitating patient self-care is an important part of the role of the NP, the use of nutritional products should be approached with caution. Herbal medications are considered nutritional supplements and are not subject to the regulatory process required for prescription and over-the-counter medications. As a result, quality control in their production can be lacking, leading to inconsistent amounts of herbs per dose. In addition, when a patient takes a nutritional supplement to treat symptoms of anxiety and depression, he or she is self-medicating a potentially life-threatening disease. Using herbs with prescription medications can lead to problems with drug interactions or additive effects, such as when St. John's wort is used concurrently with an SSRI. The NP and patient need to be aware of the effects, efficacy, and adverse effect profiles of these products (Table 15-6).

Discussion Sources

American Psychiatric Association. *Diagnostic and Statistical Manual of Mental Disorders: DSM-5.* 5th ed. Arlington, VA: American Psychiatric Association Publishing; 2013.

American Psychiatric Association. *Practice Guidelines for the Treatment of Patients With Major Depressive Disorder.* 3rd ed. Arlington, VA: American Psychiatric Association Publishing; 2010 (reaffirmed 2015). https://psychiatryonline.org/pb/assets/raw /sitewide/practice_guidelines/guidelines/mdd.pdf

TABLE 15-6 Over-the-Counter Nutritional Supplements for Mood Disorders

AGENT	MECHANISM OF ACTION	COMMENTS
St. John's wort	Like MAOI-, SSRI-, TCA-like More than 10 active compounds	Compared with TCA, less anticholinergic effect, weight gain, less efficacy in more severe depression. Compared with SSRI, similar potential for energizing such as fluoxetine, similar efficacy in mild to moderate depression with limited study. tid to qid dosing needed; 6 to 8 weeks before clinical effect. Prudent to avoid concurrent use of SSRI, TCA, MAOI because of serotonin syndrome risk. Potentially photosensitizing, peripheral neuropathy in high doses. Capable of altering activity of CYP450 enzymes extensively involved in drug metabolism and thus can interact significantly with many drugs. Can reduce serum levels of select antiretrovirals (e.g., indinavir) and cyclosporine. Use can reduce effectiveness of oral contraceptives.
Kava	Action at GABA receptors similar to BZDs	Satisfactory response compared with placebo, low-dose oxazepam (Serax®). Sedating, can potentiate effects of alcohol. Cross-allergenic with pepper. Hepatotoxicity risk with overdose, prolonged treatment, and/or comedication.
Valerian root	Action similar to BZDs	5% to 10% with paradoxical stimulating effect. Available in aromatic tea, but weaker, with shorter duration of action. Less drug "hangover" than with BZDs.

BZD, benzodiazepines; GABA, γ-aminobutyric acid; MAOI, monoamine oxidase inhibitor; SSRI, selective serotonin reuptake inhibitor; TCA, tricyclic antidepressant.

American Psychiatric Association. *Practice Guidelines for the Treatment of Patients With Bipolar Disorder.* 2nd ed. Arlington, VA: American Psychiatric Association Publishing; 2010. http://psychiatryonline.org/pb/assets/raw/sitewide/practice_guidelines/guidelines/bipolar.pdf

Department of Veteran Affairs, Department of Defense. *VA/DoD Clinical Practice Guideline for the Management of Post-Traumatic Stress Disorder and Acute Stress Reaction, 2017.* Washington, DC: Department of Veteran Affairs, Department of Defense; 2017. https://www.healthquality.va.gov/guidelines/MH/ptsd/VADoDPTSDCPGFinal012418.pdf

Posternak M, Zimmerman M. Depression: identification and diagnosis. In: Goldberg R, ed. *Practical Guide to the Care of the Psychiatric Patient.* 3rd ed. Philadelphia, PA: Elsevier Mosby; 2007:86–106.

Posternak M, Zimmerman M. Antidepressants. In: Goldberg R, ed. *Practical Guide to the Care of the Psychiatric Patient.* 3rd ed. Philadelphia, PA: Elsevier Mosby; 2007:108–136.

Truman C. Antidepressants. In: Goldberg R, ed. *Practical Guide to the Care of the Psychiatric Patient.* 3rd ed. Philadelphia, PA: Elsevier Mosby; 2007:137–157.

QUESTIONS

48. Which patient presentation is most consistent with the diagnosis of depression?

A. recurrent diarrhea and cramping

B. difficulty initiating sleep

C. diminished cognitive ability

D. consistent early morning awakening

49 to 51. When considering depression and thoughts about death, rank the following from most common (1) to least common (3):

_____ **49.** thinking it would be "OK to just die"; passive without a plan to cause self-harm

_____ **50.** having suicidal thoughts

_____ **51.** making a plan to commit suicide

52. Which of the following statements is false regarding patients with depression and hypochondriasis?

    A. About 30% of patients with depression also have hypochondriasis.

    B. A person with this condition is less likely to see a health-care provider compared with those with depression alone.

    C. A person with this condition is unable to process objective information that he/she has no particular health problem.

    D. The person with hypochondriasis perceives that an existing health problem is far more serious than it is in reality.

53. Of the following individuals in need of an antidepressant, who is the best candidate for fluoxetine (Prozac®) therapy?

    A. an 80-year-old woman with hypertension, dyslipidemia, and osteoarthritis and with persistent depressed mood 1 year after the death of her husband

    B. a 45-year-old man with mild hepatic dysfunction

    C. a 28-year-old man who occasionally "skips a dose" of his prescribed medication

    D. a 44-year-old woman with decreased appetite

54. In caring for elderly patients, the NP considers that all of the following are true except:

    A. many older patients with dementia have a component of depression.

    B. dementia signs and symptoms usually evolve over months, but depression usually has a more rapid onset.

    C. with depression and dementia, a patient is aware of difficulties with cognitive ability.

    D. treating concurrent depression can help improve symptoms of dementia.

55. Persistent depressive disorder (also known as dysthymia) is characterized by:

    A. suicidal thoughts.

    B. multiple incidents of self-harm.

    C. social isolation.

    D. low-level depression.

56. Which of the following is most consistent with the diagnosis of persistent depressive disorder?

    A. a 23-year-old man with a 2-month episode of depressed mood after a job loss

    B. a 45-year-old woman with "jitteriness" and difficulty initiating sleep for the past 6 months

    C. a 38-year-old woman with fatigue and anhedonia for the past 2 years

    D. a 15-year-old boy with a school adjustment problem and weekend marijuana use for the past year

57. Successful treatment of mood disorder typically involves:

    A. psychotherapy as the primary therapy.

    B. a psychotropic medication as the primary therapy.

    C. psychotherapy plus a psychotropic agent.

    D. electroconvulsive therapy (ECT) as an early intervention.

58. John is a 47-year-old man who reports constant sadness following the sudden death of his wife in a motor vehicle accident 3 weeks ago. He has had difficulty functioning at work, reporting, "I feel like I am just going through the motions," and avoids socializing with friends and family as "they remind me too much of my wife." You suggest a treatment plan that includes two of the following best responses.

    A. information on the anticipated course of acute grief

    B. referral for weekly psychotherapy sessions

    C. prescribing an anxiolytic to help with grief symptoms

    D. advise on local bereavement support groups

59. Successful treatment of a patient with reactive depression associated with a loss (e.g., death of a loved one) would expect all of the following results except:

A. elevated mood.

B. restored function.

C. improved decision-making ability.

D. elimination of sadness.

60. Drug treatment options for a patient with bipolar disorder with severe mania can include any of the following except:

A. lamotrigine (Lamictal®).

B. lithium carbonate.

C. risperidone (Risperdal®).

D. valproic acid (Depakote®).

61. Which of the following drugs is likely to be the most dangerous when taken in an intentional overdose equivalent to a standard adult therapeutic dose?

A. a 4-week supply of paroxetine

B. a 2-week supply of amitriptyline

C. a 3-week supply of duloxetine

D. a 5-day supply of alprazolam

62. One week into citalopram (Celexa®) therapy, a 32-year-old man complains of a new-onset recurrent dull frontal headache that is relieved promptly with acetaminophen use. Which of the following is true in this situation?

A. This is a common, transient side effect of early SSRI therapy.

B. He should discontinue the medication.

C. Fluoxetine should be substituted.

D. Desipramine should be added.

63. A 45-year-old woman has been taking sertraline for 1 week and complains of mild nausea and diarrhea that started within 48 hours of starting the medication. You advise that:

A. this is a common, long-lasting side effect of SSRI therapy.

B. she should discontinue the medication.

C. another antidepressant should be substituted.

D. she should be taking the medication with food.

64. Sally is a 34-year-old woman who is diagnosed with major depressive disorder. She feels that it is likely associated with stress resulting from her troubled marriage of the past 10 years. She is initiated on an SNRI and reports initial improvement in symptoms. However, over the following months, the medication appears to lose its effectiveness despite her insistence that she is being adherent with the dosing regimen. This is likely a result of:

A. an inadequate dose of the medication.

B. development of tolerance to the SNRI.

C. continued or escalated stress from the troubled marriage.

D. missed doses despite her insistence on compliance.

65. A 45-year-old man diagnosed with depression returns 1 month after starting antidepressant medication. He complains of anorgasmia but reports that erectile function is intact. He is most likely taking which of the following medications?

A. vilazodone (Viibryd®)

B. paroxetine (Paxil®)

C. nortriptyline (Pamelor®)

D. bupropion (Wellbutrin®)

66. Antidepressant discontinuation syndrome is best characterized as:

A. bothersome but not life threatening.

B. potentially life threatening.

C. most often seen with discontinuation of agents with a long $t_{1/2}$.

D. associated with seizure risk.

67. Which of the following SSRIs is most likely to significantly interact with warfarin?

A. citalopram

B. escitalopram

C. fluoxetine

D. sertraline

68. Which of the following SSRIs is associated with the greatest anticholinergic effect?

A. escitalopram

B. sertraline

C. fluoxetine

D. paroxetine

69. Which of the following statements is true regarding depression and relapse?

A. Without maintenance therapy, the relapse rate is typically less than 50% in the first year.

B. The risk of relapse is less for those who have experienced multiple episodes of major depressive disorder.

C. The risk of relapse is greatest in the first 2 months after discontinuation of therapy.

D. Relapse rarely occurs if there is an absence of symptoms after 9 months of treatment discontinuation.

70 to 73. Indicate (*yes or no*) whether each of these is a risk factor for depression relapse.

_____ 70. A current episode lasting more than 2 years

_____ 71. Onset of depression occurring at younger than 20 years of age

_____ 72. Poor recovery between episodes

_____ 73. Absence of persistent depressive disorder preceding the episode

74. Which of the following is most consistent with the presentation of a manic episode in a patient with bipolar I disorder?

A. increased need for sleep

B. impulsive behavior

C. fatigue

D. anhedonia

75. Which of the following is most consistent with the presentation of a patient with a depressive episode with bipolar II disorder?

A. racing thoughts

B. impulsive behavior

C. increased talkativeness

D. anhedonia

76. In general, pharmacological intervention for patients with anxiety or depression should:

A. be given for about 4 months on average.

B. continue for a minimum of 6 months after remission is achieved.

C. be continued indefinitely with a first episode of depression.

D. be titrated to a lower dose after symptom relief is achieved.

77. A 44-year-old woman has been taking an SSRI for the past 4 months and complains of new onset of sexual dysfunction and difficulty achieving orgasm. You advise her that:

A. this is a transient side effect often seen in the first weeks of therapy.

B. switching to another SSRI would likely be helpful.

C. this is a common adverse effect of SSRI therapy that is unlikely to resolve without adjustment in her therapy.

D. she should see a urologist for further evaluation.

78. The maximum recommended dose of citalopram is set at 40 mg/day in those younger than 60 years and 20 mg/day for those older than 60 years due to a risk for:

A. renal impairment.

B. nephrotoxicity.

C. QT prolongation.

D. bone marrow suppression.

79. Which of the following agents has the longest $t_{1/2}$?

A. fluoxetine

B. paroxetine

C. citalopram

D. sertraline

80. Which of the following agents should be avoided in a person who is a heavy alcohol user owing to a potential risk for hepatotoxicity?

A. duloxetine

B. desvenlafaxine

C. escitalopram

D. bupropion

81. Treatment with venlafaxine (Effexor®) can lead to dose-dependent increases in:

A. heart rate.

B. serum glucose.

C. AST/ALT.

D. blood pressure.

82. You see a 28-year-old man who has been diagnosed with moderate depression and has not responded well to SSRI therapy over the past 3 months. He was involved in a motor vehicle accident 2 years ago that resulted in head trauma and now occasionally experiences occasional tonic-clonic seizures. When considering alternative antidepressant therapy, which of the following should be avoided?

A. bupropion

B. viladazone

C. citalopram

D. duloxetine

83. When considering the use of BZDs for the treatment of GAD, the NP considers:

A. BZDs are considered first-line for long-term treatment of GAD.

B. BZDs can be used initially as adjunctive therapy to SSRIs but then tapered once a therapeutic dose of SSRI is established.

C. BZDs should only be considered with an inadequate response to SSRIs.

D. due to potential for tolerance, BZDs should be avoided in patients with GAD.

84. When using trazodone to aid sleep, the drug should be optimally taken _____ prior to sleep.

    A. immediately

    B. 15 minutes

    C. 1 hour

    D. 2 hours

85. A 50-year-old woman complains of difficulty sleeping, restlessness, and difficulty controlling worry that has occurred for the past 6 months. She denies having mood swings or feelings of hopelessness and still finds enjoyment in certain activities. The NP suspects a diagnosis of:

    A. depression.

    B. bipolar I disorder.

    C. anxiety disorder.

    D. dysthymia.

86. Which of the following describes prescriptions for psychotropic medications written by primary care providers?

    A. dose too high

    B. dose too low

    C. excessive length of therapy

    D. appropriate length of therapy

87. Anxiety in response to a challenging life event is a natural response by the body to:

    A. help a person focus on the issue at hand.

    B. diminish the fight-or-flight response.

    C. impair decision-making under duress.

    D. provide transient improvement in physical capabilities.

88. A 28-year-old woman is suspected of GAD. Which of the following signs and symptoms would be most consistent with this diagnosis?

    A. GI upset

    B. difficulty initiating sleep

    C. diminished cognitive ability

    D. consistent early morning wakening

89. Conditions that commonly mimic or can worsen anxiety include all of the following except:

    A. active opioid use.

    B. thyrotoxicosis.

    C. alcohol withdrawal.

    D. overuse of caffeine.

90. When prescribing a BZD, the NP considers that:

    A. the drugs are virtually interchangeable, with similar durations of action and therapeutic effect.

    B. the onset of therapeutic effect is usually rapid.

    C. these drugs have a low abuse potential in people who abuse other substances.

    D. elderly adults will likely require doses similar to those needed by younger adults.

91. The drug buspirone (BuSpar®) has:

A. low abuse potential.

B. significant antidepressant action.

C. a withdrawal syndrome when discontinued, similar to BZDs.

D. rapid onset of action.

92. A 24-year-old woman has a new onset of panic disorder. As part of her clinical presentation, you expect to find all of the following except:

A. peak symptoms at 10 minutes into the panic attack.

B. history of agoraphobia.

C. report of chest pain during panic attack.

D. history of thought disorder.

93. As you develop the initial treatment plan for a 34-year-old woman with panic disorder and agoraphobia, you consider prescribing:

A. carbamazepine (Tegretol®).

B. risperidone (Risperdal®).

C. citalopram (Celexa®).

D. bupropion (Wellbutrin®).

94 to 101. Indicate (*yes or no*) whether each of the following signs and symptoms is consistent with a diagnosis of GAD.

_____ **94.** difficulty concentrating

_____ **95.** consistent early morning wakening

_____ **96.** apprehension

_____ **97.** irritability

_____ **98.** constipation

_____ **99.** muscle tension

_____ **100.** hive-form skin lesions

_____ **101.** somnolence

102. The use of which of the following drugs often mimics GAD?

A. sympathomimetics

B. calcium channel blockers

C. systemic anticholinergics

D. β-antagonists

103. When considering the use of BZDs, the NP should consider that:

A. the ingestion of 3 to 4 days of therapeutic dose can be life threatening.

B. the medication must be taken at the same hour every day.

C. concomitant use of alcohol should be avoided.

D. onset of therapeutic effect takes many days.

104. A middle-aged woman who has taken a therapeutic dose of lorazepam for the past 6 years wishes to stop taking the medication. Choosing two that apply, you advise her that:

A. she can discontinue the drug immediately if she believes it no longer helps with her symptoms.

B. rapid withdrawal in this situation can lead to tremors and hallucinations.

    C. the medication should ideally be tapered over the next 3 to 4 weeks prior to discontinuation.

    D. GI upset is typically reported during the first week of BZD withdrawal.

105. The mechanism of action of BZDs is as:

    A. a mediator of γ-aminobutyric acid (GABA).

    B. an enhancer of serotonin availability.

    C. a dopamine antagonist.

    D. a norepinephrine agonist.

106. A 45-year-old man presents with a long-standing history of panic disorder who now seeks treatment. He expresses concern that he does not want to "end up addicted to drugs." While recognizing the risk versus benefit in considering the use of BZDs, the risk of misuse can be somewhat minimized by use of:

    A. agents with a shorter $t_{1/2}$.

    B. the drug as an as-needed rescue medication for acute anxiety.

    C. a more lipophilic product.

    D. products with slow onset of action.

107. Which of the following statements concerning panic disorder is false?

    A. Panic disorder rarely occurs with depression.

    B. Up to 4% of the general population suffers from panic disorder.

    C. New-onset panic disorder rarely occurs after 45 years of age.

    D. Family history of panic disorder is a risk factor for the condition.

108. Which of the following is true regarding panic disorder and agoraphobia?

    A. More men than women experience panic disorder without agoraphobia.

    B. More women than men experience panic disorder without agoraphobia.

    C. More men than women experience panic disorder with agoraphobia.

    D. More women than men experience panic disorder with agoraphobia.

109. Concomitant health problems found in a patient with panic disorder often include:

    A. irritable bowel syndrome.

    B. thought disorders.

    C. hypothyroidism.

    D. inflammatory bowel disease.

110. When initiating psychotropic therapy for a patient with panic disorder, the NP should consider all of the following except:

    A. starting with a low dose and slowly increasing to a therapeutic as is tolerated by the patient.

    B. it is preferable to use agents that are more energizing than those that are less energizing.

    C. selecting agents with a low rate of akathisia.

    D. with early psychotropic use, frequency of panic attacks is often increased but long-term use results in fewer and less severe episodes.

111. In providing primary care for a patient with PTSD, you consider that all of the following are likely to be reported except:

    A. numbing of emotions.

    B. feeling of detachment.

C. hyperarousal.

D. poor recall of the precipitating event.

112. Among the preferred first-line pharmacological treatment options for patients with PTSD are:

A. methylphenidate (Ritalin®).

B. oxazepam (Serax®).

C. lithium carbonate.

D. sertraline.

113. Which of the following therapeutic agents is commonly used to help with sleep difficulties such as insomnia associated with PTSD?

A. duloxetine

B. bupropion

C. mirtazapine

D. zolpidem

114. Which of the following is an over-the-counter nutritional supplement used to relieve symptoms of depression?

A. valerian root

B. melatonin

C. kava kava

D. St. John's wort

115. In treatment-resistant patients with panic disorder, which drug class is considered?

A. second-generation antipsychotic

B. SDRI

C. MAOI

D. neuroleptic

116. In treating a person with panic disorder using an SSRI at a therapeutic dose for a sufficient length of time, the NP should consider that there is:

A. considerable abuse potential with these medications.

B. no significant therapeutic advantage over TCAs.

C. a reduction in number and severity of panic attacks.

D. significant toxicity in overdose at the equivalent of 1 to 2 weeks of a full adult therapeutic dose.

117. Concomitant use of an SSRI with which of the following nutritional supplements can potentially lead to serotonin syndrome?

A. St. John's wort

B. kava kava

C. gingko biloba

D. valerian root

118. Use of St. John's wort is known to impact the effectiveness of all of the following oral medications except:

A. combined oral contraceptives.

B. cephalosporins.

C. cyclosporine.

D. select antiretrovirals.

119. Kava kava use has been associated with reports of:

A. renal impairment.

B. hepatotoxicity.

C. iron-deficiency anemia.

D. hyperthyroidism.

For answers and rationales, see end of chapter.

Interpersonal Violence

Overview

Interpersonal violence (IPV), also known as domestic abuse or partner violence, is defined as the intentional use of force, physical or emotional, threatened or actual, against a person or group that results in or has a significant likelihood of injury, death, and/or psychological harm. IPV among family or household members is found in all socioeconomic and ethnic groups. Because providers working with lower income and certain ethnic groups are perhaps more vigilant about this significant health and social problem, it often appears that abuse is more of a problem among certain groups.

Approximately 10 million people in the United States are victims. Current estimates project that approximately four times as many women compared to men are in abusive relationships. IPV appears to be at least as common in same-sex relationships as in opposite-sex relationships. Over their lifetime, one in four women and one in nine men will experience severe physical or emotional IPV; one in three women and one in four men will experience this misuse in a less severe form. Child abuse is present in about half of all households in which there is partner abuse.

> ### CLINICAL CONCEPT
>
> In all socioeconomic groups, access to a firearm by a perpetrator is associated with increased risk of abuse for serious or fatal injury; this is also a risk for completed suicide.

Common risk factors for IPV perpetration include a personal history of childhood physical abuse, substance abuse disorder, and sexual victimization. In addition, these are also risk factors for IPV victimization. IPV protective factors include high levels of social support from family and community. Coordination of supportive community services is also a protective factor.

Abuse can take numerous forms: psychological, financial, emotional, and physical. Acts of violence are typically thought to be against the victim but often include destruction of property, intimidation, and threats. A cycle of tension-building, including criticism, yelling, and threats, followed by violence and then a quieter period of apologies and promises to change is often seen. This cycle usually accelerates over time, however, with the violence being less predictable. Love for the perpetrator, hope that things will change, and fear of the consequences of leaving the relationship help to keep the victim in the relationship. These items also usually prevent victims from coming forth and asking for help.

Clinical Presentation

Violent behavior by a woman against a male partner is less likely to result in injury as serious as a man's violence toward a woman, in part because of the usual disparity in body size and lower likelihood of weapon use by women. A history of strangulation attempts is one of the best predictors for subsequent homicide of victims of domestic violence. The probability of becoming an attempted homicide victim increases by 700% and the probability of becoming a homicide victim increases 800% for women who have been strangled by their partner. For health-care professionals documenting domestic violence, it is important to use the correct terminology between "strangulation" and "choking." "Strangulation" refers to external neck compression, whereas the term "choking" should be reserved for internal airway blockage. It is important to note that most strangulation cases produce minor or no visible injury. Nearly all strangulation perpetrators are men, and though most abusers do not strangle to kill, they do strangle to show that they can kill.

A victim of interpersonal violence can present with variable symptoms depending on the nature of the violence. It is important to note that the batterer will often accompany the victim for treatment and will hover and answer questions for the victim. Therefore, it is critical to perform the patient history in private without intimidation or coercion. Women who are IPV victims are more likely to present with vague medical complaints, sexual problems, depression, and anxiety. The clinical presentation of a man in an abusive relationship has been less well studied. In many cases, acute or chronic pain is reported without any signs of visible injury.

The patient will often report feeling isolated or offer a history of being restrained or locked in the house.

Diagnostic Testing

Diagnostic approaches should be dictated by the type of injury presented at the time as well as the patient complaints. Screening tools are available to help identify suspected victims of interpersonal violence. These include the Partner Violence Screen (PVS) and SAFE. The SAFE questions provide an opportunity to assess the safety of the patient and can include:

- **S**tress/Safety: Assesses patient's sense of safety in a relationship (Example: Do you feel safe in your relationship?)
- **A**fraid/Abused: Assesses patient history of abuse (Example: Has your partner ever threatened or abused you or your children?)
- **F**riends/Family: Assesses social support (Example: If you have been hurt, are your friends and family aware of it?)
- **E**mergency plan: Assesses readiness in case a safe place is needed (Example: Do you have a plan of escape?)

The U.S. Department of Health and Human Services recommends that screening and counseling for IPV be performed as part of women's routine preventive health visits. Health-care providers should screen at periodic intervals during obstetric care, including the first prenatal visit, at least once per semester, and at the postpartum checkup.

> **CLINICAL CONCEPT**
>
> Other signs of interpersonal violence include multiple prior visits to the emergency department as well as a substantial delay between the time of injury and presentation for treatment.

Treatment

Health-care providers should inform the patient about mandatory reporting requirements in cases of suspected domestic violence and child abuse. Reporting to local authorities, including law enforcement, is also mandatory when a person states an intention to harm oneself or another person.

The NP is well positioned to direct the couple to the appropriate resources for help in domestic violence but should not attempt to provide this counseling because of the complexity of this type of care. Individual treatment is the rule as long as the violent behavior continues. Health-care providers should work to ensure patient safety, including providing numbers or assisting in making a call to the National Domestic Violence Hotline and local crisis intervention centers.

As with counseling and screening for other health problems, using objective statements beginning with "I" is helpful. When a patient denies that finger-shaped bruises are caused by intentional injury by another person, the NP can simply state what is seen. This statement reinforces the assessment of abuse and allows the patient to offer more information. In a situation in which a patient is verbally abused in the NP's presence, the NP should reinforce his or her role as patient advocate by stating that the behavior is unacceptable in the NP's presence. Some providers fear that this statement can possibly precipitate another episode of abuse; however, this is unlikely.

Applying the BATHE model is helpful in framing the problem, forming a therapeutic relationship, and directing intervention. Developed by Stuart and Lieberman, this model provides a guide for gathering information while helping the patient reflect on the issues at hand. See Box 15-4.

Discussion Sources

Stuart MR, Lieberman JA. *The 15-Minute Hour: Efficient and Effective Patient-Centered Consultation Skills*. 6th ed. New York, NY: CRC Press; 2018.

U.S. Department of Agriculture, Safety, Health and Employee Welfare Division. *Domestic Violence Awareness Handbook*. http://www.dm.usda.gov/shmd/handbook.htm

QUESTIONS

120. You note that a 42-year-old woman has bruises on her left forearm that appear finger shaped. She states that she does not recall how the bruises happened and denies that another person injured her. What is your best choice of statement or question in response to this?

    A. "Your bruises really look as if they were caused by someone grabbing you."

    B. "Are you sure you can't remember how this happened?"

BOX 15-4 The BATHE Model

The components of the model are as follows:

- *B* Background
  - How are things at home? At work? Has anything changed? Good or bad? Anything you wish would change?
- *A* Affect, anxiety
  - How do you feel about home life? Work? School? Life in general?
- *T* Trouble
  - What worries you the most? How stressed are you about this problem?
- *H* Handling
  - How are you handling the problems in your life? How much support do you get at home or work? Who gives you support in dealing with problems?
- *E* Empathy
  - "That sounds difficult."

You might want to add SOAAP to BATHE:

- *S* Support
  - Normalize problems, but do not minimize.
  - "Many people struggle with the same (similar) problem."
  - "What supports or resources can you use to help deal with this?"
    - Some providers may use selected self-disclosure for this. Self-disclosure usually works best in crises that are common and not of unusually tragic proportions, such as timely death or job change.
- *O* Objectivity
  - Watch your reactions to the story. Maintain your professional composure without acting stone-like, but be mindful of "recoiling" gestures.
  - Help client with objectivity.
    - "What is the worst thing that can happen?"
    - "How likely is that?"
    - "Then what would happen?"
- *A* Acceptance
  - Coach the client to personal acceptance.
    - "That is an understandable way to feel."
    - "I think you have done well considering the stress."
    - "I wonder if you are not being too hard on yourself."
- *A* Acknowledge client priorities.
  - "It sounds like family is more important to you than your work."
  - Acknowledge readiness or difficulty in making a change.
    - "Change is hard and sometimes very scary."
    - "It sounds to me like you are ready [not ready] to make a change."
- *P* Present focus
  - Assist client in focusing on the present, without minimizing concerns of the past and future.
    - "How could you cope better?"
    - "What could you do differently?"
  - What to do after you have gathered this information:
    - Negotiate a problem-focused contract for behavioral change.
    - Repeat after me, "I promise not to harm myself or anyone else in any way between now and my next visit with ____."
  - Homework assignment with "I" messages:
    - "I would like more help with the children."
    - "I feel really unimportant to you when _____."
    - "I feel angry when _____."
  - How do you keep this to 15 minutes?
    - Focus the client, using open- and closed-ended questions. Tell the client how much time you have, particularly with revisit.
    - "We have ___ minutes to chat. What would you like to focus on?"
  - If client cannot focus, ask, "If one problem in your life could just disappear, what would you choose?"

Source: Stuart MR, Lieberman JA. The 15-Minute Hour: Efficient and Effective Patient-Centered Consultation Skills. 6th ed. New York, NY: CRC Press; 2018.

C. "I notice the bruises are in the shape of a hand."

D. "I would remember if I had bruises on my arm like that."

121. Which of the following statements is true concerning domestic violence?

A. It is found largely among people of lower socioeconomic status.

B. The person in an abusive relationship usually seeks help.

C. Routine screening is indicated during pregnancy.

D. A predictable cycle of violent activity followed by a period of calm is the norm.

122 to 126. Answer the following questions true or false.

_____ 122. Access to a firearm by a male perpetrator is associated with increased risk of abuse toward women largely in lower socioeconomic income households.

_____ 123. The NP is in an ideal position to provide counseling to both members of a couple involved in domestic violence, particularly if both members of the couple are members of the NP's practice panel.

_____ 124. Women's violence against male partners is as likely to result in serious injury as men's violence toward women.

_____ 125. Interpersonal violence is uncommon in same-sex relationships.

_____ 126. Child abuse is present in about half of all homes where partner mistreatment occurs.

127. When considering characteristics of the domestic violence perpetrator, one of the best predictors of a subsequent homicide of victims of domestic violence is which of the following?

A. history of perpetrator striking victim on the face with an open hand

B. history of perpetrator attempting to strangle the victim

C. perpetrator's access to kitchen knives

D. history of victim alcohol abuse

For answers and rationales, see end of chapter.

QUESTION ANSWERS AND RATIONALES

Substance Use Disorder

1. Correct: B. administer the CAGE questionnaire.

All adults in primary care should be screened for alcohol abuse with a simple question such as "How much alcohol do you drink?" This can then be followed up with questions on type of alcohol, quantity, and frequency. For those suspected of alcohol abuse, the CAGE questionnaire offers the best sensitivity and specificity in identifying problematic drinking (B). The questionnaire consists of four questions, with a positive response for two questions indicating problem drinking.

Incorrect:

The CAGE questionnaire offers the highest specificity and sensitivity in identifying problematic alcohol use. This would be the next best step in the evaluation of this patient. An evaluation of liver enzymes can be appropriate later in his evaluation to confirm the diagnosis and detect liver damage (A), though elevated AST can be caused by other conditions. Confronting the patient and offering education on the hazards of excessive alcohol use might be appropriate at later points in his evaluation (C, D).

2. Correct: D. Have you ever engaged in a violent act while drinking?

Assessing whether an individual participated in a violent act while drinking, though important information to obtain in a person with problematic alcohol use, is not part of the CAGE questionnaire (D).

Incorrect:

The CAGE questionnaire assesses whether the individual feels that he/she should cut down on drinking (A), if the individual gets annoyed by others criticizing his/her drinking habits (B), and if the individual feels guilty about his/her drinking (C). Additionally, the questionnaire asks whether the individual ever had an eye-opener (e.g., a drink first thing in the morning) to steady his/her nerves. A positive response to two or more of these questions would suggest problematic drinking.

3 to 5. Ranking Question

3. Correct: 3

4. Correct: 2

5. Correct: 1

An alcoholic drink is defined as 12 g ethanol, which is contained in 12 oz beer, 4 oz of nonfortified wine, or 1-1.5 oz liquor (80 proof). Therefore, the 12 oz of beer is considered one alcoholic drink (3), 6 oz of wine is considered 1.5 alcoholic drinks (4), and 3.5 oz of 80-proof liquor can be counted as over two alcoholic drinks (5).

6. Correct: B. contemplation.

The stage of contemplation occurs when an individual moves beyond precontemplation and is now interested in making a behavioral change (B). Though the individual is able to identify the positive aspects of change, he/she might not be able to recognize how to move forward in making the change. This is a critical point for health-care providers to offer treatment options and support to encourage the change.

Incorrect:

An individual in the precontemplation stage is not interested in making a behavior change and might not even be aware that there is a problem (A). During the preparation stage, the individual exhibits some change behavior but might still lack the tools to proceed further (C). During the action stage, the individual takes specific steps to change but can be inconsistent with carrying through those changes (D). The final stage of maintenance/relapse encompasses the time when the individual adopts and embraces the change and deals with potential relapses. These five stages can be applied to all types of SUDs as well as other health issues.

7. Correct: D. hepatic dysfunction.

BZDs are the traditional class of agents used to manage alcohol withdrawal symptoms. However, for those with hepatic dysfunction, agents with a shorter $t_{1/2}$ (e.g., lorazepam) or agents with an absence of active metabolites (e.g., oxazepam) would be preferred to prevent a prolonged effect of these medications (D). Chlordiazepoxide and diazepam would be appropriate choices for individuals with adequate hepatic function.

Incorrect:

Short-acting BZDs (lorazepam) and agents without active metabolites (oxazepam) are preferred for individuals with hepatic dysfunction. There is no preference of these agents within the BZD class for individuals with a history of seizures (A), with folate-deficiency anemia (B), or with multiple substance abuse (C).

8. Correct: C. 24 to 36 hours

For individuals who are heavy alcohol users, alcohol withdrawal symptoms typically occur within 12 hours of the last drink. Symptoms then peak around 24 to 48 hours, with gradual abatement over the next 5 to 7 days (C). Beyond the first week, adverse effects are usually psychological and can continue for several weeks without treatment.

9 to 11. Ranking Question

9. Correct: 2

10. Correct: 1

11. Correct: 3

Stage 1 symptoms begin at 8 to 12 hours following the last drink and can include insomnia, nausea, vomiting (10), abdominal pain, and tremors. Stage 2 symptoms can begin around 24 hours after the last drink and can include hypertension, elevated and/or irregular heartbeat, hyperthermia (9), mental confusion, sweating, and irritability. In severe cases, this can be accompanied by stage 3 symptoms that include hallucinations, seizures, and severe confusion (11).

12. Correct: B. Counsel the patient that alcohol abuse is a treatable disease.

When counseling a patient with alcohol abuse, a helpful approach is to emphasize that this is a lifelong but treatable disease (B). At each visit, the patient should be asked about drinking habits and the consequences to health. Treatment options should be offered at each visit to convey the seriousness of this condition.

Incorrect:

Advising the patient to stop drinking is not effective without a more comprehensive plan that involves counseling along with pharmacotherapy (A). Similarly, the use of scare tactics, such as informing the patient about the health consequences, is not helpful as an initial approach, particularly for individuals in the precontemplation stage who do not see a need to change (C). Referral to AA would not be helpful without the patient first making a commitment to change (D).

13. Correct: C. "I am concerned about your health and safety."

When counseling patients who have a health problem with a behavioral component, the use of statements with "I" is important in emphasizing a need to change and the seriousness of the condition (C).

Incorrect:

This patient is in the precontemplation stage of behavioral change and does not see a need to change his behavior. As such, referral to a support group would not be useful (D). Using statements of how his behavior is affecting other people is not as effective as "I" statements in conveying the seriousness of his condition (B). Work is usually the last domain of life to be impacted in individuals with alcohol abuse (A).

14. Correct: B. clonidine

BZDs are the first-line agents to treat alcohol withdrawal syndrome. However, adjunctive therapy with a BZD might be needed for certain patients with refractory symptoms. The α-adrenergic agonist clonidine can be helpful in reducing blood pressure, heart rate, and tremors (B). This agent, however, does not prevent seizures or delirium observed in severe cases of alcohol withdrawal syndrome.

Incorrect:

Clonidine can be helpful as adjunctive therapy in reducing adrenergic symptoms. Verapamil, a calcium channel blocker, is not helpful in mitigating symptoms associated with alcohol withdrawal (C). Naltrexone, an opioid receptor agonist, is useful in reducing cravings for alcohol but will not alleviate symptoms of tremors and tachycardia (D). There is little evidence that barbiturates, such as phenobarbital, are helpful in mitigating symptoms of alcohol withdrawal, and they can increase the risk of respiratory depression when combined with alcohol (A).

15. Correct: D. AST 80 U/L (0 to 31 U/L), MCV 103 fL (80 to 96 fL)

Long-term alcohol abuse can result in an elevated AST level, modest or no elevation in ALT, and macrocytosis. When no other health issues are present in the patient other than alcohol abuse, the AST elevation is not dramatic. Among the answer choices, the values of AST 80 U/L and MCV 103 fL are most consistent with a patient with chronic alcohol abuse (D).

Incorrect:

Macrocytosis (i.e., MCV > 96 fL) is a common finding with long-term alcohol abuse (A, B), though a MCV of 140 fL is quite excessive (C). ALT levels will also be normal or only slightly elevated while AST levels are likely to be elevated.

16. Correct: C. helps to reduce the urge to drink

Acamprosate can be used in addition to psychosocial support and counseling to prevent relapse of alcohol abuse. Acamprosate is used to reduce cravings for alcohol (C).

Incorrect:

In addition to acamprosate, other medications used to prevent relapse include naltrexone, which modifies the intoxicating effects of alcohol (A), and disulfiram, which causes unpleasant adverse effects when combined with alcohol (B). BZDs are the traditional agents used to minimize alcohol withdrawal symptoms (D).

17. Correct: C. she likely has an underlying untreated or undertreated mood disorder.

Compared to men, women use the health-care system more frequently and have a higher rate of mood disorders. As a consequence, women are more likely to have potential drugs of abuse, such as BZDs, prescribed by a provider to manage a mood disorder (C).

Incorrect:

Individuals who misuse prescription drugs, such as BZDs, tend to abuse other substances as well (A). For those with a physical dependence of BZDs, discontinuation should occur through a slow tapering regimen to avoid severe withdrawal symptoms that can occur with rapid withdrawal (B). The long-term use of BZDs is not associated with renal or hepatic impairment or toxicity (D).

18. Correct: B. a 24-year-old female

Misuse of prescription medications is most likely to occur among young adults aged 18 to 25 years. Women are also more likely to misuse prescription medications compared to men. Among the answer choices, the 24-year-old female belongs in the demographic with the highest likelihood to misuse prescription medications (B).

19. Correct: B. SSRIs.

SSRIs are the typical first-line agent for the treatment of anxiety and panic disorders (B). These agents are generally well tolerated with the most common adverse effects being nausea, dry mouth, dizziness, and excessive sweating. Headache, nausea, and vomiting are common complaints when initiating therapy but usually resolve after 2 to 6 weeks.

Incorrect:

SSRIs are considered first-line therapy for anxiety disorders. An anxiolytic, such as BZD, is sometimes used for early management of symptoms until the SSRI exerts its therapeutic effect (A). TCAs are occasionally used to treat panic disorder but should be used selectively due to their potential toxicity with overdose and adverse effect profile (C). Barbiturates are not typically used for the treatment of anxiety or panic disorder (D).

20. Correct: C. decreasing the dose 25% per week.

Abrupt discontinuation of BZDs in an individual with physical dependence on these agents will potentially result in serious and life-threatening adverse effects including tremors, hallucinations, seizures, and a delirium tremens–like state. Discontinuation of BZDs should be done with a gradual tapering regimen, such as reducing the dose by 25% each week (C).

21. Correct: A. alcohol

BZDs generally have a favorable toxicity profile when taken alone, even in overdose. However, when combined with alcohol and barbiturates, the sedation effect is greatly enhanced and can lead to a potentially life-threatening condition (A).

Incorrect:

BZDs are generally well tolerated when taken with therapeutic doses of NSAIDs (B), beta blockers (C), or statins (D).

22. Correct: B. the development of chronic obstructive airway disease is often associated with regular smoking, particularly when combined with inhaled tobacco use.

Clinical evidence demonstrates a strong link between regular smoking of marijuana and the development of COPD, with the highest risk among those who also smoke tobacco products (B).

Incorrect:

Among daily marijuana users, physical withdrawal symptoms are frequently reported during periods of abstinence (A). Though marijuana use among teenagers remains high, with approximately 40% of 12th graders reporting use in the past year, this is still lower than alcohol use, which approached 50% use in the past year (C). Marijuana intoxication can significantly impair activities requiring concentration and physical skills, such as driving a motor vehicle (D).

23. **Correct: C. state laws should be consulted to check the legal status of medical marijuana prior to prescribing.**
A growing number of states now allow the legal use of medical and recreational marijuana. Prior to prescribing marijuana for medical purposes, the state law should be consulted (C).
Incorrect:
A growing number of states have approved the use of marijuana for medical purposes and to help relieve symptoms of many conditions, including cancer, HIV/AIDS, and chronic pain (A). Edibles can provide an alternative for those who do not wish to ingest smoke. The effect can take a longer time compared to smoking, but it will last for a longer duration (B). Inquiring about the use of marijuana is not an indication that the individual has an SUD (D).

24. **Correct: B. The effect of edibles will be faster on an empty stomach.**
Edibles can provide an alternative to ingesting smoke for cannabis treatment. Ingesting edibles on an empty stomach will hasten its effect (B). Patients should be educated on proper use and storage of edibles, including understanding what constitutes a single serving, as well as ensuring that others who are unaware of the edibles do not accidentally ingest them.
Incorrect:
Cooking cannabis will not destroy its effect as it can be infused in an edible fat such as oil or butter for cooking (A). Edibles generally take a longer time for its effect compared to smoking marijuana (C), but the effect lasts longer than smoking (D).

25. **Correct: B. hypertension.**
Common signs of opioid withdrawal include hypertension (B), tachycardia, diarrhea, nausea, fever, papillary dilation, restlessness, myalgia, lacrimation, and rhinorrhea along with an intense craving for opioids.
Incorrect:
Opioid withdrawal is commonly associated with diarrhea rather than constipation (A), and insomnia rather than somnolence (D). The individual might feel hot or cold, but there is usually no change in body temperature (C).

26. **Correct: B. buprenorphine plus naloxone.**
Methadone is a long-acting opioid that is commonly used as part of a comprehensive treatment plan to treat opioid addiction. However, methadone can only be dispensed through a qualified opioid treatment program. An alternative to methadone is the combination of buprenorphine (opioid agonist) and naloxone (opioid antagonist), which can be prescribed by qualified clinicians in a variety of settings and offers safety advantages over methadone (B).
Incorrect:
Topiramate, an anticonvulsant, has shown some benefits in reducing cravings in alcohol abuse, but evidence does not support its use in opioid addiction (D). Gabapentin is an antiepileptic drug that is used to treat neuropathic

pain, but it is not helpful in opioid addiction (A). Methylnaltrexone is a μ-opioid receptor antagonist that is used to treat opioid-induced constipation (C).

27. **Correct: C. chest pain.**
Cocaine use can cause increased heart rate, myocardial contractility, and vasoconstriction that results in increased blood pressure. This places the patient at higher risk of myocardial ischemia and infarction. Thus, inquiring about chest pain is given highest priority to evaluate for possible cardiac involvement of cocaine abuse (C).
Incorrect:
Evaluation of cardiac symptoms related to cocaine use is given highest priority. The sympathomimetic effects of cocaine use will predictably cause feelings of anxiety (A) and difficulty maintaining sleep (B). Abdominal pain is not a likely consequence of cocaine use (D).

28. **Correct: B. MDMA, or "Molly."**
Ecstasy or MDMA increases the activity of the neurotransmitters serotonin, dopamine, and norepinephrine. At high doses, the drug can induce serotonin syndrome causing dysregulation of body temperature, tachycardia, excessive sweating, shivering, and twitching (B). Severe cases are characterized by extreme hyperthermia resulting in organ failure and death.
Incorrect:
Hyperthermia and tachycardia are more likely to occur with stimulant drugs, such as amphetamines and MDMA. These are not typically observed with the use of cannabis (A), hallucinogens such as LSD (C), and barbiturates (D).

29. **Correct: B. amnesia.**
Flunitrazepam is a BZD that is not available for prescription in the United States but can be obtained in other countries as a sleep aid. Also known as "roofies" or the "date rape drug," the drug is often given without the recipient's knowledge to reduce sexual inhibition and induce amnesia, allowing for sexual assault to occur, possibly without recollection by the victim (B).
Incorrect:
Flunitrazepam is available in some countries outside of the United States and is used as a sleep aid. It would not cause agitation (A), increased appetite (C), or insomnia (D).

Eating Disorders

30. **Correct: B. PHQ-9.**
Better outcomes are achieved when eating disorders are identified and treated at early stages. Several screening tools are available to help identify those with eating disorders. However, the Patient Health Questionnaire-9 (PHQ-9) is designed to screen for depression and not eating disorders (B).
Incorrect:
The SCOFF questionnaire consists of five simple questions and provides high sensitivity for detecting AN and BN (A). The EDE involves a clinician interview and is a

preferred method for identifying specific eating disorders (C). The YBC-EDS is a semistructured interview that evaluates the preoccupation and rituals related to eating disorders (D).

31. Correct: D. all adolescents.

Age of onset of eating disorders, such as AN, is typically during the teens and early 20s. Therefore, simple screening for eating disorders should be done during annual physical examinations of all adolescents (D) and can include determination of BMI as well as an assessment of the patient's attitude on body image and dieting patterns.

Incorrect:

Eating disorders can impact individuals of all body shapes and sizes, and so BMI should not be a determinant for screening (A, B). In fact, those with BN often can have average or slightly above average BMI. Dissatisfaction with body weight and shape is not an indication of an eating disorder (C).

32. Correct: C. Depression is often found concomitantly.

Those with eating disorders typically have a high rate of comorbid depression (C). This is one explanation of why antidepression medications are frequently useful in the treatment of eating disorders.

Incorrect:

AN is predominantly found in females, who can account for over 90% of cases (A). Onset of the condition typically occurs during the teen years for females (peaks around 14 to 18 years of age), with onset in males occurring a few years later (B). Effective treatment of AN and other eating disorders will require specialty referral and an interdisciplinary approach that can include a psychiatrist and nutritionist to ensure success during the long recovery period (D).

33. Correct: B. antidepressant therapy.

Management of AN will require a comprehensive treatment plan consisting of nutritional, behavioral, and pharmacotherapy. Initial nutritional therapy should focus on correcting any fluid or electrolyte disorders, though parenteral administration would only be needed in severe cases. Pharmacotherapy should include the use of an antidepressant, such as an SSRI, since comorbid depression is a frequent occurrence in those with AN (B).

Incorrect:

Nutritional therapy should be initiated to correct electrolyte and fluid imbalances, though parenteral administration should be reserved for severe disease (A). Initial pharmacotherapy should include an SSRI rather than a psychostimulant to treat any comorbid depression (C). Pharmacotherapy should be used in combination with CBT, rather than psychoanalysis, to address perceptions of body image and disturbed eating habits (D).

34. Correct: B. dental surface erosion.

Individuals with BN are often difficult to identify as this tends to be a secretive disease and persons are frequently at normal or slightly above normal body weight. An indication for BN is the erosion of the lingual surface of the upper teeth because of excessive exposure to gastric contents during purging (B).

Incorrect:

Those with BN are frequently at normal or slightly above normal body weight (A). Hypokalemia can sometimes be found in these individuals due to excessive use of laxatives or diuretics to reduce weight. However, other physical findings, such as tachycardia (C) or hair loss (D), are not typically found.

35. Correct: B. deep cracks or splits in the corners of the mouth.

Cheilosis can occur in individuals with AN or BN and results from malnutrition and repeated episodes of vomiting. Cheilosis presents with inflammatory lesions at the corners of the mouth, which can include deep cracks and splits (B).

Incorrect:

Cheilosis is best characterized by lesions at the corners of the mouth that can include deep cracks or splits. Subconjunctival hemorrhage is defined as ruptured blood vessels in the eye (A). Cheilosis does not describe hair that is easily plucked, a finding often noted in AN (D) or the presence of lesions in the pharynx (C).

36. Correct: A. hypokalemia.

Hypokalemia is an electrolyte disturbance that can occur with excessive use of laxatives or with the use of diuretics (A).

Incorrect:

The use of these products is not typically associated with hypercalcemia (B), proteinuria (C), or hypernatremia (D).

37. Correct: B. Periods of anorexia can occur.

Individuals with BN can undergo periods of anorexia as part of the compensatory behavior following a binge episode (B). Compensatory behaviors can include fasting, excessive exercise, vomiting, or taking laxatives and diuretics.

Incorrect:

BN is a secretive disease that can present for many years before the condition is noted by a health-care provider (A). Hypokalemia, rather than hyperkalemia, can result from the use of laxatives (C). Individuals with BN are typically not obese but can have a normal or slightly above normal BMI (D), further challenging a timely diagnosis of the condition.

38. Correct: C. bupropion (Wellbutrin®).

All antidepressants can be considered in the treatment of BN except for bupropion. This agent can induce further bingeing as well as seizures in patients with BN and so should be avoided (C).

Incorrect:

Antidepressants are the first-line agent for the treatment of BN, including SSRIs such as fluoxetine (A) and paroxetine (D). TCAs, such as desipramine, can also be considered for those who do not tolerate or have an inadequate response to SSRI therapy (B).

39. **Correct: D. purging activity after an eating binge.**
BED is characterized by eating an excessive amount of food over a discrete period of time. This is not followed by purging, and thus individuals with BED are usually obese (D).
Incorrect:
BED is characterized by episodes of binge eating where the individual lacks control over the amount of food ingested during a discrete period of time (A). Binge episodes occur at least once per week for at least 3 months (B). Individuals with BED typically eat alone out of embarrassment and feel depressed, guilty, or disgusted with themselves following a binge episode (C).

40 to 42. Matching Questions

40. **Correct: C. BED**

41. **Correct: A. AN**

42. **Correct: B. BN**
Individuals with BED have one or more binge-eating episodes per week, and this is not followed by purging. As a result, those with BED are typically overweight or obese (40). The peak time of onset of AN is between 14 and 18 years and is predominantly in females. AN is associated with low body weight and malnutrition, which can lead to cheilosis (41). Those with BN are commonly at normal or slightly above normal body weight, and often cycle between binge eating and compensatory behavior, such as purging or excessive exercise (42).

43 to 47. Matching Questions

43. **Correct: BN, possible with AN if binge-purging type present**

44. **Correct: Both**

45. **Correct: AN**

46. **Correct: BN, possible with AN if binge-purging type present**

47. **Correct: Both**
Parotid (salivary) gland enlargement can occur as a result of nutritional deficiencies as well as repeated episodes of vomiting. Thus, this can be found in those with bulimia as well as those with the binge-purging type of AN (43). Electrolyte disorder can be found in both AN and BN due to malnutrition and purging, as well as the use of laxatives and diuretics, which can cause hypokalemia (44). Lanugo, or the development of soft downy hair typically on the sides of the face and along the spine, is a common finding in those with AN and might be the body's response to conserve heat (45). Esophageal tears, resulting from repeated episodes of vomiting, can be found with BN as well as the binge-purging type of AN (46). Both AN and BN are associated with cardiovascular effects that can include arrhythmia, hypotension, and bradycardia (47).

Mood Disorders

48. **Correct: D. consistent early morning awakening.**
Changes in sleep patterns are a common finding among those with depression, including excessive or insufficient amounts of sleep. Those with depression frequently report early morning awakening, such as at 3 or 4 a.m., with difficulty getting back to sleep (D).
Incorrect:
Diarrhea and cramping are not usual signs of depression, though irritable bowel syndrome is more commonly found in some mood disorders, such as anxiety (A). Sleep maintenance and early morning awakening are more common with insomnia, while difficulty with sleep initiation can be found more frequently with anxiety disorders (B). Diminished cognitive ability is a common finding for all mood disorders and is not specific for depression (C).

49 to 51. Ranking from most common (1) to least common (3)

49. **Correct: 1**

50. **Correct: 2**

51. **Correct: 3**
For those with depression, it is very common to have a passive idea of death without an actual plan (49). Suicidal ideation is occasionally present (50), though it is much less common to actually have a discrete plan to commit suicide (51). It is important to note that inquiring about suicide will not increase the risk of attempted suicide. Those with suicidal ideation should undergo a thorough safety evaluation with appropriate referral, including involuntary hospitalization for those at high risk of self-harm.

52. **Correct: B. A person with this condition is less likely to see a health-care provider compared with those with depression alone.**
A significant proportion of individuals with depression will also have hypochondriasis. These individuals are unable to come to the realization that they do not have a particular health problem, or they tend to believe an existing health problem is more serious than it actually is. As a result, those with hypochondriasis will seek medical care more frequently than those with depression alone (B).
Incorrect:
Hypochondriasis is a common finding among those with depression, affecting approximately 30% of those with depression (A). Those with hypochondriasis are unable to process objective information that there is no particular health problem (C) or they believe that an existing health problem is more serious than it actually is (D).

53. **Correct: C. a 28-year-old man who occasionally "skips a dose" of his prescribed medication.** Fluoxetine is associated with a prolonged $t_{1/2}$, and so would be advantageous for those who are prone to miss doses as the therapeutic effect will remain present (C).
Incorrect:
Given the prolonged $t_{1/2}$, fluoxetine is not recommended for those with decreased metabolism of the drug, as this can increase drug exposure. This can include the elderly (A) as well as those with decreased hepatic function (B). This agent is also energizing with anorexia and

weight loss common findings, and so would not be recommended for a patient with decreased appetite (D).

54. Correct: C. with depression and dementia, a patient is aware of difficulties with cognitive ability.
When caring for the elderly, it is important for healthcare providers to be able to differentiate depression from dementia. For those with dementia, the cognitive changes occur slowly over months to years, and individuals are not able to describe the changes in cognitive ability (C). Symptoms of depression occur over a much shorter period of time, and these patients can accurately describe the cognitive changes.

Incorrect:
For many older patients with dementia, a component of depression is commonly found (A) and should be actively treated, as this can result in improvement in cognitive function (D). Depression in the elderly is often misdiagnosed as early dementia. Symptoms of depression typically have a more rapid onset compared to symptoms of dementia, which can progress over months to years (B).

55. Correct: D. low-level depression.
Dysthymia is characterized by low-level daily depression that has lasted for at least 2 years in adults (D). Typically, treatment with an antidepressant results in a life-changing experience, and the underlying personality of the individual emerges.

Incorrect:
Dysthymia is associated with two or more depression symptoms. However, this does not include episodes of self-harm (B) or social isolation (C). Thoughts of death is a common symptom of depression, though suicidal ideation is less common and not typically expected in low-level depression characterized by dysthymia (A).

56. Correct: C. a 38-year-old woman with fatigue and anhedonia for the past 2 years
Persistent depressive disorder is characterized by low-level depression that has lasted for at least 2 years in adults. Therefore, the 38-year-old with prolonged symptoms of fatigue and anhedonia (i.e., an inability to feel pleasure) is most likely to have this diagnosis (C).

Incorrect:
A diagnosis of persistent depressive disorder requires a prolonged period (more than 2 years) of experiencing depression symptoms. The 23-year-old who had a recent job loss is likely experiencing a situational reaction to the event and not persistent depressive disorder (A). The woman with jitteriness and difficulty initiating sleep more likely describes an anxiety disorder (B). Depression is more likely associated with sleep maintenance and early morning awakening rather than sleep initiation. The 15-year-old boy possibly describes an SUD, particularly as adolescents are at high risk for these disorders (D).

57. Correct: C. psychotherapy plus a psychotropic agent.
Treatment of mood disorders is most effective with a combination of psychotherapy along with the use of a psychotropic agent (C). Medication can address the biochemical nature of the disorder, while psychotherapy and behavioral therapy can help the individual acquire the necessary skills needed to manage the disorder that is often chronic and relapsing.

Incorrect:
A combination of psychotherapy with psychotropic medications is most effective in achieving successful long-term outcomes for individuals with a mood disorder (A, B). When considering the use of a psychotropic agent, the provider should encourage psychotherapy to build skills needed to help manage the long-term condition. ECT is typically reserved for those with major depressive disorder who have not responded adequately to prior treatments (D).

58. Correct: A. information on the anticipated course of acute grief, and D. advise on local bereavement support groups
Only 3 weeks after the loss of a loved one, this individual is likely experiencing normative sadness or grief, which will likely improve with the passage of time. Health-care providers should offer support and provide information about grief and identify the difference between normative sadness of loss and depression (A). Referral to a support group can be helpful in moving through the process of grief (D). Psychotropic medications are not needed during this time.

Incorrect:
With the loss of a loved one occurring only 3 weeks ago, the individual is likely experiencing normative sadness and grief. Complicated grief can be considered if the symptoms persist beyond 1 to 3 months after the precipitating event, especially if symptoms impact normal activities of daily function. For complicated grief, treatment is similar to major depression and can consist of the use of an antidepressant in combination with psychotherapy (B). Anxiolytics are not warranted in the treatment of grief (C).

59. Correct: D. elimination of sadness.
Successful treatment of reactive depression and grief should be able to relieve the symptoms of depression. However, treatment will not relieve the normal sadness associated with the loss (D).

Incorrect:
Treatment of reactive depression is aimed at relieving the symptoms of depression that should result in restoring or elevating mood (A) and function (B) as well as improving decision-making ability (C). However, treatment should not aim to eliminate sadness, which is a normal response to the loss of a loved one.

60. Correct: A. lamotrigine (Lamictal®).
Treatment of bipolar disorder will depend on whether the patient is in a manic or depressive state. Lamotrigine, an antiepileptic medication, can be used during the bipolar depression stage, as well as quetiapine or lithium. It is less helpful during manic episodes of bipolar disorder (A).

Incorrect:

Individuals with bipolar disorder and severe mania can be treated with lithium carbonate (B), valproic acid (D), carbamazepine, or risperidone (C). Patients should be monitored closely for at least the first 6 weeks, with dose adjustments made based on serum concentrations (e.g., lithium carbonate, valproate, carbamazepine) and attainment of the desired clinical effect.

61. **Correct: B. a 2-week supply of amitriptyline**

TCAs, such as amitriptyline and nortriptyline, are associated with severe cardiovascular effects and neurotoxicity and can be fatal when taken in overdose (B). Cardiac effects can include tachycardia and prolonged QT intervals. Other agents should be considered prior to this class for the treatment of depression, particularly for individuals at risk of self-harm.

Incorrect:

SSRIs, such as paroxetine, and SNRIs, such as duloxetine, are generally safe, even when taken in overdose situations (A, C). BZDs, such as alprazolam, are also generally safe when taken alone in overdose (D). However, when combined with alcohol or a barbiturate, the sedation effect is enhanced and can be life-threatening.

62. **Correct: A. This is a common, transient side effect of early SSRI therapy.**

A dull frontal headache is a common adverse effect when initiating SSRI therapy (A). The headache should resolve within a couple of weeks and acetaminophen can be used as needed to provide relief.

Incorrect:

He should be advised to continue with treatment as the adverse effect is not serious or life-threatening and will resolve in a couple of weeks (B). This is a common adverse effect of all members of the SSRI class, so switching to another SSRI will not be helpful (C). Though TCAs, such as desipramine, are often used in headache prophylaxis, they are associated with other adverse effects and are not needed in this situation as the headache will resolve in a couple of weeks (D). Acetaminophen can be used as needed to provide headache relief.

63. **Correct: D. she should be taking the medication with food.**

GI upset is a common and usually transient adverse effect of SSRI therapy. To minimize GI upset, the medication can be taken with food (D).

Incorrect:

GI upset is a common adverse effect that usually resolves over time (A). The adverse effect is not serious or life-threatening and so the medication should be continued (B). As GI upset is usually transient and can be minimized by taking the medication with food, there is no need to switch to another antidepressant, particularly after only 1 week of treatment (C).

64. **Correct: C. continued or escalated stress from the troubled marriage.**

Initiation of antidepressant medication for an individual with major life stressors will typically show initial improvement as the medication takes effect. However, if the stressor continues, the effect of the antidepressant will diminish despite adherence to the dosing regimen (C). Ongoing interpersonal therapy is recommended to augment pharmacotherapy in these situations.

Incorrect:

The diminished effectiveness of the antidepressant is likely the result of the continued presence of the stressor and not because of an inadequate dose (A) or development of tolerance to the medication (B). This can occur even with adherence to the dosing regimen (D).

65. **Correct: B. paroxetine (Paxil®)**

Sexual dysfunction, including decreased libido and anorgasmia in either gender, are most commonly seen with use of SSRIs, such as paroxetine (B). In these cases, switching to another class can be helpful.

Incorrect:

SSRIs are most associated with sexual dysfunction, though this can be seen with other classes of agents. Patients can be switched to other agents that are associated with less sexual dysfunction, and can include bupropion (D), a TCA such as nortriptyline (C), or the dual-acting serotonergic agent vilazodone (A).

66. **Correct: A. bothersome but not life threatening.**

Symptoms of SSRI/SNRI withdrawal can include dizziness, paresthesia, anxiety, nausea, sleep disturbance, and insomnia. These symptoms can be bothersome but are not life threatening (A), unlike withdrawal from other agents, such as BZDs.

Incorrect:

SSRI/SNRI withdrawal is not a life-threatening situation but results in some bothersome symptoms that resolve over time (B). There is no seizure risk, unlike what can be observed with BZD withdrawal (D). Withdrawal symptoms are more likely to be seen when discontinuing treatment with a short $t_{1/2}$ agent, as those with a long $t_{1/2}$ (e.g., fluoxetine) will generally self-taper over time (C).

67. **Correct: C. fluoxetine**

Among the answer choices, fluoxetine exhibits the greatest inhibition of cytochrome P450 2C9, which is involved in the metabolism of warfarin (C). Concomitant use of fluoxetine with warfarin will result in enhanced action of warfarin and can increase the risk of bleeding events.

Incorrect:

Sertraline is only a mild inhibitor of CYP450 2C9 (D). Citalopram (A) and escitalopram (B) have minimal or weak inhibition of CYP450 2C9.

68. **Correct: D. paroxetine**

Among the SSRIs, paroxetine is associated with the greatest anticholinergic effect (D). This agent should generally be avoided in the elderly as it can increase the risk of anticholinergic adverse effects, such as sedation, constipation, urinary retention, dry mouth, and cognitive impairment.

Incorrect:
Though members of the SSRI class of agents can exhibit anticholinergic effect, paroxetine is associated with greater anticholinergic effect compared with escitalopram (A), sertraline (B), or fluoxetine (C).

69. Correct: C. The risk of relapse is greatest in the first 2 months after discontinuation of therapy.
As with any chronic condition, relapse is a major concern for patients with depression when discontinuing treatment. The risk of relapse is highest within the first 2 months of discontinuation (C). Health-care providers should closely monitor patients once they discontinue therapy and provide continued mental health support.

Incorrect:
Once treatment is discontinued, depression relapse can occur at high rates even if patients were successfully treated for the recommended amount of time (D). About 80% of patients with depression have a relapse within 1 year of treatment discontinuation if the patient had more than two major depressive disorder episodes (A). Relapse rates are higher for those who have experienced multiple episodes of major depressive disorder (B).

70 to 73. Yes or No

70. Correct: Yes

71. Correct: Yes

72. Correct: Yes

73. Correct: No
Several risk factors have been identified for depression relapse. These includes having dysthymia or persistent depressive disorder in the preceding episode of depression (73), poor recovery between episodes (72), a current episode lasting more than 2 years (70), onset of depression occurring at age younger than 20 years or older than 50 years (71), a family history of depression, and the presence of severe symptoms such as suicide and psychosis.

74. Correct: B. impulsive behavior
Bipolar disorder causes shifts in mood, energy, and activity levels and can impair the ability to perform normal everyday activities. Moods can range from manic episodes (i.e., extremely "up" with elation and energized behavior) to depressive episodes (i.e., "down" periods with hopelessness). In bipolar I disorder, manic episodes are characterized by impulsive behavior, which can be serious enough to warrant hospitalization (B).

Incorrect:
Manic episodes of bipolar I disorder are characterized by being extremely "up" with elation rather than anhedonia (i.e., inability to feel pleasure; D), along with energized behavior (C) and a decreased need for sleep (A). Other symptoms include increased talkativeness; increased self-esteem or grandiosity; increased goal-directed activity, energy level, and irritability; racing thoughts; poor attention; and increased risk-taking.

75. Correct: D. anhedonia
Similar to bipolar I disorder, those with bipolar II disorder experience wide mood swings ranging from hypomania to depression. The episodes of mania are relatively mild compared to those experienced in bipolar I disorder and can be productive compared to depressive episodes. The depressive episodes are characterized by the typical symptoms of depression, including anhedonia (inability to feel pleasure) (D).

Incorrect:
Racing thoughts (A), impulsive behavior (B), and increased talkativeness (C) are all symptoms of a manic episode and are likely to be exhibited by an individual with bipolar I disorder. The manic episodes of bipolar II disorder are relatively mild (hypomanic).

76. Correct: B. continue for a minimum of 6 months after remission is achieved.
Given the high rate of relapse for depression and anxiety, current recommendations for pharmacological therapy are to continue treatment for at least 6 months after remission is achieved (B). For those at high risk of relapse, continued maintenance therapy can be considered.

Incorrect:
The recommended duration of treatment is at least 6 months after remission is achieved and not 4 months of total treatment duration (A). Indefinite maintenance therapy can be considered for individuals who experience two or more episodes of depression, but generally not after the first episode (C). Once the therapeutic dose is determined for full effect, the dose should remain at that level for the duration of treatment and not titrated down (D).

77. Correct: C. this is a common adverse effect of SSRI therapy that is unlikely to resolve without adjustment in her therapy.
Sexual dysfunction, including decreased libido and anorgasmia in either gender, is a common adverse effect seen with the use of SSRIs and will continue throughout therapy. In these cases, switching to another class can be helpful (C). Patients can be switched to other agents that are associated with less sexual dysfunction, and can include bupropion, a TCA, or the dual-acting serotonergic agent vilazodone.

Incorrect:
Sexual dysfunction caused by SSRIs will likely continue throughout the duration of treatment and will not resolve on its own (A). This is a class effect of SSRIs, and so switching to another SSRI agent will not be helpful (B). Referral to a urologist is not necessary as adjustment to treatment, such as switching to another class of agents, will likely resolve the condition (D).

78. Correct: C. QT prolongation.

The maximum dose of citalopram should not exceed 40 mg/day in those 60 years and older or exceed 20 mg/day in those over 60 years due to a risk of QT prolongation (C).

Incorrect:

SSRIs are generally safe and are not associated with nephrotoxicity (B), renal impairment (A), or bone marrow suppression (D).

79. Correct: A. fluoxetine.

When prescribing medications, particularly in the elderly, it is important for health-care providers to be aware of pharmacokinetic differences among members of drug classes in order to select the safest agent. Among the SSRIs, fluoxetine has the longest $t_{1/2}$ at 24 to 72 hours, while its metabolite has a $t_{1/2}$ of 4 to 16 days (A).

Incorrect:

Paroxetine has a $t_{1/2}$ of 21 hours but should be used with caution in the elderly due to its high anticholinergic and sedation effects (B). Citalopram has a $t_{1/2}$ of 35 hours (C), while sertraline has a $t_{1/2}$ of 26 hours (D).

80. Correct: A. duloxetine

Duloxetine is associated with rare liver toxicity. However, the risk increases in the presence of other hepatic risk factors, such as heavy alcohol use (A). Patients should be cautioned against the use of alcohol when using any psychotropic medication.

Incorrect:

Liver toxicity with alcohol use is not associated with the use of desvenlafaxine (B), escitalopram (C), or bupropion (D). However, patients should be advised against the use of alcohol when taking any psychotropic medication.

81. Correct: D. blood pressure.

Due to its effect on norepinephrine reuptake, venlafaxine is associated with a dose-dependent increase in diastolic blood pressure (D). The effect is usually modest with an approximately 5 mm Hg increase on average.

Incorrect:

The use of venlafaxine, a selective SNRI, has not been associated with any clinically significant changes in heart rate (A), serum glucose (B), or serum AST/ALT levels (C).

82. Correct: A. bupropion

Bupropion should be avoided in patients with a history or at risk of seizures as well as those with closed head injury history or a history of quiescent epilepsy (A). When used in higher doses, bupropion can lower the seizure threshold, and seizure risk worsens when the dose is increased rapidly.

Incorrect:

There are no specific warnings for the use of viladazone (B), citalopram (C), or duloxetine (D) in patients with a history of seizure.

83. Correct: B. BZDs can be used initially as adjunctive therapy to SSRIs but then tapered once a therapeutic dose of SSRI is established.

First-line treatment of anxiety disorder is an SSRI. However, BZDs can be used initially as adjunctive therapy

to provide fast-onset symptom relief while the SSRI is titrated to a therapeutic level (B). Once the therapeutic level of the SSRI is reached, the BZD can be tapered over several weeks while the SSRI is continued.

Incorrect:

SSRIs are considered first-line therapy for anxiety disorder (A). BZDs can be helpful as initial adjunctive therapy while the SSRI is titrated to an effective therapeutic level (C, D). Due to the potential for physiological and psychological dependence, BZD use should be tapered as soon as the therapeutic dose of the SSRI is achieved.

84. Correct: C. 1 hour

Trazadone has a fairly long onset of action and, thus, should be taken approximately 1 hour prior to bedtime for optimal effect (C). Patients should be advised not to leave home, drive, or work for at least 8 hours after taking trazadone.

85. Correct: C. anxiety disorder.

The patient presentation is most consistent with a diagnosis of anxiety disorder (C). Major symptoms include excessive anxiety or worry, difficulty controlling worry, difficulty concentrating, as well as sleep disturbance, muscle tension, restlessness, fatigue, and irritability.

Incorrect:

Though some symptoms of anxiety disorder are common with depression, this patient lacks the key criteria for a depression diagnosis, including marked variation in mood and a lack of interest or pleasure in activities normally found to be pleasurable (A). Dysthymia is prolonged low-level depression, which does not fit this patient's description (D). Bipolar I disorder is characterized by extreme mood swings from depression to mania, which is not reported by this patient (B).

86. Correct: B. dose too low

Primary care providers write approximately 80% of all psychotropic medication prescriptions but tend to underdose the medications and prescribe them for an insufficient amount of time (B). This can lead to a poor therapeutic response, incomplete mood disorder remission, and risk for treatment failure and relapse.

Incorrect:

Primary care providers tend to prescribe psychotropic medications at too low a dose rather than too high (A). They are also more likely to prescribe these medications for too short of a duration rather than an appropriate duration (D) or too long (C).

87. Correct: A. help a person focus on the issue at hand.

Anxiety is a natural human emotion and part of the fear response that is designed to help a person focus on the issue (A). Anxiety can also help heighten senses as a protective response to danger. The response should dissipate once the issue is resolved but can be problematic if the response is exaggerated, prolonged, or interferes with normal activities.

Incorrect:

Anxiety can actually increase the fight-or-flight response in response to danger (B) and can help a person focus on the issue at hand, thereby improving decision making (C). The anxiety response will have a minimal impact on physical capabilities (D).

88. Correct: B. difficulty initiating sleep

Symptoms of GAD can often overlap with other mood disorders that are part of the continuum, such as depression. Of the findings listed, difficulty initiating sleep is most specific for a GAD diagnosis (B).

Incorrect:

GI upset and diminished cognitive ability can be common findings in mood disorders, including GAD and depression (A, C). Early morning awakening is more commonly found in depression (D), while difficulty initiating sleep is more frequently found with GAD.

89. Correct: A. active opioid use.

When making the differential diagnosis for GAD, health-care providers should be aware of other conditions that can mimic the signs and symptoms of this condition. The symptoms of opioid withdrawal syndrome can mimic GAD, including sleep disturbance, restlessness, irritability, and difficulty concentrating. However, active opioid use is more likely associated with somnolence rather than GAD-like symptoms (A).

Incorrect:

Conditions to consider when making the differential diagnosis can include thyrotoxicosis (B), alcohol withdrawal (C), and overuse of caffeine (D). Other conditions can include sleep disorders, Addison's disease, and amphetamine use.

90. Correct: B. the onset of therapeutic effect is usually rapid.

BZDs can be useful in initial treatment of GAD due to their rapid onset of action (B). These agents are typically used initially as adjunctive therapy while SSRI therapy achieves an effective therapeutic dose, and then slowly tapered. Due to the rapid onset, individuals can sense a drug versus no-drug state, possibly giving a sense of intoxication, which can lead to psychological dependence.

Incorrect:

BZDs are associated with abuse potential due to psychological and physical dependence (C). BZDs are not interchangeable and should be carefully selected based on $t_{1/2}$ and onset of action (A). Agents with a longer $t_{1/2}$, such as clonazepam, will decrease the risk of psychological dependence. Due to a decreased rate of metabolism of the drugs in the elderly, a lower dose should be considered when compared to younger adults (D), and agents with a short $t_{1/2}$ should be preferred to limit overexposure of the drug.

91. Correct: A. low abuse potential.

Buspirone is a 5-HT1A agonist that can be used as adjunctive therapy in the treatment of anxiety disorder. The agent is not associated with any abuse potential or sedating effect and will not affect performance.

Incorrect:

Buspirone only exhibits anxiolytic activity without antidepressive effects (B). It is not associated with tolerance

or withdrawal syndrome in contrast to what is seen with BZDs (C). Buspirone has a slow onset of action, typically requiring 4 to 5 weeks for full therapeutic effect (D).

92. Correct: D. history of thought disorder.

Panic disorder is characterized by recurrent and unexpected panic attacks with an age of onset typically in the 20s. The condition can occur with or without agoraphobia; however, there is no known link with a comorbid thought disorder (D).

Incorrect:

A panic attack will include feelings of intense fear or discomfort that can develop abruptly and peak within 10 minutes (A). Symptoms can include palpitations, tachycardia, sweating, trembling, chest pain (C), chills, nausea and dizziness, among others. Panic disorder with agoraphobia (fear of open spaces or where escape is difficult) is more commonly found in females compared to males (B).

93. Correct: C. citalopram (Celexa®).

First-line therapy of panic disorder includes an SSRI or SNRI due to low abuse potential and favorable adverse effects. When selecting an agent, those that are less energizing should be preferred, such as citalopram (C), paroxetine, or escitalopram, as these will lessen risk of insomnia, nervousness, and akathisia (i.e., fidgetiness).

Incorrect:

Mood stabilizers such as carbamazepine (A) and risperidone (B) can be considered for the treatment of panic disorder if there is inadequate treatment response with first-line therapy. Bupropion lacks serotonergic effect and has an energizing effect that can exacerbate symptoms of panic disorder (D).

94 to 101. Yes or No

94. Correct: Yes

95. Correct: No

96. Correct: Yes

97. Correct: Yes

98. Correct: No

99. Correct: Yes

100. Correct: No

101. Correct: No

Major symptoms of anxiety disorder include excessive anxiety or worry, difficulty controlling worry, difficulty concentrating (94), as well as difficulty initiating sleep, muscle tension (99), restlessness, fatigue, apprehension (96), and irritability (97). Consistent early morning awakening is more likely associated with depression rather than anxiety (95). Though anxiety disorder might be associated with a higher frequency of irritable bowel syndrome and diarrhea, the condition is not associated with constipation (98). Anxiety disorder is more likely associated with insomnia rather than somnolence (101), and there is no association with hive-form skin lesions (100).

102. Correct: A. sympathomimetics
Sympathomimetics are stimulant drugs that mimic the effects of sympathetic activation on the heart and circulation. These can include α-adrenoceptor agonists (e.g., clonidine, methyldopa) or β-adrenoceptor agonists (norepinephrine, dopamine), as well as illicit drugs (e.g., amphetamine, methamphetamine, cocaine). Many of the symptoms of their use are similar to the signs and symptoms of anxiety disorder.
Incorrect:
Systemic anticholinergics (e.g., doxepin, solifenacin) tend to have a sedating effect rather than an energizing effect (C). Calcium channel blockers (e.g., amlodipine, verapamil) and β-antagonists (e.g., metoprolol, propranolol) are commonly used to treat hypertension (B, D). The β-antagonists are also used to manage cardiac arrhythmias and are occasionally used to help manage anxiety symptoms.

103. Correct: C. concomitant use of alcohol should be avoided.
BZDs can be considered as initial adjunctive treatment of anxiety disorder to provide immediate relief of symptoms while the therapeutic effect of SSRI therapy takes full effect. When initiating BZD therapy, patients should be advised against alcohol use as this can increase the sedation effect of BZDs and increase the risk of a life-threatening situation (C).
Incorrect:
An overdose of BZDs by themselves is not particularly toxic (A). A life-threatening situation can occur when BZDs are used concomitantly with alcohol or barbiturates. Though patients should aim to adhere to dosing regimens, there is some flexibility with timing of doses, particularly when using agents with a longer $t_{1/2}$ (B). The therapeutic effect of BZDs is very rapid (D), with patients able to sense the drug versus no-drug states, particularly when using an agent with a short $t_{1/2}$.

104. Correct: B. rapid withdrawal in this situation can lead to tremors and hallucinations, and C. the medication should ideally be tapered over the next 3 to 4 weeks prior to discontinuation.
Physical BZD dependence is an issue for individuals with long-term use of these agents. For an individual taking an agent with a short $t_{1/2}$, such as lorazepam, symptoms can emerge within days and can include tremors, hallucinations, and seizures (B). For those desiring to discontinue treatment, the dose should be gradually tapered by 25% per week prior to discontinuation (C).
Incorrect:
Immediate discontinuation of long-term BZD treatment will result in withdrawal syndrome that can include tremors, hallucinations, and seizures (A). GI upset is not typically reported during BZD withdrawal (D).

105. Correct: A. a mediator of γ-aminobutyric acid (GABA).
Neurotransmitters involved in anxiety include GABA, norepinephrine, epinephrine, serotonin, and dopamine. GABA blocks nerve impulses between nerve cells and the brain. Serotonin has many uses in the body but is involved in a sense of well-being and happiness. Similarly, dopamine works in the brain to affect mood, sleep, memory, learning, and concentration. Dopamine deficiency is related to depression. Epinephrine or adrenaline can increase cardiac output and raise glucose levels, thus preparing the body for the fight-or-flight response. Norepinephrine can also increase heart rate but is also important in attentiveness, emotions, sleep, and dreaming. BZDs primarily work as a mediator of GABA, thereby enhancing its activity (A).
Incorrect:
SSRIs work by enhancing the availability of serotonin (B). The mechanism of second-generation antipsychotics is as a dopamine antagonist (C). Meanwhile, SNRIs are involved in serotonin and norepinephrine reuptake inhibition, increasing the action of these neurotransmitters (D).

106. Correct: D. products with slow onset of action.
Regular use of BZDs is associated with physiological and psychological dependence. Dependence is enhanced with the use of rapid-acting agents as the patient will sense a difference between the drug versus no-drug states, possibly giving a sensation of intoxication. To minimize the risk of psychological dependence, an agent with a slow onset of action, such as clonazepam, is preferred (D).
Incorrect:
Agents with a short $t_{1/2}$ and rapid onset can give a sensation of intoxication and promote psychological dependence (A). The use of BZDs on an as-needed basis is not recommended as this will heighten the patient's awareness of the drug versus no-drug state (B). As patients cycle between drug effect and withdrawal, a psychological dependence will develop to avoid development of anxiety symptoms. Lipophilic products are more rapid acting and can cause an intoxicating effect (C).

107. Correct: A. Panic disorder rarely occurs with depression.
There is strong comorbidity between panic disorder and depression (A).
Incorrect:
Panic disorder is estimated to affect 2% to 4% of the general population (B). The average age of onset is 27 years, while new-onset panic disorder rarely occurs after age 45 years (C). Genetics appear to contribute to the development of panic disorder, particularly in the development of panic disorder with agoraphobia (D).

108. Correct: D. More women than men experience panic disorder with agoraphobia.

Panic disorder can occur with or without agoraphobia, which is a fear of open spaces or feeling trapped in an area where escape would be difficult (e.g., crowded room, elevator). Panic disorder without agoraphobia occurs equally between men and women. However, women are more likely to experience panic disorder with agoraphobia compared to men, estimated at a 2:1 ratio (D).

Incorrect:

Men and women experience panic disorder without agoraphobia at a similar frequency (A, B). For panic disorder with agoraphobia, this occurs more commonly with women compared to men (C).

109. Correct: A. irritable bowel syndrome.

Common health problems associated with panic disorder include alcohol abuse, depression, chronic fatigue, and irritable bowel syndrome (A).

Incorrect:

Panic disorder is not typically associated with thought disorders (B), hypothyroidism (C), or inflammatory bowel disease (D).

110. Correct: B. it is preferable to use agents that are more energizing than those that are less energizing.

When treating anxiety disorders including panic disorder, less energizing psychotropic medications are preferred as these are less likely to exacerbate the symptoms of anxiety, including sleep disturbance, restlessness, and irritability (B).

Incorrect:

When prescribing psychotropic medications, the general rule is to start low, go slow, and get to goal (A). This will increase the chance of reaching a therapeutic level that is well tolerated by the patient. In addition to preferring agents that are less energizing, agents that have less risk of akathisia (i.e., restlessness, fidgetiness) should be preferred, as those with panic disorder can be sensitive to this adverse effect, as noted in some SSRIs (C). Initial treatment can cause an increase in the frequency of panic attacks, but this diminishes once the full therapeutic potential of the medication is achieved (D).

111. Correct: D. poor recall of the precipitating event.

PTSD can occur after experiencing a traumatic event that results in prolonged feeling of horror and helplessness. Patients have an intrusive recall of the precipitating event (D) and can lead to numbing of emotions, detachment, hyperarousal, and impaired social and occupational functioning.

Incorrect:

In addition to an intrusive recall of the precipitating event, individuals with PTSD can present with numbing of emotions (A), detachment (B), hyperarousal (C), and impaired social and occupational functioning.

112. Correct: D. sertraline.

SSRI treatment is the first-line approach for the treatment of PTSD as this can address symptoms of arousal and depression (D).

Incorrect:

Lithium carbonate, a mood stabilizer, is not indicated as a first-line treatment for PTSD but can be considered for second- or third-line treatment with inadequate response to prior treatment (C). Methylphenidate would not be recommended due to its stimulant effect (A). BZDs such as oxazepam should be avoided in PTSD due to increased habituation risk as well as increased risk of concomitant substance abuse (B).

113. Correct: C. mirtazapine

Mirtazapine, an antidepressant, can be helpful as a sleep aid as it provides sedating effects without habituation risk (C). A nighttime dose of prazosin can also be helpful in decreasing nightmares and sleep disturbances.

Incorrect:

Duloxetine and bupropion are potentially energizing and would not be helpful as sleep aids (A, B). Zolpidem can be habituating and should be avoided in general and particularly among patients with PTSD (D).

114. Correct: D. St. John's wort.

St. John's wort exhibits activity similar to MAOIs, SSRIs, and TCAs in the treatment of depression (D). It has less anticholinergic effect compared to TCAs, though it is not as effective in treating severe depression. It also exhibits similar energizing effect as fluoxetine, with similar efficacy in the treatment of mild-to-moderate depression. The supplement needs to be used as multiple doses each day for several weeks prior to therapeutic effect. However, well-controlled studies are limited in the use of St. John's wort for depression, and caution should be used with this nutritional supplement due to potential drug interactions.

Incorrect:

Kava kava exhibits action at GABA receptors similar to BZDs that might be helpful in treating anxiety (C). Similarly, valerian root demonstrates action similar to that of BZDs and is used to treat anxiety as well as insomnia (A). Melatonin is an endogenous compound that is typically used as a sleep aid but can be considered as part of overall depression management (B). Patients should be educated on the use of nutritional supplements, particularly when self-medicating a potentially life-threatening disease. This includes awareness of a lack of quality control of supplements and the potential for drug interactions.

115. Correct: C. MAOI

MAOIs are the most potent drugs available for the treatment of panic disorder. However, their use is limited due to the toxicity profile of these agents as well as a need for dietary restriction when taking these medications. Use of this class is generally limited to those

with treatment-resistant panic disorder, though expert consultation is recommended (C).
Incorrect:
Following first-line therapy with SSRI for panic disorder, TCAs are occasionally used, though concerns regarding toxicity in overdose and adverse effects can limit their use. Second-generation antipsychotics (A), SDRIs (B), and neuroleptics (D) are not typically considered for the treatment of refractory panic disorder.

116. **Correct: C. a reduction in number and severity of panic attacks.**
Successful treatment of panic disorder with an SSRI should result in a reduction in the frequency and severity of panic attacks (C). At initiation of SSRI treatment, there can be reports of a transient increase in the frequency of panic attacks. However, the number of panic attacks subsides once the SSRI attains a therapeutic level.
Incorrect:
SSRIs are not associated with abuse potential (A). When compared to TCAs, SSRIs have the advantage of a better safety profile and are generally safe even in overdose (B, D).

117. **Correct: A. St. John's wort**
St. John's wort has exhibited some efficacy in the treatment of depression. However, this nutritional supplement can interfere with the CYP450 enzyme system involved in drug metabolism via enzymatic induction. As such, its use is not recommended with concomitant use of SSRIs, TCAs, or MAOIs due to risk of serotonin syndrome (A).
Incorrect:
There are no known warnings regarding the concomitant use of SSRIs and kava kava (B), gingko biloba (C), or valerian root (D) due to increased risk of serotonin syndrome. Any patient considering the use of nutritional supplements should be made aware of a general lack of quality control of these products and the potential for clinically significant interactions when used concomitantly with other medications.

118. **Correct: B. cephalosporins.**
St. John's wort can interfere with the CYP450 enzyme system involved in the metabolism of several types of medications. However, the metabolism of cephalosporins is not significantly impacted when administered concomitantly with St. John's wort (B).
Incorrect:
Concomitant use of St. John's wort can decrease serum levels of select antiretrovirals (D; e.g., indinavir) and cyclosporine (C), and can reduce the effectiveness of combined oral contraceptives (A).

119. **Correct: B. hepatotoxicity.**
Kava kava exhibits action at GABA receptors similar to BZDs and has been used to treat anxiety. The supplement has been associated with hepatotoxicity (B) when used in overdose, for prolonged periods of time, and/or with other hepatotoxic medications, even in individuals with no prior hepatotoxicity potential.
Incorrect:
The use of kava kava has not been associated with development of renal impairment (A), iron-deficiency anemia (C), or hyperthyroidism (D).

Interpersonal Violence

120. **Correct: C. "I notice the bruises are in the shape of a hand."**
When screening and counseling patients with suspected abuse, using "I" statements can be helpful. Additionally, simply stating what is seen (e.g., "I notice the bruises are in the shape of a hand.") will reinforce the assessment of abuse and allow the patient to offer additional information (C). In this manner, the health-care provider does not seem to question the truthfulness of the patient or personalize the injury.
Incorrect:
The health-care provider should avoid statements that can be perceived as questioning the truthfulness of the patient (A, B). Additionally, statements that personalize the injury to the NP should also be avoided (D).

121. **Correct: C. Routine screening is indicated during pregnancy.**
According to the U.S. Department of Health and Human Services, health-care providers should screen for IPV at periodic intervals during obstetric care, including the first prenatal visit, at least once per semester, and at the postpartum checkup (C).
Incorrect:
Domestic violence occurs regardless of socioeconomic status (A). The majority of those in an abusive relationship do not actively seek help for various reasons, including fear, intimidation, and a belief that the situation will change (B). A typical cycle of abuse includes tension building that leads to violence that is followed by a calm period of apologies and promises to change. However, as the relationship progresses, the cycle accelerates and can become unpredictable (D).

122 to 126. True or False

122. **Correct: False**
Access to a firearm by a male perpetrator is associated with increased risk of abuse toward women in all socioeconomic classes. This is not a problem focused on lower socioeconomic households.

123. **Correct: False**
Counseling for domestic violence requires expert referral and should not be attempted by the NP due to the complexity of the situation.

124. **Correct: False**
Women's violence against men is typically less serious than a man's violence against a woman due to smaller size and strength of women compared to men, as well as a lesser likelihood of a woman using a weapon.

125. **Correct: False**

It is likely that IPV occurs at a similar frequency in same-sex relationships compared to opposite-sex relationships.

126. **Correct: True**

Child abuse is a frequent occurrence in households where partner mistreatment occurs.

127. **Correct: B. history of perpetrator attempting to strangle the victim**

A history of strangulation attempt is one of the strongest predictors for subsequent attempted homicide and homicide of victims of domestic violence (B). For women who have been strangled by a partner, the probability of a future homicide attempt increases 700% while the probability of becoming a homicide victim increases 800%. It is important to note that most strangulation cases produce little to no visible injury on the victim.

Incorrect:

Of the answer choices, a history of strangulation attempt is the strongest predictor for subsequent homicide of victims of domestic violence. A history of a perpetrator striking the victim in the face (A), access to kitchen knives (C), or a history of victim alcohol abuse (D) do not necessarily increase the risk of subsequent homicide.

Older Adults

16

Demographics in Older Adults

Overview

The current proportion of the American population in the 65 years and older age group is approximately 15%. This is projected to increase to nearly one-quarter of the population by 2060. This increase is largely attributable to the aging of the "Baby Boomers," the demographic born from 1946 to 1964, and to a sharp decline in mortality at older ages.

The older adult population is usually classified into the following groups:

- The young old, 65 to 74 years old
- The old old, 75 to 84 years old
- The oldest old, 85 to 100 years old
- The elite old, more than 100 years old

These designations are not diagnostic. At the same time, overall function, socialization, and ability to perform activities of daily living (ADLs) typically diminish as age progresses. Currently, the fastest growing group of older adults includes those older than age 85 years. At the same time, the first of the Baby Boomer cohort turned 65 years old in 2011 and will influence the U.S. older demographics for decades.

Finances

Among elderly people residing in the United States, Social Security is mentioned as the most important source of income, with upwards of 21% of couples and 43% of single older adults claiming that 90% or more of their income is from this source. Private or public pensions and income from other financial investments combined are mentioned as most important at less than half the frequency. Currently, the older adult demographic has an overall poverty rate of approximately 10%, which is a 50% drop from the rate of 20% reported in the 1970s. The old old and the elite old have often outlived savings and investment income and have a poverty rate of 20% or greater. In addition, women living alone and select ethnic groups, including Latinos and African Americans, have poverty rates double the overall older adult poverty rate. Being economically insecure, defined as living at or below 250% of the federal poverty rate, is reported as being a major source of stress for older adults, with increased concerns about housing, transportation, food, and health-care access.

CLINICAL CONCEPT

Approximately one in three older adults is considered to be economically insecure.

Discussion Source

Centers for Disease Control and Prevention, National Center for Health Statistics. National Vital Statistics System. http://www.cdc.gov/nchs/nvss/index.htm

QUESTIONS

1. In the elderly population, the current fastest-growing group is composed of those in the age range:

   A. 71 to 75 years.

   B. 76 to 80 years.

   C. 81 to 84 years.

   D. 85 years and older.

2 to 4. Match each demographic group with the correct age range.

   _____ 2. Young old

   _____ 3. Oldest old

   _____ 4. Elite old

   A. 60 to 65 years

   B. 65 to 74 years

   C. 75 to 84 years

   D. 85 to 100 years

   E. Over 100 years

5. Which of the following is most commonly reported as the largest single source of income for elderly people?

   A. Social Security

   B. public/private pension earnings

   C. asset income

   D. family financial support

6. The poverty rate among elderly people residing in the United States can best be described as:

A. at approximately the same level across ethnic and age groups.

B. highest among the old old.

C. greatest among married couples.

D. consistently increasing since the 1970s.

7. Economic insecurity causes anxiety about affording housing, food, transportation, and health care. Approximately what percentage of older adults are economically insecure?

A. 10%

B. 20%

C. 33%

D. 50%

For answers and rationales, see end of chapter.

Age-Associated Changes in the Senses

Overview

Normative aging results in changes in the senses of hearing, vision, taste, touch, and smell. In addition, certain diseases that result in changes in the senses are more common in older adults (Fig. 16-1 and Table 16-1).

Presbycusis

Presbycusis is a progressive, symmetric, high-frequency, age-related sensory hearing loss that is likely caused by cochlear deterioration. Speech discrimination is usually the primary problem; an individual with presbycusis often reports the ability to hear another person talking but has a limited ability to understand the content of the speech, particularly when in a noisy environment.

Presbyopia

Presbyopia refers to age-related vision changes caused by a progressive hardening of the lens. Patients most often complain of close vision problems, usually first manifested by difficulty with reading smaller print.

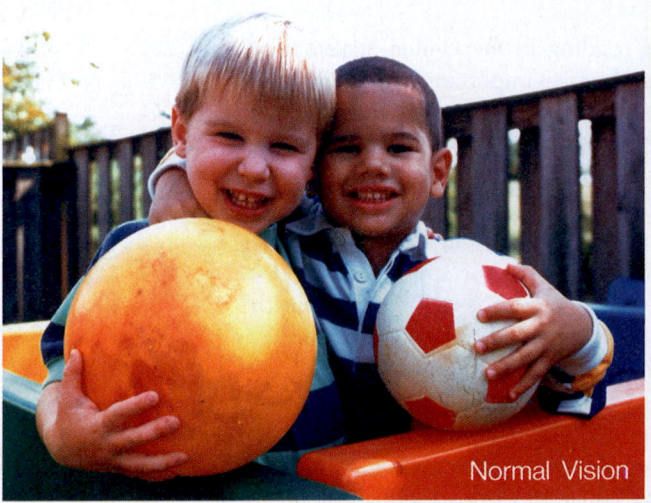

FIGURE 16-1 Normal vision.
National Eye Institute, National Institutes of Health. https://www.flickr.com /photos/nationaleyeinstitute/7544734596/in/photolist-cuGJJY-cuEJJC

TABLE 16-1 Age-Related Changes and Conditions That Result in Changes of the Senses

CONDITION	ETIOLOGY	RESULT	COMMENT
Presbyopia	Hardening of lens	Close vision problems	Nearly all adults 45 years and older need reading glasses.
Senile cataracts	Lens clouding	Progressive vision dimming, distance vision problems, close vision usually retained and can initially improve	Risk factors: Tobacco use, poor nutrition, sun exposure, corticosteroid therapy. Potentially correctable with surgery, lens implant.
Age-related maculopathy	Thickening, sclerotic changes in retinal basement membrane complex	Painless vision changes including distortion of central vision	Besides aging, risk factors include tobacco use, sun exposure, family history. Dry form: No treatment available except to minimize risk factors that worsen the condition. Wet form: Laser treatment and other therapies to obliterate neovascular membrane. Anti-angiogenic drugs injected in the eye to block new blood vessel development and leakage from abnormal vessels.
Hyposmia	Neural degeneration	Decline in sense of smell, usually gradual, resulting in fine taste discrimination (largely a function of smell)	Accelerated by tobacco use. Risk factors: Aging, head trauma, history of chronic rhinosinusitis.
Presbycusis	Multifactorial including loss of eighth cranial nerve sensitivity	Difficulty with appreciating the content of conversation in noisy environment; person can hear but cannot understand	Accelerated by excessive noise exposure. Besides aging, risk factors include family history, smoking, cardiovascular diseases, diabetes, otosclerosis, infection, and trauma. Hearing aids helpful.
Cerumen impaction	Conductive hearing loss	General diminution of hearing, easily corrected through cerumen removal	Risk factors: Ear canal hairs, use of hearing aids, bony growths secondary to osteophyte or osteoma, history of impacted cerumen. Cerumen removal.

Source: Geriatrics. Merck Manual. https://www.merckmanuals.com/professional/geriatrics.html

Additional, normal, age-related vision changes include a progressive yellowing of the lens and decreased flexibility of the sclera, in part leading to the perception of washing out of colors, difficulty seeing under low illumination, and increased sensitivity to glare.

Altered Sense of Smell and Taste

Hyposmia, characterized by a decrease in the sense of smell, or anosmia, loss of the sense of smell, is a common problem in older adults. The estimated prevalence of these disorders of smell occurs increasingly with age, with approximately one-quarter of adults in their 50s, and increasing steadily so that this is reported in nearly two-thirds of all adults 80 years and older. Its etiology is likely due to normative age-related changes in the olfactory apparatus. The condition can be worsened by tobacco or other smoke exposure, nasal polyps, or any alteration to the nasal cavity. Due to hyposmia or anosmia, the older adult often complains of lessened food enjoyment, given how much the sense of smell contributes to taste. Ageusia, or loss of sense of taste, and hypogeusia, or reduced sense of taste, are most commonly noted in older adults.

Additionally, older adults are overrepresented in food poisoning when compared to other age groups, due to an inability to detect the scent and taste of spoiled food. Reduced sense of smell also poses a safety hazard, where the older adult could miss danger cues such as the scent of smoke or a natural gas leak. There is no specific, effective therapy for age-related changes in smell and taste. Older adults should be encouraged to consult with a nutritionist for expert advice on dietary modifications to enhance food intake and enjoyment and minimize nutritional problems.

Touch

Aging can decrease the sense of pain, temperature, pressure, and vibration. This can be due to decreased blood flow to nerve endings, the brain, and the spinal cord. This places the older adult at greater risk of injury or accidents. Decreased sensitivity to temperature can lead to burns, frostbite, or hypothermia when temperature extremes are not detected. A reduced sense of pain can increase the risk of pressure ulcers or having an undetected injury. On the contrary, a thinner skin in older adults can increase sensitivity to light touches. To prevent injury, older adults should be consulted on lifestyle modifications, including lowering the water heater temperature, checking the outside thermostat to determine how to dress, and regularly inspecting the skin to check for injuries.

Cataracts

Distance vision poses the greatest problem for individuals with senile cataracts. As the lens becomes more opaque, near vision also deteriorates. Other visual changes of age-related cataracts include loss of ability to distinguish contrasts and progressive dimming of vision. Close vision is usually retained, and there are occasional improvements in reading ability.

> **CLINICAL CONCEPT**
> Excessive sun exposure has also been implicated as a risk factor for macular degeneration.

Macular Degeneration

Macular degeneration is the most common cause of newly acquired blindness and vision loss in elderly adults. Vision changes seen in macular degeneration include loss of the central vision field (Fig. 16-2). This disease is seen more often in women of European descent. A history of cigarette smoking and a family history of the disease are often found as well. The ophthalmological examination reveals hard drusen or yellow deposits in the macular area. Soft drusen can also be seen; these appear larger, paler, and less distinct (Fig. 16-3).

Discussion Source

Geriatrics. Merck Manual. https://www.merckmanuals.com/professional/geriatrics.htm

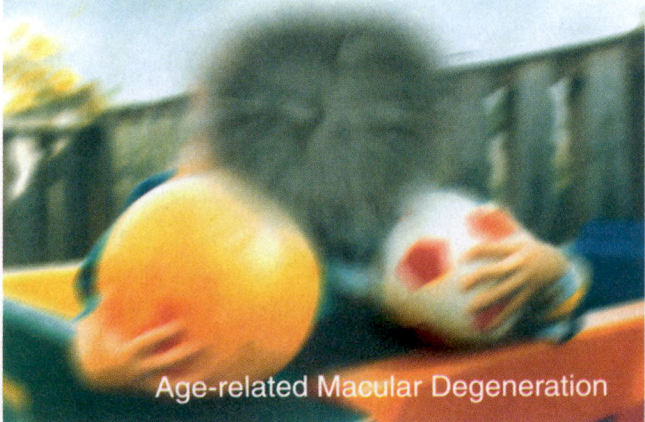

FIGURE 16-2 Age-related macular degeneration.
National Eye Institute, National Institutes of Health. https://medialibrary.nei .nih.gov/search?f%5B0%5D=category%3A8#/media/1800

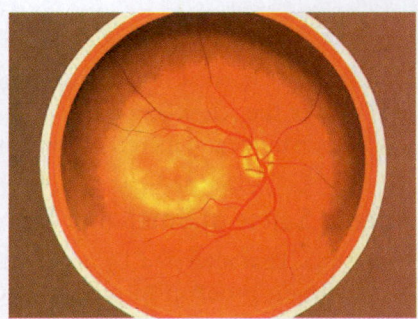

FIGURE 16-3 Macular degeneration.
National Eye Institute, National Institutes of Health. https://medialibrary.nei.nih.gov /search?f%5B0%5D=category%3A6&keywords =&items_per_page=20&page=1#/media/3527

QUESTIONS

8 to 12. Match the following age-related changes in the senses with the problem reported by the older adult.

_____ **8.** difficulty with appreciating the content of conversation in noisy environment

_____ **9.** decline in sense of smell

_____ **10.** painless vision change that includes central vision distortion

_____ **11.** results in near-vision blurriness

_____ **12.** can result in peripheral vision loss

> **A.** hyposmia
>
> **B.** presbycusis
>
> **C.** presbyopia
>
> **D.** age-related maculopathy
>
> **E.** chronic glaucoma

---

13. A 76-year-old woman is being treated for senile cataracts. The granddaughter who is accompanying the patient expresses concern that one day she could also develop cataracts. You explain that she can reduce the risk of senile cataracts by avoiding all of the following except:

A. tobacco use.

B. alcohol abuse.

C. corticosteroid therapy.

D. sunlight exposure.

---

14. An 81-year-old woman has early bilateral senile cataracts. Which of the following situations would likely pose the greatest difficulty for her?

A. reading the newspaper

B. distinguishing between the primary colors

C. following extraocular movements

D. reading road signs while driving

---

15. All of the following are consistent with normal age-related vision changes except:

A. a need for increased illumination.

B. an increasing sensitivity to glare.

C. a washing out of colors.

D. a gradual loss of peripheral vision.

---

16. Besides aging, a risk factor for age-related macular degeneration is:

A. hypertension.

B. hyperlipidemia.

C. tobacco use.

D. alcohol abuse.

---

17. An effective method to prevent presbycusis is:

A. to avoid using cotton swabs in the ear canal.

B. to use ear protection when exposed to loud noises.

C. to avoid using hearing aids for a prolonged period of time.

D. regular cerumen removal.

18. A common complaint for a person with presbycusis is:

   A. general diminution of hearing.

   B. diminution of high-frequency hearing.

   C. worsening hearing at night.

   D. inability to hear low-pitched sounds.

19. A person with cerumen impaction experiences:

   A. a general diminution of hearing.

   B. an unhampered ability to hear low-pitched sounds.

   C. pain when exposed to high-pitched sounds.

   D. an ability to hear but cannot understand a conversation in a noisy environment.

For answers and rationales, see end of chapter.

Medication Use in the Older Adult

"Start low, go slow" is geriatric prescribing advice all clinicians likely learned. Although there is wisdom in this adage, a more complete understanding of numerous age-related factors is needed for safe prescribing for elderly adults.

> **CLINICAL CONCEPT**
>
> In any given month, more than 90% of older people take at least one medication, more than 66% take three or more, and 42% take five or more.

The elderly comprise a heterogeneous group who constitutes a relatively small portion of the North American population yet use more than one-third of prescription medications and nearly three-fourths of all over-the-counter (OTC) medications.

Older adults who are prescribed multiple medications are at increased risk for adverse drug events and hospitalization from these events. Because advancing age is often accompanied by various health problems, elderly adults often have multiple health-care providers and multiple prescribers and medications. In addition, normative age-related physiological changes can influence pharmacological responses; these changes are often accentuated by illness (Table 16-2). Financial constraints commonly cause elderly adults to use a medication less often than prescribed or to attempt to substitute. The clinician must be aware of these factors to prescribe for older adults safely and effectively.

Because the term "elderly adult" is typically used to describe any person aged 65 years or older, this could imply that aging occurs only after this milestone. In reality, normal age-related changes influencing drug therapy occur gradually over decades. These changes often lead to altered pharmacokinetics; components of pharmacokinetics include drug absorption, distribution, biotransformation (metabolism), and excretion. A simple way to remember pharmacokinetic principles is that *this is what the body does to the drug*. At the same time, pharmacodynamics, the study of biochemical and physiological effects of drugs or *what the drug does to the body or disease*, does not change over the life span. Normative age-related changes, such as the loss of the β_2-receptor sites, result in less of a clinical effect with β_2-agonist use, however.

Although age alone likely does not alter the amount of the drug absorbed, age-related changes can significantly influence the rate of absorption.

■ A drug's half-life ($t_{1/2}$), defined as the time required for the amount of drug in the body to be reduced by one-half after a single dose of the medication is given, is often increased in older adults.

■ As gastric acid production decreases, stomach pH increases, potentially prolonging the initial breakdown of medications made to dissolve in low pH.

■ In addition, age-related decreases in gastrointestinal (GI) blood flow, gastric motility, and gastric emptying mean that medication stays in the gut longer, whereas decreased GI surface area can lead to erratic absorption.

Drug distribution can be altered by age-related changes. Serum albumin, an important plasma protein used to bind and distribute various medications, including warfarin (Coumadin®) and phenytoin (Dilantin®), decreases with aging. With less albumin available for drug binding, a potentially greater amount of free drug is available. These changes, coupled with altered drug elimination, often lead to a decrease in the dose needed in an aging adult. The amount of the plasma protein alpha-1-acid glycoprotein, with an affinity for

TABLE 16-2 Age-Related Changes Important to Medication Use

	AGE 20 TO 30 YEARS	AGE 60 TO 80 YEARS
Percentage of body weight as water	60%	53%
Lean muscle mass	Baseline	20% or greater reduction
Serum albumin (average)	4.7 g	3.8 g
Relative kidney weight	100%	80%
Relative hepatic blood flow	100%	55% to 60%

Source: Katzung B. Special aspects in geriatric pharmacology. In: Katzung B. Basic and Clinical Pharmacology. 14th ed. New York, NY: McGraw-Hill Medical; 2018:1058–1067.

binding with certain medications including propranolol, quinidine, and lidocaine, increases with age; as a result, less free drug is in circulation.

Age-related hepatic changes include decreased hepatic blood flow, mass, and functioning hepatocytes and diminished activity of hepatic enzymes responsible for drug metabolism. These changes contribute to a prolonged drug $t_{1/2}$ and longer duration of action than found in younger adults. In addition, the ability to recover from alcohol-induced, medication-induced, or viral-induced hepatic damage is lessened.

The Beers Criteria

Published by the American Geriatrics Society (AGS), the Beers Criteria provide an important reference to help avoid the use of potentially inappropriate medication (PIM) in the older adult population (age older than 65 years). When prescribing medications for the elderly, checking to see whether the drug is listed in the Beers Criteria is an important step in ensuring the safe use of medications.

According to Beers Criteria, medications are classified into five categories:

■ Medications to avoid in most older adults, though use in hospice and palliative care settings is likely appropriate
  • Example: Anticholinergic agents (i.e., first-generation antihistamines, amitriptyline); NSAIDs with increased risk of GI bleeding and peptic ulcer disease, potential to worsen blood pressure (BP) control and blunt the clinical effect of many hypertensive medications
■ Medications to avoid in older adults with select health problems. The use of these medications can worsen the underlying condition
  • Example: Thiazolidinediones with potential to worsen heart failure; benzodiazepines can worsen dementia and mild cognitive impairment
■ Medications that should be used with caution in older adults because of the potential for harmful adverse effects
  • Example: Aspirin due to risk of major bleeding; trimethoprim-sulfamethoxazole (TMP-SMX) due to increased risk for hyperkalemia
■ Medication combinations to avoid because of the risk for harmful drug-drug interactions
  • Example: Ciprofloxacin use in warfarin therapy, leading to a potentially dangerous increase in international normalized ratio (INR) and bleeding risk
■ Medications that should be dosed differently or avoided among those with reduced kidney function
  • Example: Dabigatran, edoxaban, duloxetine, many but not all antimicrobials

The adage "start low, go slow" in prescribing for elderly adults has an often forgotten third part: "but get to goal." Clinicians, in their zeal to provide safe pharmacotherapeutic care for older adult patients, often prescribe enough of a medication to cause anticipated adverse effects but not enough to provide the desired therapeutic effect.

CLINICAL CONCEPT
Knowledge of the safe and appropriate medication doses in older adults, keeping in mind the age-related effects on pharmacokinetics, is a critical part of safe prescriptive practice.

Discussion Sources

American Geriatrics Society. American Geriatrics Society 2019 updated AGS Beers Criteria® for potentially inappropriate medication use in older adults. *J Am Geriatr Soc.* 2019;67:674–694. https://onlinelibrary.wiley.com/doi/abs/10.1111/jgs.15767

Katzung BG. Special aspects in geriatric pharmacology. In: Katzung B. *Basic and Clinical Pharmacology.* 14th ed. New York, NY: McGraw-Hill Medical; 2018:1058–1067.

QUESTIONS

20. Age-related changes in an elderly adult include all of the following except:
    A. total body water decreases by 10% to 15% between ages 20 and 80 years.
    B. body weight as fat increases from 18% to 36% in men and from 33% to 45% in women.
    C. an increase in serum albumin.
    D. an increase in gastric pH.

21. A general principle of drug absorption in an elderly adult is best described as:
    A. amount of absorption is decreased.
    B. rate of absorption is changed.
    C. drug absorption is altered but predictable.
    D. bioavailability is altered.

22. Anticipated age-related changes that can result in less drug effect include:
    A. loss of β_2-receptor sites.
    B. lower GI pH.
    C. increased renin-angiotensin production.
    D. increased GI motility.

23. Age-related changes in the GI system include all of the following except:
    A. decreased gastric acid production.
    B. decreased gastric motility.
    C. increased GI surface area.
    D. decreased gastric emptying.

24. When dosing warfarin (Coumadin®) in older adults, it is important to consider that the dose needs to be adjusted in which of the following ways?
    A. A lower dose is usually needed due to lower serum albumin.
    B. A lower dose is usually needed due to higher serum albumin.
    C. A higher dose is usually needed due to lower serum albumin.
    D. A higher dose is usually needed due to higher serum albumin.

25 to 28. Indicate (*yes or no*) which of the following adverse effects is associated with the use of systemic anticholinergic agents in older adults.
    _____ 25. confusion
    _____ 26. hypertension
    _____ 27. urinary retention
    _____ 28. constipation

29. The process of absorption, distribution, metabolism (biotransformation), and elimination of a drug is known as:
    A. pharmacodynamics.
    B. drug interactions study.

C. pharmacokinetics.

D. therapeutic transformation.

30. The study of biochemical and physiological effects of drugs on the body or disease is called:

    A. pharmacodynamics.

    B. pharmacokinetics.

    C. biotransformation.

    D. bioavailability.

31. When considering the properties of a drug in the body, which of the following does not change as a person ages?

    A. excretion

    B. biotransformation

    C. pharmacodynamics

    D. absorption

32. When prescribing a medication, the clinician considers that half-life is the amount of time needed to decrease the serum concentration of a drug by:

    A. 25%.

    B. 50%.

    C. 75%.

    D. 100%.

33. Under ordinary circumstances, the presence of a medication in the body is needed for how many half-lives to reach steady state?

    A. 0.5 to 1

    B. 1 to 3

    C. 3 to 5

    D. 5 to 7

34. Compared with a healthy 40-year-old adult, CYP450 isoenzyme levels can decrease by _____% in elderly adults after age 70 years.

    A. 10

    B. 20

    C. 30

    D. 40

35 to 42. Match each potential drug-related adverse effect with the correct medication. An answer can only be used once.

_____ **35.** Amitriptyline

_____ **36.** Duloxetine

_____ **37.** NSAIDs

_____ **38.** Gabapentin

_____ **39.** Zolpidem

_____ **40.** TMP-SMX

_____ **41.** Pioglitazone

_____ **42.** Ranitidine

        A. sedation

        B. highly anticholinergic effect

    C. potential to worsen heart failure

    D. hyperkalemia risk

    E. delirium, falls

    F. nausea, diarrhea

    G. GI bleeding

    H. need for dose adjustment in the older adult

For answers and rationales, see end of chapter.

Elder Maltreatment

Overview

The Centers for Disease Control and Prevention (CDC) define elder maltreatment as any abuse and neglect of persons age 60 years and older by a caregiver or another person in a relationship involving an expectation of trust.

A combination of individual, relational, community, and societal factors contribute to the risk of an individual becoming a perpetrator of elder maltreatment. Understanding these factors can help identify various opportunities for prevention. Risk factors for perpetration of elder maltreatment include a current diagnosis of mental illness or alcohol abuse in the caregiver, a high level of hostility about the caregiver role, poor coping skills, inadequate preparation for caregiving responsibilities, assumption of caregiving responsibilities at an early age, and maltreatment as a child.

At the relationship level, additional risk factors emerge, including a high level of financial and emotional dependence on a vulnerable elder, past experience of disruptive behavior, and lack of social support. Elder maltreatment is likely to be more prevalent in a cultural and community milieu in which tolerance of aggressive behavior and negative beliefs about aging and elderly adults exist; formal services, such as respite care for individuals providing care to elderly adults, are limited, inaccessible, or unavailable; family members are expected to care for elderly adults without seeking help from others; and individuals are encouraged to endure suffering or remain silent regarding their pain.

At the institutional level, such as in a long-term care or assisted-living facility, unsympathetic or negative attitudes toward residents, chronic staffing problems, lack of administrative oversight, staff burnout, and stressful working conditions are considered risk factors for elder maltreatment.

In addition to elder maltreatment, self-neglect is a growing problem that often goes unreported. Self-neglect is defined as the inability of an adult to perform essential self-care, either because of physical or mental impairment or a diminished capacity to perform these tasks.

Clinical Presentation

Elder maltreatment can take various forms (Table 16-3). Neglect is the most commonly encountered type of elder maltreatment. In times of economic difficulty, the rate of financial exploitation usually increases.

Common signs of self-neglect include poor personal hygiene despite opportunity and ability to bathe, poor medication management or refusing to take medications, signs of dehydration or malnutrition, unsanitary or unclean living space, signs of unpaid bills, and lack of adequate food in the house despite finances and ability to obtain groceries.

Diagnostic Testing

Diagnostic testing in maltreatment of the older adult is directed by the resulting type of injury or condition. Current practice standards dictate that all elderly patients receive elder abuse screening as a means to prevent and detect elder abuse. Various screening tools are available that can be used in health-care settings. These include the Elder Abuse Suspicion Index (EASI), Older Adult Financial Exploitation Measure (OAFEM), the Hwalek-Sengstock Elder Abuse Screening Test (H-S/EAST), Brief Abuse Screen for the Elderly (BASE), and the Vulnerability to Abuse Screening Scale (VASS).

Visits to health-care providers are often the only opportunity to detect an abusive situation and prevent its continuation. Health-care providers should be aware of the proper interventions if elder abuse is suspected or detected.

TABLE 16-3 Forms of Elder Maltreatment

FORM OF ELDER MALTREATMENT	DESCRIPTIONS
Physical abuse	Injured by another individual, including being scratched, bitten, slapped, pushed, hit, or burned; assaulted or threatened with a weapon, including a knife, gun, or other object; or inappropriately restrained.
Sexual abuse or abusive sexual contact	Any sexual contact against elderly adult's will, including acts in which elderly adult is unable to understand the act or is unable to communicate consent.
Psychological or emotional abuse	Any event in which elderly adult experiences trauma after exposure to threatening acts or coercive tactics. Examples include humiliation or embarrassment; controlling behavior such as prohibiting or limiting access to transportation, telephone, money, or other resources; social isolation; disregarding or trivializing needs; or damaging or destroying property.
Neglect	Failure or refusal of a caregiver or other responsible person to provide for elderly adult's basic physical, emotional, or social needs, or failure to protect elderly adult from harm.
Abandonment	Willful desertion of elderly adult by caregiver or other responsible person.
Financial abuse or exploitation	Unauthorized or improper use of resources of elderly adult for monetary or personal benefit, profit, or gain by another individual.
Self-neglect	Instituted by the elderly adult, not another individual, and is the failure or refusal of elderly adult to address his or her own basic physical, emotional, or social needs. This is also characterized by the lack of intervention to halt or modify the behavior by another individual who is often in the position to recognize the problem.

Treatment

The exact intervention for mistreatment in an older adult is directed at treating the resulting physical and/or psychological injuries. As with all other illness or injury, prevention should be the first-line intervention. Certain factors have been identified as protection against elder maltreatment, including strong personal relationships, community support for the caregiver role, and coordinated resources to help serve elderly adults and caregivers. Factors within institutional settings that can be protective include effective monitoring systems in place; clear, understandable institutional policies and procedures regarding patient care; ongoing education on elder abuse and neglect for employees; education about and clear guidance on how *durable power of attorney* is to be used; and regular visits by family members, volunteers, and social workers.

Every state in the United States and the District of Columbia have enacted legislation to protect vulnerable older adults from abuse, with a requirement for health-care workers and others who come in contact with older adults to report this abuse to the appropriate protective authorities.

> **CLINICAL CONCEPT**
> Elder maltreatment is significantly underreported; for every one case reported, an estimated five other cases go unreported.

Discussion Sources

Centers for Disease Control and Prevention. Elder abuse. https://www.cdc.gov/violenceprevention/elderabuse/index.html

Elder Maltreatment Alliance. A community response to at-risk older adults: information. https://eldermaltreatment.com/information

National Center for Elder Abuse. Elder abuse screening tools for healthcare professionals. http://eldermistreatment.usc.edu/wp-content/uploads/2016/10/Elder-Abuse-Screening-Tools-for-Healthcare-Professionals.pdf

QUESTIONS

43. When making a home visit to an 89-year-old man who is bedridden, you note that he is cachectic, dehydrated, and cognitively intact. He states that he is not receiving his medications regularly and that his granddaughter is supposed to take care of him but mentions, "She seems more interested in my Social Security check." The patient is unhappy but asks that you not "tell anybody" because he wants to remain in his home. The most appropriate action would be to:

   A. talk with the patient's granddaughter and evaluate her ability to care for the patient.

   B. visit the patient more frequently to ensure that his condition does not deteriorate.

   C. report the situation to the appropriate state or local agency.

   D. honor the patient's wishes because a competent patient has the right to determine care.

44. Which of the following statements is true concerning maltreatment in the older adult?

   A. This problem is found mainly in families of lower socioeconomic status.

   B. An elderly adult who is being mistreated usually seeks help.

   C. Routine screening is indicated as part of the care of an older adult.

   D. In most instances of elder maltreatment, a predictable cycle of physical violence directed at the older adult followed by a period of remorse on the part of the perpetrator is the norm.

45. Risk factors for becoming a perpetrator of elder maltreatment include all of the following except:

   A. a high level of hostility about the caregiver role.

   B. poor coping skills.

   C. assumption of caregiving responsibilities at a later stage of life.

   D. maltreatment as a child.

46. Elder maltreatment is considered to be underreported, with an estimated _____ cases going unreported for each one case that is reported.

   A. three

   B. four

   C. five

   D. six

47. The most commonly reported form of elder maltreatment is:

   A. physical abuse.

   B. sexual exploitation.

   C. financial exploitation.

   D. neglect.

48. The daughter of a 76-year-old woman expresses concern regarding her mother's refusal of assistance in everyday living activities. The mother lives by herself and is often found with poor hygiene and reports eating one small meal a day. She also has poor adherence to her current medication regimens. This represents an example of:

   A. abandonment.

   B. self-neglect.

   C. early onset dementia.

   D. psychological abuse.

49 to 54. Indicate whether each of the following is a protective factor or risk factor for elder maltreatment within institutional settings.

   _____ 49. Frequent visits by family or volunteers

   _____ 50. Staff burnout

_____ **51.** Clear guidance on how *durable power of attorney* is to be used

_____ **52.** Stressful working conditions

_____ **53.** Chronic staffing problems

_____ **54.** Clear institutional policies on patient care

For answers and rationales, see end of chapter.

Falls

Overview

Falls are a significant source of morbidity and mortality in the elderly population; multiple falls are associated with increased risk of death. Approximately one-third of community-dwelling elderly adults and two-thirds of long-term care residents experience falls each year. Of elderly adults who fall, 20% to 30% sustain moderate to severe injuries that reduce mobility and independence and increase the risk of premature death. For adults 65 years old or older, 60% of fatal falls happen at home, 30% occur in public places, and 10% occur in health-care institutions.

> **CLINICAL CONCEPT**
> Older adults are hospitalized for fall-related injuries five times more often than they are for injuries from other causes.

Risk Factors for Falls

Comprehensive care of the older adult should focus on minimizing modifiable fall risks. Risk factors for falls are numerous and are modifiable and nonmodifiable (Box 16-1).

Polypharmacy, in particular the use of medications associated with postural hypotension, increases fall risk; this condition is present in about 20% of older adults. Although not a specific disease state, orthostatic (postural) hypotension is a manifestation of abnormal BP regulation. When these mechanisms do not work properly, BP control is not maintained with position change, usually with resulting symptoms of light-headedness, dizziness, or blurred vision that occur within seconds of changing position. The most common position change to trigger orthostasis is from sitting to standing. The condition is defined as an excessive decrease in BP when an upright position is assumed that causes the characteristic signs and symptoms; the change in BP is usually greater than 20 mm Hg systolic and greater than 10 mm Hg diastolic. The use of select medications increases orthostatic hypotension, including those that decrease circulating volume and/or peripheral vasodilation, such as diuretics, tricyclic antidepressants (TCAs), calcium channel blockers, α-adrenergic blockers, centrally acting antihypertensives such as clonidine, and nitrates. Certain disease states that alter baseline cardiac output and vascular capacity, increasing orthostatic risk, are common in older adults; these include aortic stenosis, dehydration,

---

BOX 16-1 Fall and Resulting Fracture Risk Factors in Older Adults

Postural hypotension
Sensory impairment including altered vision and hearing
Parkinsonism
Osteoporosis
Osteoarthritis
Altered gait and balance

■ Decreased proprioception
■ Increased postural sway
■ Slower righting reflexes
■ Peripheral neuropathy
■ History of stroke

Psychotropic medication use, especially products with sedating effect
Cardiac drug use, especially products with properties that cause or contribute to postural hypotension
Environmental hazards

Source: Wachel T. Falls. In: Wachel T. Geriatric Clinical Advisor. Philadelphia, PA: Mosby; 2007:77–78.

peripheral vascular insufficiency, and electrolyte disturbances. Alcohol use is also a potent contributor, as is prolonged bedrest.

Syncopal episodes can also result in falls, usually with a patient report of not remembering the fall and/or not making an effort to brace for the fall. Syncope, or fainting, can be caused by a cardiac disorder, such as cardiomyopathy (e.g., congestive heart failure), arrhythmia (e.g., supraventricular tachyarrhythmias), or valvular dysfunction. Other causes can include acute myocardial infarction, acute aortic dissection, and pulmonary embolus. Patients with a report of syncope should receive a thorough cardiac and neurological examination.

Additional fall risks include personal history of a stroke or fall; a person who has fallen is two to three times more likely to fall within the next year. Environmental hazards in the home, including poorly placed furnishings, scatter rugs, and inadequate lighting, often contribute to falls. Wearing thick, soft-soled shoes, such as jogging shoes, also increases fall risk.

Fall Prevention or Post-Fall Interventions

Interventions to prevent a fall or to initiate following a fall include the following:

- Review medications, assess doses, and eliminate high-risk drugs that can contribute to falls (Table 16-4).
- Evaluate for postural hypotension with appropriate intervention.
- Provide prevention and treatment interventions for osteoporosis.
- Recommend proper footwear, avoiding slippers, sandals, and soft-soled jogging shoes in favor of an enclosed-toe, tie shoe with a semirigid sole.
- Provide an obstacle-free, well-lit environment with removal of scatter rugs and other trip hazards.
- Raise chair heights and seat heights and add arm rests to help facilitate getting up from a seated position.
- Prescribe physical therapy as indicated to enhance conditioning.
- Counsel avoidance of quick position change and that the patient should perform multiple foot-flex maneuvers before trying to move from supine to standing or sitting to standing.
- Treat for any concomitant conditions associated with increased fall risk.

Assessment Post-Fall

When a fall does occur, the patient should be promptly and appropriately assessed. Questions should be asked to investigate for an underlying condition that could have contributed to the fall and is amenable to intervention as well as subtle age-related changes that can contribute to increased fall risk (see Box 16-1). These questions are as follows:

- What was the patient doing when he or she fell?
- Was there an aura or warning that the fall was impending?
- Was there a vision loss?
- Did the patient experience dizziness prior to falling?
- Was there a loss of consciousness prior to, during, or after the fall?
- Was the patient able to break the fall?
- Is this an isolated incident, or are falls occurring more frequently?
- What medications is the patient taking? In particular, notation should be made of newly added medications or changes in dose of existing medications.
- Was the patient drinking alcohol or taking other potentially intoxicating medications?

The assessment of an older adult after a fall should focus on identification of possible correctable fall risk factors and fall-related injury and should include, at minimum, the following:

- Vital signs with evaluation of orthostasis
- Cardiovascular assessment
- Sensory assessment
- Assessment of gait and balance, including the use of the "Get Up and Go" test, in which the elderly adult is asked to rise from a straight-backed chair, walk 10 feet using his or her usual walking aid such as a cane if applicable, turn, and return to the chair and sit down, with the clinician observing balance with sitting and on standing, pace and stability with walking, ability to turn without staggering, and time to complete the task
- Survey for fall-related injuries

The most common fall-related injuries are osteoporotic fractures of the hip, spine, or forearm.

CLINICAL CONCEPT

Of all fall-related fractures, hip fractures are the most serious and lead to the greatest number of health problems and deaths.

TABLE 16-4 Medication Use Associated With Increased Fall Risk in Older Adults

MEDICATION CLASS	EXAMPLE	COMMENT
Anxiolytics and hypnotics	Benzodiazepines, long acting and shorter acting, including lorazepam, oxazepam, alprazolam, temazepam, triazolam Nonbenzodiazepines including zolpidem	In particular, gait issues most likely to arise with onset and peak of medication's action, usually one-half to 2 hours after benzodiazepine or hypnotic is taken.
Antidepressants	Tricyclic antidepressants (TCAs), such as amitriptyline; selective serotonin reuptake inhibitors (SSRIs), such as sertraline, citalopram	Orthostatic hypotension risk, typically worse with TCA compared with SSRI use.
Neuroleptics and antipsychotics including atypical or second-generation antipsychotics (SGA)	Neuroleptics, including haloperidol; SGA including risperidone	Orthostatic hypotension and dizziness risk significant, and extrapyramidal movement risk.
Opioid analgesics/antagonists	Meperidine, morphine, codeine	Risk of sedation; meperidine particularly problematic.
Insulin, sulfonylureas	Insulins, short acting and longer acting; sulfonylureas, such as glyburide, glipizide	Fall risk most often seen in presence of drug-induced hypoglycemia (most likely noted at drug's peak of action). Glipizide preferred over glyburide and glimepiride.
Cardiac medications	Antihypertensives including diuretics, calcium channel blockers (CCBs), high-dose beta blockers, and nitrates	Orthostatic hypotension and dizziness risk

Note: This list is not intended to include all medications associated with increased fall risk in older adults but rather to highlight products with well-documented risk.

Source: Pennsylvania Patient Safety Advisory. Medication assessment: one determinant of falls risk. Pa Patient Saf Advis. 2008;5(1):16–18. http://patientsafety.pa.gov/ADVISORIES/documents/200803_16.pdf

Discussion Sources

Orthostatic hypotension. Merck Manual. https://www.merckmanuals.com/professional/cardiovascular_disorders/symptoms_of_cardiovascular_disorders/orthostatic_hypotension.html?qt=&sc=&alt

Pennsylvania Patient Safety Advisory. Medication assessment: one determinant of falls risk. *Pennsylvania Patient Safety Authority.* 2008;5(1):16–18. http://patientsafety.pa.gov/ADVISORIES/documents/200803_16.pdf

QUESTIONS

55. Most fatal falls in older adults occur in:

A. a health-care institution.

B. a public place.

C. the patient's home.

D. an outdoor setting.

56 to 60. Indicate (*yes or no*) which of the following are identifiable risk factors for falls in the older adult.

_____ **56.** negative prior history of a fall

_____ **57.** history of a stroke

_____ **58.** current diagnosis of osteoporosis

_____ **59.** osteoarthritis of the hips

_____ **60.** wearing a jogging-type shoe or sneaker

61. The nurse practitioner (NP) is asked to evaluate a 77-year-old woman who recently had an unexpected fall. The patient is normally healthy and has no mobility limitations or other obvious risk factors. During the history, the NP learns that the patient did not attempt to break the fall, "I just suddenly found myself on the floor." This statement suggests:

A. a previously undiagnosed cognitive impairment that requires further evaluation.

B. that underlying sensory deficits (visual, hearing) are the most likely cause of the fall and require physical assessment.

C. that a history of alcohol use or abuse should be explored.

D. a syncopal episode requiring a cardiovascular and neurological evaluation.

62. Orthostatic hypotension is present in about _____% of older adults.

A. 10

B. 20

C. 30

D. 40

63. The use of which of the following medications is associated with the least risk of postural hypotension in the older adult?

A. nifedipine

B. furosemide

C. clonidine

D. lisinopril

64. Lifestyle interventions for an older adult with orthostatic hypotension should include counseling about:

A. avoiding the use of compression stockings.

B. significantly restricting salt intake.

C. flexing the feet multiple times before changing position.

D. restricting fluids.

65. Orthostatic (postural) hypotension is defined as an excessive decrease in BP with position change that results in characteristic signs and symptoms. The BP change is usually greater than _____ mm Hg systolic and _____ mm Hg diastolic.

A. 10, 5

B. 15, 7

C. 20, 10

D. 30, 15

66. In an older adult, the greatest risk of long-term complication is associated with fracture of the:

A. forearm.

B. spine.

C. ankle.

D. hip.

67. A 68-year-old man is taking multiple medications for various chronic conditions. Discontinuing or finding an alternative for which of the following medications will have the greatest impact in decreasing the potential for fall risk?

A. amitriptyline

B. sitagliptin

    C. atorvastatin

    D. aspirin

68. An older adult who has recently fallen has a _____ times increased risk of falling again within the next year.

    A. 1 to 2

    B. 2 to 3

    C. 3 to 4

    D. 4 to 5

69. Which of the following is not part of the "Get Up and Go" criteria when evaluating gait and balance for a 72-year-old woman who normally uses a walker?

    A. rising from a straight-backed chair

    B. walking 10 feet without the use of a walking aid

    C. turning around after walking 10 feet

    D. returning to the chair and sitting down

70. With the use of a benzodiazepine in an older adult, the risk of fall is most likely to occur _____ of the medication.

    A. at the onset of action

    B. at the peak of action

    C. at the middle point of duration of action

    D. toward the end of anticipated duration of action

For answers and rationales, see end of chapter.

Driving Issues in Older Adults

Overview

With the aging of the population, there are more elderly drivers on the roads. By the year 2030, 70 million Americans in the United States will be age 65 years or older; 85% to 90% of them will be licensed to drive.

Clinical Considerations

Though being older does not necessarily turn a person into an unsafe driver, it is important to note that age-related changes can affect driving skills. These changes include not only diminished vision and hearing but also musculoskeletal changes that can increase the time to react to changes on the road or decrease the ability to immediately hit the brakes when necessary. Cognitive changes can decrease the attention span of older drivers, who often become more easily distracted. Those with Alzheimer's disease (AD) can have a changed way of thinking and behaving. This can include forgetting familiar routes or how to drive safely and can lead to more driving mistakes or "close calls." Though people at early stages of AD are often able to drive safely for a period of time, driving ability will be affected as the disease worsens, and caregivers should monitor driving behavior. Patients with AD typically do not stop driving for at least 3 years after the initial diagnosis.

    Older driver accidents tend to be related to diminished speed of visual processing and often involve multiple vehicle events that occur at intersections and involve left-hand turns. Common driving errors made by older adults include the following:

■ Difficulty backing up and making turns

■ Not seeing traffic signs and other cars quickly enough

■ Difficulty in locating and retrieving information from dashboard displays and traffic signs

■ Delayed glare recovery when driving at night

■ Not checking rearview mirrors and blind spots

■ Bumping into curbs and objects

> **CLINICAL CONCEPT**
>
> There is an eightfold increase in traffic accidents involving drivers with mild to moderate AD.

- Not yielding to oncoming traffic and right-of-way vehicles
- Irregular or slow vehicle speeds
- Difficulty with situations requiring quick decision making

Diagnostic Testing

Unfortunately, there are no reliable objective measures available to assess driving competency in older adults. Neuropsychiatric testing cannot be used to indicate the level of impairment at which patients are not fit to drive. Additionally, the Folstein Mini-Mental Status Examination (MMSE) has not been demonstrated to reliably predict driver risk. The Clinical Dementia Rating (CDR) can be helpful but is impractical for routine screening practice. The American Academy of Neurology advocates on-road testing for patients with dementia with a CDR score of 0.5 or higher. The American Medical Association recommends two tools for screening older drivers. The *Clinician's Guide to Assessing and Counseling Older Drivers* (3rd edition) can help health-care providers identify patients at risk for crashes, help enhance their driving safety, and ease the transition to driving retirement if and when it becomes necessary. The National Highway Traffic Safety Administration's part B of the Trail-Making Test and the Clock Drawing Test can be used to assess driving skills. There is a significant correlation with misplacement of the minute hand with the incidence of crashes, straddling of lanes during driving, and total hazardous errors.

Interventions for the Older Driver

When counseling older adults on driver safety, inform them of several steps that can be taken to improve safety:

- Exercise regularly to increase strength and flexibility.
- Review prescription and OTC medications to reduce adverse effects that can impair driving.
- Have eyes checked annually and wear glasses or corrective lenses as needed.
- Drive during daylight and good weather.
- Plan the route before you drive.
- Find the safest route with well-lit streets and ample, easy-to-locate parking.
- Maintain a large following distance behind the car in front.
- Avoid distractions in the car, such as a radio other than soft background music, talking on the cell phone, texting, and eating.
- Consider potential alternatives to driving, such as riding with a friend or using public transit.

Discussion Sources

AAA. Senior driving. https://seniordriving.aaa.com/resources-family-friends/conversations-about-driving/facts-research/
National Highway Traffic Safety Administrations (NHTSA). *Clinician's Guide to Assessing and Counseling Older Drivers*. 3rd ed.
    https://www.nhtsa.gov/sites/nhtsa.dot.gov/files/812228_cliniciansguidetoolderdrivers.pdf

QUESTIONS

71. Which of the following is a true statement with regard to driving and the elderly?

   A. The number of elderly drivers will decrease over the next decade.

   B. Crashes with elderly drivers tend to involve diminished speed of visual processing.

   C. There is a greater incidence of accidents involving right-hand turns compared with left-hand turns.

   D. There is no evidence to suggest, if the elder's health is preserved, that the skills needed for safe driving deteriorate with age.

72. Which of the following is a false statement with regard to driving and AD?

   A. Patients with AD typically continue to drive for at least 3 years following the diagnosis.

   B. Those with mild to moderate AD have an eightfold increase in the number of accidents.

   C. Those at early stages of AD can continue to drive safely, though driving should be monitored regularly.

   D. The National Transportation Safety Board (NTSB) recommends surrendering the driver's license for all individuals with an AD diagnosis.

73. Common driving errors observed with older drivers include all of the following except:

    A. difficulty backing up and making turns.

    B. delayed glare recovery when driving at night.

    C. bumping into curbs and objects.

    D. tailgating.

74. When counseling an older driver, you recommend all of the following except:

    A. reviewing current medications for potential adverse effects.

    B. having the radio on to an enjoyable talk show to enhance driving skills.

    C. predetermining the route before driving.

    D. driving during the day and in good weather.

For answers and rationales, see end of chapter.

Pressure Ulcers

Overview

Pressure ulcers (also known as bedsores or pressure sores) are injuries to the skin that result from prolonged pressure on the skin. Normally, there is a balance between pressure intensity and duration with tissue tolerability. Significant contributing factors include sustained pressure, friction, shear, and nutritional debilitation.

    Pressure ulcers are most commonly observed in individuals who have health conditions that limit their ability to change positions, require the use of a wheelchair, or are confined to a bed for prolonged periods. Other risk factors include high levels of moisture, advanced age, low BP, smoking, elevated body temperature, lack of sensory perception, weight loss, urinary or fecal incontinence, decreased mental awareness, and dehydration.

> **CLINICAL CONCEPT**
> Pressure ulcers occur when vascular pressure inhibits adequate supply of blood to the skin and underlying tissue.

Clinical Presentation

Pressure ulcers are categorized into four stages based on their severity:

- Stage 1: presence of a nonblanchable erythema on intact skin (induration can be present)
- Stage 2: presence of epidermal or dermal skin loss; can appear as an intact blister
- Stage 3: full-thickness skin loss with exposure of some amount of fat; ulcer has a crater-like appearance
- Stage 4: full-thickness skin and tissue loss; wound exposes muscle, bone, and tendons

Some conditions can mimic pressure ulcers and should be considered during evaluation, such as fungal and yeast infection, malignancy, venous and arterial ulcers, and neuropathic ulcers. Complications of pressure ulcers include sepsis, cellulitis, and bone and joint infections. Chronic, nonhealing wounds can also increase the risk of an aggressive type of squamous cell carcinoma (Marjolin's ulcer).

Diagnostic Testing

Laboratory studies should include a complete blood count (CBC) with differential to determine the presence of inflammation or invasive infection. Erythrocyte sedimentation rate (ESR) should be checked to indicate possible osteomyelitis (elevated ESR with elevated white blood cell [WBC] count). Tests to evaluate adequate nutritional stores to help with healing include serum albumin and prealbumin levels, as well as transferrin and serum protein levels. Depending on patient symptoms, other tests can be considered, such as a urinalysis and culture (in presence of urinary incontinence), stool examination for fecal WBCs or *Clostridium difficile* (in the presence of stool incontinence), and blood cultures (if bacteremia or sepsis is suspected). A plain film or bone scan can be used when osteomyelitis is suspected. A biopsy should be performed for wounds that do not heal despite adequate care (i.e., to rule out Marjolin's ulcer) or if bacterial invasion of the tissue is suspected. Culture and susceptibility testing by swabbing the pressure sore site is not typically helpful as this will not differentiate tissue invasion from simple contamination/colonization.

Treatment

The most important treatment of pressure ulcers is prevention of this condition. Prevention of pressure ulcers requires routine evaluation of patients at risk. This evaluation can involve using the Braden scale or Norton scale that measures the physical and mental condition of the patient, as well as the state of nutrition, mobility, and continence. Ongoing nutritional and hydration assessment is also important to evaluate risk for pressure ulcers. Position changes are critical in prevention. For patients with limited mobility, whether bedbound or in a wheelchair, repositioning should be done as frequently as every 15 minutes, if in a wheelchair, to at least every 2 hours of bed repositioning for those who are dependent on others. Special cushions, foam mattress pads, and air- or water-filled mattresses can be helpful in keeping a patient in a certain position and relieving pressure on vulnerable skin. The head of the bed should be elevated no more than 30° to prevent skin shearing.

Stages 1 and 2 pressure ulcers can usually heal within several weeks to months of general care that manages risks for pressure ulcers. Stages 3 and 4 ulcers are more difficult to treat, and efforts primarily focus on managing pain rather than on complete healing of the wound.

Débridement can be used to remove dead tissue, and regular cleaning and dressing of the wounds are needed to promote healing and prevent infection. Referral for surgical interventions can be considered in some cases, though underlying illnesses might limit treatment to conservative management. Surgical interventions can include skin grafts, skin flaps, myocutaneous flaps, free flaps, or direct closure (rarely a usable approach with pressure ulcers). Other approaches being studied include hyperbaric oxygen therapy, electrotherapy, growth factors, and negative-pressure wound therapy, though more research is needed to fully understand the benefits of these approaches.

To hasten healing and prevent future pressure sores, nutritional support should be used as necessary, including enteral or parenteral nutrition as well as vitamin therapy. Other measures to optimize the medical status and healing of the patient include cessation of smoking, provision of adequate pain control, maintenance of adequate blood volume, correction of anemia if present, and management of bacterial contamination or infection of the wound. Cigarette smoking in particular can lead to tissue hypoxia, which disrupts acute wound healing and increases the risk of wound infection.

Discussion Sources

Kirman CN. Pressure injuries (pressure ulcers) and wound care treatment and management. Medscape. https://emedicine.medscape.com/article/190115-overview

Mervis JS, Phillips TJ. Pressure ulcers: prevention and management. *J Am Acad Dermatol.* 2019;81(4):893–902.

QUESTIONS

75. Risk factors for pressure ulcers include all of the following except:

A. malnutrition.

B. dehydration.

C. smoking.

D. weight gain.

76. Complications of pressure ulcers include all of the following except:

A. sepsis.

B. osteoporosis.

C. bone and joint infections.

D. cellulitis.

77. A pressure ulcer that exhibits full-thickness skin loss with a crater-like appearance can be categorized as:

A. stage 1.

B. stage 2.

C. stage 3.

D. stage 4.

78 to 81. Match each pressure ulcer stage with an appropriate treatment approach. Choose all that apply.

_____ **78.** Stage 1

_____ **79.** Stage 2

_____ **80.** Stage 3

_____ **81.** Stage 4

      A. skin graft

      B. simple wound closure

      C. débridement of nonvital skin

      D. conservative (nonsurgical) approaches

82. To ensure adequate nutrition to prevent and hasten healing of pressure ulcers, all of the following are recommended except:

    A. enteral nutrition.

    B. low-fat, low-sodium diet.

    C. parenteral nutrition.

    D. vitamin therapy.

83. When evaluating a patient with a chronic pressure ulcer on the hip that has not shown signs of healing despite appropriate wound care, a possible diagnosis to consider is:

    A. zoster infection.

    B. impetigo.

    C. Marjolin's ulcer.

    D. actinic keratosis.

For answers and rationales, see end of chapter.

Delirium, Dementia, and Depression

Overview

Older adults are at higher risk for cognitive disorders that can be acute, such as delirium, or chronic, such as dementia. In addition, depression, potentially leading to cognitive issues, is common in the elderly. Adding to the complexity of evaluation and treating the older adult with a cognitive disorder is that these conditions can occur simultaneously, creating a diagnostic challenge.

In any patient with alteration in cognitive status, a thorough health history, including social and home assessment, and a physical examination should be conducted. A standardized evaluation of mental status must be included in the evaluation. The evaluation of the patient with mental status change starts with a comprehensive health history and physical examination.

DELIRIUM

Overview

Delirium is a condition in which the patient exhibits an acute onset, over hours to a few days, of reduced ability to maintain attention to external stimuli and shift attention appropriately to new stimuli. The result is disorganized thinking.

Following is the DELIRIUMS mnemonic, which can serve as a helpful memory aid regarding the most common causes of delirium.

- *D*rugs—When any medication is added or dose is adjusted. Particularly problematic medications include systemic anticholinergics (TCAs, first-generation antihistamines), neuroleptics (haloperidol, others), opioids (in particular, meperidine), long-acting benzodiazepines (diazepam, clonazepam), and alcohol.
- *E*motional—Mood disorders, loss; *E*lectrolyte disturbance, especially hyponatremia.
- *L*ow Po2—Hypoxemia from community-acquired pneumonia (CAP), chronic obstructive pulmonary disease (COPD), pulmonary embolism (PE), myocardial infarction (MI); *L*ack of drugs (withdrawal from alcohol, other habituating substances).
- *I*nfection—Urinary tract infection and CAP (the most common delirium trigger).
- *R*etention of urine or feces; *R*educed sensory input (blindness, deafness, darkness, change in surroundings).

- *I*ctal or postictal state—Alcohol withdrawal is a common reason for an isolated first seizure in an older adult.
- *U*ndernutrition—Protein/calorie, vitamin B_{12}, or folate deficiency, dehydration including postoperative volume disturbance.
- *M*etabolic (poorly controlled diabetes mellitus, undertreated or untreated hypothyroidism or hyperthyroidism); *M*yocardial problems (myocardial infarction, heart failure, dysrhythmia).
- *S*ubdural hematoma—Can be as a result of relatively minor head trauma to brain atrophy, fragile vessels.

Clinical Presentation

Two or more of the following are usually noted: an altered level of consciousness from baseline; memory impairment; perceptual disturbance, such as hallucinations; altered sleep; change in psychomotor activity; and disorientation to time, place, and person.

Diagnostic Testing

Delirium is not a diagnosis, but rather a clinical state caused by an underlying health problem. The evaluation of a patient with delirium should be focused on defining the underlying cause; there is no specific test to rule in or out the condition. Diagnostic testing should be focused to reveal the diagnosis of the underlying etiology with potentially reversible conditions (Table 16-5).

Treatment

Delirium treatment is aimed at assessing patients at greatest risk to help avoid its occurrence. When delirium occurs, treatment is focused on the condition's underlying cause. Mental status should return to baseline

TABLE 16-5 Evaluation of the Person With Mental Status Change

The evaluation of the patient with mental status change starts with a comprehensive health history and physical examination. Diagnostic testing should be focused to reveal the underlying etiology with potentially reversible conditions.

DEFINITE	AS DIRECTED BY PATIENT PRESENTATION
BUN, Cr	Brain imaging (CT versus MRI)
Glucose	PET scan
Calcium	Toxic screen
Sodium	CXR
Hepatic enzymes	ESR
Vitamin B_{12}/folate	HIV
TSH	Additional studies as needed
RPR/VDRL	
CBC with WBC differential	
UA, UC, and S	
ECG	

BUN, blood urea nitrogen; CBC, complete blood count; Cr, creatinine; CT, computed tomography; CXR, chest x-ray; ECG, electrocardiogram; ESR, erythrocyte sedimentation rate; MRI, magnetic resonance imaging; PET, positron emission tomography; RPR, rapid plasma reagin; S; TSH, thyroid-stimulating hormone; UA, urinalysis; UC, urine culture; VDRL, Venereal Disease Research Laboratory; WBC, white blood cell.

with recovery, although ongoing research suggests that perhaps this recovery is incomplete in some individuals. In about two-thirds of all patients with delirium, the condition resolves within 1 week of onset.

DEMENTIA

Overview

Dementia is defined by a chronic loss of intellectual or cognitive function of sufficient severity to interfere with social or occupational function; this condition is a symptom of an underlying diagnosis (Table 16-6). In dementia, mental status changes can evolve insidiously over months or years with a gradually worsening course. The most common causes of dementia are AD and multi-infarct or vascular dementia.

Clinical Presentation

The evaluation of a person with suspected dementia is similar to assessment in delirium; the two conditions often overlap and can mimic each other (Table 16-7). Diagnosis of AD requires a gradual onset of memory impairment plus one or more of the following: aphasia (language disturbance); apraxia (impairment of motor activities despite intact motor function); agnosia (failure to recognize objects despite intact sensory function); and executive functioning disturbance (planning, organizing, sequencing, abstracting). The deficits cause a significant impairment that represents a considerable decline from the previous level of function.

Mild cognitive impairment (MCI) can be an early sign of dementia. About 80% diagnosed with MCI will progress to AD within 7 years. MCI is characterized by memory problems that are beyond normal age-related changes. Sign of MCI include frequently losing things, forgetting to go to events or appointments, and having difficulty finding correct words in conversation.

Diagnostic Testing

AD is primarily a clinical diagnosis. Screening older adults for cognitive impairment can be important to help differentiate between reversible causes (e.g., medications, metabolic or endocrine issues) and irreversible causes (e.g., AD). Screening should be performed for all adults over 80 years of age as well as when an individual or family member expresses concerns about changes in memory or thinking, or if the healthcare provider observes issues with the patient's memory or thinking. Several screening tools are available for administration in the primary care setting, such as the GPCOG, Mini-COG, IQCODE, or AD8, and testing should be complemented with interviews with the patient and/or close family members to fully assess changes in memory, behavior, mood, and functional status. Genetic testing, neuroimaging, and biomarker testing are not useful in a diagnosis of dementia.

When diagnosing AD, guidelines identify three stages of disease:

■ *Preclinical*: Changes in the brain are progressing (such as amyloid buildup), but significant clinical symptoms are not yet evident

■ *Mild cognitive impairment*: Symptoms of memory and/or thinking problems are greater than normal for a person's age and education, but they do not interfere with the individual's independence.

■ *Alzheimer's dementia*: Symptoms are significant enough to impair a person's ability to function independently

TABLE 16-6 Dementia Etiology

DEMENTIA TYPE	COMMENT
Alzheimer's type	50% to 70%
Vascular (multi-infarct) dementia	Approximately 20%
Other: Parkinson's disease, Huntington's disease, Pick's disease, Creutzfeldt-Jakob disease	Approximately 10%
Miscellaneous causes	HIV, dialysis encephalopathy, neurosyphilis, normal pressure hydrocephalus, others

TABLE 16-7 Delirium Versus Dementia

	DELIRIUM	DEMENTIA
Definition	A sudden state of rapid changes in brain function reflected in confusion, changes in cognition, activity, and level of consciousness	A slowly developing impairment of intellectual or cognitive function that is progressive and interferes with normal functioning
Etiology	Precipitated by acute underlying cause, such as an acute illness	Various causes
Onset	Abrupt onset, over hours to days, usually a precise date, rapidly progressive change in mental status	Insidious onset that cannot be related to a precise date, gradual change in mental status
Memory	Impaired by variable recall	Memory loss, especially for recent events
Duration	Hours to days	Months to years
Reversible?	Usually reversible to baseline mental status when underlying illness resolved	Chronically progressive and irreversible
Sleep disturbance	Disturbed sleep-wake cycle, with hour-to-hour variability, often worse as the day progresses	Disturbed sleep-wake cycle but lacks hour-to-hour variability, often day-night reversal
Psychomotor	Change in psychomotor activity, either hyperkinetic (25%), hypoactive (25%), or mixed (35%); no change in motor activity in approximately 15%	No psychomotor changes until later in disease
Perceptual disturbances	Perceptual disturbances including hallucinations	No perceptual disturbances until later disease
Speech	Speech content incoherent, confused with a wide variety of often inappropriately used words such as misnamed persons and items	Speech content sparse, progressing to sparse speech content; mute in later disease

Note: Delirium and dementia often coexist. The diagnosis of delirium must be considered in the presence of sudden-onset change in mental status in the individual with dementia.

Source: Overview of delirium and dementia. Merck Manual. https://www.merckmanuals.com/professional/neurologic-disorders/delirium-and-dementia/overview-of-delirium-and-dementia#v1036234

Treatment

Early diagnosis and treatment of AD can help to slow disease progression and prolong cognitive function for as long as possible. In mild to moderate AD, mental exercises along with cholinesterase inhibitors can be used. Mentally challenging activities, such as crossword puzzles or brainteasers, can potentially reduce the risk of disease progression from MCI to AD, though this has yet to be supported in well-designed clinical studies. Patients with dementia often benefit from the use of a cholinesterase inhibitor (ChEI), such as donepezil (Aricept®), tacrine (Cognex®), rivastigmine (Exelon®), and galantamine (Razadyne®), which prevent the breakdown of acetylcholine. Though clinically significant, the effect of ChEIs in mild to moderate AD is generally minor and time limited. In moderate to severe disease, the *N*-methyl D-aspartate (NMDA)-receptor antagonist memantine (Namenda®) can help to minimize disease progression and can be used in combination with a ChEI. These classes of medications have different mechanisms of action and can be safely given together. Research has demonstrated a delay in institutionalization of patients with AD when combination therapy is used (Table 16-8). The use of any of these products to prevent dementia is currently not supported. The use of both drug classes in late disease is not advised.

For all patients with AD, regular physical activity and exercise can help slow disease progression. Exercise should be encouraged and adapted according to the individual's ability. A growing body of evidence is also suggesting a protective effect of exercise against the development of AD. A healthy diet might also

TABLE 16-8 American Academy of Neurology Standards for Care in Alzheimer's-Type Dementia (AD)

STRATEGY	COMMENT
To slow decline in AD.	Vitamin E 1,000 IU twice daily or selegiline 5 mg twice daily. No added benefit to using both products.
In mild to moderate stages of disease, the use of cholinesterase inhibitors is considered the mainstay of treatment. The use of these products in mild cognitive impairment, early AD, and severe AD is not supported, although study on these issues is ongoing.	Cholinesterase inhibitors (donepezil [Aricept®], rivastigmine [Exelon®], galantamine [Razadyne®]) have clear, although minor and time-limited, benefits by increasing availability of cholinesterase. This small effect is clinically significant.
In moderate to severe AD, further studies of multiple interventions are needed.	Approved for use in moderate to severe AD, *N*-methyl D-aspartate receptor antagonist memantine (Namenda®). Through its effect on glutamate, helps to create an environment that allows for storage and retrieval of information. Can be combined with cholinesterase inhibitor for added benefit. Rivastigmine transdermal and donepezil also approved for use in more advanced disease.
Treat agitation and depression.	Approximately 40% of individuals with dementia will also have depression. Selective serotonin reuptake inhibitors, select tricyclic antidepressants, and monoamine oxidase inhibitors are appropriate treatment options, bearing in mind potential drug-drug and drug-food interactions.
Consider reasons (noncognitive) not related to AD for behavioral issues, such as behavioral disturbances.	Evaluate for depression, pain, infection, and other clinical conditions commonly found in older adults.
If environmental manipulation fails to eliminate agitation or psychosis in the person with dementia, consider treatment with psychotropic medication.	Antipsychotics best studied for this indication, recognizing the increased risk of stroke and cardiovascular events associated with the use of this drug class in older adults with dementia.

Source: Doody RS, Stevens JC, Beck C, et al. Practice parameter: management of dementia (an evidence-based review): report of the Quality Standards Subcommittee of the American Academy of Neurology. Neurology. 2001;56:1154–1166. https://n.neurology.org/content/56/9/1154.full.pdf

prevent or delay the development of AD, though this has yet to be confirmed in clinical studies. Heavy alcohol consumption is the strongest modifiable risk factor for dementia.

DEPRESSION

Overview

Depression in older adults is common but should not be considered a normal part of aging. Some estimates of major depression in older adults range from 1% to 5% for persons living in the community but rise to 13.5% for those who require home health care.

Clinical Presentation

Signs of depression in the elderly can be wide and varied:

■ Feelings of hopelessness and/or pessimism
■ Feelings of guilt, worthlessness, and/or helplessness
■ Irritability and/or restlessness
■ Loss of interest in activities or hobbies that were once pleasurable
■ Fatigue and decreased energy
■ Difficulty concentrating, remembering details, and making decisions

CLINICAL CONCEPT

Depression in the older adult is also more common in those who have comorbid conditions (e.g., heart disease, cancer).

- Insomnia, early morning wakefulness, or excessive sleeping
- Overeating or appetite loss
- Thoughts of suicide or suicide attempts
- Persistent aches and pains, headaches, cramps, or digestive problems that do not resolve, even with treatment

Pseudodementia (also known as depressive pseudodementia) is a dementia syndrome or cognitive impairment that is associated with severe depression. Its onset is often well demarcated as compared with the gradual and insidious development of dementia. It may take patients with pseudodementia increased effort to complete a mental status examination (MSE), and they often do better on MSE questions with some encouragement and coaching. Neurocognitive testing is often needed to differentiate between pseudodementia and dementia. Treating the depression often improves memory functions in these patients, though some deficits can persist, including memory and executive functions. Thus, individuals suspected of having pseudodementia should undergo full dementia screening for early detection and treatment of AD.

Diagnostic Testing

For those suspected of depression, several screening tools are available to aid in the diagnosis or indicate when further investigation is needed (Table 16-9).

Treatment

When considering treatment for depression, the patient should be encouraged to undergo psychotherapy in addition to pharmacological treatment in order to work on building skills needed to help manage this usually long-term health problem. There are several types of antidepressant medications that can be used to treat depression, including selective serotonin reuptake inhibitors (SSRIs), serotonin-norepinephrine reuptake inhibitors (SNRIs), TCAs, and monoamine oxidase inhibitors (MAOIs). (See Chapter 15.) The choice of a psychotropic medication for depression intervention is guided by desired clinical effect and adverse effect profile. The TCAs and MAOIs are not commonly used in the older adult due to unfavorable adverse effect profiles, cardiac consideration, potential drug interactions, as well as potential systemic anticholinergic effects. The type and degree of depression as well as the adverse effect profile must be considered when selecting an appropriate antidepressant.

Some patients are candidates for other forms of intervention in addition to medications, particularly if there is an inadequate response to pharmacotherapy and/or psychotherapy; one option is electroconvulsive therapy (ECT). ECT is safe and effective for all older adults with severe depression, particularly in the presence of a psychosis and/or nutritional compromise.

TABLE 16-9 Screening Tools Used in Older Adults for Mental Health and Cognition

Geriatric Depression Scale (GDS)	Screening tool for depression in older adults 30 questions ■ Greater than 10 warrants further investigation
Cornell Scale for Depression in Dementia	Screening tool for depression in patients with dementia 19 questions ■ Greater than 12 indicates depression possibility
Mini-Mental Status Examination	Screens for cognitive impairment and used to follow cognitive function over time. High education can score falsely high. ■ 30-point questionnaire ■ Intact = 25 to 30 ■ Mild = 21 to 24 ■ Moderate = 10 to 20 ■ Severe = 9 or less

When initiating pharmacotherapy for a variety of conditions, including mood disorders in older adults, it is important to "start low, go slow, but get to goal." The latter point is important as there is a tendency to undertreat. As polypharmacy is frequent in older adults, health-care providers must consider any potential drug-drug interactions; periodic monitoring of renal and hepatic function is also recommended as dictated by comorbidity.

Discussion Sources

Melrose S. Late life depression: nursing actions that can help. *Perspect Psychiatr Care.* 2018; https://doi.org/10.1111/ppc.12341

National Institute on Aging. Assessing cognitive impairment in older patients. https://www.nia.nih.gov/health/assessing-cognitive-impairment-older-patients

Overview of delirium and dementia. Merck Manual. https://www.merckmanuals.com/professional/neurologic_disorders/delirium_and_dementia/overview_of_delirium_and_dementia.html#v1036234

QUESTIONS

84 to 88. Identify the following as most likely associated with either delirium or dementia.

_____ **84.** insidious onset over months to years

_____ **85.** acute onset of change in mental status

_____ **86.** commonly associated with use of medications with systemic anticholinergic effect

_____ **87.** mental status potentially returns to baseline prior to acute illness

_____ **88.** no perceptual disturbances (i.e., hallucinations) until later disease

89. The most common trigger for delirium is:

A. alcohol withdrawal.

B. fecal impaction.

C. head trauma.

D. acute infection.

90. The most common etiology of dementia is:

A. vascular disease.

B. AD.

C. traumatic head injury.

D. drug-drug interaction induced.

91. Medications that commonly contribute to delirium include all of the following except:

A. first-generation antihistamines.

B. cardioselective β-adrenergic antagonists.

C. opioids.

D. benzodiazepines.

92. Which of the following electrolyte disorders is commonly associated with delirium?

A. hyponatremia

B. hypernatremia

C. hyperkalemia

D. hypophosphatemia

93. Older adults are at greater risk of subdural hematoma, even with minor head trauma, because of:

A. lower bone density in the skull.

B. relatively fragile blood vessels.

C. decreased adipose tissue reserves.

D. age-related reduction in circulating clotting factors.

94. When discussing the use of a cholinesterase inhibitor with a 72-year-old woman with a recent diagnosis of AD and her family, you report that:

    A. this medication will help return memory to her pre-illness baseline.

    B. the risk associated with the use of this medication outweighs its benefits.

    C. this medication will likely afford clear, although minor and time-limited, benefits.

    D. the medication should have been started earlier to help prevent any change in cognition.

95. When managing dementia, cholinesterase inhibitors offer the greatest benefit:

    A. for prevention of AD.

    B. in patients with mild cognitive impairment.

    C. in patients with mild to moderate AD.

    D. in patients with severe AD.

96. When assessing a 76-year-old man with new-onset mental status change, all of the following diagnostic tests are essential except:

    A. serum glucose.

    B. positron emission tomography (PET) scan.

    C. CBC with white blood cell differential.

    D. ECG.

97. An 81-year-old man who was recently diagnosed with AD is accompanied by his granddaughter for an office visit. The granddaughter reports that her grandfather often acts erratically with angry outbursts that can soon be followed by a more "normal" demeanor. She reports that the grandfather recently moved in with her, and she would like for this arrangement to continue as long as possible. In counseling the granddaughter, you consider all of the following except that:

    A. behavioral difficulties often arise in patients with AD if their usual routine is disrupted.

    B. treatment with a cholinesterase inhibitor will maintain his cognitive ability to the current status for a protracted period of time.

    C. a home safety evaluation should be conducted and appropriate modification performed.

    D. any sudden change in mental status should be reported to the health-care provider as soon as possible.

98. Which of the following nutritional supplements is used to potentially slow cognitive decline in AD?

    A. vitamin B_{12}

    B. vitamin E

    C. ginkgo biloba

    D. St. John's wort

99. The NMDA-receptor antagonist memantine is recommended for use:

    A. in preventing dementia.

    B. at early stages of AD.

    C. in moderate to severe stages of AD.

    D. at any time following an AD diagnosis.

100. When considering the use of memantine with a cholinesterase inhibitor, the NP realizes:

    A. there are significant safety concerns with combination therapy.

    B. there is no additional benefit of combination therapy in AD.

    C. combination therapy can reverse cognitive decline in early stages of AD.

    D. combination therapy can have additive benefits in moderate to severe AD.

101. Potential noncognitive reasons for behavioral issues observed in older adults include all of the following except:

A. attention-deficit hyperactivity disorder (ADHD).

B. pain.

C. infection.

D. depression.

102 to 104. Match the term with its correct definition.

_____ **102.** aphasia

_____ **103.** apraxia

_____ **104.** agnosia

A. failure to recognize objects despite intact sensory function

B. language disturbance

C. impairment of motor activities despite intact motor function

105. The use of second-generation antipsychotic medications in older adults with dementia is associated with an increased risk for:

A. stroke and cardiovascular events.

B. hypoglycemia.

C. psychosis.

D. hypertension.

106. Dementia syndrome or cognitive impairment that is associated with severe depression is called:

A. delirium.

B. pseudodementia.

C. AD.

D. bipolar disorder.

107. When managing depression in older adults, all of the following should be considered except:

A. starting at the highest dose possible of antidepressant and then titrating down once symptoms resolve.

B. encouraging psychotherapy in addition to pharmacotherapy.

C. utilizing ECT for severe depression.

D. conducting a medication review to minimize potential drug-drug interactions.

For answers and rationales, see end of chapter.

Ethical and Legal Issues

Health-Care Decision Making

Advance directives are durable statements of intent based on the patient's last written wishes and can be used to help make end-of-life decisions. Advance directives can exist in several forms. Increasingly, medical orders for life-sustaining decisions (MOLST) or patient/provider/portable orders for life-sustaining decisions (POLST), forms of advance directives, are used. MOLST/POLST orders are developed after in-depth discussion between a seriously ill patient (or health-care agent if the patient cannot communicate) and health-care providers and carefully defines the life-sustaining treatments the patient wants to receive or avoid at the current time. MOLST/POLST orders include all interventions up to and including the patient's wishes on resuscitation; *Do not resuscitate (DNR)* orders are usually included in MOLST/ POLST orders.

When considering life-sustaining decisions for a terminally ill patient who cannot communicate, several approaches can be used. Often, an appointed person can make the decision based on the patient's past wishes and values. A sensible approach can make the decision based on what a "rational" person would

CLINICAL CONCEPT

Once the MOLST/POLST form is completed, it should be honored by health-care providers in all settings, including emergency health-care personnel during emergencies.

do under the circumstances. A substituted judgment approach attempts to determine what decision the patient would make if he or she were able to do so.

A *durable power of attorney for health care* authorizes another person to make decisions regarding health care when the patient is no longer able (not to be confused with a *durable power of attorney*, which covers decisions regarding property and financial matters). Alternatively, a *values history* can be a written, videotaped, or audiotaped personal discussion that can contain advance directives that can be taken into consideration when making end-of-life decisions. It is important to note that although advance directives are legally recognized by every state, they are not necessarily legally binding in all circumstances. For example, health-care providers can refuse to comply with an advance directive if they have an objection of conscience or consider the wishes to be medically inappropriate. With well-developed MOLST/POLST orders, seldom will there be confusion or disagreement in carrying out the patient's wishes.

Effects of Aging and Cognitive Changes on Decision Making

When caring for older adults, there are particular legal and ethical issues that must be considered by health-care providers. Owing to age-related diminished cognitive function in many older adults, there is the issue of patient competence to make informed decisions. The law presumes that all adults are competent to make their own decisions regarding their health care. Competence refers to the ability to make a legal decision in a rational manner. This should not be confused with capacity, which is determined by one or more health-care providers and refers to an assessment of the individual's psychological abilities to form rational decisions, specifically the individual's ability to understand, appreciate, and manipulate information and form rational decisions.

Only health-care providers have the ability to determine whether or not a patient has the ability to provide informed consent. When obtaining informed consent for health-care treatment, it is essential that the patient has knowledge of the diagnosis; understands the nature and purpose of the procedure; understands the risks, benefits, and adverse effects of the procedure; and understands reasonable alternatives, if available. A person is considered incompetent if he or she does not exhibit the mental ability and cognitive capabilities required to rationally execute a legally recognized act. Only a court can declare a person incompetent and appoint a guardian to make decisions for him or her. It is important to remember that impaired judgment does not make a person incompetent. Some patients will establish a health-care proxy, which is a legal document that appoints an agent to legally make health-care decisions on behalf of the patient when the patient is incapable of making those decisions. If an individual is determined to be incompetent and did not have a *durable power of attorney for health care* in place, then a court-appointed conservatorship might be needed. This is a time-consuming process that appoints an agent (conservator) to make health-care decisions, estate decisions, or both. The conservator is held responsible and accountable to the court. Conservatorships are mainly reserved for individuals in a coma, with advanced dementia, or with other serious illnesses or injuries.

Ageism

Despite many older adults being physically and mentally active, they are often subjected to ageism. This is defined as the process of stereotyping, prejudice, or discrimination for or against the elderly. Ageism can diminish choice, independence, and dignity and can negatively impact quality of life. Common ageism stereotypes include associating various physical or mental illnesses or disabilities with older age (e.g., memory loss or slow to understand things) as well as assuming that older persons lack knowledge of new technologies or culture (e.g., computers, social media). The consequences of ageism for an individual can be substantial, including depression, employment discrimination, lower socioeconomic status, and conforming to the stereotyped image.

Use of Restraints in the Older Adult

Physical restraints are commonly used in elderly patients in nonpsychiatric care settings, with one estimate of between 25% and 43% of residents in long-term care facilities being restrained at least once, despite statements by well-regarded authorities, backed by evidence, that physical restraints should not be used among older hospitalized patients. Chemical restraints are also frequently used to sedate an individual in an effort to prevent harming of self or others. Too often chemical restraints are used in institutionalized settings for the purpose of staff convenience, discipline, or other nonmedical reason.

The Omnibus Budget Reconciliation Act of 1987 provides that every resident of a long-term care facility has the right to be free from physical or chemical restraints imposed for the purpose of discipline or convenience and not required to treat health-care needs. Physical or chemical restraints are often seen as the only practical way to protect the safety of elderly patients and reduce the potential for liability if they injure themselves. However, when injury occurs to unrestrained individuals in the institutional setting, successful lawsuits are typically not the result of failure to restrain but a failure to meet reasonable standards of care—that is, there was negligence in duty to provide care for a wandering patient or alarm systems were not functional at the institution.

When chemical restraints are deemed necessary, the three main classes of medications used include benzodiazepines (e.g., lorazepam, diazepam), typical (first-generation) antipsychotics (e.g., haloperidol, droperidol), and atypical (second-generation) antipsychotics (e.g., risperidone, olanzapine, ziprasidone). Health-care providers and caregivers should monitor patients closely while using a chemical restraint for potentially serious adverse effects. Second-generation antipsychotics in particular have been associated with an increased risk of stroke and cardiovascular events in older adults. Many health-care institutions have banned the use of chemical restraints, though federal agencies, such as The Joint Commission, offer guidance on the use of restraints to keep the patient, staff, and others safe, though they should only be used as a last resort.

Common alternatives for physical and chemical restraints include the use of alarms, using beds or chairs that are close to the floor, and/or ensuring the unit/floor/facility is equipped to care for a patient with known behaviors. If physical restraints are needed for patient safety, it is important for health-care providers to have a thorough understanding of the risks and benefits of using restraints. This will be important in explaining the need for physical restraints to family members, who may see their use in a negative manner. Adverse effects of physical or chemical restraints include falls, pressure sores, depression, aggression, and even death. Physical restraints can also be a source of aggravation to the patient under restraint.

Discussion Sources

American Academy of Nursing. Physical restraints. http://www.aannet.org/initiatives/choosing-wisely/physical-restraints

National Institute on Aging. *Understanding Healthcare Decisions at the End of Life.* https://www.nia.nih.gov/health/understanding-healthcare-decisions-end-life

QUESTIONS

108. Which of the following statements is true with regard to decision making for the patient with cognitive impairment?

    A. Only a court or close family member can declare a person incompetent.

    B. Impaired judgment can be used to declare a person incompetent.

    C. Health-care providers have the ability to determine whether a patient can provide informed consent.

    D. Informed consent does not necessarily require disclosing the diagnosis to the patient.

109. The use of physical restraints in older adults is appropriate:

    A. as a form of reinforcement to prevent future potentially dangerous behavior.

    B. when needed to meet a health-care need.

    C. to prevent wandering outside an institution.

    D. under no circumstances.

110. When considering end-of-life decisions, which of the following statements is false?

    A. MOLST/POLST orders are considered to be forms of advance directives.

    B. A videotaped or audiotaped discussion can include advance directives.

    C. Advance directives are legally binding in all states.

    D. Advance directives are most often recognized when the patient is terminally ill where there is no clear path to recovery.

111. When considering the use of a chemical restraint in an older adult, the NP considers that chemical restraints:

  A. can include benzodiazepines and first- and second-generation antipsychotics.

  B. can be used as a form of discipline for unruly patients.

  C. are generally safe in older adults.

  D. are banned by federal agencies.

For answers and rationales, see end of chapter.

Author's Note

Please see Index for information on commonly encountered problems in older adults, including urinary tract infection, male and female genitourinary problems, endocrine disorders, pneumonia, chronic obstructive pulmonary disease, heart failure, and others.

QUESTION ANSWERS AND RATIONALES

Demographics in Older Adults

1. Correct: D. 85 years and older.
The oldest old (85 to 100 years old) and the elite old (older than 100 years) are the fastest-growing segments in the U.S. population due to the extended life spans (D). However, with the entry of the first wave of the Baby Boomers now turning 65 years, this can alter the demographics in the United States.

2 to 4. Matching Questions

2. Correct: B. 65 to 74 years

3. Correct: D. 85 to 100 years

4. Correct: E. Over 100 years
Older adults can be grouped into four demographic categories. The young old comprise those 65 to 74 years (2), the old old are those who are 75 to 84 years, the oldest old are those 85 to 100 years (3), while the elite old comprise those over 100 years of age (4). The first wave of Baby Boomers is part of the young old category.

5. Correct: A. Social Security
Social Security is identified as the most important source of income among older adults with over 40% of single recipients depending on Social Security for 90% of their income (A).
Incorrect:
Social Security is most frequently identified as the most important source of income for older adults. Private and public pensions (B) as well as income from other investments (C) are identified less than half as frequently as the most important source of income when compared to Social Security. Family financial support is not as substantial as Social Security as an income source (D).

6. Correct: B. highest among the old old.
Approximately 10% of older adults live in poverty. Those at higher risk include the old old (B), as well as women living alone and certain ethnic groups.

Incorrect:
Higher poverty rates are observed among the old old and certain ethnic groups (A). Women living alone also tend to have a higher poverty rate compared to married couples (C). Fortunately, the poverty rate among older adults has decreased by about half since the 1970s (D).

7. Correct: C. 33%
Economic insecurity is defined as living at or below 250% of the federal poverty level, currently at $29,425 for a single person in 2019. Those with economic insecurity can struggle with rising costs of housing and health care and are at risk of malnutrition. It is estimated that one in three older adults are economically insecure (C).

Age-Associated Changes in the Senses

8 to 12. Matching Questions

8. Correct: B. presbycusis

9. Correct: A. hyposmia

10. Correct: D. age-related maculopathy

11. Correct: C. presbyopia

12. Correct: E. chronic glaucoma
Normal age-related changes can affect the various senses in older adults. Hyposmia (9) is a decreased sense of smell, while anosmia is a total loss of the sense of smell. Presbycusis is a progressive loss of high-frequency sound that often makes it difficult to follow a conversation in a noisy environment (8). Vision changes are common in older age. Presbyopia results from hardening of the lens and causes close vision problems (11). Central vision loss is a typical finding with macular degeneration and can lead to permanent vision loss (10). Glaucoma, caused by increased intraocular pressure, can result in peripheral vision loss and is the second leading cause of blindness (12).

13. **Correct: B. alcohol abuse.**
Senile cataracts result in lens clouding that is often correctable with surgery and a lens implant. Several risk factors have been identified for the condition, but excessive use of alcohol is not among them (B).
Incorrect:
Risk factors for senile cataracts include tobacco use (A), poor nutrition, exposure to sunlight (D), and corticosteroid therapy (C).

14. **Correct: D. reading road signs while driving**
Senile cataracts is a progressive condition that causes dimming as well as distance vision problems. Close vision is usually retained. Thus, reading road signs while driving would present the greatest difficulty for this patient (D).
Incorrect:
Cataracts are associated with distance vision problems, while near vision is retained. Reading a newspaper would be difficult for the patient with presbyopia (A). A yellowing of the lens with aging can also lead to washing out of colors (B). Loss of peripheral vision is associated with open-angle glaucoma (C).

15. **Correct: D. a gradual loss of peripheral vision.**
A gradual loss of peripheral vision is associated with open-angle glaucoma, which is not considered a normal age-related change and should be appropriately managed to avoid permanent vision loss (D).
Incorrect:
Normal age-related changes include a hardening of the lens as well as yellowing of the lens. This can lead to close vision problems, a need for increased illumination (A), increased sensitivity to glare (B), and washing out of colors (C).

16. **Correct: C. tobacco use.**
Risk factors for macular degeneration include tobacco use (C), sun exposure, and a family history of the condition.
Incorrect:
In addition to aging, several risk factors have been identified for macular degeneration. However, hypertension (A), hyperlipidemia (B), and alcohol abuse (D) are not among these risk factors.

17. **Correct: B. to use ear protection when exposed to loud noises.**
Presbycusis is associated with difficulty following a conversation in a noisy environment. Risk factors include exposure to a noisy environment, aging, family history, tobacco use, cardiovascular disease, diabetes, otosclerosis, infection, and trauma to the ear. An effective method to prevent this condition is to use protective earwear when exposed to loud noises (B).
Incorrect:
Hearing aids can be helpful for individuals with presbycusis, and avoiding their use will not prevent the condition (C). Though avoiding the use of cotton swabs in the ear canal is important for preventing an ear injury, this will not prevent presbycusis (A). Removal of cerumen will help to improve conductive hearing loss, but this is separate from presbycusis (D).

18. **Correct: B. diminution of high-frequency hearing.**
Presbycusis is a progressive, symmetric, high-frequency, age-related sensory hearing loss that is likely caused by cochlear deterioration. A main complaint of this condition is speech discrimination, particularly in a noisy environment.
Incorrect:
Presbycusis is characterized by diminution of high-frequency hearing rather than low-pitched sounds (D). The individual can hear the surrounding sounds but has difficulty distinguishing speech and following a conversation (A). The condition does not get worse at night (C) but is usually worse in noisy environments.

19. **Correct: A. a general diminution of hearing.**
Cerumen impaction will result in conductive hearing loss and result in a general diminution of hearing (A). Regular cerumen removal will resolve the condition.
Incorrect:
Presbycusis is associated with an ability to hear but an inability to understand a conversation in a noisy environment (D). Cerumen impaction leads to a general decrease in hearing, including low- and high-pitched sounds (B). The condition is not associated with additional pain when exposed to high-pitched sounds (C).

Medication Use in the Older Adult

20. **Correct: C. an increase in serum albumin.**
Age-related changes can impact pharmacological effects and should be considered when selecting and dosing medications. Serum albumin decreases in older adults (C), and this can result in a higher proportion of free drug for medications that are normally highly protein-bound, such as warfarin and phenytoin.
Incorrect:
In older adults, percent body weight as water decreases (A), which will cause an older person to dehydrate more easily due to lower water reserves. Older adults also have a higher percentage of body weight as fat (B). This can affect the action of lipophilic medications, as they tend to remain in the body longer in older adults. Gastric acid production decreases in the elderly causing a rise in stomach pH (D). This can prolong the breakdown of medications that are designed to dissolve in low pH environments.

21. **Correct: B. rate of absorption is changed.**
Changes in the elderly GI tract can lead to changes in the rate of drug absorption (B). Stomach pH is higher in older adults, which can prolong breakdown of medications designed to dissolve in low pH environments. Additionally, decreases in GI blood flow, motility, and gastric emptying will prolong the length of time a medication stays in the gut.

Incorrect:
Though the rate of absorption can change due to age-related changes in the GI system, the total amount of drug absorption does not necessarily decrease (A). Decreased GI surface area, along with changes in stomach pH and motility, can lead to erratic and unpredictable effects on drug absorption (C). Bioavailability, or the percentage of drug that reaches systemic circulation, does not necessarily change though the rate of absorption can be altered (D).

22. **Correct: A. loss of β_2-receptor sites.**
A normative age-related change is a loss of β_2-receptor sites. This can result in a decreased clinical effect when using β_2-agonists, such as albuterol and formoterol.
Incorrect:
Aging can lead to suppressed production of renin and angiotensin, which can predispose the elderly to various fluid and electrolyte abnormalities (C). Older adults have decreased production of gastric acid leading to high stomach pH (B). Other changes in the GI system in the elderly include decreased motility (D), blood flow, and surface area.

23. **Correct: C. increased GI surface area.**
A normative age-related change in the GI system is decreased surface area in the gut (C). This can have an erratic effect on drug absorption.
Incorrect:
Other age-related changes in the GI tract include decreased gastric acid production (leading to a higher stomach pH) (A), decreased gastric motility (B), and decreased gastric emptying (D). These changes can impact the pharmacokinetics of medications, particularly in decreasing the rate of drug absorption and prolonging the amount of time that a medication remains in the gut.

24. **Correct: A. A lower dose is usually needed due to lower serum albumin.**
Warfarin is a highly protein-bound drug that has an affinity for albumin in the blood. Serum albumin decreases with age, resulting in a higher amount of free warfarin circulating and exerting its clinical effect. Thus, when dosing warfarin in the elderly, a lower dose is needed as a greater amount of the drug will be freely circulating due to a lower concentration of serum albumin (A).

25 to 28. Yes or No

25. **Correct: Yes**

26. **Correct: No**

27. **Correct: Yes**

28. **Correct: Yes**
Beers Criteria recommend avoiding medications with strong anticholinergic effect due to the potential for adverse reactions in the elderly. These effects can include confusion (25) or cognitive impairment, urinary retention (27), constipation (28), visual disturbance, and

hypotension. Hypertension is not associated with anticholinergic medications (26).

29. **Correct: C. pharmacokinetics.**
Pharmacokinetics describes what the body does to a drug and includes components of absorption, distribution, metabolism, and elimination (C).
Incorrect:
Pharmacodynamics describes the biochemical and physiological effects of a drug on the body or disease (A). For example, pharmacodynamic aspects of an antimicrobial can include C_{max}/MIC or AUC/MIC, where MIC is the minimal inhibitory concentration of the infecting organism. Drug interactions study is an unspecified term that can be used to understand drug-drug or drug-food interactions (B). Therapeutic transformation is a nondefined term (D).

30. **Correct: A. pharmacodynamics.**
Pharmacodynamics describes the biochemical and physiological effects of a drug on the body or disease (A). For example, pharmacodynamic aspects of an antimicrobial can include C_{max}/MIC or AUC/MIC, where MIC is the minimal inhibitory concentration of the infecting organism.
Incorrect:
Pharmacokinetics describes what the body does to a drug and includes components of absorption, distribution, metabolism, and elimination (B). Biotransformation refers to metabolism of a drug, typically by the cytochrome P450 system, and can convert a prodrug into its active form or convert an active form into an inactive form for elimination/excretion (C). Bioavailability refers to the percentage of an oral medication that will enter systemic circulation (D).

31. **Correct: C. pharmacodynamics**
Pharmacodynamics describes the biochemical and physiological effects of a drug on the body or disease. The pharmacodynamics of a medication do not change as a person ages (C).
Incorrect:
The components of a drug's pharmacokinetics can change as a person ages. Excretion will depend on renal function (A), while biotransformation can change depending on liver function and the CYP450 system (B). Age-related changes in the GI system can have a substantial impact on drug absorption (D).

32. **Correct: B. 50%.**
By definition, the half-life of a drug is the amount of time required to reduce the amount of drug in the body by 50% after a single dose of the drug is given (B). The half-life of medications is often increased in the elderly due to changes in drug absorption, metabolism, and excretion.
Incorrect:
A drug's half-life is the time needed to reduce the amount of drug circulating in the body by a half, or 50% (A, C, D).

33. **Correct: C. 3 to 5**

Steady state is generally defined as the time when the overall intake of a drug is approximately matched with the drug's elimination. Steady state is typically reached around three to five times the half-life of the drug after a dose (C).

Incorrect:

Under normal circumstances, steady state is typically reached after 3 to 5 half-lives of the drug (A, B, D).

34. **Correct: C. 30**

The CYP450 isoenzyme system is essential for biotransformation of medications. In the elderly, the CYP450 isoenzyme levels can be reduced by as much as 30% (C), which can have substantial impacts on the pharmacokinetics of medications, including drug half-life, C_{max}, T_{max}, and elimination from the body.

Incorrect:

Compared to a younger adult, levels of CYP450 isoenzyme can decrease by as much as 30% (A, B, D).

35 to 42. Matching Questions

35. **Correct: B. highly anticholinergic**

36. **Correct: F. nausea, diarrhea**

37. **Correct: G. GI bleeding**

38. **Correct: A. sedation**

39. **Correct: E. delirium, falls**

40. **Correct: D. hyperkalemia risk**

41. **Correct: C. increased risk of heart failure**

42. **Correct: H. need for dose adjustment in the older adult**

The Beers Criteria recommend avoiding certain potentially inappropriate medications in older adult populations. Amitriptyline is associated with highly anticholinergic effects that can cause confusion, urinary retention, and constipation, among other effects (35). Nortriptyline should be used as an alternative as it is associated with less anticholinergic effect. Duloxetine, an SNRI, is associated with GI adverse effects, such as nausea and diarrhea (36). Gabapentin is associated with sedation and should be dosed low initially and then titrated as needed (38). Zolpidem, often used to treat insomnia, can increase the risk of delirium and falls in the elderly (39). Prolonged use of NSAIDs should be avoided due to increased risk of GI bleeding (37). TMP-SMX is associated with an increased risk of hyperkalemia (40). The thiazolidinediones can potentially worsen heart failure and so should be avoided in these patients (41). Ranitidine requires dose adjustment in patients with renal impairment and can cause mental status change in the elderly (42).

Elder Maltreatment

43. **Correct: C. report the situation to the appropriate state or local agency.**

This patient clearly shows signs of neglect and possible financial abuse. Despite the patient's wish to not report the abuse, it is the mandate of the NP to look after the best interests of the patient. This will require reporting the situation to the proper state or local agency (C). Legislation from every state requires health-care workers who come in contact with older adults to report abuse to the proper authorities.

Incorrect:

As a mandate for the NP, a patient's best interest must be looked after, which includes reporting suspected abuse to the proper authorities. This should be done even if the patient expresses a desire to not report the situation (D). The granddaughter should not be confronted as this can worsen the situation (A), while planning to visit the patient more often will only delay the patient from getting the proper attention and care that he needs (B).

44. **Correct: C. Routine screening is indicated as part of the care of an older adult.**

Screening for elder abuse can be an important tool to detect and prevent abuse, and routine screening is recommended by the American Medical Association for all older adults (C). Several screening tools are available to detect elder maltreatment.

Incorrect:

Elder maltreatment occurs in all socioeconomic classes and is not focused on individuals of lower socioeconomic status (A). Elder maltreatment is significantly underreported as most elderly adults will not seek help (B). Neglect is the most common form of elder maltreatment, rather than physical abuse or violence (D).

45. **Correct: C. assumption of caregiving responsibilities at a later stage of life.**

Certain risk factors have been identified for a perpetrator of elder maltreatment. Among these is the assumption of caregiving responsibilities at an earlier, rather than later, stage of life (C). Those in their 20s or 30s might feel too young to embrace the responsibility to suddenly need to care for an elderly parent or grandparent.

Incorrect:

Other factors that increase the risk of a perpetrator for elder maltreatment can include a high level of hostility about the caregiver role (A), poor coping skills (B), a history of mental illness or alcohol abuse, and a history of maltreatment as a child (D).

46. **Correct: C. five**

Despite legislation requiring the reporting of suspected cases by health-care workers, elder maltreatment remains significantly underreported. It is estimated that for every case of elder maltreatment that is reported, there are an additional five cases that are not reported. Screening of older adults for elder maltreatment can be an important tool to detect and prevent these situations.

Incorrect:

Current estimates report that for every one case of elder maltreatment identified, there are an additional 5 cases that go unreported (A, B, D).

47. Correct: D. neglect.

Neglect is the most common form of elder maltreatment (D). Neglect is the failure or refusal of a caregiver to provide for the basic physical, emotional, and social needs of an elderly adult, or the failure to protect an elderly adult from harm.

Incorrect:

There are many forms of elder maltreatment, and neglect is the most common form. Other types of maltreatment can include physical abuse (A), sexual exploitation (B), psychological or emotional abuse, abandonment, and financial abuse or exploitation (C). Self-neglect, which is not instituted by another individual, is also a common form of maltreatment and occurs when the elderly adult fails or refuses to take care of basic physical, emotional, or social needs.

48. Correct: B. self-neglect.

Self-neglect, which is not instituted by another individual, is a common form of maltreatment and occurs when the elderly adult fails or refuses to take care of basic physical, emotional, or social needs. This patient shows clear signs of self-neglect including poor hygiene, malnutrition, and nonadherence to her medications.

Incorrect:

This is not a case of abandonment as the daughter regularly checks on her and shows concern for her well-being (A). There is also no indication of psychological abuse from this description (D). The self-neglect might be a result of depression or early onset dementia, which should be explored further (C).

49 to 54. Matching Questions

49. Correct: Protective

50. Correct: Risk

51. Correct: Protective

52. Correct: Risk

53. Correct: Risk

54. Correct: Protective

Within institutional settings, such as long-term care or assisted-living facilities, certain factors have been identified as either protective or a risk for elder maltreatment. Protective factors can include effective monitoring systems in place, clear and understandable institutional policies on patient care (54), clear guidance on *durable power of attorney* (51), and regular visits by family members, volunteers, or social workers (49). Risk factors can include unsympathetic or negative attitudes by staff toward residents, chronic staffing problems (53), lack of administrative oversight, staff burnout (50), and stressful working conditions (52).

Falls

55. Correct: C. the patient's home.

About one-third of community-dwelling elderly adults and two-thirds of residents of long-term care facilities will experience a fall each year. Most falls occur in the home as this is where elderly adults tend to spend most of their time. Approximately 60% of fatal falls will occur in the home.

Incorrect:

The majority of fatal falls will occur in the home. About 30% of fatal falls will occur in public or outdoor spaces (B, D), and 10% will occur in health-care institutions (A).

56 to 60. Indicate Yes or No

56. Correct: No

57. Correct: Yes

58. Correct: Yes

59. Correct: Yes

60. Correct: Yes

Several risk factors have been identified for falls in the elderly. A prior history of a fall is a strong predictor of a future fall (56). A person who has fallen is two to three times more likely to fall within the next year. Conditions that impact normal gait and balance will increase fall risk, including stroke (57) and peripheral neuropathy. Osteoporosis and osteoarthritis are known risk factors for falls in the elderly (58, 59). The type of shoe can also influence fall risk. Recommended footwear in the elderly is an enclosed-toe, tie shoe with semirigid sole. Slippers, flip-flops, sandals, or thick-soled jogging shoes can increase fall risk (60).

61. Correct: D. a syncopal episode requiring a cardiovascular and neurological evaluation.

A patient report of a fall where there is no memory of the fall and/or there is no attempt to brace for the fall suggests a syncopal episode (D). The patient should undergo cardiovascular and neurological evaluation to find the cause of syncope.

Incorrect:

The patient report is most consistent with a syncopal episode. Cognitive impairment would not be characterized by a fainting spell where there is no recollection of falling (A). The patient history does not reveal any significant sensory deficits that could account for the fall (B). Excessive alcohol use would be associated with other obvious signs and symptoms that are not noted in the patient description (C).

62. Correct: B. 20

Orthostatic hypotension is defined as an excessive decrease in BP with a change in body position, such as when an upright position is assumed. The effects can include light-headedness, dizziness, or blurred vision usually within seconds of changing position. The condition is present in about 20% of older adults and is a potent risk factor for falls (B).

Incorrect:

It is estimated that up to 1 in 5 older adults experience orthostatic hypotension, placing them at increased risk of injury from a fall (A, C, D).

63. **Correct: D. lisinopril**
Certain medications are associated with orthostatic hypotension in older adults that can increase fall risk. However, beta blockers and angiotensin-converting enzyme (ACE) inhibitors, such as lisinopril, are seldom implicated in orthostatic hypotension (D).
Incorrect:
Medications most often implicated in orthostatic hypotension typically cause a decrease in circulating volume or peripheral vasodilation. These can include loop diuretics (e.g., furosemide [B]), TCAs, calcium channel blockers (e.g., nifedipine [A]), α-adrenergic blockers, centrally acting antihypertensives (e.g., clonidine [C]), and nitrates.

64. **Correct: C. flexing the feet multiple times before changing position.**
Several steps can be taken to improve orthostatic hypotension and reduce fall risk. Flexing the feet multiple times before changing to an upright position will help with venous return and diminish the effects of orthostatic hypotension (C).
Incorrect:
The use of compression stockings can be helpful in increasing venous return and diminishing orthostatic hypotension (A). A certain amount of salt in the diet is needed to maintain circulating volume (B). Similarly, adequate fluid intake is also needed to maintain circulating volume and prevent dehydration (D).

65. **Correct: C. 20, 10**
Orthostatic hypotension is typically diagnosed by measuring BP in the sitting and standing positions, with the condition present when the difference exceeds 20 mm Hg systolic and 10 mm Hg diastolic. Patients with orthostatic hypotension will also report characteristic signs and symptoms when changing position, including dizziness, light-headedness, and blurred vision, which resolve within minutes of sitting down.

66. **Correct: D. hip.**
Approximately 20% to 30% of elderly adults who fall will sustain moderate to severe injuries that can reduce mobility and independence and increase the risk of premature death. Of all fall-related fractures, a fracture of the hip is most serious and most likely to lead to serious long-term health problems and mortality (D).
Incorrect:
The most common fall-related injuries are osteoporotic fractures of the hip, spine, and forearm. A hip fracture is associated with the greatest risk of long-term complications, including diminished mobility, independence, and premature death. Fractures of the forearm (A), spine (B), and ankle (C), though serious, are associated with a lower risk of long-term complications.

67. **Correct: A. amitriptyline**
The TCAs, such as amitriptyline, are associated with orthostatic hypotension that can increase fall risk (A). Amitriptyline is also highly anticholinergic and can cause sedation and confusion in the elderly and should be avoided, according to the Beers criteria.
Incorrect:
Diabetes medications associated with hypoglycemia should be avoided in the elderly as these can increase fall risk. However, sitagliptin is not associated with hypoglycemia and is an appropriate choice in the elderly (B). Statins (C) and aspirin (D) also do not increase the risk of falls, though chronic use of aspirin can increase the risk of GI bleeding.

68. **Correct: B. 2 to 3**
A prior history of a fall is a strong predictor of a future fall. An older adult who has fallen is two to three times more likely to fall within the next year (B).
Incorrect:
An older adult with a prior history of fall will have a two- to threefold increased risk of falling again within the next year (A, C, D).

69. **Correct: B. walking 10 feet without the use of a walking aid**
"Get Up and Go" is a useful test to evaluate gait and balance. For individuals who normally use a walking aid, such as a cane, the walking aid can be included as part of the test (B).
Incorrect:
Aspects of the "Get Up and Go" test include rising from a straight-backed chair (A), walking 10 feet using the usual walking aid such as a cane, if applicable, turning (C), and returning to the chair and sitting down (D). The clinician can assess gait and balance by observing balance with sitting and on standing, pace and stability with walking, ability to turn without staggering, and time to complete the task.

70. **Correct: B. at the peak of action.**
Benzodiazepines are associated with sedation when used in the elderly. The greatest amount of sedation is most likely to occur at the peak of action (B), which would correlate with the greatest risk of a fall.
Incorrect:
Fall risk with the use of benzodiazepines is associated with sedation caused by these medications. Sedation is greatest at the peak of action, and not at the onset (A) or following the peak of action (B, D).

Driving Issues in Older Adults

71. **Correct: B. Crashes with elderly drivers tend to involve diminished speed of visual processing.**
Motor vehicle accidents with elderly drivers tend to involve a slower speed of visual processing (B), which is a normal age-related change. Other age-related changes can include diminished hearing and musculoskeletal changes that can increase the time needed to react to changes in the road or to immediately brake when necessary.
Incorrect:
Due to changing demographics, the number of elderly drivers is expected to increase over the next decade (A).

Older driver accidents tend to involve multiple vehicle events and involve left-hand turns at intersections, rather than right-hand turns (C). The skills needed for safe driving will deteriorate with age, particularly with diminished vision and hearing and increased reaction time (D).

72. **Correct: D. The National Transportation Safety Board (NTSB) recommends surrendering the driver's license for all individuals with an AD diagnosis.**

Those with early stage AD can continue to drive safely for a period of time, and there is no requirement by the NTSB to surrender a driver's license following an AD diagnosis (D). Though there is an absence of reliable, objective measures to assess driving competency in older adults, several screening tools are available to determine risk for crashes among older drivers, who should be routinely evaluated and transitioned to driving retirement when it becomes necessary.

Incorrect:

Following an AD diagnosis, patients can typically drive safely for a period of time and do not stop driving for at least 3 years following the diagnosis (A). Those with mild to moderate AD have an eightfold increase in accidents (B). Older drivers with AD should be monitored regularly for driving competency and transitioned to driving retirement when necessary (C).

73. **Correct: D. tailgating.**

There are several driving errors that older drivers are more prone to make. However, since older drivers tend to drive at slower speeds, they are less likely to tailgate other drivers (D).

Incorrect:

Types of driving errors more commonly seen with older drivers include difficulty backing up and making turns (A), not seeing traffic signs, difficulty retrieving information from dashboard displays, delayed glare recovery at night (B), not checking rearview mirrors and blind spots, bumping into curbs and objects (C), and not yielding to oncoming traffic or right-of-way.

74. **Correct: B. having the radio on to an enjoyable talk show to enhance driving skills.**

An important aspect of driving among older adults is to limit distractions while driving, such as talking on a cell phone, texting, or eating. If the radio is on, it should be playing soft background music to minimize distraction (B).

Incorrect:

Several steps can be taken to improve driving safety among older drivers. Medications and OTC drugs should be reviewed to reduce adverse effects that can impair driving (A). Preference should be given to driving during daylight hours and in good weather (D). Older drivers should also plan the route before driving with a preference for the safest route with well-lit streets if driving at night (C).

Pressure Ulcers

75. **Correct: D. weight gain.**

Pressure ulcers occur when vascular pressure inhibits adequate supply of blood to the skin and underlying tissue. Contributing factors include sustained pressure, friction, shear, and nutritional debilitation. Weight loss, rather than weight gain, can increase the risk of pressure ulcers (D).

Incorrect:

Risk factors for pressure ulcers include high moisture, advanced age, low BP, smoking (C), fecal incontinence, malnutrition (A), and dehydration (B), among others.

76. **Correct: B. osteoporosis.**

Osteoporosis, identified as a loss of bone density, can lead to fractures and loss of mobility. This, in turn, can increase the risk of a pressure ulcer, particularly if confined to a bed or wheelchair. However, though osteoporosis can increase the risk of pressure ulcers, the condition is not a complication of pressure ulcers.

Incorrect:

Complications of pressure ulcers include various types of infection including sepsis (A), cellulitis (D), and bone and joint infections (C).

77. **Correct: C. stage 3.**

A stage 3 pressure ulcer is characterized by full-thickness skin loss with exposure of some amount of underlying fat (C). The ulcer has a crater-like appearance.

Incorrect:

A stage 1 pressure ulcer is identified by a nonblanchable area of erythema on intact skin (A). A stage 2 pressure ulcer can have some epidermal or dermal skin loss or appear as an intact blister (B). A stage 4 pressure ulcer involves full-thickness skin and tissue loss that exposes muscle, bone, and tendons (D).

78 to 81. Matching Questions

78. **Correct: D. conservative (nonsurgical) approaches**
79. **Correct: D. conservative (nonsurgical) approaches**
80. **Correct: A. skin graft, and C. débridement of nonvital skin**
81. **Correct: A. skin graft, and C. débridement of nonvital skin**

Stages 1 and 2 pressure ulcers can typically heal with general wound care that does not involve surgery (78, 79). This can involve special padding for vulnerable skin areas, ensuring proper nutrition and hydration, regular repositioning of the patient, and appropriate pain control when needed. In a stage 3 or 4 pressure ulcer that involves full-thickness skin loss, surgery can be considered to assist healing. Options include débridement of dead tissue as well as the use of skin grafts or skin flap (80, 81). Simple wound closure is rarely an option in pressure ulcers.

82. **Correct: B. low-fat, low-sodium diet.**

Supplemental nutrition can be helpful to address issues of malnutrition as a cause of pressure ulcers. A low-fat diet would not be preferred as caloric intake should be maximized, particularly in patients who are not feeding adequately (B). Similarly, a certain amount of sodium is needed in the diet to maintain circulating volume and prevent issues of hypotension.

Incorrect:

Supplemental nutrition can include enteral (A) or parenteral nutrition (C). Vitamin therapy can also be considered to ensure all daily requirements are met to hasten the healing of wounds (D).

83. **Correct: C. Marjolin's ulcer.**

Marjolin's ulcer refers to transformation of chronic, non-healing wounds to an aggressive form of squamous cell carcinoma (C). Though rare, the condition is associated with high mortality, and biopsy should be performed to detect Marjolin's ulcer as soon as possible.

Incorrect:

Zoster infection typically occurs in linear streaks along a dermatome with characteristic blistering lesions associated with severe pain described as burning, stabbing, and throbbing (A). Impetigo is a skin infection characterized by multiple lesions (either bullous or nonbullous) on exposed areas of the body (B). Actinic keratosis is a precancerous lesion typically found in sun-exposed areas of skin (D). The lesions are typically small and flesh colored and most easily identified by gently running a fingertip over the skin to detect small rough spots.

Delirium, Dementia, and Depression

84 to 88. Matching Questions

84. **Correct: dementia**

85. **Correct: delirium**

86. **Correct: delirium**

87. **Correct: delirium**

88. **Correct: dementia**

Delirium refers to an acute onset of mental status change (85). A number of causes can be associated with delirium, including infection, initiating a new medication or a new dose of medication (86), electrolyte disturbance, or undernutrition, among others. Typically, mental status will return to baseline level once the underlying cause is addressed (87). Dementia is mental status change that progresses over months to years (84). Changes in cognitive function are irreversible, though not usually associated with perceptual disturbances until advanced stages of disease (88).

89. **Correct: D. acute infection.**

Though there are several triggers that can cause delirium, the most common trigger is acute infection, most notably urinary tract infection and community-acquired pneumonia.

Incorrect:

Other causes of delirium include initiating a new medication or a new dose of medication, electrolyte disturbance, subdural hematoma resulting from head trauma

(C), alcohol withdrawal (A), urinary retention, or fecal impaction (B). The DELIRIUMS mnemonic can be helpful in recognizing the various causes of delirium.

90. **Correct: B. AD.**

The most common etiology of dementia is due to AD, which accounts for the majority of cases (B).

Incorrect:

Other types of dementia include vascular or multi-infarct dementia, which accounts for approximately 10% to 20% of cases (A), and Parkinson's disease, which accounts for 5% of cases. Traumatic head injury (C) and drug-drug interactions (D) would not be causes of dementia but could be triggers for delirium.

91. **Correct: B. cardioselective β-adrenergic antagonists.**

Initiation of a new medication or a new dose adjustment of a medication is a common trigger for delirium. Medications with anticholinergic activity or that cause sedation are most implicated in causing delirium. The cardioselective β-adrenergic antagonists, such as atenolol and bisoprolol, are not typically associated with causing delirium (B).

Incorrect:

Particularly problematic medications that can trigger delirium include those with high anticholinergic activity, such as the first-generation antihistamines (A), as well as opioids (C) and benzodiazepines (D).

92. **Correct: A. hyponatremia**

Electrolyte disturbance, particularly hyponatremia, can be an important trigger for delirium. Hyponatremia in the elderly can be caused by the syndrome of inappropriate antidiuretic hormone secretion (SIADH), as well as sodium loss through the GI tract or urine (A). Other symptoms can include nausea and vomiting, headache, confusion, fatigue, muscle weakness, and seizures.

Incorrect:

Hyponatremia is most commonly associated with delirium in the elderly. Hypernatremia can occur frequently in the elderly due to a greater propensity for dehydration among the older population (B). This is due to age-related decrease in thirst drive, impaired urinary concentrating ability, and reduced total body water. Symptoms include thirst, weakness, nausea, and loss of appetite. Elderly adults are also at higher risk of hyperkalemia (C), particularly in the presence of kidney dysfunction or when prescribed certain medications (e.g., spironolactone, ACE inhibitors). Symptoms can include muscle fatigue, weakness, arrhythmias, and nausea. Hypophosphatemia occurs less frequently in the elderly and is associated with alcoholism, diabetic ketoacidosis, or sepsis (D).

93. **Correct: B. relatively fragile blood vessels.**

Elderly adults are at greater risk of subdural hematoma from relatively minor head trauma due to a combination of brain atrophy along with fragile blood vessels (B).

Incorrect:

Age-related changes in bone density in the skull, as well as levels of circulating clotting factors, are relatively insignificant clinically to contribute to increased risk of subdural hematoma (A, D). Older adults typically have a higher percentage of weight as fat compared to younger adults (C).

94. **Correct: C. this medication will likely afford clear, although minor and time-limited, benefits.**
Cholinesterase inhibitors are approved for use in mild to moderate stages of disease and have been shown to slow decline in AD. However, though there is a clear benefit, the effects of these medications are minor and time limited (C).
Incorrect:
These medications will not return cognitive function to baseline levels but will more likely slow the progressive decline seen with AD (A). The benefits generally outweigh the risks in mild to moderate disease (B), but the risks will outweigh the benefits in later disease. There is no proven benefit for the use of these medications in early AD or in patients with mild cognitive impairment (D).

95. **Correct: C. in patients with mild to moderate AD.**
Cholinesterase inhibitors are approved for use in mild to moderate stages of disease and have been shown to offer a clear, though minor and time-limited, benefit (C).
Incorrect:
There is currently no definitive evidence supporting the use of cholinesterase inhibitors for the prevention of AD (A) or for those with early stage AD or with mild cognitive impairment (B). The risks of these agents generally outweigh the benefits in patients with severe AD (D).

96. **Correct: B. positron emission tomography (PET) scan.**
Triggers for new-onset mental status change in the elderly can easily go undetected. Routine laboratory tests can be used to identify the underlying cause of mental status change. A PET scan along with computed tomography, magnetic resonance imaging, or radiography would not be used routinely in the initial evaluation (B) but can be considered as an add-on diagnostic tool depending on patient presentation and initial findings. This can include a suspicion of malignancy or injury from trauma.
Incorrect:
Laboratory tests that should be routinely utilized in cases of new-onset mental status change in the elderly include serum glucose (to check for presence of hypoglycemia or hyperglycemia) (A), CBC with differential (to check for the presence of infection) (C), and an ECG (to evaluate for a cardiac event such as myocardial infarction) (D). Other tests can include blood urea nitrogen and creatinine, calcium, sodium, hepatic enzymes, and a urinalysis.

97. **Correct: B. treatment with a cholinesterase inhibitor will maintain his cognitive ability to the current status for a protracted period of time.**
Cholinesterase inhibitors are approved for use in mild to moderate stages of disease and have been shown to offer a clear, though minor and time-limited, benefit in those with AD. However, the use of these agents will not stop the progressive decline in mental status associated with AD but can slow the progression for a time period (B).
Incorrect:
It is common for behavioral issues to emerge in older adults with cognitive dysfunction with changes to their usual routine or setting (A). For the safety of the patient, a home evaluation should be performed to identify and correct safety risks (C). Though a progressive decline is expected with AD, any sudden change in mental status should be reported to a health-care provider to identify and correct the underlying cause (D).

98. **Correct: B. vitamin E**
Some evidence has suggested some improvement in slowing cognitive decline with the use of vitamin E or selegiline at early stages of disease. There is no added benefit in using a combination of these products.
Incorrect:
Vitamin E can be used to slow cognitive decline in early stages of AD. There are no recommendations supporting the use of vitamin B_{12} (A), ginkgo biloba (C), or St. John's wort (D) for AD.

99. **Correct: C. in moderate to severe stages of AD.**
NMDA antagonists, such as memantine, are approved for use in moderate to severe stages of AD (C). These can also be used in combination with a cholinesterase inhibitor for added effect, particularly in earlier disease.
Incorrect:
There is no evidence to support the use of NMDA-receptor antagonists for the prevention of dementia (A). These agents are not approved for use in early stages of disease as a solo product (B) but are reserved for moderate to severe stages (D).

100. **Correct: D. combination therapy can have additive benefits in moderate to severe AD.**
Memantine with a cholinesterase inhibitor can be safely used in the treatment of AD. Some evidence has shown added benefit with combination therapy, including delaying institutionalization of patients with AD (D).
Incorrect:
A combination of memantine and cholinesterase inhibitor can be safely used in AD patients (A). Studies suggest an added benefit of combination therapy in later disease (B), though treatment will not reverse cognitive decline at any stage of AD (C).

101. **Correct: A. attention-deficit hyperactivity disorder (ADHD).**
Several causes can contribute to behavioral issues in the elderly. However, new-onset ADHD is not a typical diagnosis made in older adults and the elderly (A).
Incorrect:
Other noncognitive reasons for behavioral issues in the elderly can include acute or chronic pain (B), infection

(C), or depression (D). Careful evaluation of the elderly with new-onset behavioral changes should include diagnostic measures to identify the underlying cause of alterations in behavior or mental status.

102 to 104. Matching Questions

102. Correct: B. language disturbance

103. Correct: C. impairment of motor activities despite intact motor function

104. Correct: A. failure to recognize objects despite intact sensory function
Safe clinical practice requires having knowledge of the correct terminology used in the clinical setting. Aphasia refers to language disturbance, typically characterized by the loss of the ability to understand or express speech (102). Apraxia is a motor disorder in which the individual has difficulty performing tasks or movements when asked despite intact motor function (103). Agnosia is the inability to interpret sensations and recognize things despite intact sensory function (104).

105. Correct: A. stroke and cardiovascular events.
Antipsychotics can be considered to help manage patients with dementia who are experiencing agitation and psychosis and who fail other approaches. However, the use of second-generation antipsychotics has been associated with an increased risk of serious adverse effects, including stroke and cardiovascular events in older adults (A).
Incorrect:
The use of second-generation antipsychotics in older adults has not been associated with an increased risk of hypoglycemia (B), psychosis (C), or hypertension (D).

106. Correct: B. pseudodementia.
Pseudodementia is the condition where the presenting symptoms are similar to dementia but is the result of depression (B). This is a reversible condition, and thus an accurate diagnosis is important to restore cognitive function of the individual.
Incorrect:
Delirium is characterized by new-onset mental status change resulting from an underlying condition, such as infection or change in medication (A). AD is an insidious, slowly progressive disease that results in irreversible mental cognition changes (C). Bipolar disorder is characterized by unusual shifts in mood, energy, activity level, and ability to perform daily tasks (D).

107. Correct: A. starting at the highest dose possible of antidepressant and then titrating down once symptoms resolve.
When initiating pharmacotherapy in the older adult population for various conditions, including depression, the general principles include "start low, go slow, but get to goal." Initiating treatment at the highest dose will increase the risk of potential drug-related adverse effects and compromise the safety of the patient (A).

Incorrect:
When managing mental health disorders such as depression, a combination of psychotherapy along with pharmacotherapy can yield better results (B). ECT in older adults with depression can be considered as an effective and safe option, particularly if there is an inadequate response to pharmacotherapy (C). Given the high frequency of polypharmacy among older adults, a careful medication review should be performed prior to adding or changing medication to avoid potential drug-drug interactions (D).

Ethical and Legal Issues

108. Correct: C. Health-care providers have the ability to determine whether a patient can provide informed consent.
Informed consent is when a patient gives authority to a health-care provider to undergo a specific medical intervention with full knowledge of the risks and benefits. Health-care providers have the ability to determine whether or not a patient is capable of providing informed consent (C).
Incorrect:
When determining competency of a patient, only a court can determine if a patient is incompetent (A). Impaired judgment does not make a person incompetent (B). When requesting informed consent, the patient should be provided information on the diagnosis, as well as understand the nature and purpose of the procedure, understand the risks, benefits, and adverse effects of the procedure, and understand reasonable alternatives, if possible (D).

109. Correct: B. when needed to meet a health-care need.
Physical restraints should not be used for staff convenience or as a form of discipline but can be considered in situations to meet a health-care need (B).
Incorrect:
The Omnibus Reconciliation Act of 1987 states that residents of long-term care facilities should be free of physical and chemical restraints in situations where they are not required to meet a health-care need. Physical restraints should not be used as a form of discipline (A) or to prevent wandering outside an institution (C), as alternative approaches can be effective (e.g., alarms). Physical restraints can be considered when required to meet a health-care need (D).

110. Correct: C. Advance directives are legally binding in all states.
Advance directives are durable statements of intent based on the patient's last written wishes that can be used to help make end-of-life decisions. Though advance directives are recognized in every state, they are not legally binding in all situations. Health-care providers can refuse to comply with an advance directive if they have an objection of conscience or consider the wishes to be medically inappropriate (C).

Incorrect:
Advance directives can include living wills, do not resuscitate orders, or a *durable power of attorney for health care* (A). A value history can be a written, video-taped, or audiotaped discussion that includes advance directives (B). Advance directives are recognized only when the patient is hopelessly and terminally ill as determined by a health-care provider (D).

111. **Correct: A. can include benzodiazepines and first-and second-generation antipsychotics.**
Chemical restraints can be considered as a last resort to ensure the safety of a patient, health providers, or others. Chemical restraints are mainly used for sedative properties, and agents can include benzodiazepines and the first- and second-generation antipsychotics (A).

Incorrect:
Similar to physical restraints, chemical restraints should not be used as a form of discipline or for staff convenience (B). Chemical restraints can cause serious drug-related adverse effects, and patients should be monitored closely (C). The Joint Commission recommends using physical or chemical restraints only as a last resort for specific situations where the safety of the patient, staff, or others is in jeopardy (D).

Pediatrics 17

Newborn and Infant Feeding

Overview

The neonatal period, defined as a baby's first month of life, is a critical period characterized by rapid growth and significant neurological development.

To ensure this growth and optimal health, adequate caloric and nutrient intake needs to be provided. Commonly shared information on the volume of liquid that the newborn in day 1 of life is able to tolerate in a feeding is as low as 5 to 7 mL. However, the more accurate amount is about 20 mL, increasing to approximately 100 mL by week 4 of life. As a result, the amount of breast milk or formula the newborn takes in at each feeding is likely more than has been previously appreciated. The infant's sole source of nutrition in the first 4 to 6 months of life should be breast milk, and if that is not possible, iron-enriched infant formula.

The newborn often takes a number of days to learn to optimally feed, while even experienced parents and caregivers take a number of days to learn about the feeding patterns for their particular baby. Consequences of inadequate feeding in the first few weeks of life can be significant, and include dehydration, hypernatremia, and/or hypoglycemia. Parents and caregivers should ensure that newborns are getting adequate caloric and fluid intake while supporting and encouraging breastfeeding optimally. Here are the cues for inadequate feeding to look for in the first days of life, using the HUNGRY mnemonic:

- **H**ypoglycemia, often characterized by protracted high-pitched cry, jitteriness, potentially seizures
- **U**nsatisfying nursing, often characterized by protracted periods of and/or more frequent (less than 2 hours) intervals of breastfeeding with the newborn continuing to exhibit hunger cues
- **N**ot waking for feeding every 2 to 3 hours, not latching appropriately, particularly after initial satisfactory latch, limpness and/or lethargy, findings that can indicate low blood sugar, dehydration, and/or electrolyte disorder
- **G**rowth or weight loss greater than 7% at any given time, particularly outside the first week of life, which increases the likelihood of neonatal jaundice and hypernatremia
- **R**educed number and frequency of wet and/or soiled diapers, especially if no wet diapers for more than 6 hours; dry, brick-colored stools, especially if the newborn has evidence of a dry mouth and/or crying without tears
- **Y**ellowing of the skin and eyes, indicating hyperbilirubinemia and jaundice, noted particularly in the first few weeks of life when feeding and fluid intake are inadequate

Whether breast- or formula-fed, the newborn should have a feeding every 2 to 3 hours. This helps minimize the risk of dehydration, hypernatremia, and neonatal jaundice. Supplemental water feedings should be avoided, even in a warmer environment, as breast milk and infant formula are nearly 90% water; proper feeding helps avoid dehydration risk. Usually, the infant will naturally increase feeding when fluid needs increase. Solid food should not be considered until at least 4 to 6 months of age and after birth weight has doubled. At this point, the baby should be consuming more than 32 oz (946 mL) of formula per day or have more than 8 to 10 feedings (breast or bottle) per day.

BREASTFEEDING

Overview

Breastfeeding provides the ideal form of nutrition during infancy. According to the Centers for Disease Control and Prevention (CDC), approximately 77% of all infants in the United States are breastfed at birth, with about 49% of all infants continuing at age 6 months. Health-care providers can help influence successful breastfeeding. Although the content of commercially prepared formula available in the developed world continues to be improved with composition closer to breast milk, infant formula still lacks critically important components.

Breast milk contains immunoactive factors that help protect infants against infectious disease and may reduce the frequency of allergic disorders. Human milk transfers the mother's antibodies to disease to the infant. About 80% of the cells in breast milk are macrophages, cells that kill bacteria, fungi, and viruses. In contrast to formula-fed infants, a breastfed infant's digestive tract contains large amounts of *Lactobacillus bifidus*, beneficial bacteria that prevent the growth of harmful organisms. Formula-fed babies typically have greater weight gain during the first few weeks of life compared to breastfed babies. However, the benefits of breastfeeding far outweigh this small difference.

Promoting Successful Infant Breastfeeding

The mother of the newborn should be advised to keep well hydrated and breastfeed every 2 to 3 hours, starting immediately after birth; one way to ensure adequate maternal hydration is to drink at minimum a 16-oz glass of fluid with each feeding. These actions help promote breast milk production. The transition from colostrum (a thick, concentrated milk produced starting around mid-pregnancy) to mature breast milk typically comes between days 2 and 5 after birth.

The baby should be well latched onto the breast to produce adequate suck and suckle, both components of successful feeding. With adequate latch, breastfeeding should be comfortable for the mother, particularly beyond the first days when nursing is often uncomfortable even with perfect latch. In addition, with adequate latch, the baby's chin and stomach should be able to comfortably rest against the mother's body, the baby's mouth is widely open, with lips flanged outward, and the areola minimally visible. While latched, the mother should be able to see or hear the baby swallowing, and the baby's ears move slightly with each suck and swallow. With inadequate latch, a problem associated with potential inability to establish adequate breast milk supply, these findings are missing; other observations with poor latch include dimpling of the baby's cheeks and/or a clicking noise with attempts at suck and swallow. Maternal factors to enhance latch include rubbing the nipple just above the baby's top lip to help trigger wide mouth opening. The newborn will generally best latch if the baby leans into the breast chin first.

Breast pumps can be particularly helpful to add flexibility with feedings as well as allow mothers to return to work or school, if necessary. There are several types of breast pumps available, and they are often covered by health insurance companies and/or state Medicaid programs. Double pumps that express milk from both breasts at the same time are particularly helpful in reducing the time needed to pump milk. In the United States, the federal Fair Labor Standards Act (FLSA) requires employers to provide a reasonable amount of break time for nursing moms to express milk as frequently as needed. Employees must also provide a functional space for expressing milk, while bathrooms are not permissible for this purpose.

The risk of developing physiological jaundice, a common problem in the first few weeks of the newborn's life, usually starting at days 3 to 5 of life, is usually the result of a normal breakdown of fetal hemoglobin and immature liver metabolism. No underlying liver disease is noted in this condition. Physiological jaundice risk, which usually starts from the head and then spreads to the body, in the breastfed neonate is reduced with adequate intake of breast milk and increased with the use of dextrose and water feedings.

During the first few days after birth, bowel movements consist of meconium, a thick black or dark-green stool that transitions to yellow-green as the intestines clear. Newborns who are breastfed often stool after each feeding or about six times per day. As the intestines mature, stooling will become less frequent, with 2- to 3-month-olds sometimes going days between stooling. Though there is no "normal" texture/consistency of stools as each baby is different, breastfed newborns tend to have loose, seedy stools (as opposed to formula-fed babies who tend to have soft, mushy to firm stools).

Whether breastfeeding in the early days of infant life comes with little effort or great challenge, most mothers benefit from assistance. Resources include La Leche League, a nursing parent-led organization that provides helpful information on a variety of topics, including lactation with adoption and support for trans and nonbinary parents, as well as the Woman, Infants, and Children (WIC) Breastfeeding Program. Most health-care systems have certified lactation consultants available, or one can be found via public registry.

Medication Use During Lactation

If a nursing mother becomes ill or has a chronic health problem, she is often erroneously advised to discontinue breastfeeding on the basis of the health-care provider's incorrect assumption that most medications are harmful to the infant. Most medications can be used during lactation, but the benefit of improved maternal health should be balanced against the risk of exposing an infant to medication.

Nearly all breastfeeding mothers use some type of medication (most often analgesic agents such as NSAIDs, acetaminophen or opioids, or antibiotics) in the first 2 weeks after giving birth. About 25% need to use medication intermittently to manage episodic disease. Such medications usually include analgesics, antihistamines, decongestants, and antibiotics.

About 5% of breastfeeding women have a chronic health problem necessitating daily use of a medication; the most common long-term medications used are for treating asthma, mental health problems, seizure disorder, and hypertension. Nursing infants usually get about 1%, often less, of the maternal dose, and only a few drugs are contraindicated. A general rule on prescribing during lactation is that medications that would be safe to use on the infant are safe to use during breastfeeding. Examples include acetaminophen, beta-lactam antibiotics, including penicillins and cephalosporins, and inhaled and short-course oral corticosteroids. Less commonly required medications by women who are breastfeeding, such as drugs for hypertension, seizure disorders, mood disorders, and other mental health conditions, are usually prescribed with expert consultation, balancing maternal-infant benefit versus risk.

The "pump-and-dump" procedure is usually not an effective means to reduce drug levels in a mother's milk because it creates an area of lower drug concentration in the empty breast. This enables the drug to diffuse from the area of high concentration (maternal serum) to the area of low concentration (breast milk). If the mother takes a medication that is problematic for the nursing infant, she needs to immediately stop taking the medication. Pumping and discarding the milk needs to continue for three to five drug-free half-lives of the medication.

Alcohol has a low molecular weight and is highly lipid soluble; both of these characteristics allow it to have easy passage into breast milk. Even in small amounts, alcohol ingestion by a nursing mother can cause a smaller amount of milk to be produced, a reduction in the let-down reflex, and less rhythmic and frequent sucking by the infant, resulting in a smaller volume of milk ingested. Cigarette smoking is similarly problematic. Nicotine, a highly lipid-soluble substance with a low molecular weight, passes easily into breast milk.

> **CLINICAL CONCEPT**
> Maternal cigarette smoking can reduce milk supply and expose an infant to passive smoke. Infant crankiness, diarrhea, tachycardia, and vomiting have been reported with high maternal nicotine intake.

FORMULA FEEDING

While breast milk provides the ideal nutrition for newborns, an iron-fortified, commercially prepared infant formula is an alternative source of nutrition for newborns and infants. In an attempt to ensure product safety and minimum nutritional standards, the U.S. Food and Drug Administration (FDA) regulates the manufacture of all infant formulas; the use of homemade infant formula, usually a mixture of cow's or goat's milk with vitamins, is discouraged due to the invariable lack of critical micronutrients and carbohydrates as well as the increased risk of contaminations. In the first year of life, infant-specific formula should be used, while toddler-specific formulas, if used, should not be started until after age 12 months. After age 1 year, most babies' nutritional needs can be met via a combination of whole cow's milk and a variety of solid foods that are able to be eaten safely by a toddler.

The majority of infant formula used is in a dry powder form that needs to be mixed with water for use. To minimize the risk of infectious contamination, the storage of the dry powder should be in a cool, dry, indoor location. Once prepared, liquid or reconstituted formula should not be left out at room temperature for more than 2 hours or more than 1 hour after the onset of feeding. If the entire amount of formula is not used during a feeding, the remainder, now a mixture of formula and the baby's saliva, should be discarded, as this combination will support bacterial growth.

If an infant is formula-fed, the parents and caregivers should be encouraged to hold the infant during feeding to have the interaction inherent in breastfeeding. Questions about frequency, amount, and type of feedings are often asked during well-baby visits. Counseling should be offered to help ensure optimal nutrition (Box 17-1 and Table 17-1).

Solid food can complement formula or breastfeeding beginning around 6 months of age. Signs that the baby is ready for solid foods include sitting with little or no support, having good head control, and opening his/her mouth and leaning forward when food is offered. Foods can include fortified infant cereals, meat or other proteins, fruits, vegetables, grains, yogurts and cheeses, among others. As the child gets older, self-feeding should be encouraged. Certain precautions should be used to prevent choking, including having the child sit up while eating, preferably in a high chair or other safe place. The child should not be lying down, and feeding in a car or stroller should be avoided. The child should be supervised by an adult who is focused on the child while eating.

BOX 17-1 Guidelines for Nutrition in the First Months of Life

- Frequency of feeding during months 1 and 2:
  - Breastfed infants: A minimum of 10 minutes at each breast every 1.5 to 3 hours
  - Bottle-fed infants: 2 to 3 oz (60 to 90 mL) every 2 to 3 hours
- Fluoride supplementation is advisable for breastfed infants or if formula is not mixed with fluoridated water in formula-fed infants
- Iron supplementation is recommended for children who are exclusively breastfed starting at 4 months of age at a dose of 1 mg/kg
- Solid foods are best introduced no sooner than age 4 to 6 months
- Signs that an infant is ready for solid food:
  - Doubled birth weight and at least 4 to 6 months of age
  - Taking more than 32 oz (946 mL) formula per day or more than 8 to 10 feedings (breast or bottle) per day

Source: Nemours Foundation. Feeding your newborn. http://kidshealth.org/en/parents/feednewborn.html

TABLE 17-1 Anticipated Weight Gain and Caloric Requirements in the First 3 Years of Life

AGE	ANTICIPATED AVERAGE WEIGHT GAIN PER DAY (G)	REQUIRED KILOCALORIE PER KILOGRAM PER DAY
0 to 3 months	26 to 31	100 to 120 kcal
3 to 6 months	17 to 18	105 to 115 kcal
6 to 9 months	12 to 13	100 to 105 kcal
9 to 12 months	9	100 to 105 kcal
1 to 3 years	7 to 9	100 kcal

Discussion Sources

Briggs GG, Freeman RK, Towers CV, Forinash AB. *Drugs in Pregnancy and Lactation.* 11th ed. Philadelphia, PA: Wolters Kluwer; 2017.
Centers for Disease Control and Prevention. Breastfeeding data and statistics. https://www.cdc.gov/breastfeeding/data/index.htm
Centers for Disease Control and Prevention. Infant formula feeding. https://www.cdc.gov/nutrition/infantandtoddlernutrition/formula-feeding/index.html
Centers for Disease Control and Prevention. What to expect while breastfeeding. https://www.cdc.gov/nutrition/infantandtoddlernutrition/breastfeeding/what-to-expect.html
Hale T. *Medications and Mothers' Milk, 2019.* 18th ed. Plano, TX: Hale Publishing; 2019.
Hansen TWR. Neonatal jaundice. Medscape. http://emedicine.medscape.com/article/974786-overview
La Leche League International. Pumping milk. https://www.llli.org/breastfeeding-info/pumping-milk/
Summary of classifications for hormonal contraceptive methods and intrauterine devices: appendix L. *MMWR.* 2010;59:76–81.
Update to CDC's medical eligibility criteria for contraceptive use, 2016. *MMWR.* 2016;65(3):1–103.
USDA. WIC Breastfeeding Support: Steps and signs of a good latch. https://wicbreastfeeding.fns.usda.gov/steps-and-signs-good-latch

QUESTIONS

1. Which of the following is appropriate advice to give to a mother who is breastfeeding her 10-day-old infant?

   A. "Your milk will come in today."

   B. "To minimize breast tenderness, the baby should not be kept on either breast for more than 5 to 10 minutes."

C. "A clicking sound made by the baby during feedings signifies a good latch and suck."

D. "The baby's urine should be light or colorless."

2. Which of the following is appropriate advice to give to a mother who is breastfeeding her 12-hour-old infant?

A. "You will likely have enough milk to feed the baby within a few hours of birth."

B. "The baby might need to be awakened to be fed."

C. "Supplemental feeding is needed unless the baby has at least four wet diapers in the first day of life."

D. "The baby will likely have a seedy, yellow bowel movement today."

3. Compared with the use of infant formula, advantages for the breastfed baby include all of the following except:

A. lower incidence of diarrheal illness.

B. greater weight gain in the first few weeks of life.

C. reduced risk of allergic disorders.

D. lower occurrence of constipation.

4. At 3 weeks of age, the average-weight, formula-fed infant should be expected to take:

A. 2 to 3 oz, or 60 to 90 mL, every 2 to 3 hours.

B. 2 to 3 oz, or 60 to 90 mL, every 3 to 4 hours.

C. 3 to 4 oz, or 90 to 118 mL, every 2 to 3 hours.

D. 3 to 4 oz, or 90 to 118 mL, every 3 to 4 hours.

5. In infants, solid foods are best introduced no earlier than:

A. 1 to 3 months.

B. 3 to 5 months.

C. 4 to 6 months.

D. 6 to 8 months.

6. Nursing infants generally maximally receive about which percentage of the maternal dose of a drug?

A. 1%

B. 3%

C. 5%

D. 10%

7. Most drugs pass into breast milk through:

A. active transport.

B. facilitated transfer.

C. simple diffusion.

D. creation of a pH gradient.

8. To remove a drug from breast milk through "pump and dump," the nursing mother should refrain from taking the offending medication and the process must be continued for:

A. two infant feeding cycles.

B. approximately 8 hours.

C. three to five drug-free half-lives of the medication.

D. a period of time that is highly unpredictable.

9. When counseling a breastfeeding woman about alcohol use during lactation, you relate that:

A. drinking a glass of wine or beer will enhance the let-down reflex.

B. because of its high molecular weight, relatively little alcohol is passed into breast milk.

C. maternal alcohol use causes a reduction in the amount of milk ingested by the infant.

D. infant intoxication can be seen with the mother having as few as one to two alcoholic drinks.

10. The anticipated average daily weight gain during the first 3 months of life is approximately:

  A. 15 g or 0.53 oz.

  B. 20 g or 0.7 oz.

  C. 25 g or 0.88 oz.

  D. 30 g or 1 oz.

11. The average required caloric intake in an infant from age 0 to 3 months is usually:

  A. 40 to 60 kcal/kg/day.

  B. 60 to 80 kcal/kg/day.

  C. 80 to 100 kcal/kg/day.

  D. 100 to 120 kcal/kg/day.

12. Regarding physiological jaundice in the newborn, select all that are correct:

  A. It occurs between the first 12 and 24 hours of life.

  B. It progresses from the abdomen toward the head of the infant.

  C. Unconjugated bilirubin is elevated.

  D. Risk of development of hyperbilirubinemia can be reduced in a breastfed infant with frequent breastfeeding every 2 to 3 hours per 24 hours.

  E. It can be avoided by supplemental water and dextrose feedings between breastfeeding in the first 3 to 4 days of life to increase infant hydration while awaiting mother's milk to come in.

13. The most likely consequence of inadequate feeding during the first few weeks of a newborn is:

  A. hypercalcemia.

  B. hypernatremia.

  C. hypokalemia.

  D. hyperkalemia

14. Which of the following would be a concern regarding weight change in a newborn?

  A. weight loss of 2% by day 2 of life

  B. no weight gain after 3 days of life

  C. weight gain of less than 3% after 1 week of life

  D. weight loss of greater than 7% at any time after the first week of life

15. A mother who has been breastfeeding her newborn is planning on returning to work and asks about the use of breast pumps. The nurse practitioner (NP) counsels on all of the following except:

  A. Some insurance companies will cover the costs of breast pumps.

  B. Breast pumps can allow flexibility in allowing mothers to return to work or school.

  C. Double pumps are not recommended as they express about half the amount of milk as single pumps.

  D. Federal law requires the employer to provide adequate breaks and a location for breast pumping.

16 to 19.   Indicate (*yes or no*) whether each of the following is expected with a good latch by a newborn.

_____   16. Areola easily visible

_____   17. Dimpling of the baby's cheeks

_____   18. Clicking noise made by baby

_____   19. Baby's mouth is widely open with lips flanged outward

20. Expected stool findings for a 2-week-old baby who is breastfeeding would most likely include:

   A. loose, seedy stools multiple times per day.

   B. black, tar-like stool about once per day.

   C. thick, blood-tinged stool after each feeding.

   D. watery stool about once every 2 to 3 days.

21. A 26-year-old mother who is breastfeeding her 4-month-old son reports a problematic cough and intermittent wheeze. She has a history of asthma that was well controlled with a medium-potency inhaled corticosteroid (ICS) and sporadic use of a short-acting beta-2 agonist (i.e., albuterol), but she stopped taking her medications during her pregnancy. The NP advises that:

   A. she should return to using the ICS on a set schedule with as-needed albuterol and continue breastfeeding.

   B. she should continue with the ICS on a set schedule with as-needed albuterol and discontinue breastfeeding.

   C. a long-acting beta-2 agonist (LABA) is recommended while breastfeeding.

   D. theophylline should be used while breastfeeding until the baby is 6 months old, then switch to an ICS.

22. The use of homemade infant formula versus commercially prepared infant formula is discouraged due to:

   A. increased risk of contaminations.

   B. increased risk of an allergic reaction.

   C. excessive amount of calcium.

   D. higher cost.

23 to 25. Indicate (*yes or no*) whether the following infant formulas should be discarded.

_____ 23. Reconstituted (unused) formula left at room temperature for 1 hour

_____ 24. Reconstituted (unused) formula stored in the refrigerator for 2 hours

_____ 25. Leftover formula following a feeding left at room temperature for 20 minutes

26 to 29. Indicate (*yes or no*) whether each would support a decision to start solid foods in an infant.

_____ 26. At least 3 months old

_____ 27. Is able to sit upright without any support

_____ 28. Has more than doubled the birth weight

_____ 29. Consumes more than 32 oz of formula each day

30. Which of the following is most accurate regarding fluoride supplementation in infants?

   A. Supplementation is not needed for any infant younger than 12 months of age.

   B. Supplementation is advised in infants 6 months and older who are exclusively breastfed.

   C. Supplementation is not needed for any formula-fed infant.

   D. All infants should receive supplementation at 4 months of age until they begin solid foods.

31. Which of the following infants would most likely require iron supplementation?

   A. a 5-month-old who is formula-fed

   B. a 2-month-old who is exclusively breastfed

   C. a 7-month-old who is exclusively breastfed

   D. an 8-month-old who is breastfed and eats a variety of solid foods

For answers and rationales, see end of chapter.

Early Childhood Development

Overview

Performing a developmental assessment is one of the most important parts of providing pediatric primary care. In addition to providing a marker for evaluating the child, the developmental assessment also affords an important learning tool for the parents. Pointing out milestones to be achieved in the near future and their impact on safety can help the family prepare appropriately for safety and activities that encourage the child's growth and development (Table 17-2). Surveillance of growth and development and determining potential lags is essential in the care of the child. Persistent delays in childhood development require additional assessment to determine etiology and to develop a plan for intervention. Initiation of early intervention improves outcomes in family and childhood developmental compromise. Examples of early interventions include audiology services, speech and language therapy, physical therapy, nutrition services, and psychological services.

TABLE 17-2 Anticipated Early Childhood Developmental Milestones

AGE	ABLE TO BE OBSERVED DURING OFFICE VISIT	REPORTED BY PARENT OR CAREGIVER

Newborn	■ Moves all extremities
	■ Spontaneous stepping
	■ Reacts to sound by blinking, turning
	■ Responds to cries of other neonates
	■ Well-developed sense of smell
	■ Cries when uncomfortable
	■ Preference for higher-pitched voices
	■ Primitive reflexes
	  • Tonic neck
	  • Palmar grasp
	  • Babinski response
	  • Rooting awake and asleep
	  • Sucking
		■ Able to be calmed by feeding, cuddling
		■ Reinforces presence of developmental tasks seen in examination room

1 to 2 months	■ Lifts head ■ Holds head erect ■ Regards face ■ Follows objects through visual field ■ Moro and palmar grasp reflexes fading	■ Social smile ■ Recognizes parents
3 to 4 months	■ Grasps cube ■ Reaches for objects ■ Brings objects to mouth ■ Raspberry sound	■ Laughs, squeals, vocalizes in response to others ■ Recognizes food by sight ■ Rolls back to side ■ Imitates others ■ Repeats interesting actions
5 months	■ Back straight when pulled to sitting ■ Bears weight on legs when standing ■ Plays with feet ■ Sits with support	■ Coughs, snorts to attract attention

Continued

TABLE 17-2 Anticipated Early Childhood Developmental Milestones—cont'd

AGE	ABLE TO BE OBSERVED DURING OFFICE VISIT	REPORTED BY PARENT OR CAREGIVER
6 to 8 months	■ Sits without support ■ Scoops small object with rake grip; some thumb use ■ Hand-to-hand transfer ■ Imitates "bye-bye" ■ Stranger and separation anxiety begins (6 months) and increases during this time period ■ Pulls feet into mouth	■ Closes lips in response to dislike of food ■ Rolls back to stomach and stomach to back ■ Recognizes "no" ■ Chains together syllables (dada, papa, mama) but does not have meaning
9 to 11 months	■ Crawls, pulling self forward by hands, then creeps with abdomen off floor ■ Stands initially by holding onto furniture, later stands solo ■ Imitates peek-a-boo and pat-a-cake ■ Picks up small object with thumb and index finger	■ Cruises ■ Follows simple command, such as "come here." Assigns meaning to words such as "mama, papa, dada"
12 to 15 months	■ Initially walks with help, progresses to walking solo ■ Neat pincer grasp ■ Places cube in cup ■ Hands over objects on request ■ Builds tower of two bricks	■ Says one to two words ■ Indicates wants by pointing ■ Scribbles spontaneously ■ Imitates animal sounds
15 to 20 months	■ Points to several body parts ■ Throws a ball overhand ■ Seats self in chair ■ Climbs	■ Uses a spoon with little spilling ■ Walks up and down steps with help ■ Understands two-step commands ■ Feeds self ■ Carries and hugs doll ■ Imitates housework ■ Speech: four to six words by 15 months, increases to 10 or more words by 18 months ■ Scribbles vigorously ■ Builds tower three cubes tall
24 months	■ Speaks in sentences of two or more words ■ Kicks ball on request ■ Jumps with both feet ■ Uses pronouns ■ Is developing handedness	■ Runs ■ Copies vertical and horizontal lines ■ Has up to a 300-word vocabulary ■ Washes and dries hands ■ Engages in parallel play ■ Puts on simple clothing
30 months	■ Walks backward ■ Hops on one foot ■ Copies circle	■ Gives first and last names ■ Uses plurals ■ Usually separates easily from parents
36 months	■ Holds crayons with fingers ■ Nearly all speech intelligible to people not in daily contact with child ■ Three-word sentences	■ Walks down stairs alternating steps ■ Rides tricycle ■ Copies circles ■ Dresses with supervision

Continued

TABLE 17-2 Anticipated Early Childhood Developmental Milestones—cont'd

AGE	ABLE TO BE OBSERVED DURING OFFICE VISIT	REPORTED BY PARENT OR CAREGIVER
3 to 4 years	■ Responds to command to place object in, on, or under a table ■ Knows gender ■ Draws circle when one is shown	■ Takes off jacket and shoes ■ Washes and dries face ■ Engages in cooperative play ■ Speech includes plurals, personal pronouns, verbs ■ Skips ■ Asks many questions
4 to 5 years	■ Runs and turns while maintaining balance ■ Stands on one foot for at least 10 seconds ■ Counts to four ■ Draws a person without torso ■ Copies (1) by imitation ■ Verbalizes activities to do when cold, hungry, tired	■ Buttons clothes ■ Dresses self (not including tying shoelaces) ■ Can play without adult input for about 30 minutes
5 to 6 years	■ Catches ball ■ Knows age ■ Knows right from left hand ■ Draws person with six to eight parts, including torso ■ Identifies best friend ■ Likes teacher	■ Able to complete simple chores ■ Understands concept of 10 items; likely counts higher by rote ■ Has sense of gender
6 to 7 years	■ Copies triangle shape ■ Draws person with at least 12 parts ■ Prints name ■ Reads multiple single-syllable words	■ Ties shoelaces ■ Counts to 30 and above ■ Able to differentiate morning from later in day ■ Generally plays well with peers ■ No significant behavioral problems in school ■ Can name intended career
7 to 8 years	■ Copies diamond shape ■ Reads simple sentences ■ Draws person with at least 16 parts	■ Ties shoelaces ■ Knows day of the week
8 to 9 years	■ Able to give response to question such as what to do if an object is accidentally broken	■ Able to add, subtract, borrow, carry ■ Understands concept of working as a team
9 to 10 years	■ Knows month, day, year ■ Gives months of the year in sequence	■ Able to multiply and do complex subtraction ■ Has increased reading fluency
10 to 12 years	■ Beginning of pubertal changes for many children	■ Able to perform simple division ■ Has complex reading skills

Source: Burns CE, Dunn AM, Brady MA, et al. *Pediatric Primary Care.* 6th ed. Philadelphia, PA: Elsevier Saunders; 2016.

Special consideration is needed when assessing development in preterm infants, typically defined as born before completing 37 weeks of gestation. For the first 24 months of life, the developmental expectations must be corrected for prematurity; for example, an 8-month-old infant born 8 weeks early, or at 32 weeks' gestation, would be expected to reach the developmental milestones of a 6-month-old.

Developmental Benchmarks and Anticipatory Guidance

Providing health advice to the growing family is a critical role of the NP. During anticipatory guidance counseling, the NP should review the normal developmental landmarks that the child is expected to reach in the near future and offer advice about how parents can cope with, adapt to, and avoid problems with these changes. This guidance is tailored to meet the needs of the family but typically follows a developmental framework and should continue through adolescence. Counseling provides an opportunity to promote healthy habits (e.g., encourage regular physical activity, encourage proper eating habits, limit screen time to 1 to 2 hours per day outside of what is needed for school work). Once a child reaches early adolescence (11 to 14 years), anticipatory guidance should include the child's emotional well-being, sexual development, and substance abuse risks.

Potential Alterations in Early Childhood Development

The NP should be aware of certain developmental "red flags" found in the young child. A persistent presence of one or more of these findings would warrant further evaluation:

- *By 6 months*: No big smiles or other warm, joyful expressions
- *By 9 months*: No back-and-forth sharing of sounds, smiles, or other facial expressions
- *By 12 months*: Lack of response to name, no babbling or "baby talk," and/or no back-and-forth gestures, such as pointing, showing, reaching, or waving
- *By 16 months*: No spoken words
- *By 24 months*: No meaningful two-word phrases that do not involve imitating or repeating

The American Academy of Pediatrics (AAP) recommends routine screening for autism between 18 and 24 months (Table 17-3). Autism spectrum disorder (ASD) affects 1 in 68 children and encompasses a range of developmental disorders and other conditions previously included in the diagnosis of pervasive developmental disorders (PDD). There are two main types of ASD behaviors: restrictive/repetitive behaviors and social communication/interaction behaviors. The behaviors cannot be explained by intellectual disability, global developmental delay, or other issue, and must be sufficient to cause difficulties with global function, including social, education, and/or occupational activities, and are present in early childhood, although quite often autism goes without being noted until social demands on the child exceed the ability to respond in what is considered to be a societally and age-anticipated manner.

Social issues in the younger child with ASD often include avoiding eye contact, having difficulty understanding personal space boundaries, avoiding or resisting physical contact, as well as having difficulty with being comforted when distressed. Activities where toddlers usually learn to interact with others through simple games like peek-a-boo, waving bye-bye, and playing pat-a-cake pose a significant challenge.

As the child ages, verbal and communication skills continue to lag. Up to 40% of children with ASD are without understandable speech, whereas approximately 25% will have some intelligible, age-appropriate speech by age 18 months but later lose this verbal ability. Some children speak later in childhood. For children with verbal skills, echolalia, where the child repeats phrases or words, is common, as is providing an unrelated answer to a question.

TABLE 17-3 Possible "Red Flags" for Autism Spectrum Disorder	
Prior to the toddler years	■ Does not respond to name **by 12 months** ■ Does not point to objects to show interest **by 14 months** ■ Does not play "pretend" games **by 18 months**
Usually toddler years and beyond	■ Avoids eye contact and wants to be alone; has obsessive interests ■ Has trouble understanding other people's feelings or expressing own feelings ■ Has delayed speech/language skills; repeats words over and over ■ Gives unrelated answers to questions ■ Gets upset by minor changes; has unusual reactions to environmental stimuli ■ Flaps hands, rocks body, or spins in circles

Source: CDC. Autism Spectrum Disorder. https://www.cdc.gov/ncbddd/autism/signs.html

TABLE 17-4 Findings of Fragile X Syndrome and XXY Male (Klinefelter's Syndrome)

DIAGNOSIS	FINDINGS
Fragile X syndrome	In males: Large testicles (macroorchidism) after the beginning of puberty, large body habitus, learning and behavioral differences (hyperactivity, intellectual disability common), large forehead and ears, prominent jaw, tendency to avoid eye contact
	In females: Significantly less common with fewer prominent findings, usually with less severe developmental/intellectual issues
	Most common known cause of autism in either gender, occurs in all racial and ethnic groups, though remains a small percentage of children with autism
	Blood testing available for carrier state (genetic risk for having a child with fragile X syndrome) or for diagnosis of the condition. Antenatal diagnosis possible.
XXY Male Klinefelter's syndrome	Only males affected, with developmental issues, most commonly language impairment. Physical habitus = low testicular volume, hip and breast enlargement.
	Blood testing available for carrier state (genetic risk for having a child with Klinefelter's syndrome) or for diagnosis of the condition. Antenatal diagnosis possible.

Sources: National Fragile X Foundation. Fragile X syndrome. https://fragilex.org/fragile-x/fragile-x-syndrome/

National Institutes of Health, U.S. National Library of Medicine. Klinefelter syndrome, https://www.ghr.nlm.nih.gov/condition/klinefelter-syndrome

Social interactions with peers pose a challenge, where the child does not, within normative age-appropriate parameters, play well with other children, having difficulty sharing toys and taking turns. Self-stimulation, with arm-flapping and other similar behaviors, may occur. A change in routine can trigger behavioral problems. At the same time, many children without ASD often have times where playing with other children or having routine disrupted is problematic. For further information, including the diagnostic criteria for ASD, please see the American Psychiatric Association's *Diagnostic and Statistical Manual of Mental Disorders, Fifth Edition* (*DSM-5*).

Occasionally, a chromosomal alteration is a contributing factor in altered childhood development. Fragile X syndrome is the most common known cause of autism in either gender and occurs in all racial and ethnic groups; at the same time, the majority of children with autism do not have fragile X syndrome. Another chromosomal anomaly, Klinefelter's syndrome (XXY male), also is associated with developmental issues, mainly verbal in nature (Table 17-4).

Discussion Sources

American Academy of Pediatrics. *Bright Futures Tool and Resource Kit.* https://brightfutures.aap.org/materials-and-tools/tool-and-resource-kit/Pages/default.aspx

American Psychiatric Association. (2013). *Diagnostic and statistical manual of mental disorders: DSM-5* (5th ed). Arlington, VA: American Psychiatric Association.

Burns CE, Dunn AM, Brady MA, Starr NB, Blosser CG, Garzon DL. *Pediatric Primary Care.* 6th ed. Philadelphia, PA: Elsevier Saunders; 2016.

Centers for Disease Control and Prevention. Learn the signs. Act early. https://www.cdc.gov/ncbddd/actearly/

Lipkin PH, Macias MM, American Academy of Pediatrics. Promoting optimal development: identifying infants and young children with developmental disorders through developmental surveillance and screening. *Pediatrics.* 2019. https://pediatrics.aappublications.org/content/pediatrics/early/2019/12/12/peds.2019-3449.full.pdf

QUESTIONS

32. Which of the following is most consistent with a normal developmental examination for a 3-month-old infant born at 40 weeks' gestation?

A. sitting briefly with support

B. experimenting with sound

C. rolling over

D. having a social smile

33. Which of the following is most consistent with a normal developmental examination for a thriving 5-month-old infant born at 32 weeks' gestation?

A. sitting briefly with support

B. experimenting with sound

C. rolling over

D. performing hand-to-hand transfers

34. A healthy full-term infant at age 3 to 4 months should be able to:

A. recognize parents.

B. grasp a cube.

C. imitate others.

D. say "dada" and "mama."

35. A healthy infant at age 9 to 11 months is expected to:

A. roll from back to stomach.

B. imitate "bye-bye."

C. play peek-a-boo.

D. hand over a toy on request.

36. A healthy 2-year-old child is able to:

A. speak in phrases of two or more words.

B. throw a ball at a target.

C. scribble spontaneously.

D. ride a tricycle.

37. At which age would a child likely start to imitate housework?

A. 18 months

B. 24 months

C. 30 months

D. 36 months

38. A healthy 3-year-old child is expected to:

A. give his or her first and last names.

B. use pronouns.

C. kick a ball.

D. name a best friend.

39. A healthy 6- to 7-month-old infant is able to:

A. roll from back to stomach.

B. confidently feed self a cracker.

C. reach for an object.

D. crawl on abdomen.

40. You examine a healthy 9-month-old infant from a full-term pregnancy and expect to find that the infant:

A. sits without support.

B. cruises.

C. recognizes "no."

D. imitates a razzing noise.

41. A healthy 3-year-old child is in your office for well-child care. You expect this child to be able to:

   A. count to four.

   B. alternate feet when climbing stairs.

   C. speak in two-word phrases.

   D. tie shoelaces.

42 to 45. Indicate (*yes or no*) whether each of the following are normal findings in a newborn.

_____ **42.** Best vision at a range of 8 to 12 inches

_____ **43.** Palmar grasp

_____ **44.** Preference for lower-pitched voices

_____ **45.** Well-developed sense of smell

46. Which of the following do you expect to find in an examination of a 2-week-old infant?

   A. a visual preference for the human face

   B. indifferent reaction in response to sounds or movements

   C. indifference to the cry of other neonates

   D. social smile

47. Which of the following is the most appropriate response in a developmental examination of a healthy 5-year-old child?

   A. being able to name a best friend

   B. giving gender appropriately

   C. naming an intended career

   D. hopping on one foot

48. You are examining an 18-month-old boy who is not speaking any discernible words. Mom tells you he has not said "mama" or "dada" yet or babbled or smiled responsively. You:

   A. encourage the mother to enroll her son in day care to increase his socialization.

   B. conduct further evaluation of milestone attainment.

   C. reassure the parent that delayed speech is common in boys.

   D. order audiogram and tympanometry.

49. The following benchmarks indicate normal development by a healthy child born at term who is now 12 months of age. *(Choose all that apply.)*

   A. talking in two-word sentences

   B. pointing to a desired object

   C. handing over objects on request

   D. walking backward

50. It is considered a possible developmental "red flag" if a child does not respond to his or her name by 9 months of age.

   A. true

   B. false

51. All of the following demonstrate possible "red flags" for ASD in a 2-year-old except:

   A. avoids eye contact.

   B. echolalia.

   C. plays pretend games while alone or with others.

   D. overreacts to unusual smells and sounds.

52. When assessing early developmental milestones in children born preterm, the developmental expectations should be corrected for prematurity until what age?

   A. 6 months

   B. 12 months

   C. 24 months

   D. 4 years

53. All of the following are consistent with a fragile X syndrome diagnosis in males except:

   A. microorchidism following onset of puberty.

   B. large body habitus.

   C. large ears.

   D. hyperactivity.

54. Which of the following chromosomal syndromes is a common etiology of social and verbal developmental delays in boys?

   A. Tay-Sachs disease

   B. cystic fibrosis

   C. fragile X

   D. trisomy 18

55. One physical sign of fragile X syndrome in males includes:

   A. large eyes.

   B. large forehead.

   C. small head.

   D. recessive jaw.

56. Klinefelter's syndrome (XXY male) is most commonly marked by:

   A. language impairment in males.

   B. fine motor delay in males.

   C. hip and breast enlargement in women.

   D. attention-deficit disorder in males.

57. Klinefelter's syndrome (XXY male) and risk for having a child with this condition can be accurately identified by which of the following? (Choose all that apply.)

   A. urine test

   B. literacy assessment

   C. amniocentesis

   D. blood testing for carrier state

58. All of the following would support a diagnosis of ASD except:

   A. a failure to initiate or respond to a social interaction.

   B. exhibiting extreme distress with small changes in routines.

   C. the symptoms are absent until the child reaches school age.

   D. excessive touching of objects.

59. At which of the following ages in a healthy infant's life is parental anticipatory guidance about teething most helpful?

   A. 1 to 2 months

   B. 2 to 4 months

C. 4 to 6 months

D. 8 to 10 months

60. At which of the following ages in a healthy young child's life is parental anticipatory guidance about temper tantrums most helpful?

A. 8 to 10 months

B. 10 to 12 months

C. 12 to 14 months

D. 14 to 16 months

61. At which of the following ages in a developmentally on-target young child's life is parental anticipatory guidance about using "time out" as a discipline method most helpful?

A. 12 to 18 months

B. 18 to 24 months

C. 24 to 30 months

D. 30 to 36 months

62. At which of the following ages in a young child's life is parental anticipatory guidance about protection from falls most helpful?

A. birth

B. 2 months

C. 4 months

D. 6 months

63. At which of the following ages in a developmentally on-target young child's life is parental anticipatory guidance about toilet-training readiness most helpful?

A. 12 months

B. 15 months

C. 18 months

D. 24 months

64. At which of the following ages in a young child's life is parental anticipatory guidance about infant sleep position most helpful?

A. birth

B. 2 weeks

C. 2 months

D. 4 months

65. At which of the following ages in a developmentally on-target young child's life is parental anticipatory guidance about sexual activity most helpful?

A. 6 years

B. 8 years

C. 11 years

D. 14 years

66. At which of the following ages in a developmentally on-target young child's life is parental anticipatory guidance about substance abuse most helpful?

A. 8 years

B. 11 years

C. 14 years

D. 16 years

67. Recommended total daily screen time (e.g., television, computer, tablet, games) for a young child is:

A. 0 to 30 minutes.

B. 1 to 2 hours.

C. 2 to 3 hours.

D. more than 4 hours.

For answers and rationales, see end of chapter.

Lead Poisoning (Plumbism)

Overview

Lead poisoning, or plumbism, remains a significant public health problem. More than 12 million children in the United States have levels above the acceptable threshold, which is estimated to cost billions of dollars in lifetime productivity associated with this exposure. Ingested lead inactivates heme synthesis by inhibiting the insertion of iron into the protoporphyrin ring. This leads to the development of a microcytic, hypochromic anemia; basophilic stippling is often noted on red blood cell morphology. In addition, lead is significantly toxic to the solid organs, bones, and nervous system.

Lead poisoning is caused by exposure to lead in the environment. The major source in children is lead-based paint. Heavily leaded paint was used in homes built up to the 1950s, with lower-level lead-based paint used into the 1970s. Lead-based paint has not been available for household use in the United States since 1978. Unless deleading procedures have been performed, however, most homes built before 1957 contain lead-based paint. A diet low in calcium, iron, zinc, magnesium, and copper and high in fat, which is a typical diet for children living in poverty, enhances oral lead absorption.

For lead poisoning to occur, there must be an intersection between the environmental hazard and the child. In older homes, the point of greatest risk is the window because the windowsills and putty have high lead concentration. Because toddlers (aged 2 to 3) are the ideal height to reach windowsills and are often drawn to open windows, they are at greatest risk, and summer is the riskiest season. Plumbism is seldom noted beyond age 4 years unless the child has an intellectual disability or disordered eating.

Children can ingest lead by inhaling paint chips, household dust, and soil contaminated by leaded paint. Inhalation of paint dust is a potent lead source for infants and for children with lead levels of less than 45 mcg/dL, although toddlers and children with lead levels of more than 45 mcg/dL are typically poisoned by also eating paint chips. The question often arises as to why children would eat a nonfood substance such as a paint chip; these chips are reported to have a slightly sweet taste. In addition to paint, other household products contain lead hazards, including traditional home health remedies such as azarcon and greta, which are used for upset stomach or indigestion in the Latino and select ethnic communities, and select imported products including candies, toys, jewelry, cosmetics, pottery, and ceramics. Additional sources include drinking water contaminated by lead leaching from lead pipes, solder, brass fixtures or valves, and consumer products, including tea kettles and vinyl blinds.

> **CLINICAL CONCEPT**
>
> Long-term complications of lead poisoning include behavior or attention problems, poor academic performance, hearing problems, kidney damage, reduced IQ, and slowed body growth.

Clinical Presentation

Clinical manifestation of lead poisoning is usually not apparent until a child's lead level is markedly elevated. Symptoms of elevated lead levels include abdominal pain and cramping, aggressive behavior, anemia, constipation, difficulty sleeping, headaches, irritability, loss of previous developmental skills in young children, low appetite and energy levels, and reduced sensations. Very high levels of lead can result in vomiting, staggering walk, muscle weakness, seizures, or coma. Because most children have low-level exposure or chronic lead exposure with few or no symptoms, periodic screening of all children is recommended. Primary prevention of lead poisoning should be the goal to reduce risk for all children. After lead risk is identified, removing the child or limiting exposure is vital.

Diagnostic Testing and Treatment

A measure of 5 mcg/dL or greater is now used to identify children with elevated blood lead levels. This value is in the highest 2.5% for children aged 1 to 5 years in the U.S. population. In the past, blood lead levels of 10 mcg/dL were defined as elevated. This lower value is being used to identify more children likely to have lead exposure, allowing parents, health-care providers, public health officials, and communities to take action earlier to reduce future exposure to lead. Most children with lead levels of 5 to 44 mcg/dL are treated with removal from the source, improved nutrition, and iron therapy. Those with lead levels of 45 to 50 mcg/dL are treated with a chelation agent such as succimer, in addition to the previously listed interventions. For children with lead levels of greater than 50 mcg/dL, hospital admission with expert evaluation is likely the most prudent course of action to avoid serious problems (including encephalopathy) associated with markedly elevated lead levels.

Discussion Sources

Centers for Disease Control and Prevention. Blood lead levels in children. https://www.cdc.gov/nceh/lead/prevention/blood-lead-levels.htm

Centers for Disease Control and Prevention. CDC's Childhood Lead Poisoning Prevention Program. http://www.cdc.gov/nceh/lead/about/program.htm

National Institute of Environmental Health Sciences. Lead. https://www.niehs.nih.gov/health/topics/agents/lead/index.cfm

QUESTIONS

68. Which of the following children is most likely to have lead poisoning?

    A. a 5-year-old child with an intellectual disability who lives in a 15-year-old house in poor repair

    B. an infant who lives in a 5-year-old home with copper plumbing

    C. a toddler who lives in an 85-year-old home

    D. a preschooler who lives near an electric-generating plant

69. Sources of lead that can contribute to plumbism include select traditional remedies such as azarcon and greta.

    A. true

    B. false

70. A diet low in the following nutrients encourages lead absorption. *(Choose all that apply.)*

    A. protein

    B. carbohydrates

    C. zinc

    D. magnesium

71. You are devising a program to screen preschoolers for lead poisoning. The most sensitive component of this campaign is:

    A. environmental history.

    B. physical examination.

    C. hematocrit level.

    D. hemoglobin electrophoresis.

72. Patients with plumbism present with which kind of anemia?

    A. macrocytic, normochromic

    B. normocytic, normochromic

    C. hemolytic

    D. microcytic, hypochromic

73. At which of the following ages should screening begin for a child who has significant risk of lead poisoning?

A. 3 months

B. 6 months

C. 1 year

D. 2 years

74. Intervention for a child with a lead level of 5 to 44 mcg/dL usually includes all of the following except:

A. removal from the lead source.

B. iron supplementation.

C. chelation therapy.

D. encouraging a diet high in vitamin C.

75. Intervention for a child with a lead level of 45 to 50 mcg/dL or greater usually includes:

A. chelation therapy.

B. calcium supplementation.

C. exchange transfusion.

D. iron depletion therapy.

For answers and rationales, see end of chapter.

Hypertension, Type 2 Diabetes, and Dyslipidemia in Children

Overview

Prevalence of hypertension, type 2 diabetes mellitus (T2DM), and dyslipidemia has increased in recent years in association with the rise in childhood obesity. Risk factors for hypertension in children and teens include a family history of heart disease, high blood pressure, elevated lipid levels, exposure to tobacco smoke, a diet low in daily recommended intake of nutrients, obesity, T2DM, and lack of physical activity. Risk factors for T2DM in children include obesity, sedentary lifestyle, race/ethnicity, family history, augmentation of growth hormone (GH) and insulin-like growth factor (IGF) secretion during puberty, polycystic ovary syndrome (PCOS), hyperandrogenism, intrauterine exposure to maternal diabetes, low birth weight, and poor infant growth. Risk factors for dyslipidemia in children include family history of lipid abnormalities and T2DM.

Screening

Hypertension, T2DM, and dyslipidemia in children, as in adults, usually are without specific clinical signs and symptoms. Screening for these conditions is an example of secondary prevention, or early detection of asymptomatic disease.

According to cardiovascular disease (CVD) screening guidelines, a child's family history for obesity should be reviewed beginning at birth. Body mass index (BMI) should be measured beginning at age 2 years. For children between 12 months and 2 years of age for whom overweight or obesity is a concern, the use of reduced-fat milk would be appropriate. Beginning at age 5 years, if BMI is at or greater than the 85th percentile, intensify dietary and activity changes to the parent. The National Diabetes Education Program provides guidelines for healthy eating choices. A diet high in nutrients, protein, and complex carbohydrates and low in sugar and saturated fat is recommended.

Increased risk for diabetes (prediabetes) in children is defined as impaired fasting glucose (glucose level greater than or equal to 100 mg/dL or 5.6 mmol/L but less than or equal to 125 mg/dL or 7 mmol/L) or impaired glucose tolerance (2-hour postprandial glucose 140 to 199 mg/dL or 7.8 to 11 mmol/L) or an A1c of 5.7% to 6.4%. Diagnosis of T2DM is confirmed if random plasma glucose level is greater than or equal to 200 mg/dL or 11.1 mmol/L in conjunction with symptoms of T2DM or an A1c 6.5% or greater.

> **CLINICAL CONCEPT**
>
> Screening for T2DM for at-risk children begins at age 10 years or at onset of puberty and continues every 2 years until adulthood; at that point, the adult guidelines from the American Diabetes Association should be followed.

Criteria for screening include a BMI greater than the 85th percentile for age and sex, weight-for-height greater than the 85% percentile, or weight of more than 120% of ideal for height, plus any two or more of the aforementioned risk factors.

The AAP screening guidelines for total cholesterol levels in children and adolescents aged 2 to 19 years old are as follows: acceptable level is less than 170 mg/dL (less than 9.4 mmol/L), borderline is 170 to 199 mg/dL (9.4 to 11 mmol/L), and high is 200 mg/dL or greater (11.1 mmol/L or greater) (Box 17-2). Definitions for elevated low-density lipoprotein (LDL), high-density lipoprotein (HDL), and triglyceride-specific levels in children and teens depend on age, gender, and percentile of height. Children should be screened for family history of CVD beginning at age 3 years and should be periodically updated annually or as required by risk factors during nonurgent health visits. As family history and/or risk factors for CVD are identified, the NP should evaluate the child's family for risk factors, including parents, grandparents, aunts, and uncles (see Box 17-2). For at-risk children, fasting lipid levels should be tested after 2 years of age (but no later than 10 years of age) and should be retested in 3 to 5 years if the values fall within the reference range.

The National Institutes of Health (NIH) CVD screening guidelines state that the child's diet should be evaluated at every visit. At the child's birth, the mother should be encouraged to breastfeed at least until the infant is 12 months of age. If the mother is not breastfeeding, iron-fortified infant formula is recommended

---

BOX 17-2 Lipid Screening and Cardiovascular Health in Childhood

1. The population approach to a healthful diet should be recommended to all children older than 2 years, according to Dietary Guidelines for Americans. This approach includes the use of low-fat dairy products. For children between 12 months and 2 years of age for whom overweight or obesity is a concern or who have a family history of obesity, dyslipidemia, or cardiovascular disease (CVD), the use of reduced-fat milk would be appropriate.

2. The individual approach for children and adolescents at higher risk for CVD and with a high concentration of low-density lipoprotein (LDL) includes recommended changes in diet with nutritional counseling and other lifestyle interventions such as increased physical activity.

3. The most current recommendation is to screen children and adolescents with a positive family history of dyslipidemia or premature CVD (55 years of age or younger for men and 65 years of age or younger for women) or dyslipidemia. It is also recommended that pediatric patients for whom family history is not known or those with other CVD risk factors, such as overweight (body mass index [BMI] greater than or equal to the 85th percentile, less than the 95th percentile), obesity (BMI greater than or equal to the 95th percentile), hypertension (blood pressure greater than or equal to the 95th percentile), cigarette smoking, or diabetes mellitus, be screened with a fasting lipid profile.

4. For these children, the first screening should take place after 2 years of age but no later than 10 years of age. Screening before 2 years of age is not recommended.

5. A fasting lipid profile is the recommended approach to screening because there is no currently available non-invasive method to assess atherosclerotic CVD in children. This screening should occur in the context of well-child and health-maintenance visits. If values are within the reference range on initial screening, the patient should be retested in 3 to 5 years.

6. For pediatric patients who are overweight or obese and have a high triglyceride concentration or low high-density lipoprotein concentration, weight management is the primary treatment, which includes improvement of diet with nutritional counseling and increased physical activity to produce improved energy balance.

7. For patients 8 years and older with an LDL concentration greater than or equal to 190 mg/dL/10.6 mmol/L (or greater than or equal to 160 mg/dL/8.9 mmol/L with a family history of early heart disease or two or more additional risk factors present or greater than or equal to 130 mg/dL/7.2 mmol/L if diabetes mellitus is present), pharmacological intervention should be considered. The initial goal is to lower LDL concentration to less than 160 mg/dL/8.9 mmol/L. However, targets as low as 130 mg/dL/7.2 mmol/L or even 110 mg/dL/6.2 mmol/L may be warranted when there is a strong family history of CVD, especially with other risk factors including obesity, diabetes mellitus, metabolic syndrome, and other higher-risk situations.

Sources: Daniels SR, Greer FR; Committee on Nutrition. Lipid screening and cardiovascular health in childhood. Pediatrics. 2008;122(1):198–208.

Expert Panel on Integrated Guidelines for Cardiovascular Health and Risk Reduction in Children and Adolescents; National Heart, Lung, and Blood Institute. Expert panel on integrated guidelines for cardiovascular health and risk reduction in children and adolescents: summary report. Pediatrics. 2011;128(Suppl 5):S213–256.

for the first 12 months; the majority of the child's caloric intake in the first year of life should come from breast milk or iron-fortified infant formula. From 12 to 24 months of age, drinking whole cow's milk or breast milk is recommended; after 24 months, children who are not breastfeeding should switch to skim or 1% milk. After 12 months, limit cow's milk to a total of 16 to 24 ounces (480 to 720 mL) a day. Fruit juice should contain 100% juice without added sugar if possible, should not replace breast milk or formula, and should be introduced no earlier than 6 months of age. Intake should be limited to 6 ounces a day for children 6 months to 5 years old. Parents and caregivers should be encouraged to use small amounts of fruit juice to flavor water, thereby increasing fluid intake while minimizing excessive juice intake. If vitamin C intake from fresh fruit is adequate, fruit juice does not need to be part of the child's diet. Dietary guidelines for children should be recommended and reinforced throughout childhood.

In the well child, check blood pressure annually beginning at age 3 years and chart for age, gender, and history. Refer to NIH guidelines when screening pediatric patients for elevated blood pressure, because definitions for elevated systolic and diastolic blood pressure vary with age, gender, and percentile of height. Blood pressure should be measured in the first 12 months only if the child has a renal, urological, or cardiac diagnosis or a history of being hospitalized in the neonatal intensive care unit.

Treatment

A weight-for-height tracking growth chart should be discussed with the parents. An age-appropriate heart healthy diet should be encouraged at every visit, with a particular emphasis on avoiding high-sodium, high-fat, and highly processed food, including products such as soda and fast foods. The NP should encourage parents to promote physical activity from the child's birth. At age 1 to 2 years, encourage active play and recommend limiting television and other screen time, including video games, to no more than a total of 2 hours or less per day. A smoke-free home should be encouraged and smoking cessation assistance offered to parents. Beginning at ages 9 to 11 years, the smoking status should be assessed and antismoking counseling offered at each visit. Smoking cessation assistance or referral should be offered when needed.

Nonpharmacological interventions in children and adolescents diagnosed with dyslipidemia, T2DM, hypertension, or more than one of these conditions include eating well, attaining or maintaining a healthy weight, and increasing physical activity. If cholesterol, glucose, and/or blood pressure goals are not reached using nonpharmacological methods, medication use is an option. Refer children to appropriate resources for treatment as needed, recognizing that lifestyle therapy, focusing on nutrition and physical activity, are typically the first-line measures.

Discussion Sources

Daniels S. Guidelines for screening, prevention, diagnosis, and treatment of dyslipidemia in children and adolescents. Endotext. 2016. https://www.ncbi.nlm.nih.gov/books/NBK395579/

Grundy SM, Stone NJ, Bailey AL, et al. AHA/ACC cholesterol clinical practice guidelines. *Circulation*. 2019;139:e1082–e1143. https://www.ahajournals.org/doi/pdf/10.1161/CIR.0000000000000625

National Institutes of Diabetes and Digestive and Kidney Diseases. Diabetes diet, eating, and physical activity. https://www.niddk.nih.gov/health-information/diabetes/overview/diet-eating-physical-activity?dkrd=hispt1153

National Institutes of Health, National Heart, Blood, and Lung Institute. Blood pressure tables for children and adolescents. http://www.nhlbi.nih.gov/health-pro/guidelines/current/hypertension-pediatric-jnc-4/blood-pressure-tables

National Institutes of Health, National Heart, Blood, and Lung Institute. *Expert Panel on Integrated Guidelines for Cardiovascular Health and Risk Reduction in Children and Adolescents: Summary Report*. https://www.nhlbi.nih.gov/node/80308

Xu H, Verre MC. Type 2 diabetes mellitus in children. *Am Fam Physician*. 2018;98:590–594

QUESTIONS

76. Which of the following are risk factors for hypertension in children and teens? *(Choose all that apply.)*

    A. obesity

    B. drinking whole milk

    C. being exposed to secondhand smoke

    D. 2 or more hours per day of screen time

77. Fruit juice intake is acceptable in children 6 months and older per which of the following recommendations? *(Choose all that apply.)*

    A. The juice is mixed in small amounts to flavor water.

    B. Only 100% juice is used.

C. Juice replaces no more than one serving of milk.

D. The juice is consumed in the morning with breakfast.

E. No more than 6 oz (177 mL) per day is recommended for children 6 months to 5 years.

78. In evaluating a 9-year-old child with a healthy BMI during a well visit, a comprehensive cardiovascular evaluation should be conducted by the following methods. *(Choose all that apply.)*

A. Obtain fasting lipid profile.

B. Screen for T2DM by measuring HbA1c.

C. Assess for family history of thyroid disease.

D. Assess diet and physical activity.

79. At what age is it appropriate to recommend dietary changes to parents if overweight or obesity in the child is a concern?

A. 12 months old

B. 5 years old

C. 10 years old

D. 18 years old

80. Which of the following is not a risk factor for T2DM in children and teens?

A. hyperinsulinemia

B. abnormal weight-to-height ratio

C. onset of nonorganic failure to thrive in the toddler years

D. Native American ancestry

81. Screening children with a known risk factor for T2DM is recommended at age 10 years or at the onset of puberty and should be repeated how often?

A. every other year

B. every year

C. every 6 months

D. every 3 years

82. Increased risk for diabetes (prediabetes) in children is defined as which of the following? *(Choose all that apply.)*

A. impaired fasting glucose (glucose level greater than or equal to 100 mg/dL or 5.6 mmol/L but less than or equal to 125 mg/dL or 7 mmol/L)

B. impaired glucose tolerance (2-hour postprandial glucose 140 to 199 mg/dL or 7.8 to 11 mmol/L)

C. HbA1c 7.5% or greater but 8.5% or less

D. random plasma glucose greater than or equal to 250 mg/dL (13.9 mmol/L)

83. Risk factors for dyslipidemia in children include which of the following? *(Choose all that apply.)*

A. blood pressure at the 70th to 80th percentile for age

B. breastfeeding into the toddler years

C. family history of lipid abnormalities

D. family history of T2DM

84. Screening cholesterol levels in children with one or more risk factors begins at what age?

A. birth

B. 2 years

C. 5 years

D. 10 years

85. An acceptable level of total cholesterol (mg/dL) in children and teens is:

   A. less than 170 mg/dL or 9.4 mmol/L.

   B. less than 130 mg/dL or 7.2 mmol/L.

   C. 110 to 130 mg/dL or 6.2 to 7.2 mmol/L.

   D. 130 to 199 mg/dL or 7.2 to 11 mmol/L.

For answers and rationales, see end of chapter.

Evaluation of the Febrile Child

Overview

Fever is a complex physiological reaction that occurs when exogenous pyrogens (microorganisms and their products, drugs, incompatible blood products) are introduced to the body. This triggers the production of endogenous pyrogens (polypeptides produced by host cells such as monocytes, macrophages, and interleukin-1). Prostaglandins activate thermoregulatory neurons and alter the hypothalamic set point. Vasomotor center reactions increase heat conservation and heat production. The result of this process is fever, defined as a rectal temperature of 100.6°F (38.1°C) or higher.

This section is focused on the evaluation and treatment of a child with fever who is age 3 months to 3 years. Infants younger than 3 months should be considered at risk for infection transmitted through the birth process and require specialized evaluation.

While parents, caregivers, and even health-care providers are fearful of fever, in the otherwise well child, an increase in body temperature has benefits. Indeed, fever is a normal physiological response, most commonly to an infectious agent, and should be thought of as a symptom rather than a disease. During fever, the viral replication rate is reduced. Increased body temperature is toxic to encapsulated bacteria, particularly *Streptococcus pneumoniae* and *Haemophilus influenzae* type B. The presence of fever has been associated with lower rates of morbidity and mortality associated with certain infectious diseases, including influenza, in both adults and children. The routine use of antipyretics including acetaminophen and ibuprofen has been associated with prolonged illness, especially when viral in origin. At the same time, a child with fever is often uncomfortable and cranky, which reinforces the perception that this is a condition that warrants treatment. However, fever also increases metabolic demands, a potential problem in a child with select chronic health problems; in these children, avoidance of fever is sometimes needed. When administering an antipyretic, caregivers should be aware of the appropriate formulation, dose, and dosing interval.

> **CLINICAL CONCEPT**
>
> Given the propensity of children to develop a number of infections, mostly the result of self-limiting viral infections, in the first years of life, fever is more commonly encountered in children than in adults.

The risk of serious illness in the presence of fever is currently significantly reduced in the advent of immunization against *H influenzae* type B and *S pneumoniae*, two bacteria that were the cause of the majority of early childhood meningitis and sepsis. The majority of cases are due to self-limiting viral infections with only 2% to 4% of febrile illnesses caused by bacterial infection. Nonetheless, the evaluation and treatment of a febrile child are an important part of providing pediatric health care. The NP needs to ascertain the febrile child's immunization status, including where in a particular series the child is or if any immunizations are missing, because this is an essential component of assessing risk of possible pathogens. Unfortunately, as more parents choose not to immunize their children, a resurgence of serious, potentially life-threatening vaccine-preventable diseases is inevitable.

Most otherwise well young children with an acute febrile illness have a self-limiting viral infection that resolves within a few days with supportive treatment only. Some children with fever have an identifiable condition where treatment with specific therapeutic agents is warranted; examples include influenza, acute otitis media (AOM), pneumonia, and urinary tract infection (UTI). On rare occasion, however, febrile young children with no obvious source of infection have serious sequelae including sepsis and death.

Fear of febrile seizure also contributes to the propensity to treat fever aggressively, with the thought that if the body temperature is reduced, seizure risk is reduced. The cause of febrile seizures is unclear but likely involves a relationship between endogenous pyrogens or cytokines and fever. Febrile seizures occur in young children when their seizure threshold is lowest. A simple febrile seizure is most likely to occur as fever is increasing rather than at its peak; however, there is no evidence that the rapidity of the rate of increase is associated with febrile seizures. A familial tendency has been noted with febrile seizure, but the condition is not predictive of the development of epilepsy. A simple febrile seizure is a benign, although frightening, common event in children 6 months to 5 years old; a child who has had one seizure is at increased risk for a recurrence. Much of what is termed "fever phobia," noted in both health-care providers and parents, arises from concerns about febrile seizure. Another unfounded concern is that even a milder fever can put the child at risk for brain damage.

Clinical Presentation

In a previously well, febrile child who is alert, able to tolerate oral fluids, aged 3 months to 3 years, the evaluation for the source of fever should start with a careful history of present illness, possible contacts with individuals with similar illness, and comprehensive physical examination. This clinical evaluation is aimed at finding an identifiable source of the fever, bearing in mind most fevers will be caused by self-limiting viral illnesses. The degree of temperature reduction in response to antipyretic therapy is not predictive of the presence or absence of bacteremia or other serious illness. Physical examination can identify worrisome findings indicating a seriously ill young child with toxic appearance that would require care in an urgent or emergent setting. Worrisome findings include pale or cyanotic skin, poor capillary refill (greater than 2 seconds), lethargy, weak or no cry, does not age-appropriately resist the examination, tachypnea (respiratory rate greater than or equal to 50% upper limit of normal [ULN] for age), tachycardia, unable to take or tolerate oral fluids, vomiting, dry mucous membranes, and no evidence of recent (within 4 hours) urinary output. Reassuring findings will include warm, dry, appropriately colored fingertips; brisk capillary refill; regards parental face; age-appropriately resists examination; has a lusty cry (or is smiling); has a respiratory rate less than 50% above ULN for age; heart rate within normal limits; tolerates oral fluids without vomiting; and adequately wet diapers. Signs of hypotension, cool skin, and/or nuchal rigidity are often absent in seriously ill young children, even in the presence of meningitis.

> **CLINICAL CONCEPT**
>
> When an identifiable source of fever is noted, such as viral upper respiratory tract infection (URI) or AOM, and the child is alert, taking fluids well, and with a nontoxic appearance, usually no particular diagnostic testing is done.

Diagnostic Testing

Diagnostic testing done, if at all, in the febrile younger child varies according to clinical presentation. In the sicker child with no identifiable source of fever and suspected sepsis, a more extensive evaluation should be initiated in an appropriate urgent or emergent setting. Testing can include:

- *Complete blood count (CBC) with white blood cell (WBC) differential*: Identify viral versus bacterial shifts and general leukocytic response
- *Blood culture*: Potentially identify causative organism in sepsis
- *Urinalysis and urine culture via transurethral catheter or suprapubic tap*: Evaluate for UTI including pyelonephritis, particularly important in child ≤2 years old or younger
- *Lumbar puncture with cerebrospinal fluid (CSF) analysis*: Evaluate for bacterial or viral meningitis, particularly important if alterations in neurological examination
- *Chest x-ray*: Rule in or out pneumonia or other respiratory tract condition that can contribute to sepsis, particularly important if dyspnea, tachypnea, decreased breath sounds, WBC ≥20,000/mm³ or greater, or other findings suggestive of lower respiratory tract infection
- *Stool culture, fecal WBC count*: Only if diarrhea present, to evaluate for possible focus of infection
- *Rapid testing for select viruses*: With suspected infection with respiratory syncytial virus (RSV), influenza virus, others
- *Laboratory markers*: Elevation in C-reactive protein (CRP), procalcitonin, lactate, others to help stratify the sickest child

Treatment

The treatment of a child with a febrile illness is dependent on its etiology. In children with suspected sepsis, inpatient admission is usually warranted or, at minimum, an evaluation in the emergency department for initiation of therapy with close follow-up care in the outpatient setting. For children with an identifiable and treatable illness, such as AOM or influenza, appropriate condition-specific medication should be initiated.

Advising the child's caregivers about the appropriate choice and use of antipyretics is an important part of providing care for a child with a non-life-threatening illness with fever. As previously mentioned, fever plays an important role in controlling infection. If a febrile child appears fairly comfortable, no specific fever treatment is needed. Even a cranky child usually is not harmed and can be helped by allowing the fever to run its course. If the child is uncomfortable with fever, commonsense measures include dressing the child lightly and increasing fluid intake. A cooling bath should not be used because the resulting shivering would drive up body temperature.

When used, the choice of an antipyretic is dictated by numerous factors, including the length of time for onset of action of the product (ideally, less than half an hour) and the duration of action (ideally, 4 to 8 hours), with no or few major reported adverse effects. Ibuprofen and acetaminophen are the most commonly prescribed antipyretics; both have onset of action within half an hour of the dose. The duration of action of acetaminophen is about 4 hours, whereas the duration of ibuprofen's action is about 6 hours. The antipyretic potential of acetaminophen is equal to that of ibuprofen. Acetaminophen has an excellent gastrointestinal (GI) adverse event profile but can be hepatotoxic with excessive use and high dose. Ibuprofen is usually well tolerated but does have the potential to cause gastric ulcer and gastritis, albeit usually with long-term high-dose use. As mentioned earlier, when administering an antipyretic, caregivers should be aware of the appropriate formulation, dose, and dosing interval. Cough-and-cold medications that contain acetaminophen or ibuprofen should not be given as there is a general lack of proven efficacy in children and use can result in overdoses when given in combination with an antipyretic. Additionally, alternating between acetaminophen and ibuprofen, so that the child gets an antipyretic every 2 to 4 hours, is not recommended, as there is a lack of evidence supporting this practice, and it can increase the risk of dosing errors and adverse effects in the infant and child. Aspirin should not be prescribed to a child with a febrile illness because of its association with Reye's syndrome. Ibuprofen should not be prescribed in varicella because its use is implicated in necrotizing fasciitis.

As mentioned, a significant concern of both parents and providers during the care of the younger child with a febrile illness is febrile seizure. Indeed, parents and caregivers often rationalize the around-the-clock use of medications such as acetaminophen and ibuprofen in an effort to avoid febrile seizures.

Daily use of common antiepileptic medications prescribed in children with seizure disorders, such as valproate and phenobarbital, appears to reduce the risk of febrile seizures. However, the risk associated with the use of these medications outweighs their minor benefit and is not recommended. In situations in which parental anxiety about febrile seizures is severe, intermittent oral diazepam (Valium®) at the onset of febrile illness is likely helpful in preventing recurrence.

> **CLINICAL CONCEPT**
>
> In reality, the use of antipyretics can improve the comfort of the child, but the use of these agents does not prevent febrile seizures, even in children with a history of this condition.

Discussion Sources

Hamilton JL, John SP. Evaluation of fever in infants and young children. *Am Fam Physician.* 2013;87:254–260.

National Institutes of Health. *Feverish Illness in Children: Assessment and Initial Management in Children Younger Than 5 Years.* http://www.ncbi.nlm.nih.gov/books/NBK45971

National Institutes of Health, National Institute of Neurological Disorders and Stroke. Febrile seizures fact sheet. https://www.ninds.nih.gov/Disorders/Patient-Caregiver-Education/Fact-Sheets/Febrile-Seizures-Fact-Sheet

Sullivan JE, Farrar HC. Fever and antipyretic use in children. *Pediatrics.* 2011;127:580–587. https://pediatrics.aappublications.org/content/127/3/580

QUESTIONS

86. Rates of sepsis in children have lowered in recent years mainly because of:

   A. more stringent screening and diagnosis of febrile illness.

   B. increased use of antipyretics.

   C. longer observation period in children with febrile illness.

   D. higher rates of select immunization.

87 to 91. When evaluating a young child with febrile illness, indicate if each is considered a *reassuring* or *concerning* finding.

_____ 87. Cyanotic skin

_____ 88. Brisk capillary refill

_____ 89. Weak or no cry

_____ 90. Respiratory rate less than 50% above ULN

_____ 91. No recent evidence of urinary output (within past 4 hours)

92. When evaluating an acutely ill febrile child with no clear cause of fever, a stool culture and fecal WBC count should most likely be performed:

    A. routinely for all febrile children.

    B. if fever has persisted for more than 48 hours despite use of antipyretics.

    C. when diarrhea is present.

    D. when fever exceeds 39.1°C (102.3°F).

93. The mechanism of action in fever includes which of the following?

    A. an increase in systemic vascular resistance

    B. endogenous pyrogens increase prostaglandin synthesis

    C. immature neutrophil forms in circulation

    D. atypical or reactive lymphocytes

94. When assessing a febrile child, the NP considers that:

    A. even minor temperature elevation is potentially harmful.

    B. nuchal rigidity is usually not found in early childhood meningitis.

    C. fever-related seizures usually occur at the peak of the temperature.

    D. most children aged 3 months to 3 years with temperatures of 38.3°C to 40°C (101°F to 104°F) have a potentially serious bacterial infection.

95. Which of the following is not seen during the body temperature increase found in fever?

    A. lower rate of viral replication

    B. toxic effect on select bacteria

    C. negative effect on *S pneumoniae* growth

    D. increased rate of atypical pneumonia pathogen replication

96. When providing care for a febrile 3-year-old who appears to have a minor, self-limiting illness, the NP bears in mind that all of the following are true except that:

    A. the use of antipyretics is potentially associated with prolonged illness.

    B. consistent use of an antipyretic provides a helpful way to shorten the course of infectious illnesses.

    C. fever increases metabolic demand.

    D. the presence of fever is associated with reduced morbidity and mortality.

97. Concerning the use of antipyretics in a febrile young child, which of the following statements is true?

    A. Ibuprofen is preferred for fever caused by viral infections.

    B. The degree of temperature reduction in response to antipyretic therapy is not predictive of the presence or absence of bacteremia.

    C. Compared with ibuprofen, acetaminophen has a delayed onset of antipyretic action.

    D. The duration of action with ibuprofen is shorter than acetaminophen.

98. When counseling the family of an otherwise healthy 2-year-old child who just had a febrile seizure, you consider which of the following regarding whether the child is at risk for future febrile seizures? *(Choose all that apply.)*

    A. The occurrence of one febrile seizure is predictive of having another.

    B. Intermittent diazepam can be used prophylactically during febrile illness to reduce risk of recurrence.

    C. A milder temperature elevation in a child with a history of a febrile seizure poses significant risk for future recurrent febrile and nonfebrile seizures.

    D. Consistent use of antipyretics during a febrile illness will significantly reduce the risk of a future febrile seizure.

99. When evaluating a child who has bacterial meningitis, the NP expects to find CSF results that include a report of an abnormal number of:

   A. neutrophils.

   B. lymphocytes.

   C. eosinophils.

   D. monocytes.

100. When evaluating a child who has aseptic or viral meningitis, the NP expects to find CSF results of:

   A. low protein.

   B. predominance of lymphocytes.

   C. glucose at about 30% of serum levels.

   D. low opening pressure.

101. Gina is 2 years old and presents with a 3-day history of fever, crankiness, and congested cough. Her respiratory rate is more than 50% of the ULN for age. Tubular breath sounds are noted at the right lung base. Skin turgor is normal, and she is wearing a wet diaper. She is alert, is resisting the examination as age appropriate, and engages in eye contact. Temperature is 38.3°C (101°F). Gina's diagnostic evaluation should include:

   A. chest x-ray.

   B. urine culture and susceptibility.

   C. lumbar puncture.

   D. sputum culture.

102. An early indicator of hypoperfusion in an acutely ill younger child is:

   A. an elevation in total WBC count.

   B. dehydration.

   C. capillary refill of more than 2 seconds.

   D. a nonresponsive child.

103. As part of the evaluation in a febrile 3-year-old boy, the following WBC count with differential is obtained:

   WBCs = 22,100/mm³

   Neutrophils = 75% (normal 40% to 70%) with toxic granulation

   Bands = 15% (normal 0% to 4%)

   Lymphocytes = 4% (normal 30% to 40%)

   Which of the following best describes this child's results?

   A. leukocytosis with neutrophilia

   B. leukopenia with lymphocytosis

   C. lymphopenia with neutropenia

   D. leukopenia with neutropenia

104. These results in question 103 increase the likelihood that the cause of the above-mentioned child's infection is:

   A. viral.

   B. parasitic.

   C. fungal.

   D. bacterial.

105. Potential adverse events with acetaminophen use in a child with fever and mild dehydration include:

   A. seizure.

   B. hepatotoxicity.

    C. petechial rash.

    D. gastric ulcer.

106. For a child with fever, a cool bath is not recommended due to:

    A. higher risk of febrile seizure.

    B. risk for development of generalized rash.

    C. an increase in body temperature resulting from shivering.

    D. increased risk of bacteremia.

107. The practice of alternating between ibuprofen and acetaminophen for a child with fever:

    A. will result in an additive effect in fever reduction.

    B. should only be performed when also giving cough-and-cold medication.

    C. is only recommended for high-grade fevers.

    D. is not recommended due to a higher potential for adverse effects.

108. The development of Reye's syndrome is associated with the administration of which of the following in children with fever?

    A. acetaminophen

    B. aspirin

    C. vitamin C supplement

    D. ibuprofen

109. The use of ibuprofen should be avoided in the child with varicella infection due to an increased risk of:

    A. seizure.

    B. Reye's syndrome.

    C. aseptic meningitis.

    D. necrotizing fasciitis.

For answers and rationales, see end of chapter.

Acute Otitis Media

Overview

AOM is among the most frequent diagnosis noted in office visits in children younger than age 15 years. Almost all cases of AOM are found to be caused by bacteria and viruses together (66%), bacteria alone (27%), or virus alone (4%). *S pneumoniae* (49% of bacterial-origin AOM), *H influenzae* (29% of bacterial-origin AOM), *Moraxella catarrhalis* (28% of bacterial-origin AOM), and various respiratory tract viruses contribute to the infectious and inflammatory processes of the middle ear.

Although AOM remains the most common childhood condition for which antibiotics are prescribed, the incidence of AOM and the resulting antimicrobial prescriptions have decreased over the past decade as a result of many factors, including increased rates of pneumococcal and influenza vaccination.

The eustachian tubes provide drainage of middle ear secretions and protection of the middle ear from pharyngeal secretions and bacterial contaminants. As a result, conditions that cause eustachian tube dysfunction or eustachian tube obstruction, such as allergic rhinitis, URI, and craniofacial abnormalities, encourage status of secretions and allow aspiration of pharyngeal flora into the middle ear, resulting in AOM. Eustachian tube obstruction caused by an upper respiratory viral illness remains the most common predisposing factor for developing AOM. Passive cigarette smoke exposure, feeding in a supine position, and pacifier use beyond age 10 months likely also predispose a child to AOM secondary to eustachian tube dysfunction or

CLINICAL CONCEPT

Nearly two-thirds of all children have at least one AOM episode by their second birthday; one-third have more than three episodes.

eustachian tube obstruction. Because children in day-care settings typically have more URIs, attendance at group child care is also a risk factor for nasopharyngeal carriage of bacteria implicated in AOM. Bottle feeding is a risk factor for AOM, with rates significantly lower among infants who were breastfed for the first 6 to 12 months of life; boys and children of Native American or Inuit ancestry are also noted to be at increased risk. An additional intervention to reduce AOM risk includes universal childhood pneumococcal and influenza immunization.

S pneumoniae causes 49% of AOM (Table 17-5); it is the least likely of the three major causative bacteria to resolve without antimicrobial intervention and causes the most significant symptoms. This organism has exhibited resistance more recently to numerous antibiotic agents, including amoxicillin, cephalosporins, and macrolides. The mechanism of resistance is an alteration of intracellular protein-binding sites, which can typically be overcome by using higher doses of amoxicillin and certain cephalosporins; on rare occasions, clindamycin is also used. The pneumococcal conjugate vaccine is effective in reducing the risk of invasive pneumococcal disease and in minimizing AOM risk when caused by serotypes included in the vaccine.

H influenzae (29%) and *M catarrhalis* (28%) are gram-negative organisms capable of producing beta-lactamase. However, cases of AOM caused by these two organisms have relatively high rates of spontaneous resolution (50% and 90%, respectively) without antimicrobial intervention. Beta-lactamase production by these organisms probably contributes less to AOM treatment failure than to prescribing an inadequate dosing of amoxicillin needed to eradicate drug-resistant *S pneumoniae*. RSV is commonly isolated from the middle ear fluid in children with AOM. Other common viral agents include human rhinovirus and coronavirus. AOM caused by these viral agents usually resolves in 7 to 10 days with supportive care alone.

Clinical Presentation

Appropriate assessment is critical to the diagnosis of AOM (Table 17-6). The AOM treatment guidelines emphasize proper diagnosis based on strict definitions of AOM and decisions regarding initial treatment.

The components of AOM include objective findings such as a bulging, erythematous tympanic membrane (TM) with limited or absent mobility on insufflation, or otorrhea unrelated to otitis externa. Presentation can also include bulging of TM and recent (48 hours or less) onset of ear pain (seen as tugging, holding, rubbing in a nonverbal child) or intense TM erythema with otalgia. Distinct otalgia with discomfort clearly referable to the ear results in interference with or precludes normal activity or sleep. Perforation of the TM can occur, often preceded by or accompanied with a purulent discharge. The child often experiences relief of pain and fever following perforation of the TM. With recovery, TM mobility

TABLE 17-5 Causative Organisms in Acute Bacterial Otitis Media (AOM)

ORGANISM	COMMENT
S pneumoniae (gram-positive diplococci) (49%)	Consider drug-resistant *S pneumoniae* risk
Treatment target in AOM	Mechanism of resistance: Altered binding sites within bacterial cells
	Low rate (approximately 10% to 20%) of spontaneous resolution without antimicrobial therapy
H influenzae (gram-negative bacilli) (29%)	Resistance via beta-lactamase production
	Moderate rate (approximately 50%) of spontaneous resolution without antimicrobial therapy
M catarrhalis (gram-negative cocci) (28%)	Resistance via beta-lactamase production
	Nearly all spontaneously resolve without antimicrobial therapy

Source: Gilbert DN, Chambers HF, Eliopoulis GM, Saag MS, Pavia AT. The Sanford Guide to Antimicrobial Therapy. *50th ed. Sperryville, VA: Antimicrobial Therapy, Inc.; 2020:11–12.*

TABLE 17-6 Diagnosis and Management of Acute Otitis Media (AOM) in Children

Diagnosis of AOM in Children	■ Moderate or severe bulging of tympanic membrane (TM) *OR* new onset of otorrhea not related to otitis externa (OE) with otalgia ■ Mild bulging of TM *AND* recent (48 hours or less) onset of ear pain (in nonverbal child– tugging, holding, rubbing) *OR* intense TM erythema with otalgia
Management of AOM should include assessment of pain, and if present, clinician should recommend treatment for pain management	Analgesics: Acetaminophen or ibuprofen is recommended Topical anesthetic agent can provide short-term (approximately 30 minutes) pain relief
Watchful waiting, consisting of analgesia without antimicrobial therapy, is an acceptable treatment option in AOM	In the otherwise well child, rationale for not immediately initiating antibiotic therapy: ■ Low risk for adverse outcome without antimicrobial therapy ■ High rate of spontaneous AOM resolution without antimicrobial therapy or worsening of symptoms ■ Watchful waiting is only appropriate for the child 6 months or older with nonsevere illness based on joint decision making with parents/caregivers for unilateral AOM ■ If watchful waiting is used, the follow-up must be ensured with the ability to start antibiotic therapy within 48 to 72 hours if symptoms do not improve or worsen
Nonsevere versus severe illness	Nonsevere illness: ■ Mild otalgia for less than 48 hours *OR* ■ Fever less than 39°C (less than 102.2°F) in the past 24 hours Severe illness: ■ Moderate to severe otalgia *OR* ■ Otalgia for more than 48 hours *OR* ■ Fever 39°C or greater (102.2°F or greater)
Treatment options **Initial treatment**	Antibiotic therapy at time of AOM diagnosis in the following: ■ Nonsevere or severe illness whether unilateral or bilateral AOM in children younger than 6 months ■ Severe illness with unilateral or bilateral AOM in children 6 months or older ■ Nonsevere illness with bilateral AOM in young children (6 to 23 months) Either prescribe antibiotic therapy *OR* offer observation with close follow-up of AOM in children 6 months or older with nonsevere illness based on joint decision making with parents/caregivers for unilateral AOM If observation is used, follow-up must be ensured with the ability to start antibiotic therapy within 48 to 72 hours if symptoms do not improve or worsen

Source: Lieberthal AS, Carroll AE, Chonmaitree T, et al. The diagnosis and management of acute otitis media. Pediatrics. 2013;31(3):e964–e999.

returns in about 1 to 2 weeks, but middle ear effusion (MEE) typically persists for 4 to 6 weeks and often up to 3 months.

Diagnostic Testing

AOM is a clinical diagnosis, arrived at via history of present illness and physical examination. No specific testing, including aspirate of middle ear exudate for culture and susceptibility, is advised unless there has been treatment failure with second- and third-line medications. Imaging studies are also seldom necessary though computed tomography (CT) scan can be used to determine if a complication has occurred. Assessing TM mobility using insufflation via a pneumatic otoscope can help determine the presence of MEE but is usually not necessary in most cases.

Treatment

Management of AOM should include assessment of pain, and if present, the clinician should recommend treatment for pain management. Acetaminophen or ibuprofen can be used as analgesics. Topical anesthetic agents, though not widely available, can provide short-term (approximately 30 minutes) pain relief.

The AOM evaluation and treatment recommendations apply only to otherwise healthy children without underlying conditions that could alter the natural course of AOM, including anatomical abnormalities such as cleft palate, certain genetic conditions such as Down syndrome, immunodeficiencies, the presence of cochlear implants, and recurrent AOM.

Observation as initial treatment is only appropriate if the child is older than 6 months, has nonsevere illness, and infection is unilateral. Placebo-controlled trials of AOM conducted during more than three decades have shown consistently that selected children who meet the criteria for observation do well, without adverse sequelae, without antibacterial therapy. Observation should include assurance of follow-up, and appropriate analgesia should be provided (Table 17-7).

Amoxicillin remains the first-line antimicrobial for AOM treatment for the majority of children who do not have penicillin allergy. Given the wide therapeutic index of this medication and the prevalence of drug-resistant *S pneumoniae*, 80 to 90 mg/kg/day is the recommended dose; in the overweight or obese child, the dose should not exceed the adult dose. Amoxicillin/clavulanate (Augmentin®), 80 to 90 mg/kg/day for the amoxicillin component, is recommended as first-line therapy in select situations. When a child is seen for AOM, measures to reduce AOM risk should be reviewed and reinforced.

Children younger than 3 months old with AOM should be seen in 1 to 2 days after diagnosis and initiation of treatment because of increased risk of treatment failure.

> **CLINICAL CONCEPT**
>
> In a child older than 3 months, otalgia, fever, and other symptoms that persist beyond 48 to 72 hours of therapy can indicate AOM initial treatment failure, and repeat evaluation is in order, and a change in therapy is recommended.

TABLE 17-7 Recommended Acute Otitis Media (AOM) Treatment Options

Length of therapy unless otherwise specified: Younger than age 2 years = 10 days, 2 to 6 years = 7 days, 6 years or older = 5 to 7 days

	RECOMMENDED	WITH PENICILLIN ALLERGY
First-line treatment	Amoxicillin (80 to 90 mg/kg/day in two divided doses) OR Amoxicillin-clavulanate (90 mg/kg/day of amoxicillin, with 6.4 mg/kg/day of clavulanate in two divided doses)	Cefdinir (14 mg/kg/day in one or two doses) OR Cefuroxime (30 mg/kg/day in two divided doses) OR Cefpodoxime (10 mg/kg/day in two divided doses) OR Ceftriaxone (50 mg IM or IV/day for 1 or 3 days)
Antibiotic treatment after 48 to 72 hours of failure of initial antibiotic treatment	Amoxicillin-clavulanate (90 mg/kg/day of amoxicillin, with 6.4 mg/kg/day of clavulanate in two divided doses) OR Ceftriaxone (50 mg IM/IV for 3 days)	Ceftriaxone for 3 days (as earlier) OR Clindamycin (30 to 40 mg/kg/day in three divided doses) with or without a third-generation cephalosporin Tympanocentesis Referral to specialist

Sources: Lieberthal AS, Carroll AE, Chonmaitree T, et al. The diagnosis and management of acute otitis media. Pediatrics. 2013;31(3):e964–e999.

Fitzgerald M. How would you prescribe cephalosporins to patients with penicillin allergies? FHEA News. 2012;12(8):13. http://fhea.com/main/content/Newsletter/fheanews_volume12_issue8.pdf

OTITIS MEDIA WITH EFFUSION: SEQUELAE OF ACUTE OTITIS MEDIA

Overview

Otitis media with effusion (OME), formerly known as serous otitis media, is defined as the presence of fluid in the middle ear in the absence of signs or symptoms of acute infection. Nearly all adults and children will have OME post AOM. OME can also occur with viral URI and un- or undertreated allergic rhinitis.

Clinical Presentation

With OME, there is usually a sensation of ear fullness, stuffiness, and itch, and the child with verbal capacity will report the same. The child who is unable to report these issues will often demonstrate ear picking or rubbing. Pain is rarely reported. On physical examination, air bubbles are noted behind the TM as air is trapped in the middle ear fluid, which is usually yellow. There is no TM redness, and the bony landmarks are usually visible. TM mobility is usually somewhat limited. In the older child who understands and can cooperate with otoscopy, the child will not complain of pain during the examination. Younger children will typically cry during otoscopy whether pain is present or absent, in part due to not understanding the examination, and needing some degree of restraint to allow the examiner to visualize the TM.

Treatment

Regardless of OME etiology, 80% of children will clear the middle ear within 8 weeks of its development without intervention. If OME is associated with an underlying cause, such as allergic rhinitis, therapy to treat the underlying cause should be initiated.

If OME persists beyond 8 weeks, particularly in the presence of communication problems and other symptoms, this dictates the need for further evaluation and treatment (Table 17-8). If persistent effusion is accompanied by language delay or suspected or documented hearing loss, intervention by tympanostomy (ventilating tube) is warranted. Current guidelines recommend that clinicians should only offer tympanostomy to children with chronic bilateral OME (3 months or longer) with documented hearing difficulty or with symptoms likely attributable to OME (e.g., balance problems, behavioral problems, ear discomfort, reduced quality of life), and also to those with recurrent AOM who have unilateral or bilateral MEE. Adenoidectomy, once the primary treatment for OME, is now used less often with greater use of tympanostomy. Evidence has demonstrated that adenoidectomy with tympanostomy achieves better results than either treatment alone in children with recurrent OME. However, adenoidectomy should be avoided in children younger than 4 years. Long-term retreatment with an antimicrobial for AOM or OME prophylaxis is not indicated, and the use of decongestants or antihistamine is not recommended (see Table 17-8).

TABLE 17-8 Otitis Media With Effusion (OME)

Defined	Fluid in middle ear without signs or symptoms of ear infection
First-line intervention	Watchful waiting in most 75% to 90% resolve within 3 months without specific treatment
Select intervention in at-risk children	Tympanostomy if chronic bilateral OME (3 months or longer) with documented hearing difficulty and recurrent AOM with unilateral or bilateral middle ear effusion. Adenoidectomy can be considered in children 4 years or older with recurrent OME.

Sources: Rosenfeld RM, Shin JJ, Schwartz SR, et al. Clinical practice guideline: otitis media with effusion (update). Otolaryngol Head Neck Surg. 2016;154(Suppl 1):S1–S41.

Rosenfeld RM, Schwartz SR, Pynnonnen MA, et al. Clinical practice guideline: tympanostomy tubes in children–executive summary. Otolaryngol Head Neck Surg. 2013;149:8–16.

Discussion Sources

Lieberthal SA, Carroll AE, Chonmaitree T, et al. The diagnosis and management of acute otitis media. *Pediatrics*. 2013; 131:e964–e999.

Rosenfeld RM, Schwartz SR, Pynnonnen MA, et al. Clinical practice guideline: tympanostomy tubes in children—executive summary. *Otolaryngol Head Neck Surg*. 2013;149:8–16.

Rosenfeld RM, Shin JJ, Schwartz SR, et al. Clinical practice guideline: otitis media with effusion (update). *Otolaryngol Head Neck Surg*. 2016;154(Suppl 1):S1–S41.

QUESTIONS

110. Which of the following is the most prudent first-line treatment choice for an otherwise well toddler without known allergies who now has AOM and requires antimicrobial therapy?

    A. oral cefdinir

    B. oral amoxicillin

    C. oral cefuroxime

    D. oral azithromycin

111. Most AOM is caused by:

    A. certain gram-positive and gram-negative bacteria and select respiratory viruses.

    B. atypical bacteria and pathogenic fungi.

    C. rhinovirus and methicillin-resistant *Staphylococcus aureus* (MRSA).

    D. predominately beta-lactamase–producing organisms.

112. The incidence of AOM in children has decreased in the past decade in part because of:

    A. earlier detection and treatment.

    B. more effective treatment options.

    C. an increase in select vaccination use.

    D. lower rates of viral infections.

113. Which of the following represents the best choice of clinical agents for a child with AOM who has had a history of penicillin allergy, with parental report of a flat, pink, slightly itchy rash without difficulty breathing during the reaction, who requires antimicrobial therapy?

    A. oral azithromycin

    B. oral cefdinir

    C. oral amoxicillin

    D. oral trimethoprim-sulfamethoxazole (TMP-SMX)

114. Which of the following does not represent a risk factor for recurrent AOM in younger children?

    A. pacifier use after age 10 months

    B. history of first episode of AOM before age 3 months

    C. exposure to secondhand smoke

    D. beta-lactam allergy

115. The main risk factor for AOM in infants is:

    A. undiagnosed dairy allergy.

    B. eustachian tube dysfunction.

    C. cigarette smoke exposure.

    D. use of soy-based infant formula.

116. In the treatment of AOM in the child, which of the following antimicrobial agents affords the most effective activity against *S pneumoniae*?
    A. oral nitrofurantoin
    B. oral clarithromycin
    C. oral TMP-SMX
    D. oral cefuroxime

117. A 3-year-old boy with AOM continues to have otalgia and fever (39°C and greater [102.2°F and greater]) after 3 days of amoxicillin 80 mg/kg/day. Which of the following is recommended?
    A. switch to high-dose oral ampicillin
    B. start antimicrobial therapy with oral azithromycin
    C. initiate therapy with oral clindamycin
    D. administer intramuscular (IM) ceftriaxone

118. Which of the following must be present for the diagnosis of AOM? *(More than one can apply.)*
    A. bulging of the TM
    B. air bubbles visible behind the TM
    C. otalgia
    D. anterior cervical lymphadenopathy

119. Which of the following signs indicates possible AOM diagnosis in a preverbal child?
    A. loss of appetite
    B. altered stooling
    C. tugging on the ear
    D. nasal discharge

120. Which of the following is usually absent in OME?
    A. fluid in the middle ear
    B. otalgia
    C. ear discharge
    D. otic itch

121. Which of the following criteria should be met for a child to be treated for AOM with observation and analgesia but no antimicrobial therapy? *(Choose all that apply.)*
    A. age greater than 6 months
    B. bilateral infection
    C. nonsevere illness
    D. presumptively caused by bacterial infection

122. Treatment of OME usually includes:
    A. "watch and wait" therapy.
    B. antimicrobial therapy.
    C. an antihistamine.
    D. a mucolytic.

123. Characteristics of *M catarrhalis* include:
    A. a high rate of beta-lactamase production.
    B. antimicrobial resistance because of altered protein binding sites.
    C. being difficult to eradicate even with antimicrobial therapy.
    D. being a gram-positive organism.

124. Characteristics of *H influenzae* include:

   A. rare beta-lactamase production.

   B. antimicrobial resistance because of altered protein binding sites.

   C. an approximate 50% spontaneous resolution rate when it is the AOM causative organism.

   D. gram-positive organism.

125. Characteristics of *S pneumoniae* include:

   A. commonly produces beta-lactamase.

   B. antimicrobial resistance because of altered protein binding sites.

   C. causative organism of skin infection associated with AOM.

   D. gram-negative organism.

126. OME typically clears by _____ after AOM.

   A. 1 week

   B. 3 weeks

   C. 8 weeks

   D. 6 months

127. A treatment option for persistent OME is:

   A. a short-term course of oral amoxicillin with clavulanate.

   B. consistent use of an oral antihistamine.

   C. use of an oral decongestant as needed.

   D. referral for tympanostomy consideration.

128. A potential complication resulting from prolonged OME includes:

   A. delay in language development.

   B. recurrent sinusitis.

   C. meningitis.

   D. development of nasal polyps.

129. The main diagnostic value of insufflation of the TM when evaluating for AOM is:

   A. detecting for a presumptive bacterial infection.

   B. assessing for potential hearing loss.

   C. measuring the severity of AOM.

   D. assessing for the presence of MEE.

130. Which of the following findings is most consistent with OME?

   A. TM erythema

   B. air trapped behind the TM

   C. bony landmarks hidden

   D. fever

For answers and rationales, see end of chapter.

Acute Bacterial Rhinosinusitis

Overview

Acute bacterial rhinosinusitis (ABRS) is a clinical condition resulting from inflammation of the lining of the membranes of the paranasal sinuses caused by bacterial infection. Risk factors include any condition that alters the normal cleansing mechanism of the sinuses, including viral infection, allergies, secondhand tobacco smoke exposure, and abnormalities in sinus structure. Inhaled tobacco smoke disturbs normal sinus mucociliary action and drainage, causing secretions to pool, and increases the risk of superimposed bacterial infection. In addition, viral URIs and poorly controlled allergic rhinitis cause similar dysfunction, increasing ABRS risk. As in adults, only a minority (6% to 7%) of children presenting with symptoms of URI will meet criteria for persistence and therefore ABRS risk. The majority of ABRS in children will spontaneously resolve without antibiotic therapy.

Clinical Presentation

As with the adult who presents with this condition, ABRS is a clinical diagnosis based on the child's presentation, largely based on health history. What presents as a challenge clinically is differentiating ABRS from a viral URI. Uncomplicated viral URI in children is marked by nasal symptoms and/or cough; nasal discharge progresses from clear to purulent to clear without antibiotics, usually within 10 days, and fever early in the illness is associated with constitutional symptoms such as headaches and myalgias that resolve in 24 to 48 hours as the respiratory symptoms worsen (Table 17-9). ABRS in children should only be considered if at least one of the following criteria are observed: worsening URI course such as double sickening,

TABLE 17-9 Diagnosis and Management of Acute Bacterial Rhinosinusitis (ABRS) in Children

Exclusions from these recommendations include children younger than 1 year of age including neonates and children with subacute and chronic sinusitis, anatomical abnormalities of the sinuses, immunodeficiencies, cystic fibrosis, and/or primary ciliary dyskinesia.

Differentiate between acute upper respiratory tract infection (URI) and ABRS diagnostic criteria	■ Uncomplicated viral URI course: • Nasal symptoms and/or cough, nasal discharge progresses from clear to purulent to clear without antibiotics, usually within 10 days • Fever early in the illness associated with constitutional symptoms such as headaches and myalgias that resolve in 24 to 48 hours as the respiratory symptoms worsen ■ ABRS should be considered only in the setting of one or more of the following: • Worsening URI course such as "double sickening," defined as acute worsening of respiratory symptoms or new fever at days 6 to 7 of URI • Persistence of URI-like symptoms without improvement after 7 to 10 days, including nasal discharge, daytime cough, fetid breath odor, fatigue, headache, decreased appetite • Acute onset: Temperature greater than 102.2°F (greater than 39°C), purulent nasal discharge, ill appearing for 3 to 4 days
Treatment options	■ Acute URI with persistent illness (nasal discharge of any quality) or daytime cough for more than 10 days without improvement • Treatment option: Antibiotic treatment or 3-day observation ■ Worsening course or new onset of nasal discharge, daytime cough, or fever after initial improvement • Treatment option: Antibiotic treatment ■ Severe onset/concurrent fever (greater than 102.2°F [greater than 39°C]) and purulent nasal discharge for more than 3 consecutive days. • Treatment option: Antibiotic treatment
Radiographic recommendations	■ In children with uncomplicated ABRS, imaging is not necessary to differentiate viral from bacterial sinusitis. ■ Contrast computed tomography of paranasal sinuses and/or magnetic resonance imaging with contrast should be obtained whenever a child is suspected of having orbital or central nervous system complications.
Likely pathogens	■ *S pneumoniae* = 30% • Decreased due to pneumococcal vaccine ■ Nontypeable *H influenzae* = 30% ■ *M catarrhalis* = 20% ■ Sterile (no pathogen isolated, likely viral) = 25%

defined as acute worsening of respiratory symptoms or new fever at day 6 or 7 of URI; persistence of URI-like symptoms without improvement after 7 to 10 days, including nasal discharge, daytime cough, fetid breath odor, fatigue, headache, decreased appetite, acute onset of a temperature of greater than 102.2°F (greater than 39°C), and purulent nasal discharge; or appearing acutely ill for 3 to 4 days (see Table 17-9). With ABRS, the rest of the physical examination is usually at the child's baseline.

Diagnostic Testing

As with the adult, ABRS is a clinical diagnosis, made by careful analysis of the patient history and physical examination. Routine sinus imaging is not recommended. Infrequently, with treatment failure using second-line medications or when the diagnosis is in question, and usually in conjunction with speciality evaluation, CT or magnetic resonance imaging (MRI) of the sinuses is warranted.

Treatment

According to the ABRS practice guidelines developed by the AAP, *S pneumoniae* and *H influenzae* (approximately 30% each) are the major causative organisms in childhood ABRS. Other pathogens that cause ABRS include *M catarrhalis* (approximately 9%), *S aureus* (approximately 10%), and anaerobes (approximately 6%). *S pneumoniae* is the least likely of the three major causative bacteria to resolve without antimicrobial intervention, and it causes the most significant symptoms. Recent antimicrobial use (i.e., within the past month) is the major risk for infection with drug-resistant *S pneumoniae*.

H influenzae and *M catarrhalis* (20%) are two organisms with relatively high rates of spontaneous resolution without antimicrobial intervention in AOM; however, infections caused by these pathogens seldom resolve without antimicrobial therapy in ABRS. Empirical antimicrobial therapy in ABRS should be aimed at choosing an agent with significant activity against gram-positive (*S pneumoniae*) and gram-negative organisms (*H influenzae, M catarrhalis*), with consideration for drug-resistant *S pneumoniae* risk and possible need for stability in the presence of beta-lactamase. Of childhood sinusitis cases, 25% are sterile, wherein the cause is likely viral.

Initial treatment options for ABRS include observation for spontaneous resolution or initiation of oral antimicrobial therapy. The use of antimicrobials should be considered if the patient experiences fever, pain, or purulent nasal discharge or if symptoms persist beyond 10 days without treatment. First-line treatment in children can include oral high-dose amoxicillin at 90 mg/kg/day or high-dose amoxicillin-clavulanate, both given as divided doses every 12 hours (Table 17-10). Children who have a penicillin allergy can be safely treated with oral clindamycin or cefpodoxime. If no improvement or worsening is seen in 3 days, treatment options include switch to oral amoxicillin-clavulanate extended release, or an oral cephalosporin (cefpodoxime, cefdinir, or cefprozil). For severe illness, a respiratory fluoroquinolone can be considered (e.g., levofloxacin, or moxifloxacin) (see Table 17-10). Doxycycline, a member of the tetracycline class, is not recommended for ABRS and should not be used in children younger than 8 years as it can lead to

TABLE 17-10 Acute Bacterial Rhinosinusitis (ABRS) Treatment in Children

INITIAL TREATMENT	NO IMPROVEMENT IN 72 HOURS	WORSE AT 72 HOURS
Observation	Additional observation OR antibiotic therapy	Amoxicillin 80 to 90 mg/kg/day with or without clavulanate
Amoxicillin* 80 to 90 mg/kg/day	Additional observation OR high-dose amoxicillin/clavulanate	High-dose amoxicillin/clavulanate
High-dose amoxicillin/clavulanate	Continue high-dose amoxicillin/clavulanate or change to clindamycin AND cefixime OR linezolid AND cefixime OR levofloxacin	Clindamycin AND cefixime OR linezolid AND cefixime OR levofloxacin

*In the case of penicillin allergy, both non–type 1 reaction (delayed or late, more than 72 hours) and type 1 (immediate, severe reaction) can safely be treated with cefdinir, cefuroxime, or cefpodoxime. Consider allergy testing for penicillin and cephalosporin in both cases prior to initiation of treatment.

Source: Wald ER, Applegate KE, Bordley C, et al. Clinical practice guideline for the diagnosis and management of acute bacterial sinusitis in children aged 1 to 18 years. Pediatrics. 2013;132;e262.

permanent staining of teeth. The use of oral decongestants or antihistamines for the treatment of ABRS is not recommended as there is a lack of evidence demonstrating any benefit of these approaches in children. Nasal decongestants might improve comfort for the child but should be restricted to 4 to 5 days to avoid rebound vasodilation. Mucolytics are also variably effective and not routinely recommended.

Discussion Sources

Gilbert DN, Chambers HF, Eliopoulos GM, Saag MS, Pavia AT. *The Sanford Guide to Antimicrobial Therapy*. 50th ed. Sperryville, VA: Antimicrobial Therapy, Inc., 2020; 51.

Wald ER, Applegate KE, Bordley C, et al. Clinical practice guideline for the diagnosis and management of acute bacterial sinusitis in children aged 1 to 18 years. *Pediatrics*. 2013;132:e262–e280.

QUESTIONS

131. Which of the following findings is most consistent with the diagnosis of ABRS in children?

　A. URI signs and symptoms persisting beyond 10 days

　B. nasal discharge progressing from clear to purulent to clear without the use of an antibiotic

　C. headaches and myalgias that resolve in 24 to 48 hours as the respiratory symptoms worsen

　D. persistent congested cough beyond 7 days of URI onset

132. "Double sickening" in the evaluation of a child with ABRS is defined as which of the following? *(Choose all that apply.)*

　A. nasal discharge progressing from clear to purulent to clear without antibiotic use

　B. acute worsening of respiratory symptoms

　C. new fever occurring 6 to 7 days after signs of URI

　D. persistent cough

133. From the list that follows, the most common causative bacterial pathogen in ABRS in children is:

　A. *M pneumoniae.*

　B. *S pneumoniae.*

　C. *M catarrhalis.*

　D. *S aureus.*

134. Risk factors for ABRS in children include all of the following except:

　A. viral respiratory tract infection.

　B. environmental allergies.

　C. tobacco smoke exposure.

　D. history of β-thalassemia minor.

135. Which of the following is a first-line therapy option for the treatment of ABRS in an otherwise well 6-year-old child?

　A. amoxicillin-clavulanate

　B. clindamycin with cefixime

　C. doxycycline

　D. levofloxacin

136. Which of the following represents a therapeutic option for ABRS in an otherwise well 7-year-old child who has not had significant clinical improvement but is not worse after 48 hours of observation?

　A. continued observation

　B. oral levofloxacin

　C. oral clindamycin and cefixime

　D. injectable ceftriaxone

137. A 5-year-old girl presents with ABRS. She has a penicillin allergy, reported by parents as "breaking out with a rash on her bottom" when she took an oral penicillin form as an infant but did not have difficulty breathing. She is otherwise well, and parents request treatment with an antimicrobial. You prescribe:

A. no medication; continue observation.

B. oral cefdinir

C. oral levofloxacin.

D. oral amoxicillin.

138. Which of the following is most accurate regarding imaging studies for ABRS diagnosis?

A. Routine imaging with CT scan is warranted for all children under 4 years of age.

B. Imaging should only be performed prior to starting antimicrobial therapy.

C. Imaging is most useful just prior to double sickening.

D. Imaging can be considered with treatment failure.

139. The mother of a 6-year-old with ABRS asks about the use of decongestants. The NP replies that:

A. oral decongestants are preferred over nasal decongestants.

B. decongestants can be safely used for up to 10 days.

C. nasal decongestants will hasten resolution of symptoms of ABRS.

D. there is little evidence that decongestants provide any benefit in children with ABRS.

For answers and rationales, see end of chapter.

Influenza

Overview

Influenza is a viral illness that typically causes many days of incapacitation and suffering and the risk of hospitalization and death. Children with influenza commonly have AOM, nausea, and vomiting in addition to the aforementioned signs and symptoms. Although the worst symptoms in most uncomplicated cases resolve in about 1 week, the cough and malaise often persist for 2 or more weeks. Individuals with ongoing health problems such as pulmonary or cardiac disease, young children, and pregnant women also have increased risk of influenza-related complications including pneumonia.

Influenza viruses spread from person to person largely via respiratory droplets from an infected person, primarily through a cough or sneeze.

Adults and children who are immunocompromised can remain infectious for up to 3 weeks. Historically, the risks for complications, hospitalizations, and deaths from influenza are higher among adults older than 65 years, young children, and individuals of any age with certain underlying health conditions than among healthy older children and younger adults. In children younger than 5 years, hospitalization rates for influenza-related illness have ranged from approximately 500/100,000 for children with high-risk medical conditions to 100/100,000 for children without high-risk medical conditions.

> **CLINICAL CONCEPT**
>
> Children remain infectious for 10 or more days after the onset of flu symptoms, a number of days longer than adults with the disease, and can shed the virus before the onset of symptoms.

Influenza Prevention

Immunization is considered to be effective in influenza prevention, with rates varying based on type of virus strain, regions of the country, and age; it also varies year to year. Historically, the influenza vaccine has been 70% to 80% effective in preventing or reducing the severity of influenza A and B viruses. This vaccine comes in a variety of forms, with the most common being inactivated influenza vaccine (IIV or flu shot) and, less commonly, live attenuated virus vaccine (LAIV, or FluMist® nasal spray). The CDC recommends that all members of the population aged 6 months and older should receive annual immunization against seasonal influenza. When a child younger than 8 years receives the influenza vaccine for the first time, two doses 4 or more weeks apart should be given. (See Chapter 2 for additional information on influenza immunization.)

Pregnant women should be immunized against influenza; the vaccine can be given regardless of pregnancy trimester. Partly because of the change in the respiratory and immune systems normally present during pregnancy, influenza is five times more likely to cause serious disease in a pregnant woman compared with a nonpregnant woman. In addition, women who are immunized against influenza during pregnancy are able to pass a portion of this protection on to the unborn child, providing important protection during the first 6 months of life. Flu vaccine is also safe to give during lactation. The influenza vaccine is recommended for household members of high-risk patients to avoid transmission of infection.

Clinical Presentation

Clinical manifestations of seasonal influenza in children can range from mild to severe. Initial symptoms can appear about 2 to 3 days after exposure to the virus and result in a high fever, chills, myalgia, headache, and fatigue. Later stage of disease can include symptoms of sore throat and pharyngitis, nasal congestion, rhinitis, a nonproductive cough, cervical lymphadenopathy, and conjunctivitis. Among infants and preschool-age children, signs of influenza and its complications can include fever without respiratory complications (i.e., a "sepsis-like syndrome"), otitis media, bronchiolitis, croup, reactive airway disease, febrile seizures, secondary bacterial pneumonia, rhabdomyolysis, myocarditis, toxic shock syndrome, Guillain-Barré syndrome, Reye's syndrome, and sudden death.

Diagnostic Testing

Children younger than 5 years of age, and especially younger than 2 years of age, are considered to be at high risk of developing complications from influenza. According to guidelines from the Infectious Diseases Society of America (IDSA), in the outpatient setting, testing for influenza should be done for high-risk patients during the flu season when testing will influence clinical management. Clinicians can also consider influenza testing for patients who are not at high risk but who present with influenza-related illness, pneumonia, or nonspecific respiratory illness if the results will influence antiviral treatment or chemoprophylaxis decisions for high-risk household contacts.

Treatment

In children, antiviral treatment should be initiated as soon as possible for those younger than 2 years of age with confirmed or suspected influenza, irrespective of influenza vaccination history. Antivirals should also be given to any patient with severe or progressive illness regardless of illness duration, those who are at high risk of complications, pregnant women, and anyone hospitalized with influenza. Postexposure antiviral prophylaxis can be considered for adults and children 3 months of age and older who are unvaccinated, and who are at very high risk of developing complications from influenza or are household contacts of a person at very high risk for complications. Current antiviral treatment options include neuraminidase inhibitors (oral oseltamivir, inhaled zanamivir, or IV peramivir) and oral baloxavir marboxil.

Discussion Sources

Centers for Disease Control and Prevention. Birth–18 years and "catch-up" immunization schedules. http://www.cdc.gov/vaccines/schedules/hcp/child-adolescent.html

Centers for Disease Control and Prevention. Influenza (flu): about flu. https://www.cdc.gov/flu/about/index.html

Centers for Disease Control and Prevention. Prevention and control of seasonal influenza with vaccines. Recommendations of the Advisory Committee on Immunization Practices—United States, 2020–21 influenza season. *MMWR*. 2020;69(8):1–24.

Uyeki TM, Bernstein HH, Bradley JS, et al. Clinical practice guidelines by the Infectious Diseases Society of America: 2018 update on diagnosis, treatment, chemoprophylaxis, and institutional outbreak management of seasonal influenza. *Clin Infect Dis*. 2019;68:e1–e47.

QUESTIONS

140. When advising parents about injectable IIV, or "flu shot," the clinician considers the following about the vaccine:

   A. The vaccine is contraindicated with a personal history of a mild hive-form reaction to eggs.

   B. Its use is limited to children older than 2 years.

   C. The vaccine contains live virus.

   D. Its use is recommended for members of households with a high-risk patient.

141. A 7-year-old child with type 1 diabetes mellitus is about to receive injectable IIV. His parents and he should be advised that:

A. the vaccine is more than 90% effective in preventing influenza.

B. use of the vaccine is contraindicated during antibiotic therapy.

C. localized immunization reactions are common.

D. a short, intense, flu-like syndrome typically occurs after immunization.

142. When giving IIV to a 7-year-old who has not received any influenza immunization in the past, the NP considers that:

A. two doses 4 weeks or more apart should be given.

B. a single dose is adequate.

C. children in this age group have the highest rate of influenza-related hospitalization.

D. the vaccine should not be given to a child with shellfish allergy.

143. With regard to seasonal influenza prevention in well children, the NP considers that:

A. compared with school-aged children, younger children (24 months old and younger) have an increased risk of seasonal influenza-related hospitalization.

B. a full adult dose of seasonal influenza vaccine should be given starting at age 4 years.

C. the use of the seasonal influenza vaccine in well children is discouraged.

D. widespread use of the vaccine is likely to increase the risk of eczema and antibiotic allergies.

144. When advising a patient about immunization with the nasal spray live attenuated influenza vaccine (LAIV, FluMist®), the NP considers the following:

A. Its use is acceptable during pregnancy.

B. Its use is limited to children younger than age 2 years.

C. It should not be given when nasal congestion is present.

D. It should not be given in the presence of egg allergy.

145. Which of the following should not receive vaccination against influenza?

A. a 19-year-old with a history of hive-form reaction to eating eggs

B. a 24-year-old woman who is 8 weeks pregnant

C. a 4-month-old infant who was born at 32 weeks' gestation

D. a 28-year-old woman who is breastfeeding a 2-week-old infant

146. The most common mode of influenza virus transmission is via:

A. contact with a contaminated surface.

B. respiratory droplet.

C. saliva contact.

D. skin-to-skin contact.

147. Which of the following is at greatest risk of having serious flu-related complications?

A. a 7-year-old with a recent previous episode of AOM

B. a 4-year-old with asthma

C. a 9-year-old living with a grandparent with chronic obstructive pulmonary disease (COPD)

D. a 6-year-old entering his first year of public school

148. When considering vaccinating a pregnant woman against influenza vaccine, the NP considers that:

A. there is a small risk of the virus spreading to the fetus.

B. immunization should not be done in the third trimester.

C. the unborn child acquires some protection against influenza up to 6 months after birth.

D. LAIV is the preferred vaccine for pregnant women.

149. Possible influenza-related complications in infants can include all of the following except:

A. bronchiolitis.

B. Reye's syndrome.

C. intussusception.

D. sudden death.

150 to 152. Indicate (*yes or no*) whether antivirals should be administered for all of the following individuals.

_____ 150. An 18-month-old unvaccinated child with a 2-day history of respiratory symptoms without fever

_____ 151. A 9-year-old otherwise healthy boy with a 5-day history of cough, fever, and myalgia and beginning to show signs of improvement

_____ 152. A 4-year-old with a history of asthma and with 24 hours of fever and headache and who tested positive for influenza

153. Indicate which of the following individuals who already received the influenza vaccine is the most likely candidate to receive antiviral chemoprophylaxis following possible exposure to the virus?

A. a 6-year-old who received two doses of the vaccine this flu season

B. a 9-year-old who lives with a mother who smokes

C. an 11-year-old who had the flu last year

D. a 2-year-old who was vaccinated less than 2 weeks ago

For answers and rationales, see end of chapter.

Croup

Overview

Croup, also called acute laryngotracheitis or acute laryngotracheobronchitis, is a common viral infection that affects about 3% of children 6 months to 3 years of age, though it can also affect older children. The most common cause of croup includes parainfluenza viruses (type 1, 2, and 3), while other viruses can include adenovirus, RSV, coronavirus, and rhinovirus, among others. Complications from croup are rare, though it can lead to secondary bacterial infection, such as pneumonia or tracheitis.

Clinical Presentation

Croup generally affects the larynx and trachea and is a common cause of fever, hoarseness, cough, and acute stridor. Fever and coryza typically last 12 to 72 hours.

These findings are due to narrowing of the larynx and trachea below the glottis. Signs can be exacerbated by emotional distress (e.g., crying) and are generally worse at night. The acute onset of a barking cough and stridor, often during the late night/early morning hours, often prompts concern from parents/caregivers that leads to a visit to urgent care or the emergency room. Though children typically recover completely, infants and young children should undergo evaluation to determine the cause of symptoms and rule out more serious conditions. Other conditions that can present similarly to croup include large airway lesion, allergic reaction, peritonsillar or retropharyngeal abscess, foreign-body aspiration, gastroesophageal reflux, or laryngeal hemangioma. Acute epiglottitis can also be considered, though this condition is becoming less prevalent with routine use of Hib vaccine in young children.

> **CLINICAL CONCEPT**
>
> The characteristic sign of croup is a seal-like barking cough, accompanied with inspiratory stridor and some degree of respiratory distress.

Diagnostic Testing

Croup is primarily a clinical diagnosis based on patient history and physical examination findings. Laboratory tests contribute little to the diagnosis.

Treatment

Most cases of mild croup can be managed with supportive care, parental guidance, and reassurance. A cool mist humidifier or sitting in the bathroom with steam from the shower can help minimize symptoms. As persistent crying can increase oxygen demand and exacerbate symptoms, the child should be engaged in calming activities, such as reading a book. Fluid intake should be encouraged to maintain hydration and loosen mucus in the oropharynx. Frozen popsicles can help alleviate sore throat pain. Acetaminophen or ibuprofen can also be used to reduce pain and fever. Exposure to irritants, such as cigarette smoke, should be avoided. Parents/caregivers should stay in close proximity to the child at nighttime to monitor if the child begins having difficulty breathing.

All children with croup, regardless of severity, should be administered a systemic corticosteroid as this can reduce disease severity by reducing laryngeal mucosal edema. A single dose of dexamethasone is preferred over budesonide or methylprednisolone as it results in faster resolution of symptoms and less frequent return to medical care. It can be given via oral, IM, or IV dose, depending on the child's age and ability to tolerate oral medication. For children with moderate to severe croup, nebulized epinephrine in conjunction with a corticosteroid is recommended to achieve faster symptom relief; administration of nebulized epinephrine is more commonly performed in the emergency department or hospital setting. Antibacterials, antivirals, or beta agonists are not warranted or helpful during croup.

Discussion Sources

Defendi GL. Croup. Medscape. https://emedicine.medscape.com/article/962972-overview

Smith DK, McDermott AJ, Sullivan JF. Croup: diagnosis and management. *Am Fam Physician.* 2018;97:575–580.

QUESTIONS

154. Common causes of croup include all of the following except:

  A. parainfluenza virus.

  B. *H influenzae.*

  C. adenovirus.

  D. rhinovirus.

155. A 2.5-year-old child with croup will most likely present with all of the following except:

  A. expiratory wheeze.

  B. stridor.

  C. bark-like cough.

  D. fever.

156. When evaluating a 3-year-old child with suspected croup, the NP realizes that:

  A. this is largely a clinical diagnosis.

  B. CBC with differential should be routinely performed.

  C. a chest radiograph is needed to confirm the diagnosis.

  D. a urine nitrite test is indicated.

157. In addition to parental guidance and reassurance, which of the following is most helpful in the management of croup?

  A. oral amoxicillin with or without clavulanate

  B. inhaled LABA

  C. oral acyclovir

  D. systemic corticosteroid

For answers and rationales, see end of chapter.

Pneumonia

Overview

In all age groups, pneumonia, an acute lower respiratory tract infection involving lung parenchyma, interstitial tissues, and alveolar spaces, is the most common cause of death from infectious disease worldwide and results in 20% of all deaths in children younger than age 5 years. The term *community-acquired pneumonia* (CAP) is used to describe the onset of the disease in an individual who resides within the community, not in a nursing home or other care facility, with no recent (within 2 weeks) hospitalization. Although numerous organisms are implicated in CAP in children, only a few seen with significant frequency.

NPs are ideally positioned to help minimize risk for pneumonia through immunization and hygienic measures. Nearly two-thirds of all fatal pneumonia is caused by *S pneumoniae,* the pneumococcal organism. Pneumococcal conjugate vaccine is recommended for all children, starting in infancy, to minimize the risk of invasive pneumococcal disease. The use of the influenza vaccine can help minimize the risk of postinfluenza pneumonia. Ensuring adequate ventilation, reinforcing cough hygiene, and proper handwashing can help minimize pneumonia risk.

Clinical Presentation

Most children with pneumonia present with a short history of cough, malaise, and fever. Compared with an adult with pneumonia, a child is less likely to complain of dyspnea, produce sputum, or report pleuritic chest pain. Tachypnea is the most sensitive, although not specific, finding. In particular, the diagnosis of lower respiratory tract disease should be considered with a respiratory rate exceeding 50/minute in children younger than 1 year and a rate exceeding 40/minute in children older than 1 year. Pulse oximetry is also informative but less so than respiratory rate. Examination of the lung fields in the child with pneumonia often fails to reveal crackles or tubular breath sounds, commonly noted in the adult with this condition, but often transmitted upper airway sounds are heard. The child should be examined for signs of respiratory distress including grunting, use of accessory muscles, nasal flaring, and retractions at the subcostal, intercostal, midsternal, or suprasternal spaces; these findings should prompt transfer of the child to the emergency department for immediate additional evaluation and consideration for hospital admission.

Diagnostic Testing

Diagnostic evaluation of a child with CAP usually includes a chest x-ray and a CBC with WBC differential. As with adults with CAP, in children with CAP, sputum specimens are usually unobtainable, and the results are unreliable, failing to reveal a causative organism. Further evaluation for invasive disease (sepsis), including procalcitonin and lactate, should be dictated by clinical presentation; typically for the child with pneumonia who is well enough to be treated at home, this additional testing is not warranted.

Treatment

Successful community-based care of a child with CAP requires many factors. The child must have intact GI function and be able to take and tolerate oral medications and adequate amounts of fluids. Parenteral antimicrobial and IV fluids are not needed in a child who is able to take and retain oral medications and fluids. A competent caregiver must be available. Also, the child should be able to be brought back for follow-up examination and evaluation.

As previously mentioned and consistent with CAP treatment in adults, antimicrobial therapy in children with pneumonia is chosen empirically (Table 17-11). Because most childhood CAP is viral in origin, watchful waiting can also be used, whereby the child is not placed on an antimicrobial regimen but rather is observed to see whether the illness improves over a few days. When antimicrobial therapy is deemed appropriate, first-line treatment includes amoxicillin 90 mg/kg per day given in two divided doses for 5 days. Alternatives can include amoxicillin/clavulanate 90 mg/kg (amoxicillin component) given in two divided doses for 5 days, or azithromycin 10 mg/kg (maximum 500 mg) for one dose followed by 5 mg/kg (maximum 250 mg) for 4 days. Azithromycin can be preferred if infection with an atypical pathogen is suspected. Given that most children with CAP will be treated at home, follow-up within 1 to 3 days of treatment initiation is advised to ensure clinical improvement.

The use of antivirals is most effective when given early in influenza infection (less than 48 hours of symptoms). However, given that the majority of children will not be seen by a health-care provider until after several days of illness, the use of these agents will have limited benefit. When deemed appropriate,

TABLE 17-11 Empirical Therapy for Pediatric Community-Acquired Pneumonia (CAP) in the Outpatient Setting in Children Aged 3 Months to 17 Years

	PRESUMED BACTERIAL PNEUMONIA	PRESUMED ATYPICAL PNEUMONIA	PRESUMED INFLUENZA PNEUMONIA
Less than 5 years old (preschool)	Amoxicillin, oral (90 mg/kg/day in two doses) Alternative: Oral amoxicillin-clavulanate (amoxicillin component, 90 mg/kg/day in two doses)	Azithromycin oral (10 mg/kg on day 1, followed by 5 mg/kg/day once daily on days 2 through 5) Alternatives: Oral clarithromycin (15 mg/kg/day in two doses for 7 to 14 days) or oral erythromycin (40 mg/kg/day in four doses)	Oseltamivir (oral) or other appropriate influenza antiviral
5 years old or older	Oral amoxicillin (90 mg/kg/day in two doses to a maximum of 4 g/day); for children with presumed bacterial CAP who do not have clinical, laboratory, or radiographic evidence that distinguishes bacterial CAP from atypical CAP, a macrolide can be added to a beta-lactam antibiotic for empirical therapy Alternative: Oral amoxicillin-clavulanate (amoxicillin component, 90 mg/kg/day in two doses to a maximum dose of 4,000 mg/day, e.g., one 2,000-mg tablet twice daily)	Oral azithromycin (10 mg/kg on day 1, followed by 5 mg/kg/day once daily on days 2 through 5 to a maximum of 500 mg on day 1, followed by 250 mg on days 2 through 5) Alternatives: Oral clarithromycin (15 mg/kg/day in two doses to a maximum of 1 g/day); erythromycin, doxycycline for children older than 7 years of age	Oseltamivir (oral) or other appropriate influenza antiviral

For children with a history of possible, nonserious allergic reactions to amoxicillin, treatment is not well defined and should be individualized. Options include a trial of amoxicillin under clinical observation; a trial of an oral cephalosporin that has substantial activity against S pneumoniae, such as cefpodoxime, cefprozil, or cefuroxime, can be provided under clinical supervision. Additional options for the child with a penicillin allergy include levofloxacin, linezolid, clindamycin, or a macrolide; close clinical follow-up and full knowledge of the use of all of these medications in children is needed.

Source: Bradley JS, Byington CL, Shah SS, et al. The management of community-acquired pneumonia in infants and children older than 3 months of age: clinical practice guidelines by the Pediatric Infectious Diseases Society and the Infectious Diseases Society of America. Clin Infect Dis. 2011;53(7):e25–e76.

antivirals to treat influenza infection in children who will be treated as outpatients include oseltamivir (oral formulation), zanamivir (inhalation powder for use in children older than 5 years), and baloxavir marboxil (oral tablets). Prudent practice dictates being aware of age-related recommendations on the use of medications in children.

Discussion Sources

Bradley JS, Byington CL, Shah SS, et al. The management of community-acquired pneumonia in infants and children older than 3 months of age: clinical practice guidelines by the Pediatric Infectious Diseases Society and the Infectious Diseases Society of America. Clin Infect Dis. 2011;53(7):e25–e76.

Gilbert DN, Chambers HF, Eliopoulos GM, Saag MS, Pavia AT. The Sanford Guide to Antimicrobial Therapy. 50th ed. Sperryville, VA: Antimicrobial Therapy, Inc.; 2020.

Messinger AI, Kupfer O, Hurst A, Parker S. Management of pediatric community-acquired bacterial pneumonia. Pediatr Rev. 2017;38:394–409.

QUESTIONS

158. When treating a 3-year-old well child with CAP, the NP realizes that the most likely causative pathogen is:

A. M pneumoniae.

B. a respiratory virus.

C. H influenzae.

D. S pneumoniae.

159. Which of the following is the most appropriate antimicrobial for treatment of CAP in a 2-year-old child who is clinically stable and able to be treated in the outpatient setting?

    A. oral amoxicillin

    B. oral doxycycline

    C. oral TMP-SMX

    D. oral levofloxacin

160. Which of the following is most likely to be noted in a 3-year-old child with CAP?

    A. complaint of pleuritic chest pain

    B. sputum production

    C. report of dyspnea

    D. tachypnea

161. Which of the following antimicrobials provides effective activity against atypical pathogens?

    A. amoxicillin

    B. cefprozil

    C. ceftriaxone

    D. clarithromycin

162. Which of the following is not a criterion for outpatient management of a child with CAP?

    A. able to tolerate oral medications

    B. able to return for follow-up evaluation

    C. adequately hydrated

    D. parenteral antimicrobial used for initial therapy

163. When evaluating a 7-year-old with suspected pneumonia, who is generally stable and likely to be treated at home, minimum diagnostic testing should include: *(More than one answer can apply.)*

    A. chest x-ray.

    B. procalcitonin.

    C. lactate.

    D. CBC with differential.

For answers and rationales, see end of chapter.

Bronchiolitis

Overview

Bronchiolitis is a common illness in early childhood; the peak incidence is in children younger than 2 years, with more than 90% of episodes occurring between November and April. The most likely bronchiolitis causative organism is RSV; it is less often caused by parainfluenza, influenza, or adenovirus. During the acute stage of infection, bronchiolar respiratory and ciliated epithelial cell function is altered, producing increased secretion of mucus, cell death, and sloughing. This stage is followed by peribronchiolar lymphocytic infiltrate and submucosal edema, leading to airway swelling and resulting symptoms. Infants and children infected with RSV usually show symptoms within 4 to 6 days of organism acquisition.

Clinical Presentation

Infants with bronchiolitis typically have rhinorrhea and a decrease in appetite. Cough usually develops 1 to 3 days later, followed by sneezing, fever, and/or wheezing.

Additional findings include tachypnea, mild fever, conjunctivitis, and pharyngitis. In most children, bronchiolitis runs a course of 2 to 3 weeks. These findings resolve as ciliary function returns. In very young infants (less than 3 months), irritability, decreased activity, and apnea may be the only symptoms of infection. Younger infants and children with weakened immune systems can be contagious for as long as 3 weeks.

Diagnosis

Bronchiolitis is usually diagnosed by clinical findings; rapid antigen tests of nasal washings provide rapid, accurate RSV detection, which can be supplemented with cell culture. Early detection can be particularly helpful in the setting of an outbreak in a day care or other similar setting. The sensitivity of RSV antigen testing can vary from 72% to 90%, whereas specificity is generally greater than 90%. Test performance decreases in older children and adults as partial prior immunity can decrease viral load in the nasal secretions used in the assay.

Treatment

Supportive therapy is usually sufficient. In infants younger than 3 months and in children with chronic health problems, hypoxemia or hypercapnia will necessitate hospital admission for hydration and oxygenation. The use of corticosteroids, ribavirin, and bronchodilators, including beta-2 agonists, remains controversial with little evidence of efficacy, although standard asthma therapies are effective in children who also have underlying reactive airway disease.

Palivizumab (Synagis®) is a monoclonal antibody that can be considered for prophylaxis against RSV infection in certain high-risk infants. The AAP recommends using palivizumab for infants born before 29 weeks' gestation, and for infants with certain chronic illnesses, such as congenital heart disease or chronic lung disease. Monthly injections should start prior to commencement of RSV season and continue throughout the RSV season. Long-term sequelae of bronchiolitis often include recurrent airway reactivity.

> **CLINICAL CONCEPT**
> Bronchiolitis, when noted in an otherwise healthy child beyond age 3 months, is often called the "disease of the happy wheezer," where the child demonstrates considerable cough and wheezing while generally appearing only mildly ill.

Discussion Sources

Centers for Disease Control and Prevention. Respiratory syncytial virus infection (RSV). http://www.cdc.gov/rsv/
National Institutes of Health. Bronchiolitis. MedlinePlus. https://medlineplus.gov/ency/article/000975.htm

QUESTIONS

164. Bronchiolitis most commonly occurs in the United States during the months of April to November.

   A. true

   B. false

165. The rate of bronchiolitis is highest in which age group?

   A. toddlers

   B. school-aged children

   C. preschool children

   D. children younger than age 2 years

166. The most common causative organism of bronchiolitis is:

   A. *H influenzae.*

   B. parainfluenza virus.

   C. RSV.

   D. coxsackie virus.

167. One of the most prominent clinical features of bronchiolitis is:

   A. fever.

   B. vomiting.

   C. wheezing.

   D. conjunctival inflammation.

168. Which of the following laboratory tests can identify the causative organism of bronchiolitis?
     A. nasal washing antigen test
     B. antibody test via blood sample
     C. urine culture
     D. a laboratory test is not available

169. In most children with bronchiolitis, intervention includes:
     A. aerosolized ribavirin therapy.
     B. supportive care.
     C. nebulized beta-2 agonist therapy.
     D. oral corticosteroid therapy.

170. Common clinical findings in a young child with bronchiolitis include all of the following except:
     A. pharyngitis.
     B. tachypnea.
     C. bradycardia.
     D. conjunctivitis.

171. Use of palivizumab (Synagis®) for the prevention of RSV infection should be considered for all of the following except:
     A. a 1-month-old born at 28 weeks' gestation.
     B. a 4-month-old with congenital heart disease.
     C. a 5-month-old born at 39 weeks' gestation who now has recurrent AOM.
     D. a 3-month-old with chronic respiratory disease.

172. The first dose of palivizumab treatment should be given:
     A. at birth.
     B. at 1 month of age.
     C. immediately prior to the RSV season.
     D. at the peak of RSV season.

For answers and rationales, see end of chapter.

Asthma

Overview

Asthma is a common chronic disorder of the airways that is complex and characterized by variable and recurring symptoms, airflow obstruction, bronchial hyperresponsiveness, underlying inflammation, and a resulting decrease in the ratio of forced expiratory volume in 1 second to forced vital capacity.

The formerly held concept in asthma was that no matter how severe the airway obstruction, the process was fully reversible. The newer disease model acknowledges that continued airway inflammation contributes to significant and potentially permanent airway remodeling and fixed obstruction. In addition, there is evidence that poorly controlled asthma can contribute to overall attenuated lung development in children.

When airway inflammatory control is poor, children with asthma typically use emergency services for treatment of frequent acute flares. With appropriate asthma family teaching to help with management of acute and chronic airway inflammation and its resulting symptoms, emergency visits can be minimized or eliminated. Asthma should not be used as an excuse to limit normal daily activities. A child with

> **CLINICAL CONCEPT**
>
> Although the condition ranks second after allergic rhinitis as the most common chronic respiratory disease in North America, many children and adults with asthma continue to be undiagnosed and untreated.

well-controlled asthma should be able and encouraged to participate in fitness and leisure activities, with the goal of having the child live as though he/she does not have asthma.

Clinical Presentation

In well-controlled asthma (the goal of therapy), cough and wheeze are noted infrequently, and activity tolerance is normal. Signs and symptoms consistent with asthma, especially with poor asthma control and flare, include recurrent cough, wheeze, shortness of breath and/or chest tightness, and evidence of air trapping. This is due to variable airflow obstruction and bronchial hyperresponsiveness triggered by underlying airway inflammation and subsequent air trapping. Symptoms often occur or worsen at night or with exercise, during viral respiratory infections, or with exposure to aeroallergens and/or pulmonary irritants (such as first- or secondhand smoke) (see Table 7-2).

The history and measurement of lung function such as forced expiratory volume at 1 second (FEV_1) or peak expiratory flow rate (PEFR) are essential and more reliable than the physical examination. That said, children under the age of 5 years are typically unable to follow directions in a way needed to provide an accurate FEV_1 or peak flow measurement.

Asthma symptoms typically follow a circadian rhythm in which bronchospasm is worse during the nighttime sleep hours. A marker of effective airway inflammation control is minimal nocturnal symptoms. With young children, parents often report awakening to the child's repeated cough while the child continues to sleep. Conversely, asthma flares are often harder to control during the nighttime hours.

Other conditions to consider when making the differential diagnosis can include alpha-1 antitrypsin deficiency, URI, gastroesophageal reflux, bronchiolitis, and cystic fibrosis.

Diagnostic Testing

As with adults, spirometry is needed to make the diagnosis of asthma; the anticipated results consistent with asthma include an increase in FEV_1 12% or greater from baseline post short-acting beta-2 agonist use. A peak flow meter should be used for monitoring, not for diagnosing, asthma. Objective evaluation for airflow obstruction should be conducted with every asthma-related visit. However, objective measure of airflow is usually only able to be obtained in children age 5 years and older. Guidelines for classifying asthma severity and initiating treatment for children aged 0 to 4 years (Fig. 17-1) and those aged 5 to 11 years (Fig. 17-2) share many commonalities with the disease's treatment in adults. The routine use of SaO_2 or chest imaging in the absence of respiratory distress is not warranted in asthma care.

Treatment

The approach to managing asthma is differentiated into two age groups: those aged 0 to 4 years (Fig. 17-3) and those aged 5 to 11 years (Fig. 17-4). Because of the wide range of asthma medications currently available, the NP, patient, and family can work together to find an age-specific lifestyle and treatment regimen that provides optimal care with minimal to few adverse medication effects.

The backbone of therapy for mild persistent, moderate persistent, or severe persistent asthma is the use of an inflammatory controller drug, such as an ICS; an additional option includes a leukotriene modifier (LTM) such as montelukast. Although all of these products have anti-inflammatory capability, ICSs have proved to be the most effective in preventing airway inflammation and are recognized as the preferred asthma controller drug. Dosing should be based on age and strength needed to control symptoms (Figs. 17-5 and 17-6). Adding an LTM to an ICS or increasing the dosage of the ICS also improves asthma outcome. The clinical effects of ICS and LTM take at least 1 to 2 weeks to be seen. Adding a LABA such as salmeterol or formoterol is also an option when ICS therapy is insufficient; as with the adult population, the FDA boxed warning about increased asthma death rate with LABA use has been removed. However, a LABA should never be used as monotherapy for a child and is only used in combination with an ICS for prevention of symptoms in moderate to severe persistent asthma. Although the inhaled mast cell stabilizers including nedocromil and cromolyn continue to be mentioned as a controller option, these products are no longer available in the United States.

Medications for asthma in children should be age and symptom specific (Table 17-12). Theophylline, a modestly effective bronchodilator, remains an option in preventing bronchospasm in children 5 years of age or older. Although inexpensive, the cost of using this medication is significant because of the required laboratory monitoring with its use. Theophylline has a narrow therapeutic index, but the dose must be closely titrated and monitored with serial serum drug levels, a particularly problematic issue in children.

Components of Severity		Classification of Asthma Severity (0–4 years of age)			
		Intermittent	Persistent		
			Mild	Moderate	Severe
Impairment	Symptoms	≤2 days/week	>2 days/week but not daily	Daily	Throughout the day
	Nighttime awakenings	0	1–2x/month	3–4x/month	>1x/week
	Short-acting beta₂-agonist use for symptom control (not prevention of EIB)	≤2 days/week	>2 days/week but not daily	Daily	Several times per day
	Interference with normal activity	None	Minor limitation	Some limitation	Extremely limited
Risk	Exacerbations requiring oral systemic corticosteroids	0–1/year	≥2 exacerbations in 6 months requiring oral systemic corticosteroids, or ≥4 wheezing episodes/1 year lasting >1 day AND risk factors for persistent asthma		
		← Consider severity and interval since last exacerbation. Frequency and severity may fluctuate over time. →			
		Exacerbations of any severity may occur in patients in any severity category.			
Recommended Step for Initiating Therapy		Step 1	Step 2	Step 3 and consider short course of oral systemic corticosteroids	
		In 2–6 weeks, depending on severity, evaluate level of asthma control that is achieved. If no clear benefit is observed in 4–6 weeks, consider adjusting therapy or alternative diagnoses.			

Key: EIB, exercise-induced bronchospasm

Notes:
- The stepwise approach is meant to assist, not replace, the clinical decision making required to meet individual patient needs.
- Level of severity is determined by both impairment and risk. Assess impairment domain by patient's/caregiver's recall of previous 2–4 weeks. Symptom assessment for longer periods should reflect a global assessment such as inquiring whether the patient's asthma is better or worse since the last visit. Assign severity to the most severe category in which any feature occurs.
- At present, there are inadequate data to correspond frequencies of exacerbations with different levels of asthma severity. For treatment purposes, patients who had ≥2 exacerbations requiring oral systemic corticosteroids in the past 6 months, or ≥4 wheezing episodes in the past year, and who have risk factors for persistent asthma may be considered the same as patients who have persistent asthma, even in the absence of impairment levels consistent with persistent asthma.

FIGURE 17-1 Classifying asthma severity and initiating treatment in children 0 to 4 years of age. *National Institutes of Health. Guidelines for the Diagnosis and Management of Asthma. http://www.nhlbi.nih.gov/health-pro/guidelines /current/asthma-guidelines/full-report*

A long-acting muscarinic antagonist (LAMA), such as tiotropium, can be used as an add-on therapy for individuals with a history of asthma flares. These agents are generally well tolerated and can improve lung function while increasing the time between flares. Tiotropium can be used in adults and adolescents but is not approved for use in children younger than 12 years of age.

Rescue medications that relieve acute superimposed bronchospasm include short-acting beta-2 agonists (SABAs), such as albuterol, levalbuterol, and pirbuterol. Compared with albuterol and pirbuterol, one of the therapeutic advantages of levalbuterol includes greater bronchodilation at a lower dose and with fewer side effects. Regardless of age or disease severity, all children with asthma should have ready access to a SABA. Prudent practice dictates that parents, caregivers, and health-care providers monitor the frequency of SABA use, as more than 2 days of use per week and/or less-than-optimal response to the bronchodilator imply persistent airway inflammation.

Children with asthma should be monitored regularly for their degree of asthma control (Fig. 17-7). Characteristics of well-controlled asthma in a 5- to 11-year-old child would include symptoms occurring

Components of Severity		Classification of Asthma Severity (5–11 years of age)			
		Intermittent	Persistent		
			Mild	Moderate	Severe
Impairment	Symptoms	≤2 days/week	>2 days/week but not daily	Daily	Throughout the day
	Nighttime awakenings	≤2x/month	3–4x/month	>1x/week but not nightly	Often 7x/week
	Short-acting beta$_2$-agonist use for symptom control (not prevention of EIB)	≤2 days/week	>2 days/week but not daily	Daily	Several times per day
	Interference with normal activity	None	Minor limitation	Some limitation	Extremely limited
	Lung function	• Normal FEV$_1$ between exacerbations • FEV$_1$ >80% predicted • FEV$_1$/FVC >85%	• FEV$_1$ ≥80% predicted • FEV$_1$/FVC >80%	• FEV$_1$ = 60%–80% predicted • FEV$_1$/FVC = 75%–80%	• FEV$_1$ <60% predicted • FEV$_1$/FVC <75%
Risk	Exacerbations requiring oral systemic corticosteroids	0–1/year (see note)	≥2/year (see note) ⟶		
		Consider severity and interval since last exacerbation. Frequency and severity may fluctuate over time for patients in any severity category. Relative annual risk of exacerbations may be related to FEV$_1$.			
Recommended Step for Initiating Therapy		Step 1	Step 2	Step 3, medium-dose ICS option	Step 3, medium-dose ICS option, or step 4
					and consider short course of oral systemic corticosteroids
		In 2–6 weeks, evaluate level of asthma control that is achieved, and adjust therapy accordingly.			

Key: EIB, exercise-induced bronchospasm; FEV$_1$, forced expiratory volume in 1 second; FVC, forced vital capacity; ICS, inhaled corticosteroids

Notes:

• The stepwise approach is meant to assist, not replace, the clinical decision making required to meet individual patient needs.

• Level of severity is determined by both impairment and risk. Assess impairment domain by patient's/caregiver's recall of the previous 2–4 weeks and spirometry. Assign severity to the most severe category in which any feature occurs.

• At present, there are inadequate data to correspond frequencies of exacerbations with different levels of asthma severity. In general, more frequent and intense exacerbations (e.g., requiring urgent, unscheduled care, hospitalization, or ICU admission) indicate greater underlying disease severity. For treatment purposes, patients who had ≥2 exacerbations requiring oral systemic corticosteroids in the past year may be considered the same as patients who have persistent asthma, even in the absence of impairment levels consistent with persistent asthma.

FIGURE 17-2 Classifying asthma severity and initiating treatment in children 5 to 11 years of age.
National Institutes of Health. Guidelines for the Diagnosis and Management of Asthma. http://www.nhlbi.nih.gov/health-pro/guidelines/current/asthma-guidelines/full-report

2 or fewer days per week (and not more than once per day), one or less nighttime awakenings per month, and SABA use 2 or fewer days per week (Fig. 17-8). This contrasts with very poorly controlled asthma, which is characterized by symptoms throughout the day, nighttime awakenings two or more times per week, and SABA use several times each day.

Due to increased risk of complications from respiratory infections in children with asthma, it is essential that children remain up to date with vaccinations, particularly pneumococcal and seasonal influenza vaccines. Other household and close contacts to the child with asthma should also be immunized annually against seasonal influenza as well as remain up to date with other vaccinations, as appropriate.

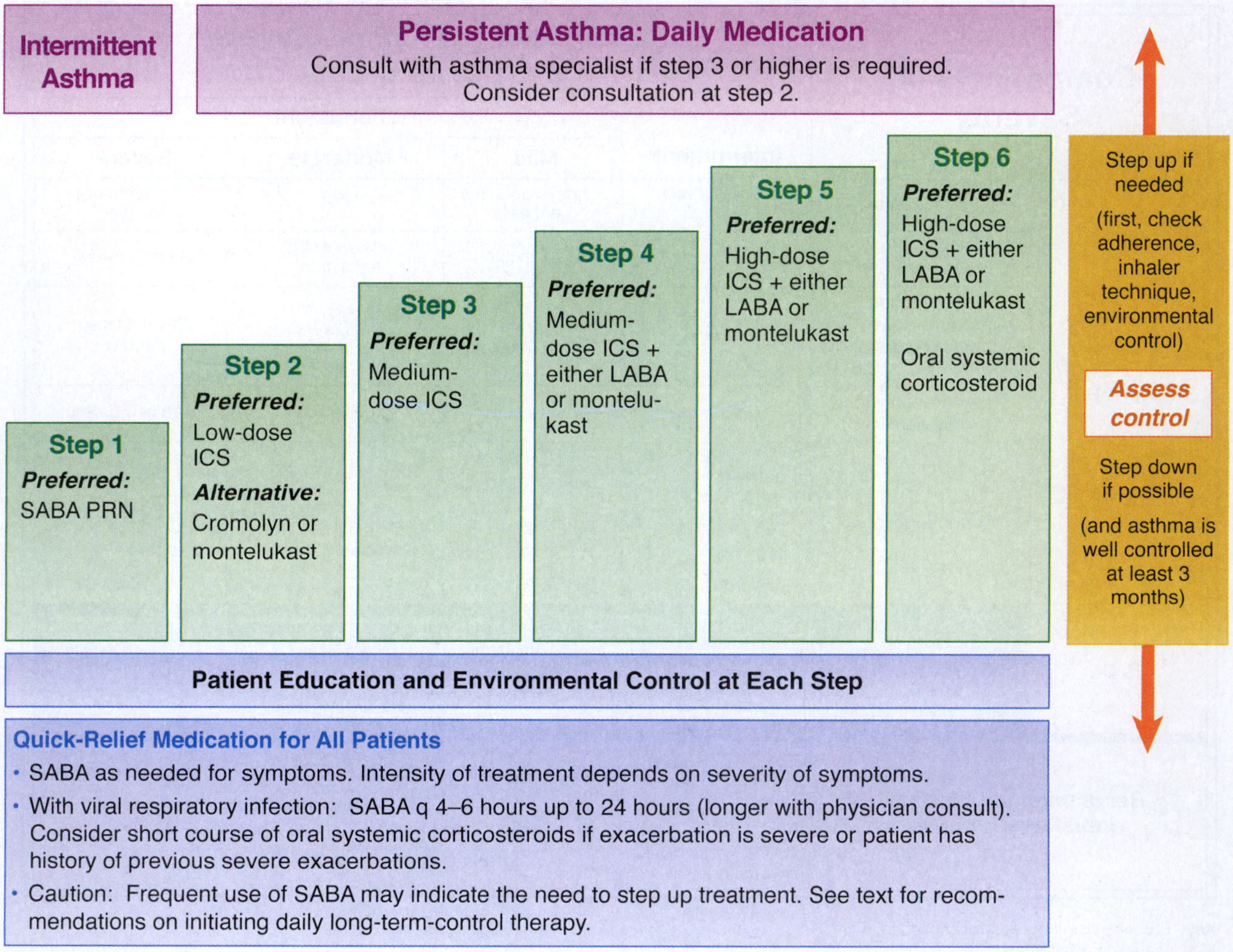

Intermittent Asthma	Persistent Asthma: Daily Medication
	Consult with asthma specialist if step 3 or higher is required. Consider consultation at step 2.

Step 1
Preferred:
SABA PRN

Step 2
Preferred:
Low-dose ICS
Alternative:
Cromolyn or montelukast

Step 3
Preferred:
Medium-dose ICS

Step 4
Preferred:
Medium-dose ICS + either LABA or montelukast

Step 5
Preferred:
High-dose ICS + either LABA or montelukast

Step 6
Preferred:
High-dose ICS + either LABA or montelukast

Oral systemic corticosteroid

Step up if needed
(first, check adherence, inhaler technique, environmental control)

Assess control

Step down if possible
(and asthma is well controlled at least 3 months)

Patient Education and Environmental Control at Each Step

Quick-Relief Medication for All Patients
- SABA as needed for symptoms. Intensity of treatment depends on severity of symptoms.
- With viral respiratory infection: SABA q 4–6 hours up to 24 hours (longer with physician consult). Consider short course of oral systemic corticosteroids if exacerbation is severe or patient has history of previous severe exacerbations.
- Caution: Frequent use of SABA may indicate the need to step up treatment. See text for recommendations on initiating daily long-term-control therapy.

Key: **Alphabetical order is used when more than one treatment option is listed within either preferred or alternative therapy.** ICS, inhaled corticosteroid; LABA, inhaled long-acting beta$_2$-agonist; SABA, inhaled short-acting beta$_2$-agonist.

Notes:
- The stepwise approach is meant to assist, not replace, the clinical decision making required to meet individual patient needs.
- If alternative treatment is used and response is inadequate, discontinue it and use the preferred treatment before stepping up.
- Theophylline is a less desirable alternative due to the need to monitor serum concentration levels.
- If clear benefit is not observed within 4–6 weeks and patient/family medication technique and adherence are satisfactory, consider adjusting therapy or alternative diagnosis.
- Studies on children 0–4 years of age are limited. Step 2 preferred therapy is based on Evidence A. All other recommendations are based on expert opinion and extrapolation from studies in older children.

FIGURE 17-3 Stepwise approach to managing asthma in children 0 to 4 years of age.
National Institutes of Health. Guidelines for the Diagnosis and Management of Asthma. http://www.nhlbi.nih.gov/health-pro/guidelines/current/asthma-guidelines/full-report

ASSESSMENT AND TREATMENT OF AN ASTHMA FLARE

Overview

An asthma exacerbation can occur in individuals with a preexisting diagnosis of asthma or as the initial presentation of asthma. Common causes for asthma flares or exacerbations are aeroallergen exposure, viral respiratory tract infections, and nonadherence to controller medications. It is important to identify triggers and develop a plan for avoiding or minimizing them. The patient should have an individualized asthma action plan to guide care during an exacerbation. Severe exacerbations can occur at all asthma severity levels.

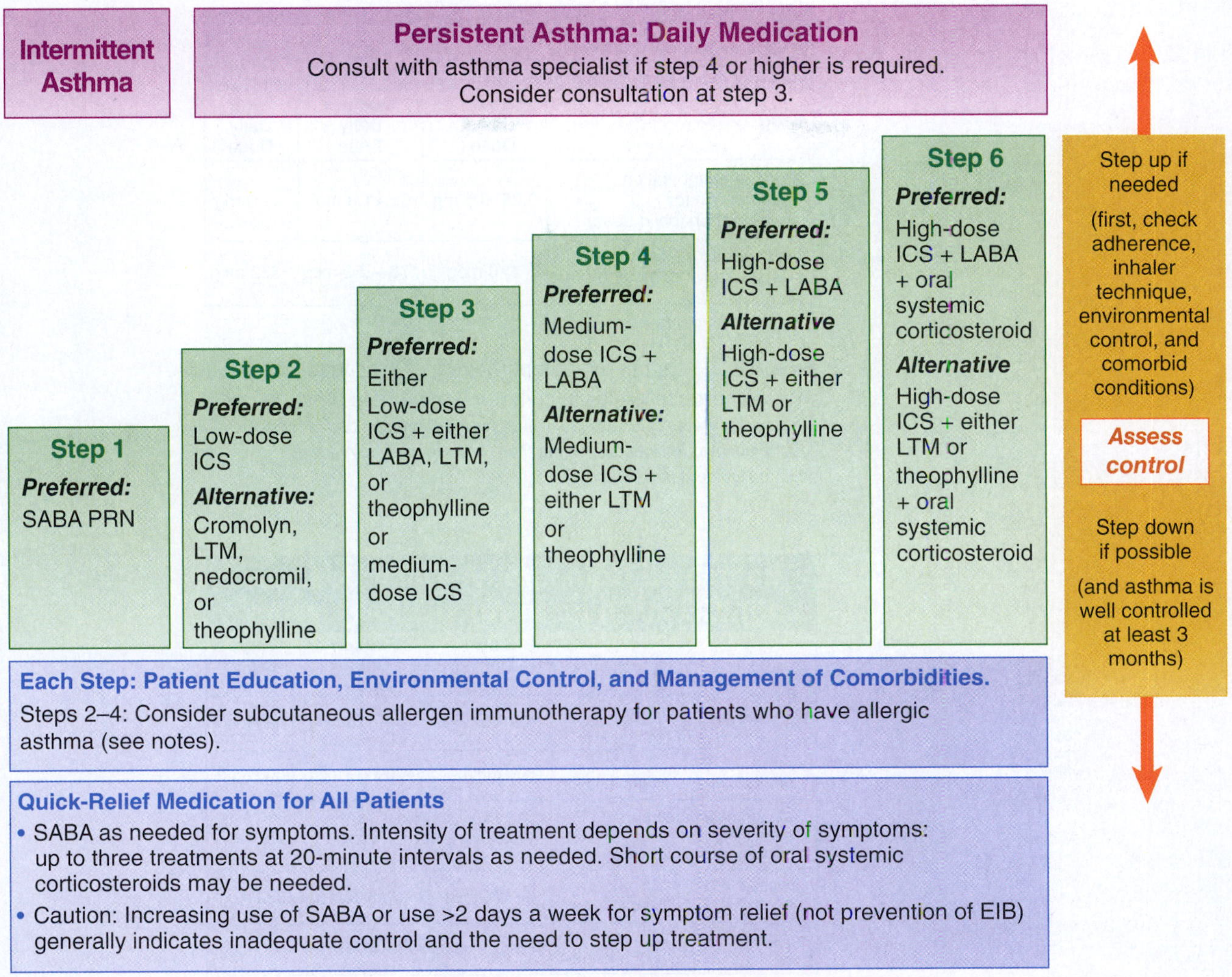

Intermittent Asthma

Persistent Asthma: Daily Medication
Consult with asthma specialist if step 4 or higher is required.
Consider consultation at step 3.

Step 1
Preferred:
SABA PRN

Step 2
Preferred:
Low-dose ICS
Alternative:
Cromolyn, LTM, nedocromil, or theophylline

Step 3
Preferred:
Either Low-dose ICS + either LABA, LTM, or theophylline or medium-dose ICS

Step 4
Preferred:
Medium-dose ICS + LABA
Alternative:
Medium-dose ICS + either LTM or theophylline

Step 5
Preferred:
High-dose ICS + LABA
Alternative:
High-dose ICS + either LTM or theophylline

Step 6
Preferred:
High-dose ICS + LABA + oral systemic corticosteroid
Alternative:
High-dose ICS + either LTM or theophylline + oral systemic corticosteroid

Step up if needed
(first, check adherence, inhaler technique, environmental control, and comorbid conditions)

Assess control

Step down if possible
(and asthma is well controlled at least 3 months)

Each Step: Patient Education, Environmental Control, and Management of Comorbidities.
Steps 2–4: Consider subcutaneous allergen immunotherapy for patients who have allergic asthma (see notes).

Quick-Relief Medication for All Patients
- SABA as needed for symptoms. Intensity of treatment depends on severity of symptoms: up to three treatments at 20-minute intervals as needed. Short course of oral systemic corticosteroids may be needed.
- Caution: Increasing use of SABA or use >2 days a week for symptom relief (not prevention of EIB) generally indicates inadequate control and the need to step up treatment.

Key: **Alphabetical order is used when more than one treatment option is listed within either preferred or alternative therapy.** ICS, inhaled corticosteroid; LABA, inhaled long-acting beta$_2$-agonist; LTM, leukotriene modifier; SABA, inhaled short-acting beta$_2$-agonist.

Notes:
- The stepwise approach is meant to assist, not replace, the clinical decision making required to meet individual patient needs.
- If alternative treatment is used and response is inadequate, discontinue it and use the preferred treatment before stepping up.
- Theophylline is a less desirable alternative due to the need to monitor serum concentration levels.
- Step 1 and step 2 medications are based on Evidence A. Step 3 ICS + adjunctive therapy and ICS are based on Evidence B for efficacy of each treatment and extrapolation from comparator trials in older children and adults—comparator trials are not available for this age group; steps 4–6 are based on expert opinion and extrapolation from studies in older children and adults.
- Immunotherapy for steps 2–4 is based on Evidence B for house-dust mites, animal danders, and pollens; evidence is weak or lacking for molds and cockroaches. Evidence is strongest for immunotherapy with single allergens. The role of allergy in asthma is greater in children than in adults. Clinicians who administer immunotherapy should be prepared and equipped to identify and treat anaphylaxis that may occur.

FIGURE 17-4 Stepwise approach to managing asthma in children 5 to 11 years of age.
National Institutes of Health. Guidelines for the Diagnosis and Management of Asthma. http://www.nhlbi.nih.gov/health-pro/guidelines/current/asthma-guidelines/full-report

Clinical Presentation

An asthma flare is characterized by a progressive increase in symptoms that can include dyspnea, cough, wheezing, or chest tightness and that are associated with decreased lung function. Oxygen desaturation is a late finding in an acute asthma flare. During a severe asthma flare with imminent respiratory arrest, a young child can appear drowsy or confused, have difficulty feeding, and/or have a softer, shorter cry.

Estimated Comparative Daily Dosages for ICS in Children Aged 0 to 4 years

Drug	Low Daily Dose	Medium Daily Dose	High Daily Dose
Budesonide inhalation suspension for nebulization (child dose)	0.25–0.5 mg	0.5–1.0 mg	>1.0 mg
Fluticasone HFA MDI: 44, 110, or 220 mcg/puff	176 mcg	176 –352 mcg	>352 mcg

Key: HFA, hydrofluoroalkane

FIGURE 17-5 Estimated comparative daily dosages for inhaled corticosteroids in children 0 to 4 years of age. *National Institutes of Health. Guidelines for the Diagnosis and Management of Asthma. http://www.nhlbi.nih.gov/health-pro/guidelines/current /asthma-guidelines/full-report*

Estimated Comparative Daily Dosages for ICS in Children Aged 5 to 11 years

	Low Daily Dose	Medium Daily Dose	High Daily Dose
Beclomethasone HFA 40 or 80 mcg/puff	80–160 mcg	>160–320 mcg	>320 mcg
Budesonide DPI 90, 180, or 200 mcg/inhalation	180–400 mcg	>400–800 mcg	>800 mcg
Budesonide inhalation suspension for nebulization (child dose)	0.5 mg	1.0 mg	2.0 mg
Fluticasone HFA MDI: 44, 110, or 220 mcg/puff	88–176 mcg	>176–352 mcg	>352 mcg
Fluticasone DPI: 50, 100, or 250 mcg/inhalation	100–200 mcg	>200–400 mcg	>400 mcg

Key: HFA, Hydrofluoroalkane

FIGURE 17-6 Estimated comparative daily dosages for inhaled corticosteroids in children 5 to 11 years of age. *National Institutes of Health. Guidelines for the Diagnosis and Management of Asthma. http://www.nhlbi.nih.gov/health-pro/guidelines/current /asthma-guidelines/full-report*

CLINICAL CONCEPT

During an asthma flare, lower airway inflammation leads to findings characteristic of air trapping, such as decreased PEF rate, prolonged expiratory phase, thoracic hyperresonance on percussion, and hyperinflation seen on chest radiographs.

Diagnostic Testing

Diagnostic testing should evaluate any change in lung function either with FEV_1 or PEFR and compare with values from the patient's previous lung function or predicted values. The frequency of symptoms can also be an important measure to determine the onset of a flare, though in some patients, symptoms can be perceived poorly, and patients can experience a substantial decline in lung function without a change in symptoms. The physical examination is often normal and does not correlate well with asthma severity. A chest x-ray is not required when evaluating a person with an asthma flare unless there is a suspicion of pneumonia. Routine measurement of arterial blood gas is not needed as abnormal findings in SaO_2 are typically seen at a late stage of the flare.

Treatment

When acute asthma flare is present with increased symptoms and objective measurement of airflow obstruction, rapidly acting, higher-potency anti-inflammatory

TABLE 17-12 Pediatric Asthma Medications

MEDICATION	MECHANISM OF ACTION	INDICATION	COMMENT
Inhaled corticosteroids	Inhibit eosinophilic action and other inflammatory mediators, potentate effects of beta-2 agonists	Controller drug, prevention of inflammation	Need consistent use to be helpful
Leukotriene modifier (montelukast [Singulair®])	Inhibits action of inflammatory mediator, leukotriene, by blocking select receptor sites	Controller drug, prevention of inflammation	Likely less effective than inhaled corticosteroids. Particularly effective add-on medication when disease control inadequate with inhaled corticosteroid, when asthma complicated by allergic rhinitis
Oral corticosteroids	Inhibit eosinophilic action and other inflammatory mediators	Treatment of acute inflammation such as in asthma flare	■ Indicated in treatment of acute asthma flare to reduce inflammation ■ In higher dose and with longer therapy ■ No taper needed if use is short term, especially less than 14 days Potential for causing gastropathy, particularly gastric ulcer and gastritis
Beta-2 agonist Albuterol (Ventolin®, Proventil®), pirbuterol (Maxair®), levalbuterol (Xopenex®)	Bronchodilation via stimulation of beta-2 receptor site	Rescue drugs for treatment of acute bronchospasm	■ Onset of action 15 minutes ■ Duration of action 4 to 6 hours
Long-acting beta-2 agonists (salmeterol [Serevent®], formoterol [Foradil®])	Beta-2 agonist; bronchodilation via stimulation of beta-2 receptor site	Prevention of bronchospasm	Example: Salmeterol ■ Onset of action 1 hour ■ Duration of action 12 hours ■ Indicated for prevention rather than treatment of bronchospasm Patient should also have short-acting beta-2 agonist as rescue drug ■ Long-acting beta-2 agonist should never be used alone but in combination with inhaled corticosteroid
Theophylline	Mild bronchodilator, helps with diaphragmatic contraction	Prevention of bronchospasm, mild anti-inflammatory	■ Narrow therapeutic index drug with numerous drug interactions ■ Monitor carefully for toxicity by checking drug levels and clinical presentation

therapy with an oral corticosteroid is needed. Treatment of an asthma exacerbation in children over 5 years is similar to treatment of adults as described in Chapter 7.

For a young child (5 years or younger) who presents in primary care with mild to moderate asthma flare, treatment should be initiated with SABA, such as albuterol 100 mcg two puffs by pressurized metered-dose inhaler (pMDI) plus spacer or 2.5 mg by nebulizer. This should be repeated every 20 minutes for the first hour if needed. Use of controlled oxygen can be considered to achieve target saturation of 94% to 98%. The child should be monitored closely for 1 to 2 hours and transferred to high-level care if there is a lack of

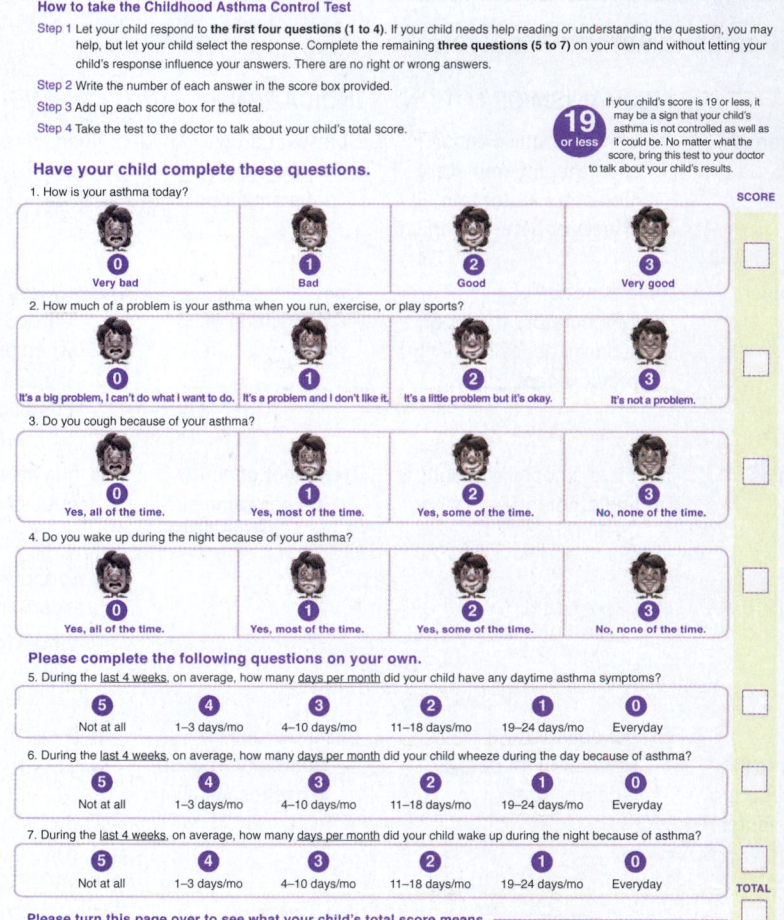

FIGURE 17-7 Childhood asthma control test for children 4 to 11 years old.
*National Jewish Health, Pediatric Asthma. Childhood Asthma Control Test. https://www
.nationaljewish.org/NJH/media/pdf/pdf-Childhood_ACT.pdf*

response to SABA therapy, any sign of severe exacerbation, increasing respiratory rate, or decreasing oxygen saturation. With improvement, SABA treatment should be continued as needed. If symptoms recur within 3 to 4 hours, extra doses of SABA can be used (two to three puffs per hour). Oral prednisolone should be given at 2 mg/kg (maximum of 20 mg for child younger than 2 years; maximum of 30 mg for 2- to 5-year-olds). Upon discharge, reliever medication should be used as needed, while controller medication can be adjusted as appropriate.

With any sign of severe or life-threatening exacerbation, immediate transfer to a high-level care facility is essential. Signs include the inability to speak or drink, central cyanosis, confusion or drowsiness, marked subcostal and/or subglottic retractions, oxygen saturation less than 92%, silent chest on auscultation, and pulse rate greater than 200 bpm (0 to 3 years) or greater than 180 bpm (4 to 5 years). While waiting to transfer, albuterol, oral corticosteroid, and oxygen therapy should be administered as soon as possible.

Discussion Sources

Global Initiative for Asthma. Global Strategy for Asthma Management and Prevention, 2020. https://ginasthma.org/gina
-reports

National Institutes of Health, National Heart, Lung, and Blood Institute, National Asthma Education and Prevention Program.
Expert Panel Report 3: Guidelines for the Diagnosis and Management of Asthma. https://www.nhlbi.nih.gov/health-topics
/guidelines-for-diagnosis-management-of-asthma

National Institutes of Health, National Heart, Lung, and Blood Institute. *Guidelines for the Diagnosis and Management of Asthma
(EPR-3).* http://www.nhlbi.nih.gov/health-pro/guidelines/current/asthma-guidelines/full-report

Components of CONTROL		Age (Years)	Level of Asthma CONTROL		
			Well Controlled	Not Well Controlled	Very Poorly Controlled
Impairment	Symptoms	0–4	≤2 days/week but ≤1x/day	>2 days/week or multiple times on ≤2days/week	Throughout the day
		5–11			
		≥12	≤2 days/week	>2 days/week	
	Nighttime awakenings	0–4	≤1x/month	>1x/month	>1x/week
		5–11		≥2x/month	≥2x/week
		≥12	≤2x/month	1–3x/week	≥4x/week
	Interference with normal activity	All	None	Some limitation	Extremely limited
	SABA use for symptoms	All	≤2 days/week	>2 days/week	Several times per day
	Lung function				
	FEV₁ (predicted) or PEF (personal best)	≥5	>80%	60%–80%	<60%
	FEV₁/FVC	5–11	>80%	75%–80%	<75%
	Validated questionnaires				
	ATAQ	≥12	0	1–2	3–4
	ACQ	≥12	≤0.75	≥1.5	n/a
	ACT	≥12	≥20	16–19	≤15
Risk	Exacerbations requiring oral corticosteroids	0–4	≤1x/year	2–3x/year	>3x/year
		5–11		≥2x/year Consider severity and interval since last exacerbation	
		≥12			
	Reduction in lung growth	5–11	Evaluation requires long-term follow-up care		
	Loss of lung function	≥12	Evaluation requires long-term follow-up care		
	Treatment-related adverse effects	All	Medication side effects can vary in intensity from none to very troublesome and worrisome.		
Recommended treatment actions		All	Maintain current step; regular follow-up at every 1–6 months; consider stepping down if well controlled for ≥3 months	Step up 1 step	Step up 1–2 steps and consider short course of oral corticosteroids
				Before stepping up, review adherence to medication, inhaler technique, environmental control, and comorbid conditions. If an alternative treatment option was used in a step, discontinue and use the preferred treatment for that step. Reevaluate the level of asthma control in 2–6 weeks and adjust therapy accordingly. For side effects, consider alternative treatment options.	

FIGURE 17-8 Assessing asthma control in children and adolescents.
EPR-3 Pocket Guide. University of Michigan Health System. Quick Reference Charts for the Classification and Stepwise Treatment of Asthma. http://www.med .umich.edu/1info/FHP/practiceguides/asthma/EPR-3_pocket_guide.pdf

QUESTIONS

173. Which of the following best describes the pathophysiology and resulting clinical presentation of asthma?

    A. intermittent airway inflammation with occasional bronchospasm

    B. a disease of bronchospasm leading to airway inflammation

    C. chronic airway inflammation with superimposed bronchospasm

    D. relatively fixed airway constriction

174. A 6-year-old boy has a 1-year history of moderate persistent asthma that is normally well controlled with budesonide via dry powder inhaler (DPI) twice a day and the use of albuterol once or twice a week as needed for wheezing. Three days ago, he developed a sore throat, clear nasal discharge, and a predominately dry cough with two episodes of production of small amounts of white sputum. In the past 24 hours, he has had intermittent wheezing, necessitating the use of albuterol two puffs with use of an age-appropriate spacer every 3 hours with partial relief of bronchospasm. Your next most appropriate action is to obtain:

  A. a chest radiograph.

  B. an oxygen saturation measurement.

  C. spirometry measurement.

  D. a sputum smear for WBCs.

175. You see a 4-year-old girl who has a 2-day history of signs and symptoms of an acute asthma flare resulting from viral URI. She is using inhaled budesonide daily and albuterol prn as directed, with excellent symptom control in the day-to-day. With her current URI, she continues to have difficulty with increased occurrence of coughing and wheezing. Her respiratory rate is within 50% of upper limit of normal for her age. Her medication regimen should be adjusted to include:

  A. daily use of oral theophylline.

  B. addition of inhaled salmeterol (Serevent®) until her acute illness is resolved.

  C. a short course of oral prednisolone.

  D. daily use of oral montelukast (Singulair®).

176. Which of the following is inconsistent with the diagnosis of asthma?

  A. a troublesome nocturnal cough

  B. cough or wheeze after exercise

  C. consistent morning sputum production

  D. colds "go to the chest" or take more than 10 days to clear

177. Celeste is a 9-year-old girl with moderate persistent asthma. She is not taking an ICS that was prescribed in the past but is using albuterol prn to relieve her cough and wheeze. According to her mother, she currently uses about six albuterol doses per day, particularly for cough and wheeze after active play. You consider that:

  A. albuterol use can continue at this level.

  B. excessive albuterol use is a risk factor for asthma death.

  C. she should also use salmeterol (Serevent®) to reduce her albuterol use.

  D. active play should be limited to avoid triggering cough and wheeze.

178. In the treatment of asthma, an LTM should be used as a:

  A. controller to prevent bronchospasm.

  B. controller to inhibit inflammatory process.

  C. reliever to treat acute bronchospasm.

  D. reliever to treat inflammation.

179. Which of the following is not a risk factor for asthma death?

  A. hospitalization or an emergency department visit for asthma in the past month

  B. current use of systemic corticosteroids or recent withdrawal from systemic corticosteroids

  C. difficulty perceiving airflow obstruction or its severity

  D. rural residence

180. A middle-school student presents, asking for a letter stating that he should not participate in physical education class because he has moderate persistent asthma. The most appropriate response is to:

  A. write the note because physical education class participation could trigger an asthma flare.

  B. excuse him from outdoor activities only to avoid pollen exposure.

    C. remind him that with appropriate asthma care, he should be capable of participating in physical education class.

    D. excuse him from indoor activities only to avoid dust mite exposure.

181. After ICS or LTM therapy is initiated, clinical effects are seen:

    A. immediately.

    B. within the first week.

    C. in about 1 to 2 weeks.

    D. in about 1 to 2 months.

182. Compared with albuterol, levalbuterol (Xopenex®):

    A. has a different mechanism of action.

    B. has the ability to provide greater bronchodilation with a lower dose.

    C. has an anti-inflammatory effect similar to an ICS.

    D. is contraindicated for use in children.

183. In caring for a child with an acute asthma flare, the NP considers that, according to current guidelines, antibiotic use is recommended:

    A. routinely.

    B. with evidence of concomitant bacterial infection.

    C. when asthma flares are frequent.

    D. with sputum production.

184. Poorly controlled asthma in children can lead to:

    A. attenuated lung development.

    B. chronic tracheitis.

    C. sleep apnea.

    D. alveolar destruction.

185. Which of the following is most consistent with asthma flare in a 4-year-old child?

    A. inspiratory stridor

    B. expiratory wheezing

    C. chronic cough with purulent sputum

    D. loud "barking" cough predominantly during the day

186. Signs of respiratory distress during an asthma flare in a 2-year-old child include all of the following except:

    A. drowsiness.

    B. confusion.

    C. respiratory rate less than 30/minute.

    D. softer, shorter cry.

187. Haley is a 6-year-old with moderate persistent asthma who presents for a follow-up visit. The NP administers the Asthma Control Test (ACT), and she scores a 22. This would indicate:

    A. well-controlled asthma.

    B. not well-controlled asthma.

    C. poorly controlled asthma.

    D. very poorly controlled asthma.

188. Which of the following would you not expect for Haley (question 187)?

    A. nighttime awakening about once a week

    B. asthma symptoms occurring about two times per week

C. asthma having little to no interference with normal activities

D. SABA use 2 days or less per week

189. All of the following are accurate regarding the use of a LAMA (e.g., tiotropium) in children with asthma except:

A. can help reduce the frequency of flares.

B. offer anti-inflammatory effect similar to ICS.

C. are usually used as add-on therapy.

D. tiotropium is not approved for use as a rescue medication.

190. Which of the following is most accurate regarding influenza vaccination in children with asthma?

A. Influenza vaccination should be delayed until 6 years of age in the presence of asthma.

B. Both the injectable and LAIV (nasal mist) vaccines are acceptable in children with asthma.

C. All children and close contacts 6 months and older should receive annual seasonal influenza vaccination.

D. Children with asthma require two doses of influenza vaccine until 10 years of age.

For answers and rationales, see end of chapter.

Urinary Tract Infection

Overview

Although often thought of as a problem primarily of women during the reproductive years, UTIs do occur in early childhood. Uncircumcised boys can have rates of UTI significantly higher than those in circumcised boys, by about 20%, but this difference decreases dramatically when normal penile growth loosens the foreskin, usually occurring by the time the boy is 1 to 2 years old. However, this potential health issue is not considered to be an indication for routine male circumcision. Commonly, the foreskin's orifice appears quite small but urine flows through it unimpeded.

> **CLINICAL CONCEPT**
> UTI rates in girls younger than 1 year are about 6.5% and at 1 to 2 years are 8.1%; the rates are lower in boys: 3.3% at younger than 1 year and 1.9% at 1 to 2 years.

Clinical Presentation

The clinical presentation of UTI in children can be without the classic symptoms such as frequency, dysuria, or flank pain. In younger children, UTI often manifests as irritability, lethargy, and fever with no obvious focal infectious source. Older children often present with abdominal pain, unexplained fever, or both; as children approach puberty, flank pain becomes more common. UTI should be considered in infants and young children 2 months to 2 years old with unexplained fever, particularly in boys younger than 6 months and girls younger than 2 years who have a temperature greater than or equal to 39°C (greater than or equal to 102.2°F). Urinary tract abnormality is a major risk factor for pediatric UTI, with vesicoureteral reflux noted in 30% to 50% of cases. Reflux nephropathy increases the risk of ascending infection that can cause pyelonephritis and renal scarring. This is a risk factor for renal failure but is largely avoidable with early reflux recognition and proper treatment.

Diagnostic Testing

Little difference is usually found in the clinical presentation and laboratory findings of cystitis or pyelonephritis in a febrile infant or younger child. A urinalysis should be obtained in a child with unexplained fever or symptoms that suggest a UTI; however, 20% of urinalyses from UTI cases return a false-negative result. Any of the following findings are suggestive, although not diagnostic, of UTI: positive leukocyte esterase, positive nitrite, more than five WBCs per high-power field in spun specimen, and bacteria present in unspun Gram-stained specimen. A positive nitrite test would indicate the presence of gram-negative bacteria as they can reduce urinary nitrate to nitrite. The most common uropathogen regardless of age or gender is gram-negative *Escherichia coli*.

The method of obtaining a urinalysis in younger children (generally younger than 5 or 6 years old) has been long debated. The "clean catch" method (catching a sample by holding a sterile specimen bottle in the urine stream) is the best noninvasive method but can be difficult with younger pre-toilet-trained children. Urine collection bags or sanitary pads offer additional noninvasive methods of collection. However, these methods likely have a high rate of skin or fecal contamination. Suprapubic bladder aspiration yields the specimen that is least likely to be contaminated; for the parent and child, this method can be fraught with fear, and it requires special provider skill. The next acceptable method is transurethral bladder catheterization.

Though hematological studies are often not helpful in the diagnosis of UTIs, a CBC and metabolic panel should be considered in children suspected of pyelonephritis. An evaluation for sepsis should also be initiated if clinical presentation warrants. Signs of sepsis include fever, tachycardia, tachypnea, cool extremities, and delayed capillary refill. A sepsis workup includes CBC, clotting function and coagulation parameters, electrolyte levels, renal and liver function tests, urinalysis, etiology-specific serology tests, tests for inflammatory markers and acute-phase reactants, and culture of blood, urine, and CSF.

Treatment

The management of a UTI in a child is dictated by the clinical severity of the illness rather than by the specific site of infection in the urinary tract. As a result, a single documented UTI in a child must be taken seriously. If an infant or young child 2 months to 2 years old with suspected UTI is assessed as toxic, dehydrated, or unable to retain oral intake, hospitalization is advised. In this circumstance, initial antimicrobial therapy should be administered parenterally, usually with a third-generation cephalosporin. Ampicillin can be added if gram-positive cocci are present in the urine or if no organism was observed. An aminoglycoside such as parenteral gentamicin can be used if there is a history of severe penicillin or cephalosporin allergy.

For a child with uncomplicated UTI who is well hydrated and able to take an antimicrobial and fluids orally, home-based care is reasonable. Other criteria for outpatient management include a caregiver with appropriate observational and coping skills, access to a telephone and automobile, and the ability to return for follow-up in 24 hours, and a patient who has no need for oxygen therapy, IV fluids, or other inpatient needs. Oral amoxicillin, TMP-SMX, or a second- or third-generation cephalosporin is recommended as an option for initial therapy; the use of TMP-SMX has a small risk of treatment failure. Although fluoroquinolone antibiotics have not been widely used in children, ciprofloxacin is approved by the FDA for use in pediatric patients for the treatment of UTI; this use is approved starting at age 1 year. Current evidence-based practice recommendations indicate a 7- to 14-day course of antibiotics because the outcomes are superior to a 1- to 3-day course in preventing spread of infection and subsequent renal scarring. Close clinical follow-up of the child and instruction of parents regarding prompt attention to recurrence of symptoms is highly recommended.

Antimicrobial treatment for prophylaxis, where a small dose of an antibiotic is used daily, to minimize future UTI is not recommended. Some experts do recommend the use of antimicrobial prophylaxis for children with high-grade reflux (grades III to V). Prophylactic agents can include nitrofurantoin, TMP-SMX, or TMP, though nitrofurantoin and sulfa drugs should not be used in infants younger than 6 weeks.

Urinary tract imaging should be considered for children with UTI, particularly in febrile children between 2 months and 2 years of age with a first documented UTI. However, whether to perform an imaging study should also be based on the clinician's judgment. The two mainstays for imaging in young children are renal-bladder ultrasound (RBUS) and voiding cystourethrography (VCUG). RBUS is an easily obtained, noninvasive test that can detect obstructive uropathy, a solitary or ectopic kidney, or moderate renal damage caused by pyelonephritis. This method can miss a small number of high-grade reflux cases. The benefits of this imaging (no radiation exposure, noninvasive, minimal discomfort for child and parents), however, outweigh the slight increase in specificity of VCUG. A renal scan, in which a small amount of radioactive material is used to visualize the kidneys, is useful for detecting renal scarring, a finding present after infection, but is not recommended for routine, initial evaluation of the young child with his/her first febrile UTI. VCUG is indicated if RBUS reveals hydronephrosis, scarring, or other findings that would suggest either high-grade vesicoureteral reflux (VUR) or obstructive uropathy, as well as other atypical or complex clinical circumstances. VCUG can also be performed if febrile UTI is recurrent. However, some parents might want to avoid VCUG even after the second UTI. These preferences should be considered. Only if high-grade (grade V) VUR or other urinary tract abnormality is noted on imaging should antimicrobial prophylaxis be continued until the abnormality is corrected.

> **CLINICAL CONCEPT**
> Current studies do not support the use of antimicrobial prophylaxis to prevent febrile recurrent UTI in infants with grades I to IV VUR.

Discussion Sources

Balighian E, Burke M. Urinary tract infections in children. *Pediatr Rev.* 2018;39:3–12.

Fisher DJ. Pediatric urinary tract infection medication. Medscape. http://emedicine.medscape.com/article/969643-medication#2/

Hatch D, Hulbert W. Pediatric urinary tract infections. American Urological Association. https://www.auanet.org/education/pediatric-urinary-tract-infections.cfm

Steering Committee on Quality Improvement and Management, Subcommittee on Urinary Tract Infection. Urinary tract infection: clinical practice guideline for the diagnosis and management of the initial UTI in febrile infants and children 2 to 24 months. *Pediatrics.* 2011;128(3):595–610.

QUESTIONS

191. Rates of UTI among uncircumcised infant boys are how much higher than those in circumcised boys?

A. as much as 10%

B. as much as 20%

C. as much as 30%

D. less than 10%

192. Which of the following is most likely to be part of the clinical presentation of UTI in a 20-month-old child?

A. urinary frequency and urgency

B. fever

C. suprapubic tenderness

D. nausea and vomiting

193. Which of the following is the most common UTI organism in children?

A. *Pseudomonas aeruginosa*

B. *E coli*

C. *Klebsiella pneumoniae*

D. *Proteus mirabilis*

194. All of the following uropathogens are capable of reducing urinary nitrates to nitrites except:

A. *E coli.*

B. *Proteus* species.

C. *K pneumoniae.*

D. *Staphylococcus saprophyticus.*

195. Which of the following is considered the ideal method for obtaining a urine sample for culture and susceptibility in an 18-month-old girl with suspected UTI?

A. suprapubic aspiration

B. transurethral bladder catheterization

C. bag collection

D. diaper sample

196. When choosing an antimicrobial agent for the treatment of UTI in a febrile female child who is 16 months old, the NP considers that:

A. gram-positive organisms are the most likely cause of infection.

B. a parenteral aminoglycoside is the preferred treatment choice.

C. the use of an oral third-generation cephalosporin is acceptable if GI function is intact.

D. nitrofurantoin use is considered first-line therapy.

197. When evaluating the urinalysis of a 10-month-old infant with UTI, the NP considers that:

A. leukocytes would be consistently noted.

B. proteinuria is usually absent.

C. the presence of urobilinogen is commonly noted.

D. up to 20% of urinalyses can be normal.

198. In children 2 months to 2 years old with UTI, antimicrobial therapy should be prescribed for:

A. 1 to 3 days.

B. 4 to 6 days.

C. 7 to 14 days.

D. 14 to 21 days.

199. A 12-month-old boy with fever who has a suspected UTI has vomited five times in the past 7 hours. His last wet diaper was approximately 6 hours ago. He is accompanied by his parents. The following action should be taken:

A. recommend continued observation at home.

B. recommend oral antimicrobial therapy.

C. conduct renal ultrasound.

D. arrange for the child to be admitted to the hospital.

200. The preferred urinary tract imaging study for a 22-month-old girl with first-time febrile UTI is:

A. RBUS.

B. renal scan.

C. VCUG.

D. IV pyelography.

201. Which of the following is the most compelling reason to use RBUS instead of VCUG?

A. This is a noninvasive test.

B. Results are available more rapidly.

C. The test is less technically demanding.

D. RBUS is less expensive.

202. VCUG is indicated:

A. after UTI diagnosis is confirmed to determine course of antimicrobial therapy.

B. when UTI is recurrent.

C. to confirm high-grade reflux.

D. as an alternative to RBUS to assure accurate detection of scarring.

203. The urinary tract abnormality most often associated with UTI in younger children is:

A. bladder neck stricture.

B. ureteral stenosis.

C. urethral stricture.

D. VUR.

For answers and rationales, see end of chapter.

Common Childhood Febrile Illness With Skin Alterations

Overview

Developing an accurate diagnosis of an acute febrile illness with associated rash or skin lesion can be a daunting task.

SCARLET FEVER

Overview

Scarlet fever is characterized by exudative pharyngitis that predominantly affects children 5 to 15 years of age, usually during winter and spring. It can affect older children and adults, though most individuals develop lifelong protective antibodies against the disease by adolescence. The causative agent of scarlet fever is *Streptococcus pyogenes* (group A beta-hemolytic streptococci [GABHS]), a gram-positive bacteria,

CLINICAL CONCEPT

Knowledge of the infectious agent, its incubation period, its mode of transmission, and its common clinical presentation can be helpful in arriving at the correct diagnosis.

which is the most common bacterial cause of pharyngitis. The incubation period of scarlet fever can range from 12 hours to 7 days, and children are contagious during the acute illness and the subclinical phase.

Clinical Presentation

Scarlet fever tends to emerge abruptly with a sudden onset of fever and sore throat. Other signs include headache and tender, localized anterior cervical lymphadenopathy. A scarlatina-form or sandpaper-like rash appears on day 2 of pharyngitis and often peels a few days later. The presence of rash does not imply a more severe or serious disease or greater risk of contagion.

Diagnostic Testing

The diagnosis is mostly based on clinical presentation. Throat culture is used for confirmation, though proper technique is critical to improve sensitivity and detect infection rather than carriage of GABHS (found in about 10% to 15% of the population). Rapid strep tests can identify GABHS in approximately 7 minutes and can allow rapid diagnosis and prompt administration of antimicrobial therapy. This is preferable to culture, which can take up to 2 to 3 days for results. Imaging studies are not indicated for scarlet fever.

Treatment

Treatment for scarlet fever is identical to that of streptococcus pharyngitis. Oral penicillin or amoxicillin is first-line therapy, while a first-generation cephalosporin can also be considered. In the case of penicillin allergy, a macrolide (azithro-, clarithro-, erythromycin) or clindamycin can be used. Treatment duration should be 10 to 14 days, with clinical improvement observed after 24 to 48 hours of effective treatment. IM penicillin can be considered if there is concern about treatment adherence for the full oral antimicrobial regimen. IM and oral penicillin formulations have identical spectrums of activity, though an oral formulation is preferred as there is a greater risk of adverse effects and serious allergic reaction with IM administration. Appropriate treatment is essential in reducing the risk of serious complications, including acute rheumatic fever and poststreptococcal glomerulonephritis.

ROSEOLA

Overview

Roseola is a common childhood disease caused by human herpesvirus-6 (HHV-6) with about 90% of cases seen in children younger than 2 years old. Once children resolve the infection, they have lifelong immunity, though the virus can remain latent in most individuals. The virus can be found in the saliva of older children during the latent phase, which is believed to be the primary source of infection in infants. The infection can result in a high-grade fever, and febrile seizures occur in about 10% of affected children.

Clinical Presentation

Roseola typically develops with abrupt onset of high-grade fever (40°C or greater [104°F or greater]). A discrete rosy-pink macular or maculopapular rash that can last hours to 3 days follows a 3- to 7-day period of fever. The presence of rash indicates the infection is no longer contagious.

Diagnostic Testing

Roseola is primarily a clinical diagnosis. Laboratory studies are not needed, though testing can be considered in the presence of high fever. Diagnostic tests can include CBC, urinalysis, blood cultures, and CSF examination. A seizure workup might be indicated in the presence of febrile seizure.

Treatment

There is currently no antiviral agent used for the treatment of HHV-6, and so treatment of roseola is largely supportive care. Use of antiseizure medication is not warranted for those with febrile seizure.

RUBELLA

Overview

Rubella is caused by the rubella virus and typically causes a mild disease in children. However, the greatest risk from this infection is during pregnancy, especially with first-trimester exposure, which confers an approximate 80% rate of congenital rubella syndrome. This can result in miscarriage, stillbirth, and severe birth defects in infants. The virus is primarily transmitted via respiratory droplet. The incubation period ranges from about 14 to 21 days with disease transmissible for approximately 1 week prior to onset of rash to approximately 2 weeks after rash appears. Fortunately, rubella is preventable via vaccination with the MMR vaccine.

Clinical Presentation

Rubella in children is generally a mild, self-limiting illness characterized by mild fever, sore throat, malaise, and nasal discharge. A diffuse maculopapular rash develops that lasts about 3 days. Posterior cervical and postauricular lymphadenopathy can occur 5 to 10 days prior to onset of rash. Arthralgia occurs in about 25% of those affected (most common in women).

Diagnostic Testing

A clinical diagnosis of rubella can be difficult, as several other conditions can mimic this infection. Laboratory confirmation is made by the presence of serum rubella IgM. A rubella diagnosis should be reported to state and/or public health authorities.

Treatment

Treatment of rubella is largely supportive as there is no antiviral therapy available for rubella. Vaccination with MMR is essential to prevent this infection.

MEASLES

Overview

Measles is caused by the rubeola virus and is one of the most contagious infectious diseases that can affect children and adults. Though endemic measles was eliminated in the United States in the early 2000s, the number of measles cases has grown recently, typically with the virus originating from a country outside the United States. Most cases of measles occur in children whose parents refused immunization.

The spread of the virus is via respiratory droplet, and it has an incubation period of 10 to 14 days. The infection is contagious from about 1 week prior to development of the rash to approximately 2 to 3 weeks after the rash appears. Central nervous system (CNS) and respiratory tract complications are common, with the possibility of permanent neurological impairment or even death.

Clinical Presentation

Measles is characterized by generalized lymphadenopathy, conjunctivitis (copious clear discharge), photophobia, and Koplik spots (appear approximately 2 days prior to onset of rash as white spots with blue rings held within red spots in oral mucosa in approximately one-third of individuals). Pharyngitis is usually mild and without exudate. Presentation can also include fever, nasal discharge, and cough. A maculopapular rash develops 3 to 4 days after the onset of symptoms, which may coalesce to a generalized erythema. The duration of illness for uncomplicated measles can last 7 to 10 days from the late prodrome period to resolution of fever and rash. Caregivers should be aware of signs of complications so appropriate interventions can be initiated.

> **CLINICAL CONCEPT**
> Measles complications are more likely to occur in children younger than 5 years of age as well as those with immune deficiencies, and include croup, encephalitis, and pneumonia.

Diagnostic Testing

The diagnosis of measles can usually be made with clinical presentation. However, confirmation is needed as cases of measles should be reported to state and/or public health authorities. Confirmation is achieved with serological testing for rubeola immunoglobulin G (IgG) and immunoglobulin M (IgM) antibodies, isolation of the virus, or reverse-transcriptase polymerase chain reaction (RT-PCR) assay.

Treatment

Management of measles largely involves supportive care for the illness and its complications. Hydration is essential to replace fluids lost through emesis and diarrhea, with IV rehydration necessary in severe cases. Vitamin A supplementation should be considered, especially in children with signs of vitamin A deficiency. Vitamin A has been shown to reduce morbidity and mortality and can help prevent eye damage and blindness. The measles vaccine should be administered to any close contacts who have not been vaccinated. The vaccine is preventive when given within 3 days of exposure. Human immunoglobulin can be given to unvaccinated individuals at high risk of complications, including immunocompromised, infants aged 6 months to 1 year, infants younger than 6 months who are born to mothers without measles immunity, and pregnant women.

VARICELLA

Overview

Varicella-zoster virus (VZV) causes the highly contagious, systemic disease commonly known as chickenpox. The virus is transmitted via respiratory droplet and contact with open lesions. Chickenpox can be serious, especially in infants or the immunocompromised. Complications of varicella infection can include bacterial infection of skin lesions, pneumonia, encephalitis, toxic shock syndrome, and Reye's syndrome (for those taking aspirin during infection). Recovery from varicella infection usually confers lifetime immunity. Reinfection can occur rarely, however, in patients who are immunocompromised. More often, re-exposure causes an increase in antibody titers without causing disease. Congenital varicella syndrome is a rare disorder that can lead to birth defects if the mother becomes infected early in pregnancy (up to 20 weeks' gestation). Varicella is a vaccine-preventable disease.

VZV can lie dormant in sensory nerve ganglia. Later, reactivation causes shingles, a painful, vesicular-form rash in a dermatomal pattern. About 15% of people who have had chickenpox develop shingles at least once during their lifetime. Shingles rates are markedly reduced in people who have received the varicella vaccine compared with people who have had chickenpox.

Clinical Presentation

This disease is characterized by an acute onset of fever, malaise, and a vesicular-form rash with intense itch. The classic skin lesions appear first on the stomach, back, and face and can spread over the entire body, causing between 250 and 500 itchy blisters (Fig. 17-9). The vesicles eventually crust over.

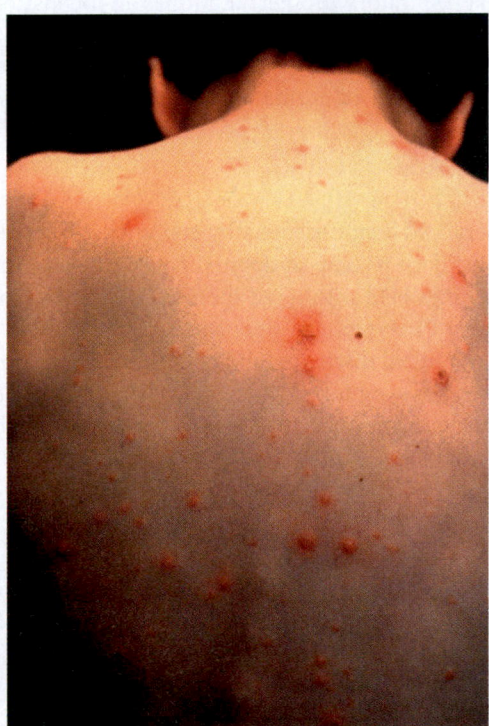

FIGURE 17-9 Distribution and appearance of skin lesions in varicella.
Centers for Disease Control and Prevention, Department of Health and Human Services, 1995. http://phil.cdc.gov /phil/details.asp?pid=6121

Diagnostic Testing

Chickenpox is usually a clinical diagnosis based on the characteristic rash. Lesions can be found in various developmental and healing stages. A Tzanck smear of vesicular fluid would reveal multinucleated giant cells and epithelial cells with inclusion bodies.

Treatment

Management in an otherwise healthy child involves largely supportive care. Pruritus can be managed with calamine lotion, pramoxine gel, oatmeal baths, or oral antihistamines. Children at higher risk of complications (e.g., immunocompromised, chronic asthma) can be treated with oral acyclovir to decrease severity and duration of infection. Antiviral therapy should not be routinely used in otherwise healthy children with varicella infection.

INFECTIOUS MONONUCLEOSIS

Overview

Infectious mononucleosis is caused by the Epstein-Barr virus (EBV; HHV-4). The infection is often referred to as the "kissing disease" as it is primarily transmitted through intimate contact with body secretions, such as saliva. Though it can affect individuals of all ages, it most frequently affects adolescents and young adults. The incubation period is quite long, ranging from 20 to 50 days, and as most individuals are asymptomatic, it is difficult to determine the source of infection. More than 90% of individuals will develop a rash if given amoxicillin or ampicillin during illness.

Clinical Presentation

Most individuals with EBV infectious mononucleosis are asymptomatic and are unaware of being infected with the virus. Symptomatic individuals can present with fever (typically low-grade), a "shaggy" purple-white exudative pharyngitis, malaise, marked diffuse lymphadenopathy, and hepatic and splenic tenderness with occasional enlargement. Nausea and anorexia (without vomiting) can also be present. Splenomegaly most often occurs between days 6 and 21 after the onset of illness and individuals are advised to avoid contact sports for at least 1 month due to an increased risk of splenic rupture; even with documented organ enlargement, splenic rupture post-EBV infection is a rare event.

Diagnostic Testing

The heterophile antibody test (i.e., the monospot test) is highly specific for infectious mononucleosis though it can be negative during the early course of EBV infection. Routine imaging of the spleen is not warranted.

Treatment

Intervention is largely supportive. Patients should be monitored closely for tonsillar enlargement that can lead to airway obstruction. The use of systemic corticosteroids can be helpful in reducing airway inflammation in these cases.

HAND, FOOT, AND MOUTH DISEASE

Overview

Hand, foot, and mouth disease (HFMD) is a highly contagious disease caused by coxsackie virus A16. The predominant mode of transmission is the oral-fecal route or via droplet, and the virus has an incubation period of 2 to 6 weeks. The infection most commonly affects children younger than 10 years of age, and subsequent outbreaks among family members and close contacts can develop.

Clinical Presentation

HFMD is characterized by fever, malaise, sore mouth, and anorexia. Conjunctivitis or pharyngitis can also develop. Skin lesions develop in the majority of patients with HFMD and present as tender macules or vesicles on an erythematous base.

> **CLINICAL CONCEPT**
> Typically 1 to 2 days following HFMD onset, oral lesions develop on the buccal mucosa, tongue, and/or hard palate.

Diagnostic Testing

HFMD is a clinical diagnosis that does not require any laboratory testing.

Treatment

There is no antiviral treatment for HFMD. Intervention is largely supportive as the illness typically lasts 2 to 7 days. Ensure an adequate intake of fluids to avoid dehydration. Antipyretics can be used to treat fever. Acetaminophen or ibuprofen are preferred to manage pain. Oral anesthetics via mouthwash or spray can be considered for oral pain along with cold drinks or ice popsicles.

FIFTH'S DISEASE

Overview

Fifth's disease, also known as erythema infectiosum, is caused by human parvovirus B19 and is common in school-aged and younger children who attend day care. The virus is transmitted to parents and siblings, typically by droplet transmission. Though the disease is relatively mild in children, there is a risk of hydrops fetalis when contracted by a woman during pregnancy that can result in pregnancy loss.

Clinical Presentation

Common findings of infection include a mild flu-like illness that begins 5 to 7 days after initial infection. Symptoms include fever, malaise, headache, nausea, myalgia, and rhinorrhea. This is followed by 7 to 10 days of a red rash that begins on the face with a "slapped cheek" appearance, which then spreads to the trunk and extremities. The onset of rash corresponds with disease immunity, and the patient is no longer viremic or contagious.

Diagnostic Testing

This is usually a clinical diagnosis, and additional laboratory testing is not needed as symptoms are mild and resolve in 5 to 7 days. If a pregnant woman is exposed to parvovirus B19, then IgG and IgM serology should be performed as soon as possible to determine risk to the fetus.

Treatment

Intervention is largely supportive care. Acetaminophen or ibuprofen can be considered to treat fever.

KAWASAKI'S DISEASE

Overview

Kawasaki's disease, also known as Kawasaki's syndrome, is a typically self-limited vasculitis of unknown etiology, although an infectious or immunological basis is suggested. Occurring primarily in the late winter and spring at 3-year intervals, Kawasaki's disease is more frequent among children of Asian ancestry, is twice as common in boys than in girls, and now surpasses rheumatic fever as the leading cause of acquired heart disease in the United States among children younger than 5 years. The development of coronary artery aneurysms can lead to coronary artery obstruction, myocarditis, heart failure, pericarditis, mitral or aortic insufficiency, and dysrhythmias. Risk of aneurysm is increased in patients who have fever for more than 16 days, have recurrence of fever after an afebrile period of at least 48 hours, are male, are younger than 1 year, and have cardiomegaly at the time of diagnosis. Some patients who do not fulfill the criteria for Kawasaki's disease have been diagnosed as having "incomplete" or "atypical" Kawasaki's disease, a diagnosis that often is based on echocardiographic findings of coronary artery abnormalities.

Clinical Presentation

Clinical presentation includes fever lasting 5 or more days and the presence of at least four of the following five symptoms: skin rash, bilateral conjunctival injection, cervical lymphadenopathy, swelling of the hands and feet, and mucocutaneous lesion. Disease implications include myocarditis (early disease stage) and development of coronary artery aneurysms (later disease stage; Box 17-3).

BOX 17-3 Diagnostic Criteria for Kawasaki's Disease

■ Fever 5 days or longer in duration, usually abrupt in onset, symptoms with no response to antibiotic therapy; if given, usually with irritability out of proportion to degree of fever or other signs

■ In addition to fever lasting at least 5 days, four or more of the following should be present:
  ■ Changes in extremities (erythema, edema, desquamation), usually with discomfort so that the child often refuses to bear weight
  ■ Bilateral, nonexudative conjunctivitis
  ■ Polymorphous rash
  ■ Cervical lymphadenopathy
  ■ Changes in lips and oral cavity (pharyngeal edema, dry/fissured or swollen lips, strawberry tongue)

Note: If fever is present with fewer than four of these symptoms, the diagnosis is established with echocardiogram to evaluate the coronary arteries to support or exclude the disease.

Source: Centers for Disease Control and Prevention. Kawasaki disease. http://www.cdc.gov/kawasaki

Diagnostic Testing

Although no specific laboratory test for Kawasaki's disease exists, the presence of certain laboratory findings can support the diagnosis when coupled with clinical presentation. Blood test often detects mild anemia, elevated WBC count, elevated sedimentation rate, and a sharp increase in the number of platelets. Urine test often reveals the presence of albumin and WBCs. In the acute stage (days 1 to 11), leukocytosis with a left shift and elevated erythrocyte sedimentation rate (ESR) are found; both are neither sensitive nor specific for the condition. In the subacute stage (days 11 to 21), the platelet count is often markedly elevated, with a measurement of more than 1 million/mm^3 being common. These values begin to normalize during the convalescent stage (days 21 to 60) but may not reach baseline values for 8 weeks.

During the acute stage of Kawasaki's disease, or if the diagnosis is in question, an echocardiogram should be obtained. If tests reveal an aneurysm or other heart or blood vessel abnormality, repeated echocardiograms or other tests are usually necessary for several years. In children who return to completely normal activity after the acute phase of the illness, the study should be repeated in the second or third week of disease and repeated 1 month after laboratory tests have resolved.

Treatment

Treatment of Kawasaki's disease includes consultation with experts in managing this condition and the use of IV immune globulin and aspirin. Confirmation of the diagnosis and treatment are likely to involve consultation with a specialist in this disease.

> **CLINICAL CONCEPT**
> Long-term prognosis in Kawasaki's disease is generally related to the degree of permanent cardiac involvement, with most patients making a full recovery.

Discussion Sources

Centers for Disease Control and Prevention. Assessing immunity to varicella. http://www.cdc.gov/chickenpox/hcp/immunity.html

Centers for Disease Control and Prevention. Group A Streptococcal (GAS) disease. Scarlet fever: all you need to know. https://www.cdc.gov/groupastrep/diseases-public/scarlet-fever.html

Centers for Disease Control and Prevention. Hand, foot, and mouth disease (HFMD). https://www.cdc.gov/hand-foot-mouth/index.html

Centers for Disease Control and Prevention. Kawasaki disease. http://www.cdc.gov/kawasaki

Centers for Disease Control and Prevention. Measles (Rubeola). https://www.cdc.gov/measles/index.html

Centers for Disease Control and Prevention. Parvovirus B19 and fifth disease. https://www.cdc.gov/parvovirusb19/fifth-disease.html

Centers for Disease Control and Prevention. Rubella (German measles, three-day measles). https://www.cdc.gov/rubella/

Centers for Disease Control and Prevention. Varicella vaccination: information for health care providers. http://www.cdc.gov/vaccines/vpd-vac/varicella/default-hcp.htm

Habif TP, Dinulos JGH, Chapman, MS, Zug KA. *Skin Disease: Diagnosis and Treatment*. 4th ed. Philadelphia, PA: Elsevier; 2017.

Newburger JW, Takahashi M, Burns JC. Kawasaki disease. *J Am Coll Cardiol*. 2016;67:1738–1749.

Scheinfeld NS. Kawasaki disease. Medscape. http://emedicine.medscape.com/article/965367-overview

Shulman ST, Bisno AL, Clegg HW, et al. Clinical practice guideline for the diagnosis and management of group A streptococcal pharyngitis: 2012 update by the Infectious Diseases Society of America. *Clin Infect Dis*. 2012;55:e86–e102.

QUESTIONS

204. You examine a 10-year-old boy with scarlet fever and a positive rapid strep screen. His mother asks if he can get a "shot of penicillin." Which of the following statements is/are true regarding the use of IM penicillin? *(Choose all that apply.)*

A. Injectable benzathine penicillin, oral amoxicillin, and cephalexin are each strongly recommended for treatment of *S pyogenes* (GAS) pharyngitis.

B. Injectable benzathine penicillin would be indicated for treatment of GAS if poor adherence to recommended therapy or inability to take a full course of oral antibiotics is anticipated.

C. The risk of severe allergic reaction with IM products is similar to that of oral preparations.

D. Injectable penicillin has a superior spectrum of antimicrobial coverage compared with the oral form of the drug.

205. The rapid strep test can be used to identify the presence of:

A. gram-positive or gram-negative bacteria.

B. gram-negative bacteria only.

C. any *Streptococcus* species.

D. group A streptococcus only.

206. You examine a 15-year-old presenting with a 1-day history of sore throat, low-grade fever, maculopapular rash, and posterior cervical and occipital lymphadenopathy. The most likely diagnosis is:

A. scarlet fever.

B. roseola.

C. rubella.

D. rubeola.

207. A 4-year-old child presents with a 2-day history of fever, sore throat, and crankiness with a 1-day history of a fine, pink rash, described by the child's parents as being "all over." The child is able to take fluids without difficulty and has a decreased appetite. Physical examination reveals an exudative pharyngitis, anterior cervical lymphadenopathy, and a generalized sandpaper-like rash. The most likely diagnosis is:

A. scarlet fever.

B. roseola.

C. rubella.

D. rubeola.

208. An 18-year-old woman has a chief complaint of "a sore throat and swollen glands" for the past 3 days. Her physical examination reveals exudative pharyngitis, minimally tender anterior and posterior cervical lymphadenopathy, and maculopapular rash. Abdominal examination reveals right and left upper quadrant abdominal tenderness. The most likely diagnosis is:

A. GABHS pharyngitis.

B. infectious mononucleosis.

C. rubella.

D. scarlet fever.

209. Which of the following is most likely to be found in the laboratory data of a child who has infectious mononucleosis?

A. neutrophilia

B. lymphocytosis

C. positive antinuclear antibody (ANA)

D. macrocytic anemia

210. The monospot test used to diagnose mononucleosis tests for the presence of:

A. viral antigen.

B. heterophile antibody.

C. viral RNA.

D. IgG.

211. You examine a 15-year-old boy who has infectious mononucleosis with marked tonsillar hypertrophy, exudative pharyngitis, significant difficulty swallowing, and a patent airway. You consider prescribing a course of oral:

A. amoxicillin.

B. prednisone.

C. ibuprofen.

D. acyclovir.

212. A 2-year-old girl presents with a 2-day history of pustular, ulcerating lesions on the hands and feet and oral ulcers. The lesions began after a number of days of fussiness with rhinorrhea. The child is cranky, well hydrated, afebrile, and age-appropriately resists the examination. The most likely diagnosis is:

A. HFMD.

B. aphthous stomatitis.

C. herpetic gingivostomatitis.

D. Vincent's angina.

213. A 6-year-old boy presents with a 1-day history of a fiery red, maculopapular facial rash concentrated on the cheeks. He has had mild headache and myalgia for the past week. The most likely diagnosis is:

A. erythema infectiosum.

B. roseola.

C. rubella.

D. scarlet fever.

214. The incubation period for measles caused by the rubeola virus is:

A. 5 to 7 days.

B. 10 to 14 days.

C. 2 to 3 weeks.

D. 1 month.

215. Most cases of roseola caused by HHV-6 occur in:

A. newborns who contracted the virus in utero.

B. infants younger than 3 months old.

C. children younger than 24 months old.

D. children older than 2 years.

216. Kawasaki's disease most commonly occurs in what age group?

A. infants

B. children aged 2 to 3 years.

C. children approaching puberty

D. children aged 1 to 8 years

217. Sam is a 4-year-old boy who presents with a 1-week history of intermittent fever, rash, and "watery, red eyes." Clinical presentation is of an alert child who is cooperative with examination but irritable, with a temperature of 38°C (100.4°F), pulse rate of 132 bpm, and respiratory rate of 38 breaths/minute.

Physical examination findings include nasal crusting; dry, erythematous, cracked lips; red, enlarged tonsils without exudate; and elevated tongue papillae. The diagnosis of Kawasaki's disease is being considered. Additional findings are likely to include:

A. vesicular-form rash.

B. purulent conjunctivitis.

C. peeling hands.

D. occipital lymphadenopathy.

218. Laboratory findings in Kawasaki's disease include all of the following except:

A. sterile pyuria.

B. elevated platelet levels.

C. blood cultures positive for offending bacterial pathogen.

D. elevated ESR.

219. The cause of Kawasaki's disease is:

A. fungal.

B. viral.

C. bacterial.

D. unknown.

220. An important part of the treatment of Kawasaki's disease includes the use of:

A. antibiotics.

B. antivirals.

C. immune globulin.

D. antifungals.

221. How is the varicella virus most commonly transmitted?

A. droplet transmission

B. contact with inanimate reservoirs

C. contact transmission

D. waterborne transmission

222. Which group is shown to have the highest rate of serious varicella disease?

A. infants

B. teenagers aged 12 to 19 years

C. adults aged 30 to 49 years

D. health-care workers

223. Potential complications of varicella infection in children include all of the following except:

A. pneumonia.

B. Crohn's disease.

C. encephalitis.

D. toxic shock syndrome.

224. At what time during pregnancy is the fetus at greatest risk of developing birth defects due to congenital varicella syndrome?

A. 8 to 20 weeks' gestation

B. 20 to 24 weeks' gestation

C. 26 to 32 weeks' gestation

D. at any time after 34 weeks' gestation

225 to 228. Match the potential complication with the most appropriate illness.

_____ **225.** hydrops fetalis

_____ **226.** coronary aneurysm

_____ **227.** birth defects

_____ **228.** permanent neurological impairment

        A. Measles

        B. Rubella

        C. Kawasaki's disease

        D. Fifth's disease

229. Supplementation with which of the following has been shown to offer some benefit for a child with the measles?

    A. vitamin A

    B. vitamin C

    C. zinc

    D. copper

230. Which of the following is most accurate regarding the need for imaging of the spleen during infectious mononucleosis?

    A. Ultrasonography is needed to confirm the diagnosis of infectious mononucleosis.

    B. Routine ultrasound should be performed to detect splenomegaly.

    C. Ultrasound should be performed 4 to 6 weeks after resolution of symptoms to confirm cure.

    D. An ultrasound of the spleen is not required for diagnosis or to confirm resolution of disease.

231. A 20-month-old child presents with a rosy-pink maculopapular rash that has developed following a 3-day period of high-grade fever (40°C [104°F]). The most likely diagnosis is:

    A. scarlet fever.

    B. rubella.

    C. roseola.

    D. rubeola.

232. A 4-year-old presents with fever, cough, and generalized lymphadenopathy. Evaluation of the oral cavity reveals a scattering of white spots with blue rings held within red spots in the oral mucosa. The most likely diagnosis is:

    A. HFMD.

    B. rubella.

    C. Fifth's disease.

    D. rubeola.

233. Treatment of roseola in a 16-month-old with a 4-day history of high-grade fever can include:

    A. acetaminophen.

    B. amoxicillin.

    C. antiseizure medication.

    D. oseltamivir.

234. Appropriate treatment options for an 8-year-old with a generalized rash due to varicella infection can include all of the following except:

    A. topical calamine lotion.

    B. oral antihistamine.

C. topical corticosteroid cream.

D. oatmeal bath.

235. When managing a child with HFMD, all of the following approaches are recommended except:

A. cold fluids or ice popsicles.

B. oral analgesic mouthwash or spray.

C. oral ibuprofen.

D. topical fluconazole on affected external surfaces.

For answers and rationales, see end of chapter.

Dermatology Conditions in Younger Children

Overview

Numerous dermatological conditions are found in infancy and early childhood. Parents understandably have concerns about these lesions. It is important for the NP to have a thorough knowledge of common conditions.

> **CLINICAL CONCEPT**
>
> As with most dermatological disorders, these conditions are diagnosed clinically, by history and physical examination. Rarely, additional diagnostics are needed.

Capillary Hemangioma

Capillary, or strawberry, hemangioma is a congenital vascular malformation. Such lesions are rarely present at birth but become evident in the first weeks of life, growing rapidly in the first year, then plateauing in size, and eventually regressing. About 90% disappear by age 9 years, usually leaving bluish vascularity over the area. If the lesion is large or involves a vital organ such as the eye or extremity, treatment by an expert in the condition is indicated. Oral propranolol is commonly used for treatment; current recommendations provide formulation, target dose, and frequency of dosing. Other treatment options include systemic corticosteroids and, less commonly, interferon-α. Vincristine, injected corticosteroids, and laser therapy are used rarely for severe cases.

Port-Wine Stain

A port-wine stain is a flat hemangioma with a stable course. These lesions usually appear on the face and are usually present at birth. Port-wine stains tend to deepen in color as time goes on and grow proportionally with the child. Although not malignant, the lesions are often cosmetically challenging and can be minimized or occasionally eliminated through the use of laser therapy. Port-wine stain is occasionally associated with other congenital or genetic syndromes (Sturge-Weber or arteriovenous [AV] malformation syndrome).

Milia

The typical presentation of milia is as white pinpoint papular lesions caused by sebaceous hyperplasia. The usual distribution is over the nose, cheeks, and other areas with an abundance of sebaceous glands. The cause is likely the maternal androgenic effect on the sebaceous glands. Benign in nature, milia resolve without special therapy by 4 weeks to 6 months of life. The infant's parents and caregivers should be advised to avoid attempting to remove or open milia as this could result in scarring.

Erythema Toxicum Neonatorum

Erythema toxicum neonatorum is a benign rash of unknown etiology that occurs in about 50% of full-term infants. Usually beginning in the first 10 days of life, the lesions look like flea bites and are widely distributed; the palms and soles are spared. The infant does not appear to be distressed by the condition. The lesions usually fade by 5 to 7 days after eruption without specific treatment.

Mongolian Spots

Mongolian spots occur in about 90% of children of African and Asian ancestries and in less than 10% of children of European ancestry. The distribution is usually over the lower back and buttocks but can occur over a wider area. Caused by an accumulation of melanocytes, these are benign lesions that typically fade by age 7 years without special therapy. Uninformed providers can misinterpret this normal finding as an ecchymotic area, raising the suspicion of child abuse. In contrast to an area of bruising or ecchymosis, when a mongolian spot is pressed or palpated, there is no discomfort.

Acne Neonatorum

Acne neonatorum consists of open and closed comedones and pustules over the forehead and cheeks, similar to the adolescent version of the condition. The etiology is likely the effect of maternal androgens on the infant's skin. It usually resolves in about 4 to 8 weeks but occasionally persists up to age 1 year. Low-dose benzoyl peroxide can be used as therapy, although the lesions typically resolve without intervention.

Eczema

Eczema or atopic dermatitis is a manifestation of a type I hypersensitivity reaction. This type of reaction is caused when IgE antibodies occupy receptor sites on mast cells, causing a degradation of the mast cells and subsequent release of histamine, vasodilation, mucous gland stimulation, and tissue swelling. There are two subgroups of type I hypersensitivity reactions: atopy and anaphylaxis.

The atopy subgroup comprises numerous common clinical conditions, such as allergic rhinitis, atopic dermatitis, allergic gastroenteropathy, and allergy-based asthma. Atopic diseases have a strong familial component and tend to cause localized rather than systemic reactions. Individuals with atopic disease are often able to identify allergy-inducing agents.

Treatment for atopic disease of eczema includes avoiding offending agents, minimizing skin dryness by limiting soap and water exposure, and consistently using lubricants. The NP should explain to the parents that the skin tends to be sensitive and needs to be treated with some care. When flares occur, the skin eruption is largely caused by histamine release. Antihistamines and topical corticosteroids can be used to control eczema flares. With an acute flare of eczema or with contact dermatitis in the older child, a topical corticosteroid with intermediate potency is likely needed to control acute symptoms. After this control is achieved, the lowest potency topical corticosteroid that yields the desired effect should be used. For eczema or contact dermatitis on the face of infants and children 3 months and older, the lowest potency (class 7) corticosteroid cream can be used, such as 1% hydrocortisone. Over-the-counter nonsteroidal moisturizing and healing ointment is recommended for frequent use.

Discussion Sources

Antaya RJ. Capillary malformation. Medscape. http://emedicine.medscape.com/article/1084479-overview

Antaya RJ. Infantile hemangioma. Medscape. http://emedicine.medscape.com/article/1083849-overview

Drolet BA, Frommelt PC, Chamlin SL, et al. Initiation and use of propranolol for infantile hemangioma: report of a consensus conference. *Pediatrics.* 2013;131:128–140.

Habif T, Dinulos JGH. *Skin Disease: Diagnosis and Treatment.* 4th ed. St. Louis, MO: Elsevier Health Sciences; 2017.

National Eczema Association. Prescription topical treatment. https://nationaleczema.org/eczema/treatment/topicals/

QUESTIONS

236. You examine a newborn with a capillary hemangioma on her thigh. You advise her parents that this lesion:

A. is likely to increase in size over the first year of life.

B. should be treated to avoid malignancy.

C. usually resolves within the first months of life.

D. is likely to develop a superimposed lichenification.

237. Treatment of capillary hemangioma includes all of the following except:

A. oral propranolol.

B. systemic corticosteroids.

C. cryotherapy.

D. interferon-α.

238. You examine a 2-month-old infant with a port-wine lesion over her right cheek. You advise the parents that this lesion:

A. needs to be surgically excised.

B. grows proportionally with the child.

C. becomes lighter over time.

D. can evolve into a malignant lesion.

239. An infant is born with a port-wine lesion on her face. You advise the parents of all of the following except that:

A. ophthalmology should be consulted if the eyelid is involved.

B. Sturge-Weber syndrome is sometimes associated with port-wine stain.

C. the lesion should resolve by 5 years of age.

D. a lesion in the vicinity of the eye can increase the risk of glaucoma.

240. Standard treatment of port-wine lesion is:

A. topical corticosteroid.

B. systemic corticosteroid.

C. vincristine injection.

D. pulsed-dye laser therapy.

241. A 10-day-old child presents with multiple raised lesions resembling flea bites over the trunk and nape of the neck. The infant is nursing well and has no fever or exposure to animals. These lesions likely represent:

A. erythema toxicum neonatorum.

B. milia.

C. acne neonatorum.

D. staphylococcal skin infection.

242. Milia is usually marked by white pinpoint papular lesions found:

A. on the back and buttocks.

B. across the chest.

C. in the underarms.

D. on the nose and cheeks.

243. Milia is typically caused by:

A. low levels of androgen.

B. enlarged sebaceous glands.

C. excessive oil production in the skin follicles.

D. an unknown etiology.

244. Milia is treated by the following method:

A. no special skin care.

B. a topical retinoid.

C. cryotherapy.

D. a topical antimicrobial.

245. Typical distribution of acne neonatorum consists of open and closed comedones and pustules:

A. on the hands and wrists.

B. on the neck and chest.

C. on the forehead and cheeks.

D. on the neck and ears.

246. Acne neonatorum treatment options include which of the following? *(More than one can apply.)*

  A. no special skin care is needed because these lesions are self-resolving

  B. topical retinoids

  C. oral antibiotic

  D. low-dose benzoyl peroxide

247. An Asian couple comes in with their 4-week-old infant, who has blue-black macules scattered over the buttocks. These most likely represent:

  A. benign mottling.

  B. mongolian spots.

  C. ecchymosis.

  D. hemangioma.

248. Standard management of mongolian spots includes:

  A. topical corticosteroids.

  B. interferon-α injection.

  C. topical or systemic antimicrobial.

  D. no treatment, as the condition resolves over time.

249. Eczema is thought to be caused by:

  A. overactive mucous glands.

  B. bacterial infection.

  C. degradation of mast cells.

  D. dry air.

250. The most important aspect of skin care for children with eczema is:

  A. frequent bathing with antibacterial soap.

  B. consistent use of medium- to high-potency topical steroids.

  C. application of lubricants.

  D. treatment of dermatophytes.

251. A common site for eczema in infants is the:

  A. dorsum of the hand.

  B. face.

  C. neck.

  D. flexor surfaces.

For answers and rationales, see end of chapter.

Gastroenteritis

Overview

Acute gastroenteritis is a common episodic disease of childhood, characterized by vomiting and diarrhea. Nearly always viral in nature, the two most common gastroenteritis organisms are norovirus or rotavirus. Given that these viral illnesses are highly contagious and easily transmitted person to person, usually there is a history of contacts with children or adults who have similar symptoms. The duration of illness is usually short, lasting fewer than 3 to 5 days and often as short as 24 hours. The major clinical concern for children with gastroenteritis is dehydration due to the significant fluid loss through vomitus and stool.

Routine vaccination of infants with rotavirus vaccine helps prevent gastroenteritis by this virus, formerly the major cause of gastroenteritis in younger children. Proper handwashing is essential in preventing the spread of virus.

Improperly handled food is a common source of the GI infection commonly known as food poisoning. The most common organisms that cause food poisoning, with incubation time and food sources, include:

- *S aureus*: Incubation period of 30 minutes to 8 hours; food sources include sliced meats, puddings, and pastries
- *Salmonella*: Incubation period of 12 to 72 hours; food sources include vegetables, chicken, pork, fruits, nuts, eggs, and beef
- *Campylobacter jejuni*: Incubation period of 2 to 5 days; food sources include unpasteurized milk, chicken, shellfish, turkey, contaminated water
- *E coli*: Incubation period of 1 to 10 days; food sources include undercooked ground beef, unpasteurized milk or juice, raw fruits and vegetables, contaminated water
- *Shigella*: Incubation period of 1 to 7 days; foodborne outbreaks most often associated with contamination by an infected food handler
- *Listeria*: Incubation period of 7 to 70 days; food sources include unpasteurized milk or dairy products made with raw milk, raw fruits and vegetables, deli meats and hot dogs, refrigerated pates and meat spreads, smoked seafood
- *Clostridium perfringens*: Incubation period of 6 to 24 hours; food sources include beef, poultry, gravies, food left at room temperature or on steam tables for prolonged periods

Clinical Presentation

A child with gastroenteritis presents with short-duration vomiting that precedes the onset of diarrhea. The vomiting and stooling episodes are usually numerous. The vomitus and stool are free of blood, and the stool is free of pus. In addition, the child usually has a low-grade or no fever. Mild URI-like symptoms are occasionally reported.

An important part of the assessment of a child with acute gastroenteritis is determining hydration status. If the child has voided within the previous few hours, the degree of dehydration is minimal. If there has been no urine output in 4 to 6 hours, then medical intervention should be considered. Many other clinical parameters are helpful in assessing for dehydration (Table 17-13).

> **CLINICAL CONCEPT**
>
> Asking about time of the last urination is a helpful way of evaluating hydration in evaluation of a child with gastroenteritis.

With a foodborne illness, the child typically presents, often along with family members and caregivers who ate the same food, with a history of sudden onset of signs and symptoms, usually within the timing of the previously mentioned problematic food ingestion, including abdominal pain, nausea, and vomiting. Lower GI signs and symptoms such as cramping and diarrhea occur a number of hours later.

Worrisome findings during acute illness in a child who has vomiting and diarrhea include protracted fever, usually quite high, coupled with bloody or pus-filled stools. If these are present, a bacterial source of infection such as shigellosis should be considered. Stool testing should be obtained, and appropriate antimicrobial therapy should be initiated.

Diagnostic Testing

In the majority of otherwise well children with viral gastroenteritis with mild to moderate dehydration, no diagnostic studies are required, as this is largely a clinical diagnosis. For children with a suspected bacterial or protozoal infection, additional testing can be considered including stool assay for occult blood, WBC count, microscopy for protozoa, *C difficile* toxin, or bacterial culture. In children with fever, nausea, vomiting, abdominal pain, and signs of dehydration, additional testing can include CBC, serum electrolytes, urea, creatinine, and amylase, with consideration for abdominal imaging studies. With high-grade fever, blood culture should be obtained.

Treatment

Most children with mild to moderate dehydration from gastroenteritis, presumed to be viral in origin, can usually be managed with frequent small-volume feedings of commercially prepared oral rehydration solution (ORS) such as Pedialyte™. In these cases, ORS is as effective as IV fluid therapy but less costly and less distressing to the child and parents/caregivers. The child should receive 50 to 100 mL/kg taken over 3 to 4 hours. A child with severe dehydration will likely need parenteral fluid in addition to small amounts of fluids orally as tolerated (Table 17-14). Because they contain inappropriate glucose and electrolyte composition, sports drinks such as Gatorade™, soda, and most fruit juices are inappropriate for rehydration.

TABLE 17-13 Assessment Criteria for Hydration Status

PARAMETER	MILD 3% TO 5%*	MODERATE 6% TO 9%*	SEVERE 10% OR GREATER*
Blood pressure	Normal	Normal to decreased	Weak, thready, not palpable
Pulse quality	Normal	Normal to slightly decreased	Moderately decreased
Heart rate	Normal	Normal to increased	Increased (sometimes bradycardia)
Turgor	Normal	Recoil less than 2 seconds	Recoil greater than 2 seconds, tenting
Fontanels	Normal	Slightly depressed	Depressed
Mucous membranes	Slightly dry lips, thick saliva	Dry lips and oral mucosa	Very dry lips, oral mucosa
Eyes	Normal, tears present	Slightly sunken, tears decreased	Deeply sunken, tears absent
Capillary refill	Normal (less than 2 seconds)	Prolonged	Minimal
Mental status	Normal	Normal, fatigued, restless, irritable	Apathetic, lethargic, unconscious
Urine output	Slightly decreased	Decreased	Minimal
Thirst	Normal, to slightly increased	Moderately increased	Very thirsty or too lethargic to assess

Source: Koyfman A. Pediatric dehydration clinical presentation. Medscape. http://emedicine.medscape.com/article/801012-clinical#a0256

* Percent body weight lost.

TABLE 17-14 Rehydration Therapy

For mild to moderate dehydration, oral rehydration therapy (ORT) with oral rehydration solution (ORS) is as effective as parenteral therapy, is easier to administer, and is more cost effective.

DEGREE OF DEHYDRATION	REHYDRATION THERAPY	REPLACEMENT OF ONGOING LOSSES
Minimal to none	Not applicable, sips of fluid frequently as tolerated to maintain circulating volume and hydration status	Less than 10 kg: 60 to 100 mL ORS for each loss; greater than 10 kg: 120 to 240 mL for each loss
Mild to moderate	ORT with ORS, 50 to 100 mL/kg over 3 to 4 hours, often best tolerated in frequent, small volumes, preferably supplied in the office or urgent-care setting	Same
Severe	Lactated Ringer's solution (LR) preferred over normal saline (NS) IV fluid therapy but used if LR not available—boluses 20 mL/kg until improvement (perfusion, LOC) then 100 mL/kg over 4 hours	Same. If unable to drink, give through nasogastric tube or give D5W1/4 NS with K⁺ 20 mEq IV

Source: Koyfman A. Pediatric dehydration treatment and management. Medscape. http://emedicine.medscape.com/article/801012-treatment#aw2aab6b6b4

For infants with mild to moderate dehydration who are breastfeeding, mothers should be encouraged to continue to breastfeed in addition to the ORS in order to provide some nutrients and calories to the infant. If the child has vomited, then the amount per feeding should be decreased initially and gradually increased as tolerated. Formula-fed infants should also receive formula feedings in addition to ORS, as tolerated. If the child has vomited, then a half-strength formula can be offered for two feedings followed by regular formula.

The use of a single dose of an oral antiemetic such as ondansetron in gastroenteritis has been demonstrated to prevent further vomiting and minimizes the need for IV fluids and hospital admission. This medication, in addition to the parenteral and oral tablet forms, is available in dissolvable tablet or film that is well tolerated even in the presence of GI upset. The use of antidiarrheal agents (e.g., kaolin-pectin) and antimotility agents (e.g., loperamide) are contraindicated in children as these medications provide no benefit and can increase the risk of adverse effects, including paralytic ileus, drowsiness, and nausea. In particular, use of antimotility agents should be avoided in children infected with *E coli* O157:H7 who are at higher risk of hemolytic uremic syndrome (HUS).

Most food poisoning episodes are short and self-limiting, resolving over a few hours to days without special intervention. In severe, protracted cases, appropriate antimicrobial therapy can be considered, particularly if stool testing reveals an offending organism.

In the majority of children with gastroenteritis, in the absence of vomiting for a number of hours, simple foods such as cooked rice, crackers, dry cereal, and bread products can be reintroduced, guided by the child's appetite and tolerance. Half-strength apple juice and simple soups are also acceptable. Fatty foods and full-fat dairy products should be avoided for a number of days as their addition often triggers lower abdominal cramping.

Discussion Sources

Brady K. Acute gastroenteritis: evidence-based management of pediatric patients. *Pediatr Emerg Med Pract*. 2018;15:1–25.
Foodsafety.gov. Bacteria and viruses. https://www.foodsafety.gov/food-poisoning/bacteria-and-viruses
Koyfman A. Pediatric dehydration overview. Medscape. http://emedicine.medscape.com/article/801012-overview

QUESTIONS

252 to 255. Indicate (*yes or no*) if each of the following can be used to determine hydration status.

_____ **252.** blood pressure

_____ **253.** heart rate

_____ **254.** skin turgor

_____ **255.** presence of dry lips and oral mucosa

256 to 259. Indicate (*yes or no*) whether the following signs can be expected during severe dehydration.

_____ **256.** anuria

_____ **257.** tears absent

_____ **258.** capillary refill of approximately 3 seconds

_____ **259.** elevated blood pressure

260. What advice should you give to a breastfeeding mother whose 4-month-old has gastroenteritis and reports two loose stools and two episodes of vomiting within the past 4 hours?

A. Switch to soy-based formula.

B. Give the infant oral rehydration solution only.

C. Continue breastfeeding.

D. Supplement with a sugar-water solution.

261. In counseling the parents of a 3-year-old with gastroenteritis who is mildly dehydrated, the NP advises to give the child:

A. 4 ounces of room-temperature ginger ale as the child requests.

B. frequent sips of an oral rehydration solution.

C. frequent sips of a sports drink such as Gatorade.

D. frequent sips of apple juice.

262. The onset of symptoms of food poisoning caused by *Staphylococcus* species is typically within what time frame of the ingestion of the offending substance?

A. within 15 minutes

B. 1 to 8 hours

C. 8 to 12 hours

D. more than 12 hours

263. The onset of symptoms in food poisoning caused by *Salmonella* species is typically how long after the ingestion of the offending substance?

A. 2 to 8 hours

B. 8 to 12 hours

C. 12 to 72 hours

D. 5 to 10 days

264. To obtain the most accurate hydration status in a 4-year-old child with acute gastroenteritis, the NP should ask about:

A. the time of last urination.

B. thirst.

C. the quantity of liquids taken.

D. the number of episodes of vomiting and diarrhea.

265. What percentage of body weight is typically lost in a child with moderate dehydration?

A. 2% to 3%

B. 3% to 5%

C. 6% to 9%

D. 10% to 15%

266. Notable clinical features of shigellosis include which of the following two findings?

A. bloody diarrhea

B. fever

C. dry cough

D. headache

267. The most common viral cause of gastroenteritis is:

A. rhinovirus.

B. norovirus.

C. coronavirus.

D. adenovirus.

268. When considering the use of an antiemetic such as ondansetron (Zofran®) for a child with gastro-enteritis, which of the following statements is true?

A. There is no demonstrated benefit for the use of antiemetics in children with viral gastroenteritis.

B. A single dose of oral antiemetic has been demonstrated to reduce vomiting and the subsequent need for IV fluids.

C. This medication class should only be used in combination with antidiarrheal agents.

D. One dose every 2 hours for the first day of the illness is the preferred regimen.

269. When considering the use of antidiarrheals and antimotility agents in young children with gastro-enteritis, which of the following statements is true?

    A. Antidiarrheals should only be used for bacterial gastroenteritis.

    B. Antidiarrheals should be dosed once after each diarrheal episode.

    C. Antimotility agents can prevent the development of HUS.

    D. These agents should be avoided in young children with gastroenteritis due to increased risk of adverse effect with use and offer of minor, if any, benefit.

270. When considering rehydration therapy for a 5-year-old with moderate dehydration from a presumed viral gastroenteritis, you consider that:

    A. IV fluid therapy is the preferred therapeutic choice.

    B. the child should be admitted immediately to the hospital.

    C. oral rehydration therapy is as effective and less costly when compared with IV fluid therapy.

    D. oral rehydration therapy should only be given once 2 hours have passed since the last diarrheal episode.

271. When caring for a 13-month-old with presumed viral gastroenteritis, you advise the parents that the best method to prevent spread of the infection is:

    A. vaccination of all household members with rotavirus vaccine.

    B. to discontinue breastfeeding if the child is nursing.

    C. proper handwashing.

    D. to bathe the child after each diarrheal episode with antibacterial soap.

272 to 275. Match each foodborne pathogen with its common food source of infection.

_____ **272.** *S aureus*

_____ **273.** *Salmonella*

_____ **274.** *C perfringens*

_____ **275.** *E coli*

    A. undercooked ground beef

    B. food left at room temperature for a prolonged period

    C. deli meats

    D. eggs

276 to 279. Indicate (*yes or no*) whether each of the following diagnostic tests is indicated for a 3-year-old with suspected bacterial gastroenteritis, high-grade fever, and multiple episodes of vomiting.

_____ **276.** Stool culture

_____ **277.** Blood culture

_____ **278.** CBC

_____ **279.** Occult blood in stool

280. For a 4-year-old with moderate dehydration, what is the recommended amount of oral rehydration solution that should be taken in the first 3 to 4 hours?

    A. 10 to 20 mL/kg

    B. 20 to 40 mL/kg

    C. 50 to 100 mL/kg

    D. 100 to 150 mL/kg

281. When advising the parents of a 5-year-old about reintroducing foods following an episode of gastro-enteritis, the NP recommends all of the following as acceptable except:

    A. cream-based soup.

    B. plain rice.

C. dry cereal.

D. diluted fruit juice.

For answers and rationales, see end of chapter.

Alterations in Puberty

Overview

Puberty consists of a series of predictable events of physical development, and the sequence of changes is commonly referred to as the Tanner stages. Alterations in puberty is boys is uncommon. Precocious puberty in girls has long been defined as the onset of secondary sexual characteristics before the child's eighth birthday. More recent study reveals that there is likely a group of girls who have the onset of slowly developing secondary sexual characteristics between ages 6 and 8 years as a benign normal variant. In particular, thelarche (the isolated appearance of breast development) is common as early as age 7 years and pubarche (the appearance of pubic hair without other signs of puberty) as early as age 8 years in otherwise healthy girls. Consequently, the most common reason for precocious puberty in girls is early onset of normal puberty. A subset of girls, particularly girls with pubertal changes noted before their sixth birthday, often has significant health problems, however, such as ovarian or adrenal tumors.

> **CLINICAL CONCEPT**
>
> The most common form of altered puberty is early onset, or precocious, puberty in girls.

Delayed puberty is defined as no evidence of secondary sexual maturation, or child is at Tanner stage 1, in girls older than age 13 years and in boys older than age 14 years. Delayed onset of puberty is multifactorial in both boys and girls. This delay can occur because the child is healthy but maturing more slowly when compared with same-age peers, a condition known as constitutional delay of puberty, which often runs in families. However, delay in puberty can be caused by hypogonadism, in which the gonads (the testes in males and the ovaries in females) produce few or no hormones. Numerous, though rarely encountered, health conditions can result in hypogonadism, including certain autoimmune disorders, developmental disorders, history of radiation exposure and/or chemotherapy, infection, surgery, or brain or pituitary tumors. Chromosomal anomalies can also result in hypogonadism, such as Kallmann's syndrome (occurring more often in boys than in girls), Turner's syndrome in girls (XO female), and Klinefelter's syndrome in boys (XXY male). For both genders, poor diet lacking in the daily recommended values of nutrients can also contribute to delayed onset. Occasionally, young girls who undergo intense physical training for a sport, such as running or gymnastics, experience delayed puberty, largely as a result of low body weight; this is not noted in males with a similar level of activity.

Clinical Presentation

In order to assess for alterations in puberty, knowledge of normative puberty is important. In boys and girls, Tanner stage 1 (prepuberty) reveals no evidence of secondary sexual maturation. Tanner stage 2 in girls is characterized by the development of breast buds with papilla elevated, as well as downy pigmented pubic hair along the labia majora. Tanner stage 3 includes breast mound enlargement along with darker, coarser, curling pubic hair the on mons and labia majora. This stage is also characterized by the onset of the growth spurt. In Tanner stage 4, the areola and papilla become elevated to form a second mound above the level of the rest of the breast; adult-type pubic hair appears with no spread to the medial surface of thighs; menarche occurs. Tanner stage 5 (full adult genitalia) is identified by recession of the areola to the mound of the breast, and extension of pubic hair to the medial thigh.

In boys, Tanner stage 2 is characterized by enlargement of the testes with scrotal skin reddening along with change in texture. There is also sparse growth of long, slightly pigmented pubic hair at the base of the penis. Tanner stage 3 results in an increase in penile length but minimal change in width; further scrotal enlargement; pubic hair becomes darker, coarser, and covers a greater area; and onset of the growth spurt. During Tanner stage 4, there is an increase in penile length and width with development of glans; further darkening of scrotal skin; and adult-type pubic hair with no spread to the medial surface of the thighs. Tanner stage 5 (full adult genitalia) incudes adult-type pubic hair with spread to the medial surface of the thighs.

For early onset puberty in girls or boys, secondary sexual characteristics are occurring before the normative age. These children are often taller than would be anticipated for age as the accelerated linear growth seen in puberty has occurred early. In delayed or late-onset puberty, the anticipated secondary sexual characteristics have not yet occurred at the normative age; these children are often shorter than would be anticipated since the typical growth spurt seen during puberty has not yet occurred. The child's physical examination is otherwise usually normal.

Diagnostic Testing

Evaluation of the child with alteration in puberty is dependent on natal or birth gender and whether early or delayed onset. In boys with suspected precocious puberty or delayed puberty, measurement of serum testosterone can be useful to determine the stage of puberty. A level of less than 30 ng/dL can be expected in prepubertal boys, while the level rises to 30 to 100 ng/dL in early puberty, and 100 to 300 ng/dL in mid- to late puberty. In girls, testing for precocious puberty is typically not needed as this is caused by early onset of normal puberty. In the subset of girls who experience pubertal changes prior to 6 years of age, this is likely caused by a significant health problem that warrants further investigation. Diagnostic testing can include measuring bone age, level of follicle-stimulating hormone and luteinizing hormone; performing abdominal ultrasound; and conducting other studies warranted by clinical presentation.

Genetic abnormalities, such as Klinefelter's syndrome (XXY in males) and Turner's syndrome (XO females), can be considered with delayed puberty along with physical and developmental findings consistent with each condition. Klinefelter's syndrome is characterized by developmental issues, mainly language impairment, along with low testicular volume and hip and breast enlargement. Signs of Turner's syndrome in adolescent girls include short height, delayed or no puberty, amenorrhea, learning disabilities, and social difficulties. Genetic testing should be performed when these conditions are suspected. Regardless of whether early or late onset, comprehensive care of the child with altered puberty warrants specialty evaluation.

Treatment

Treatment depends on the cause. For boys with early onset puberty, treatment is usually aimed at the underlying condition, since this condition rarely occurs without an identifiable cause. For girls, given early onset puberty is usually seen in an otherwise well child, counseling about the nature of the process of early puberty should be discussed with the child and family.

> **CLINICAL CONCEPT**
>
> In premature adrenarche, a condition that can be found in natal males or females, a parent usually reports that a child 5 to 6 years old has body odor, pubic hair, and (rarely) axillary hair.

Because girls typically achieve nearly all of their adult height 1 year after the first menstrual period (menarche), a girl achieving menarche at an early age often has short stature. If the child and family wish to attempt to halt the onset of puberty, a gonadotropin-releasing hormone analogue and additional therapies can be given to counteract the effects of endogenous hormones. This therapy is provided with expert consultation and appropriate informed consent.

In girls, when only premature thelarche is present, without other signs of puberty including accelerated linear growth, this is usually a benign condition. Breast development usually halts at Tanner 2 or early Tanner 3 stage and can be unilateral or bilateral. Reassurance and ongoing monitoring are the typical course of treatment.

The child in premature adrenarche has no other signs of puberty, including accelerated linear growth. Reassurance and ongoing monitoring constitute the typical course of treatment.

Discussion Sources

Kaplowitz PB. Precocious puberty. Medscape. https://emedicine.medscape.com/article/924002-overview

National Institutes of Health, Eunice Kennedy Shriver National Institute of Child Health and Human Development. What causes normal puberty, precocious puberty, and delayed puberty? http://nichd.nih.gov/health/topics/puberty/conditioninfo/Pages/causes.aspx

QUESTIONS

282. The most common reason for precocious puberty in girls is:

   A. ovarian tumor.

   B. adrenal tumor.

   C. exogenous estrogen.

   D. early onset of normal puberty.

283 to 285. Match each characteristic with the most appropriate Tanner stage.

_____ **283.** onset of growth spurt in boys or girls

_____ **284.** breast buds and papilla elevated in girls

_____ **285.** in boys, increase in penile length and width with development of glans

    A. Tanner stage 2

    B. Tanner stage 3

    C. Tanner stage 4

    D. Tanner stage 5

286. The most common reason for precocious puberty in boys is:

    A. excessive physical activity.

    B. a select number of relatively uncommon health problems.

    C. exogenous testosterone.

    D. early onset of normal puberty.

287. Which of the following is noted in a child with premature thelarche?

    A. breast enlargement

    B. accelerated linear growth

    C. pubic hair

    D. body odor

288. Which of the following is noted in a child with premature adrenarche?

    A. breast development

    B. accelerated linear growth

    C. pubic hair

    D. menstruation

289. Girls typically grow to their adult height by:

    A. menarche.

    B. 1 year before menarche.

    C. 1 year after the onset of menstruation.

    D. their 16th birthday.

290. The onset of puberty in girls is marked by:

    A. breast budding.

    B. menarche.

    C. peak of growth spurt.

    D. presence of axillary hair.

291. Which is not a known reason for the delayed onset of puberty in a 15-year-old boy?

    A. report of a high level of physical activity

    B. Kallmann's syndrome

    C. familial trait

    D. history of radiation exposure

292. Which is a possible reason for delayed onset of puberty in a 13-year-old girl?

    A. history of abdominal irradiation

    B. obesity

    C. report of asthma since age 6 years

    D. Turner's syndrome

293. Which of the following is the most appropriate diagnostic approach to assess altered puberty status in boys?

    A. serum thyrotropin (TSH) level
    B. serum testosterone
    C. serum prolactin
    D. serum aldosterone

294. When assessing a 5-year-old girl with suspected precocious puberty, each of the following tests are warranted except:

    A. serum follicle-stimulating hormone (FSH).
    B. serum luteinizing hormone.
    C. abdominal ultrasound.
    D. microscopic examination of vaginal discharge.

For answers and rationales, see end of chapter.

Car Seat Guidelines

Proper car seat use has been demonstrated to reduce the risk of injury, hospitalization, or death in children by more than 70% when compared to children who are not restrained. Advising parents and caregivers about age- and size-appropriate car restraints is one of the most important parts of providing pediatric primary care. Knowledge of appropriate child car seat restraint is an important part of practice (Table 17-15).

Discussion Source

Durbin DR, Hoffman BD, American Academy of Pediatrics Council on Injury, Violence, and Poison Prevention. Child passenger safety. *Pediatrics*. 2018;142:e20182460. https://pediatrics.aappublications.org/content/pediatrics/early/2018/08/28/peds.2018-2460.full.pdf

TABLE 17-15 Car Safety Seat Use: Most Current American Academy of Pediatrics Recommendations

AGE	TYPE OF SEAT	GENERAL GUIDELINE
Infants to toddlers	Rear-facing	Rear-facing car seat as long as possible until the child reaches the highest weight or height allowed by the car safety seat's manufacturer (usually 2 years or more).
Toddlers to preschoolers	Convertible seats and forward-facing seats with harnesses	Once child has outgrown the rear-facing weight or height limit for the car safety seat, should use a forward-facing car safety seat with a harness for as long as possible, up to the highest weight or height allowed by the car safety seat's manufacturer (usually up to 65 pounds and more).
School-aged children	Booster	All children whose weight or height is higher than the forward-facing limit for the car safety seat should use a belt-positioning booster seat until the vehicle seat belt fits properly, typically when they have reached 4 feet 9 inches (144.8 cm) in height and are between 8 and 12 years of age.
Older children	Seat belts	When children are old enough and large enough to use the vehicle seat belt alone, they should always use lap and shoulder seat belts for optimal protection. All children younger than age 13 years should be restrained in the rear seats of vehicles for optimal protection.

Source: Durbin DR, Hoffman BD, American Academy of Pediatrics Council on Injury, Violence, and Poison Prevention. Child passenger safety. Pediatrics. 2018;142:e20182460. https://pediatrics.aappublications.org/content/pediatrics/early/2018/08/28/peds.2018-2460.full.pdf

QUESTIONS

295. A young child should use a rear-facing car seat until:

A. at least age 12 months.

B. at least age 18 months.

C. at least age 30 months.

D. the child reaches the maximum height and weight allowed by the seat.

296. You anticipate that adult car seat belts fit correctly when a child is approximately _____ tall and is _____ old.

A. 51 inches (129.5 cm), 6 to 8 years

B. 53 inches (134.6 cm), 5 to 7 years

C. 57 inches (144.8 cm), 8 to 12 years

D. 59 inches (150 cm), 12 to 14 years

297. In general, children should ride in the back seat of the car until age:

A. 10 years.

B. 11 years.

C. 12 years.

D. 13 years.

For answers and rationales, see end of chapter.

QUESTION ANSWERS AND RATIONALES

Newborn and Infant Feeding

1. Correct: D. "The baby's urine should be light or colorless."
Urine that is light and colorless is a good indication that the baby is well hydrated and feeding sufficiently (D).
Incorrect:
The transition from colostrum to mature milk typically occurs between days 2 to 5 after childbirth and not 10 days after birth (A). Proper breastfeeding of the newborn should have a minimum of 10 minutes on each breast every 1.5 to 3 hours (B). A clicking sound made during nursing would indicate an improper latch (C).

2. Correct: B. "The baby might need to be awakened to be fed."
A newborn who is breastfed should feed every 1.5 to 3 hours (about 8 to 12 times per day), which may require waking the baby to ensure adequate feeding (B).
Incorrect:
The transition from colostrum to mature milk typically occurs between days 2 and 5 after childbirth (A). However, supplemental feeding with formula or dextrose and water should be avoided as this will interfere with the baby's hunger drive to breastfeed and can delay or reduce production of breast milk (C). The first bowel movements of the newborn consist of meconium, which is a thick,

black or dark green substance that eventually transitions to a yellow-green stool (D).

3. Correct: B. greater weight gain in the first few weeks of life.
Newborns that are formula-fed typically have greater weight gain during the first few weeks of life when compared to breastfed babies (B). However, the overall benefits of breastfeeding far outweigh this small difference in weight gain, and this likely represents excessive weight gain.
Incorrect:
Breastfeeding offers several benefits to the newborn as it provides the ideal form of nutrition and transfers the mother's antibodies to the infant to help prevent disease. Breastfed infants have been shown to have a lower incidence of diarrheal illness (A), a lower risk of allergic disorders (C), and a lower occurrence of constipation (D).

4. Correct: A. 2 to 3 oz, or 60 to 90 mL, every 2 to 3 hours.
During the first month of life, a formula-fed infant should be expected to consume 2 to 3 oz of formula every 2 to 3 hours (A). For breastfed infants, feeding should occur at least 10 minutes on each breast every 1.5 to 3 hours.
Incorrect:
A newborn infant that is formula-fed should be fed approximately every 2 to 3 hours (B, D) and would expect to take 2 to 3 oz at each feeding (C).

5. Correct: C. 4 to 6 months.

Solid foods should not be introduced to infants earlier than 4 to 6 months of age (C). The infant should have at least doubled the birth weight and consume at least 32 oz of formula per day or more than 8 to 10 feedings (breast or bottle) per day. Other signs would include being able to sit upright with little support, having good head control, and opening the mouth and leaning forward when food is offered.

Incorrect:

The introduction of solid foods should wait until at least 4 to 6 months of age (A, B) as certain developmental milestones are needed to be reached. Waiting up to 6 to 8 months is not needed for most infants (D).

6. Correct: A. 1%

When a nursing mother takes a medication, the nursing infant typically receives 1% or less of the maternal dose of medication from breast milk (A). Generally, if a medication is safe to give to a child, then it is safe to prescribe to a nursing mother. Only a few drugs are contraindicated in nursing mothers.

Incorrect:

Only 1% or less of a medication taken by a nursing mother will pass to the infant while nursing (B, C, D).

7. Correct: C. simple diffusion.

Most drugs pass into breast milk through simple diffusion, moving from areas of high concentration to low concentration (C). For this reason, the pump-and-dump approach is not effective in removing a medication from breast milk, as it creates an area of low concentration in the empty breast.

Incorrect:

Active transport requires the expenditure of energy to move substances or medications across membranes. Facilitated transfer utilizes transmembrane proteins to move compounds across cell membranes. Neither of these mechanisms is generally used in the movement of medication from mother's serum to breast milk (A, B). Similarly, a pH gradient is not created to facilitate movement of medications to breast milk (D).

8. Correct: C. three to five drug-free half-lives of the medication.

The pump-and-dump approach is not effective in removing a medication from breast milk as it creates an area of low concentration in the empty breast. The drug will then move from the area of high concentration (i.e., mother's serum) to the breast. To ensure a minimal amount of offending medication is present in breast milk, the mother should wait at least three to five drug-free half-lives of the medication before nursing the baby (C).

Incorrect:

The time required to ensure a minimal amount of drug is present in breast milk will depend on the medication half-life and not a set time (B) or the interval of feeding cycles (A). Half-life is a predictable pharmacokinetic property of the medication (D).

9. Correct: C. maternal alcohol use causes a reduction in the amount of milk ingested by the infant.

Small amounts of alcohol ingestion by a nursing mother can cause a reduction in the let-down reflex, decreased milk production, and less rhythmic and frequent sucking by the infant, resulting in a smaller volume of milk consumption (C).

Incorrect:

Alcohol has a low molecular weight that easily passes to breast milk (B). Alcohol consumption can reduce the let-down reflex and result in decreased milk production (A). One or two alcoholic drinks may not lead to infant intoxication as less than 1% of the alcohol will pass to breast milk. However, even small amounts of alcohol consumption can decrease the amount of milk consumption by the nursing infant (D).

10. Correct: D. 30 g or 1 oz.

During the first 3 months of life, the average daily weight gain is approximately 26 to 31 g (D). The anticipated daily weight gain will then decrease to 17 to 18 g during months 3 to 6, and 12 to 13 g daily during months 6 to 9.

Incorrect:

In a newborn up to 3 months of age, the average daily weight gain should exceed 25 g and range near 30 g (A, B, C).

11. Correct: D. 100 to 120 kcal/kg/day.

The required caloric intake for an infant between 0 and 3 months of age is approximately 100 to 120 kcal/kg/day (D). This amount does not change substantially as the child grows, with a requirement of 105 to 115 kcal/kg/day for those 3 to 6 months of age and 100 to 105 kcal/kg/day for those 6 to 9 months of age.

Incorrect:

During the first 3 months of life, the average required caloric intake ranges from 100 to 120 kcal/kg/day (A, B, C).

12. Correct: C. Unconjugated bilirubin is elevated, and D. Risk of development of hyperbilirubinemia can be reduced in a breastfed infant with frequent breastfeeding every 2 to 3 hours per 24 hours.

Physiological jaundice occurs as a result of elevated levels of unconjugated bilirubin (C). The condition can be prevented by keeping the newborn well hydrated by breastfeeding at least 8 to 12 times per day, or every 2 to 3 hours (D).

Incorrect:

Physiological jaundice typically occurs between days 3 to 5 (A) and usually starts at the head and then spreads to the body (B). Supplemental water and dextrose should be avoided as this will interfere with the infant's hunger drive to breastfeed and will delay and reduce breast milk production (E).

13. Correct: B. hypernatremia.

Consequences of inadequate feeding during the first few weeks of life can lead to dehydration, hypernatremia (B), and hypoglycemia. Hypoglycemia is often characterized by a protracted high-pitched cry, jitteriness, and potential seizures.

Incorrect:
Inadequate feeding of a newborn is not typically associated with hypercalcemia (A), while hypernatremia is more likely than hypokalemia (C) or hyperkalemia (D).

14. **Correct: D. weight loss of greater than 7% at any time after the first week of life**
A key criterion to assess for adequate feeding is slow growth or weight loss during the first few weeks of life. A weight loss of greater than 7% at any time, particularly after the first week of life, is particularly concerning as it increases the likelihood of neonatal jaundice and hypernatremia (D).

Incorrect:
Weight loss of greater than 7% at any time in a newborn is a major concern. Some weight loss can be expected during the first few days of life (A, B) before the newborn begins to gain weight (C).

15. **Correct: C. Double pumps are not recommended as they express about half the amount of milk as single pumps.**
Breast pumps can provide breastfeeding mothers with flexibility with feedings. Double pumps are particularly helpful as they reduce the time needed to pump by one-half by expressing milk from both breasts at the same time. These pumps do not differ in the amount of milk expressed compared to single pumps (C).

Incorrect:
Breast pumps can be helpful in allowing nursing mothers to return to work or school (B). Some insurance companies as well as state Medicaid will cover the costs of breast pumps (A). The FLSA requires employers to provide a reasonable amount of break time to express milk as well as a functional space in which to pump milk (D).

16 to 19. Yes or No

16. **Correct: No**

17. **Correct: No**

18. **Correct: No**

19. **Correct: Yes**
A correct latch is critical for proper breastfeeding of the newborn. With adequate latch, the baby's chin and stomach should be able to comfortably rest against the mother's body, the baby's mouth is widely open, with lips flanged outward (19), and the areola is minimally visible (16). Observations with poor latch include dimpling of the baby's cheeks (17) and/or a clicking noise with attempts at suck and swallow (18).

20. **Correct: A. loose, seedy stools multiple times per day.**
Typical stools in a healthy breastfed baby at 2 weeks of age would most likely consist of loose, seedy stools that

occur several times per day (A). As the baby matures, the frequency of stools will decrease.
Increase:
Initial stools in newborns consist of meconium, which is a thick black or dark green stool that passes during the first couple of days after birth (B). Normal stools in a newborn would not contain blood (C). A breastfed baby would produce loose stool, but it would not be considered watery, which could indicate a diarrheal condition (D).

21. **Correct: A. she should return to using the ICS on a set schedule with as-needed albuterol and continue breastfeeding.**
For this patient with a history of asthma, she should restart her asthma medication regimen to control symptoms. ICSs are generally safe to use during breastfeeding, as very little is absorbed systemically and will not concentrate in breast milk (A).

Incorrect:
ICS is not contraindicated in nursing mothers and so breastfeeding can continue with treatment (B). A LABA as monotherapy is not recommended for the treatment of asthma (C), and theophylline is not considered a first-line agent for asthma (D).

22. **Correct: A. increased risk of contaminations.**
Homemade infant formula is usually made from cow's or goat's milk with supplemental vitamins. However, the use of these homemade formulas should be discouraged as there can be an invariable lack of critical micronutrients and carbohydrates needed by the developing newborn as well as a risk of contaminations in the ingredients used (A).

Incorrect:
Though homemade infant formula can cause an allergic reaction, there is not a necessarily higher risk when compared to commercially available products (B). The concern with homemade formula is the risk of contaminants and possible lack of micronutrients and not excessive amounts of calcium (C). The cost of homemade infant formula can actually be lower than commercially produced formulas (D).

23 to 25. Yes or No

23. **Correct: No**

24. **Correct: No**

25. **Correct: Yes**
For the safety of the baby, caregivers should recognize when reconstituted formula is safe and when it should be discarded. Once formula is reconstituted, it should not be left out at room temperature for more than 2 hours (23), while storing it in the refrigerator can extend the life of liquid formula for a bit longer (24). If the entire amount of formula is not used during a feeding, the remainder, now a mixture of formula and the baby's saliva, should be discarded, as this combination will support bacterial growth (25).

26 to 29. Yes or No

26. Correct: No

27. Correct: Yes

28. Correct: Yes

29. Correct: Yes

Certain criteria can be used to help determine whether an infant can start solid foods. Typically, solid foods should not be introduced prior to age 4 to 6 months (26), and the baby should have at least doubled the birth weight (28). Other signs include the ability to sit upright without any support (27) and have good head control. Infants that consume more than 32 oz of formula each day or have more than 8 to 10 feedings (breast or bottle) per day can also be considered for solid foods (29).

30. Correct: B. Supplementation is advised in infants 6 months and older who are exclusively breastfed.

Fluoride is an important part of preventing tooth decay in children. Fluoride supplements can be considered for children 6 months and older who are at high risk of tooth decay and who are not consuming fluorinated drinking water. This would include infants who are exclusively breastfed (B).

Incorrect:

Fluoride supplements are advised for children 6 months and older who do not drink fluorinated water (A). This includes infants who are exclusively breastfed as well as formula-fed infants who use nonfluorinated water (C). Fluoride supplements are not needed for all infants at 4 months of age but would start at 6 months of age when needed (D).

31. Correct: C. a 7-month-old who is exclusively breastfed

A newborn's iron reserves typically last until 4 months of age. Breast milk contains very little iron, and so those who are exclusively breastfed should receive iron supplements beginning around 4 months and should continue until the baby begins to consume other foods that contain iron (C).

Incorrect:

Formula contains sufficient amounts of iron that will not require additional supplementation (A). A 2-month-old would not need iron supplementation since iron stores last until 4 months of life (B). For a child who eats a variety of solid foods, it is likely that the child is getting adequate amounts of iron from the food and will not require supplementation (D).

Early Childhood Development

32. Correct: B. experimenting with sound

A 3-month-old infant born at full term will most likely begin experimenting with sound, usually by making raspberry sounds (B).

Incorrect:

Sitting briefly with support is likely seen at 5 months of age (A). Rolling back to stomach and stomach to back typically occurs by 6 to 8 months of age (C). A social smile is observed by 1 to 2 months of age (D).

33. Correct: B. experimenting with sound

For preterm babies, the timing of milestones needs to be adjusted for prematurity for the first 24 months. Thus, the developmental expectations of a 5-month-old born at 32 weeks' gestation will correspond with a 3-month-old born at full term. An expected milestone for this child would be experimenting with sound, such as making raspberry sounds (B).

Incorrect:

For a 5-month-old born at 32 weeks' gestation, sitting briefly with support will be expected to occur at 7 months of age (A), while rolling over will occur by 8 to 10 months of age (C). Hand-to-hand transfer normally occurs at 6 to 8 months in an infant born at full term but will occur at 8 to 10 months in the infant born at 32 weeks' gestation (D).

34. Correct: B. grasp a cube.

By 3 to 4 months of age, the infant should be able to grasp a cube (B), reach for objects, and bring objects to the mouth.

Incorrect:

Parental recognition should be accomplished by 1 to 2 months of age (A). Imitating others is a developmental milestone reached at 5 months of age (C), while putting together syllables such as "dada" and "mama" occurs around 6 to 8 months of age (D).

35. Correct: C. play peek-a-boo.

A healthy infant born at full term will play peek-a-boo at around 9 to 11 months of age (C).

Incorrect:

The ability to roll from back to stomach (A) as well as imitate "bye-bye" (B) both occur around 6 to 8 months of age. The ability to hand over an object on request typically occurs by 12 to 15 months of age (D).

36. Correct: A. speak in phrases of two or more words.

A 2-year-old child should be able to speak in phrases of two or more words, while a 3-year-old will speak in three-word sentences (A).

Incorrect:

The abilities to scribble spontaneously (C) as well as throw a ball (B) will be expected to develop by 15 to 20 months of age. Riding a tricycle is expected to occur at 36 months of age (D).

37. Correct: A. 18 months

The ability to imitate housework is an expected milestone that occurs between 15 and 20 months of age (A).

Incorrect:

The ability to imitate housework would normally occur by 20 months of age (B, C, D).

38. Correct: A. give his or her first and last names.

A healthy 3-year-old should be able to provide first and last names upon request (A). At this age, nearly all speech should be intelligible even to those not in daily contact with the child.

Incorrect:

The ability to use pronouns (B) as well as kick a ball (C) should be achieved around 24 months of age. Having the child identify a best friend usually happens at age 5 to 6 years (D), around the time the child starts school.

39. Correct: A. roll from back to stomach.

The ability to roll from back to stomach and stomach to back is expected by age 6 to 8 months (A).

Incorrect:

Reaching for an object occurs by 3 to 4 months of age (C), while the ability to crawl on the abdomen develops by 9 to 11 months of age (D). A child will start to feed self by 15 to 20 months of age (B).

40. Correct: B. cruises.

By 9 months of age, a healthy infant should be able to crawl and cruise (B).

Incorrect:

The ability to sit without support (A) as well as recognize "no" (C) develops by 6 to 8 months of age. Making a raspberry sound develops by 3 to 4 months of age (D).

41. Correct: B. alternate feet when climbing stairs.

By 3 years of age, the child should be able to alternate feet when climbing stairs (B) as well as be able to ride a tricycle.

Incorrect:

Speaking in two-word phrases should occur by 2 years of age (C), while speaking in three-word phrases will occur by 3 years of age. The ability to count to four should occur by 4 to 5 years of age (A), and tying shoelaces will occur by 7 to 8 years of age (D).

42 to 45. Indicate Yes or No

42. Correct: Yes

43. Correct: Yes

44. Correct: No

45. Correct: Yes

Anticipated findings during the examination of a newborn include movement of all extremities and spontaneous stepping. A number of primitive reflexes can also be observed, including the Palmar grasp (43) and Babinski response. A newborn's best vision is at the range of 8 to 12 inches (42), while the newborn prefers high-pitched voices rather than low-pitched ones (44). The newborn has a well-developed sense of smell (45) and will blink in response to sound.

46. Correct: A. a visual preference for the human face

When examining the newborn, it is important to note a preference for the human face (A).

Incorrect:

A newborn will typically respond to the cries of other neonates (C) and will also respond to sudden sounds by blinking or turning the head (B). A social smile will not be apparent until about 1 to 2 months of age (D).

47. Correct: A. being able to name a best friend

A 5-year-old, who typically has started school at that age, will be able to identify a best friend (A).

Incorrect:

Identifying gender appropriately typically occurs by 3 to 4 years of age (B), while hopping on one foot is accomplished by 2.5 years of age (D). Naming an intended career is expected by 6 to 7 years of age (C).

48. Correct: B. conduct further evaluation of milestone attainment.

Typical milestones for saying "mama" and "dada" usually occur by 9 to 11 months of age, while children will begin saying a few words by 12 to 15 months of age. An 18-month-old child who is not saying any words or smiling responsibly is a cause for concern and would require further evaluation of milestone attainment to determine the next plan of action, including early interventions (B).

Incorrect:

This child is demonstrating delayed milestone attainment that requires further evaluation (C). Following a complete evaluation of milestone attainment, early intervention can be considered, which can include an audiogram and tympanometry (D). Though enrollment in day care can help develop socialization skills, the scope and cause for developmental delay should be determined first (A).

49. Correct: B. pointing to a desired object; and C. handing over objects on request

Anticipated milestones for a healthy 12-month-old child include pointing to a desired object (B), having a neat pincer grasp, having the ability to place a cube in a cup, and handing over objects on request (C).

Incorrect:

A 12-month-old child will be expected to speak a few words, while a 2-year-old child would speak in two-word sentences (A). Walking backward can be expected by 2.5 years of age (D).

50. Correct: B. false

A possible developmental "red flag" can include a lack of response to his or her name by 12 months of age and not 9 months of age (B).

51. Correct: C. plays pretend games while alone or with others.

Playing pretend games either alone or with others is a normal activity by 18 months of age. A possible red flag for ASD in a 2-year-old is not playing pretend games either alone or with others (C).

Incorrect:

"Red flags" for ASD include avoiding eye contact (A), having obsessive interests, having delayed speech/language skills, and repeating words over and over (echolalia) (B). Other signs can include getting upset by minor changes as well as having unusual reactions to smells or other environmental stimuli (D).

52. Correct: C. 24 months

For preterm babies, the timing of milestones needs to be adjusted for prematurity for the first 24 months (C). Thus, the developmental expectations of a 5-month-old born at 32 weeks' gestation will correspond with a 3-month-old born at full term.

53. Correct: **A. microorchidism following onset of puberty.**

A key sign of fragile X syndrome in males is large testicles (macroorchidism) rather than microorchidism after the beginning of puberty (A).

Incorrect:

Physical findings consistent with fragile X syndrome in males include large body habitus (B), large forehead and ears (C), and prominent jaw. Behavioral findings can include hyperactivity (D) and intellectual disability.

54. Correct: **C. fragile X**

Fragile X syndrome is the most common cause of autism in either gender and can lead to social and verbal developmental delays in boys (C). Klinefelter's disease (XXY male) is also associated with developmental issues, particularly related to verbal development.

Incorrect:

Tay-Sachs disease is a rare genetic disease that leads to nerve cell dysfunction in the brain that often leads to death in early childhood (A). Cystic fibrosis predominantly affects the pulmonary and digestive systems and does not impact social or verbal development (B). Trisomy 18, or Edwards' syndrome, can lead to developmental delays, though only about 12% of babies born with this condition will survive after 1 year (D).

55. Correct: **B. large forehead.**

Physical findings consistent with fragile X syndrome in males include large body habitus, large forehead (B) and ears, and prominent jaw.

Incorrect:

Fragile X syndrome is not associated with large eyes (A) or a small head (C) but is characterized by a prominent jaw rather than a recessive jaw (D).

56. Correct: **A. language impairment in males.**

Klinefelter's syndrome only affects males and is characterized by developmental issues, predominantly language impairment (A).

Incorrect:

Klinefelter's syndrome only affects males (C). The condition is not typically associated with fine motor delay (B) or attention-deficit disorder (D).

57. Correct: **C. amniocentesis; and D. blood testing for carrier state**

A blood test is available for diagnosis of Klinefelter's syndrome or identifying the carrier state (assesses genetic risk of having a child with the syndrome) (D). Antenatal diagnosis of Klinefelter's syndrome can also be performed via amniocentesis (C).

Incorrect:

There is no urine test (A) or literacy assessment (B) available that is able to diagnose Klinefelter's syndrome or the carrier state.

58. Correct: **C. the symptoms are absent until the child reaches school age.**

Signs of ASD can be evident in young children, and the AAP recommends routine screening for autism between 18 and 24 months of age (C).

Incorrect:

Signs of ASD can include persistent deficits in social communication and social interaction (A), hyperreactivity to sensory input or unusual interests in sensory aspects of the environment, inflexible adherence to routines (B), and repetitive use of objects or speech (D).

59. Correct: **C. 4 to 6 months**

Anticipatory guidance counseling is most helpful when it is provided near the time when the child is expected to reach the developmental landmark. In this manner, the advice can help the parents cope with, adapt to, and avoid problems with the expected changes. As teething typically starts around 6 months of age, parenteral anticipatory guidance should be given around 4 to 6 months of age (C).

60. Correct: **B. 10 to 12 months**

Anticipatory guidance counseling is most helpful when it is provided near the time when the child is expected to reach the developmental landmark. As temper tantrums typically start after 12 months of age, often peaking between 18 and 24 months, the appropriate time to provide parenteral anticipatory guidance would be between 10 and 12 months (B).

61. Correct: **B. 18 to 24 months**

Anticipatory guidance counseling is most helpful when it is provided near the time when the child is expected to reach the developmental landmark. Discipline using the "time out" method can begin around 2 years of age. Therefore, anticipatory guidance counseling on this aspect can be provided at around 18 to 24 months (B).

62. Correct: **A. birth**

Anticipatory guidance counseling is most helpful when it is provided near the time when the child is expected to reach the developmental landmark. However, falls can occur at any time in the child's life, and so anticipatory guidance should be provided as early as possible following birth to ensure the safety of the child (A).

63. Correct: **C. 18 months**

Anticipatory guidance counseling is most helpful when it is provided near the time when the child is expected to reach the developmental landmark. Though readiness for toilet training will vary for each child, the process can initially be considered around 18 months of age. Therefore, parenteral anticipatory guidance on this topic should be offered around this age (C).

64. Correct: **A. birth**

Anticipatory guidance counseling is most helpful when it is provided near the time when the child is expected to reach the developmental landmark. However, parents should be educated on appropriate sleep position for their infant at birth to ensure the safety of their child (A).

65. Correct: **C. 11 years**

Anticipatory guidance counseling is most helpful when it is provided near the time when the child is expected to reach the developmental landmark.

Parenteral anticipatory guidance regarding sexual activity should be offered prior to the child reaching puberty. The typical range of onset of Tanner stage 2 is 8 to 13 years in females and 9 to 14 years in males. Therefore, parenteral anticipatory guidance at around 11 years of age would be appropriate in most cases (C).

66. Correct: B. 11 years

Anticipatory guidance counseling is most helpful when it is provided near the time when the child is expected to reach the developmental landmark. As substance abuse can often start as early as the middle school years, parenteral anticipatory guidance on this issue should be provided by 11 years of age (B).

67. Correct: B. 1 to 2 hours.

The AAP recommends limiting screen time in young children to 1 to 2 hours per day (B). Screen media (other than video chatting) should be avoided in children younger than 18 months, while children 18 to 24 months can be introduced to digital media, though parents should choose high-quality programming, and parents should watch the programs together with their children to help them understand what they are watching. For older children, there should be strict limits set on the time spent and the types of media, and parents should make sure screen time does not interfere with adequate sleep, physical activity, and other behaviors essential to healthy living.

Lead Poisoning (Plumbism)

68. Correct: C. a toddler who lives in an 85-year-old home

The most common cause of lead poisoning is through exposure to lead-based paint that is present in older homes. Inhalation of paint dust or eating paint chips is a main source of lead in toddlers. Lead-based paint stopped being available in 1978, while heavily leaded paint was used until the 1950s, and so newer homes are not likely to contain lead-based paint as a source of lead poisoning. Therefore, the toddler living in the 85-year-old house is at greatest risk of lead poisoning (C).

Incorrect:

Children who live in newer houses without lead-based paint are at less risk of lead poisoning, including children with intellectual disabilities (A). Copper plumbing is not a source of lead poisoning, though lead pipes and brass fixtures can contribute to plumbism (B). There is no relationship between lead poisoning and living near an electric-generating plant (D).

69. Correct: A. true

In addition to lead-based paint, other household products can contain lead hazards, including imported candy, toys, jewelry, and cosmetics. Home health remedies such as azarcon and greta, which are used to treat upset stomach and indigestion in certain ethnic communities, often contain lead (A).

70. Correct: C. zinc, and D. magnesium

Increased lead absorption can occur with a diet low in calcium, iron, zinc (C), magnesium (D), and copper, as well as high-fat diets.

Incorrect:

Diets that are low in protein (A) or carbohydrates (B) do not impact lead absorption.

71. Correct: A. environmental history.

When screening young children for lead poisoning, a thorough assessment of environmental history is essential, as lead poisoning is caused by exposure to lead in the environment (A). The most obvious aspect is the presence of lead-based paint in the home, which is more commonly found in older homes.

Incorrect:

Though lead poisoning can lead to a microcytic, hypochromic anemia, screening children by checking hematocrit levels is an invasive and costly approach (C) and would not be specific for lead poisoning. Hemoglobin electrophoresis will not offer any useful information on lead poisoning but is more often used to check for genetic disorders, such as thalassemias (D). Signs of low levels of lead poisoning will not be evident upon physical examination (B).

72. Correct: D. microcytic, hypochromic

Plumbism is associated with the development of a microcytic, hypochromic anemia (D). Basophilic stippling is also often noted on red blood cell morphology.

Incorrect:

A normocytic, normochromic anemia can be found with acute blood loss or anemia of chronic disease (B). Macrocytic, normochromic anemia is most commonly caused by vitamin B_{12} deficiency and pernicious anemia (A). Hemolytic anemia can be caused by genetic conditions, such as sickle cell anemia, as well as due to infection or medication (C).

73. Correct: B. 6 months

For children at significant risk of lead poisoning, screening should begin at 6 months of age (B). This can be performed through risk assessment, which can be followed by a blood test if the assessment is positive. The risk assessment should be repeated at 9, 12, 18, and 24 months and then annually up to 6 years of age.

74. Correct: C. chelation therapy.

Several interventions can be taken for a child who is found to have elevated levels of lead in the blood. However, chelation therapy is usually reserved for children with blood lead levels of 45 to 50 mcg/dL (C).

Incorrect:

Children with elevated levels of lead in the range of 5 to 44 mcg/dL are initially treated with iron therapy (B) and improved nutrition (D), as well as removal of the child from the source of lead (A).

75. Correct: A. chelation therapy.

Chelation therapy is usually reserved for children with blood lead levels of 45 to 50 mcg/dL (A). A chelation agent such as succimer is used.

Incorrect:

Chelation therapy is the preferred intervention when blood lead level is 45 to 50 mcg/dL. Calcium supplementation (B), exchange transfusion (C), and iron depletion therapy (D) are not warranted. When blood lead levels are higher, hospitalization and expert consultation are needed to avoid serious consequences.

Hypertension, Type 2 Diabetes, and Dyslipidemia in Children

76. Correct: A. obesity, and C. being exposed to second-hand smoke

Risk factors for hypertension in children and teens include a family history of heart disease, elevated lipid levels, exposure to tobacco smoke (C), poor diet, obesity (A), and lack of physical activity.

Incorrect:

Drinking whole milk (B) and extensive screen time (D) have not been identified as substantial risk factors for hypertension in children.

77. Correct: A. The juice is mixed in small amounts to flavor water, B. Only 100% juice is used, and E. No more than 6 oz (177 mL) per day is recommended for children 6 months to 5 years.

Fruit juice does not need to be part of a child's diet, particularly if the child is receiving an adequate supply of vitamin C from fresh fruit. When fruit juice is offered to a child, it should contain 100% juice with no added sugar (B) and can be mixed in small amounts to flavor water to increase fluid intake (A). Fruit juice should be limited to 6 oz per day in young children (E).

Incorrect:

Fruit juice should not replace the recommended amount of milk or breast milk (C). If fruit juice is being offered to a child, there is no preference for when it should be consumed (D).

78. Correct: A. Obtain fasting lipid profile, and D. Assess diet and physical activity.

Screening for cardiovascular health is an important aspect in preventive care in children. A fasting lipid profile is the recommended approach, as there is no noninvasive method to assess atherosclerotic disease in children (A). An assessment of diet and physical activity is also an important indicator for future risk of CVD and should be assessed at each well-child visit (D).

Incorrect:

Screening for T2DM should be limited to children with risk factors for the disease as well as those having a BMI in the 85th percentile for age and sex, weight-for-height greater than the 85th percentile, or weight greater than 120% of that ideal for height (B). An assessment of family history for thyroid disease is not an essential component of the comprehensive cardiovascular evaluation in children (C).

79. Correct: A. 12 months old

BMI should be measured beginning at 2 years of age. However, if overweight or obesity is a concern beginning at 12 months of age, parents should be advised of dietary recommendations for the child, such as switching to reduced-fat milk, in addition to increasing physical activity (A). Dietary and activity recommendations should be intensified if BMI is greater than the 85th percentile at 5 years of age.

80. Correct: C. onset of nonorganic failure to thrive in the toddler years

Though a low birth weight and poor infant growth have been identified as risk factors for T2DM, a failure to thrive during the toddler years is not an identified risk factor (C).

Incorrect:

Risk factors for T2DM in children and teens include obesity (B), sedentary lifestyle, certain ethnicities (D), family history, PCOS, and hyperinsulinemia (A).

81. Correct: A. every other year

Current guidelines recommend screening children at risk of T2DM at age 10 years or at the onset of puberty. Screening should continue every 2 years until adulthood, at which time the adult guidelines should be followed (A).

82. Correct: A. impaired fasting glucose (glucose level greater than or equal to 100 mg/dL or 5.6 mmol/L but less than or equal to 125 mg/dL or 7 mmol/L), and B. impaired glucose tolerance (2-hour postprandial glucose 140 to 199 mg/dL or 7.8 to 11 mmol/L)

Prediabetes in children is defined as having impaired fasting glucose (glucose level greater than or equal to 100 mg/dL or 5.6 mmol/L) but less than or equal to 125 mg/dL or 7 mmol/L) (A), impaired glucose tolerance (2-hour postprandial glucose 140 to 199 mg/dL or 7.8 to 11 mmol/L) (B), or an A1c of 5.7% to 6.4%.

Incorrect:

An A1c of 6.5% or greater will result in a diagnosis of T2DM (C), as well as a random plasma glucose of 200 mg/dL or greater in conjunction with symptoms of T2DM (D).

83. Correct: C. family history of lipid abnormalities, and D. family history of T2DM

The key risk factors for dyslipidemia in children include a family history of lipid abnormalities (C) and a family history of T2DM (D).

Incorrect:

Elevated blood pressure during childhood is not a risk factor for dyslipidemia (A), and breastfeeding during the toddler years is also not a risk factor (B).

84. Correct: B. 2 years

Current guidelines recommend screening for lipid abnormalities among children with certain risk factors or whose family history is not known after 2 years of age and no later than 10 years of age (B). Lipid screening should not be performed prior to age 2 years.

85. Correct: A. less than 170 mg/dL or 9.4 mmol/L.

According to the AAP, an acceptable level of total cholesterol in children aged 2 to 19 years is less than 170 mg/dL (less than 9.4 mmol/L) (A). The borderline level is 170 to 199 mg/dL (9.4 to 11 mmol/L), while an elevated level is 200 mg/dL or greater (11.1 mmol/L or greater).

Evaluation of the Febrile Child

86. Correct: D. higher rates of select immunization.

Sepsis rates in young children have lowered in recent years predominantly as a result of increased immunization rates against select infections, particularly influenzae, *H influenzae* type B, and *S pneumoniae* (D).

Incorrect:

Rates of sepsis have not decreased because of more stringent screening and diagnosis of febrile illness (A) or a longer observation period in children with febrile illness (C). Increased use of antipyretics in children may decrease fever but would not have an impact on the development of sepsis (B).

87 to 91. Indicate Reassuring or Concerning findings

87. Correct: Concerning

88. Correct: Reassuring

89. Correct: Concerning

90. Correct: Reassuring

91. Correct: Concerning

Health-care providers should have the ability to identify reassuring or concerning findings in the febrile young child to help determine whether outpatient management is appropriate or if urgent or emergent care is needed. Reassuring findings include warm, dry, and appropriately colored fingertips, brisk capillary refill (88), lusty cry or smiling during the examination, respiratory rate less than 50% above ULN (90), and the ability to tolerate oral fluids. Concerning findings will include pale or cyanotic skin (87), poor capillary refill, weak or no cry during the examination (89), tachypnea, tachycardia, inability to tolerate oral fluids, and no evidence of recent urinary output (91).

92. Correct: C. when diarrhea is present.

When evaluating a febrile child with an uncertain cause of the fever, stool culture and fecal WBC count should be limited to only when diarrhea is present to confirm or rule out acute gastroenteritis (C).

Incorrect:

Fecal tests should not be performed routinely as part of the diagnostic process of the febrile child (A). The presence of diarrhea is the major determinant of whether stool testing is needed and not duration of fever (B) or severity of fever (D).

93. Correct: B. endogenous pyrogens increase prostaglandin synthesis

Fever can be an important part of a body's defense against infection and consists of a complex physiological reaction that occurs when exogenous pyrogens are introduced to the body. This triggers the production of endogenous pyrogens, while prostaglandins activate thermoregulatory neurons and alter the hypothalamic set point (B). Vasomotor center reactions increase heat conservation and heat production. The result of this process is fever.

Incorrect:

Fever does not involve an increase in systemic vascular resistance (which would cause increased blood pressure) (A). Fever is not the result of immature neutrophils in circulation (C) or the presence of atypical or reactive lymphocytes (D).

94. Correct: B. nuchal rigidity is usually not found in early childhood meningitis.

In seriously ill children with fever, often there is an absence of hypotension, cool skin, and/or nuchal rigidity (i.e., neck stiffness) (B). This is true even in the presence of meningitis, where older children and adults commonly report nuchal rigidity.

Incorrect:

Low- or high-grade fevers are unlikely to cause harm to the child (A). Febrile seizure is more likely to occur as body temperature increases and not at the peak (C). The most common cause of fever in the young child is due to a self-limiting viral infection and not bacterial infection, which typically comprises less than 5% of febrile illness in infants and young children (D).

95. Correct: D. increased rate of atypical pneumonia pathogen replication

Fever can provide benefits to the child in fighting infection, including reducing replication by bacteria, including atypical organisms (D).

Incorrect:

Some of the beneficial effects of fever include lowering the rate of viral and bacterial replication (A), having a toxic effect on select bacteria (B), and having a negative effect on growth by *S pneumoniae* (C).

96. Correct: B. consistent use of an antipyretic provides a helpful way to shorten the course of infectious illnesses.

The presence of fever can be helpful when trying to resolve a bacterial or viral infection. The consistent use of antipyretic agents has been shown to prolong the course of illness rather than shorten illness duration (B).

Incorrect:

The use of antipyretics will prolong the duration of illness, especially for viral infections (A). The presence of fever is associated with reduced morbidity and mortality from infection (D). One drawback of fever is that it increases metabolic demand, which can be an issue for a child with certain chronic health problems and would warrant the use of antipyretics (C).

97. Correct: B. The degree of temperature reduction in response to antipyretic therapy is not predictive of the presence or absence of bacteremia.

There is no substantial correlation between the amount of temperature reduction with use of an antipyretic and the type of infection that is present (B).

Incorrect:

Acetaminophen and ibuprofen are both appropriate for use during viral infections as they provide similar fever reduction potential and are generally safe in children (A). Ibuprofen and acetaminophen have an onset of action of within 30 minutes (C), and the duration of action of acetaminophen is 4 hours compared to 6 hours with ibuprofen (D).

98. Correct: A. The occurrence of one febrile seizure is predictive of having another, and B. Intermittent diazepam can be used prophylactically during febrile illness to reduce risk of recurrence.

Though the cause of febrile seizures is unclear, a child who experiences a first febrile seizure is at greater risk of recurrence (A). The use of antiepileptic medications is not routinely recommended, as the risk outweighs the small benefit. However, intermittent diazepam at the onset of febrile illness can be considered for prevention, particularly when parents have high anxiety about future episodes (B).

Incorrect:

Febrile seizures occur as temperature rises and not at the peak of fever. A mild temperature increase will pose little risk for febrile seizures, and a history of febrile seizure is not associated with the occurrence of nonfebrile seizures, such as epilepsy (C). The use of antipyretics during febrile illness does not reduce the risk of future febrile seizure (D).

99. Correct: A. neutrophils.

A bacterial infection is characterized by an elevation of neutrophils (A).

Incorrect:

An elevation of lymphocytes is a better indication of a viral infection rather than bacterial meningitis (B). Eosinophils are activated during a parasitic infection as well as allergic reactions (C). An elevation in monocytes is not specific to a bacterial infection but can be due to other types of infection, such as fungal infection, as well as autoimmune disorders, blood disorders, or other medical conditions (D).

100. Correct: B. predominance of lymphocytes.

An elevation in lymphocytes is an indication of viral infection and would be expected in the child with viral meningitis (B).

Incorrect:

The typical CSF response in viral meningitis includes normal glucose level (C), normal to slightly elevated protein level (A), and an elevated CSF opening pressure, which is a near universal finding in meningitis (D).

101. Correct: A. chest x-ray.

For this patient with respiratory symptoms of a congested cough and elevated respiratory rate, a chest x-ray is warranted to rule in or out pneumonia as the source of infection (A).

Incorrect:

With the presence of respiratory tract symptoms, a chest x-ray should be given priority over the other diagnostic measures to check for the presence of pneumonia. A sputum culture is not routinely needed as it can take days for the results and will not likely impact the initial management decisions (D). A sputum culture can be considered in cases of complication or treatment failure. Urine culture and susceptibility will likely not provide any useful information regarding the nature of the infection and also will require 2 to 3 days for results (B). Other tests can more rapidly detect the presence of a UTI, such as checking for the presence of urinary nitrite. The child has a number of reassuring signs and no neurological findings that would indicate meningitis, so a lumbar puncture is not warranted (C).

102. Correct: C. capillary refill of more than 2 seconds.

Hypoperfusion can be assessed by capillary refill, which is normally 2 seconds or less, and would be longer during a hypoperfusion state (C). Decreased perfusion of the skin is associated with an increase in systemic vascular resistance, which can occur early in an infant with hypovolemia.

Incorrect:

Hypoperfusion is related to blood flow and not related to the level of WBCs (A). Dehydration can be a contributor to hypoperfusion but is not an indicator for the condition (B). Nonresponsiveness in a child may be a late, rather than early, indicator of concerning findings in a seriously ill child (D).

103. Correct: A. leukocytosis with neutrophilia

An elevation in WBCs (typically greater than 11,000/mm^3) with elevated levels of neutrophils best describes leukocytosis with neutropenia (A). This is also known as a left shift and is typically observed during bacterial infection.

Incorrect:

Leukopenia is characterized by low levels of WBCs (i.e., less than 3,500/mm^3) and can place the individual at increased risk of infection or can occasionally be seen as a normal limit variant or as a result of the viral illness (D). Lymphocytosis describes an elevation in lymphocytes and typically occurs with viral infection (B). Lymphopenia and neutropenia describe the findings of low lymphocytes and low neutrophils, respectively (C).

104. Correct: D. bacterial.

A finding of leukocytosis with neutropenia is the characteristic finding in a child with a bacterial infection, as neutrophils are activated to fight these kinds of infection (D).

Incorrect:

Viral infections are more commonly associated with lymphocytosis rather than neutrophilia (A). Parasitic infections can result in eosinophilia, or elevated levels of eosinophils (B). Fungal infections result in elevated levels of monocytes (C).

105. **Correct: B. hepatotoxicity.**

Acetaminophen is generally safe to use in children when given in appropriate doses. However, excessive doses of this medication can result in hepatotoxicity (B).

Incorrect:

Acetaminophen is not associated with the development of seizure (A) or petechial rash (C). Risk for gastric ulcer is more likely observed with long-term use of ibuprofen rather than acetaminophen (D).

106. **Correct: C. an increase in body temperature resulting from shivering.**

Though caregivers may be tempted to give a cooling bath for their febrile infant or young child, the practice is not recommended as this can lead to an eventual increase in body temperature due to the child shivering as a result of the cool bath (C).

Incorrect:

Though a cooling bath is not recommended for a febrile child, it is not associated with an increased risk of febrile seizure (A), development of rash (B), or an increased risk of bacteremia (D).

107. **Correct: D. is not recommended due to a higher potential for adverse effects.**

In general, alternating between acetaminophen and ibuprofen is not recommended as there is a lack of evidence supporting this practice, and it can increase the risk of dosing errors and adverse effects in the infant and child (D).

Incorrect:

There is little clinical evidence supporting the practice of alternating between acetaminophen and ibuprofen for fever reduction (A), including those with high-grade fever (C). The use of cough-and-cold medications is also not recommended for young children as there is little evidence showing any benefit of these products, which can also contain acetaminophen or ibuprofen and lead to overdosing of the child who is also receiving antipyretic therapy (B).

108. **Correct: B. aspirin**

Aspirin use is associated with the development of Reye's syndrome when given to children with fever (B). Reye's syndrome is a rapidly progressing encephalopathy that can include symptoms of vomiting, confusion, seizures, and loss of consciousness.

Incorrect:

Reye's syndrome is not associated with the use of acetaminophen (A), ibuprofen (D), or vitamin C supplements (C) in children with fever.

109. **Correct: D. necrotizing fasciitis.**

Ibuprofen use in the child with varicella infection can increase the risk of necrotizing fasciitis (D). The anti-inflammatory effects of ibuprofen can mask the signs of a serious secondary bacterial infection. Early signs of necrotizing fasciitis include redness, swelling, and severe pain followed by sores or blisters that ooze.

Incorrect:

The use of ibuprofen is not associated with seizure (A) or aseptic meningitis (C) in children with varicella infection. Reye's syndrome is a condition that can result from the use of aspirin in children with fever (B).

Acute Otitis Media

110. **Correct: B. oral amoxicillin**

When antimicrobial therapy is deemed necessary for AOM, an agent with activity against *S pneumoniae* is needed. According to guidelines, first-line therapy would include oral amoxicillin (B) or oral amoxicillin-clavulanate.

Incorrect:

The macrolides such as azithromycin are not recommended for AOM due to elevated rates of resistance by *S pneumoniae* (D). Cephalosporins such as cefuroxime (C) or cefdinir (A) can be considered in children with a penicillin allergy and who would not be able to take amoxicillin.

111. **Correct: A. certain gram-positive and gram-negative bacteria and select respiratory viruses.**

The most common pathogens that cause AOM include the gram-positive *S pneumoniae* as well as gram-negative pathogens *H influenzae* and *M catarrhalis* (A). Certain respiratory viruses, such as RSV, human rhinovirus, and coronavirus, can also be involved.

Incorrect:

Atypical pathogens, such as *M pneumoniae* and *C pneumoniae*, and fungi are rarely implicated in AOM and are more likely to be found in lower respiratory tract infections such as pneumonia (B). Though rhinovirus has been implicated in AOM, the presence of MRSA is not a common finding (C). Though *H influenza* and *M catarrhalis* commonly produce beta-lactamase, the predominant pathogen is *S pneumoniae* (D).

112. **Correct: C. an increase in select vaccination use.**

As a greater number of children are receiving the pneumococcal and Hib vaccines, this has brought down the incidence of AOM over the years (C).

Incorrect:

Earlier detection and treatment of AOM will not affect the incidence of the disease (A) and neither will the availability of more effective treatment options (B). There has been no indication of lower rates of viral infections associated with AOM (D).

113. **Correct: B. oral cefdinir**

When antimicrobial therapy is deemed necessary for the treatment of AOM in a child with penicillin allergy, an appropriate choice would include a cephalosporin. Oral cefdinir would be the most appropriate choice for this child (B).

Incorrect:

Amoxicillin should be avoided due to the presence of a penicillin allergy (C). Azithromycin is not recommended for AOM due to the elevated rates of resistance by *S pneumoniae* against the macrolides (A). TMP-SMX is not recommended for the treatment of AOM but is more commonly used to treat UTIs (D).

114. **Correct: D. beta-lactam allergy**

AOM is one of the most common diagnoses in young children, and about one-third will have three or more episodes by the age of 2 years. Certain risk factors for recurrent AOM have been identified, though beta-lactam allergy, where a systemic allergic reaction is noted with the use of cephalosporins and/or penicillins, is not among them (D).

Incorrect:

Risk factors for recurrent AOM in young children include exposure to secondhand smoke (C), feeding in a supine position, pacifier use beyond 10 months of age (A), and history of a first AOM episode before 3 months of age (B).

115. **Correct: B. eustachian tube dysfunction.**

Knowledge of the pathophysiology of disease is critical in ensuring proper management of the disease and recognition of risk factors. Conditions that cause eustachian tube dysfunction or eustachian tube obstruction will block secretions and allow aspiration of pathogens into the middle ear, causing AOM (B).

Incorrect:

Cigarette smoke exposure is a risk factor for AOM but is not as strong a risk factor as eustachian tube dysfunction (C). A dairy allergy (A) or the use of soy-based infant formula (D) are not risk factors for AOM. However, bottle-fed babies tend to be at higher risk compared to breastfed babies.

116. **Correct: D. oral cefuroxime**

Cefuroxime is a second-generation cephalosporin that has activity against *S pneumoniae* and is recommended for the treatment of AOM in children with a penicillin allergy (D).

Incorrect:

Nitrofurantoin (A) and TMP-SMX (C) exhibit activity against gram-negative pathogens and are generally used in the treatment of UTIs, as they are effective against *E coli*. Though the macrolides do have activity against gram-positive bacteria, they are not recommended treatment options for AOM due to elevated rates of resistance by *S pneumoniae* against these agents (B).

117. **Correct: D. administer intramuscular (IM) ceftriaxone**

In cases when there is an inadequate response to oral amoxicillin treatment after 48 to 72 hours, treatment should be switched to either oral amoxicillin-clavulanate or IM ceftriaxone for 3 days (D).

Incorrect:

For an infection that is resistant to amoxicillin, it will be very likely that cross-resistance to ampicillin will occur, and so ampicillin would not be useful for this infection (A). Azithromycin (B) and clindamycin (C) are not recommended agents for the treatment of AOM, either as first-line or with treatment failure.

118. **Correct: A. bulging of the TM, and C. otalgia**

The diagnosis of AOM in children will involve moderate or severe bulging of the TM or new onset of otorrhea. Other signs can include mild bulging of the TM (A) with recent onset of otalgia (C) or a combination of intense TM erythema with otalgia.

Incorrect:

A finding of air bubbles that are visible behind the TM is more likely a sign of OME and not AOM (B). Anterior cervical lymphadenopathy can occur with AOM on the affected side; however, this is not a requirement for diagnosis (D).

119. **Correct: C. tugging on the ear**

In a nonverbal child, signs of ear pain associated with AOM can include tugging, holding, or rubbing the ear (C).

Incorrect:

The most specific sign of AOM in a nonverbal child is tugging or rubbing of the affected ear. Loss of appetite (A) and nasal discharge (D) can accompany AOM but are not specific for this particular type of infection. Similarly, altered stooling can be associated with an infection but is not specific for AOM (B).

120. **Correct: C. ear discharge**

OME results from fluid in the middle ear but without signs of acute infection. OME typically would not include signs of fever or ear discharge (C).

Incorrect:

OME can occur following an episode of AOM and results in the persistence of fluid in the middle ear (A). The condition is not associated with an acute infection but can result in limited pain (B), discomfort, or itch (D) in the affected ear.

121. **Correct: A. age greater than 6 months, and C. nonsevere illness**

For some children who present with AOM, a watchful waiting approach without antibiotic therapy can be appropriate. In these children, analgesia can be provided, and follow-up must be ensured with the ability to start antimicrobial therapy within 48 to 72 hours if symptoms persist or worsen. Key criteria for this approach include children over the age of 6 months (A) who have nonsevere (C) and unilateral AOM.

Incorrect:

Children younger than 6 months with AOM should receive antimicrobial therapy due to the risk of severe complications, including sepsis. Additionally, children with bilateral involvement (B) and severe findings should receive antimicrobial therapy. If AOM is presumptively caused by a bacterial infection, an antimicrobial should be used, as infections caused by *S pneumoniae* have a low rate of spontaneous resolution and can lead to serious complications in children (D).

122. Correct: A. "watch and wait" therapy.
Management of OME is typically a "watch and wait" approach, as the majority of cases will eventually resolve within 3 months without any specific treatment (A).
Incorrect:
As OME is typically present without an acute infection, the use of antimicrobial therapy is not warranted (B). The use of antihistamines (C) or a mucolytic (D) is not helpful for this condition.

123. Correct: A. a high rate of beta-lactamase production.
M catarrhalis is a gram-negative organism with its predominant mode of antibiotic resistance being beta-lactamase production (A). This mechanism allows resistance to beta-lactams, such as penicillin and amoxicillin, when a beta-lactamase inhibitor (e.g., clavulanate) is not used.
Incorrect:
M catarrhalis is a gram-negative bacteria (D) that produces beta-lactamase as its predominant mode of resistance, rather than utilizing altered protein binding sites (B). AOM caused by this pathogen have high rates of spontaneous resolution but can also be easily treated with a cephalosporin or beta-lactam/beta-lactamase agent, such as amoxicillin-clavulanate (C).

124. Correct: C. an approximate 50% spontaneous resolution rate when it is the AOM causative organism.
Approximately half of AOM episodes caused by *H influenzae* will resolve spontaneously without antimicrobial therapy (C).
Incorrect:
H influenzae is a gram-negative organism (D) that utilizes beta-lactamase production as the predominant form of antimicrobial resistance (A), rather than altered protein binding sites (B).

125. Correct: B. antimicrobial resistance because of altered protein binding sites.
S pneumoniae causes approximately half of AOM episodes and is the least likely pathogen to have spontaneous resolution. Its predominant mode of resistance is through altered protein binding sites (B).
Incorrect:
S pneumoniae is a gram-positive organism (D) that does not typically produce beta-lactamase (A). This pathogen is not usually associated with skin infections, which are more likely caused by group A streptococci or *S aureus* (C).

126. Correct: C. 8 weeks
OME can occur in children following AOM resulting from accumulation of fluid in the middle ear. In about 80% of children, OME will clear within 8 weeks (C). If the condition persists for a longer period, there is a risk for the development of communication problems and so further evaluation and management should be considered.

127. Correct: D. referral for tympanostomy consideration.
Persistent OME can lead to communication problems and a delay in language development. Guidelines recommend that clinicians can offer tympanostomy to children with chronic bilateral OME (3 months or longer) with documented hearing difficulty or with substantial symptoms likely attributable to OME (e.g., balance problems, behavioral problems, ear discomfort, reduced quality of life) (D).
Incorrect:
Antimicrobial therapy is not helpful in OME as there is no active infection (A). The use of antihistamines (typically used for allergic reactions) (B) or an oral decongestant (typically used for rhinosinusitis) (C) are not warranted in the management of OME.

128. Correct: A. delay in language development.
Persistent and prolonged OME can be accompanied by a language delay (A) associated with hearing loss. In these cases, tympanostomy can be considered to relieve the condition.
Incorrect:
OME is not associated with an active infection and so would not increase the risk of meningitis (C) or recurrent sinusitis (B). OME is also not associated with the development of nasal polyps (D).

129. Correct: D. assessing for the presence of MEE.
TM insufflation, usually done with a pneumatic otoscope, is not a necessary part of making an AOM diagnosis. However, it can be useful in determining the presence of MEE (D).
Incorrect:
TM insufflation is not a necessary part of the diagnostic workup for AOM and provides limited useful information other than the presence of MEE. TM insufflation cannot specifically detect a bacterial infection (A), and it cannot be used to measure the severity of AOM (C) or offer information on the potential for hearing loss (B).

130. Correct: B. air trapped behind the TM
When evaluating a child with suspected OME, physical examination will often detect air bubbles behind the TM as air is trapped in the middle ear fluid, which is usually yellow (B).
Incorrect:
During OME, there is no active infection occurring, and so there is no TM redness (A) or fever (D).

Examination will reveal the bony landmarks (C), though TM mobility is usually somewhat limited.

Acute Bacterial Rhinosinusitis

131. Correct: A. URI signs and symptoms persisting beyond 10 days

Clinicians should be able to differentiate between ABRS and a viral URI, as management of each of these conditions is very different. ABRS is characterized by a worsening URI course that can include double sickening and with symptoms that persist after 7 to 10 days (A). Symptoms can include nasal discharge, daytime cough, bad breath, fatigue, headache, and decreased appetite.

Incorrect:

A key finding in ABRS is symptoms that persist or worsen beyond 7 to 10 days. Nasal discharge that changes from clear to purulent to clear suggests improvement in symptoms and likely a viral origin (B). A short period of headache and myalgia in association with respiratory symptoms also suggests a viral infection, such as influenza (C). A persistent congested cough beyond 7 days of onset of a URI suggests the development of a lower respiratory infection and not ABRS (D).

132. Correct: B. acute worsening of respiratory symptoms, and C. new fever occurring 6 to 7 days after signs of URI

Double sickening is a common finding in ABRS in children and is defined as acute worsening of respiratory symptoms (B) or new fever at days 6 to 7 of URI (C).

Incorrect:

Nasal discharge that changes from clear to purulent to clear suggests improvement in symptoms and likely a viral origin (A). Worsening of respiratory symptoms is indicative of double sickening and not the presence of a persistent cough (D).

133. Correct: B. *S pneumoniae*

The most common pathogens to cause ABRS include *S pneumoniae* and *H influenzae*, each causing about 30% of episodes (B).

Incorrect:

Other causes of ABRS include *M catarrhalis* (C), *S aureus* (D), and anaerobes. *M pneumoniae* (A) and *C pneumoniae*, common pathogens in community-acquired pneumonia, are not normally implicated in ABRS.

134. Correct: D. history of β-thalassemia minor.

A number of risk factors for ABRS have been identified. However, β-thalassemia minor, a genetic condition that results in a mild microcytic, hypochromic anemia, is not a contributor to infectious disease such as ABRS (D).

Incorrect:

Conditions that alter the normal cleansing mechanisms of the sinuses are risk factors for ABRS. These include viral infection (A), allergy (B), exposure to tobacco smoke (C), as well as abnormalities in the sinus structure.

135. Correct: A. amoxicillin-clavulanate

First-line therapy for ABRS in an otherwise well child with no penicillin allergy can include oral high-dose amoxicillin or oral amoxicillin-clavulanate (A).

Incorrect:

In the presence of penicillin allergy, clindamycin can be used as first-line treatment, but not in combination with cefixime (B). Doxycycline is not recommended for use in children younger than 8 years as it can lead to permanent staining of teeth (C). The fluoroquinolones are not considered first-line treatment for ABRS, though they can be considered in treatment failure or when drug-resistant *S pneumoniae* is suspected (D).

136. Correct: A. continued observation

Continued observation is an appropriate choice in children with nonsevere symptoms and who are not experiencing fever, pain, or purulent discharge (A). If symptoms persist beyond 7 to 10 days or begin worsening, then antimicrobial therapy can be considered.

Incorrect:

For this patient, continued observation is an appropriate course of management. If symptoms begin to worsen, antimicrobial therapy can be considered with first-line therapy consisting of oral high-dose amoxicillin or amoxicillin-clavulanate. Levofloxacin (B) would not be considered a first-line agent. Clindamycin monotherapy can be considered in the presence of a penicillin allergy but would not be used in combination with cefixime (C). Injectable ceftriaxone is not a recommended treatment for ABRS (D).

137. Correct: B. oral cefdinir

With a diagnosis of ABRS and a parent request for antimicrobial therapy, cefdinir represents the most appropriate option in the presence of a possible penicillin allergy (B).

Incorrect:

A watchful waiting approach is appropriate with joint decision making with the parents or caregivers. Since the parents are requesting antimicrobial therapy in this case, an antimicrobial should be prescribed (A). Amoxicillin should be avoided due to a possible penicillin allergy (D). Levofloxacin is not considered a first-line agent but can be considered with treatment failure or if there is a risk of drug-resistant infection (C).

138. Correct: D. Imaging can be considered with treatment failure.

ABRS is primarily a clinical diagnosis that does not require any additional tests or imaging studies. However, CT or MRI can be considered in patients who fail therapy with second-line agents or when the diagnosis is in question (D).

Incorrect:
Routine imaging is not needed for an ABRS diagnosis for children of any age (A). Imaging can be considered following treatment failure and not prior to starting antimicrobial therapy (B). Imaging would not be performed prior to double sickening, as an ABRS diagnosis would more likely be made following double sickening (C).

139. **Correct: D. there is little evidence that decongestants provide any benefit in children with ABRS.**
The use of decongestants in children with ABRS is not recommended, as there is a lack of evidence demonstrating any benefit of these products (D).
Incorrect:
Decongestants are not generally recommended for use in children with ABRS, and oral formulations are not preferred over nasal sprays (A). Though nasal decongestants can sometimes improve comfort in a child, these medications should not be used for more than 4 to 5 days due to risk of rebound vasodilation (B). These medications offer no proven benefit in ABRS and will not hasten resolution of symptoms (C).

Influenza

140. **Correct: D. Its use is recommended for members of households with a high-risk patient.**
The injectable IIV is recommended for immunization of any individual over 6 months of age. Vaccination is particularly important for those at high risk of complications from influenza or those in close contact with high-risk individuals (D).
Incorrect:
All influenza vaccines can be given to individuals with reported mild allergic reaction to eggs (A). IIV can be used to vaccinate individuals 6 months and older (B) and does not contain live virus (C), unlike the live-attenuated virus vaccine (LAIV).

141. **Correct: C. localized immunization reactions are common.**
Similar to other injectable vaccines, a localized immunization reaction is common following vaccination with IIV that can cause redness and soreness at the site of injection (C).
Incorrect:
Vaccine effectiveness is variable and will depend on patient factors as well as the predominant flu strains during the influenza season. In healthy individuals, effectiveness can range up to 70% to 80% (A). The influenza vaccine can be administered while the patient has a mild illness and/or is taking an antimicrobial (B). A flu-like syndrome is not a typical reaction following vaccination since there is no live virus contained in the vaccine (D).

142. **Correct: A. two doses 4 weeks or more apart should be given.**
All children between the ages of 6 months and 8 years who have not received a prior influenza vaccine should receive two doses that are separated by at least 4 weeks apart (A).
Incorrect:
For this 7-year-old who has not received a prior influenza vaccination, it is recommended to administer two doses separated by at least 4 weeks for optimal effectiveness (B). Though children are at higher risk of influenza-related complications, those at highest risk of hospitalization include children younger than 2 years or older adults (65 years and older) (C). There are no warnings or precautions regarding administering the vaccine in the presence of a shellfish allergy (D).

143. **Correct: A. compared with school-aged children, younger children (24 months old and younger) have an increased risk of seasonal influenza-related hospitalization.**
Among children, those who are 24 months old and younger are at the highest risk of influenza-related complications and hospitalization (A). Therefore, it is imperative that all children 6 months and older get vaccinated as well as any other individual who has close contact with young children.
Incorrect:
For IIV vaccines, the full adult dose is usually given beginning at 3 years of age rather than 4 years (B). All children 6 months and older should be immunized, including well children (C). There is no correlation between vaccination and increased risk of eczema and antibiotic allergies (D).

144. **Correct: C. It should not be given when nasal congestion is present.**
The LAIV is available for use in individuals from 2 to 49 years of age. However, it should not be administered when the individual has nasal congestion as this can interfere with delivery of the vaccine to the nasal mucosa (C). In these cases, vaccination should be deferred or an alternative age-appropriate vaccine should be used.
Incorrect:
The LAIV vaccine should not be used in immunocompromised individuals or during pregnancy (A). The vaccine is appropriate for individuals between 2 and 49 years but not for those younger than 2 years (B). The vaccine can be used in individuals with reported egg allergy (D).

145. **Correct: C. a 4-month-old infant who was born at 32 weeks' gestation**
Influenza vaccination is recommended for all individuals 6 months and older. Therefore, vaccination would not be appropriate for the 4-month-old infant until the baby reaches 6 months extrauterine age (C). To protect the newborn, all individuals in close contact with the child should be vaccinated, including all caregivers and household contacts.

Incorrect:
Mild, hive-form reaction to eggs is not a contraindication for influenza vaccination, and any age-appropriate vaccine can be used (A). Vaccination during pregnancy is encouraged as it can transfer some protection to the newborn as well as protect the pregnant woman (B). Vaccination is strongly encouraged for any close contacts to infants under 6 months old as they cannot get vaccinated and are vulnerable to infection (D).

146. Correct: B. respiratory droplet.
The most common mode of transmission of the influenza virus is from person to person via respiratory droplet from an infected person, typically from a cough or sneeze (B).
Incorrect:
The influenza virus can live on surfaces for a limited amount of time (A) and can also be spread person to person through saliva contact (C). However, it is more likely to be transmitted through respiratory droplets from a cough or sneeze by an infected person. Skin-to-skin contact is an unlikely mode of transmission for this virus (D).

147. Correct: B. a 4-year-old with asthma
In addition to children younger than 2 years of age, those with chronic health problems, particularly chronic airway disease such as asthma, are at the highest risk of developing influenza-related complications (B).
Incorrect:
A prior history of AOM that has resolved would not necessarily increase the risk of influenza-related complications (A). The 9-year-old living with a grandparent with COPD is not at higher risk, though the individual with COPD is at high risk and should take proper precautions to prevent infection (C). The 6-year-old entering his first year of school is at higher risk of being exposed to new viruses but is not at higher risk of developing influenza-related complications (D).

148. Correct: C. the unborn child acquires some protection against influenza up to 6 months after birth.
Influenza vaccination is recommended at any stage during pregnancy as the mother is at higher risk of developing influenza-related complications. Additionally, vaccination will provide some protection to the newborn after birth (C).
Incorrect:
Use of the inactivated virus vaccines that do not contain live virus have no risk of spreading the virus to the fetus (A). Immunization can be done during any trimester of pregnancy, especially if pregnancy occurs during flu season (B). LAIV is contraindicated during pregnancy due to the theoretical risk of transmission of the virus to the fetus (D).

149. Correct: C. intussusception.
Intussusception is caused when a section of intestines invaginates into the adjoining intestinal lumen, causing

bowel obstruction. This condition is not related to influenza (C).
Incorrect:
Influenza-related complications in very young children can include otitis media, bronchiolitis (A), croup, reactive airway disease, febrile seizures, secondary bacterial pneumonia, rhabdomyolysis, myocarditis, toxic shock syndrome, Guillain-Barré syndrome, Reye's syndrome (B), and sudden death (D).

150 to 152. Yes or No

150. Correct: Yes

151. Correct: No

152. Correct: Yes
Antiviral medication should be administered as soon as possible to individuals at very high risk of influenza-related complications when they have confirmed or suspected influenza. Those younger than 2 years old are at particularly high risk of complications and should receive antiviral therapy with suspicion of influenza (150). Children with chronic respiratory conditions, such as asthma, are also at high risk of complications and should receive antiviral therapy (152). The 9-year-old is likely at the later stage of infection and showing signs of improvement and likely does not need antiviral medications (151). Additionally, antivirals are most effective when taken within 48 hours of the start of infection and would likely not provide any benefit during later stages of infection.

153. Correct: D. a 2-year-old who was vaccinated less than 2 weeks ago
Postexposure antiviral prophylaxis can be considered for children 3 months of age and older who are unvaccinated and who are at very high risk of developing complications from influenza or are household contacts of a person at very high risk for complications. Though individuals who are vaccinated do not typically require postexposure chemoprophylaxis, the immune response to immunization can take up to 2 weeks to provide protection against influenza. Therefore, the 2-year-old who was recently vaccinated and is still at high risk of complications is the most likely candidate for postexposure prophylaxis (D).
Incorrect:
Postexposure prophylaxis is typically not needed in individuals who have been vaccinated. This includes the 6-year-old who received two doses this year (due to this being the first year he is vaccinated against influenza) (A), the 9-year-old (B), or the 11-year-old who had the flu last year (C).

Croup

154. Correct: B. *H influenzae*.
Croup is caused by a variety of viruses but would not be caused by *H influenzae*, which is a gram-negative bacterium that can cause various respiratory tract infections (B).

Incorrect:
The most common cause of croup includes the parainfluenza viruses (A). Other viruses that can cause croup include adenovirus (C), coronavirus, rhinovirus (D), and RSV.

155. **Correct: A. expiratory wheeze.**
Croup is associated with upper airway obstruction that can cause stridor and a barking cough. Expiratory wheeze is more likely caused by lower airway obstruction due to conditions such as asthma or COPD (A).
Incorrect:
Common findings in the child with croup include fever (D), stridor (B), and a bark-like cough (C).

156. **Correct: A. this is largely a clinical diagnosis.**
Croup is primarily a clinical diagnosis that can be ascertained by patient history and physical examination (A). Laboratory and imaging studies are not needed or helpful unless there is a concern about an alternative diagnosis.
Incorrect:
Laboratory tests are not needed in the diagnosis of croup and are typically within normal limits (B). A chest radiograph is not needed to confirm a diagnosis of croup (C). A urine nitrite test can be used to identify a gram-negative UTI but would not detect croup (D).

157. **Correct: D. systemic corticosteroid**
All children with croup are recommended to receive systemic corticosteroid therapy, preferably a single dose of dexamethasone (D). Corticosteroid therapy is effective in rapidly diminishing symptoms and reduces the frequency of subsequent medical visits.
Incorrect:
Antimicrobial therapy is not warranted for this viral infection (A). Antiviral therapy is not helpful in the treatment of croup (C). A LABA is useful for lower airway obstruction, such as asthma, but would not be effective in upper airway disease (B).

Pneumonia

158. **Correct: B. a respiratory virus.**
Most cases of pneumonia in children 3 months to 18 years are caused by a respiratory virus (B), including RSV, metapneumovirus, rhinovirus, influenza virus, and adenovirus.
Incorrect:
Bacteria are the causative pathogen in only a minority of pneumonia cases in children. The most common bacterial pathogens include *S pneumoniae* (D), *M pneumoniae* (A), and *H influenzae* (C). *S aureus* is a rare cause of pneumonia in children.

159. **Correct: A. oral amoxicillin**
First-line treatment for a child with CAP and who will be treated in the outpatient setting is typically oral amoxicillin (A). Alternatives can include amoxicillin-clavulanate or azithromycin.

Incorrect:
The tetracyclines, such as doxycycline, should be avoided in children younger than 8 years of age due to a risk of permanent staining of teeth (B). TMP-SMX is not recommended for the treatment of respiratory tract infections but can be used for UTIs (C). Levofloxacin is not a preferred first-line agent but can be considered with penicillin allergy or in infections caused by drug-resistant *S pneumoniae* (D).

160. **Correct: D. tachypnea**
Tachypnea, or elevated respiratory rate, is the most sensitive and specific finding in children with pneumonia (D). The diagnosis of lower respiratory tract disease should be considered with a respiratory rate exceeding 50/min in children younger than 1 year and a rate exceeding 40/min in children older than 1 year.
Incorrect:
For children with CAP, a report of pleuritic chest pain (A) or dyspnea (C) would not typically be reported. Cough associated with pneumonia in children is typically dry and without sputum production (B).

161. **Correct: D. clarithromycin**
The macrolides, including azithromycin and clarithromycin (D), exhibit activity against atypical pathogens such as *C pneumoniae* and *M pneumoniae*. The fluoroquinolones are also effective against atypical pathogens.
Incorrect:
Beta-lactam agents, such as amoxicillin (A), and cephalosporins such as cefprozil (B) and ceftriaxone (C) are not effective against infections caused by atypical pathogens.

162. **Correct: D. parenteral antimicrobial therapy used for initial therapy.**
Children who are generally stable and able to tolerate oral medications do not require hospitalization and can be treated in the outpatient setting. These children would not require initial treatment with parenteral medication but can start treatment with oral formulations (D).
Incorrect:
When deciding whether a child with pneumonia can be treated in the outpatient setting, certain criteria should be fulfilled. These include the ability to tolerate oral medications (A) as well as oral fluids to remain hydrated (C). There must be a competent caregiver, and the child should also be able to return for follow-up, usually within 1 to 3 days of starting treatment (B).

163. **Correct: A. chest x-ray, and D. CBC with differential.**
The minimum diagnostic approach for a child with suspected pneumonia should include a chest x-ray (A) and CBC with differential (D). Other diagnostic tests are not typically needed for a stable child who will likely be treated in the outpatient setting.

Incorrect:

For the severely ill child who will likely be transferred to the emergency department and/or admitted for hospitalization, additional testing would be performed, particularly to check for sepsis. This can include procalcitonin (B) and lactate (C).

Bronchiolitis

164. Correct: B. false

Bronchiolitis most commonly occurs in children younger than 2 years of age with the majority of episodes occurring between November and April (B).

165. Correct: D. children younger than age 2 years

Bronchiolitis usually affects children younger than 2 years of age (D) with a peak incidence at age 3 to 6 months. RSV is the most common cause of bronchiolitis, with over half of all infants exposed to this virus by their first birthday.

166. Correct: C. RSV.

Bronchiolitis is typically caused by a viral infection. RSV is the most common cause of bronchiolitis, with over half of all infants exposed to this virus by their first birthday (C).

Incorrect:

Other common causes of bronchiolitis include parainfluenza virus (B), influenza virus, and adenovirus. Coxsackie virus is an enterovirus that is less likely to cause bronchiolitis (D). *H influenza* is a gram-negative bacterium that is not typically a cause of bronchiolitis (A).

167. Correct: C. wheezing.

A key component of bronchiolitis is the narrowing and obstruction of small airways due to secretion of mucus, peribronchiolar lymphocytic infiltrate, and submucosal edema. The main result from this is wheezing (C) and cough.

Incorrect:

Additional findings of bronchiolitis can include tachypnea, mild fever (A), conjunctivitis (D), and pharyngitis. Vomiting is not a typical sign of bronchiolitis, though this can be a result of excessive mucus production and persistent coughing (B).

168. Correct: A. nasal washing antigen test

A rapid antigen test of nasal washing can be used to identify RSV (A). This test is highly sensitive in young children but loses sensitivity in older children and adults. A real-time RT-PCR (rRT-PCR) test is also available that offers improved sensitivity to antigen testing.

Incorrect:

Early detection of RSV can be important in addressing potential outbreaks in day cares or other similar settings. Laboratory tests are available to rapidly detect RSV (D). Respiratory samples are used to detect the virus, rather than blood (B) or urine (C). Viral culture can be performed to detect the presence of virus,

though other more rapid and convenient tests are preferred.

169. Correct: B. supportive care.

In most children with bronchiolitis, supportive care is usually sufficient as the infection typically resolves in 2 to 3 weeks (B).

Incorrect:

The use of antiviral therapy (e.g., ribavirin) (A), beta-2 agonist therapy (C), and corticosteroids (D) is controversial in the treatment of bronchiolitis as there is a lack of evidence supporting their use. For children with underlying reactive airway disease, the use of asthma medications can be effective in managing symptoms.

170. Correct: C. bradycardia.

Bradycardia, or low heart rate, is not a typical finding in children with bronchiolitis (C).

Incorrect:

The most common findings in bronchiolitis include cough, wheezing, tachypnea (abnormally rapid breathing) (B), mild fever, conjunctivitis (D), and pharyngitis (A).

171. Correct: C. a 5-month-old born at 39 weeks' gestation who now has recurrent AOM.

Palivizumab is a monoclonal antibody that can be used to protect certain high-risk infants from RSV infection. This product is usually reserved for infants born before 29 weeks' gestation as well as infants with certain chronic diseases. It would not be needed for an infant born at full term with a history of AOM (C).

Incorrect:

Palivizumab can be considered for prophylaxis in infants born before 29 weeks' gestation (A) as well as those with chronic conditions, such as congenital heart disease (B) or chronic respiratory disease (D). Treatment is initiated prior to the start of the infant's first RSV season.

172. Correct: C. immediately prior to the RSV season.

Palivizumab can be considered for prophylaxis against RSV infection in high-risk infants. The medication is administered as monthly injections and should start prior to commencement of RSV season (C). Doses should continue throughout the RSV season.

Asthma

173. Correct: C. chronic airway inflammation with superimposed bronchospasm

Asthma is best described as a disease involving chronic airway inflammation that is associated with a history of respiratory symptoms that can include wheeze, dyspnea, chest tightness, and cough that can vary over time in intensity (C). Bronchospasm often results as a consequence of airway inflammation.

Incorrect:

Asthma is associated with chronic rather than intermittent airway inflammation (A). Bronchospasm is often the result of airway inflammation and not the other way around (B). Airway constriction will vary over time and will depend on disease progression, exacerbation, as well as adherence to medical treatment (D).

174. **Correct: C. spirometry measurement.**

During an asthma flare, an objective measure of airflow obstruction is needed to assess severity of the episode and help guide treatment. Spirometry is the most common lung function test used to monitor asthma and provides a rapid method to evaluate changes to the airways (C).

Incorrect:

A chest radiograph is not needed during an asthma flare unless there is a suspicion for pneumonia (such as presence of fever and/or evidence of consolidation) (A). Oxygen saturation will fall late during an asthma flare and will not be useful during the early stage of a flare (B). A sputum smear for WBC or culture and susceptibility testing is not needed for an asthma flare (D).

175. **Correct: C. a short course of oral prednisolone.**

During an asthma flare, a short course of oral corticosteroid can be helpful to relieve airway inflammation, which is evident in this patient with an elevated respiratory rate (C).

Incorrect:

Theophylline is a bronchodilator used as controller medication and is not recommended to treat an asthma flare (A). The LABA, salmeterol, does not have a role in treating an asthma flare but is used in combination with ICS to prevent bronchospasm (B). Similarly, montelukast is used as a controller agent and not a rescue medication during an asthma flare (D).

176. **Correct: C. consistent morning sputum production**

The production of sputum is not required for a diagnosis of asthma, particularly daily production of sputum (C). An alternative diagnosis should be investigated.

Incorrect:

Asthma symptoms can worsen at nighttime, including nocturnal cough in children (A). Additional common findings in asthma are cough and wheeze after exercise (B) and respiratory tract infections that become more severe and take a longer duration to clear (D).

177. **Correct: B. excessive albuterol use is a risk factor for asthma death.**

Excessive use of SABA (i.e., multiple times daily or greater than two canisters per month) suggests that asthma is not well controlled and is a risk factor for asthma-related death (B). The best approach for this patient is to initiate ICS along with a short course of oral corticosteroid therapy to control airway inflammation.

Incorrect:

Excessive use of SABA indicates that her asthma is not well controlled and is a risk factor for asthma-related death (A). An ICS would be the preferred approach to reduce airway inflammation, which can be combined with a LABA (C). LABAs should not generally be used as monotherapy but in combination with ICS. The goal of asthma therapy is to minimize symptoms so that the condition has little to no impact on normal daily activities and allows the child to fully participate in active play and recreational activities (D).

178. **Correct: B. controller to inhibit inflammatory process.**

LTMs, such as montelukast, are used as controller medications that inhibit the inflammatory actions of leukotrienes (B). These agents are generally used as add-on therapy to ICS in moderate or severe persistent asthma.

Incorrect:

LTMs are not used as reliever medications to treat acute inflammation (D) or acute bronchospasm (C). They are used as controller medications to reduce inflammation, rather than prevent bronchospasm (A).

179. **Correct: D. rural residence**

Several risk factors have been identified for asthma-related death. Though urban residence is a risk factor for more severe asthma, rural residence is not a risk factor for asthma-related death (D).

Incorrect:

Recognizing risk factors for asthma-related death can help guide management decisions. Risk factors include previous severe exacerbations, hospitalization or emergency department visit for asthma in the past month (A), greater than two canisters SABA use per month, current or recent withdrawal from systemic corticosteroids (B), poor patient perception of asthma symptoms (C), illicit drug use, low socioeconomic status, and certain comorbidities.

180. **Correct: C. remind him that with appropriate asthma care, he should be capable of participating in physical education class.**

The goal for patients with asthma is to have symptoms well controlled that will allow full participation in sports and activities as well as have minimal impact on normal activities of daily living (C). At this visit, the patient's asthma control should be evaluated, such as with the Asthma Control Test, and his medications adjusted to ensure full participation in sports and physical education class.

Incorrect:

Patients with asthma should not be routinely excused from sports participation but should be managed to attain the goal of well-controlled asthma. The patient should be evaluated for asthma control and the medications adjusted accordingly. Exercise will not typically trigger symptoms with well-controlled asthma (A). Allergic asthma is more commonly caused by indoor allergens, such as dust mites, rather than pollen exposure (B). However, only a subset of asthma patients will experience allergic asthma (D), and referral to a specialist can be considered for evaluation and potential treatment with immunotherapy.

181. **Correct: C. in about 1 to 2 weeks.**
There is often a delay of several days between the initiation of ICS or LTM therapy and improvement in asthma symptoms (C). For those with evidence of inflammation due to asthma, an improved outcome can be achieved with a short course of oral corticosteroid at the time of initiating ICS.
Incorrect:
An immediate effect from ICS or LTM therapy should not be expected as there is often a delay of 1 to 2 weeks before the full therapeutic potential is observed (A, B, D).

182. **Correct: B. has the ability to provide greater bronchodilation with a lower dose.**
Albuterol and levalbuterol are both SABAs used as rescue medications in asthma. Levalbuterol is a single isomer of the racemic mixture found in albuterol. Levalbuterol can provide greater bronchodilation at a reduced dose, thus potentially improving its tolerability (B).
Incorrect:
Albuterol and levalbuterol are both SABAs with the same mechanism of action (A). These agents cause bronchodilation and not anti-inflammatory effects as seen with ICS (C). Levalbuterol is not contraindicated in children (D).

183. **Correct: B. with evidence of concomitant bacterial infection.**
Antimicrobial therapy is not routinely recommended during acute asthma flare unless there is evidence of concomitant bacterial infection, such as pneumonia (B). Signs of infection can include fever and consolidation observed with a chest radiograph.
Incorrect:
Antimicrobial therapy should be reserved for when there is a confirmed or suspected bacterial infection and should not be used routinely (A). Frequent asthma flares would suggest poorly controlled asthma and not infection (C). Sputum production is not a good indicator for bacterial infection (D).

184. **Correct: A. attenuated lung development.**
A major concern with poorly controlled asthma in young children is the possibility of the lungs not growing to full potential, which can have permanent effects (A).
Incorrect:
There is less concern with the possibility of chronic tracheitis (B), sleep apnea (C), or alveolar destruction (D) in children with poorly controlled asthma.

185. **Correct: B. expiratory wheezing**
Characteristic findings of an asthma flare include a progressive increase in shortness of breath, cough, expiratory wheezing (B), or chest tightness, and it is associated with decreased lung function. In asthma exacerbations, breath sounds are often reduced, and hyperinflation is present because of significant air trapping.

Incorrect:
Inspiratory stridor is more associated with upper airway obstruction rather than lower airway obstruction (A). Purulent sputum is not a typical finding in asthma, even during an acute flare (C). A loud "barking" cough is not characteristic of asthma but is more likely associated with an upper airway condition such as croup (D).

186. **Correct: C. respiratory rate less than 30/minute.**
During respiratory distress, it would be expected to have an elevated respiratory rate as the child attempts to expel air out of the lungs during a flare (C).
Incorrect:
Signs of severe or life-threatening asthma flare include an inability to speak or drink, central cyanosis, confusion (B) or drowsiness (A), a softer, shorter cry (D), oxygen saturation less than 92%, silent chest on auscultation, and pulse rate greater than 200 bpm (0 to 3 years) or greater than 180 bpm (4 to 5 years).

187. **Correct: A. well-controlled asthma.**
Use of the ACT can provide a simple and convenient way for the health-care provider to evaluate how well asthma symptoms were controlled in the past 4 weeks. The total score can range from 0 to 25. A score of 20 or higher indicates asthma is well controlled (A).
Incorrect:
When conducting the ACT, a score of 20 or higher indicates well-controlled asthma. A score of 16 to 19 suggests asthma that is not well controlled (B), while a score of 15 or less indicates very poorly controlled asthma (C, D).

188. **Correct: A. nighttime awakening about once a week.**
With well-controlled asthma, nighttime awakenings should occur two or fewer times each month and not weekly (A).
Incorrect:
Other indications of well-controlled asthma include no interference with normal activities (C), use of SABA two or fewer days per week (D), and asthma symptoms occurring 2 or fewer days per week (B).

189. **Correct: B. offer anti-inflammatory effect similar to ICS.**
LAMAs can be an effective treatment option for children with a history of flares, as they provide bronchodilator effect similar to LABAs. They do not offer anti-inflammatory effect such as ICS (B).
Incorrect:
LAMAs are generally used as add-on therapy (C) to help reduce the frequency of asthma flares in children with a history of flares (A). Tiotropium is not indicated for use as a rescue medication, due to its pharmacokinetics (D).

190. **C. All children and close contacts 6 months and older should receive annual seasonal influenza vaccination.**
Children with asthma are at greater risk of complications from influenza, and so it is essential that children

with asthma along with all close contacts to the child receive annual immunization against seasonal influenza. Vaccination is recommended for all individuals 6 months and older (C).

Incorrect:

All children 6 months and older, including those with asthma, should be vaccinated annually for seasonal influenza (A). The LAIV vaccine is not recommended in children with asthma, though the injectable influenza vaccine (IIV) can be used (B). Children younger than 8 years who have not received any influenza vaccine previously should receive two doses taken at least 4 weeks apart. There are no specific guidelines for multiple doses required in children with asthma (D).

Urinary Tract Infection

191. Correct: B. as much as 20%

Rates of UTI are generally lower in boys compared to girls. Uncircumcised boys can have higher rates of UTI compared to circumcised boys, by as much as 20%, but this difference decreases dramatically by the time the boy is 1 to 2 years old (B). This potential health issue is not considered to be an indication for routine male circumcision.

Incorrect:

The rates of UTI in uncircumcised infant boys can be up to 20% higher compared to circumcised boys (A, C, D).

192. Correct: B. fever

The presentation of UTI in a young child can be without the classic symptoms observed in older children and adults. UTI in younger children typically manifests with irritability, lethargy, and fever with no obvious focal infection source (B).

Incorrect:

UTI in a young child can present without the classic symptoms of urinary frequency and urgency (A), suprapubic tenderness (C) or flank pain, or nausea and vomiting (D).

193. Correct: B. *E coli*

The most common uropathogen regardless of age and gender is *E coli* (B).

Incorrect:

Other uropathogens that can cause a UTI, though less frequently than *E coli*, can include the gram-negative organisms *P aeruginosa* (A), *K pneumoniae* (C), and *P mirabilis* (D).

194. Correct: D. *Staphylococcus saprophyticus*.

The ability to reduce urinary nitrate to nitrite is found in gram-negative bacteria. *S saprophyticus* is a gram-positive organism, and an infection caused by this organism would not result in a positive nitrite test (D).

Incorrect:

A positive nitrite test can reveal UTI caused by gram-negative pathogens such as *E coli* (A), *Proteus* species (B), and *K pneumoniae* (C).

195. Correct: A. suprapubic aspiration

The "clean catch" method is the best noninvasive method of obtaining a urine sample but can be difficult with younger pre-toilet-trained children. Suprapubic bladder aspiration yields the specimen that is least likely to be contaminated (A). However, this invasive method can cause anxiety and fear for the child and parents and requires special provider skill.

Incorrect:

When suprapubic aspiration cannot be performed, the next acceptable method is transurethral bladder catheterization (B). Urine collection bags (C) or sanitary pads offer additional noninvasive methods of collection but have a high rate of skin or fecal contamination. A diaper sample is not recommended for sample collection due to high skin and fecal contamination (D).

196. Correct: C. the use of an oral third-generation cephalosporin is acceptable if GI function is intact.

Treatment for UTI should exhibit activity against gram-negative bacteria. First-line treatment for a stable child who can tolerate oral medications and is likely to be treated in an outpatient setting can include oral amoxicillin, TMP-SMX, or a third-generation cephalosporin (C).

Incorrect:

Gram-negative bacteria, particularly *E coli*, are the most likely cause of UTI regardless of age or gender (A). A parenteral aminoglycoside can be considered if there is a history of penicillin allergy but is not the preferred first-line treatment choice (B). Nitrofurantoin is not a preferred choice in young children (D) though it is commonly used in adult UTI episodes.

197. Correct: D. up to 20% of urinalyses can be normal.

When performing a urinalysis for UTI in a young child, it is important for the health-care provider to be aware that up to 20% of results will return a false negative (D).

Incorrect:

Findings suggestive of a UTI include positive leukocyte esterase (A) as well as elevated protein level (B). However, these findings are not diagnostic. The presence of urobilinogen is an indication of hepatic dysfunction that would not be related to UTI (C).

198. Correct: C. 7 to 14 days.

Current evidence-based practice recommends antimicrobial treatment for UTI in a child for 7 to 14 days, as evidence has shown superior results when compared to shorter courses of therapy (C).

199. Correct: D. arrange for the child to be admitted to the hospital.

This child presents with signs of severe illness and dehydration and would not tolerate oral antimicrobial therapy. The best course of action is urgent admission to a hospital for IV fluids and parenteral antimicrobial therapy (D).

Incorrect:

The most urgent course of action is to begin IV fluids and parenteral antimicrobial therapy. This should not be delayed with continued observation at home (A) or diagnostic testing. The child would not tolerate oral antimicrobial therapy due to repeated vomiting (B). A renal ultrasound is not a priority at this point for the child (C) but can be useful later in confirming the diagnosis or identifying a possible structural abnormality.

200. **Correct: A. RBUS.**

With a first-time febrile UTI, the preferred imaging technique is a RBUS, as this is easily performed and noninvasive (A).

Incorrect:

Renal scan is not recommended for routine imaging of a first UTI episode and would be more helpful to detect renal scarring following an infection (B). A VCUG can be considered if abnormal findings are revealed with RBUS (C). IV pyelography is an invasive imaging technique that has largely been replaced with the use of RBUS (D).

201. **Correct: A. This is a noninvasive test.**

When considering imaging of a young child, noninvasive procedures are generally preferred as this will cause less anxiety and fear from the child and parents. In this manner, the RBUS is preferred for routine imaging of UTIs in children, while VCUG can be considered with abnormal findings from RBUS or other specific clinical situations (A).

Incorrect:

Though RBUS has certain advantages compared to VCUG, including the test is less technically demanding (C), can potentially yield more rapid results (B), and is less expensive (D), it is generally favored due to its noninvasive technique.

202. **Correct: B. when UTI is recurrent.**

There are certain situations when VCUG is indicated. These include when RBUS reveals hydronephrosis, scarring, or other findings that would suggest high-grade vesicoureteral reflux or obstructive uropathy, as well as when febrile UTI is recurrent (B).

Incorrect:

VCUG would not be used to guide antimicrobial therapy, as the infection would generally be treated empirically or based on culture and susceptibility with treatment failure (A). A high-grade reflux identified by RBUS does not need confirmation by VCUG (C). Renal scarring is best revealed by a renal scan rather than VCUG (D).

203. **Correct: D. VUR.**

VUR is the most common urinary tract abnormality associated with UTI in younger children (D). High-grade VUR can be identified by RBUS or VCUG. In some cases, the use of antimicrobial prophylaxis can be considered with high-grade VUR until the abnormality is corrected.

Incorrect:

VUR is the most common urinary tract abnormality that can cause UTI in children and not bladder neck stricture (A), ureteral stenosis (B), or urethral stricture (C).

Common Childhood Febrile Illness With Skin Alterations

204. **Correct: A. Injectable benzathine penicillin, oral amoxicillin, and cephalexin are each strongly recommended for treatment of *S pyogenes* (GAS) pharyngitis, and B. Injectable benzathine penicillin would be indicated for treatment of GAS if poor adherence to recommended therapy or inability to take a full course of oral antibiotics is anticipated.**

First-line treatment of scarlet fever is oral/IM penicillin, amoxicillin, or a first-generation cephalosporin (A). Oral and IM formulations of penicillin have similar efficacy and spectrum of activity, though the IM formulation can be considered if there is concern about adherence to the full course of oral antimicrobial therapy (B).

Incorrect:

Oral penicillin is preferred to the IM formulation as there is a smaller risk of adverse effects and severe allergic reaction with oral dosing (C). Oral and IM formulations have similar clinical effectiveness and spectrum of activity (D).

205. **Correct: D. group A streptococcus only.**

The rapid strep test provides a quick and convenient assay to detect the presence of group A streptococcus in cases of pharyngitis (D).

Incorrect:

The rapid strep test is specific for detecting group A streptococcus, a gram-positive organism (A, B). It will not be able to detect other species of streptococci that can cause respiratory tract infections, such as *S pneumoniae* (C).

206. **Correct: C. rubella.**

Rubella, caused by the rubella virus, is generally associated with mild symptoms that can include low-grade fever, sore throat, malaise, and posterior cervical and postauricular lymphadenopathy (C). A diffuse maculopapular rash appears for about 3 days.

Incorrect:

Scarlet fever is associated with a scarlatina-form or sandpaper-like rash rather than a diffuse maculopapular rash, along with exudative pharyngitis (A). Roseola is more likely associated with a high-grade fever that can last 3 to 7 days (B). Rubeola or measles is characterized by generalized lymphadenopathy, fever, conjunctivitis, and the presence of Koplik spots. A maculopapular rash will emerge that can coalesce to generalized erythema (D).

207. **Correct: A. scarlet fever**

A generalized sandpaper-like rash is most indictive of scarlet fever (A). Other signs consistent with this diagnosis include exudative pharyngitis, fever, and localized anterior cervical lymphadenopathy.

Incorrect:
Roseola is more likely associated with a high-grade fever as well as discrete rosy-pink macular or maculopapular rash (B). Rubella is characterized by mild symptoms as well as the development of a diffuse maculopapular rash (C). Rubeola or measles is characterized by generalized lymphadenopathy, fever, conjunctivitis, and the presence of Koplik spots. A maculopapular rash will emerge that can coalesce to generalized erythema (D).

208. **Correct: B. infectious mononucleosis.**
Infectious mononucleosis, caused by the Epstein-Barr virus, commonly occurs in adolescents and young adults. Though most individuals will be asymptomatic, those with clinical signs will present with a purple-white exudative pharyngitis, malaise, and marked diffuse lymphadenopathy. Hepatic and splenic tenderness can be reported with abdominal examination. A maculopapular rash develops in a minority of patients (B).

Incorrect:
Signs of scarlet fever, caused by GABHS, can include exudative pharyngitis along with fever, headache, and localized tender anterior cervical lymphadenopathy. Scarlet fever (D) and GAS pharyngitis (A) would not typically be associated with a maculopapular rash or abdominal tenderness that is more likely associated with infectious mononucleosis. Rubella is characterized by generally mild symptoms that can include a sore throat but not exudative pharyngitis (C).

209. **Correct: B. lymphocytosis**
Lymphocytosis, or an elevated level of WBCs, is an indication for the presence of a viral infection and would be an expected finding in the child with infectious mononucleosis (B).

Incorrect:
Neutrophilia, or elevated levels of neutrophils, is an expected response to an active bacterial infection and would not be anticipated in the child with infective mononucleosis caused by the Epstein-Barr virus (A). ANA is a test used to check for the presence of rheumatoid arthritis or other autoimmune diseases and would not be affected by the presence of infectious mononucleosis (C). Macrocytic anemia is not a condition associated with infectious mononucleosis (D).

210. **Correct: B. heterophile antibody.**
The monospot test is used to diagnose infectious mononucleosis by detecting the presence of heterophile antibody (B). Heterophile antibodies against Epstein-Barr virus are present in peak levels about 2 to 6 weeks after the primary infection. The test has a very high specificity, though it could be negative during the early stage of infection.

Incorrect:
The monospot test detects the presence of heterophile antibodies against EBV and does not detect viral antigen (A), viral RNA (C), or IgG (D).

211. **Correct: B. prednisone.**
During infectious mononucleosis, some individuals can experience upper airway obstruction and respiratory distress due to enlarged tonsils and lymphoid tissue. An oral corticosteroid can be used to reduce airway inflammation and obstruction (B).

Incorrect:
Ibuprofen can help with pain associated with the sore throat but will not address the airway obstruction (C). Antiviral therapy is not helpful in the treatment of infective mononucleosis (D). Amoxicillin will not be helpful in treating this viral infection and can lead to the development of rash (A).

212. **Correct: A. HFMD.**
HFMD is best characterized by the presence of lesions that can occur in the oral cavity as well as hands and feet (A). Other signs include fever, malaise, and anorexia.

Incorrect:
Aphthous stomatitis, also known as canker sores, typically occur in the mouth but would not spread to the hands or feet (B). Similarly, herpetic gingivostomatitis can cause oral lesions but would not occur in other areas of the body (C). Vincent angina, or trench mouth, is caused by a bacterial infection that can cause ulceration, swelling, and sloughing of dead tissue from the mouth and throat but would not spread to the hands or feet (D).

213. **Correct: A. erythema infectiosum.**
Erythema infectiosum, or Fifth's disease, is characterized by the presence of a red rash that begins on the face and gives a "slapped cheek" appearance (A). The rash then spreads to the trunk and extremities. The rash is typically preceded by a period of mild flu-like illness that can include headache and myalgia.

Incorrect:
Roseola is characterized by a discrete rosy-pink macular or maculopapular rash and a high-grade fever (B). Rubella is associated with mild symptoms and a diffuse maculopapular rash rather than the "slapped cheek" appearance (C). Scarlet fever is characterized by exudative pharyngitis as well as a sandpaper-like rash (D).

214. **Correct: B. 10 to 14 days.**
Measles is a highly contagious disease with an incubation period of about 10 to 14 days (B). Disease transmission can occur for about 1 week prior to the onset of rash and then 2 to 3 weeks following the development of rash.

215. **Correct: C. children younger than 24 months old.**
Knowing a disease's epidemiology is important when making the differential diagnosis. About 90% of roseola

cases occur in children less than 2 years of age (C). Due to high-grade fever typically associated with this infection, there is a risk for febrile seizures.

216. Correct: D. children aged 1 to 8 years

Kawasaki's disease is a disease of unknown origin that results in fever, skin rash, bilateral conjunctival injection, cervical lymphadenopathy, swelling of the hands and feet, and mucocutaneous lesions. The disease most commonly affects children between 1 and 8 years of age (D).

217. Correct: C. peeling hands.

In addition to the observed findings in this child, Kawasaki's disease is also associated with edema and erythema of the hands and feet with peeling skin occurring at late stages of disease, usually 1 to 2 weeks after the onset of fever (C).

Incorrect:

Kawasaki's disease is associated with bilateral conjunctivitis but without discharge (B). Edema and erythema of the hands and feet can be observed with eventual skin peeling, though a vesicular-form rash is not typically noted (A). Cervical lymphadenopathy is more common rather than occipital lymphadenopathy (D).

218. Correct: C. blood cultures positive for offending bacterial pathogen.

There is no known cause for Kawasaki's disease and so a blood culture would not identify the offending organism (C).

Incorrect:

There is no specific laboratory test to confirm a diagnosis of Kawasaki's disease, though certain findings can support this diagnosis when coupled with clinical presentation. Urine tests will reveal the presence of albumin and WBCs, or pyuria (A). Blood test will reveal mild anemia, elevated WBCs, elevated ESR (D), and elevated platelets (B).

219. Correct: D. unknown.

The exact cause of Kawasaki's disease is unknown (D) though there is a belief that the disease is triggered by an infectious or immunological factor.

Incorrect:

An exact infectious cause of Kawasaki's disease has not been determined, including a fungal (A), viral (B), or bacterial (C) cause.

220. Correct: C. immune globulin

Treatment of Kawasaki's disease involves the use of IV immunoglobulin as well as oral aspirin (C). Treatment during the acute phase of the disease has been shown to reduce coronary abnormalities. Expert consultation is warranted for these patients.

Incorrect:

Without an identified infectious cause of Kawasaki's disease, the use of antibiotics (A), antivirals (B), or antifungals (D) is not warranted and will not provide any benefit.

221. Correct: A. droplet transmission

Varicella is a highly contagious disease also known as chickenpox. The virus is most commonly transmitted via respiratory droplets from the infected individual who coughs or sneezes (A).

Incorrect:

In addition to respiratory droplets, the virus can be transmitted through contact with an open pox lesion (C), though this occurs less frequently. Waterborne transmission (D) and contact with inanimate reservoirs (B) are not likely modes of transmission.

222. Correct: C. adults aged 30 to 49 years

Although most cases of varicella are seen in children younger than 18 years of age, the greatest risk of serious infection and mortality occurs in individuals 30 to 49 years old (C).

223. Correct: B. Crohn's disease

Serious complications can occur as a result of varicella infection in children. However, Crohn's disease, an autoimmune disorder that predominantly affects the GI tract, is not associated with varicella (B).

Incorrect:

Serious complications from varicella infection can include pneumonia (A), encephalitis (C), and toxic shock syndrome (D).

224. Correct: A. 8 to 20 weeks' gestation

Congenital varicella syndrome is a rare condition that can lead to birth abnormalities. This occurs when the mother becomes infected with varicella early during pregnancy, typically before 20 weeks' gestation (A).

Incorrect:

The risk of birth defects due to congenital varicella syndrome decreases after 20 weeks' gestation (B, C, D).

225 to 228. Matching Questions

225. Correct: D. Fifth's disease

226. Correct: C. Kawasaki's disease

227. Correct: B. Rubella

228. Correct: A. Measles

When managing children with infection, it is important for the clinician to be aware of potentially serious complications from disease, either for the child or close contacts who may be vulnerable to disease. Fifth's disease typically results in a mild disease for the child but can cause hydrops fetalis and pregnancy loss if contracted by a woman during pregnancy (225). Kawasaki's disease can lead to coronary abnormalities, including coronary artery dilatation and coronary aneurysm (226). Rubella is characterized by a mild illness in children but can lead to congenital rubella syndrome if a woman is infected during pregnancy, which can lead to developmental abnormalities including cardiac and ocular lesions, deafness, and microcephaly (227). Complications from measles include CNS and respiratory tract disorders that can lead to permanent neurological impairment and death (228).

229. Correct: A. vitamin A

Vitamin A supplementation has been shown to reduce morbidity and mortality in children with the measles and can help prevent eye damage and blindness (A). Vitamin A supplementation should be considered for all children with the measles, especially in children with signs of vitamin A deficiency.

Incorrect:

There is no evidence supporting the use of vitamin C (B), zinc (C), or copper (D) to improve clinical outcomes in children with the measles.

230. Correct: D. An ultrasound of the spleen is not required for diagnosis or to confirm resolution of disease.

Approximately 50% to 60% of patients with infective mononucleosis will develop splenomegaly. Though splenic rupture is a rare occurrence, patients are advised to avoid contact sports for at least 4 weeks after resolution of symptoms. However, routine ultrasound of the spleen is not needed to confirm the diagnosis, which is usually made with the monospot test along with clinical presentation (D).

Incorrect:

A diagnosis of infectious mononucleosis is made with a positive finding on the monospot test, which is highly specific, and not imaging of the spleen (A). Splenomegaly occurs in about half of patients with infectious mononucleosis, but routine imaging is not required as it will not impact management of the disease (B). Splenomegaly will normally resolve about 4 weeks after resolution of symptoms, and a confirmatory ultrasound is not routinely warranted (C). For those who participate in contact sports, if there is a concern of splenic rupture, then an ultrasound could be considered to confirm the absence of splenomegaly prior to returning to sports participation.

231. Correct: C. roseola.

Roseola occurs most commonly among children younger than 2 years of age and is characterized by a rosy-pink macular or maculopapular rash that follows a period of high-grade fever (C). About 10% of children will experience a febrile seizure during the illness.

Incorrect:

Scarlet fever is characterized by a sandpaper-like rash and exudative pharyngitis (A). Rubella is associated with mild symptoms that can include low-grade fever and a diffuse maculopapular rash (B). Rubeola or measles is characterized by a maculopapular rash that can coalesce to generalized erythema (D). Other findings include fever, nasal discharge, cough, and the presence of Koplik spots prior to the onset of rash.

232. Correct: D. rubeola.

The presence of Koplik spots, described as white spots with blue rings held within red spots in the oral mucosa, is an indication of rubeola or measles (D). The Koplik spots appear about 2 days prior to the onset of rash.

Incorrect:

HFMD can cause lesions in the oral mucosa as well as the hands and feet. The lesions would not be similar to the Koplik spots described in cases of measles (A). Rubella results in mild symptoms with posterior cervical lymphadenopathy and a diffuse maculopapular rash and will not result in the development of Koplik spots (B). Fifth's disease is characterized by a rash starting on the cheeks and then extending to the trunk and extremities (C).

233. Correct: A. acetaminophen.

Treatment of roseola is largely with supportive care, as the fever will pass after a few days. Acetaminophen or ibuprofen can be used to manage fever as appropriate (A).

Incorrect:

Roseola is caused by HHV-6 and so antimicrobials such as amoxicillin will not be effective (B). Antivirals are also not particularly helpful, especially oseltamivir which is used to treat influenza (D). Though about 10% of children with roseola will develop febrile seizures, the use of antiseizure medication is not recommended (C).

234. Correct: C. topical corticosteroid cream.

Treatment of varicella infection, or chickenpox, is largely supportive, and certain measures can be used to minimize symptoms and discomfort. However, the use of a topical corticosteroid is not warranted for this condition (C).

Incorrect:

The use of a topical calamine lotion (A) or oatmeal baths (D) can be helpful in reducing discomfort associated with the rash and skin lesions. An oral antihistamine can also be considered to minimize symptoms and discomfort (B).

235. Correct: D. topical fluconazole on affected external surfaces.

Treatment of HFMD is largely supportive and aimed at minimizing discomfort and pain. The infection is caused by the coxsackie virus A16 and not due to a fungal infection. Thus, the antifungal fluconazole would not be warranted (D).

Incorrect:

Supportive treatment can include the use of cold fluids and ice pops to help alleviate pain and discomfort from mouth sores as well as maintain hydration (A). Oral anesthetic mouthwash or spray can also be useful to alleviate oral pain (B). Ibuprofen or acetaminophen is also appropriate for pain relief and to reduce fever if present (C).

Dermatology Conditions in Younger Children

236. Correct: A. is likely to increase in size over the first year of life.

A capillary hemangioma is rarely present at birth but becomes evident during the first week of life. The hemangioma will rapidly grow in the first year before plateauing and then regressing (A).

Incorrect:

Capillary hemangioma will likely resolve by 9 years of age rather than the first few months of life (C). This dermatological condition is not associated with malignancy (B) and will not develop a super-imposed lichenification such as seen with plaque psoriasis (D).

237. **Correct: C. cryotherapy.**

Most cases of capillary hemangioma will not require treatment. However, treatment can be considered for large lesions or if it involves a vital organ or extremity. Cryotherapy is not used to treat these conditions (C).

Incorrect:

Treatment options for capillary hemangioma include the use of oral propranolol (A) as well as systemic corticosteroids (B) and interferon-α (D).

238. **Correct: B. grows proportionally with the child.**

Port-wine stains typically appear at birth and most commonly appear on the face. Port-wine stains will tend to deepen in color over time and grow proportionally with the child (B).

Incorrect:

Port-wine stains are not malignant and do not have the capacity to evolve into malignant lesions (D) but can be cosmetically challenging. The color will tend to deepen rather than become lighter over time (C). Treatment of port-wine stains will use laser therapy rather than surgical excision (A).

239. **Correct: C. the lesion should resolve by 5 years of age.**

Port-wine lesions will tend to get darker and often become nodular as the child grows. The lesion will not regress over time (C).

Incorrect:

When port-wine lesions involve the eyelid, it is important to consult ophthalmology (A) as the condition is associated with the development of glaucoma (D). Port-wine lesions are occasionally associated with other congenital or genetic conditions such as Sturge-Weber syndrome (B), which is a condition that affects the development of blood vessels and can impact normal brain, eye, and skin development.

240. **Correct: D. pulsed-dye laser therapy.**

The standard treatment of port-wine lesions is pulsed-dye laser therapy (D). The expected result of therapy is a lightening of the lesion but not necessarily complete removal of the lesion.

Incorrect:

Topical or systemic corticosteroids (A, B) or vincristine injection (C) are not used in the treatment of port-wine lesions.

241. **Correct: A. erythema toxicum neonatorum.**

Erythema toxicum neonatorum is a rash that is commonly found in newborns that appears within the first

10 days of life (A). The rash has the appearance of flea bites that are widely distributed throughout the body, though sparing the palms and soles of feet.

Incorrect:

Milia presents as pinpoint papular lesions typically on the nose, cheeks, and other areas with high concentration of sebaceous glands (B). Acne neonatorum consists of open and closed comedones and pustules on the forehead and cheeks (C). Staphylococcal skin infections can have varying presentations but can consist of red, swollen, and painful lesions often mistaken for a spider bite (D).

242. **Correct: D. on the nose and cheeks.**

The most common location of milia is on the nose, cheeks, and other areas with a high concentration of sebaceous glands (D).

Incorrect:

Milia typically form on areas where there is an abundance of sebaceous glands. This would not typically include the chest (B), underarms (C), or back and buttocks (A).

243. **Correct: B. enlarged sebaceous glands.**

The likely cause of milia is enlarged sebaceous glands, possibly caused by maternal androgenic effect (B).

Incorrect:

Milia likely result from maternal androgenic effect rather than low levels of androgen (A). This leads to enlarged sebaceous glands that cause milia (D). Milia is not caused by excessive oil production in the skin follicles (C).

244. **Correct: A. no special skin care.**

Milia will normally resolve without any special treatment by 4 weeks to 6 months (A). Caregivers should be advised to avoid trying to remove or open the milia as this can cause scarring of the skin.

Incorrect:

No special treatment is needed for milia. Thus, the use of a topical retinoid (B) or antimicrobial (D) is not warranted, nor is the use of cryotherapy (C).

245. **Correct: C. on the forehead and cheeks.**

Similar to the adolescent version of acne, the distribution of acne neonatorum typically includes the forehead and cheeks (C). The lesions typically resolve in about 4 to 8 weeks without any intervention.

Incorrect:

Acne neonatorum is most likely to affect the forehead and cheeks rather than the extremities (A), neck and chest (B), or neck and ears (D).

246. **Correct: A. no special skin care is needed because these lesions are self-resolving, and D. low-dose benzoyl peroxide**

Acne neonatorum will typically resolve by 4 to 8 weeks without any intervention (A). In some cases, the condition can persist for up to 1 year. The use of low-dose benzoyl peroxide can be considered for treatment (D).

Incorrect:

If treatment of acne neonatorum is warranted, then a low-dose benzoyl peroxide is preferred. A topical retinoid (B) or oral antibiotic (C) is not warranted for this condition.

247. **Correct: B. mongolian spots.**

Mongolian spots can present similar to bruising that is typically distributed over the lower back and buttocks. The condition occurs in about 90% of children of African or Asian ancestries (B).

Incorrect:

Hemangioma presents as a benign tumor-like lesion of the endothelium (D). Mongolian spots present similarly to ecchymosis or bruising, though there is no discomfort when a mongolian spot is pressed (C). In infants of African or Asian ancestry, clinicians should be aware of the high prevalence of mongolian spots rather than misinterpret these findings as bruising and possible child abuse. Bluish mottling of an infant's skin can occur when exposed to cold temperatures and will usually resolve when the skin is warmed (A).

248. **Correct: D. no treatment, as the condition resolves over time.**

Mongolian spots will normally resolve by age 7 years and thus no treatment is needed (D).

Incorrect:

No treatment is needed for mongolian spots, as the condition will resolve with time. The use of topical corticosteroids (A), interferon-α injection (B), or antimicrobial therapy (C) is not warranted.

249. **Correct: C. degradation of mast cells.**

Eczema results from a type I hypersensitivity reaction that is caused by IgE antibodies occupying receptor sites on mast cells, causing degradation of the mast cells, releasing histamines, and resulting in vasodilation and tissue swelling (C).

Incorrect:

Eczema results from the degradation of mast cells and subsequent release of histamine. This is due to a type I hypersensitivity reaction rather than a bacterial infection (B). A consequence of histamine release is mucus gland stimulation. However, eczema is not caused by overactive mucus glands (A). Intervention in eczema involves minimizing skin dryness and the use of lubricants. Dry air can contribute to symptoms of the condition but is not the cause of eczema (D).

250. **Correct: C. application of lubricants.**

The main approach in the treatment of eczema is avoiding any offending agents and minimizing skin dryness, usually with the application of lubricants (C).

Incorrect:

Treatment of eczema includes minimizing skin dryness. This can involve limiting skin exposure to soap and water rather than frequent bathing (A). Topical corticosteroids can be used during an eczema flare, though

the lowest potency corticosteroid that yields the desired effect should be used (B). The presence of dermatophytes, typically caused by a fungal infection on the skin, is not a frequent concern when managing eczema (D).

251. **Correct: B. face.**

A common site for eczema in infants is on the face (B). In these cases, the lowest potency corticosteroid cream can be used for treatment, in addition to frequent use of a nonsteroid moisturizing ointment.

Incorrect:

Eczema can occur on numerous sites on the infant, though eczema on the face is a common site. Less common sites of eczema include the dorsum of the hand (A), neck (C), and flexor surfaces (D).

Gastroenteritis

252 to 255. Yes or No

252. **Correct: Yes**

253. **Correct: Yes**

254. **Correct: Yes**

255. **Correct: Yes**

When evaluating a young child, several aspects can be used to help determine hydration status. Blood pressure will be normal to decreased with moderate dehydration and will be weak, thready, and impalpable with severe dehydration (252). Heart rate will be elevated with moderate to severe dehydration, with bradycardia occurring sometimes in severe cases (253). In severe dehydration, assessment of skin turgor will demonstrate recoil requiring more than 2 seconds along with tenting (254). Evaluation of mucous membranes will reveal dry lips and oral mucosa with dehydration (255).

256 to 259. Yes or No

256. **Correct: Yes**

257. **Correct: Yes**

258. **Correct: Yes**

259. **Correct: No**

Severe dehydration in a young child is a serious and life-threatening condition, and the clinician should be aware of particular signs of this condition. Anuria, or no urine output, for 4 to 6 hours is a concern and is indicative of severe dehydration (256). The eyes will appear as deeply sunken with tears absent (257). Capillary refill will be prolonged to minimal, which typically requires less than 2 seconds under normal conditions (258). Blood pressure will be decreased, weak, and/or impalpable with severe dehydration, rather than elevated (259).

260. **Correct: C. Continue breastfeeding.**

Continued breastfeeding should be encouraged during episodes of gastroenteritis to maintain hydration and provide some needed calories for the infant (C). This can be supplemented with ORS if mild to moderate dehydration is noted. With vomiting, the breastfeeding amount should be reduced initially and then gradually increased over time as tolerated by the infant.

Incorrect:

The infant should continue to breastfeed and not be switched to a soy-based formula (A). ORS can be used to supplement breast milk when needed, especially in the presence of mild to moderate dehydration (B). Sugar-water solution, sports drinks, or sodas are not recommended and can exacerbate diarrheal episodes (D).

261. **Correct: B. frequent sips of an oral rehydration solution.**

The optimal treatment for mild to moderate dehydration in a child is oral rehydration solution, which is specially formulated to replace the electrolytes in the young child (B).

Incorrect:

The use of soda (A), sports drinks (C), or fruit juice (D) is not recommended to treat dehydration in children as they contain inappropriate glucose and electrolyte composition when compared to ORS. Additionally, drinks with a high sugar content can exacerbate diarrheal episodes in the child.

262. **Correct: B. 1 to 8 hours**

Recognizing the incubation time of pathogens that cause food-borne illnesses can be imperative in identification of the offending food source and management of the illness. The incubation period for *Staphylococcus* is generally short, ranging from 1 to 8 hours before the onset of symptoms (B).

263. **Correct: C. 12 to 72 hours**

Recognizing the incubation time of pathogens that cause food-borne illnesses can be imperative in identification of the offending food source and management of the illness. The incubation period for *Salmonella* species can range from 12 to 72 hours before the onset of symptoms (C).

264. **Correct: A. the time of last urination.**

Among the answer choices, urination provides the most accurate measure of dehydration, as urine will only be produced if the body has an adequate amount of fluid available (A). If the child has voided in the previous few hours, then dehydration is likely minimal. However, if there has been an absence of urination for 4 to 6 hours, then dehydration is likely that will require intervention.

Incorrect:

Thirst is not a highly measurable parameter that can be used to assess hydration status (B). The impact of the quantity of liquids taken on hydration status can be affected by the number of episodes of vomiting or diarrhea (C). Similarly, the impact of the number of episodes of vomiting and diarrhea on hydration status can be affected by the amount of liquids taken by the child (D). Thus, these are not reliable measures to assess hydration status.

265. **Correct: C. 6% to 9%**

Moderate dehydration typically results in the loss of 6% to 9% of body weight (C).

Incorrect:

Mild dehydration results in a loss of body weight between 3% and 5% (B), while severe dehydration results in a loss of 10% or more of body weight (D). Minimal dehydration can result in less than a 3% loss in body weight (A).

266. **Correct: A. bloody diarrhea, and B. fever**

Shigellosis, a serious bacterial infection, is associated with worrisome symptoms including fever (B), vomiting, and diarrhea that contains copious amounts of blood or pus (A).

Incorrect:

Shigellosis is not typically associated with the development of respiratory tract symptoms, such as cough (C), or with headache (D).

267. **Correct: B. norovirus.**

The most common causes of viral gastroenteritis are norovirus (B) and rotavirus. However, routine vaccination of infants against rotavirus has helped to reduce the incidence of gastroenteritis by this pathogen.

Incorrect:

Norovirus is the most common cause of viral gastroenteritis. Rhinovirus (A), coronavirus (C), and adenovirus (D) are more commonly associated with respiratory tract infections.

268. **Correct: B. A single dose of oral antiemetic has been demonstrated to reduce vomiting and the subsequent need for IV fluids.**

The use of ondansetron or similar medication can be considered for the child with gastroenteritis and vomiting episodes (B). Studies have shown that a single dose can reduce vomiting, thereby increasing tolerability of oral fluid intake and reducing the need for IV fluids and hospitalization.

Incorrect:

Studies have shown the benefit of ondansetron use in the child with gastroenteritis, namely, reducing vomiting and a need for IV fluids (A). Antidiarrheal agents are not recommended during gastroenteritis due to the potential for adverse effects (C). Only a single dose of ondansetron is needed for its benefit, and it should not be administered every 2 hours (D).

269. **Correct: D. These agents should be avoided in young children with gastroenteritis due to increased risk of adverse effect with use and offer of minor, if any, benefit.**

The use of antidiarrheal and antimotility medications is contraindicated in children with gastroenteritis. These medications provide no benefit and can increase the risk of adverse effects, including paralytic ileus, drowsiness, and nausea (D).

Incorrect:

Antidiarrheals should not be used in any child with gastroenteritis (B), particularly children with bacterial gastroenteritis due to a risk of adverse effects and little benefit (A). Antimotility agents can actually increase the risk of HUS in children infected with *E coli* O157:H7 (C).

270. Correct: **C. oral rehydration therapy is as effective and less costly when compared with IV fluid therapy.**

For the child with mild to moderate dehydration, oral rehydration therapy is preferred as it is as effective as parenteral therapy, easier to administer, and a more cost-effective treatment (C).

Incorrect:

IV therapy is preferred for severe dehydration, while ORS is preferred for mild to moderate dehydration (A). Hospitalization is not needed for moderate dehydration with ORS (B), and oral rehydration therapy does not have to be delayed until a set time since the last diarrheal episode (D). The best approach is to encourage small, frequent sips of ORS.

271. Correct: **C. proper handwashing.**

Viral gastroenteritis is a highly contagious disease that is most often spread by the fecal-to-oral route. Proper handwashing is essential in preventing the spread of this infection (C).

Incorrect:

The rotavirus vaccine is only administered during infancy and offers protection of young children from this specific virus but not other viruses that can cause gastroenteritis, such as norovirus (A). Breastfeeding should be continued during an episode of gastroenteritis as it can help maintain hydration and provide calories to the infant (B). Proper diaper hygiene is advised during gastroenteritis, as frequent bathing can lead to skin irritation in the infant (D).

272 to 275. Matching Questions

272. Correct: **C. deli meats**

273. Correct: **D. eggs**

274. Correct: **B. food left at room temperature for a prolonged period**

275. Correct: **A. undercooked ground beef**

Understanding common sources of foodborne pathogens and incubation periods can help the clinician identify the potential pathogen and food involved in food poisoning. *S aureus* has a quick incubation time of between 30 minutes and 8 hours with common food sources including sliced meats, puddings, and pastries (272). *Salmonella* is commonly found in eggs, chicken, pork, fruits, and vegetables and has an incubation time of between 12 and 72 hours (273). *C perfringens* is found in beef, poultry, and gravies as well as food left at room temperature or on steam tables for prolonged periods of time. Its incubation period is between 6 and 24 hours (274). *E coli* is found in a variety of food sources including undercooked ground beef, raw fruits and vegetables, and

unpasteurized milk. *E coli* has an incubation time of 1 to 10 days (275).

276 to 279. Yes or No

276. Correct: **Yes**

277. Correct: **Yes**

278. Correct: **Yes**

279. Correct: **Yes**

For children with suspected viral gastroenteritis, a clinical diagnosis is usually sufficient without additional laboratory testing. However, for suspected bacterial infection, additional testing can be considered including stool assay for occult blood (279), WBC count, and stool bacterial culture (276). In children with fever, nausea, vomiting, abdominal pain, and signs of dehydration, additional testing can include CBC (278), serum electrolytes, urea, creatinine, and amylase, with consideration for abdominal imaging studies. With high-grade fever, blood culture should be obtained (277).

280. Correct: **C. 50 to 100 mL/kg**

The recommended amount of ORS that should be administered to a child with mild to moderate dehydration is 50 to 100 mL/kg over a span of 3 to 4 hours. The child should be encouraged to take frequent, small sips of the fluid.

281. Correct: **A. cream-based soup.**

When attempting to reintroduce foods to a child following gastroenteritis, it is best to avoid fatty foods and full-fat dairy products for the first few days as this can trigger lower abdominal cramping. Thus, cream or cream-based soups would not be an appropriate choice (A).

Incorrect:

Following gastroenteritis, simple foods such as cooked rice (B), crackers, dry cereal (C), and bread products can be reintroduced, guided by the child's appetite and tolerance. Half-strength apple juice (D) and simple soups are also acceptable.

Alterations in Puberty

282. Correct: **D. early onset of normal puberty.**

Most cases of precocious puberty result in developmental changes occurring as early as 8 years of age. This is typically a benign condition caused by early onset of normal puberty (D).

Incorrect:

Precocious puberty that occurs in girls before the age of 6 years typically indicates a more serious condition that could be the result of ovarian (A) or adrenal (B) tumors. Expert consultation and referral are typically needed in these cases. Exogenous estrogen is not a usual cause of precocious puberty (C).

283 to 285. Matching Questions

283. Correct: **B. Tanner stage 3**

284. Correct: A. Tanner stage 2

285. Correct: C. Tanner stage 4

It is important for the health-care provider to be familiar with normative changes during puberty in order to identify alterations in development. For both boys and girls, the onset of growth spurt occurs during Tanner stage 3 (283). In girls, Tanner stage 2 is characterized by the development of breast buds with papilla elevated, as well as downy pigmented pubic hair along labia majora (284). In boys during Tanner stage 4, there is an increase in penile length and width with development of glans; further darkening of scrotal skin; and adult-type pubic hair with no spread to medial surface of thighs (285).

286. Correct: B. a select number of relatively uncommon health problems.

In boys, precocious puberty occurs less commonly than in girls and is typically associated with relatively uncommon health problems (B), such as gonadal or adrenal tumors or a select number of genetically based diseases. Prompt referral and expert care are warranted in these situations.

Incorrect:

Precocious puberty in boys occurs much less frequently than in girls and is likely attributed to an uncommon health condition rather than early onset of normal puberty (D). Precocious puberty would not be triggered by excessive physical activity in boys (A), and exogenous testosterone is not a common cause of this condition (C).

287. Correct: A. breast enlargement

Premature thelarche is a relatively common, benign condition that results in breast enlargement in female toddlers (A). The child would have no other signs of puberty.

Incorrect:

With premature thelarche, breast enlargement will occur without other signs of puberty including accelerated linear growth (B). Premature adrenarche is associated with the development of body odor (D), pubic hair (C), and sometimes axillary hair in a 5- to 6-year-old child.

288. Correct: C. pubic hair

Premature adrenarche is associated with the development of body odor, pubic hair (C), and sometimes axillary hair in a 5- to 6-year-old child. There are no other signs of puberty, and reassurance and ongoing monitoring are the usual course of action.

Incorrect:

Premature adrenarche is not associated with accelerated linear growth (B) or menstruation (D). Premature thelarche is associated with breast development in the young child (A).

289. Correct: C. 1 year after the onset of menstruation.

In both boys and girls, the onset of the growth spurt occurs during Tanner stage 3, while menarche occurs

in Tanner stage 4. A girl will typically achieve her full adult height about 1 year following the start of menstruation (C).

290. Correct: A. breast budding.

In girls, the onset of puberty, or Tanner stage 2, is noted by the development of breast buds with papilla elevated (A), as well as downy pigmented pubic hair along the labia majora.

Incorrect:

The onset of growth spurt occurs during Tanner stage 3 (C), menarche occurs during Tanner stage 4 (B), and the development of axillary, adult-type hair occurs late in puberty (D).

291. Correct: A. report of a high level of physical activity

Several conditions can contribute to delayed puberty in boys. However, unlike girls, there is no correlation with increased physical activity and delayed onset of puberty (A).

Incorrect:

Delayed onset of puberty in boys can be due to genetic disorders, such as Kallmann's syndrome or Klinefelter's syndrome (B), a prior history of radiation exposure (D), or constitutional delay that runs in families (C).

292. Correct: D. Turner's syndrome

Turner's syndrome (XO female) is associated with delayed or absent puberty, short height, amenorrhea, learning disabilities, and social difficulties (D). Genetic testing should be performed when this condition is suspected.

Incorrect:

Obesity and overweight are not associated with a delayed onset of puberty (B). Certain medications used in asthma have been associated with a small decrease in height attained but would not delay the onset of puberty (C). A history of abdominal irradiation is not a typical reason for delayed onset of puberty but is potentially more likely to result in early onset of puberty with an increased risk of adrenal or ovarian tumors (A).

293. Correct: B. serum testosterone

In boys with suspected precocious or delayed puberty, measurement of serum testosterone can be useful to determine the stage of puberty (B). A level of less than 30 ng/dL can be expected in prepubertal boys, while the level rises to 30 to 100 ng/dL in early puberty, and 100 to 300 ng/dL in mid- to late puberty.

Incorrect:

TSH level offers no useful information in determining puberty status (A) nor does evaluation of serum prolactin (C) or aldosterone (D).

294. Correct: D. microscopic examination of vaginal discharge.

For a child with precocious puberty younger than 6 years of age, diagnostic tests are needed to identify the cause of the condition, which can include adrenal

or ovarian tumors. However, microscopic evaluation of vaginal discharge would not be warranted (D).
Incorrect:
Testing that can be included in the evaluation of precocious puberty in a 5-year-old includes measurement of FSH (A) and luteinizing hormone (B), measuring bone age, and performing an abdominal ultrasound (C).

Car Seat Guidelines

295. **Correct: D. the child reaches the maximum height and weight allowed by the seat.**
Current guidelines from the AAP recommend keeping the infant and toddler in a rear-facing car seat for as long as possible. This would be until the child reaches the maximum height and weight allowed by the car seat manufacturer and would not normally be until the child is at least 2 years old (D).

296. **Correct: C. 57 inches (144.8 cm), 8 to 12 years**
A child can stop using a belt-positioning booster seat once the vehicle's lap and shoulder belt fits properly on the child. This typically occurs when the child reaches a height of 4 feet 9 inches (57 inches) and is between 8 and 12 years of age (C).

297. **Correct: D. 13 years.**
Though a child may no longer need a belt-positioning booster seat, the child should continue to be positioned in the rear seat until age 13 years for optimal protection (D).

Childbearing

18

Normative Changes During Pregnancy

Overview

Pregnancy is a physiological condition marked from conception to childbirth. Knowledge of appropriate terminology and recognizing the normative changes to the woman during pregnancy are critical components in providing prenatal care.

Several terms are used to describe the various stages of growth. The fertilized egg forms a *zygote*. During the first 2 weeks of growth, the group of rapidly dividing cells is known as a *blastocyst*. An *embryo* reflects growth during weeks 2 to 8, while a *fetus* refers to the offspring from weeks 8 to 10 until term.

Full-term pregnancy generally refers to birth occurring between 39 weeks 0 days and 40 weeks 6 days. *Early term* pregnancy occurs between 37 weeks 0 days and 38 weeks 6 days. A *late-term* pregnancy refers to birth occurring between 41 weeks 0 days and 41 weeks 6 days, while *post-term* pregnancy occurs with birth after 42 weeks.

Uterine Size During Pregnancy

Knowledge of normal pregnancy development is a critical component to providing prenatal care. One of the major changes during pregnancy is uterine size, which increases from about 10-mL capacity and 70-g weight in prepregnancy to 5,000-mL capacity and 1,100-g weight at term. Uterine size and changes during the various stages of pregnancy are as follows:

- *Nongravid*: The size of a lemon; mobile, firm, and nontender.
- *8 weeks*: The size of a tennis ball or orange. Common signs occurring during this time include the Hegar sign (softening of the uterine isthmus), Goodell sign (softening of vaginal portion of the cervix), and Chadwick sign (blue-violet vaginal color).
- *10 weeks*: The size of a baseball. The first fetal heart tone can be heard via abdominal ultrasound around 10 to 12 weeks.
- *12 weeks*: The size of a softball or grapefruit. The uterine fundus is palpable through the abdominal wall as it rises above the symphysis pubis.
- *16 weeks*: Uterine fundus located halfway between the symphysis pubis and umbilicus. Quickening (fetal movement) is first noted in a woman who has been pregnant previously (second trimester or beyond) during 16 to 17 weeks; quickening noted around 18 weeks during a first pregnancy.
- *20 to 36 weeks*: About 1-cm gain in fundal height per week. Uterine fundus is located at the umbilicus at 20 weeks; usually concordant with gestational age, plus or minus 1 cm.
- *At term*: Uterus dips into the pelvis with fetal head engagement, and fundal height decreases. The fetus is in the vertex position (cephalic) in 95% of pregnancies by 36 weeks.

Other Physiological Adaptations During Pregnancy

A woman's body undergoes significant changes during pregnancy. These changes are normative, allowing the body to adapt to the increased fetal needs. Knowledge of these changes is critical to providing counseling and care during pregnancy. Notable changes include:

- *Cervix*: Its color and texture change, becoming cyanotic (Chadwick's sign) and less firm (Goodell's sign).
- *Skin*: Striae (stretch marks) appear in approximately 50% of women; melasma (pregnancy mask) is also commonly present. Linea nigra (hyperpigmented line on abdomen) appears or darkens as melanocytes are stimulated.
- *Breast*: Nipples and areolae darken and increase in size. Venous congestion is noted. Breast tissue becomes more nodular because of proliferation of lactiferous glands.
- *Blood*: Blood volume increases by 40% to 50%, peaking at week 32. Red blood cell (RBC) production increases by 33% but still results in dilutional physiological anemia of pregnancy.
- *Cardiovascular*: A decrease in systolic blood pressure (BP) occurs throughout pregnancy, with a decrease in diastolic BP being most notable during the second trimester. Cardiac output is dependent on maternal position, with a noted decrease if in the supine position because of reduced venous return caused by vena cava compression to an increase of 30% to 50% with lateral recumbent position. The S_1 heart sound becomes louder, and physiological systolic ejection murmur is usually evident. The heart is displaced, resulting in a left axis deviation that resolves post birth.
- *Renal*: Increased renal blood flow, glomerular filtration rate (GFR), and dilation of the renal collecting system

occur. Physiological glucosuria and proteinuria occur partly because of an increase in GFR and resulting inability of renal tubules to reabsorb glucose and protein.

- *Respiratory*: Partly because of increased abdominal content, there is an increase in transverse thoracic diameter and diaphragmatic contraction, and the costal angle widens. Tidal volume increases with reduced residual volume in later pregnancy.
- *Digestive*: The lower esophageal sphincter is more relaxed while corresponding pressures increase, resulting in increased esophageal reflux. Decreased stomach and intestinal motility is seen, allowing for greater nutrient absorption but increased risk for constipation. (Increased progesterone levels influence the aforementioned changes.) The gallbladder doubles in size with more dilute bile and less-soluble cholesterol, increasing the risk of stones.
- *Metabolic/endocrine*: Insulin levels increase by twofold to 10-fold over prepregnancy levels. Fasting plasma glucose decreases slightly. The thyroid and pituitary glands increase in size. Maternal weight changes account for weight gain in the first half of pregnancy, whereas uterine contents account for most weight gain in the second half.

Discussion Sources

American College of Obstetricians and Gynecologists. Definition of term pregnancy. Committee Opinion No. 579. *Obstet Gynecol.* 2013;122:1139–1140. http://www.acog.org/Resources_And_Publications/Committee_Opinions/Committee_on_Obstetric _Practice/Definition_of_Term_Pregnancy

Datta S, Kodali BS, Segal S. Maternal physiologic changes during pregnancy, labor, and the postpartum period. In: Datta S, Kodali BS, Segal S, eds. *Obstetric Anesthesia Handbook.* 5th ed. New York, NY: Springer; 2010:1–14.

QUESTIONS

1 to 4. Match the stage of pregnancy with the appropriate term.

_____ **1.** Fertilized ovum

_____ **2.** Up to 2 weeks' postconception

_____ **3.** Up to 8 to 10 weeks

_____ **4.** 10 weeks to term

      A. embryo

      B. fetus

      C. blastocyst

      D. zygote

5 to 17. Identify the following changes in a normal pregnancy as true (normal, anticipated finding) or false (not associated with normal pregnancy):

_____ **5.** Blood volume increases by 40% to 50%, peaking at week 32.

_____ **6.** A decrease in diastolic BP is most notable during the second trimester.

_____ **7.** The S_1 heart sound becomes louder.

_____ **8.** A physiological systolic ejection murmur is usually evident and resolves post birth.

_____ **9.** Dilation of the renal collecting system occurs.

_____ **10.** Physiological glucosuria and proteinuria are common.

_____ **11.** There is a decrease in transverse thoracic diameter and diaphragmatic contraction.

_____ **12.** The lower esophageal sphincter is more relaxed.

_____ **13.** There is increased intestinal motility.

_____ **14.** The gallbladder doubles in size.

_____ **15.** Insulin levels increase by twofold to 10-fold over prepregnancy levels.

_____ **16.** Fasting plasma glucose increases slightly.

_____ **17.** The thyroid decreases in size.

18 to 23. Match uterine size with stage of pregnancy.

_____ **18.** nongravid

_____ **19.** 8 weeks

_____ **20.** 10 weeks

_____ **21.** 12 weeks

_____ **22.** 16 weeks

_____ **23.** 20 weeks

     A. size of a baseball

     B. size of a softball or grapefruit

     C. size of a large lemon

     D. size of a tennis ball or orange

     E. uterine fundus at umbilicus

     F. uterine fundus halfway between symphysis pubis and umbilicus

24 to 26. Match each sign with its correct characteristic.

_____ **24.** Hegar's sign

_____ **25.** Goodell's sign

_____ **26.** Chadwick's sign

     A. blue-violet vaginal color

     B. softening of uterus isthmus

     C. softening of vaginal portion of the cervix

27. Approximately ____% of fetuses are in vertex position by the 36th week of pregnancy.

     A. 30

     B. 50

     C. 75

     D. 95

For answers and rationales, see end of chapter.

Health and Nutrition Counseling During Pregnancy

The nurse practitioner (NP) needs to have knowledge of nutritional requirements during pregnancy to provide appropriate counseling. In particular, ensuring that maternal nutrition is optimized either preconception or as early as possible during pregnancy is critical to optimal outcomes for both mother and baby.

Folic Acid Deficiency

While the terms *folate deficiency* and *folic acid deficiency* are used interchangeably, there is a subtle difference. When vitamin B$_9$ occurs naturally in food, this micronutrient is known as folate. The synthetic form of vitamin B$_9$ is known as folic acid. The term *folic acid deficiency* (FAD) is most often used to describe the condition when this important micronutrient is not found in sufficient amounts.

FAD during pregnancy is a teratogenic state, resulting in an increased risk of neural tube defects (NTDs) and other potentially serious problems in the developing pregnancy. Examples of NTDs include anencephaly, spina bifida, and encephalocele.

Dietary-associated FAD is rare unless severe malnutrition is present. This micronutrient is added to most wheat and other flours. Folate naturally occurs in large amounts in legumes, leafy greens, eggs, as well as many fruits and additional vegetables. Women who eat less nutritious diets should be encouraged to adopt a folate-rich diet, ideally prior to pregnancy.

Correcting FAD before pregnancy by increased dietary and supplement intake dramatically reduces NTD risk, and continuing this increased intake throughout pregnancy minimizes the mother's risk of developing folate-deficiency anemia. As a result, the Centers for Disease Control and Prevention (CDC) recommend that all women of reproductive age take a folic acid 400 mcg supplement daily, even if not

CLINICAL CONCEPT

Women who eat typical amounts of bread, pasta, and other flour-based foods with these folate-rich fruits and vegetables are unlikely to have FAD.

attempting to conceive. The rationale behind this advice in part stems from the fact that at least 50% of all pregnancies are unplanned.

While folic acid supplementation is demonstrated to reduce NTD risk, the risk has not been eliminated. A genetic contribution to NTDs is likely and is thought to be the result of a complex interaction of environment and heredity. As a result, if a woman has carried a pregnancy with an NTD, or there is a family history of NTD, recommended folic acid intake increases to 4 mg/day for 1 month before pregnancy and during the first 3 months of gestation. Most prescription prenatal multivitamins contain 1 mg of folic acid. In a woman with a reported NTD pregnancy in her family, consideration should be given for preconception specialty counseling.

Calcium Intake During Pregnancy

Increased calcium intake is important for the development of fetal bones and teeth; the required amount can usually be met by ensuring three to four servings of high-quality dairy products per day. Examples of a single dairy serving include 8 oz (240 mL) of milk, 1 to 1.5 oz (28 to 43 g) of cheese, 1 cup (240 mL) of yogurt, or 1 cup (240 mL) of calcium-fortified juice. Although dietary sources of calcium are best, supplementation is sometimes required if a woman is lactose intolerant or is otherwise unable to meet these goals. The recommended daily intake of calcium for women 19 to 50 years of age is 1,000 mg. Women 14 to 18 years of age have an increased calcium requirement of 1,300 mg daily.

Maternal Iron Requirements During Pregnancy

Maternal iron requirements increase in the second and third trimesters of pregnancy, in part because of the fetus's need to build iron stores during this time. Iron deficiency is the most common form of maternal anemia during pregnancy, with most cases occurring because the woman enters pregnancy with iron deficiency, rather than develops this problem because of increased iron requirements due to fetal needs. Pregnancy-related iron requirements, given in terms of elemental iron, are as follows: in the absence of iron deficiency, 30 mg/day; with iron deficiency or in a multiple-gestation pregnancy, 60 to 100 mg/day. A 325-mg ferrous sulfate tablet contains 65 mg of elemental iron, whereas most prescription prenatal vitamins contain 30 to 65 mg. There is ongoing debate about the helpfulness of prenatal vitamin use, in particular the iron content, for women who eat a well-balanced diet.

Weight Gain During Pregnancy

Specific guidelines for recommended total and rate of weight gain during pregnancy have been developed, based on studies of optimal fetal and maternal outcomes (Table 18-1). Excessive total weight gain during pregnancy is associated with higher rates of postpartum weight retention and increased birth weight. Inadequate total weight gain during pregnancy is associated with lower birth weight. Excessive and inadequate total weight gain are associated with a variety of pregnancy-related complications.

As would be expected, the weekly rate of weight gain in the second and third trimesters of pregnancy is higher than in the first trimester, related to increased maternal circulating volume, uterine enlargement,

TABLE 18-1 Weight Gain Recommendations During Pregnancy

PREPREGNANCY WEIGHT CATEGORY	BODY MASS INDEX (KG/M²)	RECOMMENDED RANGE OF TOTAL WEIGHT LB (KG)	RECOMMENDED RATES OF WEIGHT GAIN IN THE SECOND AND THIRD TRIMESTERS LB/WEEK (MEAN RANGE LB/WEEK) (KG/WEEK [MEAN RANGE KG/WEEK])
Underweight	Less than 18.5	28 to 40 (12.7 to 18.14)	1 (1 to 1.3) (0.45 [0.45 to 0.59])
Normal weight	18.5 to 24.9	25 to 35 (11.34 to 15.88)	1 (0.8 to 1) (0.45 [0.36 to 0.45])
Overweight	25 to 29.9	15 to 25 (6.8 to 11.34)	0.6 (0.5 to 0.7) (0.27 [0.23 to 0.32])
Obese (includes all classes)	30 and greater	11 to 20 (4.99 to 9.07)	0.5 (0.4 to 0.6) (0.23 [0.18 to 0.27])

Source: American College of Obstetricians and Gynecologists. Committee Opinion #548: Weight gain during pregnancy. January 2013. https://www.acog.org/clinical/clinical-guidance/committee-opinion/articles/2013/01/weight-gain-during-pregnancy

and rising fetal weight. The energy requirements for a pregnant woman during the first trimester are the same as those for a nonpregnant woman. As a result, there is no need for a woman to increase caloric intake in early pregnancy, but she should consume a well-balanced diet. In the second and third trimesters, her caloric needs typically increase by about 340 to 450 calories a day. Therefore, the average daily calorie intake during pregnancy in an otherwise healthy woman carrying a single fetus is an increase of approximately 300 calories per day. Protein intake is increased in pregnancy from approximately 46 g/d, recommended intake for a woman who is not pregnant, to at least 60 g/d. The fat and carbohydrate intake needs during pregnancy are largely unchanged.

Avoiding Potentially Harmful Substances and Practices

Providing appropriate advice and counseling to women before and during pregnancy on avoiding potentially harmful substances is critical to optimize pregnancy outcomes. In particular, given that many substances are used without immediate harm by women who are not pregnant, it is critical to ensure that pregnant women are aware of potential and often devastating consequences of substance use to the mother and developing child.

> **CLINICAL CONCEPT**
> A safe level of maternal ingestion during pregnancy for marijuana and other intoxicating substances has not been established, and abstinence should be encouraged.

Women who are pregnant should be counseled about avoiding the use of recreational drugs, both prescription and nonprescription, alcohol, tobacco, and caffeine. It is estimated that up to 5% of pregnant women use one or more addictive substances. Opioid use disorder at labor and delivery has increased fourfold in the past three decades. While the negative effects of fetal alcohol, tobacco, and opioid exposure are well documented, the impact of other substance misuse during pregnancy is emerging.

The effects to the mother and developing child from use of some of the most common substances during pregnancy include the following:

- *Tobacco use in any form*: It is well established that smoking tobacco products increases the risk of several types of cancer, cardiovascular disease, and chronic respiratory diseases, among other health conditions. Tobacco use during pregnancy can increase the risk of preterm birth, low birth weight, and birth defects of the mouth and lips, and can increase the risk of sudden infant death syndrome (SIDS) in newborns. E-cigarettes and tobacco products with nicotine can also damage brain and lung development. Though not fully studied, flavorings used in e-cigarettes can contain toxic chemicals that can be harmful to the baby.
- *Alcohol*: There is no safe amount of alcohol to consume during pregnancy. Alcohol use during pregnancy can cause miscarriage, stillbirth, and a range of fetal alcohol spectrum disorders (FASDs) that include abnormal facial features, small head size, reduced height, poor coordination, learning disabilities, speech and language delays, and vision and hearing problems, among others. For the mother, alcohol use can cause sedation, mood alteration, loss of memory, delayed motor reactions, and impaired judgment.
- *Opioids*: Use of opioids during pregnancy can increase the risk of preterm birth and stillbirth as well as neonatal abstinence syndrome (NAS), which comprises a group of withdrawal symptoms in newborns. Risks to the mother include sedation, respiratory depression, and possible death with overdose.
- *Stimulants (e.g., cocaine and methamphetamines)*: Use of stimulant drugs can increase the risk of preterm birth and low birth weight. Children born to women who used methamphetamines during pregnancy are also found to have neurobehavioral problems that can lead to long-lasting motor deficits, decreased arousal, and attention impairments. Maternal effects include extremes in emotion, hypervigilance, impaired judgment, tachycardia, and psychomotor agitation. Overdose can lead to arrhythmias, confusion, coma, and seizures.

Pica

Pica is the ingestion of nonfood substances, such as clay, cornstarch, laundry starch, dry milk of magnesia, paraffin, coffee grounds, paper, or ice. Occasionally, pica will take the form of eating a food, but not in a form typically ingested, such as uncooked rice. Pica is found in all socioeconomic and ethnic groups. Certain pica habits are likely harmless, such as sucking on ice chips, but do little to replace intake of more nutritious substances. Most other pica forms contain potential risk, however, because nonfood substances are taken in preferably over more nutritious food sources. In addition, some pica forms, such as eating cornstarch, come with a high caloric burden, leading to weight gain; one cup of cornstarch contains approximately 600 calories.

With the ingestion of clay, starches, and paraffin, there is risk of constipation, bowel obstruction, and nutritional deficiency. In particular, many common pica substances can be contaminated with heavy metals

CLINICAL CONCEPT

During pregnancy, women should be frequently screened for pica by asking about food and nonfood intake.

such as lead or mercury and other industrial pollutants that are particularly toxic to the mother and the developing fetus. The issue of pica should be raised with all pregnant women. Some women believe that pica is normal, or they are encouraged to eat substances such as clay by well-meaning friends and family members as a way of relieving tension. Recognize this, but inform the woman about the potential risks of pica.

Iron-deficiency anemia is more common in women who have pica during pregnancy. Fetal outcomes are variable, dependent on the substance ingested and maternal nutritional status. In particular, maternal ingestion of heavy metals such as lead can potentially result in a negative impact of fetal neurodevelopment. Information should be offered about the possible negative pregnancy outcomes with pica.

Discussion Sources

American College of Obstetricians and Gynecologists. Committee Opinion #548: Weight gain during pregnancy. January 2013. https://www.acog.org/Clinical-Guidance-and-Publications/Committee-Opinions/Committee-on-Obstetric-Practice/Weight-Gain-During-Pregnancy

Centers for Disease Control and Prevention. Substance use during pregnancy. https://www.cdc.gov/reproductivehealth/maternalinfanthealth/substance-abuse/substance-abuse-during-pregnancy.htm

Institute for Clinical Systems Improvement. Prenatal care, routine. https://www.icsi.org/guidelines__more/catalog_guidelines_and_more/catalog_guidelines/catalog_womens_health_guidelines/prenatal/

Kominiarek MA, Rajan P. Nutrition recommendations in pregnancy and lactation. *Med Clin North Am*. 2016;100:1199–1215.

March of Dimes. Nutrition, weight and fitness. http://www.marchofdimes.org/pregnancy/nutrition-weight-and-fitness.aspx

Pregnancy: staying healthy and safe. Womenshealth.gov. https://www.womenshealth.gov/pregnancy/you-are-pregnant/staying-healthy-safe.html

Young SL. Pica in pregnancy: new ideas about an old condition. *Annu Rev Nutr*. 2010;30:403–422.

QUESTIONS

28. The recommended weight gain during pregnancy for a woman with a desirable or healthy prepregnancy body mass index (BMI) is:

    A. 15 to 25 lb (6.8 to 11.3 kg).

    B. 11 to 20 lb (5.0 to 9.1 kg).

    C. 25 to 35 lb (11.3 to 15.9 kg).

    D. 35 to 45 lb (15.9 to 20.4 kg).

29. For a healthy woman with a desirable or healthy prepregnancy BMI, the average daily caloric requirements during pregnancy are typical baseline caloric needs plus ____ kcal.

    A. 100

    B. 300

    C. 600

    D. 1,000

30. When counseling a woman entering her second trimester of pregnancy about increased caloric intake, the NP emphasizes there should be a greater intake of:

    A. carbohydrates.

    B. unsaturated fats.

    C. protein.

    D. water.

31. The recommended rate of weight gain per week during the second and third trimesters of pregnancy for a woman who was overweight prepregnancy is approximately:

    A. 0.25 lb (0.1 kg).

    B. 0.6 lb (0.3 kg).

    C. 1 lb (0.45 kg).

    D. 2 lb (0.9 kg).

32. For a healthy woman with a healthy or desirable prepregnancy BMI, daily caloric requirements during lactation are typical baseline caloric needs plus ___ kcal.

A. 250

B. 500

C. 750

D. 1,000

33. Recommended calcium intake for a woman during pregnancy is _____ mg of elemental calcium per day.

A. 400 to 600

B. 600 to 800

C. 800 to 1000

D. 1,000 to 1,300

34. Increased folic acid intake before conception is likely to reduce the risk of which of the following birth defects?

A. congenital cataract

B. pyloric stenosis

C. clubfoot

D. open NTDs

35. Maternal iron requirements are greatest during what part of pregnancy?

A. first trimester

B. second and third trimesters

C. equal throughout pregnancy

D. preconception

36. The most common form of acquired anemia during pregnancy is:

A. iron deficiency.

B. folate deficiency.

C. vitamin B_{12} deficiency.

D. primary hypoproliferative.

37. Concerning the use of alcohol during pregnancy, which of the following statements is most accurate?

A. Although potentially problematic, maternal alcohol intake does not increase the risk of miscarriage.

B. Risk to the fetus from alcohol exposure is greatest in the third trimester.

C. No level or time of exposure is considered safe.

D. Risk of fetal alcohol syndrome is present only if alcohol exposure has occurred throughout the pregnancy.

38. Pica (ingestion of nonfood substances) during pregnancy should be considered:

A. a harmless practice common in certain ethnic groups.

B. problematic only if more nutritious food sources are left out of the diet and are replaced by the nonfood substance.

C. a way of providing select micronutrients not usually found in food products.

D. potentially dangerous because of contaminants in the nonfood substance.

39. Examples of NTDs include all of the following except:

A. anencephaly.

B. spina bifida.

C. encephalocele.

D. omphalocele.

40 to 43. Match each of the following substances of abuse with the most appropriate expected effect on the developing fetus during pregnancy.

_____ **40.** Alcohol

_____ **41.** Tobacco

_____ **42.** Opioids

_____ **43.** Stimulants

A. SIDS

B. neurobehavioral disorders

C. neonatal abstinence syndrome

D. abnormal facial features

44 to 46. Match each of the following substances of abuse with the most appropriate expected maternal effects.

_____ **44.** Tobacco

_____ **45.** Opioids

_____ **46.** Stimulants

A. seizures

B. chronic respiratory disease

C. respiratory depression

For answers and rationales, see end of chapter.

Prenatal Care and Screening

Overview

Numerous recommendations exist regarding the frequency of prenatal care and associated laboratory and other testing (Table 18-2 and Table 18-3). These are simply guidelines for the care that is needed for a well woman with a pregnancy with low physiological and psychosocial risk.

> **CLINICAL CONCEPT**
>
> More frequent visits and testing are often indicated during pregnancy, but a minimum of 8 to 10 visits should be scheduled.

Prepregnancy and Antenatal Screening

The goal of preconception and prenatal care is to optimize pregnancy outcome. Preconception care, provided prior to pregnancy, focuses on reducing maternal and fetal mortality and morbidity. This care provides the health-care provider the opportunity to work with the woman to optimize her health prior to becoming pregnant. For example, approximately 50% of women in North America are overweight or obese, conditions well known to increase pregnancy complications, including gestational diabetes, hypertension, macrosomia, birth trauma, increased caesarean and induced birth rates, as well as preterm labor. In addition, approximately 20% of women of reproductive age have asthma, about 10% have primary hypertension, and about 3% have diabetes. Uncontrolled asthma can cause fetal hypoxia, which can impair growth and lead to preterm birth and low birth weight. Uncontrolled diabetes during pregnancy can increase the risk of stillbirth as well as macrosomia and respiratory distress. While none of the conditions prevents a woman from having a healthy pregnancy and childbirth, the treatment and control of these chronic conditions should be optimized prior to conception.

In addition, preconception care should optimally include screening for genetically based maternal conditions that potentially impact the fetus' or infant's health. Select testing constitutes an important part of prenatal care. Testing for Tay-Sachs' disease should be performed prior to pregnancy among high-risk populations including Ashkenazi Jews, French Canadians, and those of Cajun ancestry. Cystic fibrosis testing

TABLE 18-2 Frequency of Prenatal Visits

TIME IN PREGNANCY	FREQUENCY OF VISITS
Up to 28 weeks	Every 4 weeks
28 to 36 weeks	Every 2 weeks
36 weeks or more	Every week

Source: Akkerman D, Cleland L, Croft G, et al.; Institute for Clinical Systems Improvement. Routine prenatal care. https://www.bmchp.org/~/media/23e81f82425240699b6a73c9582fc84c.pdf

TABLE 18-3 Testing as Part of Prenatal Care

TIME OF TESTING	PRENATAL TEST
10 to 13 weeks	First-trimester screen with plasma protein A (PAPP-A) and β-hCG and ultrasound of nuchal translucency (NT) and calculated with maternal age, weight, and race for early detection of Down/trisomy 18. Sequential screening: Patient gets results and then proceeds with Quad at 15 to 21 weeks. Integrated first-trimester screen done but no results until Quad is done in second trimester.
15 to 21 weeks (ideal 16 to 18 weeks)	Quad/AFP4/Tetra marker/screen to screen for Down/trisomy 18, neural tube defect, ultrasound (little evidence of improved pregnancy outcomes with routine obstetric ultrasound in low-physiological-risk pregnancy).
24 to 28 weeks	One-hour glucose load to screen for gestational diabetes mellitus, Rh neg—Get antibody screen and give RhIg (RhoGAM) 300 mcg IM at 28 weeks if indicated.
28 to 32 weeks	Hb, sexually transmitted infection testing as indicated (VDRL, HIV, HBsAg, GC, chlamydia), RhoGAM as indicated.
32 to 36 weeks	Fetal presentation, kick count (fetal movements: four or more in 1 hour, 10 or more in 2 hours).
35 to 37 weeks	Group B strep culture (rectal and vaginal)—Treat intrapartum with appropriate antibiotic to reduce risk of neonatal infection.
40 to 42 weeks	Vaginal examination to assess cervical ripeness, fetal station (little evidence results are predictive of labor onset).
41+ weeks	Nonstress test, biophysical profile (BPP) to check fetal status. The BPP consists of five components, including fetal breathing movements, gross body movements, tone, amniotic fluid index, and a nonstress test. Each component is scored as either 0 or 2, with a maximum score of 10. Modified BPP: amniotic fluid index greater than 5 cm and reactive nonstress test.

Source: U.S. Department of Veterans Affairs. Clinical practice guideline for pregnancy management. https://www.healthquality.va.gov/guidelines/WH/up/

can be performed prior to or early in pregnancy for high-risk groups consisting of those with Northern European or Ashkenazi Jewish heritage and less commonly those with African ancestry. The sickle cell trait can also be tested for prior to or early in pregnancy among those with African, Latino, Arabic, Greek, Maltese, Italian, Sardinian, Turkish, and Indian ancestry.

One point of confusion is the difference between screening and diagnostic tests. Commonly offered prenatal tests include maternal serum analysis for alpha-fetoprotein (AFP), human chorionic gonadotropin (hCG), inhibin-A, and unconjugated estriol levels, also known as the "quad (quadruple) screen." When the amounts of these substances are analyzed, increased risk of open NTDs, trisomy 21 (Down syndrome), and trisomy 18 (Edwards' syndrome) can be detected. An abnormal "quad screen" result is not diagnostic of any condition, however, and further testing is recommended, including amniocentesis and level II ultrasound. Consultation with a perinatology specialist and/or genetic counseling is also indicated.

Fetal aneuploidy is defined as an abnormal number of chromosomes present in the fetus. A single additional chromosome is called trisomy and is an important cause of congenital anomalies and developmental disability. Down syndrome (trisomy 21), Edwards' syndrome (trisomy 18), and Patau's syndrome (trisomy 13) are the most common types. Initially, screening for fetal aneuploidy involved offering amniocentesis to higher-risk mothers. However, noninvasive methods are available for initial screening. All women regardless of age should be offered prenatal assessment for aneuploidy either by screening or invasive prenatal diagnosis techniques. In addition to the quad screen, the cell-free fetal DNA test that assesses fetal DNA derived from the plasma of pregnant women offers a noninvasive method to screen for fetal aneuploidy. The cell-free fetal DNA test can be used as a primary screening test in women at increased risk of aneuploidy. These risks include the following:

■ Maternal age 35 years and older at delivery
■ Fetal ultrasonographic findings indicating an increased risk of aneuploidy
■ History of a prior pregnancy with a trisomy
■ Positive test result for aneuploidy, including first trimester, sequential, or integrated screen, or a quad screen
■ Parental balanced Robertsonian translocation with increased risk of fetal trisomy 13 or trisomy 21

Noninvasive prenatal testing (NIPT) can detect fetal DNA in maternal serum at greater than 10 weeks' gestation. Women should be counseled on the limitations of the cell-free fetal DNA test, which should include a discussion that this test may not be as accurate as diagnostic tests such as amniocentesis or chorionic villi sampling.

Ongoing Evaluation During Pregnancy

Prenatal care is not just an issue of serial testing and screening. Ongoing evaluation of maternal well-being, coaching, and counseling are essential components of care of the woman during pregnancy, with a goal of enhancing the likelihood of a healthy mother and infant (Table 18-4).

> **CLINICAL CONCEPT**
>
> In particular, ongoing screening, and when needed, intervention for substance misuse, substance abuse disorder, and interpersonal violence are critical components of prenatal care.

TABLE 18-4 Health Guidance in Pregnancy

TOPIC	RECOMMENDATIONS
Travel	Avoid prolonged sitting (increases risk of embolism); walk q 2 hours × 10 minutes
	Can fly up to 36 weeks if low risk (ACOG); airlines have own restrictions
	Wear seat belt (under abdomen as pregnancy progresses)
Work	Safe to work throughout pregnancy
	Exceptions: Avoid repetitive lifting, prolonged standing, activities that increase risk of falling/trauma, hazardous chemicals
Dental care	Gum disease linked to preterm birth
	Maintain excellent oral hygiene, seek routine dental care (cleaning) and immediate care if problems arise; most dental treatment acceptable in pregnancy
Exercise	Maintain prepregnancy fitness routines
	Stop exercising if extreme fatigue, dizziness, shortness of breath
	Avoid overheating, stay well-hydrated
	Avoid supine position in second and third trimesters

Continued

TABLE 18-4 Health Guidance in Pregnancy—cont'd

TOPIC	RECOMMENDATIONS
Sexual activity	No need to restrict unless rupture of membranes or placenta previa Unclear if increased risk if at risk of preterm labor
Immunizations	Recommended: Influenza vaccine for women in first, second, third trimesters during flu season (acceptable to administer in first trimester but often preferred to wait until after 14th week) Tdap in third trimester with each pregnancy, regardless of when last Tdap given
Warning signs in pregnancy	Contact provider if: ■ Vaginal bleeding ■ Abdominal pain/pelvic pressure ■ Severe nausea/vomiting ■ Signs/symptoms of infection: Fever, rash, persistent diarrhea ■ Severe headache, dizziness, visual changes ■ Abnormal vaginal discharge or fluid from vagina ■ Decreased or absent fetal movement (after quickening)

Discussion Sources

American College of Obstetricians and Gynecologists. Practice bulletin No. 162: Prenatal diagnostic testing for genetic disorders. *Obstet Gynecol.* 2016;127:e108–122.

American College of Obstetricians and Gynecologists. Practice bulletin No. 163: Screening for fetal aneuploidy. *Obstet Gynecol.* 2016;127:e123–137.

American Pregnancy Association. Chorionic villus sampling: CVS. https://americanpregnancy.org/prenatal-testing/chorionic-villus-sampling/

American Pregnancy Association. Quad screen test. https://americanpregnancy.org/prenatal-testing/quad-screen/

Centers for Disease Control and Prevention. Treating for Two: a national strategy for safer medication use in pregnancy. https://www.cdc.gov/pregnancy/meds/treatingfortwo/index.html

March of Dimes. Amniocentesis. http://www.marchofdimes.org/pregnancy/amniocentesis.aspx

QUESTIONS

47. The recommended frequency of prenatal visits in weeks 28 to 36 of pregnancy is every:
    A. week.
    B. 2 weeks.
    C. 3 weeks.
    D. 4 weeks.

48. Testing for sexually transmitted infection should be initially obtained:
    A. as early as possible in pregnancy.
    B. during the second trimester.
    C. during the third trimester.
    D. as close to the anticipated date of birth as possible.

49. Which of the following is considered the most accurate study for antenatal diagnosis?
    A. cell-free fetal DNA test
    B. serum AFP
    C. serum inhibin-A
    D. amniocentesis

50. The quad screen should be obtained at about _____ weeks of pregnancy.

    A. 6 to 10

    B. 11 to 15

    C. 16 to 20

    D. 21 to 25

51. Aneuploidy is defined as:

    A. a physical malformation of the fetus of unknown origin.

    B. a birth defect originating from the use of a teratogenic drug.

    C. the presence of an abnormal number of chromosomes.

    D. a birth defect originating from a nutritional deficiency.

52. The quad screen is used to help detect increased risk for which of the following conditions in the fetus?

    A. trisomy 21 and open NTDs

    B. cystic fibrosis and Angelman's syndrome

    C. Tay-Sachs' disease and trisomy 18

    D. sickle cell anemia and β-thalassemia major

53. Prenatal assessment for aneuploidy should be offered:

    A. only to women older than 35 years of age.

    B. only to women younger than 21 years of age.

    C. only to women either younger than 21 years or older than 35 years of age.

    D. to all women regardless of age.

54. Tina is a 26-year-old woman who is pregnant and has an abnormal quad screen. The test was done at an appropriate time during her pregnancy. When sharing this information with Tina, you consider that:

    A. this testing is diagnostic of specific conditions.

    B. further testing is recommended.

    C. the testing should be repeated.

    D. no further testing is required.

55. The rate of spontaneous fetal loss related to amniocentesis that is done at a facility that performs these procedures on a regular basis is approximately 1 in _____ procedures.

    A. 75

    B. 200

    C. 500

    D. 800

56. Women at high risk for aneuploidy include all of the following except those with:

    A. a maternal age of 35 years or older at anticipated time of giving birth.

    B. a history of prior pregnancy with trisomy.

    C. fetal ultrasonographic findings indicating an increased risk of aneuploidy.

    D. a history of multiparity.

57. All of the following can cause an elevated maternal AFP except:

    A. underestimated gestational age.

    B. open NTD.

    C. meningomyelocele.

    D. Down syndrome.

58. Edwards' syndrome is the clinical manifestation of trisomy _____.

    A. 13

    B. 15

    C. 18

    D. 21

59. In Edwards' syndrome, which of the following statements is true?

    A. Edwards' syndrome is more common than Down syndrome.

    B. Most affected infants with Edwards' syndrome die during the first year of life.

    C. Edwards' syndrome is unlikely to cause developmental disability.

    D. Edwards' syndrome is associated with elevated AFP.

60. In Down syndrome, which of the following is true?

    A. Most infants affected with Down syndrome are born to women older than age 35 years.

    B. Down syndrome is noted in about 1 in 10,000 live births.

    C. Down syndrome is associated with a decreased maternal serum AFP level.

    D. Antenatal serum analysis is sufficient to make the diagnosis.

61. Down syndrome is the clinical manifestation of trisomy _____.

    A. 13

    B. 15

    C. 18

    D. 21

62. Components of the antenatal screening test known as the "quad screen" include all of the following except:

    A. AFP.

    B. hCG.

    C. unconjugated estriol.

    D. progesterone.

63. Elevated inhibin-A is noted when a pregnant woman is at increased risk of carrying a fetus with:

    A. Down syndrome.

    B. Edwards' syndrome.

    C. open NTD.

    D. hemolytic anemia.

64. A 25-year-old woman presents in the 10th week of gestation requesting antenatal screening for Down syndrome. What advice should the NP give?

    A. Because of her age, no specific testing is recommended.

    B. She should be referred for second-trimester ultrasound.

    C. Screening that combines nuchal translucency measurement and biochemical testing and/or free cell DNA is available.

    D. She should be referred to a genetic counselor.

65 to 67. Match the following at-risk ethnic groups to the following genetically based conditions.

_____ **65.** Tay-Sachs' disease

_____ **66.** cystic fibrosis

_____ **67.** sickle cell trait

    A. French Canadian

    B. northern European ancestry

    C. African ancestry

68. A possible pregnancy-related complication for a woman with poorly controlled asthma can include:

    A. macrosomia.

    B. low birth weight.

    C. trisomy 21.

    D. cystic fibrosis.

69. Possible pregnancy-related complications due to poorly controlled type 2 diabetes mellitus can include all of the following except:

    A. stillbirth.

    B. respiratory distress.

    C. anencephaly.

    D. macrosomia.

For answers and rationales, see end of chapter.

Medication Use During Pregnancy

Overview

According to the CDC, 90% of American women take at least one medication during their pregnancy, and about 70% take at least one prescription medication. Pregnant women have similar incidence of acute and chronic illnesses to age-matched women who are not pregnant.

> **CLINICAL CONCEPT**
>
> Though ideally no woman would take any medication during pregnancy, pregnant women often need drug therapy to optimize maternal health. This optimizes pregnancy outcomes.

Potentially Teratogenic Medications

Certain medications are potentially teratogenic, or capable of inducing congenital anomalies, and should be avoided or used with great caution during pregnancy. By definition, a teratogenic drug is a substance that has the potential to create a characteristic set of malformations in the fetus. The classic teratogenic period occurs in a specific time of fetal development, usually between day 31 and day 81, following the last menstrual period (LMP) when organogenesis is occurring. For a teratogen to exert its effect, the product must be taken at the point in the pregnancy when the affected organ system is developing. For example, lithium can cause a characteristic teratogenic cardiac defect when taken as the cardiac tube is forming; taken earlier or later in the organ development process, the drug likely has no effect on the heart. Before day 31 post-LMP, the pregnancy exists as a group of poorly differentiated cells with no discrete organ systems to damage. A teratogen could be taken at that point and no damage would result because there are no organ systems to disrupt. After day 81 post-LMP, the organs are formed but are still growing and developing. The likelihood of a substance exerting a teratogenic effect decreases. At the same time, no medication exerts a teratogenic effect every time it is used.

Drug Transfer Across the Placenta

Many factors influence drug transfer across the placenta, including the molecular weight of the substance, lipid solubility, and duration of exposure. Medications usually pass by passive diffusion, where the maternal drug level is greater than that of the fetus; more drug is passed when maternal levels are greatest. The degree of diffusion is influenced by many factors besides maternal drug levels, including the drug's molecular weight and degree of lipophilicity. Drugs with a low molecular weight (500 daltons or less) cross the placental barrier more easily than drugs with a molecular weight greater than 500 daltons, whereas drugs with a molecular weight greater than 1,000 daltons cross the placenta infrequently or in very small amounts. The lower the molecular weight, the greater the potential becomes for passage of the drug through the placenta. Alcohol and cocaine have low molecular weights (100 daltons or less) and are easily passed. Insulin and heparin (molecular weight greater than 5,000 daltons) are examples of drugs that are poorly transported to the fetus and can be given with relative safety in pregnancy. Most oral over-the-counter and prescription medications have molecular weights of less than 500 daltons and pass easily through the placenta. The placenta preferentially allows highly lipophilic drugs to pass through to the fetus. Fetal liver maturity also plays a role because 40% to 60% of fetal blood circulation goes through the liver. With increasing maturity, the fetus' hepatic enzymes become more capable of metabolizing drugs.

Not all drugs within the same therapeutic class have the same lipid solubility. Diphenhydramine (Benadryl®) is a highly lipophilic antihistamine and penetrates the placenta and maternal central nervous system easily, causing sedation. In contrast, loratadine (Claritin®) is more hydrophilic and has fewer fetal or maternal effects. Drugs with a long half-life or with extended-release formulations are usually held in maternal circulation for protracted periods and have the potential to have a greater effect on the fetus than similar drugs with shorter half-lives or drugs that are metabolized more rapidly.

Classifying Medication Use During Pregnancy

The U.S. Food and Drug Administration (FDA) established standards in product labeling for information about using medicines during pregnancy and breastfeeding. The letter categories that have been long used to classify medication use during pregnancy (i.e., A, B, C, D, X) have been replaced with three detailed subsections (i.e., pregnancy, lactation, and females/males of reproductive potential) that describe risks within the real-world context of use for pregnant and nursing women who need medication. The Pregnancy and Lactation Labeling Rule (PLLR) is now in effect for prescription drugs and biological products submitted for FDA approval. Labeling changes for prescription medications approved in the past will be phased in gradually.

Even with these changes in labeling, many clinicians continue to use the older classification of medication use during pregnancy and lactation as a clinical reminder of which drugs to use and avoid. A quick way to remember the categories (also see Table 18-5) is as follows:

■ *Category B for Best* because very few products are category A.
■ *Category C for Caution* because these products have been shown to have risk in animal models.
■ *Category D for Danger* because these products have been shown to have risk when used in human pregnancy but are used occasionally in life-threatening maternal disease.
■ *Category X for "Cross these drugs off the list"* because these products have shown teratogenic risk and have no therapeutic indication for use during human pregnancy.

Medication Use for Commonly Encountered Health Issues During Pregnancy

Asthma

Up to 8% of pregnant women have asthma, with a documented increase in maternal morbidity and mortality during pregnancy for women with the most severe asthma before conception. Most pregnant women with asthma have no change in their symptoms or experience an improvement in symptoms.

Bronchospasm symptoms are usually worse between 29 and 36 weeks of gestation because of esophageal irritation from gastroesophageal reflux disease (GERD). Symptoms usually improve late in gestation when gradual fetal descent occurs. Lifestyle changes that help improve symptoms of GERD help with asthma management. Generally, the risk of fetal hypoxia is greater than the risk of medication exposure, so standard asthma medications should be continued. Most inhaled corticosteroids (ICSs) are FDA risk category C (with budesonide [Pulmicort®] being the exception as risk category B), a designation that is based on high oral or parenteral doses given to laboratory animals, but this appears to have little applicability in human use. As such, use of ICSs in pregnant women is generally acceptable as the inhaled medication has a low rate of systemic absorption. Oral corticosteroids have the same designation but should be used only to treat an asthma flare. Beta-2 agonist bronchodilators are also category C, based on studies of high oral doses in laboratory animals, and should be prescribed as a rescue drug for a pregnant woman with asthma. Leukotriene modifiers (e.g., montelukast) have not been studied as extensively in pregnant women and carry a risk category B.

Nausea and Vomiting During Pregnancy

Nausea and vomiting in pregnancy (NVP) is reported by up to 80% of all women during pregnancy. While often called "morning sickness," the condition can occur at any time of the day. NVP's onset is usually around weeks 5 to 6 of pregnancy and usually resolves by approximately week 12. Its severity ranges from mild nausea in response to certain scents or triggers to debilitating vomiting that precludes participating in daily activities. In its most extreme form, hyperemesis gravidarum, the pregnant woman is sufficiently ill to be unable to maintain hydration and nutrition.

TABLE 18-5 Medication Use During Pregnancy

An FDA risk category is assigned to all drugs based on risk of drug exposure to the human fetus: A, B, C, D, or X. New drugs undergo animal studies, and perhaps a small number of inadvertent human exposures during clinical trials are considered.

RISK CATEGORY	OUTCOMES	EXAMPLE
Category A	Well-controlled human study: No fetal risk in first trimester No evidence of risk in second and third trimesters Risk to fetus appears remote	Vitamins at recommended daily allowance ■ Vitamin A caution (risk factor X in doses 8,000 IU/day or more) Levothyroxine
Category B B: *Best because nothing is A*	Animal studies do not show fetal risk, but no controlled study in humans, *or* Animal studies show adverse effect not shown in human study	Beta-lactam antimicrobials ■ The penicillins, cephalosporins Select macrolides ■ Azithromycin, erythromycin Acetaminophen
Category C C: *Use with caution*	No controlled study in humans available Animal studies reveal adverse fetal effects	Approximately two-thirds of all prescription medications Select antimicrobials ■ Clarithromycin ■ Fluoroquinolones (-*floxacin* suffix) ■ TMP-SMX Commonly prescribed medications ■ Most selective serotonin reuptake inhibitors, corticosteroids, antihypertensives, others
Category D D: *Danger is known*	Positive evidence of human fetal risk Use in pregnant women occasionally acceptable despite risk	Gentamicin Angiotensin-converting enzyme inhibitors (-*pril* suffix), angiotensin receptor blocker (-*sartan* suffix) Tetracyclines ■ Doxycycline, minocycline Paroxetine
Category X *Cross these off your list of medications to use during pregnancy*	Animal or human studies show fetal abnormality Evidence of fetal risk based on human study No therapeutic indication in pregnancy	Isotretinoin (Accutane®), misoprostol (Cytotec®), thalidomide

Source: Briggs G, Freeman R. Drugs in Pregnancy and Lactation. 11th ed. Philadelphia, PA: Lippincott Williams & Wilkins; 2017.

CLINICAL CONCEPT

Taking vitamin B$_6$, 25 mg twice a day, has been noted to prevent future nausea and vomiting.

For the majority of women with NVP, successful management is targeted toward relieving nausea by increasing rest, decreasing stress, eating frequent small meals, avoiding high-fat foods, and avoiding symptom trigger situations. Ginger or lemon aromatherapy is often helpful and can be facilitated by making a "kit" by placing five ginger or lemon teabags in an airtight plastic tub. When nausea occurs, the patient opens the tub and sniffs the vapors. Treating the concomitant gastric irritation that often accompanies severe nausea and vomiting during pregnancy with a chewable calcium antacid tablet every 2 hours for 2 to 3 days can be helpful.

A 5-HT$_3$-receptor antagonist, such as ondansetron (Zofran®), can offer a therapeutic option for preventing severe morning sickness but is not effective in managing acute symptoms, albeit with conflicting studies on the risk of birth defects. In hyperemesis gravidarum, expert consultation is advised to manage dehydration and possibly initiate parenteral nutrition.

Primary Hypertension

For women being actively treated for primary hypertension prior to pregnancy, angiotensin-converting enzyme inhibitors and angiotensin receptor blockers are risk category D and should be avoided during pregnancy. The use of beta blockers is also associated with fetal risks, including decreased placental perfusion (leading to slower fetal growth), bradycardia, and hypoglycemia. Select calcium channel blockers, select alpha-beta blockers, and certain centrally acting antihypertensives are usually used to treat primary hypertension during pregnancy. Expert consultation should be sought in the care of the woman with primary hypertension during pregnancy.

Migraine

Among women with a migraine history, most note fewer and less intense headaches during pregnancy; however, about 5% to 10% have worsening headaches. Treatment options are limited and include acetaminophen. NSAIDs are category C, and their use during pregnancy is controversial. NSAID use in the first half of pregnancy is correlated with higher miscarriage rate. At the same time, NSAIDs should generally be avoided after 30 to 32 weeks of pregnancy because of a potential for rare and serious fetal abnormalities (i.e., premature closure of ductus arteriosus and persistent fetal circulation). Acetaminophen use during pregnancy has been associated with a higher rate of attention-deficit hyperactivity disorder in the offspring. Triptans are risk category C, partly because of the theoretical risk of vasoconstriction as well as evidence of embryo-lethality and fetal abnormalities observed in animal studies. However, no teratogenic effect has been observed in human pregnancy. The medications commonly used to prevent migraine, including beta blockers, tricyclic antidepressants, and select antiepileptic drugs, are risk category C or D and should not be used during pregnancy. Given these limitations, helping a woman with migraine during pregnancy poses a challenge. Localized measures during the headache such as ice packs to the affected area and resting in a cool, dark, and quiet place are often helpful but also difficult to access. Avoiding headache triggers such as hunger and thirst is important. Lidocaine 4% used as a nasal spray, applied to the nostril on the affected side of the head, can help attenuate headache symptoms with minimal systemic drug absorption.

Mood Disorders

Women are twice as likely as men to experience major depressive disorder. Consequently, many women enter pregnancy in a depressed state or develop depression during the course of the pregnancy. Therapy for any mood disorder usually includes lifestyle changes, counseling, and drug therapy. Mood disorder treatment options include serotonin, norepinephrine, dopamine receptor modulators, tricyclic antidepressants, and benzodiazepines. Although selective serotonin reuptake inhibitors (SSRIs) are in risk category C (with the exception of paroxetine, which is risk category D), the link between SSRI use and birth defects is still unfolding. Though some risk has been observed with SSRI use during pregnancy, it is important to note that the overall risk of birth defects remains very low.

Bupropion is a dopamine receptor modulator and is also pregnancy risk category C. Serotonin and norepinephrine reuptake inhibitors (SNRIs) such as venlafaxine (Effexor®) and duloxetine (Cymbalta®) are risk category C. Although few clinical studies have investigated the effects of these drugs during pregnancy, safety surveillance studies indicate the frequency of abnormal outcomes while taking these agents during pregnancy is consistent with historic rates in the general population.

If a patient wishes to discontinue psychotropic therapy during pregnancy, she should be counseled about the risk of mood disorder recurrence. A slow taper of approximately 25% of the total dose per week is required to avoid SSRI withdrawal syndrome. The withdrawal syndrome is bothersome but not life-threatening. Symptoms include jitteriness, nausea, and sleep disturbance and are more severe with SSRIs with a shorter half-life such as paroxetine (half-life 26 hours) and less severe with SSRIs with a longer half-life such as fluoxetine (half-life 24 to 72 hours and metabolite half-life up to 26 hours). If SSRIs are used late in the third trimester, fetal withdrawal can also occur, which is the reason for the common recommendation to taper, with a goal of discontinuation prior to giving birth, a pregnant woman's SSRI dose over the last month of pregnancy. Neonatal effects are similar to maternal withdrawal and include irritability, protracted crying, and shivering; the timing of the onset of neonatal SSRI withdrawal symptoms is related to the drug's half-life and can occur within days to weeks of birth. This neonatal withdrawal syndrome is also noted with the maternal use of SNRIs if taken throughout the pregnancy.

Tricyclic antidepressants and benzodiazepines are risk category C or D and are rarely prescribed during pregnancy. If an expectant mother has been on long-term benzodiazepine therapy, it is critical to taper doses gradually (25% per week) to avoid withdrawal syndrome. Rapid withdrawal can lead to tremors, hallucinations, seizures, and a delirium tremens–like state that is most common with the use of products with a shorter half-life. The onset of withdrawal symptoms occurs a few days after the last dose in a benzodiazepine with a shorter half-life (e.g., lorazepam) and up to 3 weeks in one with a longer half-life (e.g., clonazepam).

Urinary Tract Infection

Pregnancy-related anatomical changes in the urinary tract, such as pressure on the bladder from the enlarging uterus and increase in the size of the ureters, contribute to urinary reflux. Asymptomatic bacteriuria occurs in 5% to 9% of nonpregnant and pregnant women. If left untreated in pregnancy, progression of asymptomatic bacteriuria to symptomatic UTI, including acute cystitis and pyelonephritis, occurs in 15% to 45%, or fourfold higher than in nonpregnant women. This progression largely results from the lower interleukin-6 levels and serum antibody responses to *Escherichia coli* antigens that occur during pregnancy, resulting in a less robust immune response.

> **CLINICAL CONCEPT**
> Urinary tract infection (UTI) in a pregnant woman, especially if recurrent, is a significant risk factor for low-birth-weight infants and prematurity.

Because asymptomatic bacteriuria, usually caused by aerobic gram-negative bacilli or *Staphylococcus saprophyticus,* can lead to UTI, a urine culture should be obtained from all women early in pregnancy, even in the absence of UTI symptoms. Approximately 20% to 40% of women with asymptomatic bacteriuria develop UTI during the course of the pregnancy; only 1% to 2% of women with a negative urine culture develop UTI. Asymptomatic bacteriuria should be treated with a 3- to 7-day course of antimicrobials, which reduces the risk of symptomatic UTI by 80% to 90%. Options for the treatment of asymptomatic bacteriuria and symptomatic UTI during pregnancy are guided by pathogen susceptibility, and preferred antimicrobials include those with FDA pregnancy risk category B. Antimicrobials in pregnancy risk category B include beta-lactams (amoxicillin, cephalexin, cefpodoxime, cefixime, and amoxicillin-clavulanate) and nitrofurantoin. Nitrofurantoin has the advantage of sparing disruption of normal vaginal flora and consistent efficacy against *E coli* and *S saprophyticus.* Nitrofurantoin should be avoided after the 36th week of gestation because of the potential (although unlikely) risk for hemolysis if the fetus is glucose-6-phosphate dehydrogenase–deficient and for infections caused by *Proteus mirabilis.* Beta-lactam use usually fails to eradicate the offending pathogen from the periurethral and perivaginal areas, increasing the risk of reinfection.

Women with symptomatic UTI during pregnancy should be treated for 7 days. When UTI is documented, monthly screening of urine cultures should be obtained for the duration of the pregnancy. Daily antimicrobial prophylaxis with an appropriate agent should be considered with evidence of 2 days of a symptomatic UTI or persistent, unresolved bacteriuria despite effective antimicrobial therapy. Urological evaluation should also be considered to rule out structural abnormality.

Discussion Sources

Antonucci R, Zaffanello M, Puxeddu E, et al. Use of non-steroidal anti-inflammatory drugs in pregnancy: impact on the fetus and newborn. *Curr Drug Metab.* 2012;13(4):474–490.

Briggs G, Freeman R, Yaffe S. *Drugs in Pregnancy and Lactation: A Reference for Fetal and Neonatal Risk.* 11th ed. Philadelphia, PA: Lippincott Williams & Wilkins; 2017.

Centers for Disease Control and Prevention. Treating for Two: a national strategy for safer medication use in pregnancy. http://www.cdc.gov/ncbddd/birthdefects/documents/ncbddd_birth-defects_medicationuseonepager_cdcrole.pdf

Gilbert DN, Chambers HF, Eliopoulos GM, Saag MS, Pavia AT. *The Sanford Guide to Antimicrobial Therapy.* 50th ed. Sperryville, VA: Antimicrobial Therapy, Inc.; 2020.

Ogunyemi DA. Hyperemesis gravidarum. Medscape. http://emedicine.medscape.com/article/254751-overview

QUESTIONS

70. Medications most commonly pass through the placenta via:

A. facilitated transport.

B. passive diffusion.

C. capillary pump action.

D. active diffusion.

71. During pregnancy, the most intense organogenesis occurs how many days following the LMP?

A. 12 to 30 days

B. 31 to 81 days

C. 92 to 120 days

D. 121 to 150 days

72. A drug with demonstrated safety for use in all trimesters of pregnancy is categorized as FDA risk category:

A. A.

B. B.

C. C.

D. D.

73. A drug shown to cause teratogenic effects in human study but that has benefits that could outweigh the risks of use in a life-threatening situation is assigned FDA risk category:

A. A.

B. B.

C. C.

D. D.

74. A drug that has not been shown to be harmful to the fetus in animal studies, but for which no human study is available, is assigned FDA risk category:

A. A.

B. B.

C. C.

D. D.

75. A drug shown to cause teratogenic effect in animal studies but for which no human study is available, is assigned FDA risk category:

A. A.

B. B.

C. C.

D. D.

76. Prior to day 31 post-LMP, the embryo is best described as:

A. a single, undifferentiated cell.

B. a group of poorly differentiated cells.

C. a conglomerate of highly differentiated cells and primitive organs.

D. a small fetus with developed organs.

77. What is the molecular weight requirement for a drug to easily pass through the placental barrier?

A. less than 250 daltons

B. less than 500 daltons

C. less than 1,000 daltons

D. less than 5,000 daltons

78. What is the molecular weight requirement for a drug to be unable to pass through the placental barrier?

A. greater than 250 daltons

B. greater than 500 daltons

C. greater than 1,000 daltons

D. greater than 5,000 daltons

79. When treating a woman with a urinary tract infection who is 28 weeks' pregnant, the NP considers prescribing:
    A. trimethoprim-sulfamethoxazole (TMP-SMX).
    B. cephalexin.
    C. ciprofloxacin.
    D. doxycycline.

80. In a pregnant woman with asthma, in what part of her pregnancy do symptoms and bronchospasm often worsen?
    A. 6 to 14 weeks
    B. 15 to 23 weeks
    C. 24 to 33 weeks
    D. 29 to 36 weeks

81. In treating a pregnant woman with acute bacterial rhinosinusitis, the NP would likely avoid prescribing:
    A. amoxicillin.
    B. cefuroxime.
    C. cefpodoxime.
    D. levofloxacin.

82. The duration of antimicrobial therapy for treatment of symptomatic urinary tract infection in a pregnant woman is:
    A. 3 days.
    B. 5 days.
    C. 7 days.
    D. 10 days.

83. SSRI withdrawal syndrome is best characterized as:
    A. bothersome but not life threatening.
    B. potentially life threatening.
    C. most often seen with medications with a longer half-life.
    D. associated with seizure risk.

84. The placenta is best described as:
    A. poorly permeable.
    B. an effective drug barrier.
    C. able to transport lipophilic substances.
    D. capable of impeding substances with molecular weight 300 daltons or less.

85. Preferred treatment options for a pregnant woman in the second trimester with migraine include:
    A. sumatriptan.
    B. codeine.
    C. aspirin.
    D. acetaminophen.

86. In counseling women about SSRI use during pregnancy, the NP considers that studies reveal that:
    A. a clear teratogenic pattern has been identified for all drugs in this class.
    B. the drugs have a negative effect on intellectual development.

    C. the use of paroxetine during pregnancy is associated with an increase in risk for congenital cardiac defect.

    D. there is an increased rate of seizure disorder in exposed offspring.

87. Among the most commonly used medications by women in the first trimester of pregnancy are:

    A. antiepileptic drugs.

    B. antibiotics.

    C. antihypertensives.

    D. opioids.

88. Benzodiazepine withdrawal syndrome is best characterized as:

    A. bothersome but not life threatening.

    B. not observed during pregnancy.

    C. most often seen with agents that have a long half-life.

    D. associated with seizure risk.

89. The cornerstone controller therapy for moderate persistent asthma during pregnancy is the use of:

    A. oral theophylline.

    B. mast cell stabilizers.

    C. leukotriene receptor antagonist.

    D. inhaled corticosteroids.

90. You examine a 24-year-old woman with mild intermittent asthma who is 24 weeks' pregnant and has an acute asthma flare. Her medication regimen should be adjusted to include:

    A. titration to a therapeutic theophylline level.

    B. addition of timed salmeterol (Serevent®) use.

    C. a short course of oral prednisone.

    D. use of montelukast (Singulair®) on a regular basis.

91. For a pregnant woman with asthma, bronchospasm symptoms are often reported to improve during _____weeks of gestation.

    A. 8 to 13

    B. 20 to 26

    C. 29 to 36

    D. 36 to 40

92. The FDA has replaced the letter categories (i.e., A, B, C, D, X) of pregnancy risk with detailed subsections in the prescribing information sheets to describe risks within real-world context of use. These new subsections include all of the following except:

    A. females attempting to conceive.

    B. pregnancy.

    C. lactation.

    D. females and males of reproductive age.

93. For a pregnant woman who is on long-term benzodiazepine treatment, an appropriate course of action is to:

    A. increase the dose by 25% during the course of pregnancy.

    B. discontinue treatment immediately.

    C. taper the dose down 25% each week.

    D. switch to paroxetine therapy.

94. The use of NSAIDs during later pregnancy can potentially increase the risk for:

    A. premature birth.

    B. NTDs.

    C. premature closure of ductus arteriosus.

    D. ventricular septal defects.

95. The use of NSAIDs during early stages of pregnancy can potentially increase the risk for:

    A. premature birth.

    B. miscarriage.

    C. premature closure of ductus arteriosus.

    D. aneuploidy.

96. A 26-year-old woman has been taking an SSRI for depression during the entire course of her pregnancy. She gives birth to a full-term healthy girl. Five days after the birth, she reports that the baby is irritable with protracted periods of crying. This is likely a result of:

    A. increased intracranial pressure from in utero SSRI exposure.

    B. SSRI withdrawal.

    C. colic.

    D. impending sepsis.

97. Which of the following antimicrobials, when used as indicated, is preferred during pregnancy?

    A. clarithromycin

    B. doxycycline

    C. azithromycin

    D. ofloxacin

98. Which of the following antimicrobials is preferred for the treatment of a UTI during pregnancy?

    A. doxycycline

    B. levofloxacin

    C. cephalexin

    D. TMP-SMX

99. Which of the following antimicrobials should be avoided after the 36th week of pregnancy because of increased risk of fetal hemolysis?

    A. gentamicin

    B. nitrofurantoin

    C. clarithromycin

    D. ciprofloxacin

100. In a pregnant woman, asymptomatic bacteriuria:

    A. should be treated only if bladder instrumentation or surgery is planned.

    B. needs to be treated to avoid complicated UTI.

    C. is a common, benign finding.

    D. is a risk factor for the development of hypertension.

101. Which of the following is the most common UTI organism in pregnant women?

    A. *Pseudomonas aeruginosa*

    B. *E coli*

    C. *Klebsiella pneumoniae*

    D. *P mirabilis*

102. Recommended length of antimicrobial therapy for a pregnant woman with asymptomatic bacteruria is:

A. 1 to 3 days.

B. 3 to 7 days.

C. 8 to 10 days.

D. 2 weeks.

For answers and rationales, see end of chapter.

Conditions Encountered in Later Pregnancy

HYPERTENSIVE DISORDERS

Hypertensive disorders occur in 12% to 22% of all pregnancies. These disorders are usually divided into the following categories: chronic hypertension, or high BP diagnosis that predates the pregnancy, and hypertensive disorders acquired during pregnancy. Hypertensive disorders acquired during pregnancy include gestational hypertension, preeclampsia, and eclampsia.

Preeclampsia Overview

Preeclampsia is a condition found exclusively during the latter half (20 weeks' gestation or greater) of pregnancy or the early postpartum period; preeclampsia affects about 5% to 8% of all pregnancies. While its etiology remains poorly understood, the more common preeclampsia risk factors include age (40 years or older, 16 years or younger), first pregnancy or first pregnancy with a new partner, pregestational or gestational diabetes mellitus, presence of collagen vascular disease, prepregnancy or primary hypertension, presence of maternal renal disease, a family history of pregnancy-induced hypertension, or multiple gestation pregnancy. Additional risk factors include maternal obesity and select autoimmune diseases including antiphospholipid syndrome and systemic lupus.

Clinical Presentation and Diagnostic Testing

The presentation of preeclampsia can include headache, right upper quadrant or epigastric pain, and edema occurring after the 20th week of gestation. Diagnostic criteria for preeclampsia include elevated BP (140/90 mm Hg or higher on two readings at least 4 hours apart, or 160/110 mm Hg or higher for one reading) and proteinuria (300 mg or greater per 24-hour urine collection, or protein/creatinine ratio of 0.3 mg/dL or more, or dipstick reading of 2+). In the absence of proteinuria, other criteria can include any of the following: (1) thrombocytopenia (less than 100,000 platelets/mm^3), (2) renal insufficiency (serum creatinine greater than 1.1 mg/dL or a doubling of serum creatinine concentration in the absence of other renal disease), (3) impaired liver function (liver transaminases greater than two times the upper limit of normal [ULN]), (4) pulmonary edema, or (5) new-onset headache unresponsive to medication and not accounted for by another diagnosis. Additional findings, usually with more severe disease, include right upper quadrant abdominal pain, nausea, and vomiting. Preeclampsia can progress to the syndrome of hemolysis with resulting anemia, elevated liver enzymes indicating hepatocellular damage, and low platelet count and eclampsia; this constellation is known as HELLP and is noted in 5% to 10% of patients with preeclamptic symptoms (Table 18-6). Typical criteria for the diagnosis of HELLP include lactate dehydrogenase (LDH) elevated to 600 IU/L or more, AST and ALT elevated greater than two times ULN, and platelets less than 100,000/mm^3.

Treatment

The most important intervention in preeclampsia is maintaining a high index of suspicion in women with considerable risk and prompt recognition of the condition when it occurs.

When preeclampsia is recognized, expert obstetrics consultation should be obtained. Intervention includes rest, ongoing maternal and fetal monitoring, and antihypertensive or anticonvulsant medications, or both; all of these measures have only a small effect on outcome. Birth is the definitive intervention and is usually the treatment of choice in later pregnancy. In severe cases of preeclampsia, induction of delivery should be considered after 34 weeks' gestation. Though many studies have investigated strategies to prevent preeclampsia, to date there is no intervention that has been proven

> **CLINICAL CONCEPT**
>
> Women with higher preeclampsia risk should be evaluated in early pregnancy by a high-risk obstetrics provider team.

TABLE 18-6 Hypertensive Disorders During Pregnancy

CATEGORY OF HYPERTENSIVE DISORDER DURING PREGNANCY	DEFINING CHARACTERISTICS OF DISORDER
Chronic hypertension	High blood pressure diagnosed before pregnancy, present before 20th week of pregnancy, and/or persisting ≥6 weeks' postpartum
Gestational hypertension	High blood pressure diagnosed after 20th week of pregnancy but resolving within 6 weeks' postpartum, without significant proteinuria or other signs of preeclampsia
Preeclampsia	High blood pressure diagnosed after 20th week of pregnancy, accompanied by significant proteinuria (300 mg protein or more in 24-hour urine collection) or other findings (thrombocytopenia, elevated liver enzymes, renal insufficiency, headache) that cannot be attributed to another cause; usually accompanied by increased edema
Eclampsia	Presentation as in preeclampsia with tonic-clonic seizures or other alteration in mental status that cannot be attributed to another cause
HELLP syndrome	Preeclampsia accompanied by elevated lactose dehydrogenase and hepatic enzymes, and low platelets

Source: ACOG. Practice bulletin no. 202: gestational hypertension and preeclampsia. Obstetrics Gynecol. 2019;133:e1–e25. https://journals.lww.com/greenjournal/Fulltext/2019/01000 /ACOG_Practice_Bulletin_No__202__Gestational.49.aspx

to unequivocally reduce the risk of this condition. These studies included vitamin supplements, folic acid, low-sodium diets, and fish oil. A study on the use of aspirin (150 mg daily) from weeks 11 to 14 of gestation until 36 weeks' gestation in a high-risk population resulted in a significant decrease in preterm preeclampsia but no difference in term preeclampsia when compared to placebo.

GROUP B STREPTOCOCCUS

Overview

Neonatal infection with group B streptococci (GBS) is a leading cause of newborn morbidity and mortality, resulting in an estimated 7,600 cases of neonatal sepsis and approximately 300 neonatal deaths per year. Maternal lower genitourinary tract colonization with this organism is a major risk factor for early onset GBS infection, usually in the first week of life. The transmission of the organism from mother to fetus usually occurs after the onset of labor or membrane rupture. The lower gastrointestinal (GI) tract is the natural reservoir for this organism; this most likely contributes to GBS vaginal or rectal colonization in about 10% to 30% of pregnant women. This rate varies geographically.

Clinical Presentation

GBS colonization is not considered to be a sexually transmitted infection and can be transient, chronic, or intermittent. As a result, the pregnant woman with GBS carriage is typically without specific signs and symptoms.

Diagnostic Testing

GBS screening should be performed in all women at 35 to 37 weeks of pregnancy. The culture should be obtained by swabbing the lower vagina and vaginal introitus, followed by the rectum; insertion of the swab into the anal sphincter is needed for optimal results. The patient or health-care provider can obtain the culture. No vaginal speculum is needed, and cervical cultures should not be obtained because these can be negative in the presence of heavy lower vaginal GBS colonization. Women with scheduled caesarean births should be cultured as well.

Treatment

Intrapartum IV antimicrobial chemoprophylaxis is currently the most effective intervention to help prevent infant GBS disease. Oral or intramuscular (IM) formulations have not been shown to be as effective as IV administration of intrapartum antimicrobial prophylaxis. Antimicrobial treatment should begin at the onset of labor and continue through delivery. IV penicillin is the first-line option, while IV ampicillin is an acceptable alternative. For those with penicillin allergy and low risk of anaphylaxis, treatment with a first-generation cephalosporin (e.g., cefazolin) can be used. For women at high risk of anaphylaxis due to penicillin allergy, clindamycin can be considered if the GBS isolate is susceptible to this agent. If the isolate is not susceptible to clindamycin, then vancomycin remains the only acceptable choice in those situations. It is important to note that women with a positive prenatal GBS culture who undergo a cesarean birth before the onset of labor and with membranes intact do not require antimicrobial prophylaxis.

Discussion Sources

ACOG. Prevention of group B streptococcal early-onset disease in newborns. No. 797, February 2020. https://www.acog.org/clinical/clinical-guidance/committee-opinion/articles/2020/02/prevention-of-group-b-streptococcal-early-onset-disease-in-newborns

ACOG. Practice bulletin no. 202: gestational hypertension and preeclampsia. *Obstetrics Gynecol.* 2019;133:e1–e25. https://journals.lww.com/greenjournal/Fulltext/2019/01000/ACOG_Practice_Bulletin_No__202__Gestational.49.aspx

Akkerman D, Cleland L, Croft G, et al. *Routine Prenatal Care.* Bloomington, MN: Institute for Clinical Systems Improvement (ICSI); 2012, https://www.bmchp.org/~/media/23e81f82425240699b6a73c9582fc84c.pdf

Lim K-H. Preeclampsia. Medscape. http://emedicine.medscape.com/article/1476919-overview

QUESTIONS

103 to 107. Match each hypertensive disorder with its characteristic.

_____ **103.** chronic hypertension

_____ **104.** gestational hypertension

_____ **105.** preeclampsia

_____ **106.** eclampsia

_____ **107.** HELLP syndrome

    A. high BP diagnosed after the 20th week of pregnancy

    B. presence of tonic-clonic seizures or other alteration in mental status

    C. high BP diagnosed before pregnancy

    D. preeclampsia accompanied by elevated LDH and hepatic enzymes and low platelets

    E. high BP diagnosed after the 20th week of pregnancy and accompanied by significant proteinuria

108. Risk factors for preeclampsia include all of the following except:

    A. low maternal weight.

    B. age younger than 16 years or older than 40 years.

    C. collagen vascular disease.

    D. first pregnancy with a new partner.

109. For a woman who was normotensive before 20 weeks of gestation, an indication of preeclampsia is BP of more than ___ mm Hg systolic and more than ___ mm Hg diastolic measured on two occasions separated by at least 4 hours.

    A. 130, 80

    B. 140, 90

    C. 150, 95

    D. 160, 100

110. Preeclampsia presentation is noted after the ____ week of pregnancy.

A. 10th

B. 15th

C. 20th

D. 25th

111. The components of HELLP syndrome include all of the following except:

A. hepatic enzyme elevations.

B. thrombocytosis.

C. elevated lactate dehydrogenase.

D. preeclampsia.

112. Which of the following is the most important part of care of a woman with preeclampsia?

A. antihypertensive therapy

B. anticonvulsant therapy

C. prompt recognition of the condition

D. induction of labor

113. Which of the following is most accurate regarding prevention of preeclampsia?

A. There have been no definitive strategies identified to prevent preeclampsia.

B. Sodium restriction is effective in preventing preeclampsia when initiated during the first trimester.

C. Low-dose aspirin is effective in preventing preeclampsia throughout pregnancy.

D. Bedrest is the best prevention strategy for high-risk women.

114. Regarding the risk for neonatal GBS disease, the NP considers that:

A. about 50% to 70% of all pregnant women harbor this organism.

B. there is no risk of disease with cesarean birth with ruptured membranes.

C. the organism is most often acquired by vertical transmission in the second trimester of pregnancy.

D. intrapartum antimicrobials should be given to nearly all women with evidence of GBS colonization.

115. GBS cultures should be obtained from:

A. the cervix.

B. the urethra.

C. urine.

D. the lower vagina and rectum.

For answers and rationales, see end of chapter.

Early Pregnancy Loss

Overview

About 25% to 30% of women experience some vaginal bleeding in the first trimester of an intrauterine pregnancy (IUP), and at least 50% of these women have pregnancy loss. Spontaneous abortion is defined as the natural ending of a pregnancy before 20 weeks of gestation; the majority of these pregnancies will be lost prior to 10 weeks' gestation. In about 60% of spontaneous abortions, chromosomal anomalies of maternal or paternal origin are responsible for the pregnancy loss. Maternal factors such as trauma, illness, or infection lead to the loss in about 15% of cases. In the remaining cases, no obvious cause can be found. Ectopic pregnancy, or a pregnancy occurring outside the uterus, is less common but critically important to recognize.

With all forms of pregnancy loss, significant emotional support should be offered. Referral to pregnancy-loss support groups is often helpful. As with any clinical condition, evaluation of hemodynamic stability is crucial.

SPONTANEOUS ABORTION

Risk factors for spontaneous abortion (SAB) include prior history of spontaneous abortion, maternal age older than 35 years, and poorly controlled chronic health problems such as diabetes, hypertension, and thyroid disease. Additional risk factors include maternal use of select stimulants including cocaine, and excessive use of alcohol and caffeine. For women with recurrent early pregnancy loss, usually characterized by two to three consecutive SABs, expert consultation is advised to investigate an underlying, potentially treatable, condition.

> **CLINICAL CONCEPT**
> Autoimmune disorders, thrombophilia, and uterine factors are among the more common contributors to recurrent early pregnancy loss.

Four terms are usually used to modify the majority of spontaneous abortions: threatened, inevitable, incomplete, and complete.

■ Threatened abortion
  • *Clinical presentation*: Vaginal bleeding or brown spotting during early pregnancy with or without cramping or discomfort but without cervical dilation or change in cervical consistency.
  • *Diagnostic testing*: Ultrasound evaluation shows a viable pregnancy, and serum quantitative β-hCG is consistent for gestational age.
  • *Intervention*: Barring other complications, the pregnancy in threatened abortion progresses without problems. A few days of rest, then resumption of normal activities, are usually recommended, although even this common-sense treatment likely makes little difference in the pregnancy outcome.
■ Inevitable abortion
  • *Clinical presentation*: The cervix is open, and the uterine contents are in the process of being expelled. The patient has cramping, abdominal pain, and usually brisk vaginal bleeding.
  • *Diagnostic testing*: Ultrasound evaluation reveals that the uterine contents are in the process of or have been expelled. Serum quantitative β-hCG is low for gestational age.
  • *Treatment*: Usually no surgical intervention is needed. Ongoing evaluation for hemodynamic stability is critical, with prompt referral for emergency care if hemodynamic instability is noted.
■ Complete abortion
  • *Clinical presentation*: The pregnancy-related uterine contents have been completely expelled. The patient has minimal cramping, though likely reports a period of significant discomfort during the products of conception passing. The cervical os is likely still slightly open, and the uterine size is returning to normal.
  • *Diagnostic testing*: Ultrasound evaluation reveals that the uterine contents have been expelled. Serum quantitative β-hCG is low for gestational age.
  • *Treatment*: Further medical or surgical intervention is usually not needed. As with all pregnancy loss, considerable emotional support is needed to help the woman and her family deal with this significant event.
■ Incomplete or missed abortion
  • *Clinical presentation*: Some portion of the products of conception remains in the uterus, but the pregnancy is no longer viable. The cervical os is usually closed, and minimal cramping is reported. Uterine size is often smaller or consistent with gestational age.
  • *Diagnostic testing*: Ultrasound fails to reveal a viable pregnancy, though products of conception remain. Serum quantitative β-hCG is low for gestational age.
  • *Treatment*: Expectant management, or "watch and wait," while the uterus completes the emptying process. Medical therapy to encourage uterine emptying is also an appropriate option. Evacuation of the uterine contents by dilation and aspiration is often required. Expert consultation should be sought.

Overview

Ectopic pregnancy is defined as any gestation that occurs outside of the uterus. Although reports of cervical, abdominal, and interstitial pregnancies exist, approximately 95% of all ectopic pregnancies are located in a fallopian tube; the term *tubal pregnancy* is nearly synonymous with ectopic pregnancy. Because the physiological and physical needs of the fetus cannot be met when pregnancy occurs outside the uterus, the pregnancy cannot progress beyond the earliest stages and will be lost. Most ectopic pregnancies resolve without intervention via miscarriage or involution of the gestational sac and reabsorption. Ectopic pregnancies that do not resolve pose a significant risk to the mother; often the woman is unaware that she was carrying an ectopic pregnancy.

Risk factors for ectopic pregnancy include factors that can influence normal tubal motility and patency, such as a history of pelvic inflammatory disease, prior ectopic pregnancy, current intrauterine device (IUD) use, pregnancy achieved by means of in-vitro fertilization or fertility drugs, prior tubal surgery (reconstruction or tubal ligation), and cigarette smoking. Increased maternal age (35 years of age or greater) also appears to be a risk factor for ectopic pregnancy.

Clinical Presentation

The classic clinical triad of ectopic pregnancy—abdominal pain, vaginal bleeding, and adnexal mass—is found in only 50% of women with the condition. Commonly, the woman presents with irregular menstrual-like flow and lower abdominal cramping. Rarely, the woman with ruptured ectopic pregnancy will present with hemodynamic instability. Consequently, careful clinical assessment to support or disprove the diagnosis is critical and expert consultation sought when evaluating the woman with suspected ectopic pregnancy. Differential diagnoses include ovarian torsion, appendicitis, pelvic inflammatory disease, and ruptured corpus luteum.

Diagnostic Testing

Diagnostic testing in ectopic pregnancy includes obtaining a quantitative β-hCG value. Urine and serum tests are usually positive, and a negative test rules out the diagnosis. Usually the serum quantity of β-hCG in ectopic pregnancy at gestational weeks 6 to 10, the most common time for clinical presentation, is approximately 1,000 to 6,000 mIU/mL; this compares with 40,000 mIU/mL or greater for a viable IUP. The normal rapid increase in serum quantitative β-hCG noted in a viable IUP is missing, and the value tends to stall. With a positive β-hCG level of 1,500 mIU/mL or greater, a gestational sac should be identifiable within the uterus on transvaginal ultrasound with an IUP; the presence of an intrauterine gestational sac effectively excludes the diagnosis of ectopic pregnancy. If ectopic pregnancy is suspected, a serum progesterone level is often obtained, though its usefulness is debated. Progesterone is a hormone produced by the developing chorion. A progesterone level less than 15 ng/mL is seen in only 11% of viable intrauterine pregnancies but is noted in most ectopic pregnancies or with inevitable abortion. Some have proposed a cutoff of greater than 25 ng/mL to exclude ectopic pregnancy and 5 ng/mL or less for a nonviable pregnancy, including ectopic pregnancy. However, a significant number of results will fall between these two values.

Pelvic/transvaginal ultrasound is a critical part of the evaluation of the woman with suspected ectopic pregnancy. Of women with ectopic pregnancy, approximately 15% to 26% have a nondiagnostic ultrasound; thus, a normal ultrasound scan does not rule out the condition. Occasionally, pelvic computed tomography or magnetic resonance imaging is indicated, recognizing the limitations of these studies in ectopic pregnancy but their utility in identifying other reasons for abdominal pain.

Treatment

When the diagnosis of ectopic pregnancy is established, treatment depends on the patient's condition. If the patient is stable, surgical or medical intervention is warranted according to the availability of treatment options.

Medical therapy with methotrexate, a medication that inhibits cell division and causes the pregnancy to regress and resolve, is an option when ectopic pregnancy is diagnosed while the tube is intact, the patient is hemodynamically stable, there is no ultrasound evidence of fetal cardiac activity or free fluid in the cul-de-sac, and there are no contraindications for methotrexate use. A quantitative β-hCG of greater than 6,000 mIU/mL, evidence of fetal cardiac activity, and free fluid in the cul-de-sac (a common finding in tubal rupture) are all contraindications to methotrexate use. Close follow-up is critical with medical management of ectopic pregnancy to ensure pregnancy resolution; surgical intervention is sometimes needed if this therapy fails. Compared with surgical therapy, tubal patency is usually better preserved with medical management. Evaluation for a concurrent (heterotopic) IUP should also be done as this can be found in 10% of women presenting with ectopic pregnancy.

If the patient is hemodynamically unstable, immediate surgical intervention is warranted. Surgical treatments include salpingostomy, in which the tube is opened and the pregnancy contents are removed. The tube is then repaired. Salpingectomy is usually performed when the tubal rupture has occurred or tubal damage is severe and repair is not possible. After surgical intervention, β-hCG levels should be monitored weekly until they reach 0 to ensure the treatment was complete.

> **CLINICAL CONCEPT**
>
> Regardless of the treatment modality in ectopic pregnancy, considerable emotional support is also needed because the woman has faced a potentially life-threatening illness and the loss of a pregnancy.

Discussion Sources

Prine LW, MacNaughton H. Office management of early pregnancy loss. *Am Fam Physician*. 2011;84(1):75–82. http://www.aafp.org/afp/2011/0701/p75.html

Sepilian VP. Ectopic pregnancy. Medscape. http://emedicine.medscape.com/article/2041923-overview

Tulandi T. Ectopic (tubal) pregnancy: beyond the basics. UpToDate. http://www.uptodate.com/contents/ectopic-tubal-pregnancy-beyond-the-basics

QUESTIONS

116. Approximately ___% of all clinically recognized pregnancies end in spontaneous abortion.

A. 5

B. 15

C. 30

D. 40

117. Approximately ___% of spontaneous abortions are associated with chromosomal defects.

A. 20

B. 40

C. 60

D. 80

118. Risk factors for spontaneous abortion include all of the following except:

A. maternal age older than 35 years.

B. BMI greater than 30 kg/m².

C. excessive use of alcohol.

D. poorly controlled hypertension.

119. Which of the following best describes a woman with recurrent early pregnancy loss?

A. woman with one medical pregnancy termination followed by one spontaneous abortion at 17 weeks' gestation

B. woman with one spontaneous abortion followed by two full-term pregnancies

C. woman who reports three consecutive pregnancy losses under 10 weeks' gestation

D. woman with two medical pregnancy terminations followed by one full-term pregnancy

120. The classic clinical triad of ectopic pregnancy includes all of the following except:

A. abdominal pain.

B. vaginal bleeding.

C. large-for-gestational-age uterus.

D. adnexal mass.

121. The classic clinical triad of ectopic pregnancy is found in no more than ___% of women presenting with this condition.

A. 10

B. 25

C. 50

D. 75

122. In the first weeks of a viable IUP, serum quantitative hCG levels usually double every ___ hours until approximately 10,000 to 20,000 mIU/mL.

A. 24

B. 48

C. 72

D. 96

123. For a woman who presents with symptoms consistent with ectopic pregnancy, the NP should also consider all of the following conditions when making a differential diagnosis except:

A. pelvic inflammatory disease.

B. ruptured corpus luteum.

C. urinary tract infection.

D. appendicitis.

124. In ectopic pregnancy, all of the following statements are true except:

A. hCG is low for gestational age and is not increasing normally.

B. Ultrasound evaluation fails to reveal abnormality in 20% to 30% of cases.

C. Location of the pregnancy is often on the ovary or cervix.

D. Risk factors include current pregnancy via assisted reproduction.

125 to 128. Match the clinical presentation to the following description:

_____ **125.** complete abortion

_____ **126.** inevitable abortion

_____ **127.** threatened abortion

_____ **128.** incomplete abortion

    A. Uterine contents include a nonviable pregnancy that is in the process of being expelled.

    B. Some portion of the products of conception remains in the uterus, although the pregnancy is no longer viable.

    C. The products of conception have been completely expelled.

    D. Ultrasound evaluation shows a viable pregnancy, although vaginal bleeding is present.

For answers and rationales, see end of chapter.

Labor, Birth, and Recovery

Overview

The NP must have knowledge of the normal process of labor to provide appropriate counseling. Numerous theories exist as to why labor starts. These theories include factors related to placental aging and uterine distention. At the normal pregnancy term, a time between 37 and 42 weeks of gestation, the process of labor begins.

Stages of Labor

The stages of labor are outlined here.

■ *Early labor*, also called the *latent phase of labor*, is often the longest part, sometimes lasting 2 to 3 days, and is characterized by mild to moderate contractions that last about 30 to 45 seconds and are 5 to 20 minutes apart, often starting and stopping. During this time, the cervix usually dilates to about 3 cm, and the membranes are intact.

■ The first stage of *active labor* starts when the cervix is about 3 to 4 cm dilated and is complete when the cervix is fully dilated. Contractions become closer and more intense, culminating in transition, when contractions occur every 2 to 3 minutes and last 50 to 70 seconds or more. The pregnant woman should be instructed to go to the hospital or birthing center when contractions are every 5 minutes apart and lasting 1 minute. During active labor, the woman often feels restless and excited by the impending birth but is usually communicative between contractions. In transition, the final stage of active labor with the cervix dilated from 7 to 10 centimeters, the woman is usually quite focused on getting through the birthing process and is often distracted by the comments of others. The presence of a support person is important throughout the birthing process.

■ The *second stage of labor* is the actual birth, a stage that can last a few minutes or a few hours. The mother often passes through this stage with a variety of emotions, from exhaustion to elation.

■ The *third stage of labor* occurs when the placenta detaches and is expelled from the uterus.

First-time mothers usually have an average of 9 to 12 hours of first-stage labor, and second-stage labor lasts approximately 30 minutes to 2 hours. For women who have previously given birth, the first and second stages of labor usually last approximately 6 to 8 hours in total. The pregnant woman and her labor support person should be encouraged to attend childbirth and infant care classes. Referral to these classes usually occurs during the second trimester of pregnancy.

> **CLINICAL CONCEPT**
> The pregnant woman is usually able to be up and around during this period and is often frustrated by the apparent slow progress of early labor.

Labor Induction

Induction of labor, through the use of either medications or other methods (e.g., stripping the membranes, cervical ripening, others), can stimulate contractions to promote a vaginal birth. Induction can be recommended if the health of the mother or fetus is at risk. Elective induction can be offered under special circumstances (i.e., living a long distance from the hospital) and is gaining popularity for a variety of reasons, including patient and provider convenience. Additionally, a recent study noted that elective induction of labor at 39 weeks can lead to a reduced number of caesarean births, reduced rate of stillbirth, and reduced severe complications to the mother and neonate. Elective induction should not be performed prior to 39 weeks of pregnancy; if the pregnant woman does not go into naturally occurring labor by week 41 of pregnancy, she will be encouraged to have labor induction. Carrying a pregnancy beyond 41 weeks is associated with increased maternal and fetal risks. A failed attempt at induction will require another method of induction or having a caesarean delivery. Helpful information on labor induction for patients is available at the American College of Obstetricians and Gynecologists Web site.

Cesarean Birth

A cesarean birth (or C-section) is the delivery of the baby through incisions made in the mother's abdomen and uterus. A cesarean birth can be recommended in certain situations, such as twin or higher-order multiples pregnancy, failure of labor to progress, fetal macrosomia (large baby), breech presentation, and certain maternal infections. Cesarean delivery is associated with a longer hospital stay and certain medical risks (e.g., infection, blood loss, blood clots, and injury to bowel and bladder). Cesarean birth can also increase the risk of complications in subsequent pregnancies. In the absence of medical circumstances, cesarean delivery should not be routinely offered to pregnant women.

Vaginal delivery should be recommended as safe and appropriate when there are no indications for a cesarean delivery. Patients who request a cesarean mainly because of fear of pain in childbirth should be counseled about options during pregnancy, including analgesia and emotional support during labor. When a cesarean delivery has been decided, it should not be performed prior to 39 weeks of gestation. Women should be educated on the potential consequences of repeat cesareans, including placenta previa, placenta accrete spectrum, and gravid hysterectomy.

Discussion Sources

ACOG. Committee Opinion No. 761. Cesarean delivery on maternal request. December 2018. https://journals.lww.com/greenjournal
/FullText/2019/01000/ACOG_Committee_Opinion_No__761__Cesarean_Delivery.52.aspx

ACOG. Practice Advisory: Clinical guidance for integration of findings of The ARRIVE Trial: Labor induction versus expectant
management in low-risk nulliparous women. August 2018. https://www.acog.org/clinical/clinical-guidance/practice-advisory
/articles/2018/08/clinical-guidance-for-integration-of-the-findings-of-the-arrive-trial

American Pregnancy Association. Labor and birth. http://americanpregnancy.org/labor-and-birth/

U.S. Department of Health and Human Services, Office on Women's Health. Pregnancy. Womenshealth.gov.
https://www.womenshealth.gov/pregnancy/childbirth-and-beyond/labor-and-birth

QUESTIONS

129. First-time mothers usually have an average of _____ hours of active first-stage labor.

   A. 6 to 8

   B. 9 to 12

   C. 13 to 15

   D. 16 to 18

130. For women who have previously given birth vaginally, the first and second stages of labor usually last a total of _____ hours.

   A. 3 to 5

   B. 6 to 8

   C. 9 to 10

   D. 11 to 13

131. Which of the following statements is most accurate regarding early labor?

   A. The mother is instructed to go to the hospital at the start of early labor.

   B. Early labor ends once the cervix reaches 5-cm dilation.

   C. The mother should be encouraged to remain physically active as she tolerates during early labor.

   D. Contractions are typically absent during early labor.

132. The actual birth occurs during which stage of labor?

   A. stage 1

   B. stage 2

   C. stage 3

   D. latent stage

133. A woman who is at 37 weeks' gestation of her first pregnancy asks about induction. Her pregnancy is unremarkable, but she is concerned because she lives a long distance away from the hospital. The NP responds:

   A. an induction can be scheduled after 39 weeks of gestation.

   B. an induction is only recommended for high-risk pregnancies.

   C. there is a greater risk of cesarean births with induction.

   D. there is less need for analgesia during labor with induction.

For answers and rationales, see end of chapter.

Postpartum Mood and Anxiety Disorders

Overview

Postpartum mood and anxiety disorders can include the postpartum blues ("baby blues"), depression, or psychosis (Table 18-7).

TABLE 18-7 Postpartum Mood Disorders

DISORDER	INCIDENCE (%)	PRESENTATION	TREATMENT
Postpartum blues	26 to 85	Often begins within a few days of giving birth	Support and reassurance including recruiting helpers so mother can get more rest
Postpartum depression	10 to 20	Most common at 2 to 4 months' postpartum	Psychotherapy, psychopharmacological, medication therapy as indicated, recognizing all will be secreted in breast milk; hospitalization as needed
Postpartum psychosis	0.2	Early onset usually by day 3 postpartum; characterized by delusions	Hospitalization usually needed for safety of mother and infant. Psychopharmacological medication therapy as indicated (antipsychotics, mood stabilizers, benzodiazepines, antidepressants, others)

Source: Cohen LS, Wang B, Nonacs R, et al. Treatment of mood disorders during pregnancy and postpartum. Psychiatr Clin North Am. 2010;33(2):273–293.

Postpartum Blues

Postpartum blues is the most common condition and generally begins within a few days after giving birth. Symptoms include weepiness or crying for no apparent reason, impatience, irritability, restlessness, anxiety, fatigue, insomnia, sadness, mood changes, and poor concentration. The condition is likely linked to hormonal changes that occur during pregnancy and following birth. The symptoms generally lessen within 14 days after delivery. Mothers should receive support, reassurance, and assistance in taking care of the newborn so the mother can get needed rest.

One contributor to postpartum blues is the sleep deprivation that follows childbirth. While postbirth sleep is usually erratic, the new mother should aim for at least 6 to 8 hours of every 24 hours devoted to sleep. This is best attained by having support so the mother can sleep during times when the newborn is asleep.

> **CLINICAL CONCEPT**
> With postpartum blues, the mother is able to continue to care for the newborn, albeit greatly benefiting from social and family support.

Postpartum Depression

Postpartum depression can occur in up to 20% of new mothers and presents at about 2 to 4 months following birth. The signs and symptoms are more intense than the postpartum blues and last longer, which can interfere with the mother's ability to care for the baby. Symptoms include loss of appetite, insomnia, intense irritability and anger, overwhelming fatigue, lack of sexual drive, lack of joy in life, severe mood swings, withdrawal from friends and family, and thoughts of harming oneself or the baby. Risk factors include having and/or experiencing a history of depression or postpartum depression, stressful events during the past year, problems in the relationship with a spouse or significant other, a weak support system, financial problems, or a pregnancy that was unplanned or unwanted. With this condition, there is a risk for maternal suicide. Treatment usually includes counseling, psychotropic medications, and/or hormone therapy (e.g., estrogen supplementation). With appropriate treatment, postpartum depression usually resolves within a few months. Usually, breastfeeding should be encouraged with the use of select psychotropics. Expert consultation is warranted.

Postpartum Psychosis

Postpartum psychosis is a rare condition that typically develops within a few weeks following delivery. Symptoms include confusion and disorientation, hallucinations and delusions, paranoia, and attempts to harm herself or the baby. Women with bipolar disorder are at higher risk of postpartum psychosis. Those with this disorder require immediate treatment, often in the hospital, in part to ensure the safety of mother and baby. Treatment involves a combination of antidepressants, antipsychotics, and mood stabilizers. Electroconvulsive therapy also is commonly used. Expert consultation is warranted.

Discussion Sources

Joy S. Postpartum depression. Medscape. http://reference.medscape.com/article/271662-overview

Meltzer-Brody S, Howard LM, Bergink V, et al. Postpartum psychiatric disorders. Nat Rev Dis Primers. 2018;4:18022.

Smith B, Dubovsky SL. Pharmacotherapy of mood disorders and psychosis in pre- and post-natal women. Expert Opin Pharmacother. 2017;18:1703–1719.

QUESTIONS

134. Postpartum "baby blues" typically begin:

  A. 1 to 2 weeks prior to the birth.

  B. within a few days following the birth.

  C. 1 to 2 weeks following the birth.

  D. approximately 1 month following the birth.

135. Risk factors for postpartum depression include all of the following except:

  A. history of depression.

  B. financial problems.

  C. history of carrying two or more pregnancies to term.

  D. unplanned pregnancy.

136. Symptoms of postpartum depression include which of the following? *(Choose all that apply.)*

  A. hallucinations

  B. overwhelming fatigue

  C. insomnia

  D. severe mood swings

  E. disorientation

137 to 140. Rank each of the following treatments for postpartum depression from most effective (1) to least or not effective (4).

  _____ **137.** Psychotherapy

  _____ **138.** Antidepressants

  _____ **139.** Electroconvulsive therapy

  _____ **140.** Hormone therapy

141. The risk of infanticide is greatest in a woman with which of the following conditions?

  A. postpartum depression

  B. postpartum "baby blues"

  C. postpartum psychosis

  D. There is little risk of infanticide with any of the above conditions.

142. A risk factor for postpartum psychosis is:

  A. history of depression.

  B. multiple births (i.e., twins, triplets).

  C. history of bipolar disorder.

  D. illegal drug use.

143. Treatment of postpartum psychosis typically includes all of the following except:

  A. hospitalization.

  B. estrogen replacement therapy.

  C. antipsychotic therapy.

  D. electroconvulsive therapy.

For answers and rationales, see end of chapter.

QUESTION ANSWERS AND RATIONALES

Normative Changes During Pregnancy

1 to 4. Matching Questions

1. Correct: D. zygote

2. Correct: C. blastocyst

3. Correct: A. embryo

4. Correct: B. fetus

Using appropriate terminology is a key component of providing prenatal care. A fertilized ovum is called a *zygote* (1). The zygote rapidly undergoes cell division during the first 2 weeks, during which this group of cells is called a *blastocyst* (2). The blastocyst is a precursor to the *embryo*, when the baby's major systems and structures develop, which lasts up to 8 to 10 weeks (3). Following the embryonic stage, the baby is now referred to as a *fetus* until term (4).

5 to 17. True or False

5. Correct: True

6. Correct: True

7. Correct: True

8. Correct: True

9. Correct: True

10. Correct: True

11. Correct: False

12. Correct: True

13. Correct: False

14. Correct: True

15. Correct: True

16. Correct: False

17. Correct: False

There are a number of physiological changes that can be expected during pregnancy. In the cardiovascular system, blood volume increases by up to 50%, and RBC production can increase by 33% (5). Systolic and diastolic BP will decrease (6), while the S_1 heart sound becomes louder (7) and physiological ejection murmur is usually evident (8). In the renal system, there is an increase in renal blood flow with dilation of the renal collecting system (9). Due to an increase in GFR, this can lead to physiological glucosuria and proteinuria (10). In the respiratory system, there is an increase in the transverse thoracic diameter and diaphragmatic contraction (11). In the GI system, the lower esophageal sphincter is more relaxed (12), which can cause esophageal reflux. Intestinal motility is decreased (13) to improve nutrient absorption but can lead to constipation. The gallbladder doubles in size with more dilute bile (14) and less-soluble cholesterol that can increase the risk of gallstones. Endocrine changes include insulin levels increasing several-fold (15), while fasting plasma glucose decreases slightly (16), and the thyroid and pituitary increase in size (17).

18 to 23. Matching Questions

18. Correct: C. size of a large lemon

19. Correct: D. size of a tennis ball or orange

20. Correct: A. size of a baseball

21. Correct: B. size of a softball or grapefruit

22. Correct: F. uterine fundus halfway between symphysis pubis and umbilicus

23. Correct: E. uterine fundus at umbilicus

Knowledge of normal pregnancy development is important in providing prenatal care. When considering uterine size, the typical size in a nongravid woman is approximately the size of a lemon (18), which grows to the size of a tennis ball by 8 weeks (19) and a baseball by 10 weeks (20). By 12 weeks, the uterus is the size of a grapefruit, and the uterine fundus is palpable through the abdominal wall (21). By 16 weeks, the uterine fundus is located halfway between the symphysis pubis and umbilicus, and quickening is usually noted between 16 and 18 weeks (22). At 20 weeks, the uterine fundus is at the umbilicus (23).

24 to 26. Matching Questions

24. Correct: B. softening of uterus isthmus

25. Correct: C. softening of vaginal portion of the cervix

26. Correct: A. blue-violet vaginal color

By 8 weeks of pregnancy, certain signs can be evident on the uterus and cervix. The Hegar sign is characterized by a softening of the uterine isthmus (24). The Goodell sign is observed with a softening of the vaginal portion of the cervix (25), while the Chadwick sign is present when the cervix and vagina becomes cyanotic, having a blue-violet color (26).

27. Correct: D. 95

By the 36th week of pregnancy, approximately 95% of fetuses are in the vertex position (cephalic) (D), which is the head-first position and facing the mother's back. This is the ideal position for a vaginal delivery. An occiput posterior position is head-first and facing the mother's abdomen. This can lead to problems during delivery including a prolonged labor.

Incorrect:

By late pregnancy, the vast majority (approximately 95%) of fetuses are in the vertex position (A, B, C).

Health and Nutrition Counseling During Pregnancy

28. Correct: C. 25 to 35 lb (11.3 to 15.9 kg).
For women with a healthy weight and within the normal BMI range of 18.5 to 24.9 kg/m², the recommended weight gain during pregnancy is between 25 and 35 lbs (C).
Incorrect:
For expectant mothers who are underweight (BMI less than 18.5 kg/m²), the recommended weight gain is 28 to 40 lb. Those who are overweight (BMI of 25 to 29.9 kg/m²), the recommended weight gain is 15 to 25 lb. (A), while obese women (BMI 30 kg/m² or greater) should gain between 11 and 20 lb during pregnancy (B). A weight gain of 35 to 45 lb exceeds recommendations regardless of BMI prepregnancy (D)

29. Correct: B. 300
The energy requirement for a woman early in pregnancy is the same for a nonpregnant woman, and so caloric intake should not change. However, weight gain is expected during the second and third trimesters, and so caloric intake should increase with a well-balanced diet. During the latter stages of pregnancy, caloric intake should increase by about 340 to 450 kcal per day. The average daily caloric intake throughout pregnancy should be an increase of about 300 kcal per day (B).
Incorrect:
For women with a healthy prepregnancy BMI, daily caloric intake should increase by about 300 kcal (A), but should not substantially exceed this amount (C, D).

30. C. protein.
Women in their second and third trimesters of pregnancy should increase caloric intake to support the growing fetus. Increased caloric intake should largely come from an increase in protein (C), where recommended amounts should increase from 46 grams per day to at least 60 grams per day.
Incorrect:
During the latter stages of pregnancy, fat (B) and carbohydrate (A) needs are unchanged, as increased caloric intake should largely be due to increased protein intake. Though it is important for expectant mothers to stay hydrated with plenty of water and other fluids, water is not a source of needed calories (D).

31. Correct: B. 0.6 lb (0.3 kg).
Weight gain is expected and recommended during the second and third trimesters of pregnancy. For women who are overweight prepregnancy, the recommended rate of weight gain is approximately 0.6 lb per week (B).
Incorrect:
For women who are normal or underweight in prepregnancy, the recommended rate of weight gain during the second and third trimesters is approximately 1 lb per week (C). For those who are obese (BMI 30 kg/m² or greater) in prepregnancy, the rate of weight gain should be about 0.5 lb per week. A gain of 2 lb per week exceeds the normal recommendations for

an expectant mother (D), while a gain of only 0.25 lb per week is too low (A).

32. Correct: B. 500
Lactating women should increase caloric intake in order to support milk production and breastfeeding. For a woman with a healthy prepregnancy BMI, the recommended increase in caloric intake is approximately 500 kcal per day (B).
Incorrect:
In healthy women, lactating women should increase their daily caloric intake by 500 kcal (A), but should not exceed this amount (C, D).

33. Correct: D. 1,000 to 1,300
Increased calcium intake during pregnancy is critical for the normal development of fetal bones and teeth. Dietary sources of calcium are preferred, though supplementation can also be considered. The recommended intake of calcium ranges from 1,000 mg daily for women 19 to 50 years of age to 1,300 mg daily for women 14 to 18 years of age (D).
Incorrect:
Daily calcium intake for pregnant women should be in the range of 1000 to 1300 mg (A, B, C).

34. Correct: D. open NTDs
FAD results in a teratogenic state that can lead to the development of open NTDs including anencephaly, spina bifida, and encephalocele. Though the nutrient is found in large amounts in several types of foods, folic acid supplementation is generally recommended by the CDC for all women of reproductive age.
Incorrect:
FAD is associated with the development of NTDs and not congenital cataracts (A), pyloric stenosis (B), or clubfoot (C).

35. Correct: B. second and third trimesters
Iron needs are greatest during the second and third trimesters as the fetus is building iron stores (B). In the absence of iron deficiency, the recommended iron requirement for a pregnant woman is 30 mg per day.
Incorrect:
Though it is important to maintain healthy levels of iron throughout pregnancy (A, C), the greatest maternal need is during the second and third trimesters. Low iron stores in prepregnancy can result in the development of iron-deficiency anemia later in pregnancy (D).

36. Correct: A. iron deficiency.
The most common form of anemia during pregnancy is iron-deficiency anemia (A). This is typically not as a result of increased iron requirements during pregnancy but is more likely to occur in a woman who enters pregnancy with iron deficiency.
Incorrect:
Folate-deficiency anemia is relatively rare among women who eat a balanced diet and are not genetically predisposed to the condition (B). Vitamin B_{12}–deficiency anemia (C) and anemia due to hypoproliferation of RBCs (D) are rare conditions acquired during pregnancy.

37. Correct: C. No level or time of exposure is considered safe.

It is generally recommended to abstain from all alcohol use during pregnancy, as no amount of alcohol exposure is considered safe to the developing baby (C).

Incorrect:

Alcohol use during pregnancy can increase the risk of miscarriage, stillbirths, and FASD (A). FASD can result from alcohol consumption at any stage of pregnancy (B), and alcohol exposure does not have to occur throughout the pregnancy for the condition to manifest (D). Light or moderate use of alcohol during pregnancy can lead to lesser degrees of alcohol-related problems. However, FASD remains the leading preventable cause of developmental disability in children.

38. Correct: D. potentially dangerous because of contaminants in the nonfood substance.

Though pica is sometimes viewed as a harmless practice that is common in certain ethnic groups, the ingestion of nonfood substances can have serious and potentially dangerous consequences to the mother and developing baby (D). This is particularly true when the substance being ingested is contaminated with heavy metals or industrial pollutants that are toxic.

Incorrect:

Pica can be a dangerous practice when the substance being ingested can potentially contain toxic chemicals and heavy metals (A). The risk of toxicity is compounded when nutritious food is being replaced by nonfood substances (B). Pica can also replace nutritious foods with high-calorie foods that can then lead to excessive weight gain. A well-balanced diet should be able to provide all of the micronutrients needed without the need to consume nonfood substances (D).

39. Correct: D. omphalocele.

FAD is a teratogenic state that can lead to the development of NTDs. However, omphalocele is not an NTD but occurs when the infant's intestines or other abdominal organs are outside of the body due to a hole in the abdominal wall (D).

Incorrect:

NTDs that can develop due to FAD can include anencephaly (i.e., the absence of a major portion of the brain, skull, and cap) (A), spina bifida (i.e., the spine and spinal cord do not develop properly) (B), and encephalocele (i.e., a sac-like protrusion of the brain and membranes through an opening in the skull) (C).

40 to 43. Matching Questions

40. Correct: D. abnormal facial features

41. Correct: A. SIDS

42. Correct: C. neonatal abstinence syndrome

43. Correct: B. neurobehavioral disorders

Substance abuse during pregnancy can have permanent or long-lasting effects on the unborn child, and expectant mothers should be made aware of the consequences of this practice. The use of many of these substances during pregnancy can increase the risk of miscarriage, stillbirth, preterm birth, and low birth weight. Consumption of alcohol can lead to FASD that includes abnormal facial features (40), small head size, and learning disabilities. Smoking tobacco products can increase the risk of SIDS (41), while stimulant use can cause long-term neurobehavioral problems in children (43). Neonatal abstinence syndrome can occur when the newborn has been exposed to addictive drugs during pregnancy, such as opioids, and the newborn undergoes subsequent withdrawal symptoms (42).

44 to 46. Matching Questions

44. Correct: B. chronic respiratory disease

45. Correct: C. respiratory depression

46. Correct: A. seizures

Substance abuse can have adverse effects that put the mother and baby at risk. Tobacco products have long been associated with increased risk of several types of cancer and cardiovascular disease as well as chronic respiratory diseases such as chronic obstructive pulmonary disease (44). Opioid abuse can cause sedation and respiratory depression that can eventually lead to death (45). Use of stimulants such as cocaine or methamphetamines can cause psychomotor agitation, tachycardia, arrhythmias, coma, and seizures (46).

Prenatal Care and Screening

47. Correct: B. 2 weeks.

Approximately 8 to 10 visits are scheduled during a pregnancy, though more may be needed if indicated. Up to 28 weeks, the frequency is about every 4 weeks, which then increases to every 2 weeks during weeks 28 to 36 (B). After week 36, scheduled visits should occur every week.

Incorrect:

Weekly visits are recommended after week 36 (A) while visits occurring every four weeks is recommended prior to week 28 (D). Visits every 3 weeks is not a usual schedule for prenatal visits at any period during a pregnancy (C).

48. Correct: A. as early as possible in pregnancy.

Initial testing for sexually transmitted infections should occur as early as possible in the pregnancy (A). Testing should include HIV, syphilis, hepatitis B, gonorrhea, and chlamydia. Testing should be repeated in the third trimester, especially for women at higher risk.

Incorrect:

Testing for STIs should not be delayed once a pregnancy is confirmed and should be repeated in the third trimester for high-risk women (B, C, D).

49. Correct: D. amniocentesis

Prenatal screening tests are useful in detecting the potential risk of aneuploidy or open NTD. When a screening test is positive, additional testing is needed to confirm the diagnosis. For antenatal screening tests, an amniocentesis is the most accurate study to make a diagnosis (D).

Incorrect:

Common prenatal screening tests include maternal serum analysis of AFP (B) and serum inhibin-A (C). A cell-free fetal DNA test can also be used to screen for aneuploidy (A). However, with an abnormal finding with these tests, confirmation is needed with follow-up testing, such as amniocentesis.

50. **Correct: C. 16 to 20**

The quad screen is used to screen for aneuploidy as well as open NTDs. The test is ideally performed during 16 to 20 weeks of pregnancy (C). The test can provide an inaccurate result if performed too early or too late during the pregnancy.

Incorrect:

The quad screen should not be performed prior to week 16 as this can lead to an inaccurate result (A, B). Delaying the test past week 20 of pregnancy is not recommended (D).

51. **Correct: C the presence of an abnormal number of chromosomes.**

Fetal aneuploidy is defined as an abnormal number of chromosomes present in the fetus (C). Aneuploidy is an important cause of congenital malformations and mental impairments. The most common types of aneuploidy include Down syndrome (trisomy 21), Edwards' syndrome (trisomy 18), and Patau's syndrome (trisomy 13).

Incorrect:

Aneuploidy is not caused by the use of a teratogenic drug (B) or nutritional deficiency (D). Aneuploidy is also not defined as a congenital malformation of unknown origin (A).

52. **Correct: A. trisomy 21 and open NTDs**

The quad screen tests for maternal serum levels of hCG, inhibin-A, AFP, and unconjugated estriol levels. The screen is effective in detecting the possible presence of open NTDs as well as trisomy 21 (Down syndrome) and trisomy 18 (Edwards' syndrome) (A).

Incorrect:

The quad screen is used to test for open NTDs and certain types of aneuploidy. It will not be able to screen for cystic fibrosis or Angelman's syndrome (B), Tay-Sachs' disease (C), sickle cell anemia, or β-thalassemia major (D).

53. **Correct: D. to all women regardless of age.**

Though women who will be 35 years or older at the time of delivery are at higher risk of aneuploidy, prenatal assessment should be offered to all women regardless of age (D). The quad screen as well as the cell-free fetal DNA test both offer noninvasive techniques to screen for aneuploidy.

Incorrect:

Though certain women are at higher risk of aneuploidy, the test should be offered to all women regardless of age (A, B, C).

54. **Correct: B. further testing is recommended.**

It is important to remember that screening tests are not diagnostic as they detect for the presence of risk for a condition, and further testing is recommended to confirm a diagnosis (B). With an abnormal quad screen result, follow-up testing can include amniocentesis or a level II ultrasound.

Incorrect:

The quad screen is not diagnostic (A), and additional testing is needed (D) to make a diagnosis, such as amniocentesis or level II ultrasound. The quad screen should not be repeated, but the patient should be offered a diagnostic test (C).

55. **Correct: C. 500**

Though amniocentesis can be an important diagnostic tool, women should be counseled that the procedure does have risk. Spontaneous fetal loss related to amniocentesis occurs in approximately 1 of every 500 procedures (C) when performed at a facility that does these procedures on a regular basis.

Incorrect:

The procedure for amniocentesis is associated with a certain risk to the fetus and can ead to spontaneous fetal loss in about 1 in 500 procedures (A, B, D).

56. **Correct: D. a history of multiparity.**

All women should be offered prenatal assessment of aneuploidy regardless of age or risk. Screening is particularly important for those at higher risk. However, a history of multiparity is not a risk factor for aneuploidy (D).

Incorrect:

Risk factors for aneuploidy include a maternal age 35 years or older at the time of giving birth (A), a history of prior pregnancy with trisomy (B), or a fetal ultrasonographic finding indicating an increased risk of aneuploidy (C).

57. **Correct: D. Down syndrome.**

AFP is part of the quad screen used to detect for possible fetal abnormalities, including aneuploidy and open NTDs. However, the presence of Down syndrome will cause a decrease in maternal AFP level (D).

Incorrect:

AFP is produced by the fetal yolk sac, GI tract, and liver, and maternal levels can be elevated for a number of reasons, including the presence of an open NTD (B) such as meningomyelocele (C), anencephaly, or spina bifida. An underestimated gestational age can also lead to a misinterpreted level of AFP as the level is typically higher in early pregnancy (A).

58. **Correct: C. 18**

Trisomy is the presence of a single additional chromosome and can be an important cause of congenital malformations and mental impairments. Edwards' syndrome is due to trisomy 18 and occurs approximately 1 in every 6,000 births (C). Clinical manifestations of the condition include low birth weight, developmental disability, and cranial, cardiac, and renal malformations.

Incorrect:

Trisomy 21 is Down syndrome that occurs approximately 1 in every 1,000 births (D). Patau's syndrome is trisomy 13 (A) and occurs 1 in every 8,000 to 12,000 births. Clinical manifestations of Patau's syndrome include microcephaly, omphalocele, NTDs, and polydactyly. Trisomy 15 or mosaic trisomy 15 is an extremely rare occurrence (B).

59. Correct: B. Most affected infants with Edwards' syndrome die during the first year of life.

Edwards' syndrome (trisomy 18) can lead to complex and serious clinical manifestations in the newborn. Stillbirth and death in the first week are common, while most affected infants will die in the first year of life (B).

Incorrect:

Edwards' syndrome occurs less frequently when compared with Down syndrome (about 1 in every 6,000 births compared to 1 in every 1,000 births with Down syndrome) (A). Edwards' syndrome causes complex and serious clinical manifestations including developmental disability and malformation in the heart, kidney, and cranium (C). Trisomy 18 will cause a decrease in maternal AFP levels during pregnancy (D).

60. Correct: C. Down syndrome is associated with a decreased maternal serum AFP level.

When performing the quad screen in pregnancy, the presence of Down syndrome will typically result in elevated levels of hCG and inhibin A and decreased levels of AFP (C) and unconjugated estriol.

Incorrect:

Though women 35 years and older are at higher risk of having an infant born with Down syndrome, approximately 75% of all children with Down syndrome are born to women younger than age 35 years (A). Down syndrome occurs in approximately 1 in every 1,000 births, though this increases to 1 in every 270 births in women 35 to 40 years old (B). An indication of Down syndrome from antenatal serum analysis would require follow-up testing to make the diagnosis, such as with amniocentesis (D).

61. Correct: D. 21

Trisomy is the presence of a single additional chromosome and can be an important cause of congenital malformations and mental impairments. Trisomy 21 is Down syndrome that occurs in approximately 1 in every 1,000 births (D).

Incorrect:

Edwards' syndrome is due to trisomy 18 and occurs in approximately 1 in every 6,000 births (C). Clinical manifestations of the condition include low birth weight, developmental disability, and cranial, cardiac, and renal malformations. Patau's syndrome is trisomy 13 (A) and occurs in 1 in every 8,000 to 12,000 births. Clinical manifestations of Patau's syndrome include microcephaly, omphalocele, NTDs, and polydactyly. Trisomy 15 or mosaic trisomy 15 is an extremely rare occurrence (B).

62. Correct: D. progesterone.

Progesterone, a hormone that is important in the menstrual cycle and plays a role in the early stages of

pregnancy, is not part of the quad screen used to screen for open NTDs or aneuploidy (D).

Incorrect:

The four components of the quad screen include maternal serum levels of AFP (A), hCG (B), unconjugated estriol (C), and inhibin-A.

63. Correct: A. Down syndrome.

When a quad screen reveals elevated levels of maternal inhibin-A, this would suggest a higher-risk situation for Down syndrome (A). Additional testing is needed to make the diagnosis, such as with amniocentesis.

Incorrect:

Pregnancies at higher risk of Edwards' syndrome (B) or open NTD (C) would not cause an elevation in maternal inhibin-A levels. Hemolytic anemia is not revealed with the use of the quad screen and would not impact maternal inhibin-A levels (D).

64. Correct: C. Screening that combines nuchal translucency measurement and biochemical testing and/or free cell DNA is available.

The quad screen is ideally performed in the second trimester between 16 and 18 weeks. Prenatal tests available at 10 weeks include biochemical tests with plasma protein A and β-hCG along with an ultrasound of nuchal translucency that can be used for early detection of Down syndrome (C).

Incorrect:

Prenatal testing is recommended for all women during pregnancy regardless of age (A). Tests are available during the first trimester for early detection of Down syndrome, and follow-up screening should be performed during the second trimester to determine risk of aneuploidy and open NTDs (B). Genetic counseling as well as follow-up testing should be considered for women who are found to be at higher risk of having an infant with Down syndrome. However, counseling prior to results from a screening test is likely not warranted (D).

65 to 67. Matching Questions

65. Correct: A. French Canadian

66. Correct: B. northern European ancestry

67. Correct: C. African ancestry

It is important for clinicians to recognize at-risk ethnic groups when considering testing for genetically based conditions. Ethnic groups at higher risk for Tay-Sachs' disease include Ashkenazi Jews, French Canadians, and those of Cajun ancestry (65). Cystic fibrosis testing can be considered among those with Northern European or Ashkenazi Jewish heritage (66). The sickle cell trait can be tested among those with African, Latino, Arabic, Greek, Maltese, Italian, Sardinian, Turkish, and Indian ancestry (67).

68. Correct: B. low birth weight.

Expectant mothers should be counseled on ensuring chronic medical conditions are well controlled during pregnancy due to a risk of complications to the mother and baby. A woman with uncontrolled asthma during pregnancy can limit the amount of oxygen reaching the growing fetus (fetal hypoxia) and can impair development and growth, increasing the risk of a preterm birth and low birth weight (B).

Incorrect:
Trisomy 21 (C) and cystic fibrosis (D) are genetically based conditions that would not result from uncontrolled asthma during pregnancy. Macrosomia, or an abnormally large newborn, is more likely to occur with uncontrolled diabetes mellitus (A).

69. **Correct: C. anencephaly.**
Anencephaly is an NTD that can occur with FAD during pregnancy. The development of NTDs is not associated with poorly controlled diabetes mellitus during pregnancy (C).

Incorrect:
Poorly controlled diabetes mellitus during pregnancy can lead to an increased risk of stillbirth (A) as well as other pregnancy-related complications. Respiratory distress for the newborn can result as the lungs may not develop fully (B). Macrosomia, or a larger than average newborn, can lead to a difficult labor and delivery (D).

Medication Use During Pregnancy

70. **Correct: B. passive diffusion.**
Medications typically pass through the placenta by passive diffusion, when the medication moves from areas of higher concentration to areas of lower concentration (B). The degree of diffusion is influenced by a variety of factors including molecular weight and lipophilicity. The highest concentration of drug in the fetus is usually when maternal serum concentrations are highest.

Incorrect:
Facilitated transport occurs when the movement of substances across a cell membrane is facilitated by specific transmembrane proteins (A). Capillary action is the ability of liquids to flow in narrow spaces, though capillary pump action as it pertains to diffusion is not defined (C). Active diffusion involves the expenditure of energy by a cell to move substances across cell membranes (D).

71. **Correct: B. 31 to 81 days**
The most intense period of organogenesis occurs 31 to 81 days following LMP and is the period of time when teratogenic drugs can have the greatest effect in development (B). Prior to this period, the embryo consists of a group of poorly differentiated cells with no discrete organs. Following day 81 post-LMP, the organs are essentially formed and are then growing and developing.

Incorrect:
The most intense period of organogenesis occurs after the first month past LMP (A) and prior to 3 months past LMP (C, D).

72. **Correct: A. A.**
FDA pregnancy risk category A is best described as having demonstrated safety for use in all trimesters of pregnancy (A). Few if any drugs are given FDA pregnancy risk category A.

Incorrect:
FDA pregnancy risk category B is described as a drug that has not been shown to be harmful to the fetus in animal studies but for which no human study is available (B). Pregnancy risk category C is a drug shown to cause teratogenic effect in animal studies but for which no human study is available (C). Pregnancy risk category D is described as shown to cause teratogenic effects in human study, but the benefit could outweigh the risk of use in a life-threatening situation (D).

73. **Correct: D. D.**
Pregnancy risk category D is described as shown to cause teratogenic effects in human study, but the benefits could outweigh the risks of use in a life-threatening situation (D).

Incorrect:
FDA pregnancy risk category A is best described as having demonstrated safety for use in all trimesters of pregnancy (A). FDA pregnancy risk category B is described as a drug that has not been shown to be harmful to the fetus in animal studies but for which no human study is available (B). Pregnancy risk category C is a drug shown to cause teratogenic effect in animal studies but for which no human study is available (C).

74. **Correct: B. B.**
FDA pregnancy risk category B is described as a drug that has not been shown to be harmful to the fetus in animal studies but for which no human study is available (B).

Incorrect:
FDA pregnancy risk category A is best described as having demonstrated safety for use in all trimesters of pregnancy (A). Pregnancy risk category C is a drug shown to cause teratogenic effect in animal studies but for which no human study is available (C). Pregnancy risk category D is described as shown to cause teratogenic effects in human study but may have benefits that could outweigh the risks of use in a life-threatening situation (D).

75. **Correct: C. C.**
Pregnancy risk category C is a drug shown to cause teratogenic effect in animal studies but for which no human study is available (C).

Incorrect:
FDA pregnancy risk category A is best described as having demonstrated safety for use in all trimesters of pregnancy (A). FDA pregnancy risk category B is described as a drug that has not been shown to be harmful to the fetus in animal studies but for which no human study is available (B). Pregnancy risk category D is described as shown to cause teratogenic effects in human study, but the benefits may outweigh the risks of use in a life-threatening situation (D).

76. **Correct: B. a group of poorly differentiated cells.**
Prior to day 31 post-LMP, the embryo is best described as a group of poorly differentiated cells with no discrete

organ systems (B). At this stage, teratogenic agents will typically not cause significant damage as there are no organs to disrupt.

Incorrect:

A single, undifferentiated cell, or the zygote, is what is formed immediately following fertilization (A). A conglomerate of highly differentiated cells and primitive organs is formed between 31 and 81 days post-LMP, and teratogenic agents taken at this stage can cause significant damage to the developing embryo (C). After 81 days post-LMP, the pregnancy consists of a small fetus with differentiated organs that will continue to grow and develop (D).

77. Correct: B. less than 500 daltons

When considering drugs passing through the placenta, it is important to recognize that the lower the molecular weight, the greater the potential for passage. For a drug to easily pass through the placenta via passive diffusion, it should generally be less than 500 daltons in size (B). Drugs that are greater than 1,000 daltons will pass through the placenta infrequently.

Incorrect:

The size limit of a drug to easily pass through the placenta is approximately 500 Da (A). Drugs that are larger will be less likely to pass (C, D).

78. Correct: C. greater than 1,000 daltons

When considering drugs passing through the placenta, it is important to recognize that the lower the molecular weight, the greater the potential for passage. For a drug to easily pass through the placenta via passive diffusion, it should generally be less than 500 daltons in size. Drugs that are greater than 1,000 daltons will pass through the placenta infrequently (D).

Incorrect:

Drugs that are 500 Da or smaller can easily pass through the placenta (A, B). Drugs that are 1000 Da or larger will be unable to pass the barrier (D).

79. Correct: B. cephalexin.

In considering the use of antimicrobials during pregnancy, the beta-lactams including the penicillins and cephalosporins are pregnancy risk category B and provide a safe option. Cephalexin would be the best choice among the options for the treatment of a UTI during pregnancy (B).

Incorrect:

The fluoroquinolones (C) and TMP-SMX (A) are pregnancy risk category C and should be used with caution during pregnancy. Doxycycline is pregnancy risk category D and should only be considered in life-threatening situations when other safer options are not available (D).

80. Correct: D. 29 to 36 weeks

Appropriate control of asthma during pregnancy is essential to prevent fetal hypoxia that can slow growth and development. Though most pregnant women with asthma show no change in symptoms and sometimes

have an improvement in symptoms, symptoms of bronchospasm tend to worsen between 29 and 36 weeks of gestation (D). This can be attributed to esophageal irritation from GERD in the latter stages of pregnancy. Symptoms improve a bit once fetal descent occurs late in pregnancy.

Incorrect:

Though women can experience asthma symptoms throughout pregnancy, symptoms tend to worsen towards the end of pregnancy, after week 29 (A, B, C).

81. Correct: D. levofloxacin.

Clinicians must consider the risk of medications to both the mother and fetus during pregnancy. The fluoroquinolones such as levofloxacin are pregnancy risk category C and so should be used with caution as there are no controlled studies in humans available and/or animal studies reveal adverse fetal effects (D).

Incorrect:

Beta-lactam antimicrobials are generally preferred during pregnancy as they are pregnancy risk category B, where animal studies do not show fetal risk though there is no controlled study done in humans, or animal studies show adverse effect of the medication, but this is not revealed in human study. The beta-lactams include penicillins (e.g., amoxicillin [A]) and cephalosporins such as cefuroxime (B) and cefpodoxime (C).

82. Correct: C. 7 days.

UTIs during pregnancy are particularly concerning due to increased risk of low-birth-weight babies and premature delivery. Screening and treating for asymptomatic bacteriuria are important as this can progress to symptomatic UTIs including pyelonephritis. Treatment of asymptomatic bacteriuria typically involves a 3- to 7-day course of antimicrobials. For those with symptomatic UTI during pregnancy, a 7-day course is needed to ensure eradication of the infection (C).

Incorrect:

Those with asymptomatic bacteriuria during pregnancy can use a shorter course of antimicrobial therapy (A, B). Ten days of antimicrobial therapy is not typically warranted in cases of symptomatic bacteriuria (D).

83. Correct: A. bothersome but not life threatening.

Serotonin syndrome can occur with rapid termination of SSRI therapy after taking the medication for a prolonged period of time. The symptoms are best described as bothersome and can include jitteriness, nausea, and sleep disturbances (A).

Incorrect:

Serotonin syndrome is not considered a life-threatening condition, though the symptoms can be bothersome (B). Symptoms are generally more severe when using SSRIs with a shorter half-life when compared to agents with a longer half-life (C). There is no increased risk of seizure with serotonin syndrome (D), unlike what is observed with rapid discontinuation of long-term use of benzodiazepines.

84. **Correct: C. able to transport lipophilic substances.**

Several factors can influence the transport of medications through the placenta including molecular size and lipophilicity. The placenta preferentially allows highly lipophilic drugs to pass through (C). Medications that are more hydrophilic are less inclined to pass through the placenta and will result in fewer fetal effects.

Incorrect:

The placenta is not considered an effective drug barrier (B), particularly for drugs that are smaller than 500 daltons, which can easily cross the placental barrier (D). The placenta is fairly permeable, as it allows substances and nutrients to flow between the mother and fetus (A).

85. **Correct: D. acetaminophen.**

For pregnant women in the *second trimester* of pregnancy, preferred treatment of migraine is acetaminophen, as this is pregnancy risk category B (D). NSAIDs should be avoided as they are pregnancy risk category C.

Incorrect:

The use of full doses of aspirin during pregnancy should be avoided as it poses various risks depending on the stage of pregnancy (C). NSAIDs and aspirin during late stages of pregnancy can lead to premature closure of the ductus arteriosus and persistent fetal circulation. Sumatriptan is pregnancy risk category C and should be avoided because of a possible risk of vasoconstriction (A). Opioid medications, such as codeine, should generally be avoided during pregnancy and are mostly given pregnancy risk category C (the exception is oxycodone, which is category B) (B).

86. **Correct: C. the use of paroxetine during pregnancy is associated with an increase in risk for congenital cardiac defect.**

Most SSRIs are placed in pregnancy risk category C. The exception to this is paroxetine, which is pregnancy risk category D. This is due to evidence demonstrating an increased risk of congenital cardiac defects when this medication is taken during pregnancy (C).

Incorrect:

Though caution should be used when using SSRIs during pregnancy, there has been no clear teratogenic pattern from observational studies of children born to women taking these medications (A). There has been no indication of a negative effect on intellectual development with SSRI use during pregnancy (B), and there is no association with an increased rate of seizure disorder (D).

87. **Correct: B. antibiotics.**

Data from the CDC reveal that about 90% of women take at least one medication during pregnancy and 70% take at least one prescription medication. The most common medications taken by pregnant women are antibiotics (B). This can be contributed by an increased risk of UTIs during pregnancy as well as a need to treat for asymptomatic bacteriuria.

Incorrect:

Though a large majority of pregnant women will take at least one prescription medication, the most common type of medication are antimicrobials and not antiepileptic drugs (A), antihypertensives (C) or opioids (D).

88. **Correct: D. associated with seizure risk.**

Benzodiazepines are pregnancy risk category C or D and should be discontinued during pregnancy. Because of severe withdrawal symptoms with rapid discontinuation, the dose should be tapered gradually, such as a 25% reduction per week. Rapid withdrawal can lead to tremors, hallucinations, seizures, and delirium tremens (D).

Incorrect:

Rapid withdrawal of benzodiazepines for pregnant and nonpregnant women can lead to serious and life-threatening symptoms, including seizures (A, B). The onset of symptoms will occur more rapidly with agents having a short half-life, while there will be a longer delay in symptoms when using agents with a longer half-life (C).

89. **Correct: D. inhaled corticosteroids.**

Similar to nonpregnant populations, the primary treatment for moderate persistent asthma during pregnancy is the use of an inhaled corticosteroid (D). These agents are considered to be generally safe during pregnancy as they have low rates of systemic absorption.

Incorrect:

Theophylline is not indicated as controller therapy for moderate persistent asthma but is used for prevention of bronchospasm. It is pregnancy risk category C and should be used with caution (A). Mast cell stabilizers such as cromolyn are no longer available in the United States due to more effective treatment options and are not considered first-line therapy for moderate persistent asthma (B). Leukotriene receptor antagonists are generally less effective than inhaled corticosteroids as controller medication, and these agents have not been studied extensively in pregnant women (C).

90. **Correct: C. a short course of oral prednisone.**

An asthma flare is best treated with a short course of an oral corticosteroid, such as prednisone (C). This offers the most effective approach in achieving baseline status and returning to controller therapy.

Incorrect:

Theophylline is pregnancy category C and should only be used with caution during pregnancy (A). The beta-agonists are also pregnancy risk category C and can be considered as a rescue drug during pregnancy, particularly if there is an inadequate response with oral corticosteroid therapy (B). The addition of a leukotriene modifier will not be helpful in managing an asthma flare (D).

91. **Correct: D. 36 to 40**

During pregnancy, bronchospasm symptoms typically peak between weeks 29 and 36 of gestation, possibly due to esophageal irritation from GERD during this time.

Bronchospasm symptoms improve following week 36 of gestation when gradual fetal descent occurs (D).
Incorrect:
Bronchospasm symptoms peak at weeks 29 to 36 of gestation (C). Symptoms do not improve during earlier stages of pregnancy (A, B).

92. **Correct: A. females attempting to conceive.**
The FDA has replaced the letter categories that have long been used to classify medication use during pregnancy (i.e., A, B, C, D, X) with three detailed subsections that describe risks within the real-world context of use for pregnant and nursing women who need medication. However, there is not a subsection that specifically focuses on women attempting to conceive (A).
Incorrect:
Prescribing information sheets of newer medications are now required to include subsections of the effects of the medication in pregnancy (B), lactation (C), and females and males of reproductive age (D).

93. **Correct: C. taper the dose down 25% each week.**
Benzodiazepines are pregnancy risk category C or D and should be discontinued during pregnancy. Because of severe withdrawal symptoms with rapid discontinuation, the dose should be tapered gradually, such as 25% reduction per week (C). Rapid withdrawal can lead to tremors, hallucinations, seizures, and delirium tremens.
Incorrect:
Benzodiazepines should be slowly tapered when attempting to discontinue therapy to avoid severe withdrawal symptoms when discontinued immediately (B). The dose should not be increased during pregnancy as these agents pose a risk to the fetus (A). Paroxetine should also be avoided in pregnancy due to an associated increased risk for cardiac malformations in the newborn (D).

94. **Correct: C. premature closure of ductus arteriosus.**
The use of NSAIDs during pregnancy should be avoided as it poses various risks depending on the stage of pregnancy. NSAIDs during late stages of pregnancy (particularly after week 32) can lead to premature closure of the ductus arteriosus and persistent fetal circulation (C). NSAID use in early pregnancy is associated with an elevated risk of miscarriage.
Incorrect:
Use of NSAIDs during the later stages of pregnancy is not associated with ventricular septal defects (D) or premature birth (A). NTDs are more likely associated with FAD and not NSAID use (B).

95. **Correct: B. miscarriage.**
Clinical evidence has demonstrated that the use of NSAIDs at the early stage of pregnancy can increase the risk of an early miscarriage by up to fourfold (B).
Incorrect:
NSAID use during the later stages of pregnancy should be avoided due to premature closure of the ductus arteriosus (C). NSAID use is not associated with premature

birth (A) and is not associated with genetically based abnormalities such as due to aneuploidy (D).

96. **Correct: B. SSRI withdrawal.**
Newborns who are born to mothers who were taking SSRIs during pregnancy will undergo withdrawal syndrome within days to weeks, depending on the half-life of the SSRI. Neonatal symptoms will include irritability, protracted crying, and shivering (B). Therefore, it is recommended to taper SSRI use during the last month of pregnancy to avoid fetal withdrawal.
Incorrect:
The most likely cause of symptoms in this baby is SSRI withdrawal. The use of SSRI during pregnancy is not associated with increased intracranial pressure in the newborn (A). Though a colicky child will present with similar symptoms, colic peaks around 6 weeks of age (C). Signs of sepsis can include elevated temperature, breathing difficulty, reduced movements, and tachycardia, which were not reported in this newborn (D).

97. **Correct: C. azithromycin**
Among the answer choices, azithromycin is pregnancy risk category B and would offer the safest antimicrobial during pregnancy (C).
Incorrect:
The fluoroquinolones (D) and clarithromycin (A) are pregnancy risk category C and should be used with caution. Doxycycline is pregnancy risk category D and should be avoided during pregnancy (B).

98. **Correct: C. cephalexin**
The beta-lactams or nitrofurantoin are the preferred antimicrobials to use for the treatment of a UTI during pregnancy. Cephalexin is pregnancy risk category B and considered safe for the fetus (C). Nitrofurantoin should be avoided after the 36th week of gestation due to a possible risk of hemolysis.
Incorrect:
The fluoroquinolones (B) and TMP-SMX (D) are pregnancy risk category C and should be used with caution. Doxycycline is pregnancy risk category D and should be avoided during pregnancy (A).

99. **Correct: B. nitrofurantoin**
Nitrofurantoin is pregnancy risk category B and a preferred antimicrobial to use for the treatment of UTIs during pregnancy. However, this medication should be avoided after the 36th week of gestation due to a possible (though unlikely) risk of fetal hemolysis (B). This can occur if the fetus is glucose-6-phosphate dehydrogenase-deficient as well as in infections caused by *P mirabilis*.
Incorrect:
Gentamicin (A), clarithromycin (C), and ciprofloxacin (D) are not associated with fetal hemolysis when used during pregnancy. However, these agents are generally not recommended due to potential adverse effects to the fetus.

100. Correct: B. needs to be treated to avoid complicated UTI.

UTI during pregnancy is a significant risk factor for low birth weight and premature delivery. Due to anatomical changes during pregnancy, asymptomatic bacteriuria is more likely to progress to a symptomatic UTI as well as pyelonephritis when compared to nonpregnant women. Therefore, all women should have urine cultures performed early in pregnancy and be treated with an appropriate antimicrobial (B) when asymptomatic bacteriuria is detected.

Incorrect:

Asymptomatic bacteriuria is found in less than 10% of pregnant and nonpregnant women. Though this is typically not treated in nonpregnant women, treatment is recommended during pregnancy to reduce the risk of complicated UTI (C). This is true for all pregnant women with asymptomatic bacteriuria and not just for those with bladder instrumentation or planned surgery (A). Asymptomatic bacteriuria increases the risk of UTI and complicated UTI, such as pyelonephritis, and can increase the risk of low birth weight or premature delivery, though not hypertension (D).

101. Correct: B. *E coli*

E coli is the most common uropathogen found in both pregnant and nonpregnant women (B), and antimicrobial selection should focus on activity against this pathogen.

Incorrect:

Though *E coli* is the predominant uropathogen in UTIs, other gram-negative pathogens could include, to a lesser degree, *P aeruginosa* (A), *K pneumoniae* (C), and *P mirabilis* (D), as well as the gram-positive pathogen *S saprophyticus*.

102. Correct: B. 3 to 7 days.

UTIs during pregnancy are particularly concerning due to increased risk of low birth weight and premature delivery. Screening and treating for asymptomatic bacteriuria are important as this can progress to symptomatic UTIs including pyelonephritis. Treatment of asymptomatic bacteriuria typically involves a 3- to 7-day course of antimicrobials (B). For those with symptomatic UTI during pregnancy, a 7-day course is needed to ensure eradication of the infection.

Conditions Encountered in Later Pregnancy

103 to 107. Matching Questions

103. Correct: C. high BP diagnosed before pregnancy

104. Correct: A. high BP diagnosed after the 20th week of pregnancy

105. Correct: E. high BP diagnosed after the 20th week of pregnancy and accompanied by significant proteinuria

106. Correct: B. presence of tonic-clonic seizures or other alteration in mental status

107. Correct: D. preeclampsia accompanied by elevated LDH and hepatic enzymes and low platelets

Hypertensive disorders are a common condition during pregnancy, and clinicians should maintain a high degree of suspicion for women at increased risk in order for prompt recognition and management when needed. Chronic hypertension refers to elevated BP that occurs prior to pregnancy, prior to the 20th week of gestation, and/or persists after 6 weeks' postpartum (105). Gestational hypertension occurs after the 20th week of pregnancy without proteinuria or other signs of preeclampsia and resolves within 6 weeks' postpartum (106). Preeclampsia is hypertension diagnosed after the 20th week of gestation along with proteinuria and/or other signs of more severe disease (107). HELLP syndrome consists of preeclampsia that is also accompanied by thrombocytopenia, elevated LDH, and elevated liver enzymes (109). Eclampsia presents similarly as preeclampsia along with the possibility of tonic-clonic seizures or other change in mental status (108).

108. Correct: A. low maternal weight.

Several risk factors have been identified for preeclampsia. Among these include prepregnancy overweight (BMI greater than 30 kg/m²) rather than low maternal weight (A).

Incorrect:

Risk factors for preeclampsia include maternal age 16 years or younger or 40 years or older (B), a first pregnancy or first pregnancy with a new partner (D), pregestational or gestational diabetes, collagen vascular disease (C), chronic hypertension, and prior history of preeclampsia.

109. Correct: B. 140, 90

The latest criteria from ACOG on diagnosing preeclampsia are to have a BP reading higher than 140/90 mm Hg on two occasions separated by at least 4 hours, or to have one measurement of greater than 160/110 mm Hg on one occasion. Other conditions will also need to be present for a diagnosis, including proteinuria, thrombocytopenia, elevated liver enzymes, or renal insufficiency, among other criteria.

Incorrect:

A blood pressure of 130/80 mm Hg is at the high end of normal during pregnancy (A). A blood pressure that exceeds 140/90 mm Hg is an indication of preeclampsia (C, D).

110. Correct: C. 20th

A diagnosis of preeclampsia can be made after the 20th week of gestation (C). If hypertension is detected prior to the 20th week, an alternative diagnosis should be investigated.

Incorrect:

A preeclampsia diagnosis should not be considered prior to the 20th week of gestation (A, B), but can be considered prior to the 25th week (D).

111. Correct: B. thrombocytosis.

HELLP syndrome is preeclampsia that is accompanied by thrombocytopenia, or low platelet counts, rather than thrombocytosis, which is an elevation of platelet counts (B).

Incorrect:

HELLP syndrome is characterized as preeclampsia (D) that is accompanied by elevation in liver enzymes (AST and ALT) (A), thrombocytopenia, and elevated levels of lactate dehydrogenase (C).

112. Correct: C. prompt recognition of the condition

Clinicians should be aware of risk factors for preeclampsia in order to have a high level of suspicion at the first signs of the condition (C). Prompt recognition of preeclampsia should be immediately followed by expert obstetrical consultation.

Incorrect:

Treatment with antihypertensive medications (A) and anticonvulsant therapy (B) can be important parts of care during preeclampsia but will likely only have a small effect on outcome. Birth is the definitive intervention, and induction of labor should be considered after the 34th week of gestation in severe cases (D).

113. Correct: A. There have been no definitive strategies identified to prevent preeclampsia.

Though many studies have attempted to identify interventions to prevent preeclampsia, there have been no strategies identified to date that definitively prevent this condition (A).

Incorrect:

Several clinical studies have evaluated nutritional supplements or sodium restriction on the effect in preventing preeclampsia, though none have shown to be effective for this purpose (B). A study with low-dose aspirin demonstrated a reduction in preterm preeclampsia but did not result in a significant reduction in full-term preeclampsia (C). Evidence does not support bedrest for preventing or managing preeclampsia and so it should not be recommended (D).

114. Correct: D. intrapartum antimicrobials should be given to nearly all women with evidence of GBS colonization.

For women with evidence of GBS colonization, the use of intrapartum antimicrobials is recommended in nearly all cases (D). An exception to the use of intrapartum antimicrobials would be for women who undergo a cesarean delivery and the membranes are intact. IV penicillin and ampicillin are the recommended first-line options. In cases of penicillin allergy, a first-generation cephalosporin or clindamycin are additional options, depending on the severity of allergic reaction.

Incorrect:

GBS colonization is found in approximately 10% to 30% of pregnant women (A). There is little risk in women undergoing cesarean birth with membranes intact. However, with ruptured membranes,

antimicrobial prophylaxis is needed (B). The transmission of the organism most frequently occurs during the onset of labor or membrane rupture and not during the second trimester (C).

115. Correct: D. the lower vagina and rectum.

The lower GI tract is the natural reservoir for GBS, while vaginal and rectal colonization occurs in 10% to 30% of pregnant women. When screening for GBS, usually during weeks 35 to 37 of gestation, culture should be obtained by swabbing the lower vagina and vaginal introitus followed by the rectum (D).

Incorrect:

Screening for GBS during pregnancy should not include urine (C) or the urethra (B). Cervical cultures should also not be obtained as these are usually negative, even in the presence of heavy GBS colonization of the lower vagina (A).

Early Pregnancy Loss

116. Correct: B. 15

Spontaneous abortion is defined as the natural ending of a pregnancy before the 20th week of gestation. Up to 30% of women experience some form of vaginal bleeding in the first trimester of pregnancy, and about half of these women will have pregnancy loss (B). The most common cause of spontaneous abortion is chromosomal defects.

117. Correct: C. 60

Chromosomal defects of paternal or maternal origin are the leading cause of spontaneous abortion, accounting for approximately 60% of cases (C). Maternal factors such as trauma, illness, or infection account for about 15% of cases, while there is no obvious cause for the remaining cases of spontaneous abortion.

118. Correct: B. BMI greater than 30 kg/m².

Several factors have been identified that increase the risk of spontaneous abortion. However, overweight is not a demonstrated risk factor (B).

Incorrect:

Risk factors for spontaneous abortion include a previous history of spontaneous abortion, age older than 35 years (A), excessive use of alcohol or caffeine (C), and poorly controlled chronic medical conditions such as diabetes mellitus, thyroid disease, and hypertension (D).

119. Correct: C. woman who reports three consecutive pregnancy losses under 10 weeks' gestation

Recurrent early pregnancy loss is usually characterized by two to three consecutive SABs. For these women, expert consultation is advised to investigate an underlying and potentially treatable condition. Among the answer choices, the woman with three consecutive pregnancy losses best describes recurrent early pregnancy loss.

Incorrect:

Medical pregnancy termination is not considered a criterion for early recurrent pregnancy loss, as these procedures are not spontaneous events (A, D). Two or more consecutive SABs are needed for recurrent early pregnancy loss (B).

120. **Correct: C. large-for-gestational-age uterus.**
Ectopic pregnancy is one that occurs outside of the uterus. A clinical presentation finding in ectopic pregnancy is a uterus size that is less than the anticipated size for gestational age, and not larger than expected (C).
Incorrect:
The classic clinical triad for ectopic pregnancy is abdominal pain (A), vaginal bleeding (B), and adnexal mass (D). However, it is important to note that this triad of findings occurs in only about 50% of women with ectopic pregnancy; therefore, follow-up evaluation is needed to confirm the diagnosis. These include an ultrasound as well as levels of progesterone and β-hCG.

121. **Correct: C. 50**
The classic triad for ectopic pregnancy is abdominal pain, vaginal bleeding, and adnexal mass. However, it is important to note that this triad of findings occurs in only about 50% of women with ectopic pregnancy (C); therefore, follow-up evaluation is needed to confirm the diagnosis.

122. **Correct: B. 48**
During a viable IUP, hCG levels rapidly rise and double every 48 hours until a level of 10,000 to 20,000 mIU/mL is reached (B). When the hCG level is greater than 1,500 mIU/mL, a gestational sac is visible on transvaginal ultrasound. The gestational sac is visible on transabdominal ultrasound when the hCG level exceeds 6,000 mIU/mL.

123. **Correct: C. urinary tract infection.**
When making a differential diagnosis for ectopic pregnancy, it is important for the clinician to recognize other conditions that can present similarly. The most common signs of ectopic pregnancy include abdominal pain, adnexal tenderness and adnexal mass, and vaginal bleeding. UTI would not present in this manner but would more likely be associated with dysuria, urinary urge, pelvic pain, and blood in the urine.
Incorrect:
Other conditions that present with one or more symptoms of abdominal pain, adnexal mass, adnexal tenderness, and vaginal bleeding can include pelvic inflammatory disease (A), ruptured corpus luteum (B), appendicitis (D), and ovarian torsion.

124. **Correct: C. Location of the pregnancy is often on the ovary or cervix.**
The most common location of ectopic pregnancies is within the fallopian tube, accounting for approximately 95% of cases (C).
Incorrect:
A key finding in ectopic pregnancy is a low level of hCG for gestational age, reaching about 1,000 to 6,000 mIU/mL by weeks 6 to 10, compared to about 40,000 mIU/mL or higher in a viable IUP (A). A normal ultrasound does not rule out the condition, as an abnormality is not observed in a substantial portion of these procedures (B). Pregnancy achieved via in-vitro fertilization or fertility drugs is a risk factor for ectopic pregnancy (D).

125 to 128. Matching Questions

125. **Correct: C. The products of conception have been completely expelled.**

126. **Correct: A. Uterine contents include a nonviable pregnancy that is in the process of being expelled.**

127. **Correct: D. Ultrasound evaluation shows a viable pregnancy, although vaginal bleeding is present.**

128. **Correct: B. Some portion of the products of conception remains in the uterus, although the pregnancy is no longer viable.**
There are four terms used to describe spontaneous abortion. A threatened abortion presents with vaginal bleeding or brown spotting with or without cramping and without cervical dilation, while ultrasound reveals a viable pregnancy (129). An inevitable abortion presents with an open cervix, and uterine contents are in the process of being expelled (128). An incomplete abortion occurs when some portion of the products of conception remain in the uterus though the pregnancy is no longer viable (130). Evacuation of the uterine contents by dilation and aspiration is sometimes needed in these cases. A complete abortion occurs when the products of conception have been completely expelled (127).

Labor, Birth, and Recovery

129. **Correct: B. 9 to 12**
The first stage of labor starts when the cervix is about 3 to 4 cm dilated and ends when the cervix is fully dilated. For first-time mothers, this stage of pregnancy lasts about 9 to 12 hours (B), while second-stage labor that ends with birth can last from 30 minutes to 2 hours.

130. **Correct: B. 6 to 8**
For women who have previously given birth, the combined time for the first and second stages of labor lasts about 6 to 8 hours (B). This will encompass the time when the cervix is about 3 to 4 cm dilated until birth.

131. **Correct: C. The mother should be encouraged to remain physically active as she tolerates during early labor.**
Early labor is characterized by mild to moderate contractions that occur between 5 and 20 minutes apart. This stage of labor can last up to 2 to 3 days, and the mother is encouraged to remain physically active as is tolerated (C), though she may be frustrated by the slow progress of labor.
Incorrect:
Mothers are instructed to go to the hospital during the first stage of labor, when contractions are occurring about every 5 minutes and lasting for 1 minute (A).

Early labor ends when the cervix dilates to about 3 cm, which then begins the first stage of pregnancy (B). Contractions are present during the early labor, though they are typically mild to moderate and spaced by up to 20 minutes, sometimes starting and stopping (D).

132. Correct: B. stage 2

The second stage of labor begins when the cervix is fully dilated and ends with the actual birth (B).
Incorrect:
Stage 1 begins with the cervix dilated to between 3 and 4 cm and ends when the cervix is fully dilated (A). Contractions occur more frequently and are more intense during this stage. The third stage of labor occurs when the placenta detaches and is expelled from the uterus (C). There is no latent stage of labor (D).

133. Correct: A. an induction can be scheduled after 39 weeks of gestation.

Elective induction can be considered under certain circumstances, such as living a far distance from the hospital. However, it is recommended that induction should not be performed prior to 39 weeks of gestation (A).
Incorrect:
Induction of labor can be considered under certain circumstances that do not necessarily involve high-risk pregnancies (B). One study demonstrated that there was a lower risk of cesarean births, stillbirths, and complications to the mother and fetus with induction (C). As the mother will still experience the three stages of labor with induction, there should not be any difference on the need for analgesia with or without induction (D).

Postpartum Mood and Anxiety Disorders

134. Correct: B. within a few days following the birth.

Postpartum blues is the most common mood disorder following childbirth and typically occurs within a few days after giving birth (B). This is possibly linked to hormonal changes that occur during pregnancy and immediately following childbirth and can include symptoms of unexplained weepiness or crying, impatience, irritability, restlessness, anxiety, fatigue, and insomnia.
Incorrect:
Postpartum blues occur within a few days following delivery and not prior to delivery (A) or a week or later following delivery (C, D).

135. Correct: C. history of carrying two or more pregnancies to term.

Postpartum depression is more severe than postpartum blues and typically occurs 2 to 4 months following childbirth. Several risk factors have been identified for postpartum depression; however, a history of multiple pregnancies is not a risk factor for this condition (C).
Incorrect:
Risk factors for postpartum depression include a prior history of depression or postpartum depression (A), stressful events in the past year, relationship problems

with the partner, a weak support system, financial problems (B), or a pregnancy that was unplanned or unwanted (D).

136. Correct: B. overwhelming fatigue, C. insomnia, and D. severe mood swings

The most common symptoms of postpartum depression include loss of appetite, insomnia (C), intense irritability and anger, overwhelming fatigue (B), lack of sexual drive, lack of joy in life, and severe mood swings (D).
Incorrect:
Symptoms of hallucinations (A) and disorientation (E) are characteristic of postpartum psychosis. For these individuals, hospitalization is needed for the safety of the mother and newborn.

137 to 140. Ranking Question

137. Correct: 1

138. Correct: 2

139. Correct: 4

140. Correct: 3

For new mothers experiencing postpartum depression, first-line treatment should include counseling and psychotherapy (139). Pharmacotherapy can be considered if there is an inadequate response to psychotherapy, though keeping in mind that any medication will be present in breastmilk for nursing mothers. SSRIs are typical first-line antidepressant treatment for postpartum depression (140). Hormone therapy, such as estrogen replacement therapy, can also be effective if postpartum depression is caused by hormonal changes associated with pregnancy and childbirth (142). This approach can be considered if there is an inadequate response to antidepressant therapy or if there is concern about medication in breastmilk. Electroconvulsive therapy is not a typical approach for the treatment of postpartum depression (141).

141. Correct: C. postpartum psychosis

Though a rare condition, postpartum psychosis is associated with hallucinations, delusions, and paranoia and can result in attempts to harm themselves or the baby (C). Hospitalization is usually needed for the safety of both the mother and the infant.
Incorrect:
Postpartum depression (A) and "baby blues" (B) are characterized by irritability, anxiety, fatigue, insomnia, and mood changes. Postpartum depression can also include thoughts of harming oneself or the baby. However, this risk is much smaller when compared to postpartum psychosis (D).

142. Correct: C. history of bipolar disorder.

A prior history of bipolar disorder is a key risk factor for the development of postpartum psychosis (C).
Incorrect:
A history of depression would be a risk factor for the development of postpartum depression but not

postpartum psychosis (A). Having multiple births (B) or illegal drug use (D) are not risk factors for postpartum psychosis.

143. **Correct: B. estrogen replacement therapy.**
Postpartum psychosis is a severe mental health disorder that requires hospitalization along with pharmacotherapy. Estrogen replacement therapy, though often useful in the treatment of postpartum

depression, would not be effective in managing postpartum psychosis (B).
Incorrect:
Those with postpartum psychosis will often require hospitalization for the safety of the mother and the infant (A). Treatment options will also include pharmacotherapy with antipsychotic medications (C) and mood stabilizers as well as electroconvulsive therapy (D).

Professional Issues 19

Medicaid

Overview

The Medicaid program was started in 1965 and is the major source of health-care insurance for low-income Americans. Medicaid is an entitlement program; that is, its benefits are granted by federal law to citizens and select noncitizens legally residing in the United States.

This program covers a broad population, including pregnant women, children, and some parents in both working and jobless families, and children and adults with physical and mental health conditions and disabilities; nearly all live below or near the poverty line. Additionally, Medicaid provides assistance to low-income Medicare beneficiaries, known as "dual eligible" beneficiaries, providing assistance with Medicare premiums and cost-sharing and covering key services, particularly in long-term care (e.g., nursing homes), that Medicare excludes or limits.

Medicaid currently covers approximately 20% of the U.S. population, including nearly 40% of all children. This includes coverage for those with Down syndrome, cerebral palsy, and autism, among other conditions. Medicaid can provide access to a broader range of services needed by the disabled, including in-home therapy, speech and occupational therapy, as well as assistance to maximize independence.

Medicaid is the main source of coverage and financing for long-term services and supports (LTSS; e.g., nursing home care) because Medicare and private insurance largely do not provide coverage for these services. Of the nearly 10 million Americans who utilize LTSS, about half are elderly and about half are children and working-age adults with disabilities.

Funding for Medicaid

The cost of Medicaid is shared by the federal government and the states. The federal government matches state Medicaid spending based on a specified formula that varies for each state, but the federal match rate is at least 50% in every state. Though state participation in Medicaid is voluntary, all states participate. The states administer Medicaid within broad federal guidelines. States must cover federal core groups of low-income individuals including pregnant women, children, parents, elderly individuals, and individuals with disabilities.

The Centers for Medicare and Medicaid Services (CMS) provides oversight of each state to ensure that the core requirements are met. Beyond these core requirements, each state has flexibility regarding eligibility, benefits, provider payment, delivery systems, and other aspects. Thus, Medicaid programs can vary considerably from state to state.

Medicaid Services

In addition to the federal core groups to which states must provide coverage in order to receive federal matching funds, states must also cover a set of mandatory services defined by federal law (Box 19-1). These services include benefits typically covered by private insurance but can also include additional services, such as transportation and nursing and community-based long-term care. Services provided by federally qualified health centers (FQHCs) and rural health clinics (RHCs) are included, reflecting the role of these providers in serving the low-income population. In addition to these services, states have the flexibility to cover optional services, which tend to be vital for individuals with chronic conditions or disabilities and the elderly.

States are allowed to charge premiums and cost-sharing for Medicaid in accordance with federal limitations. Out-of-pocket costs can include copayments, coinsurance, and deductibles. Cost-sharing is largely prohibited for Medicaid-insured children and pregnant women and can vary for adults based on income level. Certain services are exempt from cost-sharing, such as preventive services for children, emergency services, select family planning services, and pregnancy-related services. Copayments are often used by states to encourage cost-effective use of prescription medications (i.e., generics versus brand-name drugs). States can also

> **CLINICAL CONCEPT**
>
> Only American citizens and specific categories of lawfully present noncitizens can qualify for Medicaid; lawfully present noncitizens typically must have a specified waiting period before enrollment in Medicaid.

> ### BOX 19-1 Mandatory Services Defined by Federal Law for Medicaid
>
> *Mandatory Services*
>
> - Health-care services provided by nurse practitioners, physician assistants, nurse midwives, and medical physicians
> - Nursing facility services for individuals 21 years old and older
> - Hospital services (inpatient and outpatient)
> - Laboratory and x-ray services
> - Early and periodic screening, diagnostic, and treatment (EPSDT) services for individuals under the age of 21 years
> - Select family planning services and supplies
> - Home health care for persons eligible for nursing facility services
> - Transportation related to health-care services
> - Federally qualified health center (FQHC) and rural health clinic (RHC) services
> - Tobacco cessation counseling for pregnant women
> - Free-standing birth center services

Source: Centers for Medicare and Medicaid Services. Mandatory & Optional Medicaid Benefits. https://www.medicaid.gov/medicaid/benefits/mandatory-optional-medicaid-benefits/index.html

impose higher copayments for nonemergency use of the emergency department (ED). States can terminate Medicaid coverage if premiums are not paid and can permit providers to deny care in certain circumstances if Medicaid patients do not pay their cost-sharing amounts.

Over half of the Medicaid spending for long-term care is used to provide services in the home or community to enable the elderly or disabled to live independently rather than in institutional care.

> **CLINICAL CONCEPT**
>
> Medicaid provides care for approximately 60% of all nursing home residents and covers approximately half of all long-term care costs in the United States.

Impact of Medicaid on Community Health

Medicaid improves access to health care for children. When compared to children with private insurance, children with Medicaid and the Children's Health Insurance Program (CHIP) demonstrated comparable levels of several core measures of preventive and primary care. However, working-age adults with Medicaid have greater difficulty in accessing health care compared with adults with private insurance. Medicaid patients use ED services at higher rates than those with private insurance. However, only about 10% of Medicaid ED visits are for nonurgent symptoms, compared with 7% for those with private insurers. Adults with Medicaid tend to have a higher burden of illness and disability and are more likely to have a secondary diagnosis of a mental disorder; a larger share of their visits involves more than one major diagnosis.

Discussion Sources

Centers for Medicare and Medicaid Services. Medicaid. https://www.medicaid.gov/medicaid/index.html

Rudowitz R, Garfield R, Hinton E. 10 Things to Know About Medicaid: Setting the Facts Straight. The Henry J. Kaiser Family Foundation. https://www.kff.org/medicaid/issue-brief/10-things-to-know-about-medicaid-setting-the-facts-straight/

QUESTIONS

1. Medicaid is best defined as:

   A. an entitlement program to provide health-care coverage for unemployed families.

   B. publicly financed coverage of health care and long-term care for low-income people.

   C. free acute care coverage for those who meet special criteria.

   D. publicly supported health care for low-income people under the age of 65 years.

2. Which of the following is not an entitlement program in the United States?

   A. Medicaid

   B. Social Security

   C. 401K programs

   D. Medicare

3. A "dual eligible" beneficiary is an individual who receives Medicaid and:

   A. private insurance.

   B. Social Security.

   C. government welfare benefits.

   D. Medicare.

4. Concerning long-term care coverage such as nursing home care, Medicaid:

   A. does not provide any coverage of long-term care expenses.

   B. only covers eligible individuals younger than 65 years of age.

   C. finances approximately 50% of all long-term care spending.

   D. provides coverage primarily for individuals with physical disabilities.

5. Which of the following statements concerning funding for Medicaid is accurate?

   A. Federal funding of Medicaid for each state is based primarily on the state population size.

   B. The federal government matches at least 50% of state Medicaid spending.

   C. States are not required to provide funding for Medicaid as long as they meet guidelines to receive federal funding.

   D. Federal funding typically accounts for less than 20% of all Medicaid funding.

6. Along with CHIP, Medicaid provides coverage for approximately what percentage of all children in the United States?

   A. 10%

   B. 20%

   C. 40%

   D. 60%

7. Federal core groups that states must cover to receive federal matching Medicaid funding include all of the following except:

   A. pregnant women.

   B. elderly.

   C. children.

   D. undocumented persons residing in the United States.

8. Concerning individuals who are disabled, Medicaid funding can assist in all of the following except:

   A. funding educational opportunities (i.e., tuition).

   B. providing a fuller range of health-care services.

   C. maximizing independent living opportunities.

   D. obtaining speech and occupational therapy services.

9. "Mandatory services" defined by federal law for inclusion in Medicaid include all of the following except:

   A. laboratory and x-ray services.

   B. select family planning services.

   C. rehabilitation therapy.

   D. nurse practitioner (NP) services.

10. Coverage of services from all of the following health-care centers is considered mandatory for inclusion in Medicaid by federal law except:

    A. RHC.

    B. acute care hospital.

C. hospice.

D. FQHC.

11. Which of the following statements is false regarding Medicaid premiums and cost-sharing?

A. States have limited flexibility to charge Medicaid premiums based on income level.

B. Preventive services for children are exempt from cost-sharing.

C. States can terminate Medicaid coverage if premiums are not paid by an individual.

D. All ED visits are exempt from copayments.

12. When compared with children with private insurance, those with Medicaid and CHIP are:

A. comparable in access to health care and meeting several core measures in preventive care.

B. more deficient in several core measures of preventive care.

C. less likely to see primary care providers (PCPs).

D. more likely to receive mandatory immunizations.

13. Which of the following statements is most accurate regarding the use of ED services by Medicaid patients?

A. The majority of ED visits by Medicaid patients is for nonurgent symptoms.

B. Those with Medicaid are more than twice as likely to use the ED for nonurgent symptoms compared with those with private insurance.

C. Medicaid patients use EDs at a similar rate when compared with people with private insurance.

D. ED visits by Medicaid patients more often involve multiple diagnoses compared with those with private insurance.

For answers and rationales, see end of chapter.

Medicare

Overview

Medicare was initially established in 1965 to provide health insurance for individuals older than age 65 years regardless of income or medical history. The program has subsequently been expanded to include individuals younger than 65 years with certain medical conditions and disabilities.

> **CLINICAL CONCEPT**
>
> Recently reported numbers show that approximately 60 million people receive Medicare coverage, including about 9 million people younger than age 65 years with disabilities.

The Components of Medicare

Medicare is divided into four parts, each providing different health-care benefits:

- *Part A (Hospital Insurance Program)*: Covers inpatient hospital services, skilled nursing facilities, home health, and hospice care. This is funded by a tax of 2.9% of earnings paid by employers and workers.
- *Part B (Supplemental Medical Insurance Program)*: Helps pay the outpatient, home health, and preventive services of the health-care provider. This is funded by general revenues and beneficiary premiums.
- *Part C (Medicare Advantage Program)*: Allows beneficiaries to enroll in a private plan, such as a health maintenance organization, preferred provider organization, or private fee-for-service plan, as an alternative to the traditional fee-for-service plan. These plans receive payments from Medicare to provide Medicare-covered benefits, such as hospital and physician services.
- *Part D*: Provides prescription drug benefits delivered through private plans that contract with Medicare. A monthly premium is typically paid by beneficiaries who enroll in these plans.

In addition to funding from payroll taxes and Medicare premiums, other sources of funding include taxation of Social Security benefits, payments from states, and interest.

Individuals aged 65 years and older are eligible for Medicare if they are a U.S. citizen or permanent legal resident regardless of prior medical history, comorbidities, income, or assets. Persons younger than 65 years with permanent disabilities are eligible for Medicare after receiving Social Security Income (SSI) payments for 24 months. Select health conditions, such as end-stage renal disease or Lou Gehrig's disease, allow immediate eligibility for Medicare without waiting through 24 months of SSI payments.

Most beneficiaries of Part A do not pay a monthly premium but are often responsible for a deductible before Medicare coverage begins. Some individuals who are not entitled to Part A coverage (such as those who did not pay enough Medicare taxes during their working years) have the option to pay a monthly premium for Part A benefits. There are also several limitations in Medicare coverage that are commonly needed by the elderly or those with permanent disabilities. These include coverage for long-term care services either at home (i.e., home health to individuals who could otherwise not safely reside outside of a care facility) or in a facility (such as a nursing home or assisted living facility), routine dental care and dentures, routine vision care and eyeglasses, or hearing examinations and hearing aids. Medicare also has significant deductibles and cost-sharing requirements for covered benefits.

Medicare Advantage (Part C) allows beneficiaries to enroll in private health plans to receive Medicare-covered benefits. These plans tend to provide all benefits covered under traditional Medicare and can offer additional benefits, including Part D prescription coverage. Medicare contracts with various types of private plans to offer benefits, including HMOs, preferred provider organizations (PPOs), provider-sponsored organizations (PSOs), private fee-for-service (PFFS) plans, high deductible plans linked to medical savings accounts (MSAs), and special needs plans (SNPs), for those eligible for both Medicare and Medicaid, individuals residing in select long-term care facilities, or those with chronic conditions. Enrollment in Medicare Advantage plans has steadily increased since its inception with approximately one-third of all Medicare beneficiaries participating in these plans.

Discussion Source

The Henry J. Kaiser Family Foundation. An Overview of Medicare. https://www.kff.org/medicare/issue-brief/an-overview-of-medicare/

QUESTIONS

14. Medicare is best defined as:

  A. an entitlement program to provide health-care coverage for low-income elderly persons.

  B. a publicly supported health insurance program for elderly persons and younger persons with permanent disabilities.

  C. a health insurance program for persons ineligible for private insurance.

  D. the nation's insurance program for long-term care coverage in elderly persons.

15. Persons eligible for Medicare include all of the following except:

  A. individuals age 65 and older.

  B. individuals younger than 65 years of age with certain permanent disabilities.

  C. certain individuals concurrently receiving Medicaid.

  D. healthy individuals younger than 65 years with income below 150% of the federal poverty line.

16 to 19.   Match the Medicare part with its appropriate benefits.

_____ 16. Part A

_____ 17. Part B

_____ 18. Part C

_____ 19. Part D

  A. allows beneficiaries to enroll in a private plan as an alternative to the traditional fee-for-service (FFS) plan

  B. covers inpatient and hospital services

  C. provides outpatient prescription drug benefits

  D. helps pay for physician, NP, outpatient, home health, and preventive services

20 to 22. Indicate (*yes or no*) if each of the following is eligible for Medicare.

_____ 20. a 67-year-old man with multiple comorbidities and high income

_____ 21. a 72-year-old permanent legal resident (non–U.S. citizen) who has been a member of the paid workforce in the United States for more than 25 years

_____ 22. a 68-year-old undocumented, noncitizen resident

23. Funding for Medicare includes all of the following sources except:

    A. payroll taxes.

    B. monthly premiums from beneficiaries.

    C. sales taxes on alcohol and tobacco products.

    D. taxes from Social Security benefits.

24. All of the following are not typically covered by Medicare except:

    A. long-term care services.

    B. preventive care.

    C. hearing exams and hearing aids.

    D. routine vision care and eyeglasses.

For answers and rationales, see end of chapter.

Malpractice

Overview

Malpractice is the failure of a person with specialized education and training to act in a reasonable and prudent manner. There are four elements of malpractice, which a plaintiff must prove in order to win a case in court:

1. Duty of care

2. Breach of the standard of care

3. Injury

4. Proximal cause (i.e., that the injury was caused by the breach of standard of care)

Duty of Care

A duty of care is established when there is a provider-patient relationship. A visit to an NP by a patient establishes an NP's duty to a patient. Duty can also be established outside of an office visit, such as via a telephone conversation. In addition, duty can be established with an individual who is not officially a patient.

> **CLINICAL CONCEPT**
>
> If an NP gives professional advice or treatment, in any setting, duty, and therefore a provider-patient relationship, is viewed as being established.

For example, a friend of the NP missed an appointment with her PCP and has now run out of her antihypertensive medications. She asks the NP to renew her prescription as she awaits her next appointment; the NP agrees to provide the antihypertensive prescription but encourages her friend to keep her appointment with her PCP. Although this appears on the surface as a personal favor, in fact the NP's actions have now helped to establish a provider-patient relationship for health care with her friend.

Breach of Standard of Care

Though the definition of standard of care can differ among jurisdictions, it generally refers to the care that a reasonable, similarly situated professional would have provided for an individual. NPs are duty bound to use such reasonable, ordinary care, skill, and diligence as NPs in good standing in the same geographic area and in the same general type of practice in similar cases. When an NP is sued for malpractice, the standard of care is argued in court. The attorneys hire expert witnesses, usually other NPs, who will give testimony describing the actions a reasonably prudent NP would have taken in the situation. An NP in a specialty practice will not usually be called as an expert witness in a case that occurred in primary care, and alternatively, a primary care NP will not be called to comment on a specialty practice situation. The plaintiff's expert's testimony may conflict with the defense's expert's testimony. A judge or jury will accept either the plaintiff's or the defendant's expert's explanation of the standard of care and will then decide whether the defendant NP met that standard.

Injury

A provider could be negligent, but if there is no injury, there is no malpractice. For example, an NP prescribes penicillin for a patient who has a known allergy to that antibiotic. If the patient takes the penicillin but has no adverse reaction that injures the patient, then there is no malpractice, even though the standard of care has been breached.

Proximal Cause

For malpractice to have occurred, a breach of the standard of care must have caused an injury to the plaintiff; this is known as proximal cause. For example, the NP diagnoses acute otitis media and prescribes amoxicillin to a patient with documented penicillin allergy. The patient takes the medication and develops an anaphylactic reaction and requires hospitalization. Clearly, there is a connection between the act of the NP, the prescription, the breach in standard of care, the avoidance of amoxicillin prescribing in a person with a documented allergy, and the resulting severe allergic reaction. At the same time, there can be a breach in standard of care, an injury, but no proximal cause, or connection of the breach and an injury. For example, a patient visits an NP and is diagnosed with otitis media. The NP prescribes amoxicillin, though the patient's chart indicates a penicillin allergy. The patient leaves the clinic with the prescription filled, but before the patient takes any of the potentially problematic medication, the patient falls on the front steps of the clinic, sustaining a laceration that results in a scar on her face. The patient sues the clinic and the NP, claiming the NP had a duty to the patient, the NP breached the standard of care (by prescribing a penicillin form for a penicillin-allergic patient), and the patient suffered an injury. All of these claims are true, but there is no malpractice, because the breach of the standard of care—prescribing amoxicillin to a penicillin-allergic patient—did not cause the injury.

Avoiding Malpractice

The following recommendations should be followed to avoid malpractice:

■ Comply with the state nurse practice act.
  • This ensures that the NP is practicing within his/her scope of practice, which is dictated by the state's Board of Nursing (BON) and NP practice act. For example, an NP practicing in a full practice authority (FPA) state, where no physician collaborator is required, could be informed that, per employer policy, he/she must have a physician collaborator. Conversely, the NP who practices in a state where NPs do not have FPA cannot be made to practice without a physician collaborator as dictated by the state's BON.
■ Maintain effective collaboration, based on state regulations and prudent practice.
  • For NPs in FPA states, he/she must maintain effective collaborator relationships with other clinicians, as is prudent to all health-care providers, whether medical doctor (MD), NP, physician assistant (PA), doctor of osteopathy (DO), or other preparation.
■ Participate in periodic peer review and comply with protocols and/or guidelines.
  • Peer review is a process whereby health-care providers evaluate the quality of colleagues' work. Its purpose is to ensure standards of care are being met. This activity is usually viewed as part of a health-care agency's overall commitment to quality improvement. A reviewer should truly be the clinician's peer, where a primary care NP would review the practice of another NP in a similar practice setting.
■ Ensure that collaborating professionals and facilities maintain appropriate insurance.
  • Medical professional liability insurance, also known as medical malpractice insurance, can protect health-care professionals from liability related to breaches in the standard of care that result in injury, medical expenses, and property damage as well as the cost of defending lawsuits related to malpractice claims. Ensuring an adequate and appropriate insurance is in place requires the NP to be a voice in the business side of the practice.
■ Maintain current and accurate patient records.
  • This includes an up-to-date problem list and medication list, test results, telephone communications, consultations, and referrals. Systems and policies should be in place that allow for effective patient follow-up, particularly for high-risk diagnoses.
  • This is an important professional responsibility for all health-care providers.
■ Release information in accordance with the Health Insurance Portability and Accountability Act (HIPAA) regulations.
  • This is standard for all practices. Violating HIPAA regulations, even if by error and not purposeful action, carries the potential for significant financial penalties and possibly even loss of license, arrest, and/or incarceration.

> **CLINICAL CONCEPT**
> Keep in mind, an employer can restrict an NP's practice to less than, but not more than, state law.

■ Ensure a system is in place to assist with follow-up diagnostic tests and clinical/specialty referrals. This system should be able to easily answer the following questions about diagnostic and clinical/specialty referrals.
- Was it done?
- Are results on record?
- If the test results were abnormal, was the condition followed up to a diagnosis or ruled out?
- If this was a referral to another health-care provider, was appropriate follow-up advised and completed?
- Ensure revisit on an unresolved problem is possible until the issue is resolved.

Off-Label Medication Use

Off-label drug use is the practice of prescribing a medication to be used in a manner different from what is approved by the U.S. Food and Drug Administration (FDA). This is a legal practice used by prescribing health-care providers (e.g., MDs, PAs, NPs, and DOs), and it is estimated that up to 20% of prescriptions are written off-label. Prescribing off-label is predominantly done in two manners: (1) use of a medication for an unapproved indication, such as gabapentin for bipolar disorder, or (2) use of a medication for an unapproved population (e.g., a medication approved in adults is used in pediatrics).

Though there is no legal requirement to inform patients about off-label use of prescription medications, it is best to inform them when off-label use is not supported in the literature, can involve risk to the patient, and/or will not be covered by insurance.

> **CLINICAL CONCEPT**
>
> Professional associations, including the American Medical Association, approve off-label use in certain situations as long as it is based on sound scientific evidence and medical opinion and is done in the patient's best interest.

Discussion Sources

Buppert C. *Avoiding Malpractice: 10 Rules, 5 Systems, 20 Cases.* 3rd ed. Law Office of Carolyn Buppert; 2010. http://buppert.com/publications/

Buppert C. *The Nurse Practitioner's Business Practice and Legal Guide.* Sudbury, MA: Jones & Bartlett Learning; 2018.

Saleh N. Do's and don'ts for off-label prescribing. https://www.mdlinx.com/internal-medicine/article/3743

QUESTIONS

25 to 28. Match each element of malpractice with its characteristic.

_____ **25.** duty of care

_____ **26.** breach of the standard of care

_____ **27.** injury

_____ **28.** proximal cause

    A. failure of a provider to adhere to current practice standards

    B. the existence of damages that flow from an injury such that the legal process can provide redress

    C. results from the establishment of a provider-patient relationship

    D. a causal relationship between a failure to provide standard of care and harm to a patient

29. All of the following establish a provider-patient relationship except:

    A. professional advice given over the phone to a person who is not officially a patient of the clinic.

    B. observing an accident victim being attended to by paramedics.

    C. helping a neighbor select an over-the-counter (OTC) cough medicine in the local pharmacy.

    D. covering patients for a colleague who had to leave the clinic for a personal emergency.

30. Which of the following statements about standard of care is true?

    A. Standard of care is rarely argued in court during malpractice claims.

    B. Standard of care generally refers to the care that a reasonable, similarly educated and situated professional would provide to a patient.

    C. Standard of care is constant regardless of geographic area.

    D. Standard of care does not typically apply to NPs.

31. In a malpractice case involving the family NP care of a 4-year-old previously well boy with acute otitis media who is seen in a family practice primary care setting, the most appropriate expert the plaintiff may use to establish standard of care would be:

A. a pediatrician.

B. a family NP.

C. an infectious disease (ID) physician assistant.

D. an NP specializing in ethical and legal dilemmas.

32. Which of the following examples represents a potential malpractice scenario?

A. A patient with type 2 diabetes mellitus is prescribed an inappropriate dose of insulin and experiences a severe hypoglycemic episode.

B. A patient with a known sulfa allergy is prescribed trimethoprim-sulfamethoxazole (TMP-SMX) but no reaction occurs.

C. A patient with acute bacterial sinusitis does not see any improvement in signs and symptoms 3 days after being given a dose-appropriate prescription for amoxicillin-clavulanate.

D. Prior to taking a medication, a patient realizes that the wrong drug was dispensed at the pharmacy.

33. A main goal of peer review within a health-care setting is to:

A. recognize NPs for possible promotion or demotion.

B. allow physicians and PAs an opportunity to review NP practice.

C. document corrections recently put in place in case of malpractice litigation.

D. ensure standards of care are met.

34. Which of the following is best suited to provide peer review for an NP who sees many patients with acute bacterial rhinosinusitis in the primary care setting?

A. NP in ENT specialty practice

B. NP in similar primary care practice

C. NP in urgent or emergency care

D. medical physician

For answers and rationales, see end of chapter.

Billing for Professional Services

Overview

An important part of practice is understanding how the services the NP delivers are reimbursed. Reimbursement follows proper billing. If services of an NP are not billed, or not billed correctly, the practice or employer can miss a significant source of revenue. However, overbilling or "upcoding" (assigning, for billing purposes, a higher than justified billing code) can lead to charges of health-care fraud. Therefore, NPs must have a thorough understanding of the requirements to receive third-party payments.

Reimbursement for Nurse Practitioner Services

NPs seeking reimbursement by third-party payers (Medicare, Medicaid, and commercial health plans and insurers) will require a "yes" response to each of the following questions:

■ Does the service include a medical evaluation and medical decision making that the NP is prepared to provide?

■ Does the clinician have the legal authority to perform this level of service?

■ Does the clinician have the legal authority to receive reimbursement for these services?

■ Is the clinician enrolled with the payer, such as the insurer?

■ Is the patient's health plan or insurance coverage current?

■ Is the service covered by the patient's health plan or insurance?

■ Is the service medically necessary?

■ Is there a CPT code (*Current Procedural Terminology*, a compendium of codes for every medical procedure, published and maintained by the American Medical Association) for the service? Has the appropriate CPT code been submitted on the claim form?

■ Is there a diagnosis code (*International Classification of Diseases* or *ICD*) for the patient's illness or condition? Has the appropriate *ICD* code been submitted on the claim form?

■ If the NP works for or is a specialist, has the PCP authorized the visit or procedure?

■ Has a "clean claim" been submitted—that is, has the practice filled out the claim form fully and appropriately?

■ Has the payer's process been followed?

■ Have the payers' rules been followed?

NPs' legal authority to bill for their services comes from various sources, depending on the payer. For Medicare, the authority comes from federal law. For Medicaid, the authority comes from federal and state law. Regarding commercial insurers and health plans, the authority usually comes from state law or is not specifically excluded by state law. In the latter case, the commercial payers make their own decisions about whether or not to reimburse NPs. Whether the payer is Medicare, Medicaid, or a commercial insurer or health plan, there are rules and policies about what can be reimbursed, and these policies can differ significantly from company to company.

Third-party payers reimburse NPs when they are performing these services requiring a high level of clinical skill and decision making, but not when they are performing nursing services. Nursing services are typically defined as those services that would fall under the practice of the registered nurse. NPs' authority to perform high-level services is derived from state law, and that legal authority is called "scope of practice." Some state laws are more explicit than others in describing an NP's scope of practice. For example, in select state law, what the NP can do is provided in great detail, whereas in other states, the law tends to be more broadly stated.

At minimum, an NP would need the scope of practice under state law to bill for "evaluation and management" services. The components of evaluation and management, according to CPT, are taking a history; physical examination; medical (clinical) decision making at the NP, MD, DO, or physician assistant level; counseling; and coordination of care. Medical (clinical) decision making is defined as diagnosing, deciding on a course of treatment, and ordering and performing treatments.

The first requirement for reimbursement is having a scope of practice under state law that authorizes the NP to perform services that would historically be considered physician services. States' laws are worded so that there is little question that an NP can perform evaluation and management services (taking a history, performing a physical examination, and making medical decisions about further diagnosis and treatment).

Payment for NP services can come in several forms—FFS, capitation, or pursuant to a contract between the practice and another entity. A practice often receives payments under a mixture of fees-for-services, capitation, and contracts.

In the FFS payment system, every procedure performed has an associated payment. A procedure might be a visit for evaluation and management, a consultation, or excising a lesion. Under an FFS payment system, the more services that are billed, the more revenue the practice, agency, or institution will make. As a result, it is important to know which services will be reimbursed and to bill all reimbursable services.

Under a capitated system of reimbursement, the agency, institution, or practice gets a set amount, per month, for all services needed by the patient and covered under a contract between the payer company and the practice company. Capitated rates are often negotiable. The rates are based on profit projections and actuarial data (i.e., data on past utilization of services by males, females, and age cohorts). If a patient's services are reimbursed under a capitated schedule, the practice generates revenue by signing up large numbers of patients, negotiating favorable capitation rates, and keeping expenses to a minimum by providing as few face-to-face visits and services as possible, while providing an acceptable level of care. When payment is capitated, practices want to take care of as much as possible through telephone calls, electronic communication, mailings, or visits with staff other than NPs, MDs, DOs, or PAs.

The type of payment system will impact how an NP provides care on a day-to-day basis. If a patient's services are reimbursed under an FFS schedule, a practice receives more revenue with an increasing number of visits and procedures performed. An NP who wants to generate more revenue will see more patients and code comprehensively and at the highest level of service justified by the work performed and the medical necessity of the services. A practice that excels at FFS reimbursement will negotiate favorable fee schedules and be adept at following up unpaid or denied claims.

Coding for Reimbursement for Nurse Practitioner Services

Under the CPT system, there are five levels of evaluation and management visits performed in an office. For an office visit with an established patient, the most frequently billed visit for Medicare patients is a level 3 visit (CPT 99213). However, many evaluation/management visits with NPs are at level 4 (CPT 99214). Medicare reimbursement for a level 4 visit is significantly greater than for a level 3 visit. As a result, if the NP can meet the requirements for a level 4 visit, he or she will receive additional reimbursement. Conversely, the NP who bills a level 4 visit but only documents enough work to meet the requirement of a level 3 visit will be in danger of failing an audit, which can result in a demand from the payer for money already paid, fines, mandated education and auditing, and even possible dismissal as a reimbursable provider. If billing errors are frequent, a clinician could be charged with health-care fraud.

Certain criteria must be met to distinguish between a level 3 and a level 4 visit. A level 3 office visit for an established patient requires meeting two of the following three levels of medical work:

■ At least one element of history of present illness and at least one positive or negative response to review-of-systems questions.
■ At least six elements of physical examination.
■ Medical decision-making of low complexity.

A level 4 office visit for an established patient requires meeting two of the following three levels of work:

■ At least four elements of history of present illness, positive or negative responses to at least two review-of-systems questions, and at least one notation about past history, family history, or social history.
■ At least 12 elements of physical examination.
■ Medical decision making of moderate complexity.

The difference between the levels is a matter of more extensive history taking, more medical decisions, and higher risk of morbidity and mortality with the higher-level code.

Proper coding is essential for the individual and the practice. A clinician who erroneously codes a level higher than is documented could be exposing the individual and the practice to a charge of false claims. However, coding a level lower than the documentation supports is failing to recover full reimbursement to the practice. Documentation and coding need to be appropriate for the specific visit.

"Incident-to" Billing for Registered Nurse and Nurse Practitioner Services

"Incident-to" billing under Medicare is the most misunderstood concept in billing. "Incident-to" services are defined as those that are "an integral, although incidental, part of the physician's personal professional services in the course of diagnosis or treatment of an injury or illness." The purpose of "incident-to" billing is to allow a physician to bill for services provided by an assistant or delegate in the office. For example, if a patient being treated by a physician for hypertension comes in for a blood pressure check, the physician is able to have a licensed nurse check the blood pressure, and the physician or practice can bill Medicare for CPT 99211 (a level 1 visit). To accomplish this, the physician must be in the office suite at the time of the patient visit, the physician must have documented the plan of care, the physician must employ the nurse (or they both must be employed by the same entity), and the physician must remain involved in the care of the patient. NPs, like physicians, are able to bill the services of another health-care provider such as an RN if the rules of "incident to" billing are followed.

Practice owners or managers often prefer to bill all NP services "incident to" the physician's service. This is legal, but only if Medicare's rules or the commercial payer's rules are followed. Medicare's rules for a physician billing "incident to" are the following:

■ Services of the NP must be rendered under a physician's "direct personal supervision."
■ The NP must be an employee or independent contractor of a physician or physician group.
■ Services must be furnished "during a course of treatment where a physician performs an initial service and subsequent services of a frequency which reflect the physician's active participation in and management of a course of treatment."

Medicare administrators have interpreted this last rule as meaning:

■ The physician must conduct the initial visit and any visit in which there is a new episode of illness or a change in the plan of care. Note that NPs can evaluate and manage new episodes of illness, but in those cases, the service must be billed under the NP's name.
■ The physician must be in the suite of offices, though not in the same room, when the NP performs the service.
■ The physician must remain involved in the care of the patient.

"Incident-to" billing can only be used for services provided during office visits, with two exceptions. It is permissible to bill "incident-to" for a home visit under most circumstances, but both the physician and NP must be present in the home. It is permissible to bill "incident to" in a nursing home, but only if care is provided in an office space rented by the physician, and the physician, NP, and patient all are present. Prudent practice dictates that the NP keeps abreast of current regulations and advisories.

"Incident-to" billing does not apply to services provided in a hospital. However, NPs and physicians are able to "share" evaluation and management visits to inpatients, ED patients, and outpatients. NP visits for evaluation and management can be billed under a physician employer's number if the physician provides any face-to-face service on the same day. The rules on shared visits are complicated; prior to billing in this fashion, the NP should be well informed on the appropriate regulations.

There are certain monetary advantages for physicians to bill all NP services under the physician's provider number. In this manner, the practice will get 100% of the physician's fee schedule rather than the 85% rate if billing is done under the NP's provider number. However, "incident-to" billing cannot be used at all times, such as when the physician is not present in the practice (e.g., out to lunch, visiting hospitalized patients, or on vacation). During these times, visits to patients covered by Medicare and conducted by an NP must be billed under the NP's name.

It is important for NPs to be familiar with when their services can be billed under either the physician's provider number or the NP provider number. A practice can bill some NP services under a physician's number when "incident-to" or "shared visit" rules are followed. Other services can be billed under the NP's number, such as when the physician is out of the office, the patient is a new patient, or the patient has a new problem. To optimize reimbursement, NPs must understand the rules on "incident-to" and "shared" billing. The NP should preferably bill under the physician's name when the criteria for "incident-to" or shared billing are met and under the NP's name when the criteria are not met.

Medicaid prefers clinicians to bill under their own names. However, each commercial payer (e.g., Blue Cross/Blue Shield and Cigna) develops its own rules and policies, with some following Medicare's "incident-to" rules and some that do not insist on following those rules.

Discussion Sources

American Medical Association. *Current Procedural Terminology 2019 Professional Edition*. Chicago, IL: American Medical Association; 2018.

Buppert C. *Productivity Incentive Plans for Nurse Practitioners: How and Why*. Law Office of Carolyn Buppert; 2016. http://buppert.com/publications/

Buppert C. *Billing Physician Services Provided by Nurse Practitioners in Specialist's Offices, Hospitals, Nursing Facilities, Homes and Hospice*. Law Office of Carolyn Buppert; 2017. http://buppert.com/publications/

Buppert C. *Safe, Smart Billing and Coding: Evaluation and Management: An Educational Program on CD*. Law Office of Carolyn Buppert; 2017. http://buppert.com/publications/

Buppert C. *The Nurse Practitioner's Business Practice and Legal Guide*, 6th ed. Sudbury, MA: Jones & Bartlett Learning; 2018. https://www.jblearning.com

Centers for Medicare and Medicaid Services. Evaluation and Management Services. https://www.cms.gov/Outreach-and-Education/Medicare-Learning-Network-MLN/MLNProducts/Downloads/eval-mgmt-serv-guide-ICN006764.pdf

QUESTIONS

35 to 39. Which of the following questions must be answered yes in order for an NP to be reimbursed by a third-party payer (i.e., Medicare, Medicaid, private insurance)?

_____ **35.** Does the service include a medical evaluation and medical decision making?

_____ **36.** Does the clinician have legal authority to receive reimbursement for these services?

_____ **37.** Does the service involve procedures the clinician cannot perform?

_____ **38.** Is the clinician enrolled with the payer?

_____ **39.** Is the service covered by the patient's health plan or insurance?

40. In medical coding, the abbreviation CPT stands for:

    A. Current Pricing Tier.

    B. Current Procedural Terminology.

    C. Clinical Practice Terminology.

    D. Compendium of Procedures and Therapy.

41. In medical coding, the abbreviation *ICD* stands for:

    A. *Insurance Code for Diagnoses.*

    B. *Integrated Clinical Dilemmas.*

    C. *International Classification of Diseases.*

    D. *Initial Classification of the Diagnosis.*

42. When billing Medicaid, an NPs' authority to bill for their services comes from:

    A. state law only.

    B. federal law only.

    C. state and federal law.

    D. neither state nor federal law.

43. When billing commercial insurance, NPs' authority to bill for their services comes from:

    A. state law only.

    B. federal law only.

    C. state law and/or the commercial payers.

    D. federal law and/or commercial payers.

44. All of the following are components of medical decision making according to CPT except:

    A. patient history taking.

    B. diagnosing.

    C. deciding a course of treatment.

    D. performing treatments.

45. An FFS system is best defined as which of the following?

    A. Up-front payments are made prior to any service.

    B. A practice gets a set amount each month for all services needed by a patient.

    C. Payment for each service is based on a sliding scale according to patient income.

    D. For every procedure, there is an associated payment.

46. Which of the following statements is false regarding a capitated system of reimbursement?

    A. The institution or practice gets a set amount per month for all services needed by the patient and covered under a contract between the payer and practice.

    B. Capitated rates are not negotiable.

    C. Capitated rates are based on profit projections and actuarial data.

    D. When payment is capitated, clinics prefer to take care of patients as much as possible through phone calls and mailings rather than seeing an NP or MD.

47. Potential consequences of failing an audit because of upcoding, that is, applying an artificially high-level code to a visit, include all of the following except:

    A. repaying the money to the payer.

    B. a malpractice lawsuit.

    C. a dismissal as a reimbursable provider.

    D. a mandated education.

48. All of the following criteria can be used to distinguish a level 3 office visit for an established patient except:

    A. at least six elements of physical examination.

    B. at least one element of history of present illness and at least one positive or negative response to review-of-systems questions.

    C. medical decision making of low complexity.

    D. at least one new prescription or a prescription refill.

49. All of the following criteria can be used to help determine whether a level 4 office visit occurred for an established patient except:

    A. at least four elements of physical examination.

    B. at least four elements of history of present illness.

    C. medical decision making of moderate complexity.

    D. positive or negative responses to at least two review-of-systems questions and at least one notation about past history.

50. Services that are an integral, although incidental, part of the physician's personal professional services in the course of diagnosis or treatment of an injury or illness can be classified as:

    A. capitated services.

    B. "incident-to" services.

    C. mandatory services.

    D. shared services.

51. Criteria for an "incident-to" office visit include all of the following except that:

    A. all prescriptions must be written by the physician.

    B. the physician must conduct the initial visit and any visit in which there is a new episode of illness or a change in the plan of care.

    C. the physician, in most instances, must be in the suite of offices, though not in the same room, while the NP performs the service.

    D. the physician must remain involved in the care of the patient.

52. "Incident-to" billing does not apply to services provided:

    A. in home care.

    B. in a nursing home.

    C. in the physician's office.

    D. in a hospital.

For answers and rationales, see end of chapter.

Privacy Issues

Overview

A number of decades ago, the U.S. Department of Health and Human Services (HHS) established for the first time a set of national standards for the protection of certain health information ("Privacy Rule") that implemented the requirement of the Health Insurance Portability and Accountability Act of 1996 (HIPAA). A major goal of the Privacy Rule is to protect an individual's health information but still allow the flow of health information needed to provide and promote high-quality health care. The Privacy Rule addresses the use of "protected health information" by "covered entities" as well as sets standards for individuals' privacy rights to understand and control how their health information is used.

> **CLINICAL CONCEPT**
>
> A major purpose of the Privacy Rule and HIPAA is to define and limit the circumstances in which an individual's protected health information can be used or disclosed by covered entities.

HIPAA-Covered Entities

A covered entity encompasses every health-care provider who electronically transmits health information in connection with certain transactions. These transactions can include claims, benefit eligibility inquiries, referral authorization requests, or other transactions identified by HHS under HIPAA. Health-care providers include any other person or organization that furnishes, bills, or is paid for health care. These can include "providers of services" (e.g., institutional providers such as hospitals) or "providers of medical or health services" (e.g., noninstitutional providers such as physicians, dentists, nurse practitioners, or others) as defined by Medicare.

Individually Identifiable Health Information

The Privacy Rule protects information held or transmitted by a covered entity or its business associates in any form of media, such as electronic, paper, or oral. "Individually identifiable health information" protected by the Privacy Rule consists of information that identifies the individual or for which there is a reasonable basis to believe the information can be used to identify the individual, including the following:

■ The individual's past, present, or future physical or mental health or condition
■ The provision of health care to the individual
■ The past, present, or future payment for the provision of health care to the individual

There are no restrictions on the use of health information that has been de-identified. De-identified health information does not identify an individual, and it cannot provide a reasonable basis to identify an individual. Information can be de-identified by either (1) having a formal determination made by a qualified statistician or (2) removing specified identifiers of the individual as well as any relatives, household members, and employers, and is adequate only if the covered entity has no actual knowledge that the remaining information could be used to identify the individual.

Disclosing Protected Health Information

A covered entity cannot use or disclose protected health information except either (1) as the Privacy Rule permits or requires or (2) as the individual who is the subject of the information authorizes in writing. A covered entity is allowed to disclose protected health information without the individual's authorization under certain circumstances, including the following:

■ To the individual
■ Treatment, payment, and health-care operations
■ Opportunity to agree or object
■ Incident to an otherwise permitted use and disclosure
■ Public interest and benefit activities
■ Limited data set for the purpose of research, public health, or health-care operations

Covered entities can use and disclose protected health information without individual authorization as required by law in certain situations. This includes disclosure of information to public health authorities authorized by law to collect or receive such information for preventing or controlling disease, injury, or disability and to public health or other government authorities authorized to receive reports of child abuse or neglect. Additionally, covered entities are able to disclose protected health information to appropriate government authorities regarding victims of abuse, neglect, or domestic violence. Disclosure is also permitted when a covered entity believes it is necessary to prevent or lessen a serious and imminent threat to a person or the public, when the disclosure is made to someone they believe can prevent or lessen the threat. Covered entities can also disclose to law enforcement if the information is needed to identify or apprehend an escapee or violent criminal.

When disclosing information, the covered entity must make reasonable efforts to use, disclose, and request only the minimum amount of protected health information needed to accomplish the intended purpose of the request. This central aspect of the Privacy Rule is called the principle of "minimum necessary" use and disclosure.

Penalties for Violation of HIPAA Regulations

Failure to comply with Privacy Rule requirements by a covered entity can result in a fine of $100 per failure. A person who knowingly obtains and discloses individually identifiable health information can face a fine of $50,000 and up to 1 year of imprisonment. The penalty increases to $100,000 and up to 5 years of imprisonment if the wrongful conduct involves false pretenses. If the wrongful conduct involves the sale, transfer, or use of individually identifiable health information for commercial advantage, personal gain, or malicious harm, the penalty increases to $250,000 and up to 10 years of imprisonment.

Discussion Source

U.S. Department of Health and Human Services (HHS). Summary of the HIPAA Privacy Rule. http://www.hhs.gov/hipaa/for
-professionals/privacy/laws-regulations/index.html

QUESTIONS

53. HIPAA stands for:
    A. Health Information Planning and Accessibility Amendment.
    B. Health Information Protection and Accountability Act.
    C. Health Insurance Portability and Accountability Act.
    D. Healthcare Initiative for Patient Access Amendment.

54. A major purpose of the Privacy Rule is to:
    A. define and limit the circumstances in which an individual's protected health information can be used or disclosed by covered entities.
    B. set standards for the distribution and selling of health information to third parties.
    C. define accountability by health-care providers that can be used in courts when there is suspected breach of information.
    D. protect individuals' health information when access to electronic medical records (EMRs) is illegally obtained.

55 to 58. A covered entity as defined by the Privacy Rule includes which of the following? *(Answer yes or no.)*
    _____ 55. hospitals
    _____ 56. private health-care insurance companies
    _____ 57. NPs
    _____ 58. medical assistants

59. Examples of "individually identifiable health information" can include all of the following except:
    A. an individual's past history of schizophrenia.
    B. the type of prescription written for an individual.
    C. a patient's diagnosis of prostate cancer.
    D. the percentage of patients with type 2 diabetes at a clinic.

60. When specific identifiers have been removed from protected health information so that it no longer can be used to identify an individual, the information is said to be:
    A. cleansed.
    B. de-identified.
    C. deprivatized.
    D. HIPAA certified.

61. Written authorization by the individual is not needed prior to disclosure of protected health information in all of the following circumstances except:
    A. cases of child abuse or neglect.
    B. domestic violence incidents.
    C. when a covered entity believes it is necessary to prevent a serious and imminent threat to the public.
    D. a request of information from a family member.

62. The principle of "minimum necessary" disclosure relates to which of the following?
    A. Covered entities must provide the requested protected health information in as short a time as possible.
    B. Covered entities can only charge a nominal fee for providing requested protected health information.
    C. Covered entities must make reasonable efforts to use, disclose, and request only the minimum amount of protected health information needed to accomplish the purpose of the request.
    D. Covered entities must make reasonable efforts to provide electronic records, including medical images, of protected health information in as small a file as possible.

63. The penalty for the sale of individually identifiable health information for personal gain is a:

   A. $100 fine and up to 1 year of probation.

   B. $5,000 fine and up to 60 days of imprisonment.

   C. $25,000 fine and up to 1 year of imprisonment.

   D. $250,000 fine and up to 10 years of imprisonment.

For answers and rationales, see end of chapter.

Select Issues Related to the Role of the Nurse Practitioner

In addition to the role of clinician, the NP can play a variety of roles as an advocate for patient health at the individual, local, or national level. These roles include mentor, educator, researcher, and leader.

Leadership

Leadership is defined as a process by which a person influences a group of individuals to achieve a common goal. Examples of leadership can include involvement in health-based initiatives aimed at addressing practice gaps (e.g., improving vaccination rates of the elderly) or becoming involved in policymaking designed to promote the role of the NP. Advocacy for the role of the NP is an important part of NP practice and can include involvement in legislative processes as well as national, regional, or local initiatives.

Research

As a researcher, the NP is able to evaluate and integrate research findings into evidence-based practice (EBP) as well as directly participate and lead research initiatives. EBP aims to optimize decision making by emphasizing current best evidence from well-designed and well-conducted clinical studies. In establishing EBP, it is important to recognize the evidence hierarchy when evaluating the quality of research available for making medical decisions. The hierarchy from greatest weight (highest quality) to least weight (lowest quality) is as follows:

- *Systematic reviews and meta-analysis*: Review of high-quality published research (e.g., randomized controlled trials) for a specific clinical issue and drawing of conclusions based on the overall data.
- *Randomized controlled trials*: Designed to evaluate the effectiveness or safety of a medical intervention (e.g., medication or clinical procedure) in carefully selected patients who are randomly assigned into groups to receive the intervention or act as a control (either placebo or active comparator).
- *Cohort study (prospective or retrospective)*: Follows subjects who are either exposed or not exposed (not in a randomized manner) to a particular variable (e.g., medication) and followed over time for development of a stated outcome (e.g., cure of disease, death).
- *Case-control study*: Retrospective analysis that matches cases (patients with a particular variable) and controls (patients without the variable) by specific characteristics (e.g., age, gender) and compares them for the development of a particular outcome.
- *Case series and case reports*: A retrospective analysis of a single patient or group of patients with a particular condition or disease and/or treated with a specific medication or procedure.
- *Editorial or expert opinion*: An essay authored by a qualified individual or group of individuals that addresses a specific clinical topic.

Informatics

In addition to EBP, informatics can be used to help achieve patient-centered care and improve outcomes. *Health-care informatics* is a term used to describe the acquiring, storing, retrieving, and analyzing of patient health-care information in order to refine clinical processes and medical decision making to improve efficiency and quality of care. Nursing informatics integrates nursing science with information management and analytical sciences to identify, define, manage, and communicate data and information in nursing practice. Informatics can be more readily utilized with the expansion of EMRs and computerized clinical documentation (rather than handwritten notes). Clinicians working with information technology (IT) professionals can utilize the clinical information to develop health informatics tools that can be used to promote patient care that is safe, efficient, effective, timely, and patient centered.

EBP and informatics can help support quality improvement efforts in nursing. Quality and performance improvement initiatives have become a significant part of health-care systems nationwide. The goals of quality improvement include improving the patient care experience, improving the population's health, and reducing health-care costs. To achieve these goals, efforts are needed in four areas: care coordination and patient safety, increased access to and use of preventive services, improved care for at-risk populations, and enhanced patient and caregiver experience of care. To ensure performance measures are met within health-care institutions, the CMS require the monitoring and reporting of specific quality core measures, such as certain hospital-acquired conditions. These reports are made public, and thus, poor scores can tarnish an institution's reputation as well as impact reimbursement rates by CMS and other payers. As nurses are an integral part of patient care, they are also pivotal in efforts to improve quality. The NP can play an essential part in an institution's quality and performance improvement initiative by participating as leaders on committees and helping to develop and implement the tools needed to provide quality patient care.

Discussion Sources

American Nurses Association. *Nursing Informatics: Scope and Standards of Practice*. 2nd ed. Silver Spring, MD: American Nurses Association; 2014.

Draper DA, Felland LE, Liebhaber A, Melichar L. *The Role of Nurses in Hospital Quality Improvement*. Center for Studying Health System Change; March 2008. HSC Brief no. 3. http://www.hschange.org/CONTENT/972/

Ho PM, Peterson PN, Masoudi RA. Evaluating the evidence: is there a rigid hierarchy? *Circulation*. 2008;118:1675–1684.

QUESTIONS

64. Which of the following best illustrates the leadership role of NPs?

   A. Discussing with a pharmacist the selection of the most appropriate hypertension medication for a 72-year-old man

   B. Collaborating with public health officials to develop a community initiative to improve childhood vaccination rates

   C. Volunteering to teach a group of high school students about substance abuse

   D. Teaching an expectant mother on proper nutrition during her pregnancy

65 to 68. Rank each type of study from highest quality (1) to lowest quality (4).

   _____ **65.** retrospective case-control study

   _____ **66.** prospective cohort study

   _____ **67.** case series

   _____ **68.** meta-analysis

69. The goals of quality and performance improvement initiatives in health-care institutions include all of the following except:

   A. identifying poor-performing institutions.

   B. improving the patient care experience.

   C. improving population health.

   D. reducing health-care costs.

70. A primary goal of informatics is to utilize health-care data in order to:

   A. determine cost and reimbursement for health-care services.

   B. guide medical decision making to improve patient care and efficiency.

   C. guide selection of medications for hospital formulary.

   D. determine premiums for individuals by private insurance companies.

For answers and rationales, see end of chapter.

Acknowledgment

The contributions of Carolyn Buppert, JD, NP, to this chapter are gratefully acknowledged.

QUESTION ANSWERS AND RATIONALES

Medicaid

1. Correct: B. publicly financed coverage of health care and long-term care for low-income people.

Medicaid is an entitlement program that provides medical assistance and other services to low-income individuals and families (B). Medicaid also provides long-term care for the elderly and disabled populations.

Incorrect:

Employment status is not a criterion for Medicaid eligibility, as the program is available for those near or below the federal poverty line regardless of employment (A). Medicaid can provide both acute and long-term care services, though cost-sharing with the patient is possible in certain situations (C). Individuals over the age of 65 years who are receiving Medicare can also be eligible for Medicaid, particularly for coverage of long-term care (D).

2. Correct: C. 401K programs

Entitlement programs provide benefits that are granted by federal law to citizens and select noncitizens legally residing in the United States. The 401K program is a retirement program that is regulated by the federal government, but the federal government does not guarantee benefits to individuals participating in 401K programs (C). The benefits depend on contributions from the employee and employer as well as investment returns.

Incorrect:

Entitlement programs that are granted by the federal government to individuals who meet certain criteria include Medicaid (A), Social Security (B), and Medicare (D). These programs guarantee certain benefits to citizens and certain noncitizens who meet specific criteria.

3. Correct: D. Medicare.

"Dual eligible" beneficiaries are individuals who receive both Medicaid and Medicare (D). Medicaid can provide assistance for low-income individuals in paying Medicare premiums and cost-sharing as well as covering key services, such as long-term care.

Incorrect:

"Dual eligible" recipients refer to those receiving both Medicaid and Medicare and not private insurance (A), Social Security (B), or government welfare benefits (C).

4. Correct: C. finances approximately 50% of all long-term care spending.

Medicaid is an important source for providing long-term care, including nursing home care, in the United States. Medicaid supports about 60% of nursing home residents and finances about half of all long-term care costs (C).

Incorrect:

Medicaid provides long-term care, while Medicare does not (A). Medicaid can be used for low-income individuals younger and older than 65 years, while Medicare is primarily reserved for those over 65 years (B). Medicaid provides coverage for low-income individuals and can include the elderly and physically disabled (D).

5. Correct: B. The federal government matches at least 50% of state Medicaid spending.

Medicaid is funded jointly by the federal and state governments. The match rate is based on a federal formula and can range from 50% to as high as 75% in the poorest states (B). Though states are not required to participate in Medicaid, all states do participate in the program.

Incorrect:

The federal match rate is based on a formula that is generally based on state need rather than the state population size (A). States are required to provide funding for Medicaid and must meet certain guidelines to receive the federal match (C). The federal matching rate can range from 50% to up to 75% based on state need (D).

6. Correct: C. 40%

Medicaid provides coverage for approximately 20% of the total U.S. population and nearly 40% of all children (C). This can include children in low-income families as well as children with disabilities, such as Down syndrome, cerebral palsy, and autism.

Incorrect:

Medicaid provides coverage for nearly half of all children in the US (A, B), though not as high as 60% (D).

7. Correct: D. undocumented persons residing in the United States.

In order to obtain federal matching funds for Medicaid, states are required to meet certain criteria and provide coverage to core groups of low-income individuals. However, the federal core groups do not include undocumented persons who reside in the United States (D).

Incorrect:

Federal core groups include pregnant women (A), children (C), parents, elderly individuals (B), and individuals with disabilities with income below specified minimum thresholds.

8. Correct: A. funding educational opportunities (i.e., tuition).

Medicaid can provide a variety of support opportunities for children and adults with disabilities, including those with autism, Down syndrome, and cerebral palsy. However, Medicaid does not help fund educational opportunities for these individuals (A).

Incorrect:

Some of the support available through Medicaid for disabled individuals includes providing access to a broader range of health-care services (B), obtaining speech and occupational therapy services (e.g., children with autism) (D), and obtaining services that help to maximize opportunities to support independent living (C).

9. Correct: C. rehabilitation therapy.

States must provide a set of mandatory services in order to qualify for federal matching funds for Medicaid. However, rehabilitation services are not included among the mandatory services (C).

Incorrect:

A variety of services are mandatory in order for states to receive federal matching funds for Medicaid. Mandatory services include physician and NP services (D), hospital services (both inpatient and outpatient), laboratory and x-ray services (A), transportation services, and select family planning services and supplies (B).

10. Correct: C. hospice.

Medicaid provides health-care services from various types of health-care centers. However, hospice services are not considered mandatory for inclusion in Medicaid by federal law (C).

Incorrect:

In addition to providing hospital services (both inpatient and outpatient) (B), Medicaid ensures support of health-care settings that serve low-income populations. These include RHCs (A) and FQHCs (D).

11. Correct: D. All ED visits are exempt from copayments.

States can impose cost-sharing by individuals in the form of copayments, coinsurance, and deductibles. To discourage the use of the ED for nonemergency services, states can impose a higher copayment for these visits when an ED visit is deemed to be a nonemergency, and the services are accessible at other health-care centers (D).

Incorrect:

States are allowed to charge premiums and cost-sharing for Medicaid based on federal guidelines that are largely based on income level (A). Certain services are exempt from cost-sharing, such as preventive services in children and family planning services (B). States are allowed to terminate Medicaid coverage if premiums are not paid by the individual (C).

12. Correct: A. comparable in access to health care and meeting several core measures in preventive care.

Medicaid has been shown to improve access to health care for children. When compared to children with private insurance, those with Medicaid and CHIP have comparable access to health care as measured by several core measures of preventive and primary care services (A).

Incorrect:

Children with Medicaid and CHIP have not been shown to be more deficient in core preventive care measures (B) or less likely to see a PCP (C) when compared to those with private insurance. There is no notable difference in receiving mandatory immunizations when comparing children with Medicaid and CHIP with those with private insurance (D).

13. Correct: D. ED visits by Medicaid patients more often involve multiple diagnoses compared with those with private insurance.

Adults with Medicaid tend to have a higher burden of illness and disability and are more likely to have a secondary diagnosis of a mental health disorder. As such, ED visits by Medicaid patients more frequently involve multiple diagnoses compared to those with private insurance (D).

Incorrect:

Only a small percentage of ED visits by Medicaid patients are for nonemergency reasons (A), and this rate is only slightly higher (10% versus 7%) compared to those with private insurance (B). Because Medicaid patients tend to have a higher frequency of multiple diagnoses compared to those with private insurance, Medicaid patients tend to use the ED at a higher rate (C).

Medicare

14. Correct: B. a publicly supported health insurance program for elderly persons and younger persons with permanent disabilities.

Medicare was originally designed to provide health-care coverage for individuals 65 years and over. Since its inception, coverage has expanded to include younger individuals with certain conditions and permanent disabilities (B).

Incorrect:

Medicaid is best described as an entitlement program to provide health-care coverage for low-income individuals (A). Medicare is not limited to individuals who cannot get private insurance (C) and will not cover long-term care (e.g., nursing homes) for the elderly (D).

15. Correct: D. healthy individuals younger than 65 years with income below 150% of the federal poverty line.

Individuals younger than age 65 years can be eligible for Medicare if they have certain medical conditions and permanent disabilities. Healthy individuals would not be eligible for Medicare regardless of income level (D).

Incorrect:

All U.S. citizens and permanent legal residents are eligible for Medicare at 65 years of age (A). Certain individuals younger than 65 years can be eligible for Medicare if they have certain permanent disabilities (B). "Dual eligible" beneficiaries are able to receive both Medicare and Medicaid (C).

16 to 19. Matching Questions

16. Correct: B. covers inpatient and hospital services

17. Correct: D. helps pay for physician, NP, outpatient, home health, and preventive services

18. Correct: A. allows beneficiaries to enroll in a private plan as an alternative to the traditional FFS plan

19. Correct: C. provides outpatient prescription drug benefits

Medicare is divided into four parts that each offer different health-care benefits. Part A covers inpatient hospital services as well as services at skilled nursing facilities, home health, and hospice care (16). Part B pays for outpatient, home health, and preventive services (17). Part C allows beneficiaries to enroll in a private plan that covers all Medicare Part A and Part B services and sometimes Part D services as well (18). Part D provides coverage of outpatient prescription drugs (19).

20 to 22. Yes or No

20. Correct: Yes

21. Correct: Yes

22. Correct: No

All individuals 65 years and over who are U.S. citizens or permanent legal residents (21) are eligible for Medicare regardless of prior medical history, comorbidities (20), income, or assets. Undocumented residents are not eligible for Medicare benefits (22).

23. Correct: C. sales taxes on alcohol and tobacco products.

Medicare is funded through variable sources including certain taxes as well as premiums paid by the beneficiary. However, sales taxes of any products are not used to fund Medicare (C).

Incorrect:

Funding of Medicare includes payroll taxes (A) and taxes on certain Social Security benefits (D). Additionally, beneficiaries pay monthly premiums for Medicare (B).

24. Correct: B. preventive care.

Preventive care is a key component of Medicare that is covered by Part B (B).

Incorrect:

Though Medicare covers a wide variety of health-care services, there are certain aspects of health care that are not covered by this program. This includes hearing exams and hearing aids (C) as well as vision care and eyeglasses (D). Long-term care is not covered by Medicare (A), though Medicaid provides some long-term care coverage for certain beneficiaries.

Malpractice

25 to 28. Matching Questions

25. Correct: C. results from the establishment of a provider-patient relationship

26. Correct: A. failure of a provider to adhere to current practice standards

27. Correct: B. the existence of damages that flow from an injury such that the legal process can provide redress

28. Correct: D. a causal relationship between a failure to provide standard of care and harm to a patient

There are four elements that must be present for a plaintiff to win a malpractice case in the court of law. A duty of care must be demonstrated where there is the establishment of a provider-patient relationship (25). A provider-patient relationship does not necessarily require an office visit but can occur in other ways, such as a telephone conversation, where professional advice or treatment is given. A breach in the standard of care is demonstrated when the health-care provider fails to provide the quality of care that a reasonable, similarly situated professional would have provided for the individual (26). Some type of injury must have occurred (27), and there must be a causal relationship between the breach in the standard of care and the injury to the patient, known as the proximal cause, to support a malpractice claim (28).

29. Correct: B. observing an accident victim being attended to by paramedics.

A provider-patient relationship is established when a health-care provider gives professional advice or treatment to an individual. This does not necessarily have to be in the office setting. However, in the situation of observing paramedics providing care without direct involvement, there is no provider-patient relationship (B).

Incorrect:

A provider-patient relationship is established when a health-care provider gives professional advice or treatment to an individual. This can occur in the office, over the phone (A), or with a friend/neighbor outside of the office setting (C). A provider-patient relationship is established when direct care is given in the health-care setting, even when covering for another provider's patients (D).

30. Correct: B. Standard of care generally refers to the care that a reasonable, similarly educated and situated professional would provide to a patient.

The definition of standard of care can differ among jurisdictions, but it largely refers to the care that a reasonable, similarly educated and situated professional would provide to a patient (B). During malpractice claims, lawyers would typically argue that there was a breach in the standard of care.

Incorrect:

The standard of care is a major point argued by lawyers during malpractice suits (A). Standard of care applies to all health-care providers, including NPs (D), who are duty bound to use reasonable, ordinary care, skill, and diligence as other NPs in good standing in the same geographic area (C) and same general type of practice.

31. Correct: B. a family NP.

When establishing the standard of care in court, it is essential to use expert witnesses who are at the same professional level as the defendant, as the standard of care can vary greatly between an NP in primary versus specialist care. In this case involving a family NP, the most appropriate expert witness to establish the standard of care would be another family NP (B).

Incorrect:

When trying to establish the standard of care in court for a family NP, the use of a pediatrician (A) or ID physician assistant (C) would not be helpful, as they are expected to have a different standard of care compared to the family NP. An NP specializing in ethical and legal dilemmas would also not be an appropriate choice to establish the standard of care in this situation (D).

32. Correct: A. A patient with type 2 diabetes mellitus is prescribed an inappropriate dose of insulin and experiences a severe hypoglycemic episode.

A malpractice scenario will require a *breach in the standard of care* as well as injury directly related to that breach. In the patient with type 2 diabetes, there is a breach in the standard of care when an incorrect dose of insulin is prescribed. This directly results in injury to the patient via a severe hypoglycemic episode (A).

Incorrect:

For the patient with a sulfa allergy, there was a breach in standard of care but no injury to the patient (B). Similarly, for the patient given the wrong medication at the pharmacy: a breach in standard of care is evident but there is no injury resulting from this breach as the mistake is realized prior to taking the medication (D). For the patient with sinusitis, it seems that standard of care was provided for the patient as a dose-appropriate prescription was given. Treatment failure is not a valid reason for malpractice in this scenario (C).

33. Correct: D. ensure standards of care are met.

Routine peer review within a health-care setting can be a useful practice to evaluate the quality of care provided by colleagues and to ensure that standards of care are being met (D).

Incorrect:

Though peer review can be helpful in reducing the risk of malpractice by ensuring standards of care are met, a main goal is not to document the corrections in practice in case of a malpractice suit (C). A review of a colleague's work should be truly done by a professional peer and would not have a physician or PA review an NP's work (B). A main goal of peer review is not to identify candidates for promotion or demotion (A).

34. Correct: B. NP in similar primary care practice

Peer review should be performed by colleagues who are in a similar position and clinical practice. Thus, the work performed by a primary care NP should be reviewed by NPs in a similar practice to ensure standards of care are being met for those patients in that particular health-care setting (B).

Incorrect:

Peer review should be truly done by professional peers in similar practice settings. Thus, a primary care NP should be reviewed by other primary care NPs and not specialty NPs (A, C) or medical physicians (D).

Billing for Professional Services

35 to 39. Yes or No

35. Correct: Yes

36. Correct: Yes

37. Correct: No

38. Correct: Yes

39. Correct: Yes

When an NP is seeking reimbursement from a third-party payer, there are certain criteria that must be met. These include ensuring that the service includes a medical evaluation and medical decision making (35) and that the clinician actually has a legal authority to receive reimbursement for those services (36). Depending on the payer, legal authority can come from federal law (e.g., Medicare), state law (e.g., Medicaid along with federal law), or commercial payers. The clinician must be enrolled with the payer to receive reimbursement, (38) and the service should be covered by the patient's health plan or insurance (39). The service should not involve procedures that cannot be performed by the clinician (37).

40. Correct: B. Current Procedural Terminology.

CPT stands for Current Procedural Terminology and is the system of codes for every medical procedure (B). The CPT codes are published and maintained by the American Medical Association.

41. Correct: C. *International Classification of Diseases*.

ICD stands for *International Classification of Diseases* and provides a diagnosis code for every illness or condition (C). An *ICD* code is needed when submitting a claim form for reimbursement.

42. Correct: C. state and federal law.

When billing Medicaid, the NP gets the legal authority to bill from both federal and state law, as Medicaid is funded by federal and state governments (C).

Incorrect:

The authority to bill Medicare is from federal law only, as this program is funded through the federal government (B). Medicaid is funded through the state with federal matching funds and so both federal and state law determine the authority to bill (A, D).

43. Correct: C. state law and/or the commercial payers.

The legal authority to bill commercial payers can vary by the payer but generally follows state law with or without additional policies set by the payer (C). Commercial payers can make their own decisions about whether to reimburse services performed by NPs, and these policies can vary significantly from company to company.

Incorrect:

The NP's authority to bill comes from both state law and commercial payers (A). Federal law does not impact the NP's authority to bill for services (B, D).

44. Correct: A. patient history taking.

Taking a patient's history is not included in the medical decision-making process according to CPT (A).

Incorrect:

Medical (clinical) decision making according to CPT can involve making a diagnosis (B), deciding on a course of treatment (C), or ordering or performing treatment (D).

45. Correct: D. For every procedure, there is an associated payment.

There are different payment systems that can be utilized in the health-care setting. In the FFS system, every procedure performed during a visit is charged a fee (D). Procedures can involve evaluation, diagnostics, or medical intervention.

Incorrect:

Under a capitated system for reimbursement, the practice gets a set amount per month for all of the services needed by the patient covered under a contract between the payer and the practice (B). In this system, it would be favorable for the practice to minimize face-to-face visits and services and maximize patient management via phone calls, online, or utilizing staff other than NPs, MDs, or PAs. An up-front payment made prior to any service during an office visit best describes a copayment (A). The practice of payments based on a sliding scale according to patient income is not typical (C). However, Medicaid can determine monthly premiums based on income.

46. Correct: B. Capitated rates are not negotiable.

Under a capitated system for reimbursement, the practice gets a set amount per month for all of the services needed by the patient covered under a contract between the payer and the practice. The capitated rates are negotiable and generally based on profit projections and actuarial data (B).

Incorrect:

Providers under a capitated system will get a set amount each month to provide all of the services needed by covered individuals (A). The capitated rates are generally determined by profit projections and actuarial data that analyze past utilization of services among males, females, and age cohorts (C). In this system, it would be favorable for the practice to minimize face-to-face visits and services and maximize patient management via phone calls, mailings, online communication, or by utilizing staff other than NPs, MDs, or PAs (D).

47. Correct: B. a malpractice lawsuit.

The NP must be aware of proper billing practices in order to ensure all services are properly reimbursed as well as avoid billing errors that can lead to an audit. For practices that fail an audit, there are several possible consequences. However, a malpractice lawsuit is not a consequence, as this does not meet the criteria for malpractice, namely, a breach in the standard of care that causes injury to the patient.

Incorrect:

Consequences of failing an audit can include repaying money to the payer (A), payment of fines, mandated education (D), and possible dismissal as a reimbursable provider (C). If billing errors occur frequently, a clinician could be charged with health-care fraud.

48. Correct: D. at least one new prescription or a prescription refill.

Under the CPT system, certain criteria are set to distinguish a level 3 office visit. However, a requirement for at least one new prescription or a prescription refill is not included in these criteria (D).

Incorrect:

Criteria for a level 3 office visit include at least six elements of physical examination (A), at least one element of history of present illness and at least one positive or negative response to review-of-systems questions (B), and medical decision making of low complexity (C).

49. Correct: A. at least four elements of physical examination.

Under the CPT system, certain criteria are set to distinguish a level 4 office visit. One of the criteria is to have at least 12 (not 4) elements of physical examination (A).

Incorrect:

Criteria for a level 4 office visit include at least four elements of history of present illness (B), medical decision making of moderate complexity (C), positive or negative responses to at least two review-of-system questions (D), and at least one notation about past history, family history, or social history.

50. Correct: B. "incident-to" services.

By definition, "incident-to" services are those that are an integral, although incidental, part of the physician's personal professional services in the course of diagnosis or treatment of an injury or illness (B). "Incident-to" billing allows the physician to bill for services provided by an assistant or delegate in the office as long as certain criteria are met.

Incorrect:

Under a capitated system for reimbursement, the practice gets a set amount per month for all of the services needed by the patient covered under a contract between the payer and the practice (A). Mandatory (C) and shared (D) services are not defined when regarding billing by clinicians.

51. Correct: A. all prescriptions must be written by the physician.

In order to utilize "incident-to" billing, the physician must still be integrally involved in the care of a patient. However, it is not necessary for the physician to write all of the prescriptions for patients (A).

Incorrect:

Certain criteria must be met to utilize "incident-to" billing for services provided in the office setting. These include that the physician must conduct the initial visit as well as any visit in which there is a new episode of illness or a change in the plan of care (B). The physician should also be present in the suite of offices, though not necessarily in the same room as the patient, when an NP performs the service (C). The physician must also remain involved in the care of the patient (D).

52. Correct: D. in a hospital.

"Incident-to" billing can be used for certain services that occur outside of the office setting. However, this type of billing cannot be used for any services performed in the hospital setting (D).

Incorrect:

In addition to office visits (C), "incident-to" billing can be used for services performed in home care when the NP and physician are both present during the visit (A). This billing can also be used for services in a nursing home when the care is performed in an office rented by the physician, and the physician, NP, and patient are all present (B).

Privacy Issues

53. Correct: C. Health Insurance Portability and Accountability Act.

The set of national standards for the protection of certain health information is implemented through the

Health Insurance Portability and Accountability Act (HIPAA) (C).

54. **Correct: A. define and limit the circumstances in which an individual's protected health information can be used or disclosed by covered entities.**
The Privacy Rule addresses the use of health information by covered entities and sets standards for individuals' privacy rights to understand and control how their health information is used. A major goal of the Privacy Rule is to define and limit circumstances in which a patient's health information is used or disclosed by covered entities (A).
Incorrect:
The Privacy Rule does not offer any standards for the selling of health information (B), and it does not define accountability by health-care providers when there is a suspected breach of information (C). The Privacy Rule cannot protect individual's health information when the information has been illegally obtained (D), though it does provide standards on de-identifying health information.

55 to 58. Yes or No

55. Correct: Yes

56. Correct: Yes

57. Correct: Yes

58. Correct: Yes
A covered entity includes all health-care providers who electronically transmit health information in connection with certain transactions, which can include claims, benefits eligibility inquiries, and referral authorization requests, among others. Therefore, covered entities can include hospitals (55), private health-care insurance companies (56), NPs (57), and medical assistants (58), among other clinicians.

59. **Correct: D. the percentage of patients with type 2 diabetes at a clinic.**
Individually identifiable health information consists of information that can identify an individual or that there is a reasonable basis to believe the information can be used to identify the individual. However, general patient data at a clinic, such as the percentage with type 2 diabetes, cannot be used to specifically identify an individual and would not be considered to be individually identifiable health information (D).
Incorrect:
Examples of individually identifiable health information can include a patient's past, present, or future physical or mental health condition (A, C); the provision of health care to an individual (B); or the past, present, or future payment for the provision of health care to the individual.

60. **Correct: B. de-identified.**
Health information that has been de-identified cannot be used to identify an individual, and it cannot be used to provide a reasonable basis to identify an individual. Health information can be de-identified by having a formal determination by a qualified statistician, or by

removing specific identifiers of the individual, relatives, family members, and employers.
Incorrect:
Health information that can no longer be used to identify an individual is said to be "de-identified" and not cleansed (A), deprivatized (C), or HIPAA certified (D).

61. **Correct: D. a request of information from a family member.**
Covered entities are allowed to share health information without the written authorization of the individual in certain circumstances. However, sharing information with family members will still require authorization by the individual (D).
Incorrect:
Situations where written authorization is not needed to share health information include providing information to appropriate government authorities regarding victims of abuse or neglect (A), domestic violence (B), or when there is a belief that it is necessary to prevent a serious and imminent threat to a person or the public (C).

62. **Correct: C. Covered entities must make reasonable efforts to use, disclose, and request only the minimum amount of protected health information needed to accomplish the purpose of the request.**
When disclosing health information, the covered entity must follow the principle of "minimum necessary." This helps to ensure that reasonable efforts are made to use, disclose, and request only the minimum amount of protected health information needed to accomplish the purpose of the request (C).
Incorrect:
The principle of "minimum necessary" does not relate to the amount of time used (A) or fee charged (B) to provide the health information. It also does not relate to the size of the file when providing the information electronically (D).

63. **Correct: D. $250,000 fine and up to 10 years of imprisonment.**
The Privacy Rule stipulates serious consequences for individuals who knowingly obtain and disclose individually identifiable health information. Wrongful conduct of knowingly obtaining and disclosing individually identifiable health information can be punished by a fine of $50,000 and up to 1 year in jail. Those found guilty of wrongful conduct that involves the sale, transfer, or use of individually identifiable health information for personal gain can face a fine of $250,000 and up to 10 years in jail (D).

Select Issues Related to the Role of the Nurse Practitioner

64. **Correct: B. Collaborating with public health officials to develop a community initiative to improve childhood vaccination rates**
The nursing leadership role is best defined when a nurse is able to influence a group of individuals to achieve a common goal. This is best illustrated by the example of

working with public health officials to improve child-hood vaccination rates within a community (B).

Incorrect:

Volunteering to teach a group of high school students on substance abuse is an important role as an educator (C). Similarly, teaching an expectant mother about nutrition demonstrates the role of counselor and educator (D). Working with a pharmacist to select the most appropriate medication is a key role as a clinician (A). Though all of these are essential roles of the nurse, they are not examples of the leadership role.

65 to 68. Rank from highest (1) to lowest (4) quality

65. Correct: 3

66. Correct: 2

67. Correct: 4

68. Correct: 1

The ability to evaluate quality of research is important in determining evidence-based medicine. The highest quality of research is derived from meta-analyses and systematic reviews (68), followed by well-designed randomized controlled trials. Lower on the hierarchy are prospective or retrospective cohort studies, which follow a group of subjects over time for the development of a specified outcome (66). Next would be a retrospective case-control study that matches patients with controls to see if there is a relationship between a specified variable with an outcome (65). Lowest-quality evidence includes case studies or case series (67) followed by editorials or expert opinion pieces.

69. Correct: A. identifying poor-performing institutions.

The implementation of quality and performance initiatives, such as those developed by the CMS, is aimed to improve overall patient care while also providing cost-efficient patient care. Reports on how well institutions are able to meet certain core measures are made public. As a consequence, poorly performing health-care institutions are made public, and this can impact reimbursement for services by the CMS (A), though this is not a major goal of these initiatives.

Incorrect:

Quality and performance improvement initiatives have been developed to improve the patient care experience (B), improve overall population health by increasing access to and use of preventive services (C), and reduce health-care costs by promoting cost-efficient health-care measures (D).

70. Correct: B. guide medical decision making to improve patient care and efficiency.

Health-care informatics involves the process of acquiring, storing, retrieving, and analyzing patient health-care information with the purpose of using this data to guide clinical processes and medical decision making to improve patient care and efficiency (B). As more and more health-care institutions are utilizing EMRs, informatics can be a powerful tool in refining how clinicians provide care for optimal outcomes in a cost-efficient manner.

Incorrect:

Though informatics can be used to help support decisions on health-care costs by providers and payers (A, D), this is not a main goal of these studies, as they are aimed to improve efficiency and quality of patient care. Similarly, formulary decisions can include input from informatics analyses, but this is not a main goal of these studies (C).

Index

Note: Page numbers with f, t, or b indicate figures, tables, or boxes, respectively.